EMERGENCY RADIOLOGY

EMERGENCY RADIOLOGY

Editors

David T. Schwartz, MD, FACEP

Assistant Professor of Clinical Emergency Medicine
New York University School of Medicine
Bellevue Hospital and New York University Medical Center
New York, New York

Earl J. Reisdorff, MD, FACEP

Associate Professor
Program Director, Michigan State University Emergency Medicine Residency
Ingham Regional Medical Center and Sparrow Hospital
Lansing, Michigan

McGraw-Hill
Health Professions Division

New York St. Louis San Francisco Auckland Bogotá Caracas Lisbon London Madrid
Mexico City Milan Montreal New Delhi San Juan Singapore Sydney Tokyo Toronto

McGraw-Hill

A Division of The McGraw-Hill Companies

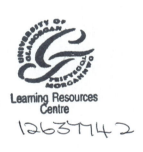
EMERGENCY RADIOLOGY

456789 QPKQPK 0654

ISBN 0-07-050827-5

This book was set in Times Roman by York Graphic Services. The editors were John J. Dolan, Susan R. Noujaim, and Peter J. Boyle; the production supervisor was Richard C. Ruzycka; the text and cover designer
was Marsha Cohen/Parallelogram Graphics; the indexer was Jerry Ralya.
Quebecor Printing/Kingsport was printer and binder.

This book is printed on acid-free paper.

Cataloging-in-publication data is on file for this title at the Library of
Congress.

*To all physicians who are dedicated to
the care of the acutely ill and injured patient.*

CONTENTS

CONTRIBUTORS

Bobby Abrams, M.D.
Attending Physician
Department of Emergency Medicine
Utah Valley Regional Medical Center
Provo, Utah
Chapter 21

Tom P. Aufderheide, M.D.
Associate Professor of Emergency Medicine
Department of Emergency Medicine
Medical College of Wisconsin
Milwaukee, Wisconsin
Chapter 18

Michael S. Beeson, M.D., M.B.A., F.A.C.E.P.
Program Director, Department of Emergency Medicine
Summa Health System
Akron, Ohio
Associate Professor of Clinical Emergency Medicine
Northeastern Ohio Universities College of Medicine
Rootstown, Ohio
Chapter 4

William J. Brady, Jr., M.D.
Department of Emergency Medicine
University of Virginia Health Sciences Center
University of Virginia Hospital
Charlottesville, Virginia
Chapter 18

Ken Butler, D.O.
Assistant Director, Division of Emergency Medical Services
University of Maryland School of Medicine
Baltimore, Maryland
Chapter 22

Diane B. Chaney, M.D.
Assistant Professor of Clinical Medicine
Section of Emergency Medicine
University of Chicago
Chicago, Illinois
Chapter 16

David M. Chuirazzi, M.D.
Assistant Professor of Emergency Medicine
Allegheny University of the Health Sciences
Assistant Residency Director
Department of Emergency Medicine
Allegheny General Hospital
Pittsburgh, Pennsylvania
Chapter 5

James E. Cisek, M.D.
Associate Professor of Emergency Medicine
Medical College of Virginia
Medical Director of Virginia Poison Center
Virginia Commonwealth University
Richmond, Virginia
Chapter 20

Ross S. Cohen, D.P.M.
North Arandel Hospital
Glen Burnie, Maryland
Chapter 8

Tanvir Dara, M.D.
Attending Physician
Department of Emergency Medicine
Erie County Medical Center
Clinical Instructor of Emergency Medicine
State University of New York at Buffalo
Buffalo, New York
Chapter 21

Timothy C. Evans, M.D.
Associate Professor of Emergency Medicine
Emergency Medicine Residency Director
Medical College of Virginia Hospitals
Department of Emergency Medicine
Virginia Commonwealth University
Richmond, Virginia
Chapter 11

Carlos Flores, M.D.
Director, Department of Emergency Medicine
Lawrence Hospital
Bronxville, New York
Assistant Professor of Emergency Medicine/Surgery
New York University School of Medicine
New York, New York
Chapter 15

Mark Glazer, M.D.
Attending Neuroradiologist
Department of Radiology
St. Luke's South Shore Hospital
Milwaukee, Wisconsin
Chapter 16

Dennis P. Hanlon, M.D.
Residency Director, Emergency Medicine
Assistant Professor of Emergency Medicine
Department of Emergency Medicine
Allegheny General Hospital
Pittsburgh, Pennsylvania
Chapter 11

Brian S. Hartfelder, M.D.
Attending Physician, Saint Mary's Hospital
Saginaw, Michigan
Assistant Clinical Professor, Program in Emergency Medicine
Michigan State University, College of Human Medicine
Saginaw Cooperative Hospitals, Inc.
Saginaw, Michigan
Chapter 17

Daniel C. Huddle, D.O.
Department of Diagnostic Radiology
Yale University School of Medicine
New Haven, Connecticut
Chapter 16

Frederic M. Hustey, M.D.
Attending Physician
Department of Emergency Medicine
Cleveland Clinic Foundation
Assistant Professor of Clinical Emergency Medicine
Department of Emergency Medicine, The Ohio State University
Cleveland, Ohio
Chapter 12

Dietrich Jehle, M.D.
Associate Professor and Vice Chairman, Department of Emergency Medicine
State University of New York at Buffalo
Director of Emergency Medicine
Erie County Medical Center
Buffalo, New York
Chapter 21

Phoebe A. Kaplan, M.D.
Professor of Radiology
Co-Director, Musculoskeletal Imaging
Department of Radiology
University of Virginia Health Sciences Center
Charlottesville, Virginia
Chapter 18

Terry Kowalenko, M.D.
Detroit Medical Center/Grace Hospital
Department of Emergency Medicine
Grace Hospital
Detroit, Michigan
Chapter 10

Richard Levitan, M.D.
Assistant Professor, Department of Emergency Medicine
Hospital of the University of Pennsylvania
Philadelphia, Pennsylvania
Chapter 14

William M. Maguire, M.D.
Assistant Professor in Clinical Emergency Medicine
Education Coordinator
University of Minnesota Hospitals
Minneapolis, Minnesota
Chapter 6

Stephen W. Meldon, M.D.
Assistant Professor, Emergency Medicine
Case Western Reserve University
Cleveland, Ohio
Department of Emergency Medicine
Metro Health Medical Center
Cleveland, Ohio
Chapter 3

Renu Chawla Mital, M.D.
Instructor in Emergency Medicine
New York Hospital/Cornell University
Joan and Sanford I. Weill Medical College
Cornell University Medical Center
New York, New York
Chapter 4

David T. Overton, M.D., F.A.C.E.P.
Emergency Medicine Program Director
Michigan State University, Kalamazoo Center for Medical Studies
Professor and Chairman, Emergency Medicine
Michigan State University College of Human Medicine
Kalamazoo, Michigan
Chapter 24

Martin V. Pusic, M.D.
Fellowship Director, Pediatric Emergency Medicine
Assistant Professor, Department of Emergency Medicine
Montreal Children's Hospital
Montreal, Quebec, Canada
Chapter 22

Rodolfo Querioz, M.D.
University of Rochester Medical Center
Department of Emergency Medicine
Rochester, New York
Chapter 7

Earl J. Reisdorff, M.D., F.A.C.E.P.
Associate Professor
Program Director, Michigan State University Emergency Medicine Residency
Ingham Regional Medical Center and Sparrow Hospital
Lansing, Michigan
Chapters 1, 2

Corinna Repetto, M.D.
EMS Medical Director, Department of Emergency Medicine
Bloomington Hospital
Bloomington, Indiana
Chapter 24

Ralph Riviello, M.D.
Attending Physician, Department of Emergency Medicine
Assistant Professor of Emergency Medicine
Ohio State University
Columbus, Ohio
Chapter 5

Brent Ruoff, M.D.
Associate Chief, Department of Emergency Medicine
Barnes-Jewish Hospital
Associate Professor of Emergency Medicine
Washington University School of Medicine
St. Louis, Missouri
Chapter 13

Daniel L. Savitt, M.D.
Program Director
Brown University Emergency Medicine Residency Program
Associate Professor of Medicine
Department of Emergency Medicine
Rhode Island Hospital
Providence, Rhode Island
Chapter 19

David T. Schwartz, M.D., F.A.C.E.P.
Assistant Professor of Clinical Surgery/Emergency Medicine
New York University School of Medicine
Attending Physician
Bellevue Hospital and New York University Medical Center
New York, New York
Chapters 1, 2, 6, 8, 9, 10, 15, 17, 19, 23

Matthew J. Spates, M.D.
Attending Physician and Clinical Instructor
Department of Emergency Medicine
Robert Wood Johnson University Hospital
New Brunswick, New Jersey
Chapter 19

Andrew Sucov, M.D.
Assistant Professor of Medicine
Medical Director, Department of Emergency Medicine
Rhode Island Hospital
Providence, Rhode Island
Chapter 7

Mary Josephine Wagner, M.D.
Associate Director, Department of Emergency Medicine
Saginaw Cooperative Hospitals
Associate Professor, Emergency Medicine
Michigan State University College of Human Medicine
Saginaw, Michigan
Chapter 17

John Douglas Wartella, M.D.
Assistant Chief of Emergency Services
David Grant Medical Center
Travis AFB, California
Chapter 8

O. Clark West, M.D.
Chief, Emergency Radiology
Hermann Hospital, Memorial Hermann Healthcare System
Assistant Professor of Radiology
University of Texas–Houston Medical School
Houston, Texas
Chapter 13

Laila Moettus Wilber, M.D.
Attending Physician
Department of Emergency Medicine
University of Colorado
Boulder, Colorado
Chapter 12

Keith Wilkinson, M.D.
Residency Program Director, Emergency Medicine
William Beaumont Hospital
Assistant Professor of Emergency Medicine
Department of Emergency Medicine
Wayne State University School of Medicine
Royal Oak, Michigan
Chapter 20

Matthew Wilks, M.D.
Attending Physician
Chandler Regional Hospital
Chandler, Arizona
Chapter 3

Brandt H. Williamson, M.D.
Clinical Instructor
West Virginia University School of Medicine
Robert C. Byrd Health Sciences Center
Martinsberg, West Virginia
Chapter 9

Robert W. Wolford, M.D.
Associate Professor and Vice-Chair
Program in Emergency Medicine
Michigan State University College of Human Medicine
Residency Director, Saginaw Cooperative Hospitals, Inc.
Michigan State University Emergency Medicine Residency
Saginaw, Michigan
Chapter 17

PREFACE

Over three decades ago, emergency medicine emerged as an organized discipline. With more than 100 residency training programs now in existence, emergency medicine has evolved into a sophisticated and broad-based arena of medical practice. The radiograph is an important tool for the evaluation of many acutely ill or injured patients, and understanding the use and interpretation of radiographic studies is an essential skill of the emergency physician. In addition, advanced imaging modalities such as computed tomography and ultrasonography are frequently used in the care of emergency department patients.

This text was developed to teach emergency radiology from the vantage point of the clinical emergency physician. The book is intended to serve as an instructional guide for the emergency medicine resident, practicing clinician, and medical student, as well as a reference text in the busy emergency department. Most chapters follow a similar format. The chapters begin with a discussion on *clinical decision making*—reviewing the indications for radiographic studies. This is followed by a discussion of *anatomy and physiology*, including the biomechanics needed to understand radiographic patterns of injury. The *radiographic technique* section illustrates the standard and supplementary radiographic views for each anatomical region and describes how these views are obtained. The core section of each chapter is entitled *radiographic analysis*. In this section, we present a step-by-step approach to interpreting the radiographs. This information is presented in a table and in drawings of each standard radiographic view. *Common abnormalities* reviews those injuries and pathologic conditions that are most frequently encountered in the emergency department, as well as those that have substantial associated morbidity. *Errors in interpretation* focuses attention on injuries that are easily missed. *Common variants* discusses anatomical variants such as accessory bones that can cause difficulty in radiographic interpretation. The *controversies* section addresses issues that are currently being debated or represent evolving practice patterns in emergency medicine.

Highlighting the text are illustrations and tables that reinforce key points. A figure appearing in most chapters focuses attention on *sites prone to injury and easily missed injuries.*

These figures provide rapid visual cues to radiograph interpretation. A corresponding table summarizes a systematic way to review the radiographs. Each standard radiographic view is shown with an accompanying line drawing that details the radiographic anatomy. An additional table describes all of the standard and supplementary views. Finally, examples of both obvious and subtle radiographic abnormalities are illustrated. Where applicable, tables describing injury patterns and radiographic findings are included.

Key concepts in the use of the radiography as a diagnostic tool for the emergency physician are presented in Chapters 1 and 2—Introduction to Emergency Radiology and Fundamentals of Skeletal Radiology. These chapters provide an introduction to the principles of radiographic analysis that are used throughout the book. Chapters 3 through 12 address the skeletal radiology of the extremities and pelvis. Chapter 13 is an extensive review of the cervical spine, while Chapter 14 continues with a discussion of the thoracolumbar spine. Facial imaging (plain film and CT) is covered in Chapter 15. An introduction to cranial CT appears in Chapter 16. Chapters 17 and 18 are devoted to pulmonary and cardiovascular radiography. Chapter 19 discusses abdominal radiography, including plain film interpretation and advanced imaging studies such as computed tomography, enteric contrast studies, and ultrasonography. The radiographic evaluation of the trauma victim is covered in Chapter 20. An introductory overview of emergency department ultrasonography is provided in Chapter 21. Pediatric considerations, including the developing skeleton, abdominal and respiratory tract emergencies, and the radiology of child abuse, are reviewed in Chapter 22. Chapter 23 addresses the role of radiology in the evaluation of the poisoned patient, a topic unique to emergency medicine. Finally, a discussion of quality improvement completes the text.

It is our hope that this book will assist physicians dedicated to the care of the acutely ill and injured patient.

David T. Schwartz, MD, FACEP
Earl J. Reisdorff, MD, FACEP

ACKNOWLEDGMENTS

The authors are pleased to acknowledge the many efforts of those who helped in the development of this book. Their contributions richly enhanced the quality of this text.

At McGraw-Hill Health Professions Division, John Dolan (Executive Editor) provided consistent encouragement for the project. Susan Noujaim (Assistant Editor) graciously assumed many of the necessary editorial tasks. Peter Boyle (Editing Supervisor) ably steered the book through the complex production process. Thanks are also given to our copy editor, Heidi Thaens, and the layout artists Marsha Cohen, Paul Lacy, Mary McDonnell, Joan O'Connor, and Wanda Lubelska, whose skill and dedication are evident throughout the book.

A special thank you is offered to Karen Jury, who served as secretary, typist, and consultant. Her cheerfulness and never-waning support proved to be beyond value. Jon Lee, M.D., and Tony Jones contributed their artistic skills to many of the line drawings of the book.

At Ingham Regional Medical Center, the Chi Medical Library staff (under the direction of Ms. Judith Barnes) satisfied numerous requests for information. David Courey kindly surrendered his dark room and taught one slow novice darkroom techniques so that this project could proceed. The staff in the radiology file room tracked down countless films on a need-it-now basis. Finally, the entire Department of Radiology at Ingham Medical Center and specifically Drs. Archambeau, Leago, Tai, Cimmerer, Dorfman, Patel, and Lindgren were quick to share their knowledge and expertise. They serve as a model of service and commitment to patient care. My hope for emergency physicians everywhere is that they have the opportunity to work with a similarly dedicated group of colleagues in the specialty of radiology.

I would also like to thank my colleagues in the Michigan State University Department of Emergency Medicine and the emergency medicine residents for their understanding. A project of this enormity diverted resources and energies away from their specific interests. (EJR)

At Bellevue Hospital and New York University Medical Center, I would like to express my gratitude to the residents (past and present), fellow faculty, and students who provide a continuing stimulus to grow and learn, and who share in the excitement of the practice of emergency medicine. Their devotion to the care of patients in the emergency department is truly an inspiration. I offer my most sincere thanks to Dr. Lewis R. Goldfrank for his unfailing encouragement and support throughout the years of work on this project. The outstanding radiology faculty at New York University serve both as excellent educators and provide invaluable assistance in the care of emergency department patients. Special thanks are given to Drs. Barry Leitman (chest radiology), Emil J. Balthazar (abdominal radiology), Cornelia Golumbo and Mahvash Rafii (skeletal radiology), Richard Siegman (emergency radiology), Richard Pinto (neuroradiology), and Albert Keegan (Director of Radiology, Bellevue Hospital). Finally, Leon Yost helped in making many high quality photographic prints that appear throughout the book. (DTS)

We also extend our sincere appreciation to Dr. Brandt Williamson. Dr. Williamson provided the original impetus for the book, contacted and obtained commitments from contributing authors, and wrote the initial draft of the sample chapter (The Ankle). The ankle chapter served as a template for the other chapters in the book. We are indebted to his contributions.

Above all, we wish to thank the many contributing authors. Their knowledge and gift of instruction were freely given.

Special Acknowledgments

Thanks to my wife, Jane—your boundless measure of kindness is a testament to your spirit. You are the finest person I know. To my daughters Rebecca and Hannah—you continue to provide the energy in my life that allows me to serve others. (EJR)

My most sincere thanks to Harriet for her kind support and assistance over the countless hours needed to bring this project to fruition. (DTS)

CHAPTER 1

INTRODUCTION TO EMERGENCY RADIOLOGY

EARL J. REISDORFF / DAVID T. SCHWARTZ

In 1895, Wilhelm Conrad Roentgen discovered x-rays, revolutionizing medicine. Although many modifications of diagnostic imaging have since developed [e.g., computed tomography (CT)], plain radiography remains the cornerstone of diagnostic radiology for emergency medicine. Of all patients seen in the emergency department (ED), 35 to 61% undergo radiographic evaluation.[1-3] Of one hospital's radiologic evaluations in ED patients, 89% were plain film studies and 11% were advanced studies (e.g., contrast study, CT) (Table 1-1).[2] Moreover, 22% of patients required multiple studies. The ED is a significant source of activity for the radiology department. Of all plain film studies done in the radiology department, 44% are ordered through the ED.[2]

CLINICAL DECISION MAKING IN EMERGENCY RADIOLOGY

The emergency physician must understand the clinical indications for various diagnostic radiographic studies. For example, the inability to walk, or localized tenderness over the posterior aspect of the distal fibula, is an indication to obtain ankle radiographs. A mild, isolated antalgic gait (limp) without bony tenderness probably does not constitute a clinical indication to obtain radiographs. However, the decision to obtain radiographic evaluation must consider the patient's age and other clinical factors, such as the history of the injurious event. The patient's expectation can also modify the physician's approach to ordering radiographs.

Ideally, radiographs should provide clinically relevant information that helps to direct the patient's care. The radiograph usually provides an extraordinary measure of information for both defining the presence of disease and excluding disease. For some situations, radiographic findings have an extremely high positive predictive value (e.g., tibial shaft fracture, lobar pneumonia). In other conditions, radiographic findings correlate poorly with the final diagnosis and add little to the patient's care (e.g., abdominal radiographs for appendicitis). Once radiographic information is obtained, the physician must revisit the differential diagnosis and decide whether any additional imaging studies would be of benefit.

The timing of diagnostic studies must also be considered. At times, stabilization of the patient requires that the diagnostic evaluation be deferred until a therapeutic action is complete.[4] For example, in the case of a tension pneumothorax, the need for a tube thoracostomy (therapeutic) outweighs the importance of getting a chest radiograph (diagnostic) to document the condition. Delaying treatment is not justified by the desire to obtain diagnostic information.

Emergency physicians must insist on receiving quality radiographs. However, it is not always necessary that the emergency physician obtain "perfect" radiographs in every setting. Nonetheless, the images must be adequate for the diagnosis in question. For example, it is of little consequence if, on a chest film, the lung apex is "cut off" on the side of a large pneumothorax. At times the patient cannot be positioned perfectly or must be imaged through an immobilization backboard. However, the emergency physician should never accept a film that does not completely visualize all critical areas. For example, the patient's nameplate must not be placed over the fifth metatarsal on an ankle film.

There is great variation among physicians in their approaches to ordering radiographs.[5-9] As compared with generalists, specialists order more radiographs. With the acquisition of experience, physicians tend to order fewer radiographs.[5,7] In addition to addressing a specific diagnostic concern, radiographs are obtained for "baseline screening," medicolegal reasons, patient reassurance, and patient demands. The number of ED radiographs ordered for medicolegal "protection" ranges from 10 to 46%.[7,8]

TABLE 1-1

Radiologic Evaluation of Emergency Department Patients*

Total patients	315
Patients receiving a study	192 (61%)
Patients with no radiologic evaluation	123 (39%)
Total number of studies performed	254
Plain radiographs	227
Advanced studies†	27
Patients receiving multiple studies	43
Patients receiving single studies	149

*Random sample of 315 ED patients seen during January 1996 at Ingham Regional Medical Center, Lansing, MI.
†Advanced studies include CT of the head (13), CT of the abdomen (3), intravenous pyelogram (5), ultrasound of the abdomen (1), leg Doppler studies for deep venous thrombosis (4), and ventilation/perfusion scan (1).

EMERGENCY PHYSICIANS AND RADIOGRAPH INTERPRETATION

The emergency physician must have expertise in the interpretation of radiographs. In fact, experienced emergency physicians have high levels of agreement with radiologists (83 to 99.6%) in radiographic interpretation.[3,10–18] In one study of 1417 patients, there were 102 (7.2%) discordant readings, yet only 38 (2.7% of patients) required any change in their treatment.[1] In another study, emergency physicians correctly interpreted 99.2% of radiographs.[19] Less than half (46%) of misread films warranted any change of therapy. Therefore, only 4 patients per 1000 required a change in treatment.[19] Among emergency medicine residents, accuracy in interpretation is related to their experience. As compared with senior-level residents, more inexperienced residents tend to overread radiographs.[20]

Errors in radiograph interpretation tend to occur in specific anatomic areas. One study found the highest error rate (12%) in studies involving the face.[3] Another study found that most missed fractures involved the ribs, elbow, and periarticular region of the phalanges. These three regions accounted for 72 of 162 missed fractures (44%).[21] A high rate of discordance also occurs in the interpretation of skull radiographs.[1,18]

At most hospitals, emergency physicians and radiologists share responsibility for the primary interpretation of radiographs. At some hospitals, radiologists interpret all films (12 to 21%).[22] At other hospitals, emergency physicians interpret all radiographs first (12 to 26%). In most settings, radiologists provide first-reading services during daytime hours; emergency physicians interpret all radiographs during the evening and overnight (62 to 67%). The in-hospital presence of a radiologist is variable in hospitals throughout the country. Nonetheless, it is essential to have radiologic consultation available on a 24-hour basis. The absence of an on-site radiologist means that the emergency physician must have substantial expertise in interpreting radiographs.

MALPRACTICE

The emergency physician must use the knowledge and skill that a reasonable clinician would employ under similar circumstances. Failure to obtain a radiologic consultation can also result in liability. The clinical reasons for ordering or not ordering radiographs should be documented. One is liable for negligence when the accepted standards of professional care are not maintained and, as a result, the patient is directly harmed.

Approximately 12% of all malpractice is radiology-related.[23] The most common causes are missed fractures and dislocations. Excellent radiographic technique and careful interpretation of the radiographs are the best safeguards against error. In one study, 20% of malpractice suits (Pennsylvania Hospital Insurance Company) from 1977 to 1981 involved the ED. Of these 200 cases involving the ED, 38 (19%) were due to failure to interpret radiographs correctly.[24] The Physician Insurance Association of American (PIAA) identified claims involving myocardial infarction and fractures of the cervical vertebrae as representing the largest dollar amounts paid in emergency malpractice medicine cases. The greatest *number* of claims in the PIAA data involved missed fractures.

Fractures and orthopedic injuries represented the third largest segment of malpractice costs (14% of all monies paid) in a study by the American College of Emergency Physicians.[25] Of these fractures, 44% were vertebral or pelvic and 22% involved the extremities.

As many as 46% of all radiographic studies are obtained because of physician concern for potential malpractice.[7,8,26] The use of clinical decision rules can provide protection for clinicians as well as guidance in clinical decision making. These are being developed for the evaluation of the cervical spine, knee, and ankle.[27–29] Similar criteria have also been developed for skull radiography.[30]

BIOLOGICAL EFFECTS OF X-RAYS

The primary risk to patients undergoing x-ray evaluation is radiation-induced malignancy, such as leukemia, thyroid cancer, breast cancer, lung cancer, and gastrointestinal cancer. Radiation exposure to the gonads has a risk of inducing genetic alteration in offspring. In addition, x-rays can cause teratogenic defects in the developing fetus and can predispose to the future development of certain malignancies after birth.

Radiation exposure to patients should be minimized. This is most easily accomplished by limiting the number of examinations. Obtaining good-quality images initially eliminates the need to retake views. Restricting the x-ray beam to those areas requiring study also reduces exposure. The gonadal areas should be shielded with a lead apron whenever they may be exposed to x-rays and do not lie in the field of interest.

TABLE 1-2

Irradiation Skin Exposures for Routine Studies

EXAMINATION	SKIN EXPOSURE, MRADS PER PROJECTION
Chest (PA)	12–26
Skull (lateral)	105–240
Abdomen (AP)	375–698
Retrograde pyelogram	475–829
Cervical spine (AP)	35–165
Thoracic spine (AP)	295–485
Extremity	8–327
Dental (bitewing and apical)	227–425
Head and body CT (total images)	3400–5500*

*The skin exposure for the CT is reported as the total dose for the entire study, not for a single image.
SOURCE: Modified from *Merrill's Atlas of Radiology,* 7th ed. St. Louis: Mosby-Year Book, 1991. With permission.

TABLE 1-3

Approximate Gonadal Doses with Various Radiographic Examinations

EXAMINATION	GONADAL DOSE, MRAD	
	MALE	FEMALE
Skull	<1	<1
Cervical spine	<1	<1
Full-mouth dental	<1	<1
Chest	<1	<1
Stomach and upper gastrointestinal	2	40
Gallbladder	1	20
Lumbar spine	175	400
Intravenous pyelogram	150	300
Abdomen	100	200
Pelvis	300	150
Upper extremity	<1	<1
Lower extremity	<1	8

SOURCE: From *Merrill's Atlas of Radiology,* 7th ed. St. Louis: Mosby–Year Book, 1991. With permission.

The standard unit of radiation exposure is the *rad* (radiation absorbed dose). This is the amount of radiation absorbed per volume of tissue. Another unit is the *rem* (radiation equivalent in man). For x-irradiation, the rad and the rem are equal. For other types of radiation (e.g., alpha-particle irradiation from a radioactive substance), the rad and the rem are not equal.

The quantity of radiation exposure to the patient is expressed in three different ways. One way is as the amount of radiation delivered to the area exposed—the *skin dose* (Table 1-2). Another way is the radiation exposure to the gonads (or fetus)—the *gonadal dose* (Table 1-3). The gonadal dose is calculated

TABLE 1-4

Estimated Whole-Body Radiation Doses from Common Diagnostic Procedures

PROCEDURE	WHOLE-BODY DOSE, MREM
Dental	2
Chest	10
Skull	40
Cervical spine	50
Cholecystogram	70
Intravenous pyelogram	120
Lumbar spine	130
CT head	200
Thoracic spine	240
Kidneys, ureters, bladder (KUB)	450
Mammogram	450
Upper GI*	750
Barium enema*	1100

*Includes fluoroscopy.
SOURCE: From Juhl JH, Crummy AB: *Essentials of Radiologic Imaging,* 5th ed. Philadelphia: Lippincott, 1987. With permission.

even if the pelvic region lies outside of the radiographic field, such as with a chest radiograph. This measure is used to assess the radiation exposure to the gonads for genetic or teratogenic effects. Finally, the *total-body radiation dose* is used to determine the risk of inducing such malignancies, as leukemia, or of causing bone marrow suppression (Table 1-4). This measure is usually used in the setting of exposure to radioactive materials.

The Pregnant Patient

Prior to ordering an elective radiographic examination, the emergency physician should determine if a woman is pregnant, especially if the examination involves the pelvis or abdomen (Table 1-5). When a patient is pregnant, alternative imaging procedures such as ultrasound and magnetic resonance imaging (MRI) should be considered. No risk of fetal malformation has been implicated in human exposures less than 1 rad.[31] Fewer than 0.1% of all properly performed radiographic examinations (not including fluoroscopy) subject the fetus to a radiation dose of 1 rad or more.[32] Fetal risk depends on the stage of pregnancy.[33] For example, in the first 2 weeks after conception, radiation does not cause malformation, but it can cause spontaneous abortion. Later in fetal development risks include cancer, malformation, and mental retardation.

The National Council on Radiation Protection states that "the risk (to the fetus) is negligible at 5 rad or less when compared to the other risks of pregnancy, and the risk of malformation is significantly increased above control levels only at doses above 15 rad."[34] In nearly all forms of diagnostic radiology performed in the ED, fetal doses are below 5 rad. Even if the fetus is in the direct path of the x-ray beam, the fetal dose is typically between 1 and 4 rad, depending on the number of films. For doses lower than 5 rad, it is unlikely that an increase in fetal malformation is measurable in human populations.

TABLE 1-5

Guidelines for Radiating the Pregnant or Potentially Pregnant Patient

1. Do not irradiate the abdomen, pelvis, lumbar spine, or hips of a woman in the first trimester of pregnancy unless it is clearly medically indicated.
2. Whenever possible, defer the examination or choose an alternative imaging modality (e.g., ultrasound).
3. In evaluating a pregnant woman with modalities that use ionizing radiation, limit the number of images or views obtained to those required to ensure adequate care.
4. If the abdomen or pelvis of a pregnant patient is accidentally irradiated, the radiology department needs to be notified. The radiation safety officer can establish the radiation dose to the fetus, and this calculation can be used to determine the potential effects on the fetus.

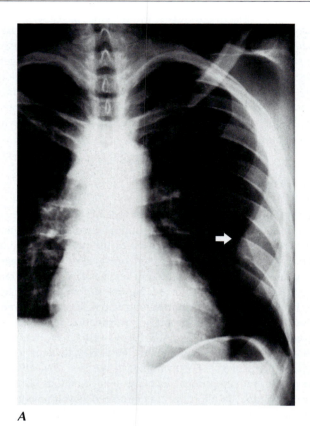

A

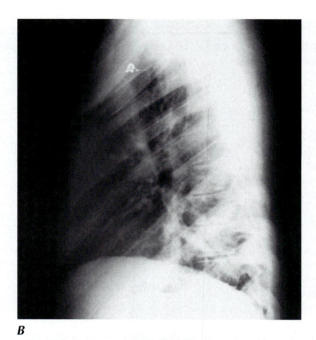

B

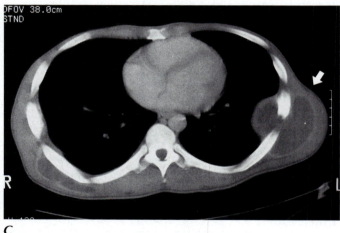

C

IMAGING MODALITIES

Conventional Plain-Film Radiography

Because of its ready availability, relatively low cost, and great diagnostic potential, plain-film radiography is the chief imaging modality in emergency medicine. Plain-film radiographic imaging depends on differences in radiographic density between air, soft tissues, bone, and metal. In addition, the shadow that an object makes on the radiographic film is a function of its thickness. Finally, an object is more apparent on the radiograph if its border is sharp and well-defined. If there is a gradual change in tissue density, the object casts an indistinct shadow on the radiograph and, in some instances, the object is "invisible" (Fig. 1-1). A nondisplaced fracture is radiographically obvious if the fracture line is parallel to the x-ray beam, whereas if the fracture lies at an angle to the x-ray beam, it will not be apparent (Fig. 1-2).

When examining a radiograph, it must be remembered that the radiograph is a two-dimensional image of a three-dimensional object. Overlapping structures are superimposed on the radiographic image. One must mentally subtract overlapping structures from the structures upon which they are superimposed (Fig. 1-3).

Standardized radiographic views have been devised for all regions of the body. These views are grouped into a radiographic series—e.g., a shoulder or abdominal series. The physician must be familiar with the positioning of the patient and the anatomy depicted on each of these radiographic views. The interpretation of a radiograph begins with the identifica-

FIGURE 1-1. Without a well-defined border, an anatomical structure can be invisible. *A.* A pleural-based mass is easily seen on the PA radiograph because it has a distinct border with the adjacent air-filled lung (*arrow*). *B.* On the lateral radiograph, the pleural-based mass is invisible because its margins are indistinct. *C.* A CT scan clearly demonstrates the nature of the lesion. The pleural-based mass tapers gradually as it intersects with the chest wall. In addition, there is a contiguous mass on the outer surface of the chest wall (*arrow*). The lesion proved to be extrapulmonary tuberculosis. (Copyright David Schwartz, MD)

tion of the particular view and assessment of its technical adequacy.

Frontal radiographs are designated by the x-ray beam's direction as it passes through the patient, either from anterior to posterior (AP) or posterior to anterior (PA). For lateral radiographs, the direction of the x-ray beam is usually not specified. The terminology for oblique radiographs is variable. For extremities in which the frontal view is an AP view, such as the ankle or elbow, an internal (medial) oblique view is obtained when the x-ray beam is directed medially, from front to back. An external (lateral) oblique is obtained when the beam is directed laterally.

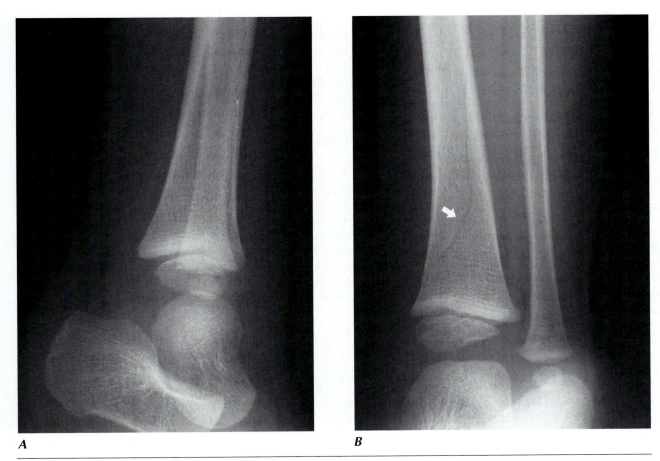

A

B

FIGURE 1-2. *A.* A nondisplaced fracture is not seen on this lateral view because the fracture line is not parallel to the x-ray beam. *B.* Another view at a different orientation shows the fracture clearly (*arrow*). This is known as a *toddler's fracture* of the tibial shaft.

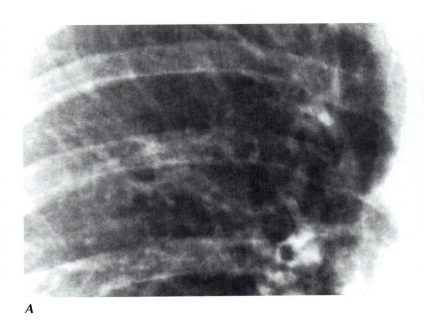

A

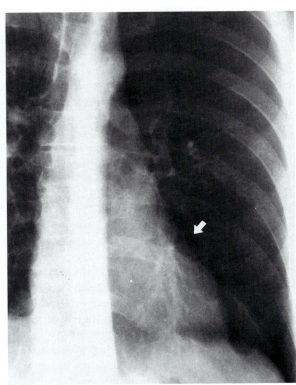

B

FIGURE 1-3. A radiograph is a two-dimensional image of a three-dimensional object. Overlapping shadows can create the appearance of structures that do not exist. *A.* The confluence of normal pulmonary vascular markings creates cyst-like shadows. *B.* The left heart border appears to have a radiolucent depression (*arrow*). This apparent concavity is caused by superimposition of the left-lower-lobe pulmonary artery and the upper margin of a rib.

PORTABLE RADIOGRAPHY. When the unstable patient cannot leave the ED, portable radiographs are obtained. The films must be developed and promptly returned to the treating physician to review. Disadvantages of portable radiography include the technical inferiority of the image, increased exposure of ED personnel to ionizing radiation, and increased patient irradiation. Only those portable radiographs that are essential should be performed when the ED staff is in an unprotected area. The ED personnel should wear protective garments (lead aprons) or position themselves behind protective shields. Increasing one's distance from the radiation source effectively decreases radiation exposure. The radiation exposure (dose) diminishes inversely with the square of the distance from the x-ray tube.[35]

RADIOGRAPHIC CONTRAST MATERIAL. Contrast studies are used to evaluate the gastrointestinal tract, urinary tract, central nervous system, and vascular system. In the ED, intravenous contrast agents are most often used for intravenous pyelograms and CT. Emergency angiography is used to evaluate the aorta, pulmonary arteries, and peripheral blood vessels. To opacify the lumen of the gastrointestinal (GI) tract, either water-soluble contrast or a suspension of barium is used.

A prior allergic reaction to intravenous contrast material is a relative contraindication to its use. Numerous pretreatment protocols have been developed to decrease allergic reactions to contrast agents. Protocols involve the administration of steroids and antihistamines 12 hours prior to the study. Because of the time delay, studies requiring pretreatment are best performed on an elective basis, not as an ED study. If needed, an alternative study or noncontrast study can often be substituted.

In a patient with suspected renal disease (e.g., diabetes, multiple myeloma, connective tissue disease), serum creatinine levels should be determined prior to contrast administration. In addition, the patient should be well hydrated prior to the study. Renal insufficiency (serum creatinine ≥ 1.7 mg/dL) increases the risk of contrast-induced renal failure. In most cases, contrast-induced renal failure is transient. In addition, the hypovolemic patient given a contrast agent is at increased risk for developing renal disease. The amount of contrast material that is given to a hypotensive patient should be limited.

Both ionic (high-osmolality) and nonionic (low-osmolality) agents are available for intravascular use. Nonionic agents produce fewer adverse reactions—either allergic or renal.[36–39] However, the cost of nonionic contrast is ten to twenty times greater than that of ionic contrast.[40,41] The issue of cost will become considerably less important in the near future, when the patents of some nonionic contrast agents expire. The price of nonionic agents will then be only about three times that of conventional ionic agents.

The contrast agent most often used to evaluate the bowel is barium, a high-density compound suspended in water. It is administered either orally or rectally. Barium should be avoided when a perforated viscus is suspected because it is irritating to exposed tissues and is not resorbed. Water-soluble contrast agents (e.g., Gastrografin) are used when GI perforation is suspected because they are readily absorbed by the peritoneum. Water-soluble contrast agents are hypertonic, producing a

cathartic effect. Because this may lead to hypovolemia and hypotension, water-soluble contrast agents must be used cautiously in dehydrated, malnourished, elderly, or debilitated patients. If aspirated, water-soluble contrast material causes a chemical pneumonitis. Owing to this, barium is preferred when the patient is at risk for aspiration.

Computed Tomography

In CT, a narrowly collimated x-ray beam rotates 360° around the patient (Fig. 1-4). With current CT scanners, the acquisition time for each slice (time for the x-ray source to rotate around the patient) is about 2 sec. A ring of x-ray detectors encircles the patient. These detectors measure the attenuation of the x-ray beam as it passes through the patient in a great number of directions. From these data, a computer generates the CT image on a rectilinear grid made up of picture elements (pixels) (Fig. 1-5). Each pixel is assigned a density number in

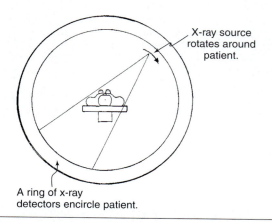

FIGURE 1-4. Diagram of a fourth-generation CT scanner. The x-ray source rotates around the patient. The attenuation of the x-ray beam is measured by a fixed ring of detectors surrounding the patient. A different set of measurements is made for each position of the x-ray source. (Redrawn from Ballinger PW: *Merrill's Atlas of Radiology*, 7th ed. St. Louis, Mosby-Year Book, 1991, with permission.)

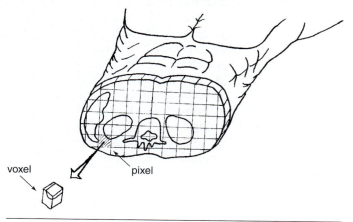

FIGURE 1-5. The CT image is constructed on a grid. Each square on the grid is termed a picture element or *pixel*. Each pixel represents a volume of tissue (*voxel*) that corresponds to the thickness of the CT slice. (Redrawn from Ballinger PW: *Merrill's Atlas of Radiology*, 7th ed. St. Louis, Mosby-Year Book, 1991, with permission.)

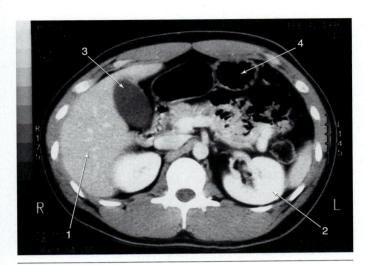

FIGURE 1-6. An abdominal CT scan demonstrates the great ability of CT to distinguish differences in radiodensity. Intravenous and oral contrast have been administered. The intraabdominal organs are readily differentiated from surrounding fat tissue. The liver is moderately enhanced; there is greater enhancement of intrahepatic blood vessels (*arrow 1*). The kidneys are intensely enhanced (*arrow 2*). The gallbladder contains unenhanced fluid that appears medium gray (*arrow 3*). Enteric contrast is within bowel loops in the mid-abdomen. Mesenteric and perinephric fat is nearly black. Gas within the intestinal lumen appears black (*arrow 4*).

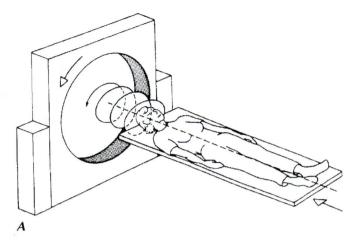

A

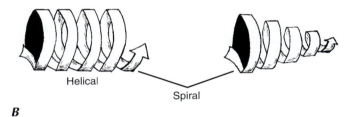

B

FIGURE 1-7. *A.* A helical (spiral) CT scanner. As the x-ray tube continuously rotates around the patient, the patient is simultaneously advanced through the scanner on the scanner gantry. (From Brink JA: Technical aspects of helical CT. *Radiol Clin North Am* 33:826, 1995. With permission.) *B.* Comparison of the terms *spiral* and *helical*. The term *helix* is limited to a cylindrical configuration, whereas *spiral* is a broader term that applies to both cylindrical and conical shapes. Both terms are appropriately applied to this CT technology.

Hounsfield units. The pixel actually represents a volume of tissue, the thickness of which is equal to the thickness of the CT slice. The thickness of CT slices ranges from the standard 10-mm slice, to 5-mm slices for detailed imaging of the brain or abdomen, to 1.5-mm slices that provide fine detail of bone.

There are two key advantages to CT scanning. First, it provides tomographic slices. This eliminates the overlap of structures inherent in conventional radiography improving anatomical resolution. Second, CT is better able than conventional radiography to discriminate slight differences in soft tissue density. This, for example, allows the CT to distinguish intraabdominal organs from their surrounding fat (Fig. 1-6). Contrast material is injected intravenously and administered enterally to enhance visualization of certain anatomic structures.

Helical (spiral) CT is a significant advance in imaging technology. The x-ray source rotates continuously around the patient as the patient is slowly advanced through the scanner (Fig. 1-7). This eliminates time delay and patient movement between slices. An entire chest or abdominal study can be performed in 20 to 30 sec. during a single held breath. The alignment between slices is improved, providing greater accuracy for reformatted images in the coronal or sagittal planes. Reformatted images with three-dimensional surface rendering improve visualization of complex fractures such as those of the face or pelvis. Rapid imaging after a bolus of intravenous contrast permits excellent visualization of major arterial structures such as the aorta or pulmonary arteries.

Uses of CT. CT scanning is used in the emergency evaluation of traumatic and nontraumatic disorders of the central nerv-

ous system (CNS) and abdomen. CT is performed electively to determine the anatomy of complex fractures of the spine, face, and pelvis. CT of the spine is occasionally used in the ED to clarify a questionable abnormality seen on plain films.

In emergency cranial CT scanning, detection of hemorrhage or mass effect is the main diagnostic concern and a scan without administration of intravenous contrast is usually sufficient. If additional information is needed about mass lesions such as tumors, abscesses, or vascular malformations, a contrast infused scan is performed after the noncontrast study.[42]

In imaging the abdomen, an optimal CT study employs both intravenous and oral contrast. To opacify the lumen of the entire intestinal tract, oral contrast material should be administered over a 2-hour period. If a 2-hour delay is not practical, as is often the case in patients with blunt abdominal trauma, this time period can be shortened with only a limited loss of information. Intravenous contrast is used in abdominal CT studies to better detect lesions of solid organs (liver, spleen, kidneys), such as infarction or intraparenchymal hemorrhage. Vascular lesions and abnormalities of the bowel wall are also better detected using intravenous contrast. If there is a contraindication to intravenous contrast (allergic history, asthma, renal insufficiency) and a delay of 12 hours for steroid pretreatment is not possible, a noncontrast abdominal CT can be useful. For detecting ureteral calculi in the setting of flank pain, a noncontrast helical CT study is used.

Emergency thoracic CT is used to assess major vascular disorders such as aortic dissection and thoracic aortic aneurysms. Recently, helical CT with bolus intravenous contrast has been used to detect pulmonary embolism and traumatic aortic injury.

Ultrasonography

Ultrasonography is a noninvasive imaging technique that uses ultra-high frequency sound waves. Ultrasound image formation depends on echogenicity rather than radiodensity. Ultrasound is especially valuable in visualizing soft tissues such as solid organs and vascular structures that are poorly seen by conventional radiography. The abdomen, pelvis, and heart are the main regions where ultrasound is used. Ultrasound does not employ ionizing radiation and can scan the body in any plane. The primary disadvantages of ultrasound are its dependence on the technical skill of the operator and its inability to penetrate gas and bone.

Current ultrasound technology generates two-dimensional real-time gray-scale images. These are usually recorded as static two-dimensional pictures. A videotape recording is sometimes used with cardiac imaging. The incorporation of Doppler technology into the ultrasound transducer (duplex ultrasound) allows detection of blood flow within vascular structures. Color Doppler provides a two-dimensional image of flow within a major blood vessel or the heart.

Ultrasonography is performed in the radiology department, at the bedside in some emergency departments, and in certain office settings. In the radiology department, the imaging is usually performed by an ultrasound technician and interpreted by a radiologist. A limited bedside ultrasound can be performed in the ED by clinicians to rapidly acquire information related to particular clinical questions. There are six specific uses for ED ultrasound. In suspected acute cholecystitis or biliary colic, gallstones can be readily detected. Hydronephrosis can be seen in patients with suspected renal colic. An abdominal aortic aneurysm is quickly and reliably diagnosed or excluded. Transvaginal ultrasound reliably detects an intrauterine gestation early in pregnancy, considerably reducing the likelihood of an ectopic pregnancy. In blunt abdominal trauma, the ultrasound can quickly detect hemoperitoneum and obviate the need for diagnostic peritoneal lavage in an unstable patient. Finally, bedside ultrasound can readily identify a pericardial effusion due to trauma or an inflammatory process. In the setting of nontraumatic cardiac arrest, the presence or absence of cardiac contractions can be helpful in assessing cardiac resuscitation.

Radiology department ultrasound provides more complete evaluation. Complete abdominal ultrasonography visualizes the liver, biliary tree, pancreas, and kidneys. Special graded-compression technique is used to diagnose appendicitis. Pelvic ultrasound studies using a Doppler probe can detect reduced or absent blood flow due to ovarian torsion. Scrotal duplex ultrasound can likewise distinguish testicular torsion from epididymitis. Lower extremity duplex ultrasound is used to diagnose deep venous thrombosis, especially if the thrombus is proximal to the calf. Transthoracic echocardiography is used to assess heart chamber size, wall motion, and valvular lesions. Transesophageal echocardiography can examine the thoracic aorta for evidence of dissection or traumatic laceration.

Nuclear Scintigraphy

Nuclear imaging uses radioactively labeled materials that are injected intravenously or inhaled. A particular organ selectively absorbs the isotope. The patient is then studied with a detector that measures radioactive emission from the isotope. Nuclear medicine studies are used in emergency medicine to detect pulmonary embolism (lung ventilation/perfusion scanning) and acute cholecystitis (hepatobiliary scanning).

Magnetic Resonance Imaging

In many areas of clinical medicine, MRI has become the definitive diagnostic imaging study. This includes imaging of the brain and spine, orthopedic trauma involving soft tissues, and great vessels of the thorax (Fig. 1-8).[43] Nevertheless, in the emergency setting, the role of MRI remains limited. In many institutions there is limited availability of MRI on an emergency basis. Image acquisition time is slow, requiring a stable and cooperative patient. Moreover, access to life-support equipment is limited. For cranial imaging, CT is in fact preferable to MRI for many acute disorders, such as traumatic and nontraumatic hemorrhage.[42]

In two situations, MRI is the preferred imaging modality in the ED. With acute spinal cord compression, MRI provides evaluation of the entire spinal cord without the hazardous intrathecal injection of contrast needed for myelography or CT myelography. MRI can also diagnose an occult femoral neck fracture in an individual with osteoporosis.[44] The alternative study, bone scintigraphy, is not diagnostic for 5 or more days after the injury.

MRI does not use ionizing radiation. The patient is placed in a chamber and subjected to a strong magnetic field, causing alignment of the minute magnetic poles of hydrogen nuclei (protons). A brief radiofrequency stimulus is applied to the area of the body part being studied. This causes a perturbation in the magnetic alignment of the protons. The protons then return to their baseline state, during which they emit a signal. This signal is used to form the magnetic resonance image. Differing radio-signal stimuli and detection protocols determine the different signal strengths for various tissues.

MRI provides even greater discrimination of various soft tissues than CT. It has excellent anatomic resolution and can generate images in any anatomic plane (axial, coronal, sagittal, oblique). The image is not degraded by bone artifacts, which is important in imaging the posterior fossa and brainstem. How-

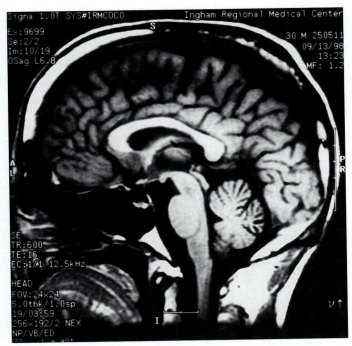

A

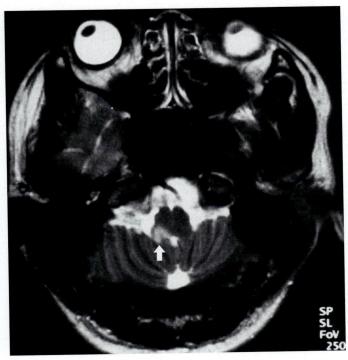

B

FIGURE 1-8. *A.* A midsagittal cranial MRI demonstrates that MRI provides far greater discrimination of soft tissues than does CT. Images can be obtained in any plane, such as sagittal, coronal, or oblique. *B.* An MRI showing a brainstem infarction (*arrow*) due to vertebral artery dissection. The dense surrounding bone is not visible and, unlike CT, does not cause degradation of the image. In this T2-weighted image, fluid has a very strong signal, and the CSF and brainstem edema both appear white. The patient presented with mild vertigo 2 days after twisting her neck. She had ipsilateral facial numbness, pupillary dilation, and contralateral arm paresthesia. (*B.* Copyright David Schwartz, MD)

ever, MRI is less sensitive than CT in detecting calcified lesions and acute intracranial hemorrhage. Certain radiofrequency pulse sequences are used to generate MR angiographic images.

REFERENCES

1. Mayhue FE, Rust DD, Aldag JC, et al: Accuracy of interpretations of emergency department radiographs: effects of confidence levels. *Ann Emerg Med* 18:826, 1989.
2. Reisdorff EJ: Radiologic studies in the ED at Ingham Regional Medical Center, Lansing, Michigan (unpublished data), January 1996.
3. Gratton MC, Salomone JA III, Watson WA: Clinically significant radiograph misinterpretations at an emergency medicine residency program. *Ann Emerg Med* 19:497, 1990.
4. Walls RM, Connell DG: Multiple trauma, in Rosen P, Doris PE, Barkin RM, et al (eds): *Diagnostic Radiology in Emergency Medicine.* St. Louis: Mosby–Year Book, 1992.
5. Childs AW, Hunter ED: Non-medical factors influencing the use of diagnostic x-ray by physicians. *Med Care* 10:323, 1972.
6. Cummins RO: Clinicians' reasons for overuse of skull radiographs. *AJR* 135:549, 1980.
7. de Lacey GJ, Barker A, Wignall V, et al: *AJR* for requesting radiographs in an accident department. *BMJ* 1:159, 1979.
8. Eliastam M, Rose E, Jones H, et al: Utilization of diagnostic radiologic examinations in the emergency department of teaching hospitals. *J Trauma* 20:61, 1980.
9. Pineault R: The effect of medical training factors on physician utilization behavior. *Med Care* 15:51, 1977.
10. Fleisher G, Ludwig S, McSorley M: Interpretation of pediatric x-ray films by emergency department pediatricians. *Ann Emerg Med* 12:153, 1983.
11. Nolan TM, Oberklaid F, Boldt D: Radiological services in a hospital emergency department: An evaluation of service delivery and radiograph interpretation. *Aust Paediatr J* 20:109, 1984.
12. McLain PL, Kirkwood CR: The quality of emergency room radiograph interpretations. *J Fam Pract* 20:443, 1985.
13. Overton DT: Quality assurance assessment of radiograph reading accuracy by emergency medicine faculty (abst). *Ann Emerg Med* 16:503, 1987.
14. Quick G, Podgorny G: An emergency department radiology audit procedure. *JACEP* 6:247, 1977.
15. Masel JL, Grant PJF: Accuracy of radiological diagnosis in the emergency department of a children's hospital. *Aust Paediatr J* 20:221, 1977.
16. Galasko CSB, Monahan PRW: Value of re-examining x-ray films of outpatients attending accident services. *BMJ* 1:643, 1971.
17. de Lacey G, Barker A, Harper J, et al: An assessment of the clinical effects of the clinical effects of reporting accident and emergency radiographs. *Br J Radiol* 53:394, 1980.
18. Rhea JT, Potsaid MS, DeLuca SA: Errors of interpretation as elicited by a quality audit of an emergency radiology facility. *Radiology* 132:277, 1979.
19. Brunswick JE, Ilkhanipour K, Seaberg DC: Radiographic interpretation in the emergency department. *Am J Emerg Med* 14:346, 1996.
20. Ilkanipour K, Seaberg DC: Emergency department radiograph interpretation: Effect of education level. *Ann Emerg Med* 25:159, 1995.

21. Freed HA, Shields NN: Most frequently overlooked radiographically apparent fractures in a teaching hospital emergency department. *Ann Emerg Med* 13:900, 1984.

22. O'Leary MR, Smith M, Olmsted WW, Curtis DJ: Physician assessments of practice patterns in emergency department radiograph interpretation. *Ann Emerg Med* 17:1019, 1988.

23. Berlin L: Malpractice and radiologists, update 1986: An 11.5-year perspective. *AJR* 147:1291, 1986.

24. Trautlein JJ, Lambert RL, Miller J: Malpractice in the emergency department—Review of 200 cases. *Ann Emerg Med* 13:709, 1984.

25. Fastow JS: Medical legal risks: Identification and reduction, in American College of Emergency Physicians (eds): *Comprehensive Guide to Effective Practice Management.* Dallas: ACEP, 1986.

26. Twine EH, Potchen EJ: *A Dynamic Systems Analysis of Defensive Medicine.* Cambridge, MA: MIT, June 1973.

27. Cadoux CG, White ST, Hedberg MC: High yield roentgenographic criteria for cervical spine injuries. *Ann Emerg Med* 16:738, 1997.

28. Stiell IG, Greenburg GH, McKnight D, et al: Decision rules for the use of radiography in acute ankle injuries. *JAMA* 269:1127, 1993.

29. Stiell IG, Greenburg GH, Wells GA, et al: Prospective validation of a decision rule for the use of radiography in acute knee injuries. *JAMA* 275:611, 1996.

30. Masters SJ, McClean PM, Arcarese JS, et al: Skull x-ray referral criteria panel: skull x-ray examinations after head trauma; Recommendations for multi-disciplinary panel and validation study. *New Engl J Med* 316:84, 1987.

31. Wagner LK, Lester RG, Saldana LR (eds): *Exposure of the Pregnant Patient to Diagnostic Radiation: A Guide to Medical Management.* Philadelphia: Lippincott, 2nd ed., 1997.

32. Bureau of Radiologic Health: *Population Exposure to X-Rays, U.S. 1970.* DHEW Publications (FDA) 73-8047. Washington, DC: U.S. Government Printing Office, 1973.

33. Graham S, Levin ML, Lilienfeld AM, et al: Preconception, intrauterine, and post-natal irradiation as related to leukemia, in *Epidemiologic Approaches to the Study of Cancer and Other Chronic Diseases,* W Haenszel (ed). National Cancer Institute, monograph #19 Washington, DC: U.S. Government Printing Office, 1966.

34. *Medical Radiation Exposure of Potentially Pregnant Women.* NCRP Report #54. Bethesda, MD: National Council on Radiation Protection and Measurements, July 15, 1977.

35. Tominaga GT, Ingegno M, Nahabedian M, et al: Radiation exposure from cervical spine radiographs. *Am J Emerg Med* 12:15, 1994.

36. Widrich WC, Beckman CF, Robins AH, et al: Iopamidol and meglumine diatrizoate: Comparison of effects on patient discomfort during aortofemoral angiography. *Radiology* 148:61, 1983.

37. Ciuffo AA, Fuchs RM, Guzman PA, et al: Benefits of nonionic contrast in coronary arteriography: Preliminary results of a ran-

domized double-blind trial comparing iopamidol with Renografin-76. *Invest Radiol* 19:S197, 1984.

38. Gwitt DG, Nagle RE: Contrast media for left ventricular angiography: A comparison between Cardio-Conray and iopamidol. *Br Heart J* 51:427, 1984.

39. Bettman MA, Higgins CB: Comparison of an ionic contrast agent for cardiac angiography: Results of a multicenter trial. *Invest Radiol* 20:S70, 1985.

40. Fischer HW, Spataro RF, Rosenberg PM: Medical and economic considerations in using a new contrast medium. *Arch Intern Med* 146:1717, 1986.

41. Wolf GF: Safer, more expensive iodinated contrast agents: How do we decide? *Radiology* 159:557, 1986.

42. Gilman S: Imaging of the brain. *New Engl J Med* 338:812, 1998.

43. Edelman RR, Warach S: Magnetic resonance imaging. *New Engl J Med* 328:708, 1993.

44. May DA, Purins JL, Smith DK: MR imaging of occult traumatic fractures and muscular injuries of the hip and pelvis in elderly patients. *AJR* 166:1075, 1966.

BIBLIOGRAPHY

American College of Emergency Physicians: *Cost Effective Diagnostic Testing in Emergency Medicine.* Dallas: ACEP, 1994.

Ballinger PW: *Merrill's Atlas of Radiographic Positions and Radiographic Procedures,* 7th ed. St. Louis: Mosby–Year Book, 1991.

Harris JH, Haris WH, Novelline RA: *The Radiology of Emergency Medicine,* 3d ed., Baltimore: Williams & Wilkins, 1993.

Keats TE: *Emergency Radiology,* 2d ed. Chicago: Year Book, 1989.

Langston CS, Squire LF: *Exercises in Diagnostic Radiology:* Vol 7. *The Emergency Patient.* Philadelphia: Saunders, 1975.

Levy RC, Hawkins H, Barsan WG: *Radiology in Emergency Medicine.* St. Louis: Mosby, 1986.

McCort JJ, Mindelzan RE: *Trauma Radiology.* New York: Churchill-Livingstone, 1990.

Mirvis SE, Young JWR: *Imaging in Trauma and Critical Care.* Baltimore: Williams & Wilkins, 1992.

Nicholson DA, Driscoll PA: *ABC of Emergency Radiology.* London: BMJ Press, 1995.

Novelline RA: *Squire's Fundamentals of Radiology,* 5th ed. Cambridge, MA, Harvard University Press, 1997.

Redman HC, Purdy PD, Miller GL, Rollins NK: *Emergency Radiology.* Philadelphia: Saunders, 1993.

Rosen P, Doris PE, Barsan RM, Barsan SZ, Markovchick VJ: *Diagnostic Radiology in Emergency Medicine.* St. Louis: Mosby, 1992.

Wiest P, Roth P: *Fundamentals of Emergency Radiology.* Philadelphia: Saunders, 1996.

CHAPTER 2

FUNDAMENTALS OF SKELETAL RADIOLOGY

DAVID T. SCHWARTZ / EARL J. REISDORFF

Skeletal studies are the most commonly ordered radiographs in the emergency department (ED). In most cases, they are obtained to evaluate traumatic injuries. Less commonly, nontraumatic skeletal lesions are seen. The emergency clinician must be proficient in interpreting these radiographic images. In addition, the physician must understand the indications for ordering these radiographic studies and the clinical implications of the results.

THE CLINICAL DIAGNOSIS OF A FRACTURE

The diagnosis of a fracture is based on the findings on clinical examination. Radiography provides diagnostic confirmation and anatomic detail about the injury. The clinical diagnosis of a fracture is based on three factors: (1) the mechanism of injury, (2) the findings on physical examination, and (3) the age of the patient. These three clinical factors can predict the patient's injury. For example, after a fall on an outstretched hand resulting in an injured elbow, the adult is most likely to have a radial head fracture, whereas a child is likely to have a fracture of the supracondylar region of the distal humerus. The diagnosis of soft tissue injuries of the extremities rests on clinical rather than radiographic examination. Such soft tissue injuries as neurovascular, ligamentous, or tendon injuries can be of greater clinical importance than the associated skeletal lesions. Finally, the clinical examination will determine which radiographic studies to obtain and when radiographs can be safely avoided. However, only when a fracture can be confidently excluded should radiographs be omitted.

Occasionally, a fracture is present without any radiographic abnormality. In these cases, the diagnosis rests solely on the clinical findings. For example, stress fractures and some nondisplaced fractures of the scaphoid are not shown on the initial radiographic examination. Likewise, some nondisplaced growth plate fractures in children can be difficult or impossible to detect radiographically. In these cases, the clinical diagnosis of a "probable fracture" should be made and the patient treated with adequate immobilization and follow-up care. Subsequent radiographs in 1 to 2 weeks reveal the fracture by showing signs of healing, such as resorption at the fracture site or periosteal reaction.

THE RADIOGRAPHIC DIAGNOSIS OF A FRACTURE

There are three radiographic signs that indicate a fracture: (1) identification of the fracture line, (2) changes in the surrounding soft tissues, and (3) alterations in skeletal contour or alignment. These three radiographic findings are used in the "ABC'S" approach to skeletal radiograph interpretation, in which "A" stands for *alignment,* "B" represents fracture lines disrupting the *bone,* "C" directs attention to *cartilage* (joint spaces) and "S" stands for *soft tissue* abnormalities.

Visualization of the Fracture

Demonstration of a break in the cortex or trabecular network of a bone is the most direct radiographic sign of a fracture. To characterize a fracture adequately, radiographs in at least two perpendicular planes (usually frontal and lateral views) are necessary. In areas of complex anatomy such as the wrist and foot, a third view, usually an oblique view, is included in the standard radiographic series. The views included in a "standard" series vary from institution to institution; the clinician must be aware of these differences (Table 2-1).

Occasionally, *supplementary views* are needed to demonstrate the fracture. This is especially true for nondisplaced fractures in which the fracture line is not parallel to the x-ray beam in the standard views (Fig. 2-1). Supplementary views are also used to confirm a questionable abnormality seen on the standard views and to more fully define an injury that is evident on the standard views. The supplementary view is often an oblique view. Supplementary oblique views are used, for example, to diagnose a tibial plateau fracture of the knee or a radial head fracture at the elbow. Sometimes, a supplementary view is taken in the third perpendicular plane, usually an axial view. For example, a "sunrise" view of the patella can detect a vertical patellar fracture; the axial view of the calcaneus is obtained to detect a longitudinal fracture of the posterior tuberosity of the calcaneus; and an axillary view of the shoulder is used to detect a posterior shoulder dislocation. Some supplementary views entail special positioning, such as the "scaphoid"

TABLE 2-1

Standard and Supplementary Radiographic Views of the Extremities

	STANDARD VIEWS*	SUPPLEMENTARY VIEWS
Shoulder	AP views: External rotation Internal rotation	Y view of scapula Axillary view
Clavicle	Straight AP Angled AP	Steeply angled sternoclavicular view
Elbow	AP Lateral	Oblique views (2) Olecranon view
Wrist	PA Lateral Pronation oblique	Scaphoid view Supination oblique Carpal tunnel view
Finger	PA Lateral Pronation oblique	
Thumb	PA (thumb is oblique) Lateral	True AP (Robert view)

Pelvis	AP	Judet views (oblique views of acetabulum) Inlet and outlet views
Hip	AP (pelvis) "Frog-leg"	Cross-table lateral Oblique view
Knee	AP Lateral	Oblique views (2) "Sunrise" patellar view Notch view (tunnel view)
Ankle	AP Lateral Mortise	Oblique views (2) "Poor" lateral
Foot	AP Lateral Internal oblique	Calcaneal axial view External oblique

*The specific radiographic views that are "standard" often vary from institution to institution.

view of the wrist. The scaphoid view is a posteroanterior (PA) view with the wrist in ulnar deviation. This positioning reduces the foreshortening of the scaphoid present on the standard PA view and can reveal a fracture through the midportion of the scaphoid that is not seen on the standard wrist series.

Fracture Mimics. Certain radiographic findings mimic fracture lines. These include an accessory ossicle, a growth plate (physis) or an unfused apophysis in a child, a nutrient artery foramen, and a Mach band due to radiographic shadows that overlie the bone (Fig. 2-2). These "pseudofractures" are distinguished from fractures by their characteristic location, smooth and well-corticated margins, and the absence of a cortical defect on the adjacent bone. Moreover, acute fractures are tender on examination, whereas pseudofractures are not tender.

Soft Tissue Abnormalities

Soft tissue findings provide indirect evidence of a fracture and may be more radiographically prominent than the fracture itself (Table 2-2). In some instances, soft tissue signs should be considered presumptive evidence of a fracture and the patient should be managed accordingly. For example, a hemarthrosis of the el-

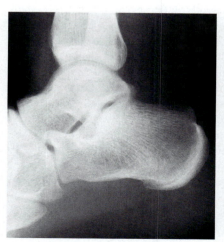
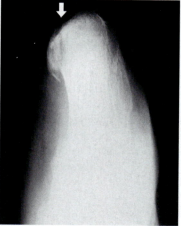
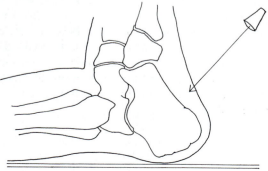

FIGURE 2-1. A supplementary radiographic view is sometimes necessary to visualize a nondisplaced fracture. *A.* The standard lateral view of the foot does not show this posterior calcaneal fracture. The posterior portion of the calcaneus is not seen on an AP view of the foot or ankle. *B.* An axial view reveals the longitudinal fracture of the posterior tuberosity of the calcaneus. *C.* Positioning for the axial calcaneal view. (Copyright David T. Schwartz, MD)

A   *B*   *C*

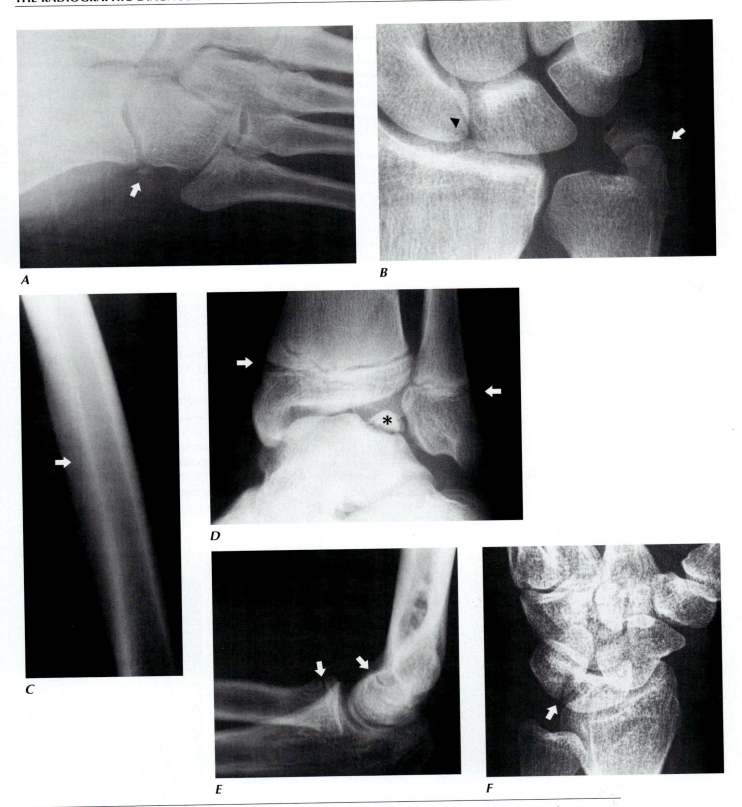

FIGURE 2-2. Pseudofractures should not be misinterpreted as acute injuries. *A.* Accessory ossicles of the foot are common. The os peroneum is adjacent to the cuboid. *B.* An accessory ossicle of the ulnar styloid is distinguished from a fracture by its smooth, well-corticated margins (*arrow*). *C.* The foramen of a nutrient artery is an interruption in the cortex with well corticated margins; it has a typical location and an oblique orientation. Nutrient artery foramena are present on only one side of the bone. *D.* Growth plates in children can have an irregular appearance that mimics a fracture. An osteochondral fracture of the talar dome is also present (*asterisk*). *E.* Partially fused growth plates at the elbow. *F.* Overlying bones or soft tissue shadows can create an illusory dark *Mach band* that looks like a fracture. In a wrist radiograph, the overlying lunate creates a Mach band on the triquetrum (*arrow*). A Mach band is also seen in *B* (*arrowhead*).

TABLE 2-2

Soft Tissue Signs of Fracture

SOFT TISSUE SIGN	RADIOGRAPHIC VIEW	COMMON FRACTURES

Elbow fat pads:
    Posterior fat pad
    Anterior "sail" sign
	Lateral elbow	Radial head (adult)
		Supracondylar humerus,
		   lateral condyle (child)

Supinator fat stripe	Lateral elbow	Proximal radius or ulna
Pronator quadratus fat stripe	Lateral wrist	Distal radius
Scaphoid fat stripe	PA wrist	Scaphoid
Knee lipohemarthrosis	Cross-table lateral knee	Tibial plateau, intercondylar eminence, osteochondral fracture
Ankle effusion	Lateral ankle	Distal tibial or fibular articular surface, talar dome
Cervicocranial prevertebral soft tissue swelling	Lateral cervical spine	Cervicocranial injuries

Maxillary sinus air/fluid
level
	Waters view (upright)	Orbital floor fracture
		   (blowout fracture, tripod
		   fracture, LeFort fracture)

Orbital emphysema	Waters view	Fracture into maxillary
		   sinus, ethmoid sinus, or
		   frontal sinus (uncommon)

Scalp swelling	Head CT	Skull fracture: coup injury
		   (brain contusion, epidural
		   hematoma, subdural
		   hematoma)

bow due to an intraarticular fracture causes a distinctive elevation of fat tissue normally hidden within the olecranon and coronoid fossae of the distal humerus (Fig. 2-3). In an adult, a displaced anterior or posterior fat-pad on the lateral elbow radiograph is most often due to a fracture of the radial head. In a child, a supracondylar or lateral condylar fracture of the distal humerus is most common.

In the upper cervical spine, prevertebral soft tissue swelling seen on the lateral radiograph is an important clue to a fracture. On facial radiographs, orbital emphysema and an air-fluid level in the maxillary sinus are soft tissue signs that indicate an orbital fracture. An air-fluid level in the sphenoid sinus seen on a cross-table lateral radiograph of the cervical spine or a head CT scan suggests a basilar skull fracture.

Changes in Skeletal Contour or Alignment

When an actual break in a bone is not seen, changes in the *contour* of the bone or in *alignment* between adjacent bones are signs of a fracture, dislocation, or subluxation (Fig. 2-4). Changes in contour or alignment can be difficult to recognize and familiarity with normal radiographic anatomy is required. For example, an abnormal angle between the femoral

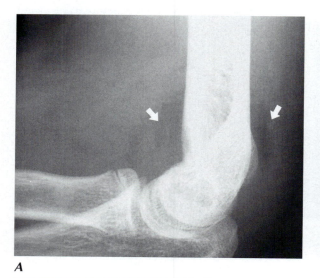 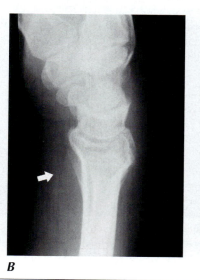 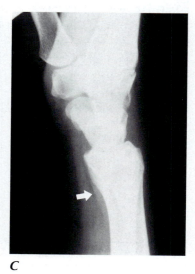

A   *B*   *C*

FIGURE 2-3. Changes in nearby soft tissues are sometimes more easily seen than the fracture itself. *A.* Displaced anterior and posterior fat pads indicate an intraarticular fracture about the elbow (*arrows*). *B.* The pronator quadratus fat stripe is bowed forward and partly obliterated (*arrow*) by hemorrhage due to a nondisplaced fracture of the distal radius (*arrowhead*). (Copyright David T. Schwartz) *C.* A normal pronator quadratus fat stripe lies close to the volar surface of the distal radius (*arrow*).

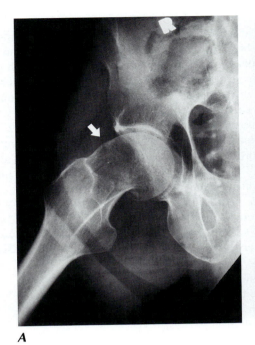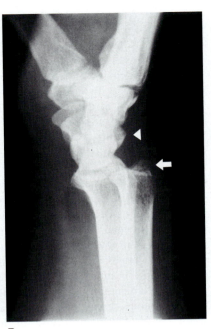

A   *B*

FIGURE 2-4. Abnormalities in skeletal contour or alignment are indicative of a fracture or dislocation. *A*. In this impacted fracture of the femoral neck, there is an abnormal angle between the femoral head and the femoral neck. *B*. Dislocation of the distal radioulnar joint was initially missed. Although the dorsal surfaces of the distal radius and ulna are usually superimposed on a lateral radiograph, they will not overlap if the positioning is rotated. However, the tip of the ulnar styloid (*arrow*) should "point" to the dorsal surface of the triquetrum (*arrowhead*), even if the view is rotated. Knowledge of normal radiographic anatomy is necessary to detect subtle abnormalities. (Copyright David T. Schwartz)

neck and femoral head is a sign of a subcapital fracture of the proximal femur. Malalignment of the carpal bones on the lateral view of the wrist is usually the clearest radiographic finding of a perilunate dislocation.

SYSTEMATIC INTERPRETATION OF SKELETAL RADIOGRAPHS

The accurate interpretation of a radiographic study depends on knowing normal radiographic anatomy, and characteristic abnormalities that occur the region being examined. Characteristic abnormalities include fracture patterns (both obvious and subtle) and anatomic variants. Two complementary approaches are used to analyze skeletal radiographs in the setting of trauma.

An *ABC'S approach* sequentially examines alignment, bones, cartilage, and soft tissue (Table 2-3). With a *targeted approach*, common sites of injury are first examined and then sites of frequently missed abnormalities are scrutinized.

The ABC'S Approach to Radiograph Interpretation

Adequacy. The correct patient's name, date, and proper left-right labeling are on the film. All of the appropriate views are included and all important anatomic structures are shown (e.g., the C7-T1 interface on cervical spine films, the fifth metatarsal base on ankle films). The patient is positioned properly and there is correct penetration (exposure) to ensure sufficient radiographic detail of the important area.

Alignment. All the bones have their normal anatomic relationships to adjacent bones. For instance, abnormal alignment of the inferior margins of the acromion and the clavicle suggests an injury to the acromioclavicular joint. On the PA radiograph of the wrist, the carpal bones are aligned in a continuous arc.

Bones. In examining the bones for fractures, the cortical margins are carefully inspected throughout the entire length of the bone. Most fractures are obvious, yet small breaks in the cortex can be difficult to see. One must be particularly careful in examining overlapping or foreshortened bones because fractures there can

TABLE 2-3

ABC'S Approach to Interpreting Skeletal Radiographs

Adequacy	All views are included Positioning and penetration (exposure) are correct
Alignment	Anatomic relationships between all bones are normal

Bones	Look for fracture lines or distortion of cortex and trabeculae
	Supplementary views may be needed to detect nondisplaced fractures
	Pseudofractures can mimic a fracture:
	    Accessory ossicles, growth plates, nutrient artery foramina, and
	    Mach bands

Cartilage	Joints should be of normal width and have uniform spacing Fracture fragments may be seen within joint space
Soft tissues	Soft tissue swelling, joint effusions, and distortion of fat planes may be easier to see than the fracture itself

be masked. Abrupt angulation of the cortex may be the only indication of a fracture. For example, in a child, a torus fracture of the distal radius may show no break in the cortex, although there will be an abnormal abrupt angulation in the cortex of the metaphysis. Impacted fractures also often have abrupt angulations rather than lucent breaks in the cortex. The trabecular network of the metaphysis is carefully evaluated for disruption or impaction. Finally, not every break in the cortex represents a fracture. For example, a nutrient foramen can be confused with a small, nondisplaced cortical fracture.

Cartilage.   "C" stands for cartilage which prompts an examination of the joint spaces; the cartilage itself is not directly seen on conventional radiographs. A widened uneven joint space generally results from severe ligamentous injury between the bones forming the joint. For example, in the ankle, a nonuniform mortise joint space indicates instability of the joint due to ligamentous disruption. An uneven joint space can also result from arthropathies that erode the articular cartilage.

Soft Tissues.   In certain regions, soft tissue abnormalities serve as important clues to fractures (Table 2-2). Some specific soft tissue signs (fat-pad signs of the elbow and prevertebral swelling of the cervical spine) are highly significant. A blood fat level (lipohemarthrosis) in the knee on the cross-table lateral radiograph suggests an intraarticular fracture. A soft tissue defect over the distal femur occurs with a complete disruption of the patellar tendon.

Overlying soft tissue swelling generally does not assist in distinguishing a fracture from an isolated soft tissue injury. For example, soft tissue swelling over the lateral malleolus is frequently seen with ankle sprains and has a limited role in detecting a fracture. Although soft tissue swelling will direct the radiologist's attention to a specific area of the film, the clinician already knows the region of likely injury based on the physical examination.

The Targeted Approach to Radiograph Interpretation

Although the ABC'S approach provides a general method for interpreting radiographs, each skeletal region has characteristic abnormalities that should be specifically sought when examining the radiographs. In using a *targeted approach,* common sites of injury are examined first. This is followed by scrutiny of areas where injuries are easily missed and areas

where there may be uncommon injuries that have considerable clinical implications (Table 2-4). Radiographic interpretation is most accurate and efficient when attention is directed to those areas with a high probability of abnormality. The targeted approach described here for skeletal radiography is also applicable to other regions, such as the chest and abdomen.

For example, with the shoulder, attention is first focused on the humeral neck and greater tuberosity. The relationship between the humeral head and the glenoid fossa is checked for evidence of dislocation. Next, easily missed injuries are sought, such as injury to the acromioclavicular joint and rib fractures.

TABLE 2-4

Easily Missed Fractures and Dislocations

Shoulder
    Posterior dislocation and fracture-dislocation (humeral neck fracture)
    Distal clavicular fracture (elderly) or acromioclavicular separation (young adults)
Elbow
    Radial head fracture (adults)
    Children: supracondylar, lateral epicondylar, medial epicondylar fractures
Forearm
    Monteggia and Galeazzi fracture-dislocations
Wrist
    Distal radius fracture (nondisplaced)
    Carpal fractures: scaphoid, triquetrum, etc.
    Dislocations/instability: perilunate, scapholunate dissociation
    Proximal metacarpal fractures and intraarticular fractures
Hand
    Phalangeal avulsion fracture

Pelvis
    Acetabular fractures
    Public ramus fractures
    Iliac wing fractures
    Avulsions fractures (anterior iliac spine, ischial tuberosity)
Hip
    Femoral neck fractures and intertrochanteric fractures (elderly, osteoporosis)
Knee
    Tibial plateau fracture
    Patellar fractures
    Soft tissue injuries
Ankle
    Tibiofibular syndesmosis tear—Maisonneuve fracture
    Fifth metatarsal tuberosity ("pseudo-Jones fracture")
Foot
    Calcaneus and talus (hindfoot) fractures
    Navicular and other midfoot fractures
    Tarsometatarsal fracture-dislocation (Lisfranc)

Missed fractures in the multiple-trauma victim (requires complete secondary survey)
Soft tissue foreign bodies
Fractures in children
    Growth-plate fractures (Salter-Harris)
    Torus (buckle) fractures, acute plastic bowing

These relatively common injuries can present with subtle clinical and radiographic findings. The radiographs should be scrutinized for these injuries. The corresponding physical signs should likewise be specifically sought when examining the patient. Additional radiographic views are sometimes needed to visualize these injuries.

With the elbow, common sites of injury include the radial head, the supracondylar area, and the olecranon. Easily missed injuries include a nondisplaced fracture of the radial head or, in a young child, a supracondylar fracture. Abnormalities of the anterior or posterior fat pad can be easier to see than the fracture itself. Detecting an injury to the epiphyseal growth plates can be difficult, and comparison views may be required. Injuries that have significant consequences include, in children, a supracondylar fracture and a displaced medial epicondylar fracture that has migrated into the joint space.

THE LANGUAGE OF FRACTURES

Some general terms apply to most long bones. The *diaphysis* is the shaft of the bone. It has a thick cortex and few trabeculae within the medullary cavity. The outer margin of the cortex should be smooth except at sites of tendon or ligament insertion. The inner margin of the cortex should also be well demarcated. The *metaphysis* is continuous with the ends of the diaphysis where the bone flares outward toward the articular surfaces. The metaphysis has a thin cortex and an abundant trabecular network. The trabeculae follow lines of stress within the bone and gradually fan out from the cortical margins of the diaphysis. The *epiphysis* at the end of a long bone forms the articular surface. In adults, the epiphysis is continuous with the metaphysis. In children, the *physis* or *epiphyseal growth plate* is located between the epiphysis and metaphysis. Many bones have anatomic regions that bear specific names, such as *the greater tuberosity of the proximal humerus.*

In describing fractures, it is important to use accurate terms (Table 2-5). Features that must be mentioned include the anatomic location and direction of the fracture, the alignment of the fragments, intraarticular involvement, and associated soft tissue injuries. The shaft of a long bone is divided into the proximal, middle, and distal thirds. Terms such as *head, neck, base,* and *condyle* are used when appropriate. Specific terms (e.g., *greater trochanter*) are used where ever applicable. In describing skeletal injuries, one does not refer to joints as being fractured (e.g., a "fractured ankle"); only bones (forming joints) can be fractured.

The direction of the fracture is determined by the direction of forces causing the fracture. The direction of the fracture is described in relation to the long axis of the bone. A *transverse* fracture is perpendicular to the long axis of the bone and is caused by tension opposite a direct blow. A *spiral* fracture results from torsional forces encircling the shaft of a long bone.

TABLE 2-5

Fracture Terminology

Alignment: the angular or rotational relationship between the proximal and distal fragments of a fracture

Apophysis: similar to an epiphysis but it does not articulate with another bone

Apposition: the amount of end-to-end contact of the fracture

Avulsion fracture: a small fracture (piece of bone, usually near a joint, that is pulled off by a ligamentous or tendonous attachment)

Closed fracture (also called a *simple fracture*): there is no cutaneous wound near the fracture site

Comminuted fracture: a fracture with multiple pieces

Dislocation: disruption of the continuity of the joint where articular surfaces are not in relationship to one another. (Note that fractures do not *dislocate;* they *displace.*)

Displaced fracture: a fracture whose ends are not normally apposed

Epiphyseal fracture: a fracture of the growth plate, usually in the long bone

Epiphysis: that part of a bone which is beyond the growth plate

Fracture: any break in the cortex of a bone

Fracture-dislocation: a dislocation that occurs in conjunction with a fracture

Greenstick fracture: an incomplete fracture, often where one side of the cortex is involved and not the other, usually occurring in children

Impaction fracture: a fracture whose ends are forced into one another

Intraarticular fracture: a fracture that involves a joint surface of the bone

Malunion: healing of bones in an unsatisfactory position

Nonunion: failure of bones to heal

Occult fracture: a fracture that is not readily apparent on initial radiologic evaluation. Radiographs taken 2 to 3 weeks later can show the fracture line or periosteal formation.

Open fracture (also called a *compound fracture*): a fracture for which there is an open wound in the skin overlying the fracture

Pathologic fracture: a fracture that occurs because the bone is weakened by some abnormal conditions, such as bone cancer

Rotation: rotation of fracture fragments is often difficult to characterize radiographically but is usually easier to determine clinically.

Stress fracture: a fracture that occurs from repeated minor stressors

Subluxation: the partial disruption of a joint where bones only partially articulate with one another

Torus or buckle fracture: caused by compression of the cortex, most often involving the metaphysis of the long bone occurring in children

An *oblique* fracture runs diagonally across the diaphysis and is caused by shear forces. This type of fracture is most common in the medial malleolus of the ankle. An *impacted* fracture is due to compressive forces. With an impacted fracture, trabecular bone is compressed, causing it to appear to have increased density (*sclerosis*). A *butterfly* fragment is a small, triangular fragment that results from compression along one side of a fracture caused by bending of the bone. An *avulsion* fracture is a fragment of bone pulled away at the attachment of a tendon or ligament. A *comminuted* fracture has multiple fragments.

A *closed* (simple) fracture is one where the overlying skin is intact. An *open* (compound) fracture is where the overlying skin is broken and the fracture communicates with the outside environment. Skin breaks include puncture wounds and full-thickness lacerations. A *complicated* fracture is associated with neurovascular, ligamentous, or muscular injury.

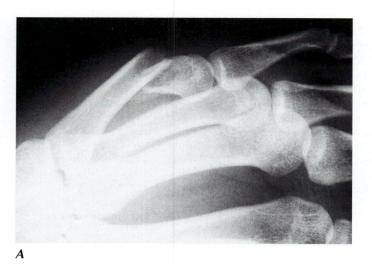

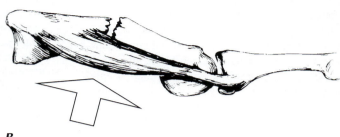

A   *B*

FIGURE 2-5. Angulation of a fracture is due to the pull of muscles that attach to the fracture parts. In a fracture of the metacarpal shaft, pull of the interosseus and lumbrical muscles causes *dorsal* angulation of the fracture (i.e., the arrow points in a dorsal direction). (*B.* From Rockwood CA, Green DP: *Fractures in Adults,* 2d ed. Philadelphia: Lippincott, 1984. With permission.)

In children, a fracture can be *complete* (through and through); *incomplete* ("greenstick") in which only one cortex is visibly broken; or *buckled* without a visible break in the cortex (torus). Fractures in children can also involve the growth plate (physis).

If the ends of the fracture fragments are not normally apposed, the fracture is *displaced*. The amount of displacement is described relative to the thickness of the shaft of the bone. For example, a fracture could be displaced "one-third the thickness of the bone." Complete displacement with overlapping of the fracture ends is called a *bayonette* deformity. If the fragments are separated, the fracture is *distracted*.

Angulation occurs when the long axes of the two fracture fragments are not in normal alignment. The direction of angulation is described by imagining the two fracture fragments as forming the head of an arrow. This arrow "points" in the direction of angulation (Fig. 2-5). (This is the conventional terminology used in the United States.) Angulation is caused by the pull of muscles attached to the fracture fragments. In the lower extremity, two additional terms are used to describe angulation: *valgus* and *varus*. A *valgus* deformity occurs when the distal bone fragment is shifted away from the midline of the body (laterally). A *varus* deformity denotes displacement of the distal part toward the midline (medially).

Pathologic fractures occur in bone weakened by a pathologic process. The term is most often used in the setting of metastatic malignancy but can also be applied to a fracture associated with benign cysts or tumors (such as enchondromas), osteomyelitis, Paget's disease, and osteogenesis imperfecta. *Insufficiency fractures* occur in pathologically weakened bone that is subjected to the stresses of normal activity, most often in elderly women with osteoporosis. *Stress fractures* occur in normal bone that is subjected to abnormal activity levels, such as in military recruits on long marches and in athletes.

NONTRAUMATIC SKELETAL RADIOLOGY

Nontraumatic skeletal lesions are occasionally seen in patients presenting to the ED, although these disorders are generally not of an acute nature. The pathologic lesions include neoplasia (primary and metastatic), bone infections, inflammatory arthropathies, degenerative changes, metabolic bone diseases, and developmental disorders. In an ED patient, the bone lesion may be the underlying condition that results in an acute event (e.g., a pathologic fracture). The skeletal lesion may cause subacute or chronic pain that leads to the ED visit. Finally, a bone lesion may simply be an incidental finding on a radiograph obtained for other reasons.

Localized Bone Lesions

There are a wide variety of localized skeletal lesions and it is often difficult or impossible to make an exact diagnosis based on the radiograph alone. Clinical information—such as the patient's age, a history of malignancy, and clinical signs of infection—are needed to narrow the differential diagnosis. In some cases, the radiographic appearance is virtually pathognomonic. Most focal skeletal lesions cause lucent defects in the involved bone. Usually bone destruction (lysis) is accompanied by some degree of new bone formation (sclerosis). The principal diagnostic concern is to distinguish benign from malignant disorders. However, because this is usually not possible based solely on the radiographic picture, it is preferable to use the terms "aggressive" and "nonaggressive" bone lesions. The principal radiographic features used to distinguish aggressive from nonaggressive lesions are the margin of the lesion (well-defined versus ill-defined) and the type of periosteal reaction (Table 2-6) (Figs. 2-6 and 2-7). Both benign and malignant disorders

TABLE 2-6

Characteristics of Bone Focal Lesions

Benign (nonagressive) bone lesions
    Sclerotic margins, narrow and well-defined
    Smooth, continuous (noninterrupted) periosteal reaction
    Expansion of an intact cortex
Solitary malignant bone lesions
    Margins wide and ill-defined (may or may not be sclerotic)
    Permeative or moth-eaten bone destruction
    Interrupted, irregular or spiculated periosteal reaction
    Metaphyseal location
    Extraosseous extension with soft tissue mass and occasional
        fluffy calcifications
Metastatic lesions
    Margins wide and ill-defined (may or may not be sclerotic)
    Moth-eaten destruction of medulla and cortex
    Absence of periosteal reaction
    Diaphyseal location
    Pathologic fractures
    Multiple bone involvement
Infection
    Interrupted, irregular periosteal reaction, no spiculation
    Bone destruction variable
    Diaphyseal involvement, often involving long segments
    Destruction of adjacent cartilage, crossing joints (most malignant
        lesions do not)
    Sequestration and involucrum formation

TABLE 2-7

Malignant Bone Tumors

TISSUE OF ORIGIN	TUMOR
Bone	Osteosarcoma
Cartilage	Chondrosarcoma
Marrow elements	Ewing's sarcoma Multiple myeloma, plasmacytoma Lymphoma
Fibrous tissue	Fibrosarcoma
Metastatic	Lung, breast, prostate, kidney, thyroid

can have an aggressive or a nonaggressive radiographic appearance. The patient's age plays a key role in determining the most likely etiology. For example, any skeletal lesion in a patient older than 40 years of age can represent metastatic disease, even though it has a nonaggressive appearance. Osteomyelitis also has an aggressive radiographic appearance and is often difficult or impossible to distinguish from malignancy without clinical information.

Both malignant and benign skeletal lesions are grouped according to their tissue of origin: bone, cartilage, marrow elements, or fibrous tissue (Tables 2-7 and 2-8). Primary malignancies occur in children, young adults, and the elderly depending on the particular tissue type. Metastatic disease oc-

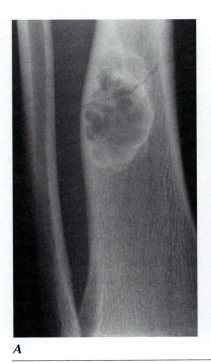

A

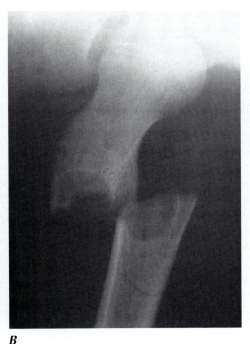

B

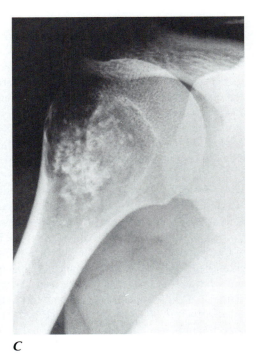

C

FIGURE 2-6. The thin, well-defined margins of these lytic bone lesions are characteristic of benign lesions. Pathologic fractures are present in patients A and B. *A.* A geographic lesion with a "bubbly" appearance that is characteristic of nonossifying fibroma. *B.* A simple (unicameral) bone cyst. *C.* A proximal humerus lesion with stippled calcification typical of an enchondroma. This lesion should be further evaluated electively to exclude a low-grade chondroblastoma.

TABLE 2-8

Benign Bone Lesions*

ORIGIN	LESION	
Bone	Osteoid osteoma	Dense cortical bone with a small central lucency. Causes deep, boring pain.
Cartilage	Enchondroma	Occurs in midlife. Affects small tubular bones of hands and feet (also femur and humerus). Due to rests of cartilaginous tissue within medullary cavity. Causes speckled calcifications.
	Osteochondroma (exostosis)	Cartilaginous outgrowth at physis, with encasing bone cap.
Marrow elements	Eosinophilic granuloma	Lytic lesion. With healing, sclerotic rim forms. Affects the skull, spine, long bones.
Fibrous tissue	Nonossifying fibroma	Thin sclerotic rim around lytic area. Bubbly appearance.
	Fibrous dysplasia	Lytic area containing fibrous tissue (ground-glass appearance).
Cystic	Simple (unicameral) bone cyst	Fluid-filled cyst. Treatment: aspirate and inject with steroids.

*Most of these lesions occur in children and adolescents and appear as a lytic area with a thin rim of surrounding bone. They are usually solitary and occur in the metaphysis or shaft of larger long bones. Less common lesions not listed include osteoblastoma, chondroblastoma, giant cell tumor, aneurysmal bone cyst.

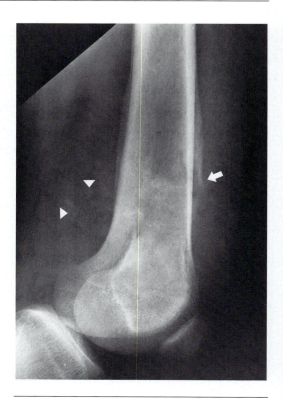

FIGURE 2-7. In this aggressive bone lesion, there is a wide, ill-defined transition zone. The periosteum is raised and periosteal new bone formation is interrupted where the tumor is growing rapidly (*arrow*). Extraosseus calcification is characteristic of osteogenic sarcoma (*arrowheads*).

curs primarily in individuals over the age of 50 years. Most benign skeletal lesions occur in children and adolescents and represent anomalies in skeletal development. With aging, they involute or stabilize. Most of these lesions appear as a lytic area with a thin rim of surrounding bone. They are usually solitary and occur in the metaphysis or shaft of larger long bones such as the femur, tibia, or humerus. Many have distinguishing radiographic features. They are usually asymptomatic and are discovered as an incidental radiographic finding. Occasionally, they are responsible for a pathologic fracture.

Margins of the Lesion. The principal radiographic feature distinguishing a nonaggressive from an aggressive bone lesion is its margin (zone of transition). Nonaggressive lesions grow slowly and have a thin, well-defined, sclerotic border. The shape of the lesion can be cystic or it can have a serpiginous margin, giving it a "geographic" appearance (Fig. 2-6). Aggressive lesions have ill-defined transition zones. When the lesion has many small, ill-defined lytic regions, the radiographic pattern is called *permeative* or *moth-eaten* (Fig. 2-7). Most malignant bone tumors—such as osteosarcoma and Ewing's sarcoma in children and young adults, and chondrosarcoma in patients above age 40—have an aggressive radiographic appearance. A sclerotic, wide, poorly defined border is characteristic of an aggressive lesion that incites considerable new bone formation, such as osteoblastic metastases (breast, prostate, and gastrointestinal cancers) (Fig. 2-8). In other cancers, bone lysis pre-

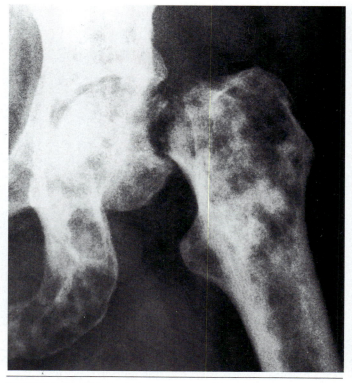

FIGURE 2-8. Metastatic breast cancer with pathologic fracture. Extensive lytic and osteoblastic changes are seen. There is no periosteal reaction.

dominates and there is no sclerotic margin (multiple myeloma and metastatic lung cancer).

With a well-defined, nonaggressive skeletal lesion, the differential diagnosis depends on the age of the patient. In patients below 30 years of age, a nonaggressive lytic lesion is likely to be a benign entity such as a unicameral bone cyst, a nonossifying fibroma, enchondroma, fibrous dysplasia, or eosinophilic granuloma. Many of these disorders have distinguishing radiographic characteristics (Table 2-8), which are described in the reference texts on bone radiology (Helms, Edeiken, Resnick) listed in the bibliography. Occasionally, osteomyelitis or chondroblastoma has a nonaggressive radiographic appearance. On the other hand, some nonmalignant lesions can have an aggressive radiographic appearance (eosinophilic granuloma and osteomyelitis). In patients above 40 years of age, lesions with a nonaggressive radiographic appearance are potentially due to malignancy (especially metastasis or multiple myeloma).

Periosteal Reaction. A second radiographic feature of skeletal lesions that distinguishes aggressive from nonaggressive lesions is the periosteal reaction. When the outer periosteal membrane is irritated, osteoblastic cells produce new bone. Periosteal new bone can have a solid or an interrupted appearance (Table 2-9). Solid osteoreactions generally suggest a benign process, an indolent infection, or fracture healing (Fig. 2-9). Interrupted periosteal reactions are usually associated with aggressive malignant disease or infection. The sunburst pattern of osteogenic sarcoma and the laminated onionskin periosteal reaction of Ewing's sarcoma are interrupted forms of periosteal reaction (Fig. 2-10). Another characteristic radiographic sign of an aggressive periosteal process is a short spicule of bone at the edge of the lesion where the periosteum is lifted from the cortical surface. This is known as a *Codman's triangle.* It is a characteristic of aggressive processes, such as malignancy or osteomyelitis. Unfortunately, in many patients, the differentiation between a benign and an aggressive osteoreaction is difficult to make radiographically. Metastatic lesions often do not incite a periosteal reaction.

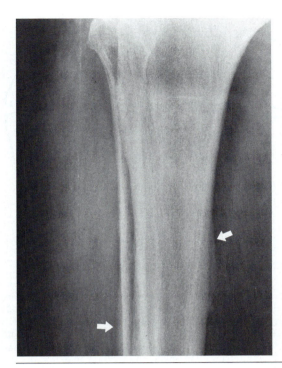

FIGURE 2-9. Continuous formation of new, smooth periosteal bone is characteristic of a benign (nonaggressive) bone lesion. This patient has chronic cellulitis of the lower extremity. Periosteal elevation is also a sign of osteomyelitis. However, in a patient with cellulitis of long duration, osteomyelitis would be expected to also cause cortical changes (erosion and thickening). The periosteal reaction in this patient represents "periostitis" caused by overlying cellulitis.

FIGURE 2-10. An aggressive periosteal reaction is seen in the femur of a 14-year-old boy with Ewing sarcoma. There is laminated ("onionskin") formation of periosteal new bone and a slight amount of spiculated ("sunburst") formation of periosteal new bone. Codman triangles are seen at the superior margins of the tumor. Within the bone, there is reactive sclerosis. A large soft tissue mass extends beyond the bone margins. (From Berman CG, Brodsky NJ, Clark RA: *Oncologic Imaging.* New York: McGraw-Hill, 1998. With permission.)

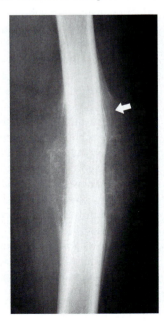

TABLE 2-9

Periosteal Reactions

Solid periosteal reaction (nonaggressive)	
Thin	Eosinophilic granuloma, osteoid osteoma
Thin, undulating	Hypertrophic pulmonary osteoarthropathy
Dense, undulating	Vascular
Dense, elliptical (with destruction)	Osteoid osteoma
Cloaking	Long-standing malignancy
	Chronic infection
Interrupted periosteal reaction (aggressive)	
Perpendicular (spiculated or sunburst)	Osteosarcoma, Ewing sarcoma, infection
Lamellated (onion skin)	Osteosarcoma, Ewing sarcoma, infection
Amorphous	Malignant tumors
Codman triangle	Malignant tumors, infection, hemorrhage

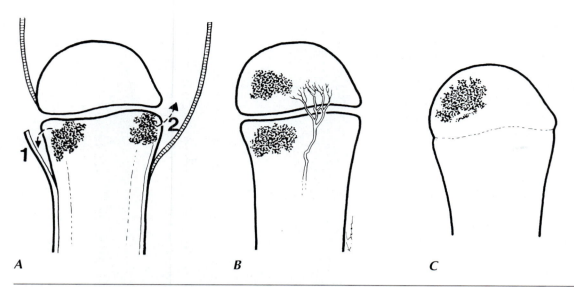

A   *B*   *C*

FIGURE 2-11.   Sites of hematogenous osteomyelitis in the long bones of the child, infant, and adult. The focus of hematogenous osteomyelitis in tubular bones is dependent on its blood supply. *A.* In a child, the focus of infection is in the metaphysis. Blood flow is usually stopped at the growth plate. Spread to the periosteum can result in a subperiosteal abscess if the growth plate is extracapsular (1) or septic arthritis if the growth plate is intraarticular (2). *B.* In an infant, the focus of infection is typically both metaphyseal and epiphyseal because the arterial blood supply crosses the growth plate. *C.* In adults, the focus of infection occurs in the highly vascular subchondral bone of the epiphysis. (From Resnick D, Niwayama G: *Diagnosis of Bone and Joint Disorders,* Philadelphia: Saunders, 1981. With permission.)

Osteomyelitis

Infection of bone occurs in a variety of clinical settings and is caused by different pathologic events. Osteomyelitis is grouped into two broad categories: hematogenous and exogenous. The time course of osteomyelitis can be acute, subacute, or chronic. Hematogenous seeding usually occurs in children and affects the metaphysis of a long bone (Fig. 2-11). In neonates, the infection is often multifocal and spreads to involve the epiphysis. Hematogenous osteomyelitis also occurs in the elderly, the debilitated, and injection drug users. In these patients, the infection usually involves the vertebral column. Exogenous osteomyelitis occurs from direct inoculation of the bone, as with an open fracture or surgical procedure. Exogenous osteomyelitis also occurs by spread from a contiguous focus of infection, such as cellulitis (Fig. 2-12). Finally, osteomyelitis occurs in areas of poor blood supply, as in the feet of diabetic patients.

Early in the disease process, *acute hematogenous osteomyelitis* produces swelling of surrounding soft tissues without changes in the bone itself. After 7 to 12 days, destruction of the bone cortices begins to appear (Table 2-6). Periosteal elevation and new bone formation also appears (Table 2-9). Plain radiographs do not clearly demonstrate changes in bone until at least 50% of the bone has been destroyed. This usually takes 2 to 4 weeks (Fig. 2-13).

Chronic osteomyelitis usually appears as irregular, sclerotic bone with multiple isolated areas of radiolucency. Irregular areas of destruction are frequently present. The periosteum is thickened.

In the *spine,* infection begins in the intervertebral disk and spreads to the adjacent vertebral bodies. Isolated disk space infection (diskitis) is uncommon and is usually seen in children. Radiographically, there is erosion of the vertebral body end plates and narrowing of the intervertebral disk space. With disease progression, there is further destruction of the bone and loss of vertebral body height. Spinal cord compression occurs when the infection spreads to form an epidural abscess.

Other Disorders Affecting the Skeleton

Gout.   Early in its course, gout arthritis has a normal radiographic appearance. Ultimately, destructive changes develop with a characteristic "punched out" appearance. Rapid destruction and degeneration of the articular cartilage follows (Fig. 2-14).

Degenerative Osteoarthritis.   Degenerative changes in bones and joints are common in the elderly and begin to appear after 40 years of age. Degenerative changes are seen in the extremities and axial skeleton and are felt to be caused by long-standing "wear and tear." Degenerative changes are characterized by asymmetrical joint space narrowing, marginal osteophyte formation, and increased bone density, especially in bone adjacent to the articular cartilage (subchondral sclerosis or *eburnation*). Ligament calcifications (also called bone spurs or *enthesophytes*) are also common (Fig. 2-15).

Osteoporosis.   Osteoporosis is the most common cause of osteopenia, which is the loss of bone density. Osteoporosis is pri-

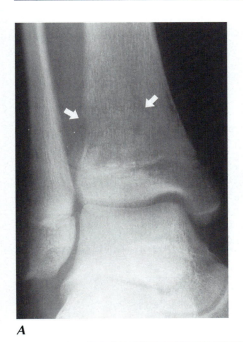
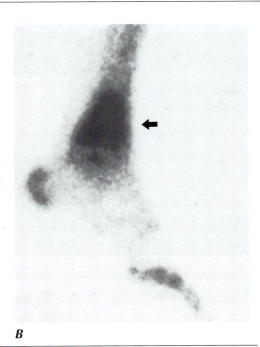
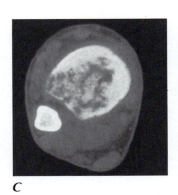
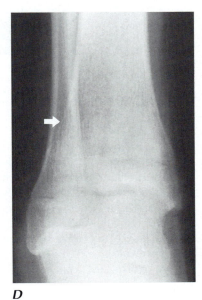
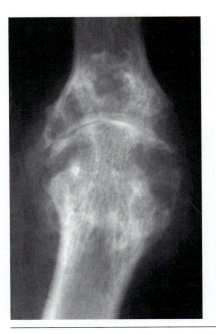

A

B

C

D

FIGURE 2-13. Acute hematogenous osteomyelitis. *Staphylococcus aureus* osteomyelitis of the distal tibia. *A.* The initial radiograph of the ankle shows areas of slight lucency of the distal tibial metaphysis. *B.* A bone scan reveals marked uptake over the distal tibia. *C.* CT scan of the distal tibia shows mottled lucencies within the medullary cavity and cortical erosion. Periosteal reaction and formation of new subperiosteal bone has not yet occurred. *D.* A radiograph of the ankle obtained several days later shows a mottled appearance due to mixed bone resorption and formation of new bone (sclerosis). This appearance is not specific for osteomyelitis. It can also be seen in neoplastic disorders such as Wilms tumor. (Courtesy of Ellen Cavenagh, M.D., Sparrow Hospital, Lansing, MI.)

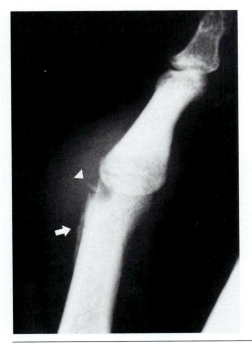

FIGURE 2-12. Acute exogenous osteomyelitis from a contiguous focus of soft tissue infection. The patient presented 10 days after a minor crush injury over the proximal interphalangeal joint. The radiograph shows soft tissue swelling and focal erosion of the cortex and medullary cavity *(arrowhead)*. There is an irregular pattern of periosteal new bone formation *(arrow)*. The fragment of cortical bone within the region of osteomyelitis is either a fracture fragment or a sequestrum (devitalized bone surrounded by infected tissue).

FIGURE 2-14. Advanced gouty arthritis of the first metatarsophalangeal joint. There are "punched out" subchondral and marginal erosions, joint space narrowing, and periarticular calcified tophi. (From Wilson FC, Lin PP: *General Orthopedics.* New York: McGraw-Hill, 1997. With permission.)

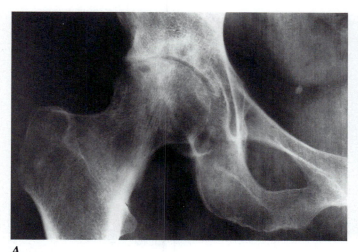 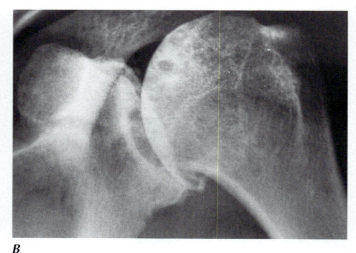

A   *B*

FIGURE 2-15. Osteoarthritis (degenerative joint disease) causes asymmetrical joint space narrowing, marginal osteophytes, and subchondral sclerosis (eburnation). These changes are seen in the hip and shoulder of two patients.

marily a disease of the elderly women. It also occurs during prolonged disuse, as from immobilization of a fracture in a cast. Radiographically, osteoporosis is characterized by cortical thinning, although this can be difficult to discern unless it is pronounced. The trabecular bone also becomes thinned. The interconnecting trabeculae are lost and there is a paradoxical accentuation of the primary structural trabeculae (Fig. 2-16). These patients are a high risk for insufficiency fractures, which, when nondisplaced, can be difficult to detect on plain-film radiographs.

Paget's Disease. Paget's disease is characterized by a thickened cortex and thickened, disordered trabeculae (Fig. 2-17). It is most often seen in the pelvis and proximal femur. There is excessive bone destruction and repair. Bone pain is common with Paget's disease, which must be differentiated from osteogenic sarcoma, multiple myeloma, metastatic carcinoma (es-

pecially of the prostate), and osteitis fibrosa cystica. The radiographic appearance of Paget's disease differs from that of osteoblastic prostate cancer in that Paget's disease often causes expansion of the bone, whereas prostatic metastases do not.

BIBLIOGRAPHY

Ballinger PW: *Merrill's Atlas of Radiographic Positions and Radiographic Procedures,* 7th ed. St. Louis: Mosby–Year Book, 1991.

Browner BD, Jupiter JB, Levine AM, Trafton PG: *Skeletal Trauma.* Philadelphia: Saunders, 1992.

Edeiken J, Dalinka M, Karasick D (eds): *Edeiken's Roentgen Diagnosis of Disease of Bone,* 2d ed. Baltimore: Williams & Wilkins, 1990.

Harris JH, Harris WH, Novelline RA: *The Radiology of Emergency Medicine,* 3d ed. Baltimore: Williams & Wilkins, 1993.

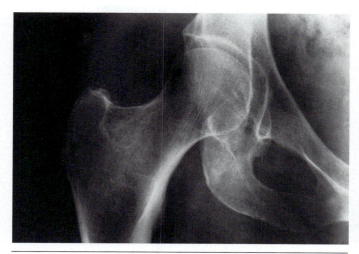 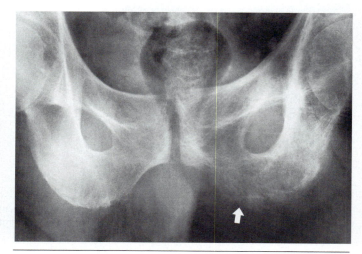

FIGURE 2-16. Osteoporosis causes accentuation of the primary supportive trabeculae. This paradoxical effect is due to loss of secondary interconnecting trabeculae. There is also cortical thinning.

FIGURE 2-17. Paget's disease causes thickening and irregularity of the cortex and trabeculae with expansion and distortion of the bone. This patient has mild changes of Paget's disease in the pelvis (*arrow*).

Helms CA: *Fundamentals of Skeletal Radiology,* 2d ed. Philadelphia: Saunders, 1995.

Keats TE: *Atlas of Normal Roentgen Variants That May Simulate Disease,* 6th ed. St. Louis: Mosby, 1996.

McCort JJ, Mindelzan RE: *Trauma Radiology.* New York: Churchill Livingstone, 1990.

Nicholson DA, Driscoll PA: *ABC of Emergency Radiology.* London: BMJ Press, 1995.

Resnick D: *Diagnosis of Bone and Joint Disorders,* 3d ed. Philadelphia: Saunders, 1995.

Riddervold HO: *Easily Missed Fractures and Corner Signs in Radiology.* Mt. Kisco, NY: Futura, 1991.

Rockwood CA, Green DP, Bucholz RW, Heckman JD: *Rockwood and Green's Fractures in Adults,* 4th ed. Philadelphia: Lippincott-Raven, 1996.

Rogers LF: *Radiology of Skeletal Trauma,* 2d ed. New York: Churchill Livingstone, 1992.

Ruiz E, Cicero JJ: *Emergency Management of Skeletal Injuries.* St. Louis: Mosby, 1995.

Simon RR, Koenigsknecht JJ: *Emergency Orthopedics: The Extremities,* 3d ed. Norwalk, CT: Appleton & Lange, 1995.

Swischuk LE: *Emergency Radiology of the Acutely Ill or Injured Child,* 3d ed. Baltimore: Williams & Williams, 1994.

Weissman BN, Sledge C: *Adult Orthopedic Radiology.* Philadelphia: Saunders, 1986.

SUGGESTED READINGS

Cone RO: Clues to the initial radiographic evaluation of skeletal trauma. *Emerg Med Clin North Am* 2:245, 1984.

Daffner RH: Skeletal pseudofractures. *Emerg Radiol* 2:96, 1995.

Freed HA, Shields NN: Most frequently overlooked radiographically apparent fractures in a teaching hospital emergency department. *Ann Emerg Med* 13:900, 1984.

Moore MN: Orthopedic pitfalls in emergency medicine. *South Med J* 81:371, 1988.

Weissman BN: The radiographic diagnosis of subtle extremity injuries. *Emerg Med Clin North Am* 2:245, 1984.

CHAPTER 3

THE HAND

MATTHEW WILKS / STEPHEN MELDON

Hand injuries significantly reduce one's functional ability, especially if the injury involves the dominant hand. Early recognition and appropriate management are key in preventing disability. Many hand injuries, such as simple lacerations, do not require radiographs. However, radiography of the hand is essential to provide precise anatomic definition of fractures and dislocations. Radiographs define the degree of intraarticular fracture involvement and measure the amount of fracture displacement. Radiographs are also required for evaluation of other conditions, such as osteomyelitis. Wounds with a high potential for foreign-body retention also need radiographic evaluation.

Hand films show more bones (29 in all) than any other extremity radiograph. Despite this, interpretation of hand films usually poses little difficulty because the skeletal anatomy of the hand and the associated injury patterns are relatively simple. In addition, the physical examination is helpful in guiding the emergency physician in radiographic interpretation. Although the skeletal anatomy of the hand is relatively simple, its function and soft tissue anatomy are quite complex. Minor structural injuries can cause significant functional compromise.

CLINICAL DECISION MAKING

No well-defined guidelines exist to determine when to obtain radiographs of the hand. Clinical factors that suggest the need to obtain radiographs include deformity; a severe mechanism of injury; soft tissue swelling, ecchymosis; an altered range of motion (either increased or decreased); and a loss of neurovascular integrity (Table 3-1).

Certain mechanisms of injury—such as a crush, fall, hyperextension, or hyperflexion—carry a significant risk of radiographically identifiable injury. Forced flexion of the tip of the finger can result in a small proximal avulsion of the distal phalanx (mallet finger). Rapid forced abduction of the thumb can cause a ligamentous avulsion at the thumb metacarpophalangeal (MCP) joint.

Any gross deformity warrants radiographic evaluation. Soft tissue indicators of potential injury include the "three E's": edema, erythema, and ecchymosis. Edema and erythema may also be due to soft tissue infection and osteomyelitis. Ecchymosis over the volar plate may be associated with a small periarticular avulsion fracture.

Bone tenderness and range of motion are assessed. Bone tenderness may indicate a fracture. Decreased range of motion of a joint may result from soft tissue swelling or a soft tissue or bone fragment that is entrapped within the joint. Increased range of motion of a joint may represent a ligamentous tear or a fracture. Although ligamentous injuries are undetectable on routine radiographs, they are sometimes associated with an avulsion fracture. Finally, any neurovascular deficit warrants radiologic study.

Radiographs should be ordered liberally in children. Metaphyseal and growth-plate fractures of bones in the hand are frequent. Comparison views are considered when the radiographic findings are uncertain, especially with a Salter-Harris type 1 fracture.

In most cases, a standard hand series should be requested. Specific finger views should be obtained, rather than a hand series, when injuries are isolated to the proximal interphalangeal (PIP) joint, the distant interphalangeal (DIP) joint, or the middle or distal phalanx. When the injury is centered in the wrist,

TABLE 3-1

Considerations for Obtaining Hand Radiographs

Severe mechanism
    Fall
    Crush injury
    Severe hyperextension
    Severe hyperflexion
Deformity
Soft tissue changes
    Complex laceration
    Marked erythema
    Marked edema
    Ecchymosis (especially over volar plate)
Functional changes
    Decreased range of motion
    Increased range of motion (consider stress views)
    Vascular impairment
    Neurologic deficit
Immature skeleton
    Fractures may involve the physis
    Consider comparison views if findings uncertain
Foreign body
    Suspected retained foreign body
    High-pressure injection injury
Infection suspicious for osteomyelitis

radiographs of the wrist, rather than the hand, should be obtained. Stress views can help identify ligamentous injuries; however, these are rarely obtained in an acute hand injury.

When a retained foreign body is suspected, a radiograph should be obtained. If the physician can perform an adequate exploration of an open injury that essentially excludes a foreign body, then radiographic evaluation can be deferred. Nonetheless, a high index of suspicion for a retained foreign body should be maintained with lacerations or puncture wounds. Glass larger than 1 mm in diameter is usually visible on plain radiographs. Organic material such as wood is usually not visible. Computed tomography (CT) and ultrasound are sometimes able to detect such nonradiopaque foreign bodies.

High-pressure injection injuries require radiography and frequently need extensive surgical exploration and debridement.

ANATOMY AND PHYSIOLOGY

The back of the hand is referred to as the *dorsum*. The palmar surface is also called the *volar aspect*. The "thumb side" is called the *radial aspect*; the *ulnar aspect* is bordered by the little finger. *Flexion* occurs in the direction of fist formation, whereas *extension* is movement of the fingers in a dorsal plane. Bringing the fingers together is referred to as finger *adduction*; spreading them apart is finger *abduction*.

TABLE 3-2

Standard and Supplementary Views of the Hand

STANDARD VIEWS	POSITION	EVALUATION OF ADEQUACY	LIKELY FINDINGS
PA	Palm placed on film cassette. Fingers spread slightly. The x-ray beam perpendicular to middle digit MCP.	All carpals, metacarpals, and phalanges from thumb to little finger seen. Articulation between carpals and distal radius and ulna seen. Trabeculae are well defined.	Most fractures of metacarpals, phalanges, and carpals. Subtle injuries to the phalanges and carpals may not be seen.
Lateral	Ulnar surface of hand placed on film cassette. Thumb is perpendicular to the palm. Fingers are fanned using a foam form. (Fanned positioning not routine at all institutions.)	Metacarpals are superimposed. Distal radius and ulna are superimposed. Phalanges are individually seen. The IP joints are open. Thumb does not overlap other digits.	Angulation of metacarpal fractures and dislocations. With the fingers fanned, fractures at the IP joints are detected.
Pronation oblique	Ulnar surface of hand placed on cassette. Palm raised to 45° angle. Fingers are fanned.	Middle and fourth MC shafts have minimal overlap. Slight overlap of MC bases and heads. The second and third MC separated. Articulation with distal radius and ulna seen.	Angulation of MC fractures. Nondisplaced MC and phalanx fractures.
SUPPLEMENTARY VIEWS			
Supination oblique (ball-catcher's view)	Ulnar surface of hand placed on film cassette, palm rotated to semi-supinated position. The fingers are fanned as if to catch a ball, thumb is abducted.	Ulnar side of hand is seen, especially little and ring fingers and corresponding metacarpals.	Subtle fractures of little and ring finger MC bases.
Brewerton view	Hand placed dorsal side down. X-ray beam angled 30° from ulnar side of hand.	MC bases seen with less overlap.	Fractures at MC bases.

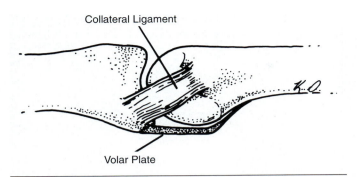

FIGURE 3-1. Volar plate and collateral ligaments of the interphalangeal and metacarpophalangeal joints.

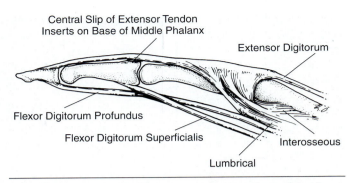

FIGURE 3-2. Flexor and extensor tendon insertions of the finger.

The hand consists of 14 phalanges and 5 metacarpal bones in addition to the carpal bones of the wrist. All hand bones have a similar structure: a shaft, a proximal end (the base), and a distal end (the head). The thumb has only two phalanges while the other digits each have three. Practical nomenclature refers to the digits by name: the *thumb, index, middle, ring,* and *little* fingers. Referring to the digits by number (e.g., the thumb as digit I and the little finger as digit V) can lead to confusion.

The IP and the MCP joints are supported by the fibrocartilaginous *volar plate* and bilateral *collateral ligaments*. These structures are easily disrupted by dislocations and hyperextension injuries. Understanding the anatomy of the volar plate and tendon insertions is important in recognizing radiographic findings (Figs. 3-1 and 3-2). Each finger has two flexor tendons: the *flexor digitorum superficialis* and the *flexor digitorum profundus*. The flexor digitorum superficialis is responsible for flexion of the MCP joint and PIP joint. The flexor digitorum profundus is responsible for isolated flexion of the DIP joint. The *extensor tendon* of the finger divides at the PIP joint into a central slip and two lateral bands. The central slip inserts on the base of the middle phalanx. The two lateral bands reunite distally over the shaft of the middle phalanx into a single tendon that inserts on the base of the distal phalanx.

PRINCIPLES OF RADIOGRAPHIC TECHNIQUE

The standard radiographic projections of the hand are the *posteroanterior (PA)*, the *lateral*, and the *pronation oblique views* (Table 3-2). A finger study also usually includes three views (Table 3-3). Additional views may be necessary to define certain injuries—for example, a *ball-catcher's view*[1] (supination oblique) for an injury of the little finger. If an injury to the carpal bones or carpo-metacarpal (CMC) joint is suspected, then wrist films should be obtained.

Hand Posteroanterior (PA). The PA view is obtained by placing the palmar surface of the hand on the film cassette with the fingers spread slightly apart (Fig. 3-3*A* and *B*). The x-ray beam is centered over the third metacarpophalangeal joint.

Hand Lateral. The lateral view is obtained by placing the ulnar surface of the hand against the film cassette and centering the x-ray beam over the MCP joints (Fig. 3-3*C* and *D*). With a "straight lateral," all of the metacarpals and phalanges are su-

TABLE 3-3

Radiographic Views of the Digits

	POSITION	EVALUATION OF ADEQUACY	LIKELY FINDINGS
Finger study	Digit placed in position for PA, lateral, and semipronation oblique views.	Cortex, trabeculae, and articular surfaces clearly seen. Proximal portion of metacarpal shaft seen.	Fractures of middle and distal phalanges Injuries to PIP and DIP joints.
Thumb study	PA, lateral, and oblique views. Lateral of thumb requires additional 15° pronation of the hand.	Cortex, trabeculae, and articular surfaces clearly seen. Thumb PA view is usually slightly oblique.	Fractures of thumb phalanges and metacarpal.
AP thumb (Robert view)	Hand is hyperpronated with anatomic snuff box placed against film cassette.	True AP view without rotation. Articular surfaces have no overlap.	A true frontal projection of metacarpal and CMC joint of thumb.

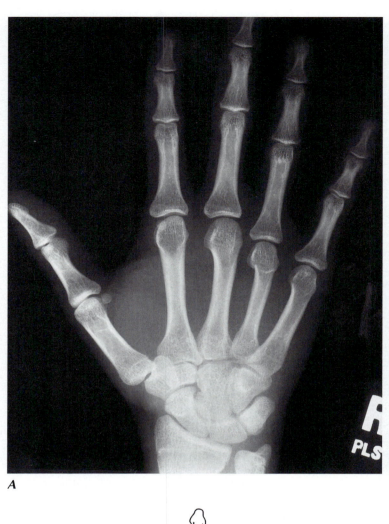

A

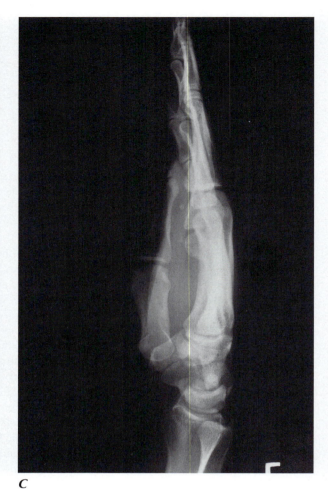

C

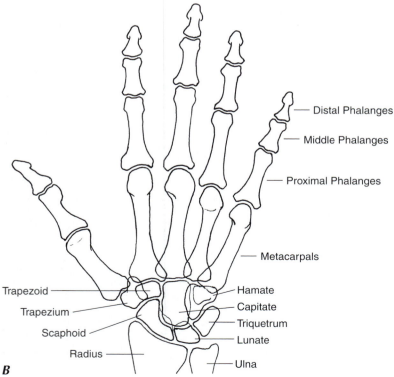

- Distal Phalanges

- Middle Phalanges

- Proximal Phalanges

- Metacarpals

Trapezoid ——

Trapezium ——

Scaphoid ——

Radius ——

—— Hamate

—— Capitate

—— Triquetrum

—— Lunate

—— Ulna

B

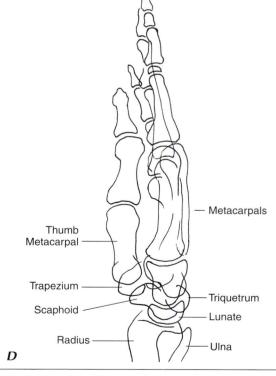

Thumb
Metacarpal ——

Trapezium ——

Scaphoid ——

Radius ——

—— Metacarpals

—— Triquetrum

—— Lunate

—— Ulna

D

FIGURE 3-3. *A an*d *B*. PA view.

FIGURE 3-3. *C* and *D*. Lateral view.

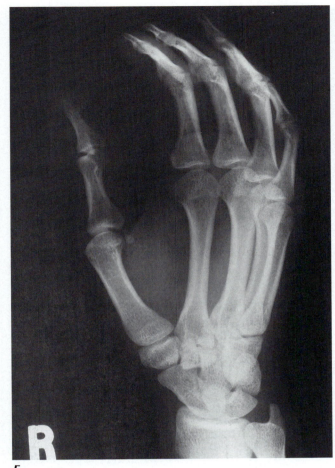

E

perimposed. Placing the fingers in varying degrees of flexion ("fanning") eliminates the overlap of the middle and distal phalanges. This fan view is preferred when a phalangeal injury is suspected.

Hand Pronation Oblique. The pronation oblique view is obtained by placing the hand in a semipronated position with the ulnar side against the cassette. The fingers are then fanned. The MCP joints are in a plane that is 45° above the plane of the film cassette (Fig. 3-3*E* and *F*). The x-ray beam passes from posterior to anterior through the hand. This view is also called a *PA oblique.*

Hand Supination Oblique. The supination oblique is usually a supplementary view. It is obtained by placing the dorsal surface of the hand on the film cassette and moving the hand into a semi-supinated position (Fig. 3-4). The x-ray beam passes from anterior to posterior. This view, also called the *ball-catcher's view,* clearly shows the little finger metacarpal and is useful in demonstrating subtle fractures in this area.

Brewerton View. Occult fractures at the base of the metacarpals are sometimes seen using the *Brewerton view.*[2] In this view, the hand is placed dorsal-surface down with the beam angled 30° from the ulnar side of the hand.

Finger Views. The standard views for a finger study are the PA, lateral, and, in some institutions, pronation oblique (Fig. 3-5). Finger views provide improved cortical and trabecular detail. They should be used if the injury involves the area distal to and including the shaft of the proximal phalanx. The individual finger is placed directly against the film cassette and the x-ray beam is centered on the finger. This provides better detail and less magnification distortion than hand radiographs.

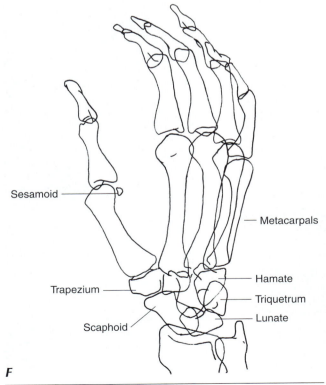

Sesamoid

Metacarpals

Trapezium

Hamate

Triquetrum

Lunate

Scaphoid

F

FIGURE 3-3. *E* and *F.* Pronation oblique view.

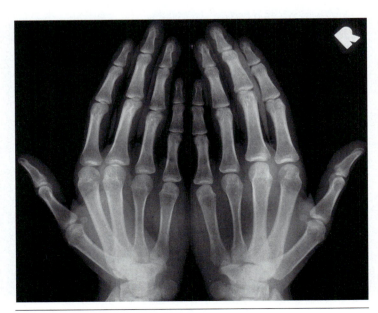

FIGURE 3-4. Supination oblique view ("ball-catcher" view).

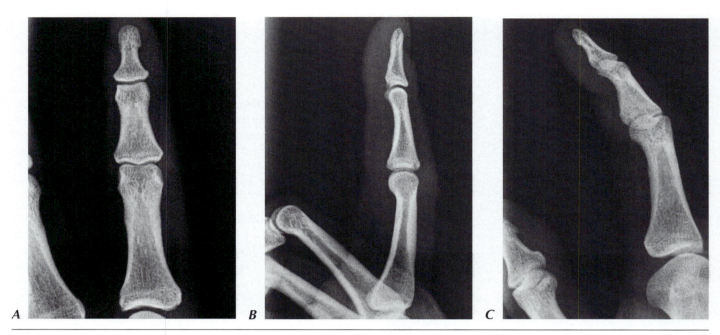

FIGURE 3-5.   Finger radiographs (*A*. PA view. *B*. Lateral view. *C*. Oblique view.)

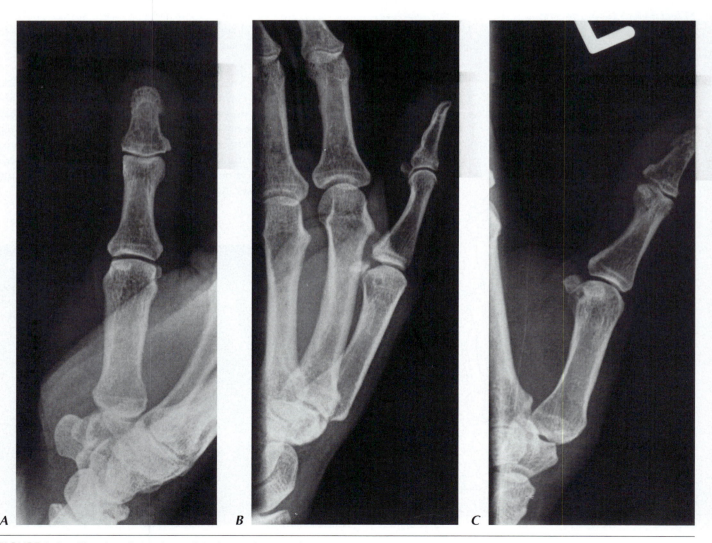

FIGURE 3-6.   Thumb radiographs (*A*. PA view. *B*. Lateral view. *C*. Oblique view.)

Thumb Views. The standard views include a PA, oblique, and lateral (Fig. 3-6). However, the PA view is at a slightly oblique angle. If a true frontal view is essential, the *anteroposterior (AP) Robert view* is obtained by placing the "anatomic snuffbox" against the cassette and extending the thumb (hyperpronation). The primary advantage of this view is that it shows the CMC joint of the thumb more clearly than the PA view.

RADIOGRAPHIC ANALYSIS

An adequate history is obtained and physical examination performed before reviewing radiographs. This information focuses attention on a particular area of the radiograph and heightens suspicion for certain injuries. Evaluation of the radiograph should integrate an approach that is both targeted and systematic. Attention is directed to sites prone to injury and frequently missed injured sites (Fig. 3-7). Then the entire radiograph must be inspected in a systematic manner so as not to miss any injuries (Table 3-4).

TABLE 3-4

Systematic Analysis of Hand and Finger Radiographs

Adequacy	Three views included Radiographs correctly labeled and technically adequate in position and penetration

Focus on region of likely injury
   based on clinical examination
	Diaphysis (shaft)
	     Displaced fractures are obvious
	     Nondisplaced fractures are subtle and seen
	         on only one view
	 End portion (base and head)
	     Displaced fractures are obvious
	     Nondisplaced fractures are subtle and seen
	         on only one view
	 Joint
	     Avulsion fractures at site of tendon or
	         ligament attachment
	     Proper alignment at joint and uniform
	         joint space

Look for abnormalities outside region of likely injury	Same digit Adjacent digits Elsewhere in hand Wrist
Reevaluate patient in light of the radiographic findings	Rotational malalignment Ligament laxity Tendon malfunction Joint subluxation

Consider additional radiographic
   studies if the injury is not
   entirely elucidated
	Supination oblique, if the fourth or
	     fifth metacarpal injured
	 Finger films, if hand films initially ordered
	 Hand films, if only finger films initially ordered
	 Wrist films
	 Stress views—physical examination is the
	     primary means of assessing joint instability

Adequacy. First, the adequacy of the image is assessed (Tables 3-2 and 3-3). There should be minimal overlap of bones. All relevant structures should appear on the image. Adequate penetration clearly displays the cortex and trabecular structure of each bone.

Examine the Region of Likely Injury. The region of suspected injury (based on the physical examination) is reviewed. Adjacent soft tissue swelling can suggest the site of injury. Within this area of interest, the bones are examined for particular fracture types. Displaced fractures of the shaft (diaphysis) are usually obvious. Any angulation, shortening, or rotation is noted. For metacarpal fractures, the oblique view is reviewed. Nondisplaced fractures can be difficult to see and may be seen on only one view. Metacarpal fractures are seen on the PA and oblique views. They are difficult to see on the lateral view because of the overlap of osseous structures. Displaced and comminuted fractures are usually easily identified. Intraarticular involvement is noted. Avulsion fractures from either end of the phalanges indicate ligament or tendon injury. Alignment of the articular surfaces must be evaluated carefully. The joint space should have uniform width. Any possible joint subluxation seen on the radiographs must be confirmed by physical examination, because alignment may falsely appear abnormal on a radiograph. Full range of motion without pain indicates that the apparent radiographic malalignment does not exist.

Examine Other Regions of Possible Injury. Next, the radiographs are examined for abnormalities outside the region of likely injury. The entire digit, adjacent digits, and the rest of the hand and wrist are evaluated.

Reexamine the Patient. The patient is then reevaluated using the radiographic findings to guide the physical examination. Rotational malalignment, ligamentous laxity, tendon malfunction, and joint subluxation are tested.

Additional radiographic studies might be considered. For example, the supination oblique (ball-catcher's) view is obtained if a metacarpal injury of the ring or little finger is suspected but not seen on the standard hand series. If a wrist injury is suspected, then wrist films should be obtained. One may want to order a finger series if only hand radiographs were ordered. Stress views may also be considered.

COMMON ABNORMALITIES

The classification of hand injuries is similar for each of the bones of the hand

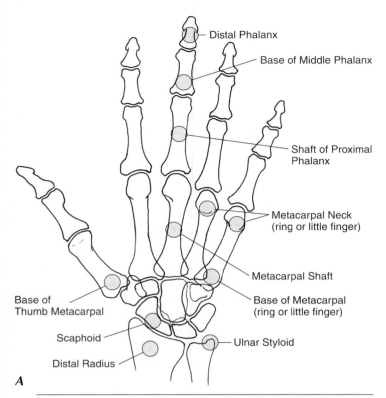

A

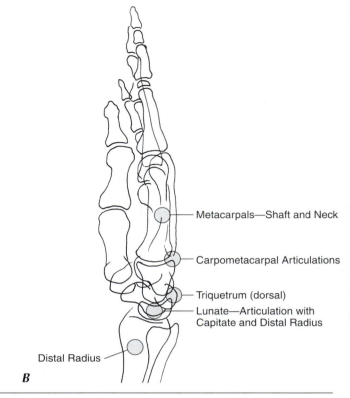

B

FIGURE 3-7.   Sites prone to injury and easily missed injuries. *A*. PA.

FIGURE 3-7.   *B*. Lateral.

(metacarpals, and proximal, middle, and distal phalanges). There are fractures of the shaft, base, neck, and head of these bones. The fractures may have intraarticular extension, rotation, or foreshortening. There may be associated injury to the ligaments or tendons. Injuries to the distal phalanges are most common, followed by the proximal phalanges and the metacarpals.

Metacarpal Fractures

Metacarpal fractures occur at four distinct fracture locations: the base, shaft, neck, and head. The location and displacement of the fracture dictate treatment.

METACARPAL BASE FRACTURES.   Fractures at the base of the metacarpals may be difficult to detect radiographically because of overlap with the adjacent bones (Fig. 3-8). Fractures of the base of the little-finger metacarpal are common. These may be

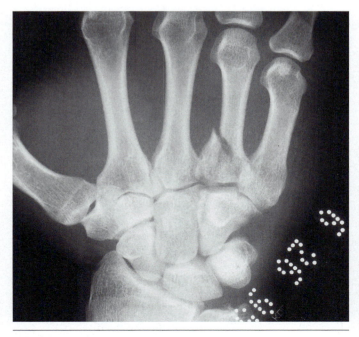

FIGURE 3-8.   Fracture at base of ring finger metacarpal.

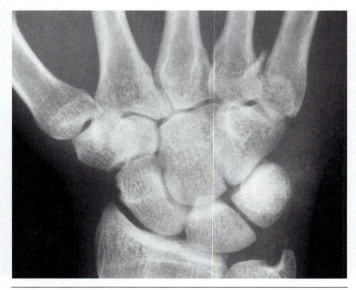

FIGURE 3-9.   Fracture at base of little finger metacarpal.

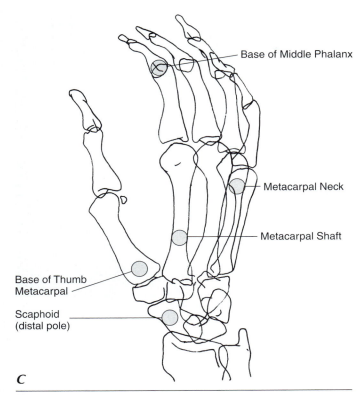

Base of Middle Phalanx

Metacarpal Neck

Metacarpal Shaft

Base of Thumb
Metacarpal

Scaphoid
(distal pole)

C

FIGURE 3-7. *C.* Oblique.

complicated by subluxation of the metacarpohamate joint (Fig. 3-9). A supination oblique (ball-catcher's) view may be needed to visualize this fracture.[1] Open reduction and internal fixation are often required.

THUMB METACARPAL BASE FRACTURES. Fractures involving the metacarpal at the base of the thumb are common and can result in significant disability.

Bennett Fracture. This injury is a fracture-dislocation involving the articular surface of the base of the thumb metacarpal.[3] The metacarpal base is displaced dorsally and radially by the abductor pollicus longus tendon (Fig. 3-10). This intraarticular fracture usually requires operative fixation.[4] Provisional emergency department (ED) management includes immobilization with a thumb spica splint and early referral to a hand specialist.

Rolando Fracture. This is a Y-shaped fracture of the base of the thumb metacarpal.[5] It can be considered an intraarticular, comminuted Bennett fracture (Fig. 3-11). ED management requires a thumb spica splint and referral. The prognosis is worse than that of a Bennett fracture, and operative fixation is usually necessary.

Extraarticular Fractures. Extraarticular fractures of the base of the thumb metacarpal are either transverse or spiral (Fig. 3-12). Healing of these fractures is affected by the degree of displacement and comminution. These extraarticular fractures should be distinguished from the intraarticular Bennett or Rolando fracture. A thumb spica splint and early referral are appropriate.

METACARPAL SHAFT FRACTURES. Fractures of the metacarpal shaft occur anywhere along the length of the diaphysis. Shaft fractures are generally *transverse* (Fig. 3-13) or *spiral* (Fig. 3-14). Marked angulation can occur. Angulation is most frequently seen with the ring finger, little finger, or thumb. These fingers are more mobile and lack the rigid ligamentous support that prevents angulation. A fracture of the shaft of the ring or little finger should be distinguished from a *boxer's fracture*, which is a fracture through the metacarpal neck (see below). Metacarpal shaft fractures generally angulate dorsally. The oblique view is helpful for identifying angulation and shorten-

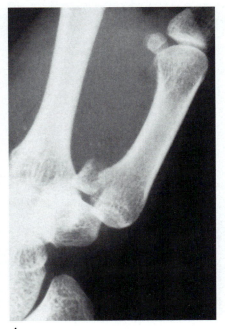

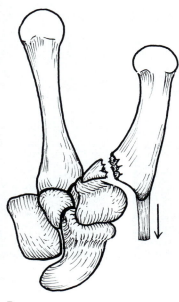

FIGURE 3-10. Bennett fracture. An intraarticular fracture at the base of the thumb metacarpal. The pull of the abductor pollicis tendon displaces the thumb carpometacarpal joint. (*B.* From Wilson FC, Lin PP: *General Orthopedics.* McGraw-Hill, 1997, with permission.)

A   *B*

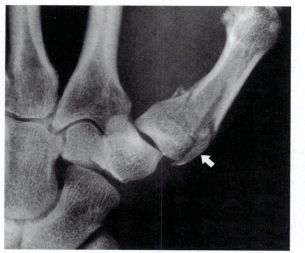
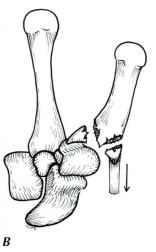
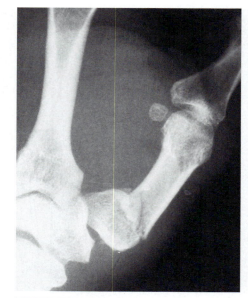

FIGURE 3-11.   Rolando fracture. A comminuted intraarticular fracture at the base of the thumb metacarpal. Because of the fracture comminution, only the insertion site of the abductor pollicis tendon is displaced. (*B*. From Wilson FC, Lin PP: *General Orthopedics*. McGraw-Hill, 1997, with permission.)

FIGURE 3-12.   Extraarticular fracture at base of thumb metacarpal.

ing. Up to 5 mm of shortening is tolerated without a significant decrease in function. However, any degree of rotation will greatly affect function because the rotational deformity is amplified distally at the fingertip. Therefore, almost any rotational malalignment requires correction. Fractures with rotational deformity and irreducible fractures require internal fixation.

METACARPAL NECK FRACTURES.   Fractures of the metacarpal neck are commonly referred to as *boxer's fractures* because they typically occur when the patient forcefully strikes his or her fist against a solid object, such as a mandible or a wall. The impact occurs at the metacarpal head with the MCP joint in flexion. These are the most common metacarpal fractures and

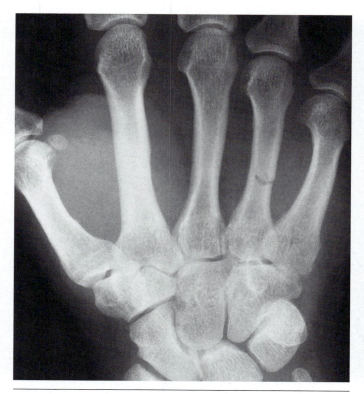

FIGURE 3-13.   Transverse fracture of metacarpal shaft of the ring finger.

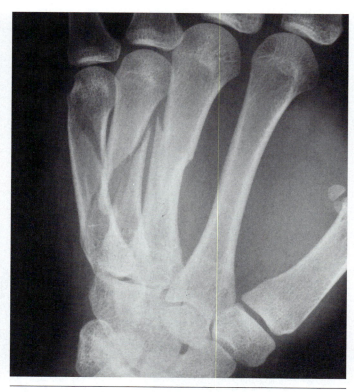

FIGURE 3-14.   Spiral fractures of middle, ring and little finger metacarpals. There is slight foreshortening, angulation, and rotation.

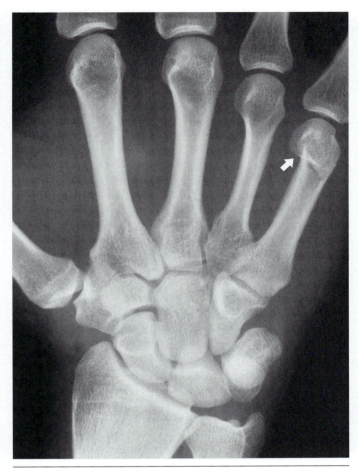

FIGURE 3-15. Boxer's fracture. Fracture of the neck of the little finger metacarpal.

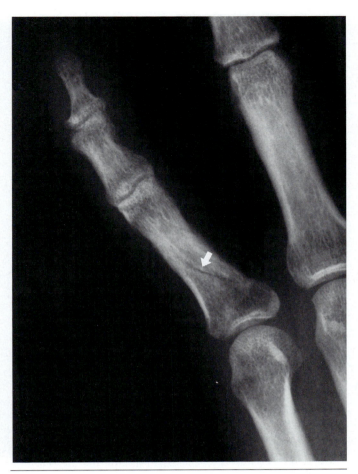

FIGURE 3-16. Subtle, nondisplaced oblique fracture of proximal phalanx of little finger.

usually involve the ring or little finger. The degree of angulation that is allowable varies depending on which metacarpal is involved (see "Controversies," below). These fractures are typically unstable because of comminution of their volar aspect (Fig. 3-15).

METACARPAL HEAD FRACTURES. Fractures of the metacarpal head are uncommon. They usually result from extension of metacarpal neck fractures. The involved joint has a high risk of dysfunction. It is important to distinguish correctly between metacarpal neck and head fractures.

Proximal Phalanx Fractures

A direct blow to the finger is the usual cause of this fracture. Transverse fractures of the proximal phalanges typically angulate in a volar direction because of the action of the interosseous muscles on the phalanges that flex the proximal segment. Stable, nondisplaced transverse fractures are treated by "buddy taping" the finger to the adjacent digit. In contrast, oblique fractures are usually unstable because of foreshortening and rotation (Fig. 3-16). Fractures of the base and neck of the proximal phalanx are uncommon and may be subtle. The oblique view often reveals the fracture more readily than the PA view.

GAMEKEEPER'S (SKIER'S) THUMB. Gamekeeper's thumb was first described as a chronic overuse injury seen in gamekeepers. Ulnar collateral ligament injury is caused by the repetitive breaking of rabbits' necks between the thumb and index finger.[6] Today, the most common mechanism is an acute hyperextension of the thumb MCP joint that occurs from falling with a ski pole in the hand. Some 50 percent of all skiing injuries to the hand are of this type.[7] The injury is usually entirely ligamentous—a tear in the ulnar collateral ligament of the thumb MCP joint. In some cases, there may be an avulsion fracture of the ulnar collateral ligament insertion site (Fig. 3-17). The injuries range from partial to total disruption of the ligament. Total ligament disruption results in greater than 30° of angulation at the MCP joint. Operative repair may be necessary.

Middle Phalanx Fractures

TRANSVERSE FRACTURE. Transverse fractures of the middle phalanx are less common than proximal and distal phalangeal fractures. These fractures exhibit dorsal angulation because of the extensor tendon's insertion on the dorsal base of the middle phalanx and the flexor tendon's insertion on the distal volar surface.

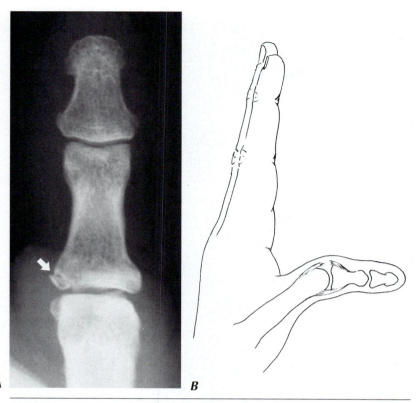

A   *B*

FIGURE 3-17. Gamekeeper's thumb (skier's thumb). A tear of the ulnar collateral ligament of the thumb MCP joint occurs with either chronic repetitive trauma (gamekeeper's thumb) or an acute injury (skier's thumb). A small avulsion fracture is sometimes seen at the base of the phalanx. (*B.* From Scaletta TA, Schrader JJ: *Emergent Management of Trauma.* McGraw-Hill, 1997, with permission.)

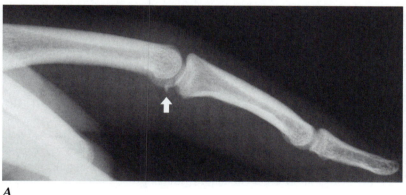

A

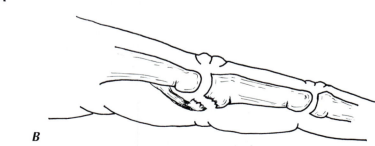

B

FIGURE 3-18. Volar plate avulsion. Hyperextension of the PIP joint tears the volar plate. A small avulsion fracture is often seen at the volar surface of the base of the middle phalanx. In some cases a larger fracture is produced by concomitant impaction and shearing. If a large portion of the articular surface is fractured, operative fixation with pins is necessary.

VOLAR PLATE AVULSION. Although there are volar plates at each DIP and MCP joint, the only common volar plate injury is at the PIP joint. Hyperextension at the PIP is the mechanism of injury. Complete rupture of the volar plate is necessary for dorsal dislocation to occur. Volar plate disruption is frequently a purely ligamentous injury (Fig. 3-1). Occasionally, there is a small chip avulsion off the volar surface of the base of the middle phalanx (Fig. 3-18). The avulsed chip may be the only radiographic clue to a volar plate injury. When the intraarticular avulsion fracture involves more than 30% of the articular surface, the joint is unstable and operative fixation is necessary. Because these injuries are often reduced before the patient arrives at a medical facility, the diagnosis must be made by the history and physical examination.

PIP DISLOCATION. In most PIP dislocations, the distal element is dorsally displaced (Fig. 3-19). If the dislocation is not reducible, there may be entrapment of the volar plate or the flexor tendons.[8,9] An unstable joint or an irreducible dislocation requires operative repair. A "stable" volar plate injury or a reduced dorsal PIP dislocation should be splinted in 15 to 20° of flexion.

BOUTONNIERE INJURY. Disruption of the central slip of the extensor tendon causes the lateral bands of the tendon to slide below the axis of the PIP joint during flexion. The lateral bands then function as PIP flexors instead of extensors. There is hyperextension at the DIP joint due to the pull of the displaced lateral bands. This creates the characteristic *boutonniere deformity,* with the PIP flexed and the DIP extended (Fig. 3-20). The injury is usually limited to soft tissues, but there may be an avulsion fracture from the insertion site of the central slip at the base of the middle phalanx. Identification of the avulsed fragment and assessment of its size are important because a large fragment requires open reduction and internal fixation. The characteristic deformity, which may not be evident at the time of initial injury, often progresses over time and causes significant disability. Lack of an immediate deformity can make the diagnosis difficult. Identification of the avulsion fracture or tenderness over the area increases suspicion for this injury.

Distal Phalanx Fractures

Distal phalanx fractures are the most common fractures of the hand and account for more than half of all hand fractures.[10-12] Most distal phalanx fractures are produced by crush injuries. Soft tissue

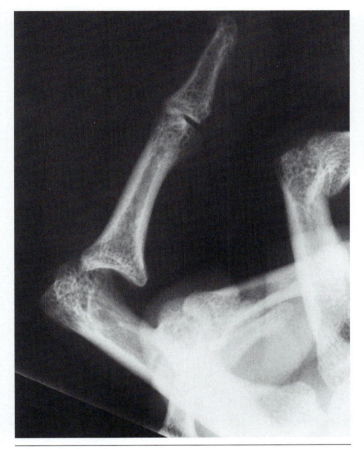

FIGURE 3-19. Volar PIP dislocation.

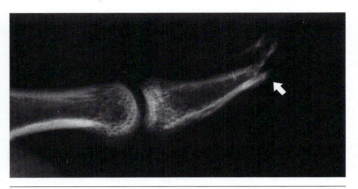

FIGURE 3-21. Displaced transverse fracture of thumb distal phalanx.

avulsion or disruption results in an open fracture. The most frequent type of distal phalanx fracture is the *tuft* ("crushed eggshell") *fracture.* Longitudinal and transverse fractures of the shaft are less common.

TUFT FRACTURE.   A crush injury is the most common cause of a tuft fracture. The fracture can be transverse (Fig. 3-21), spiral, or comminuted (eggshell) (Fig. 3-22). It is important to identify these injuries whenever there is concomitant soft tissue injury. Antibiotic therapy is often recommended for open tuft fractures. The presence of a large subungual hematoma (50% or greater) usually signifies a significant nailbed injury. Such injuries can result in deformity of the nail if the nailbed is not repaired.

SHAFT FRACTURE.   Transverse and longitudinal fractures are seen as lucencies transecting the bone. They are usually caused by a direct blow. When there is significant angulation, transverse fractures require pin fixation. Shaft fractures should be assessed for intraarticular extension because this alters management.

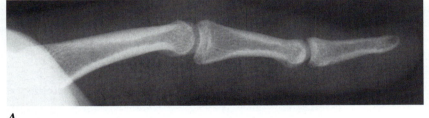

A

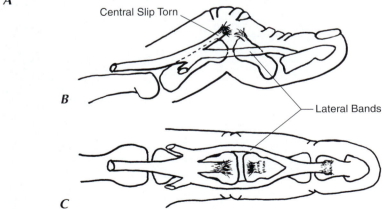

Central Slip Torn

B

Lateral Bands

C

FIGURE 3-20.   Boutonniere deformity. *A.* Slight flexion of the PIP joint and extension of the DIP joint is seen. There is soft tissue swelling over the PIP joint. *B, C.* An extensor tendon injury at the PIP joint results in a boutonniere deformity. The central slip of the extensor tendon inserts on the base of the middle phalanx. It is torn by trauma to the dorsal surface of the PIP joint. The lateral bands of the extensor tendon then migrate volarly causing flexion of the PIP joint and extension of the DIP joint.

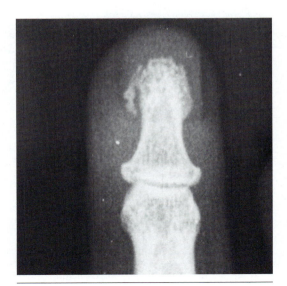

FIGURE 3-22.   Distal phalanx tuft fracture.

MALLET FINGER.   A direct blow to the tip of the finger while the DIP is in flexion causes the mallet finger injury. There is hyperflexion of the DIP joint, which results in either stretching or complete rupture of the insertion of the extensor tendon from the base of the distal phalanx. Many mallet finger deformities are entirely tendonous. It is also common to see an intraarticular avulsion fracture at the base of the distal phalanx that involves one-third or more of the articular surface (Fig. 3-23). If less than one-third of the articular surface is involved, the extensor tendon usually remains intact.

This injury is usually treated by splinting in slight hyperextension at the DIP joint. If the avulsion fracture involves greater than 50% of the articular surface, then percutaneous K-wire fixation is often required.

Epiphyseal Growth Plate Fractures

Children frequently have fractures that involve the growth plate (Fig. 3-24). In the hand, epiphyses occur only at one end of the phalanges (as opposed to both ends in long bones). The most common epiphyseal fracture in the hand involves the base of the proximal phalanx (Fig. 3-25). The Salter-Harris classification is useful for description, treatment, and prognosis of these injuries.

Other Abnormalities

OSTEOMYELITIS.   Although the radiographic signs of osteomyelitis are fairly specific, they are late findings. Plain radiographs have limited use in early detection of osteomyelitis. The classic radiographic findings are periosteal elevation and lucent lytic areas of cortical bone destruction (Fig. 3-26). These

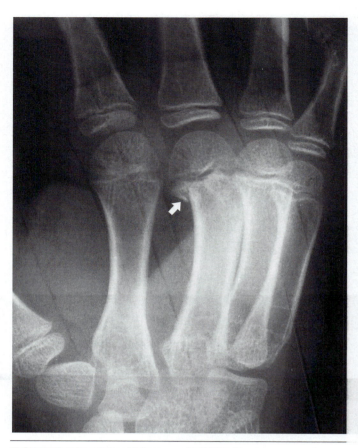

FIGURE 3-24.   Salter II fracture of middle finger metacarpal.

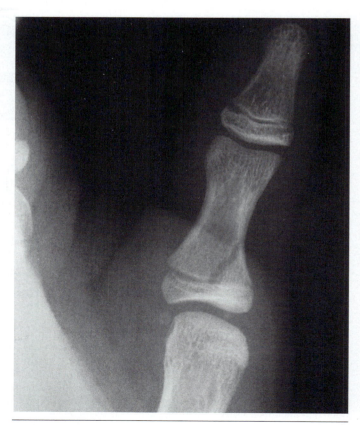

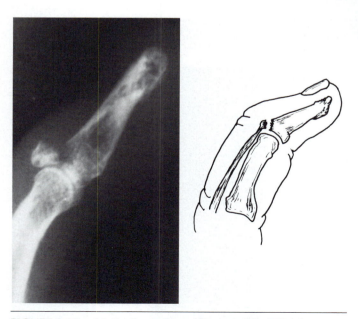

FIGURE 3-23.   Mallet finger. Forced flexion of the DIP joint causes avulsion of the extensor tendon from the base of the distal phalanx. An associated avulsion fracture is sometimes seen.

FIGURE 3-25.   Salter II fracture at proximal phalanx of thumb.

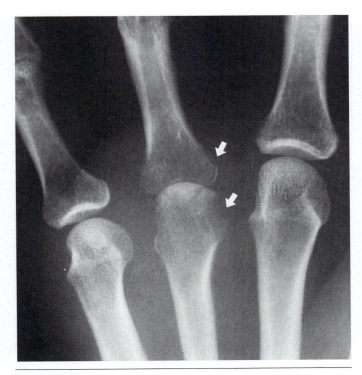

changes begin to appear a week or more after the infection has begun and are commonly noted 4 weeks after onset of the infection. Bone scans provide earlier evidence of osteomyelitis.

FOREIGN BODY. Contaminated wounds should be explored directly. Radiographs are most useful for wounds that are difficult to explore. Plain radiographs, however, are limited in their ability to detect foreign bodies. The foreign material must be either radiopaque (e.g., metal or glass) relative to the surrounding soft tissues or radiolucent (Figs. 3-27 and 3-28). Most deep wounds of the hand involving broken glass or metallic projectiles should be radiographed.

HIGH-PRESSURE INJECTION. The hand is a common site of injection injuries due to a high-pressure gas, grease, or paint gun. Radiographs are used to determine the extent and distribution of the injury (Fig. 3-28). High pressure injection injuries are surgical emergencies.

HUMAN-BITE/CLENCHED-FIST INJURY. Lacerations of the hand over the MCP or PIP joints occur during a fistfight when the clenched fist strikes teeth. The radiograph may show an intraarticular fracture or a tooth fragment. These injuries have an extremely high incidence of infection.

OSTEOARTHRITIS. Osteoarthritis is most common in postmenopausal women and usually affects the IP joints and thumb

FIGURE 3-26. Osteomyelitis. There is cortical erosion of the metacarpal head and base of proximal phalanx of the ring finger. The MCP joint space is narrowed.

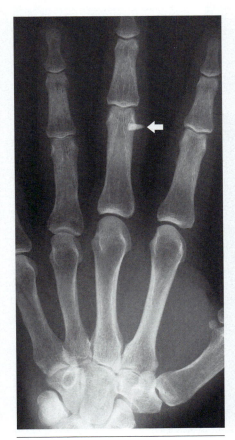

FIGURE 3-27. Glass foreign body overlying proximal phalanx of middle finger.

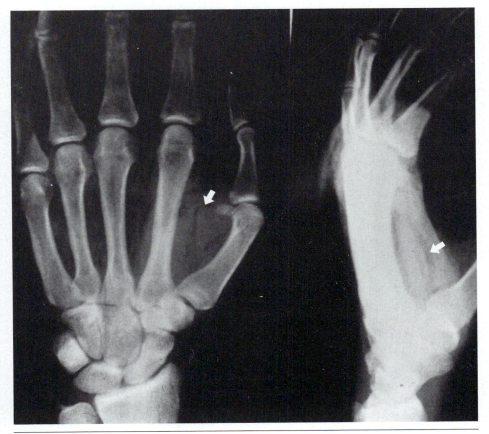

FIGURE 3-28. High-pressure injection injury. A grease gun accidentally injected into the hand of this worker. Multiple radiolucent streaks are seen throughout the soft tissues of the palm. (Courtesy of David Effron, MD. MetroHealth Medical Center, Cleveland, OH).

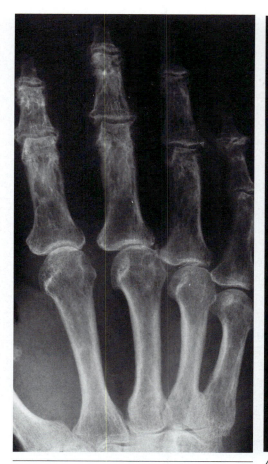

FIGURE 3-29. Osteoarthritis. There is joint space narrowing and marginal osteophyte formation at the DIP and PIP joint.

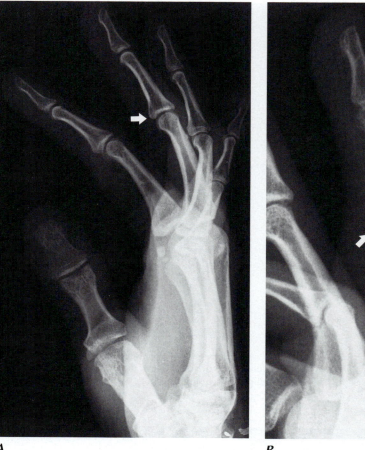

A   *B*

FIGURE 3-30. Finger injury not visible on hand radiographs. *A.* No fracture was visible on the hand radiographs. *B.* The volar plate avulsion fracture was seen on the lateral finger radiograph. (Copyright David T. Schwartz, MD.)

MCP. Radiographic findings include joint space narrowing, subchondral sclerosis, and marginal osteophytes (Fig. 3-29). Other findings include bony spurs of the DIP joint (Heberden's nodes) and hook-like osteophytes at the MCP joints.

RHEUMATOID ARTHRITIS.   Rheumatoid arthritis (RA) results in periarticular soft tissue swelling, uniform joint space narrowing, demineralization (periarticular osteopenia), and articular destruction. The articular erosions are irregular and jagged. Ulnar deviation at the MCP joints is common. In contrast to osteoarthritis, with RA the DIP joints are relatively spared.

PSORIATIC ARTHRITIS.   Psoriatic arthritis affects approximately 7% of patients with psoriasis. Characteristic radiographic findings include diffuse soft tissue swelling of the digits, extensive proliferative erosions, and marked involvement of the DIP joints.

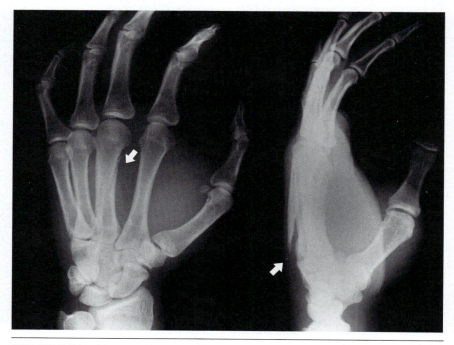

FIGURE 3-31. Fracture seen best on only one view. Subtle middle finger metacarpal fracture on the oblique view. Displacement is seen on lateral view.

ERRORS IN INTERPRETATION

Missed Fractures.   Fractures may be overlooked because they lack displacement and are visible on only one view. A small nondisplaced fracture at the base of the middle phalanx is often seen only on the lateral finger projection (Fig. 3-30). Even large or displaced fractures may be surprisingly subtle on one view yet obvious on another (Fig. 3-31). An impaction fracture at the metacarpal neck or base can be particularly difficult to identify (Figs. 3-32 and 3-33). Soft tissue swelling noted on the radiograph and physical examination add significance to a questionable radiographic abnormality. Multiple injuries are common. Each radiograph must be completely inspected, because it is easy to identify one abnormality and neglect the remainder of the film.

Metacarpal Base Fractures.   A fracture at the base of the metacarpal can be difficult to identify because of overlying shadows from adjacent bones (Fig. 3-34). If clinical suspicion is high and no abnormality is identified on the standard radiographs, a Brewerton view[2] depicts the CMC region more clearly. A supination oblique view shows the base of the fourth or fifth metacarpals.

Impacted Boxer's Fracture.   Impaction can mask the cortical disruption of a fracture (Fig. 3-32). Often the best image for identifying an impacted boxer's fracture is the lateral view. However, because of overlying shadows from the other metacarpals, the lateral view can be difficult to interpret. The ball-catcher's view[1] reveals the head and neck of the little-finger metacarpal more clearly.

Rotational Misalignment.   Rotational misalignment is difficult to assess radiographically. It occurs in fractures of the metacarpals, proximal phalanges, and middle phalanges. Examining the patient's hand with fingers flexed will best assess rotational misalignment. If one of the flexed digits does not point toward the scaphoid area or overlaps an adjacent digit, rotational misalignment is present. On the radiograph, one sees different projections of the bone proximal and distal to the fracture. For example, the proximal portion of the involved bone is seen in a true lateral projection, whereas its distal portion appears oblique.

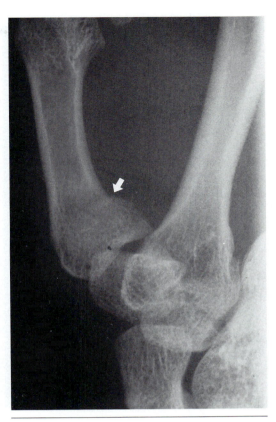

FIGURE 3-33.   Subtle metacarpal base fracture. An impacted fracture at base of thumb metacarpal was not seen on the hand radiograph.

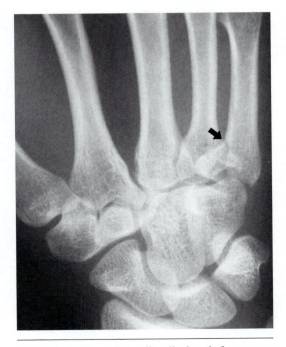

FIGURE 3-34.   Minimally displaced fracture at base of small finger metacarpal. The fracture is difficult to see because of overlap with the adjacent metacarpal base. The fracture extends to the articular surface. A supination oblique view (ball-catcher's view) can better define this fracture.

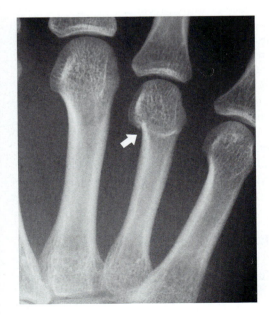

FIGURE 3-32.   Subtle boxer's fracture. An impacted fracture of the neck of the ring finger metacarpal. Only slight cortical interruption is seen.

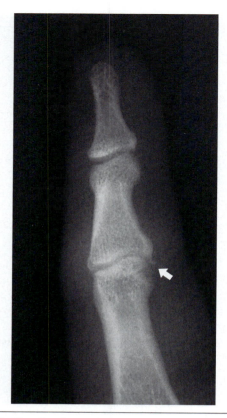

FIGURE 3-35. Small avulsion fracture at PIP joint. The fracture was seen only on the oblique finger view.

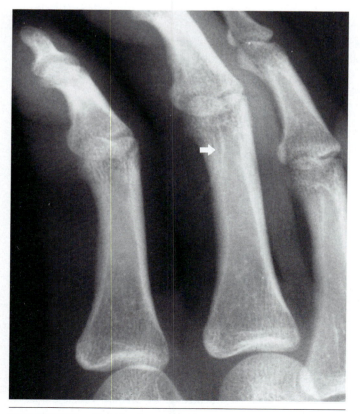

FIGURE 3-36. Vascular foramen in the proximal phalanx of the middle finger. It has a characteristic oblique orientation, smooth well-corticated margins, and involves only one side of the cortex.

Joint Involvement. A critical issue in the management of a hand injury is deciding whether the fracture extends intraarticularly. Although it is obvious in some fractures that the fracture line extends into the joint, it is unclear in others. The use of multiple views can often confirm intraarticular extension. Finger views, if not already obtained, are often helpful.

Tendon and Ligament Injuries. Most injuries of tendons and ligaments are diagnosed on physical examination. Sometimes the physical signs can be subtle and must be specifically sought, such as a thumb ulnar collateral ligament tear (gamekeeper's or skier's thumb) or avulsion of the central slip of the extensor tendon (boutonniere deformity). In some cases, a small bone chip representing an avulsion fracture at the site of the tendon or ligament insertion can provide a radiographic clue to the injury (Fig. 3-35).

COMMON VARIANTS

Sesamoid Bones. Five sesamoid bones, small bones imbedded in the flexor tendons, are commonly found in the hand. Typical locations include the volar thumb MCP joint, where two are often found; the volar thumb IP joint; and the volar aspect of the MCP joints of the index and little fingers. These bones are distinguished from small avulsion fractures by their spherical shape; smooth, intact cortex; distance from the site of injury; and lack of tenderness. When in doubt, comparison radiographs from the other hand are helpful because the sesamoids are usually bilateral (Fig. 3-3A).

Joint Angulation. Joints in the hand naturally possess some degree of radioulnar laxity. Depending on the position of the joint at the time of the radiograph, the angulation may appear more or less pronounced. This can be misinterpreted as joint subluxation. If injuries to the ligaments of the joint are suspected clinically, then comparison radiographs or stress views may be appropriate. One radiographic indication of an unstable joint may be a small avulsion fracture.

Vascular Grooves. Vascular grooves can be misinterpreted as fractures. Nutrient artery canals are common and are located near the middle of the phalangeal and metacarpal shafts. They have an oblique orientation, smooth sclerotic margins, and do not cause cortical disruption. They do not cross the bone entirely, and never cause displacement (Fig. 3-36).

Epiphyseal Lines. In children, open epiphyseal lines can be confused with fractures. Open physes appear as lucent sclerotic, parallel, undulating lines. Fracture lines are irregular and show cortical disruption (Fig. 3-24).

CONTROVERSIES

Stress Views. Purely ligamentous injuries may appear normal on static views; therefore dynamic or stress views will be required for diagnosis. Stress views are rarely ordered in the ED

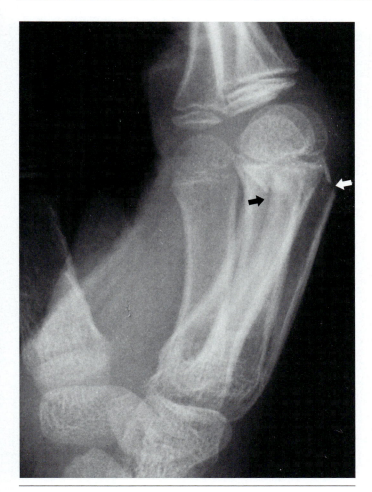

FIGURE 3-37.   Angulated (35°) metacarpal neck fracture.

and add little to the emergent management of these injuries. If a ligamentous injury is suspected based on physical examination, appropriate immobilization and follow-up should be arranged.

Amount of Fracture Angulation.   Metacarpal neck fractures of the ring and little fingers (boxer's fractures) can have up to 70° of angulation with little or no decrease in function after healing because of the mobility at the CMC joint.[13,14] Some hand surgeons suggest that angulation less than 40° does not require reduction.[13,15] Others believe that with greater than 30° of angulation there is increased pain and decreased function of the digits.[16] They recommend reduction of all metacarpal neck fractures with angulation of greater than 30°. Although this controversy is unresolved, it does emphasize the need to measure the degree of angulation accurately. The clinician can then make an informed decision regarding reduction and splinting versus simply splinting. There is little controversy about metacarpal

neck fractures in the middle and index fingers. It is generally agreed that angulation greater than 10 to 15° requires reduction (Fig. 3-37).

Postreduction Films.   Postreduction radiographs of dislocations occasionally reveal small avulsion fractures that were not evident in the initial radiographs. Although postreduction radiographs rarely change the emergent management of these injuries, they do confirm adequate reduction and may show findings that influence definitive management, such as need for operative intervention for large, unstable avulsion fragments. For this reason, post-reduction radiographs of hand dislocations are generally recommended.

REFERENCES

1. Stapczynski JS: Fracture of the base of the little finger metacarpal: Importance of the "ball-catcher" radiographic view. *J Emerg Med* 9:145, 1991.
2. Brewerton DA: A tangential radiographic projection for demonstrating involvement of metacarpal heads in rheumatoid arthritis. *Br J Radiol* 40:233, 1967.
3. Bennett EH: Fractures of the metacarpal bones. *Dublin J Med Sci* 73:72, 1882.
4. Timmenga EJ, Blokhuis TJ, Raaigmakers EL: Long-term evaluation of Bennett's fracture: A comparison between open and closed reduction. *J Hand Surg Br* 19:373, 1994.
5. Rolando S: Fracture de la base de premier metacarpien: et principalement surg une variete non encore decrite. *Presse Med* 18:303, 1910.
6. Campbell CS: Gamekeeper's thumb. *J Bone Joint Surg* 37B:148, 1955.
7. Benke GJ, Stableforth PG: Injuries of the proximal interphalangeal joint of the fingers. *Hand* 11:263, 1979.
8. Green SM, Posner MA: Irreducible dorsal dislocations of the proximal interphalangeal joint. *J Hand Surg Am* 10:85, 1985.
9. Kjeldal I: Irreducible compound dorsal dislocations of the proximal interphalangeal joint of the finger. *J Hand Surg Br* 11:49, 1986.
10. McNealy RW, Lichtenstein ME: Fractures of the metacarpals and phalanges. *J Surg Obstet Gynecol* 43:156, 1935.
11. McNealy RW, Lichtenstein ME: Fractures of the bones of the hand. *Am J Surg* 50:563, 1940.
12. Browne EZ Jr: Complications of fingertip injuries. *Hand Clin* 10:125, 1994.
13. Hunter JM, Cowen NJ: Fifth metacarpal fractures in a compensation clinic population: A report on one hundred and thirty-three cases. *J Bone Joint Surg Am* 52:1159, 1970.
14. Holst-Neilsen F: Subcapital fractures of the four ulnar metacarpal bones. *Hand* 8:290, 1976.
15. Eichenholtz SN, Rizzo PC: Fracture of the neck of the fifth metacarpal bone: Is overtreatment justified? *JAMA* 178:151, 1961.
16. Smith RJ, Peimer CA: Injuries of the metacarpal bones and joints. *Adv Surg* 11:341, 1977.

CHAPTER 4

THE WRIST AND FOREARM

RENU CHAWLA MITAL / MICHAEL BEESON

Wrist injuries account for 2.5% of all emergency department (ED) visits.[1] The spectrum of wrist injuries ranges from simple contusions to disabling fractures, dislocations, and ligamentous injuries. Because most occupational and recreational activities rely on functional use of the wrist, injuries to this region can be debilitating.

The complete and accurate diagnosis of forearm and wrist injuries requires a thorough history, physical examination, and radiographic studies. The physical examination often provides clinical signs of a specific injury that is verified by radiographic examination. Many wrist injuries have subtle radiographic findings and can even have normal radiographs. Minor distortions of radiographic anatomy can represent significant injury. Failing to diagnose injuries on the initial presentation can result in a poor functional outcome. Therefore, early and accurate diagnosis is imperative to avoid future disability.

The anatomic extent of the wrist includes the distal radius and ulna, the two rows of carpal bones, and the proximal metacarpals. There are two major zones of wrist injury: the distal radius and the carpus. Injuries to the forearm include fractures of the shaft of the radius or ulna and associated injuries to the elbow or wrist.

CLINICAL DECISION MAKING

In many patients with wrist trauma, it is difficult to differentiate between soft tissue and skeletal injury solely on the basis of the history and physical examination. As a result, radiographs are usually necessary to make a diagnosis. To the contrary, the most common wrist fracture, a displaced distal radius fracture, is easy to diagnose clinically. Yet, radiographs are even necessary in the patient with a displaced distal radius fracture to completely define the anatomic extent of the injury, the degree of comminution, and the presence of articular involvement. These considerations are important for orthopedic management of the injury, especially in determining whether closed reduction is adequate or operative fixation is necessary.

Other wrist injuries, such as nondisplaced distal radius fractures and carpal injuries, can have subtle clinical and radiographic findings. There are no studied clinical guidelines for ordering wrist films. Therefore, in deciding when to obtain radiographs, the physician must rely on clinical judgment and the knowledge of wrist injury patterns. The bones of the wrist lie close to the skin surface, so that focal tenderness due to a fracture is usually evident on clinical examination. Swelling and

limitation of motion suggest a fracture, although these signs are also seen with soft tissue injuries such as sprains and contusions. If pain, tenderness, swelling, and limitation of movement are minimal, then radiographs can probably be omitted. However, in attempting to be selective in ordering radiographs, it is important to remember that the consequences of misdiagnosis of certain wrist injuries can result in prolonged morbidity. For instance, a fractured scaphoid is subject to nonunion and avascular necrosis, which leads to considerable long-term disability. The risk of such complications is increased if the fracture is misdiagnosed and inadequately immobilized. It is therefore advisable to be liberal in ordering wrist radiographs.

Normal wrist radiographs do not definitively exclude a fracture. About 10 to 20% of scaphoid fractures have normal radiographs at the time of ED evaluation. Other wrist injuries can also present with "negative" radiographs. Therefore, the patient suspected of having a fracture based on clinical examination should be managed as though a fracture were present. The clinical signs of a scaphoid fracture include tenderness in the "anatomic snuff box," pain with supination against resistance, and pain with longitudinal (axial) compression of the thumb.[2]

Findings on physical examination assist in radiographic interpretation by calling attention to areas of focal tenderness. Some fractures are better seen on supplementary views, and the decision to obtain these views is directed by the physical examination findings. For example, tenderness over the ulnar side of the volar surface of the wrist suggests a fracture of the hook of the hamate. This injury is best seen on a carpal tunnel view.

In summary, the diagnosis of the most common wrist fracture, a displaced distal radius fracture, is usually straightforward. For nondisplaced fractures and carpal fractures, the physical examination findings can be similar to those of soft tissue injuries. Because the consequences of a missed wrist fracture can be great, radiographs are ordered liberally in ED patients with wrist injuries.

The situation for the forearm is different from that of the wrist. Fractures of the shaft of the radius and ulna are readily identified by pain, tenderness, and deformity. Soft tissue contusions are reliably distinguished by physical examination, therefore clinical findings can be confidently used in selecting patients for radiographic examination. Patients with forearm fractures may have associated injuries to the elbow or wrist. These areas must be carefully examined to detect injuries that can be less obvious than the forearm fracture. If there is pain, tenderness, or limited range of motion, the involved joint requires radiographic examination.

ANATOMY AND PHYSIOLOGY

Wrist Anatomy

The wrist is a complex mechanical system providing motion and transmitting force between the hand and the forearm. The proximal portion of the wrist is formed by the distal radius and ulna. The distal end of the radius is expanded and forms the articular surface of the radiocarpal joint. The lateral process of the distal radius is called the *radial styloid*. The radiocarpal joint surface is tilted slightly in a volar direction. The medial surface of the distal radius has a concave notch that articulates with the distal ulna. The ulna ends in a rounded articular surface and a pointed projection, the *ulnar styloid*.

Between the distal radius and ulna and the metacarpals, there are eight carpal bones divided into two rows; these are collectively called the *carpus* (Fig. 4-1). Each carpal bone has two names; the preferred names are given first in the figure and the secondary names in parentheses. For example, the term *scaphoid* is preferred to *navicular*. The proximal carpal row includes the scaphoid, lunate, and triquetrum. The pisiform is a sesamoid of the flexor carpiulnaris tendon. The distal carpal row consists of the trapezium, trapezoid, capitate, and hamate. The scaphoid, which bridges both rows, provides a stabilizing link for the midcarpal joint.

The proximal and distal carpal rows form two major articulations—the *radiocarpal* and *midcarpal* joints. The radiocarpal joint provides approximately 62% of wrist extension while the midcarpal joint provides approximately 62% of wrist flexion. About 55% of radial and ulnar deviation is provided by the midcarpal joint.[3]

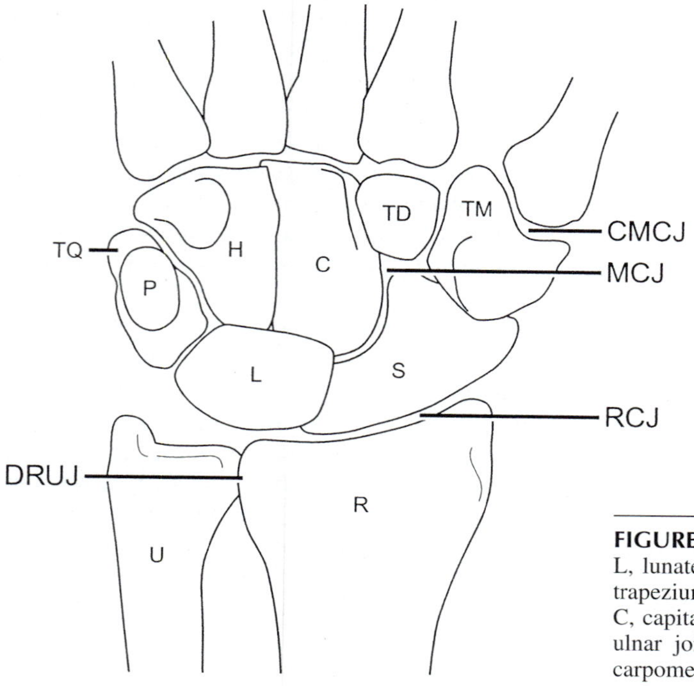

The carpal bones are linked to each other, the metacarpals, and the forearm by a complex set of ligaments.[4,5] The carpal ligaments are grouped into two main categories—extrinsic and intrinsic. The extrinsic ligaments join the carpus to the radius, ulna, and metacarpals. The intrinsic ligaments link the carpal bones themselves. The carpal ligaments are also classified as dorsal, volar, and interosseous. Both the dorsal and volar ligaments have extrinsic and intrinsic components.

The dorsal ligaments are less developed and weaker than the volar ligaments. The dorsal radiocarpal ligaments originate from the dorsal rim of the radius and insert onto the scaphoid, lunate, and triquetrum, forming the radioscaphoid, radiolunate, and radiotriquetral ligaments (Fig. 4-2*A*). The dorsal extrinsic ligaments prevent ulnar translation of the carpus down the slope of the radiocarpal articular surface.

The volar ligaments are relatively strong and stabilize the carpus with respect to the radius and ulna (Fig. 4-2*B*). One set of ligaments originates on the distal radius and inserts on the proximal and distal carpal rows. A second set of ligaments originates on the ulna and inserts on the proximal carpal row. A third set of ligaments originates on the scaphoid and triquetrum and inserts on the capitate. This third set of ligaments has an inverted V configuration and is also known as the *deltoid ligament*. Between these three sets of volar ligaments is an area relatively devoid of ligamentous support known as the *space of Poirier*. It overlies the articulation between the lunate and capitate and is a common site of carpal dislocation.

The ulnotriquetral articulation is a ligamentous complex known as the *triangular fibrocartilage complex* (TFCC) (Fig. 4-2*C*). The function of the TFCC is to stabilize the distal radioulnar joint and support the ulnocarpal joint. The TFCC consists of the triangular fibrocartilage (articular disk), the ulnocarpal meniscus homologue, dorsal and volar radioulnar ligaments, and the extensor carpi ulnaris tendon sheath.

The interosseus ligaments link adjacent carpal bones (Fig. 4-2*D*). The interosseus ligaments of the proximal row are the scapholunate, scaphotrapezial, lunotriquetral, and triquetrohamate ligaments. The distal carpal row is joined into one functional unit by strong, short connecting ligaments.

FIGURE 4-1. Wrist anatomy (volar view). S, scaphoid (navicular); L, lunate (semilunar); TQ, triquetrum (cuneiform); P, pisiform; TM, trapezium (greater multangular); TD, trapezoid (lesser multangular); C, capitate (os magnum); H, hamate (unciform); DRUJ, distal radioulnar joint; RCJ, radiocarpal joint; MCJ, midcarpal joint; CMCJ, carpometacarpal joint.

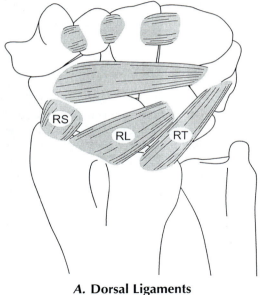

A. Dorsal Ligaments

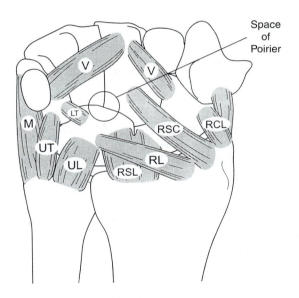

Space of Poirier

B. Volar Ligaments

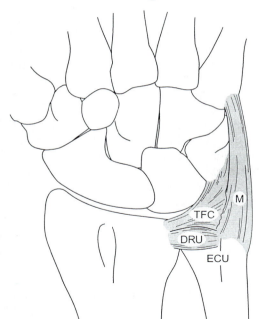

C. Triangular Fibrocartilage Complex

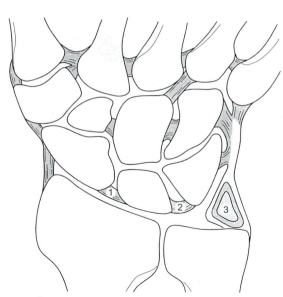

D. Interosseous Ligaments

FIGURE 4-2. Wrist ligaments. *A.* Dorsal wrist ligaments: RT, radio-triquetral; RL, radiolunate; RS, radioscaphoid. *B.* Volar wrist ligaments: RSC, radioscaphocapitate; RSL, radioscapholunate; RL, radiolunate; V-V, deltoid ligament; M, ulnocarpal meniscus homologue; UT, ulno-triquetral; UL, ulnolunate; LT, lunotriquetral; RCL, radial collateral. The *space of Poirier* is the region relatively devoid of ligamentous support between the lunate and the capitate on the volar surface of the wrist. *C.* Triangular fibrocartilage complex (TFCC): M, ulnocarpal meniscus homologue; articular disk or TFC, triangular fibrocartilage; DRU, dorsal radioulnar ligaments; ECU, extensor carpi ulnaris tendon sheath. *D.* Interosseous ligaments: (1) scapholunate, (2) lunotriquetral; (3) TFCC.

DEVELOPMENTAL ANATOMY. The distal radius and ulna each have a single primary epiphyseal ossification center. The ulnar styloid does not have a distinct ossification center. Therefore, a bone fragment separate from the rest of the epiphysis signifies an ulnar styloid fracture. A smooth, well-corticated ulnar styloid fragment is seen with nonunion of an old fracture. A fine osseous line traversing the distal radius represents the remnant of the growth plate and can persist into adulthood. This should not be misinterpreted as an impaction fracture.

Each of the carpals has a single primary ossification center, although the scaphoid rarely has two centers. The carpals begin to ossify at 3 months of age, starting with the hamate and capitate. The scaphoid and trapezoid are the last to appear and may not be visible until 5 to 6 years of age.

Forearm Anatomy

The forearm consists of the radius, the ulna, and their proximal and distal articulations. The radius and the ulna articulate at their ends and remain essentially parallel in the forearm. The shaft of the radius has a lateral bow, whereas the ulna is relatively straight. The radius and ulna are bound proximally at the elbow by the *annular ligament* and the joint capsule of the elbow (see chap. 5, fig. 5-2). The annular ligament allows rotation of the radial head on the ulna. Distally, the forearm bones are bound by the capsule of the wrist joint, the radioulnar ligaments, and the TFCC.

The forearm is divided into anterior and posterior compartments by the interosseous membrane. The anterior compartment contains the flexor muscles and associated neurovascular structures (radial and ulnar arteries and ulnar and median nerves). The posterior compartment contains the extensor muscles and associated neurovascular structures. The interosseous membrane is a strong fibrous sheet that runs between the interosseous borders of the radius and the ulna. The bones of the forearm are thus tightly bound together. A displaced fracture of one of the forearm bones is often accompanied by a second injury at the elbow or wrist.

At the elbow, the ulnohumeral joint creates a hinge or ginglymus joint. A ginglymus joint allows motion only in a single plane, such as flexion and extension of the forearm. The radiohumeral and proximal radioulnar joints allow pronation and supination of the forearm.[6]

Distally, the ulna articulates with both the radius and the carpus. The distal radioulnar joint (DRUJ) is the articulation between the head of the ulna and the sigmoid notch of the radius. The DRUJ allows forearm rotation.

RADIOGRAPHIC TECHNIQUE

A routine radiographic series of the wrist consists of at least three views: a posteroanterior (PA) view, a lateral view, and a semipronated oblique view (Fig. 4-3). In some institutions, a fourth view, the ulnar-deviated PA view, also called the scaphoid view, is included. In other institutions, this view is obtained only in patients clinically suspected of having a scaphoid fracture, especially if a fracture is not seen on the initial three views. All of the wrist views must include the distal 5 to 6 cm of the radius and ulna as well as the proximal metacarpal bones (Table 4-1).

A hand radiographic series includes views similar to those of the wrist series; however, if a wrist injury is suspected, one should obtain wrist films. Hand radiographs do not include the full extent of the distal radius and ulna. In addition, the x-ray beam in wrist radiographs is centered on the carpals, whereas the x-ray beam in a hand series is centered on the metacarpals.

This slightly distorts the image of the carpal bones on hand radiographs, making subtle injuries difficult to detect.

PA View

The *PA view* shows the full extent of the proximal and distal carpal rows and the distal radius and ulna (Fig. 4-3*A* and *B*). The radiograph is taken with the wrist pronated and its volar surface lying flat against the film cassette. There should be no ulnar or radial deviation of the carpus at the radiocarpal joint. The long axis of the third metacarpal should be parallel with the long axis of the radius. The lunate is located adjacent to the distal radioulnar joint. The distal radioulnar joint is clearly seen, with a joint-space width of 1 to 2 mm. The ulnar styloid should project along the ulnar margin of the wrist.

Lateral View

The *lateral view* is most useful for visualizing distal radius fractures and carpal dislocations (Fig. 4-3*C* and *D*). This view is taken with the wrist in midposition between pronation and supination. The ulnar margin of the wrist is placed against the film cassette. The wrist should not be flexed or extended, such that the dorsal surfaces of the metacarpal shafts are in line with the dorsal surface of the radius.

In a correctly positioned lateral view, the dorsal surface of the ulnar shaft either overlies or is 1 to 3 mm dorsal to the radial shaft. Correct positioning can also be determined by observing that the radial styloid appears as a triangular shadow overlying the lunate, with its apex located in midposition between the volar and dorsal surfaces of the distal radius.

Pronation Oblique View

The *pronation oblique view* shows the radial portions of the wrist to better advantage, since this region is foreshortened on the PA view (Fig. 4-3*E* and *F*). This includes the thumb and index finger carpometacarpal area and the distal pole of the scaphoid. The pronation oblique view is taken with the wrist in 45° pronation. The radial side of the hand is raised from the cassette and the ulnar margin of the wrist remains against the film cassette. When correctly positioned, there is a good view of the proximal first and second metacarpals, the joint space between the trapezium and trapezoid, and the joint space between the scaphoid and trapezium.

Scaphoid View

The *ulnar-deviated PA view*, or *scaphoid view,* detects scaphoid fractures that are not visible on the PA view (Fig. 4-4*A*). This view reduces the foreshortening of the scaphoid seen on a neutral-position PA view and the entire length of the scaphoid is clearly displayed. The volar surface of the wrist is placed flat

TABLE 4-1

Radiographic Views of the Wrist

Projection	Position	Adequacy*	Likely Findings
PA	Hand pronated, volar surface against the film. Ulnar styloid projects along ulnar border of wrist.	Radiocarpal joint in neutral position without ulnar or radial deviation; third metacarpal shaft in line with the shaft of radius. Lunate straddles the distal radioulnar joint.	Most carpal fractures. Alignment of proximal and distal carpal rows. Displaced distal radius, radial styloid, and ulnar styloid fractures.
Lateral	Wrist in midposition between pronation and supination; ulnar border of hand against film.	True lateral position shows the dorsal surface of the ulna located 1 to 3 mm dorsal to the radius. Dorsal surfaces of metacarpals are parallel to the dorsal surface of radius (no flexion or extension at wrist).	Distal radius fractures and direction of displacement. Carpal dislocations. Dorsal chip fracture of triquetrum.
Pronation oblique	Wrist 45° semi-pronated. Ulnar margin of hand against film.	Joint space between the trapezium and trapezoid is visible. Minimal overlap between the proximal first and second metacarpals.	Fractures of the scaphoid tuberosity (distal pole), trapezium, first and second metacarpal bases. Fractures of the triquetrum and hamate.
Supplementary views			
Scaphoid view	PA view with wrist in ulnar deviation.	Full length of scaphoid is seen. Lunate entirely overlies the distal radius.	Fractures of the waist of the scaphoid.
Supination oblique	Wrist 45° semi-supinated. Ulnar margin of hand against film.	No overlap at the base of the fifth metacarpal. Joint space between pisiform and triquetrum is clearly seen.	Pisiform fractures. Fractures of the base of the fifth metacarpal.
Carpal tunnel view	Wrist hyperextended. X-ray beam tangential to volar surface of wrist.	Carpal tunnel seen without overlap.	Fractures of the hook of the hamate, pisiform, and volar ridge of the trapezium. Occasional scaphoid tuberosity and capitate fractures.

*All views should include the proximal metacarpals and the distal 5 to 6 cm of the radius and ulna.

on the film cassette and the wrist is positioned with maximal ulnar deviation. The long axis of the third metacarpal is ulnarly deviated with respect to the radius, and the lunate entirely overlies the distal radial articular surface.

Supination Oblique View

The *supination oblique view* more clearly demonstrates the pisiform, the palmar aspects of the triquetrum and the hamate (the hook of the hamate), and the base of the little finger metacarpal (Fig. 4-4*B*). This is an AP view obtained with the wrist in 45° of supination and the ulnar surface of the hand resting against

the film cassette. The *ball catcher's view* (Norgaard view) of the hand is similar but with greater supination (Fig. 4-4*C*).

Carpal Tunnel View

The *carpal tunnel view* is an axial view of the carpal tunnel (Fig. 4-4*D*). It is obtained with the wrist hyperextended and the x-ray beam directed tangentially across the volar surface of the wrist. This view shows the hook of the hamate and pisiform on the ulnar side of the wrist, the volar ridge of the trapezium and the scaphoid tubercle on the radial side of the wrist, and the volar surface of the capitate at the base of the carpal tunnel.

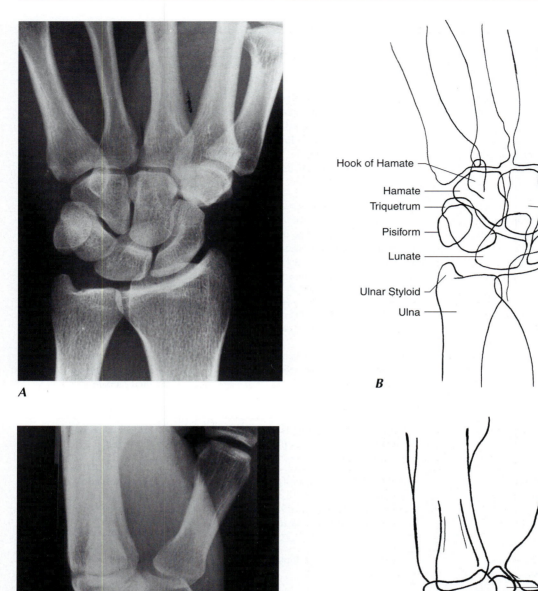

A

B

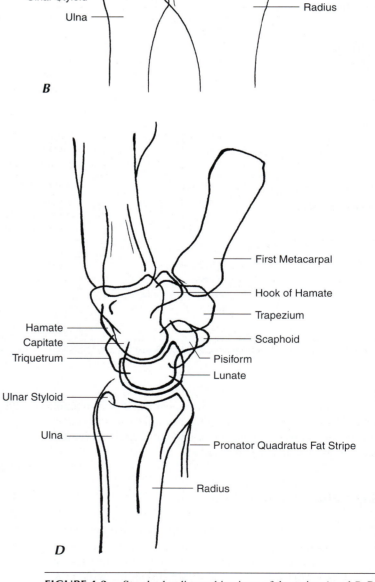

C

D

FIGURE 4-3.   Standard radiographic views of the wrist. *A* and *B*. PA wrist radiograph. *C* and *D*. Lateral wrist radiograph. *E* and *F*. Pronation oblique radiograph.

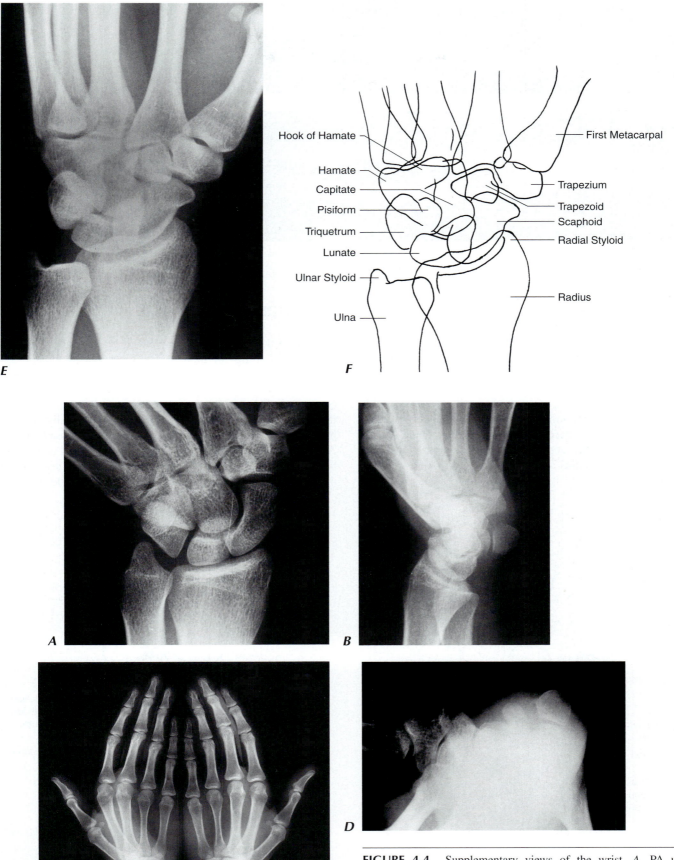

Hook of Hamate

Hamate

Capitate

Pisiform

Triquetrum

Lunate

Ulnar Styloid

Ulna

First Metacarpal

Trapezium

Trapezoid

Scaphoid

Radial Styloid

Radius

E

F

A

B

C

D

FIGURE 4-4. Supplementary views of the wrist. *A.* PA ulnar-deviated radiograph, "scaphoid view." *B.* Supination oblique view. *C.* Ball-catcher's (Norgaard) view of hand. *D.* Carpal tunnel view.

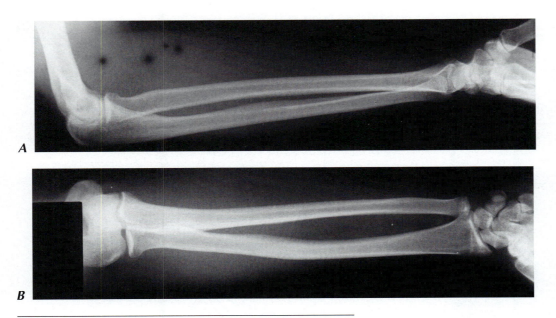

FIGURE 4-5. Lateral (*A*) and AP (*B*) radiographs of the forearm.

Forearm Radiographs

The standard radiographic series of the forearm consists of anteroposterior (AP) and lateral radiographs (Fig. 4-5). The AP view is obtained with the forearm in supination and the elbow maximally extended, so that the shafts of the radius and ulna are parallel. The lateral view is obtained with the elbow in 90° flexion and the forearm in a position midway between supination and pronation. Forearm radiographs must include the entire length of the radius and ulna, the DRUJ, and the proximal articulations of the radius and ulna with the humerus at the elbow.

RADIOGRAPHIC ANALYSIS

Because of the complex anatomy of the wrist and the subtle radiographic findings of many wrist injuries, a systematic approach is necessary when one is interpreting wrist radiographs. It is important to examine each view individually and thoroughly, then compare any abnormality seen on one view with the corresponding portions of the others. One easily remembered device to employ in reviewing wrist radiographs is the ABC'S—sequentially examining the adequacy and alignment, bones, cartilage (joint spaces), and soft tissues (Table 4-2). A detailed analysis of each view focuses on sites of com-

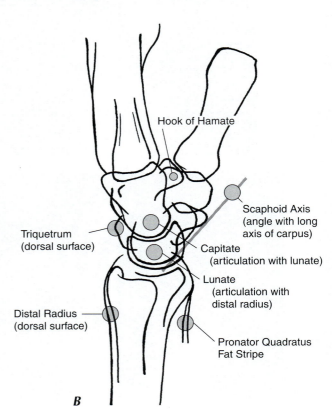

FIGURE 4-6. Sites prone to injury and easily missed injuries. *A*. PA view. *B*. Lateral view. *C*. Pronation oblique view.

TABLE 4-2

Systematic Analysis of Wrist Radiographs

Two regions are examined in each view—the carpus (and proximal metacarpals) and the distal radius (and ulna).

PA view	Adequacy	No radial or ulnar deviation of the carpals—long axis of third metacarpal is parallel with the long axis of radial shaft; lunate overlies the distal radioulnar joint.
	Alignment	Three arches of the articular surfaces of the proximal and distal carpal rows form smooth curves.
	Bones	Carpal bones—especially the scaphoid. Scaphoid "ring" sign indicates rotary subluxation (scapholunate dissociation). Lunate has trapezoidal appearance (not triangular). Proximal metacarpals. Distal radius and ulna.
	Cartilage	Intercarpal joint spaces should be uniform (2 mm). Especially examine the scapholunate joint space. Distal radioulnar joint—radial and ulnar articular surfaces separated by 1 to 2 mm.
	Soft tissues	Navicular fat stripe—displaced or obliterated by scaphoid fracture.
Lateral view	Adequacy	Dorsal surface of the ulnar shaft overlaps or is 1 to 2 mm dorsal to the radial. No flexion or extension at the wrist; long axis of the metacarpals is parallel to the radius.
	Alignment	Sequence of adjacent Cs—articular surfaces of the distal radius, lunate, capitate are aligned. Longitudinal axes of radius, lunate, and capitate are nearly parallel. Axis of the scaphoid makes an angle of 30 to 60° relative to the long axis of the wrist. Distal radioulnar joint—ulnar styloid should point to the dorsal surface of the triquetrum.
	Bones	Distal radius. Triquetrum (dorsal surface)—chip fracture.
	Soft tissues	Pronator quadratus fat stripe—bulging or obliterated with a nondisplaced distal radius fracture.
Oblique view	Adequacy	Trapezium and trapezoid joint space seen with minimal overlap.
	Bones	Bases of I and II metacarpals; trapezium and trapezoid. Scaphoid—distal pole (tuberosity). Triquetrum (the most ulnar bone of proximal carpal row). Distal radius—oblique fracture may only be seen on this view.
Supplementary views Obtain additional views if no fracture is seen on standard views depending on site of tenderness.		Scaphoid view—tenderness in "anatomic snuff-box." Supination oblique view—tenderness over fifth metacarpal base or pisiform. Carpal tunnel view—tenderness over volar surface of the carpals.

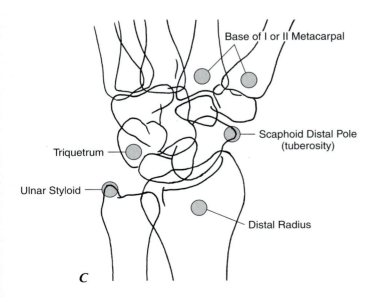

Base of I or II Metacarpal

Scaphoid Distal Pole (tuberosity)

Triquetrum

Ulnar Styloid

Distal Radius

C

mon injury and sites of frequently missed injuries (Fig. 4-6). Interpretation of the radiographs is assisted by correlating the radiographic images with the findings on physical examination.

There are two distinct regions of injury in the wrist—the distal radius and the carpals. Fractures of the distal radius are better seen on the lateral view, and carpal fractures are better seen on the PA view. Both the distal radius and the carpal region must be examined in each view, because simultaneous injuries to these two areas can occur.

Adequacy

On the PA view, there should be no overlap of the radius and ulna. The long axis of the third metacarpal should be parallel with the long axis of the radius, indicating that there is no radial or ulnar deviation of the wrist (Table 4-1) (Fig. 4-2).

On a correctly positioned lateral view, the dorsal surface of the distal ulna is superimposed or 1 to 3 mm dorsal to the surface of the radius. The dorsal surface of the metacarpals should be parallel to the long axis of the radius, indicating that there is no flexion or extension of the wrist.

A correctly positioned oblique view clearly shows the distal pole of the scaphoid, the bases of the first and second metacarpals, and the trapezium and trapezoid.

All wrist radiographs must include at least 5 to 6 cm of the distal radius and ulna as well as the proximal portion of the metacarpals.

PA View

The examination begins with the carpal region and then proceeds to the distal radius and ulna (Figs. 4-2A and B, 4-6A, and 4-7A). The articular surfaces of the proximal and distal carpal rows are normally aligned in three smooth arcs (Fig. 4-7). The first arc is the proximal joint surface of the proximal carpal row; the second arc is the distal joint surface of the proximal carpal row; and the third arc is the proximal surface of the distal carpal row. Disruption of any one of these arcs is a sign of carpal dislocation or fracture. All of the intercarpal joint spaces should be of uniform width (about 1 to 2 mm). The scapholunate joint is most frequently injured.

Each of the carpal bones is examined for fracture lines or impaction, focusing especially on the scaphoid. If the distal portion of the scaphoid is foreshortened and has a ring appearance, then there is either rotary subluxation of the scaphoid

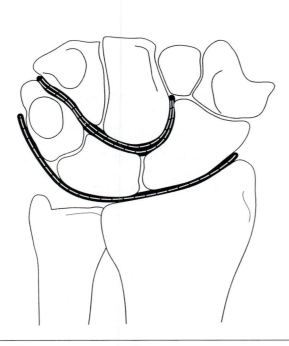

FIGURE 4-7. The three carpal arches seen on the PA radiograph: the proximal articular surfaces of the proximal carpal row, the distal articular surfaces of the proximal carpal row, and the proximal articular surfaces of the distal carpal row.

or the view is incorrectly positioned with radial deviation of the wrist. The lunate should have a trapezoidal shape. If the lunate has a triangular appearance, there is either a volar lunate dislocation or incorrect positioning with the wrist in flexion. Finally, the bases of the metacarpals are examined.

Next, the distal radius and ulna are examined for evidence of fractures, although these are more easily seen on the lateral view. Comminution and intraarticular extension should be noted. Ulnar styloid fractures are readily apparent. The distal radioulnar joint space should be clearly seen and is normally 1 to 2 mm wide. There should be no overlap of the distal radius and ulna.

One soft tissue sign seen on the PA view is the *scaphoid fat stripe*.[7] This is a thin, slightly concave, radiolucent stripe along the radial margin of the scaphoid. A bright light is often needed to see this shadow. A normal fat stripe suggests that there is no scaphoid fracture, whereas a scaphoid fracture is likely if the stripe is bowed outward or obliterated.

Lateral View

Much of the wrist anatomy is overlapping in this projection (Figs. 4-2C and D, 4-6B). The distal radius and ulnar are well seen, and fractures of the distal radius are best discerned on the lateral view. The cortical margins of the radius and ulna are carefully traced, looking for breaks or abrupt angulation indicative of a fracture.

The carpal bones are difficult to visualize because of overlap. Nevertheless, certain landmarks are important to identify. The lunate is a cup-shaped bone whose proximal surface articulates with the curved surface of the distal radius. The concave distal articular surface of the lunate articulates with the proximal end of the capitate. The capitate is difficult to identify in its entirety because of the multitude of overlapping shadows. These four articular surfaces (the distal radius, the proximal and distal lunate, and the proximal capitate) form a sequence of adjacent C's (Fig. 4-8). The longitudinal axes of the radius, lunate, and capitate should be nearly parallel.

The scaphoid has a dumbbell or peanut shape. The distal pole (tuberosity) projects anteriorly. The proximal portion of the scaphoid parallels the curved proximal articular surface of the lunate. The long axis of the scaphoid normally makes an angle of 30 to 60° with the long axis of the carpus. Because the entire outline of the scaphoid is not often visible, the axis of the scaphoid is more easily determined by drawing a line that connects the distal and proximal convexities of the volar surface of the scaphoid (Fig. 4-6B).

The dorsal surface of the triquetrum is readily identified on the lateral view. The triquetrum projects dorsally in the midcarpal region. This is a common site of fracture. The ulnar styloid normally "points" to the dorsal surface of the triquetrum. If not, there is dislocation of the distal radioulnar joint.

Soft tissue signs of a fracture include soft tissue swelling, especially over the dorsal surface of the wrist. Of greater importance is the *pronator quadratus fat stripe*. This is a thin, radiolucent stripe representing a layer a fatty tissue overlying the

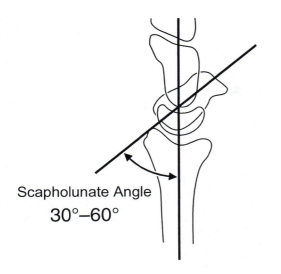

Scapholunate Angle
30°–60°

FIGURE 4-8. The "four C's" seen on the lateral radiograph: the sequential curved articular surfaces of the distal radius, proximal and distal articular surfaces of the lunate, and the proximal articular surface of the capitate. The long axes of the distal radius, lunate, and capitate are collinear. The scapholunate angle is normally between 30 and 60°.

pronator quadratus muscle. It normally extends from the volar lip of the distal radius articular surface and runs parallel to the surface of the radius (Fig. 4-9).[8] When this stripe is bulging outward or obliterated, a fracture of the distal radius must be considered.

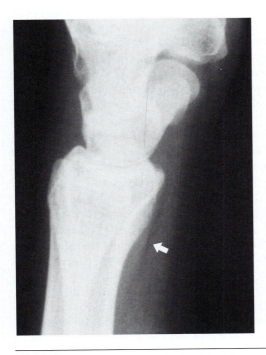

FIGURE 4-9. Normal pronator quadratus fat stripe. The thin radiolucent stripe closely parallels the volar surface of the distal radius *(arrow)*.

Oblique View

This projection provides a good view of the radial aspect of the wrist, including the trapezium and trapezoid, the metacarpal bases of the thumb and index finger, and the distal pole (tuberosity) of the scaphoid. On the ulnar side, the triquetrum and body of the hamate are seen (Figs. 4-2*E* and *F,* 4-6*C*).

Supplementary Views

When certain injuries are suspected based on the physical examination, additional views are obtained if the injury is not seen on the standard views. For example, if there is tenderness in the "anatomic snuff box," a fracture of the scaphoid can be seen on a *scaphoid view* (ulnar-deviated PA view) (Fig. 4-3*A*). If there is tenderness over the ulnar margin of the carpus, a *supination oblique view* may show a fracture of the pisiform, hook of the hamate, or base of the fifth metacarpal (Fig. 4-3*B*). If there is tenderness on the volar aspect of the carpus, a *carpal tunnel view* can detect a fracture of the hook of the hamate, pisiform, volar ridge of the trapezium, or scaphoid tubercle (Fig. 4-3*D*).

COMMON ABNORMALITIES

The two zones of injury to the wrist are the carpals and the distal radius. Fractures of the distal radius are approximately ten times more frequent than carpal fractures. The most common mechanism of injury is a fall on an outstretched hand that impacts the volar surface of the hyperextended wrist. Although a fall on an outstretched arm can cause injuries from the hand to the shoulder, injury to the wrist is most frequent. The resulting injury is partly dependent on the patient's age. In children, injuries include a torus (buckle) or greenstick fracture of the distal radius or a fracture through the growth plate. In young adults, a scaphoid fracture is a common injury. In the elderly, the most frequent injury is a fracture of the distal radius.

Carpal Fractures

SCAPHOID FRACTURES. The scaphoid is the most commonly fractured carpal (60 to 80% of carpal injuries). Fractures of the scaphoid are usually caused by a fall onto the hyperextended wrist. The distal pole of the scaphoid along with the distal carpal row translate dorsally. With forced hyperextension, the volar aspect of the scaphoid fails in tension, the dorsal aspect fails in compression, and a fracture results.[9–11]

Scaphoid fractures are classified as proximal third, middle third (waist), and distal third (tuberosity) (Fig. 4-10). Seventy percent of fractures involve the middle third. Middle-third and proximal fractures have a higher incidence of nonunion and avascular necrosis than do distal fractures because of the nature of the scaphoid blood supply. Most of the blood supply of the scaphoid comes from the dorsal scaphoid branch of the radial artery, which enters the scaphoid distally.[12] Therefore a

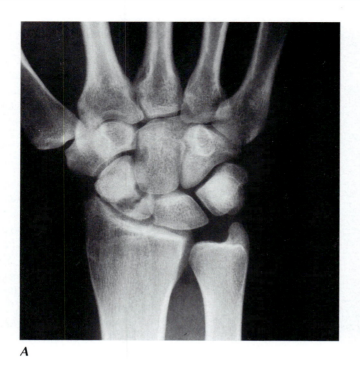

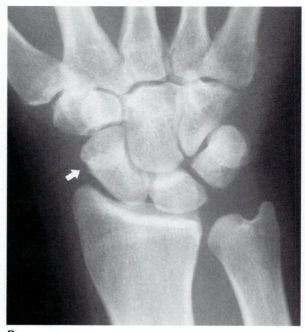

A   *B*

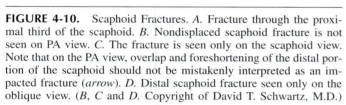

FIGURE 4-10.   Scaphoid Fractures. *A.* Fracture through the proximal third of the scaphoid. *B.* Nondisplaced scaphoid fracture is not seen on PA view. *C.* The fracture is seen only on the scaphoid view. Note that on the PA view, overlap and foreshortening of the distal portion of the scaphoid should not be mistakenly interpreted as an impacted fracture (*arrow*). *D.* Distal scaphoid fracture seen only on the oblique view. (*B, C* and *D.* Copyright of David T. Schwartz, M.D.)

fracture through the midportion of the scaphoid interrupts the blood supply to the proximal part.

Although displaced scaphoid fractures are usually obvious radiographically, a nondisplaced fracture can be subtle. In one series, 13% of radiographically visible scaphoid fractures were missed when the film was initially read in the ED.[13]

Because the long axis of the scaphoid is tilted 40 to 50° volar to the frontal plane, the scaphoid is foreshortened on the PA view. In addition, a patient with a scaphoid fracture tends to hold the wrist in slight radial deviation because of pain. This further foreshortens the scaphoid on an improperly positioned PA view, making a fracture even more difficult to see. With the wrist positioned in ulnar deviation, the axis of the scaphoid is fully elongated. A PA radiograph with ulnar deviation (*scaphoid view*) can detect fractures not seen on the straight PA view (Fig. 4-10*B* and *C*). Some distal scaphoid fractures may be seen only on the pronation oblique view (Fig. 4-10*D*).

Difficulty in the radiographic diagnosis of scaphoid fractures is further compounded by variations in the appearance of the scaphoid that mimic a fracture. In one series, 20% of normal films were misinterpreted as showing a scaphoid fracture.[14] The radial articular surface of the scaphoid often ends with a slight "bump" that looks like a cortical irregularity due to a fracture (see below, Fig. 4-37). Foreshortening and overlap of the distal pole of the scaphoid can mimic the increased trabecular density of an impacted fracture (Fig. 4-10*B*). These errors are avoided by obtaining good-quality radiographs and a scaphoid view. One finding

that distinguishes a fracture from a fracture mimic is that a fracture line extends through to the medial surface of the scaphoid.

The standard wrist radiographic series, including a scaphoid view, is negative in 10 to 20% of scaphoid fractures. Because the radiographic diagnosis of a scaphoid fracture is unreliable, management is based on clinical findings. With a scaphoid fracture, there is tenderness in the anatomic snuffbox and pain with axial loading of the thumb.

Scaphoid fractures are complicated by malunion and avascular necrosis, causing chronic pain and dysfunction. The situation is compounded in patients who are misdiagnosed as having a "wrist sprain" and are inadequately immobilized. Scaphoid fractures often occur in young working persons, and failure to diagnose is accompanied by a high risk of disability. If a fracture is clinically suspected on the basis of snuff-box tenderness, the patient must be immobilized in a thumb spica splint or cast. Early follow-up is mandatory for proper casting and continuing care. Prompt immobilization may reduce the rate of nonunion and avascular necrosis.

With a clinically suspected scaphoid fracture, immobilization is used for 10 to 14 days, after which a repeat examination is conducted and radiographs are obtained. During this time, the initial stages of fracture healing result in bone resorption at the fracture line and the scaphoid fracture is more reliably detected. However, only 10% to 20% of patients immobilized for an occult scaphoid fracture actually have a fracture.

Other imaging modalities can make an earlier diagnosis. A bone scan can be done on the fourth day after the injury. If negative, a bone scan reliably excludes a scaphoid fracture.[15] A positive bone scan, however, does not necessarily indicate a scaphoid fracture, because soft tissue injuries and other fractures cause abnormal scintigraphic uptake. In fact, fractures of the distal radius and triquetrum are common in patients with snuff-box tenderness and negative initial radiographs.

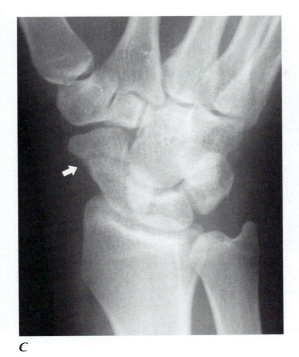

C

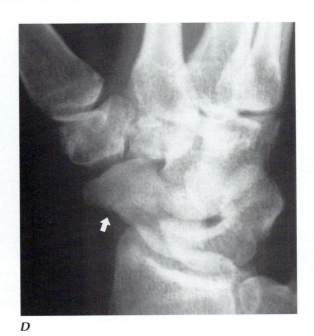

D

Magnetic resonance imaging (MRI) has also been used to detect occult carpal fractures. MRI demonstrates the fracture immediately and provides exact anatomic diagnosis.[16]

A thumb spica cast is recommended for nondisplaced scaphoid fractures. Open reduction and internal fixation (ORIF) is recommended for scaphoid fractures that are displaced 1 mm or more.[17] The frequency of nonunion increases from 5 to 45% if treatment is delayed longer than 4 weeks.[18] Factors that increase the likelihood of a poor result include delayed diagnosis and treatment, proximal sites of fracture, and fracture displacement.[19]

Scapholunate advanced collapse (SLAC) of the wrist is a late complication of a scaphoid fracture, scapholunate dissociation, or lunate injury (Fig. 4-11A). The proximal pole of the scaphoid and the lunate undergo avascular necrosis with collapse (volume loss). There is proximal migration of the capitate. The patient presents with chronic pain as long as 10 to 20 years after the injury. Treatment includes wrist fusion or proximal-row carpectomy, in which the entire proximal carpal row is surgically removed (Fig. 4-11B). It is therefore essential to diagnose scaphoid fractures early and to manage suspected scaphoid fractures conservatively.

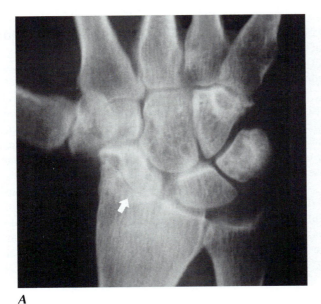

A

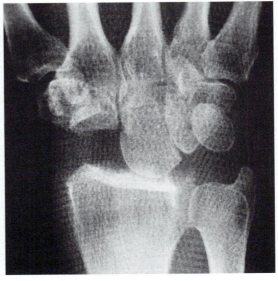

B

FIGURE 4-11. *A.* SLAC (scapholunate advanced collapse) wrist due to long-standing avascular necrosis of the scaphoid. *B.* Proximal-row carpectomy used to treat SLAC wrist.

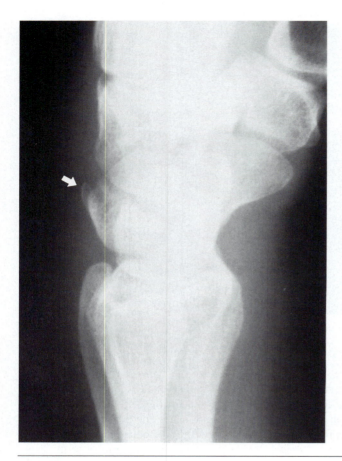

FIGURE 4-12.   Dorsal chip fracture of the triquetrum *(arrow)*.

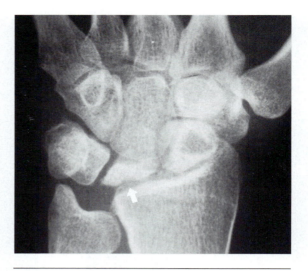

FIGURE 4-13.   Kienböck disease—avascular necrosis of the lunate *(arrow)*.

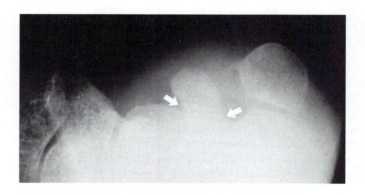

FIGURE 4-14.   Fracture of the hook of the hamate seen only on the carpal tunnel view *(arrows)*.

OTHER CARPAL FRACTURES.   Dorsal chip fractures of the *triquetrum* are common, accounting for 10 to 20% of carpal fractures.[20] They are caused by a fall on the outstretched hand. The patient has tenderness of the dorsoulnar aspect of the wrist. On the lateral radiograph, the triquetrum is the most dorsal carpal bone seen. This region should be examined on all wrist radiographs, especially in patients with tenderness or swelling on the dorsum of the wrist (Fig. 4-12).

Avascular necrosis of the *lunate,* known as *Kienböck disease,* is secondary to loss of blood supply to the lunate. This may be due to fracture, repetitive trauma, or ligamentous injury. Patients with avascular necrosis of the lunate have central dorsal wrist pain, swelling, limited motion, and decreased grip strength (Fig. 4-13).[21,22]

Fractures of the *hook of the hamate* occur in sports such as golf, tennis, racquetball, and baseball. Patients have dull pain in the volar-ulnar region of the palm. Ulnar nerve palsy or flexor tendon rupture can occur with this fracture. The fracture is best seen with the carpal tunnel view, bone scintigraphy or CT. The carpal tunnel radiograph shows the palmar aspects of the trapezium, the scaphoid tuberosity, the trapezoid, the capitate, the hook of the hamate, the triquetrum, and the pisiform (Fig. 4-14). Other fractures of the carpal bones are seen less frequently.

Carpal Dislocations and Ligamentous Injuries

Subluxations and dislocations make up 10% of carpal injuries. The most common injuries are known as *perilunate injuries,* which involve the ligamentous attachments of the lunate. The volar aspect of the lunate is an area of weakness owing to the relative lack of ligamentous support at the *space of Poirier* (Fig. 4-2B). The spectrum of perilunate injury includes tears of the scapholunate ligament, perilunate dislocations, lunate dislocations, and perilunate fracture/dislocations.[23]

Perilunate injuries result from hyperextension of the wrist. Limited tears of the intercarpal ligament are usually caused by a fall on an outstretched hand, and these patients complain of poorly localized wrist pain. Carpal dislocations are due to high-energy trauma resulting from motorcycle- or motor vehicle–related injury or falls from a great height. There is considerable swelling and deformity of the wrist, although the deformity may be masked by swelling. Neurovascular status, especially median nerve function, must be checked.

Three discrete injury patterns are described: scapholunate dissociation, perilunate dislocation, and lunate dislocation.

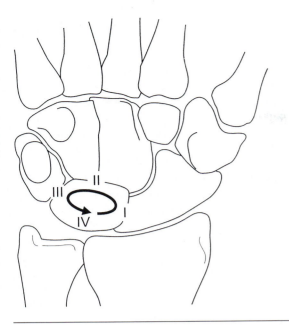

FIGURE 4-15. The four successive stages of perilunate injury.

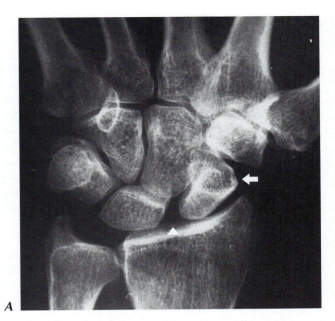

A

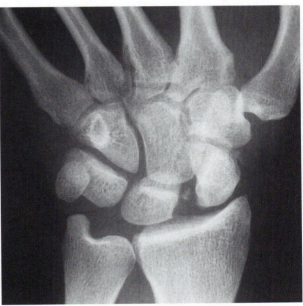

B

However, these injury patterns are actually part of a continuous spectrum, and intermediate injuries are seen.

Mayfield describes four stages of perilunate instability (Fig. 4-15).[24] Stage I is a tear of the scapholunate interosseous ligament and the radioscapholunate ligament, resulting in scapholunate dissociation. Stage II results in scaphoid and capitate instability due to injury to the volar capitolunate joint. Stage III involves injury to the triquetrolunate interosseous ligament and the volar lunate triquetral ligament, resulting in instability of the scaphoid, capitate, and triquetrum with respect to the lunate. This can result in dorsal perilunate dislocation. Stage IV is lunate dislocation due to injury to the dorsal radiolunate ligaments. The volar radiolunate ligaments remain intact.

SCAPHOLUNATE DISSOCIATION. With scapholunate dissociation, the scapholunate joint space is wider than 4 mm (Fig. 4-16). This is known as the *Terry-Thomas sign,* named after the British comic actor with dental diastema (separation between the two front teeth).[25] This diastasis is exaggerated and better seen with a clenched-fist view or a PA view in ulnar deviation.[26] Scapholunate dissociation is also known as *rotary subluxation of the scaphoid* because, when the attachment between the scaphoid and the lunate is disrupted, the scaphoid tends to rotate into a more transverse orientation. On the lateral radiograph, the scapholunate angle is greater than 60° (Fig. 4-17). On the PA view, the scaphoid is foreshortened and has the appearance of a "signet ring" because the distal pole is viewed end-on (Fig. 4-16).[27]

FIGURE 4-16. Scapholunate dissociation. *A.* The "Terry-Thomas" sign (*arrowhead*) and "signet ring" appearance of rotary subluxation of the scaphoid (*arrow*) are seen. *B.* An avulsion fracture is seen within the scapholunate joint space.

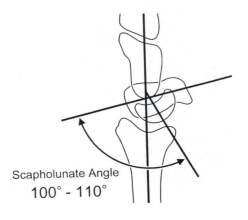

Scapholunate Angle
100° - 110°

FIGURE 4-17. Rotary subluxation of the scaphoid (scapholunate angle, >60°) and dorsal intercalated segment instability (DISI—the lunate is dorsally angulated relative to the long axis of the distal radius.)

PERILUNATE AND LUNATE DISLOCATIONS.   Dorsal perilunate dislocations and volar lunate dislocations are more severe injuries.[28] In a perilunate dislocation, the capitate is dislocated dorsal to the lunate (Fig. 4-18). In a lunate dislocation, the lunate is anteriorly dislocated and rotated relative to the distal radius (Fig. 4-19).

In a perilunate dislocation, all of the volar ligaments connecting the lunate to the carpus are disrupted except the volar radiolunate ligament. In a lunate dislocation, the dorsal radiolunate ligament is also disrupted. Carpal fractures and injuries to the median nerve are seen with these dislocations.

On the PA view in both perilunate and lunate dislocations, there is disruption of the smooth carpal arcs and "crowding" of the proximal and distal carpal rows (Fig. 4-7). The lunate appears triangular (rather than quadrilateral), depending on the amount of volar dislocation and rotation (Figs. 4-18*A* and 4-19*A*).

On the lateral view, the sequence of adjacent C-shaped articular surfaces is disrupted and the axes of the radius, lunate, capitate, and third metacarpal are not collinear. With perilunate dislocation, the capitate is dorsally dislocated with respect to the lunate, while the lunate is in its normal position in the lunate fossa of the distal radius (Fig. 4-18*B*). With a lunate dislocation, the lunate is volarly dislocated and rotated with respect to the distal radius, resembling a "spilled teacup." The capitate is close to its normal alignment to the distal radius (Fig. 4-19*B*). The long axis of the scaphoid may be rotated volarly > 60° with respect to the long axis of the wrist due to rotary subluxation of the scaphoid (Fig. 4-8).

PERILUNATE FRACTURE/DISLOCATIONS.   With perilunate fracture/dislocations, the force of injury is transmitted to the bones surrounding the lunate. In a *transscaphoid perilunate fracture/dislocation,* the injury is through the scaphoid rather

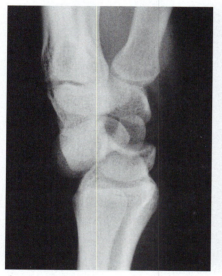
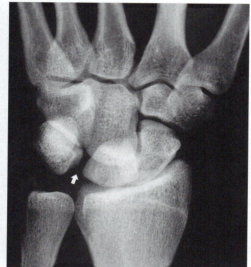

A   *B*

FIGURE 4-18.   Dorsal perilunate dislocation. *A.* On the lateral view, the capitate is dislocated dorsal to the lunate. *B.* On the PA view, there is disruption of the carpal arcs with "crowding" of the proximal and distal carpal rows. The space between the lunate and triquetrum is wide due to lunotriquetral ligament tear *(arrow).* (A. Copyright David T. Schwartz, M.D.)

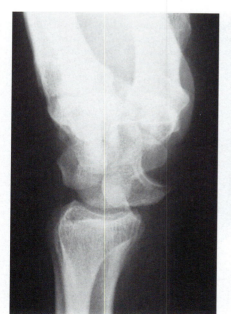
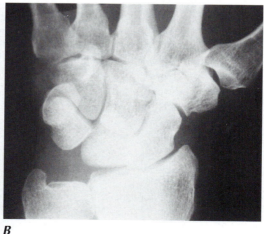

B

A

FIGURE 4-19.   Volar lunate dislocation. *A.* On the lateral film, the lunate is volarly dislocated and tilted like a "spilled teacup." The capitate has migrated volarly and has reassumed alignment with the distal radius. *B.* On the PA film, the lunate has a triangular shape. (Copyright David T. Schwartz, M.D.)

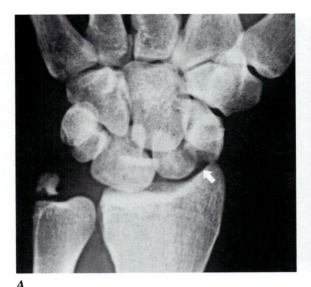

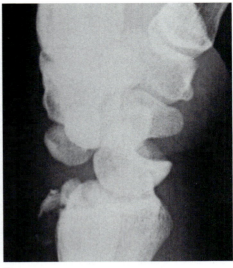

A

B

FIGURE 4-20. Transscaphoid perilunate fracture/dislocation with an associated ulnar styloid fracture. The scaphoid fracture is widely displaced *(arrow)*.

than the scapholunate ligament (Fig. 4-20). The clinical findings are identical to those of a perilunate dislocation, and the diagnosis is made by radiographic examination. In other cases, the fracture is through the capitate or triquetrum.

Distal Radius Fractures

Fractures of the distal radius are among the most common fractures seen in the ED.[29] These injuries usually occur after a low-velocity fall, but they can also result from high-energy trauma. Fractures of the distal radius occur in both children and adults. The peak incidences are in 6- to 10-year-old children and in 60- to 69-year-old adults.

A number of eponyms are applied to various distal radius fractures. Although in common usage, eponyms are occasionally applied incorrectly and can be a source of confusion. One should describe the fracture accurately using proper medical terminology rather than relying on these eponyms. Nevertheless, some eponyms conveniently describe common injury patterns.

COLLES FRACTURE. A Colles fracture occurs at the distal metaphysis of the radius with dorsal displacement and radial shortening. The eponym is commonly used to describe all fractures of the distal radius with dorsal displacement—both intraarticular and extraarticular.[30]

Fractures of the distal radius most often result from a low-velocity fall on an outstretched hand. The volar surface of the distal radius is fractured under tension; the fracture propagates dorsally, causing compression and comminution of the dorsal surface of the radius.[31] Patients have deformity of the wrist with dorsal displacement, the "silver-fork" deformity. The patient with a Colles fracture must be carefully examined for injuries elsewhere in the upper extremity, especially for a scaphoid fracture and an elbow injury.

The diagnosis is confirmed with radiologic studies (Fig. 4-21). The fracture may be difficult to discern on the PA view, especially the direction of displacement. A Colles fracture is obvious on the lateral view.

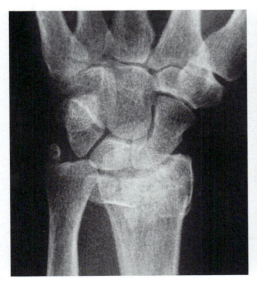
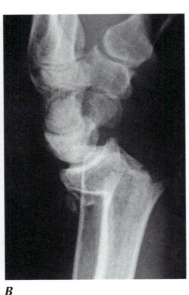

A   *B*

FIGURE 4-21. Colles fracture. A fracture through the metaphysis of the distal radius with dorsal displacement.

A number of different classification systems exist for fractures of the distal radius.[32] Frykman's classification is based on involvement of the radiocarpal and radioulnar joints (Fig. 4-22).[33] Unfortunately, this classification system fails to identify initial displacement, comminution, shortening, and bone quality, all of which affect the final functional result.

One specific intraarticular distal radius fracture is the *die-punch fracture,* which is also known as a radiolunate fracture or lunate load fracture (Fig. 4-23). The die-punch fracture is an intraarticular fracture of the distal radius with impaction of the dorsal aspect of the lunate fossa.

Management Considerations. Anatomic restoration and functional outcome are directly related. In postreduction radiographs, close attention is given to five measurements: radial inclination, radial volar tilt, radial length, radial shift, and ulnar variance. Radial inclination is measured on the PA view. It is the angle between a line drawn from the tip of the radial styloid to the ulnar edge of distal radial articular surface and a line

perpendicular to the long axis of the radius. The average radial inclination is 22 to 23° (Fig. 4-24A).[34] Radial volar tilt is measured on the lateral view and is the angle between a line extending from the dorsal and volar lip of the distal radius and a line perpendicular to the long axis of the radius. The average volar tilt is 11 to 12° (Fig. 4-24B). Radial length, measured on the PA view, is the distance between two lines drawn perpendicular to the long axis of the radius, one at the tip of the radial styloid and the other at the distal articular surface of the ulna. Normal radial length is 11 to 12 mm (Fig. 4-24C).[35] Radial shift, measured on the PA view, is the distance between the longitudinal axis, drawn down the center of the radius, and the lateral tip of the radial styloid. This value is compared with that of the contralateral wrist.[36] Ulnar variance, measured on the PA view, is the distance between two lines that are perpendicular to the longitudinal axis of the radius; one line is tangent to the lunate fossa of the distal radius and the other tangent to the distal ulnar articular fossa. With normal ulnar variance, the ulna is even with or 1 to 2 mm shorter than the radius (Fig. 4-24C).[37]

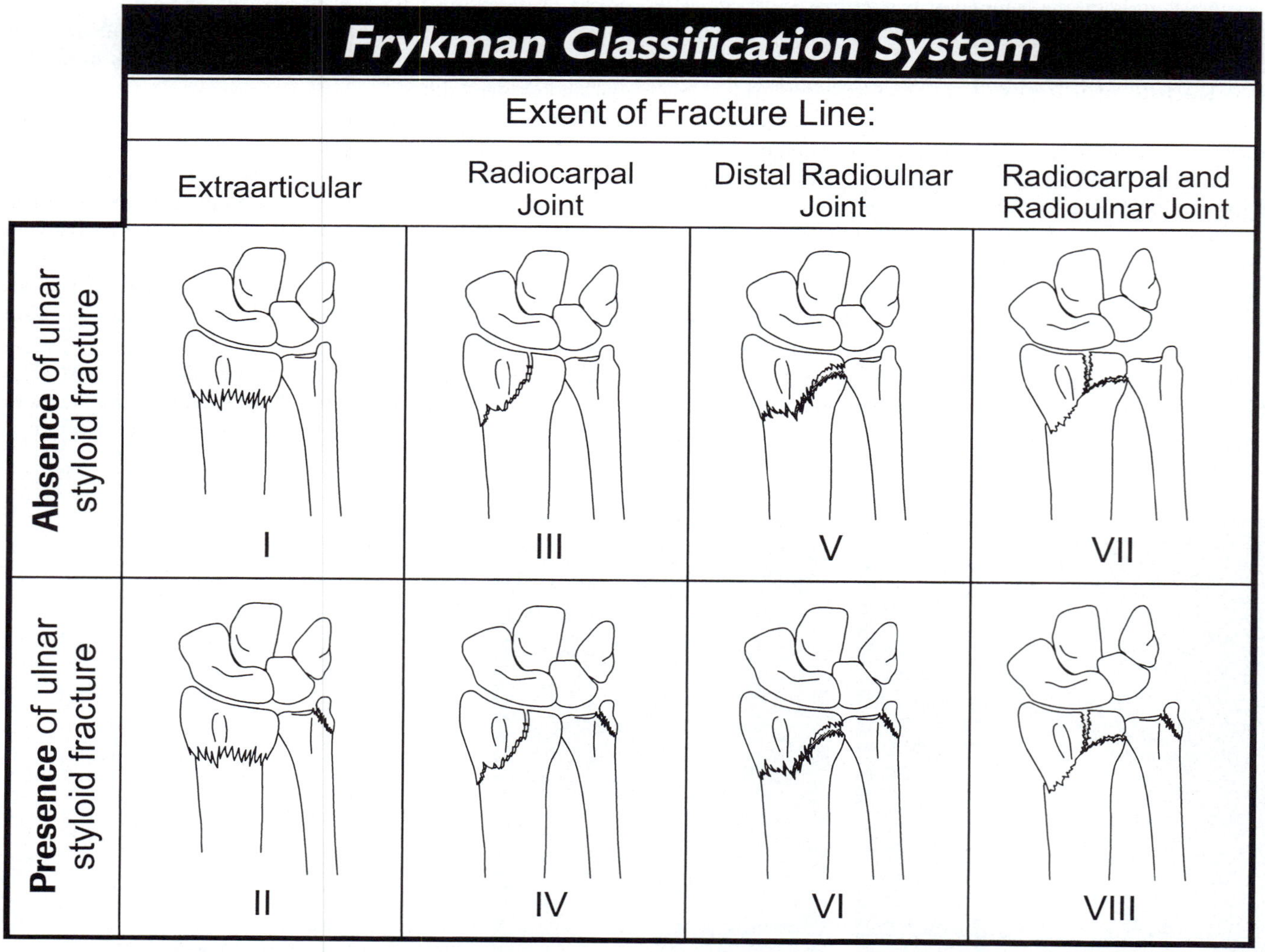

Frykman Classification System

	Extent of Fracture Line:			
	Extraarticular	Radiocarpal Joint	Distal Radioulnar Joint	Radiocarpal and Radioulnar Joint
Absence of ulnar styloid fracture	I	III	V	VII
Presence of ulnar styloid fracture	II	IV	VI	VIII

FIGURE 4-22. Frykman classification system of distal radius fractures.

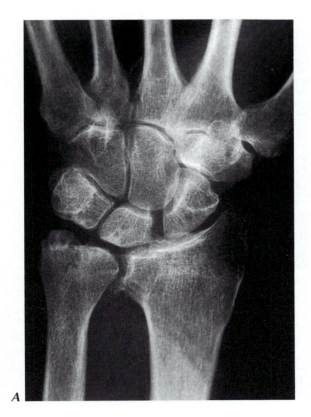

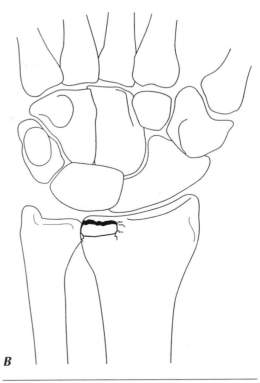

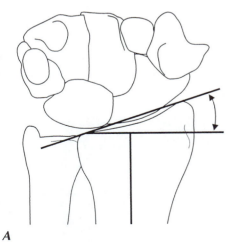

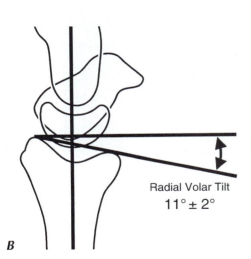

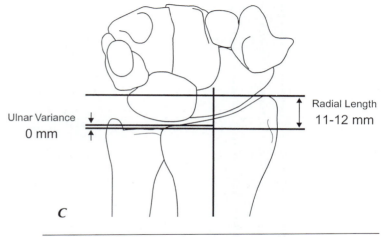

FIGURE 4-23.   Die-punch or lunate-load fracture.

FIGURE 4-24.   *A.* Radial inclination. *B.* Radial volar tilt. *C.* Radial length and ulnar variance.

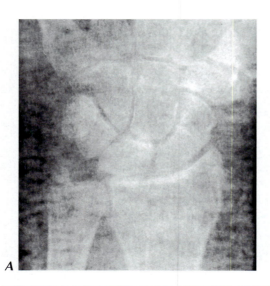

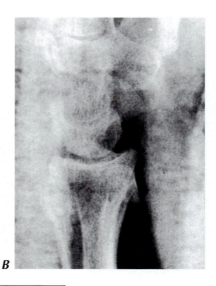

FIGURE 4-25.   Colles fracture, postreduction. There is good restoration of the radiocarpal articulation.

Closed reduction and casting is adequate with many fractures of the distal radius (Fig. 4-25). Operative treatment is usually necessary in unstable extraarticular fractures with severe comminution and shortening, intraarticular fractures, and fractures that have failed closed therapy.

Injuries to the triangular fibrocartilage complex are seen in some fractures of the distal radius. A fracture through the base of the ulnar styloid disrupts the attachment of this cartilage complex. Fractures of the ulnar styloid that are displaced 2 mm or more warrant surgical repair to maintain the stability of the distal radioulnar joint.

Patient management is individualized based on age, occupation, lifestyle, functional requirements, and patient expectations. Consideration must also be given to conditions that ad-

versely affect a good result, such as bone quality, associated medical problems, and poor compliance (Table 4-3). "What would be considered a good result in an elderly arthritic patient might be deplored as a comparative failure in a young working man."[38]

NONDISPLACED FRACTURE OF THE DISTAL RADIUS.   A nondisplaced fracture of the distal radius can be subtle radiographically (Fig. 4-26). The pronator quadratus fat pad sign suggests that a fracture is present. With a fracture, there is anterior displacement or obliteration of the pronator quadratus fat stripe on the lateral view. Although this finding is nonspecific, the fat pad is abnormal in 85% of nondisplaced fractures of the distal radius.[39]

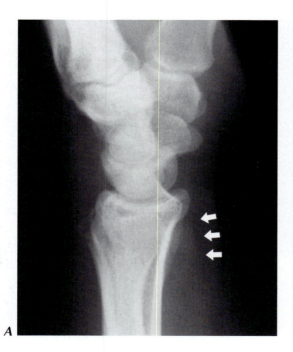

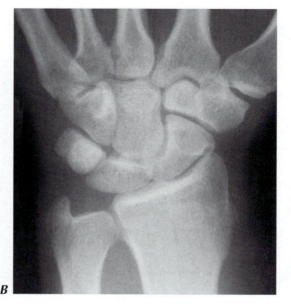

FIGURE 4-26.   Nondisplaced distal radius fracture. These fractures can be subtle. *A.* The fracture itself is not visible on this view. However, the pronator quadratus fat stripe is bowed forward and partially obliterated *(arrows). B.* Jagged disruption of the distal radius's trabeculae is seen. (Copyright David T. Schwartz, M.D.)

TABLE 4-3

Important Features of Fractures of the Distal Radius

Open versus closed fracture
Intraarticular versus extraarticular fracture
Dorsal versus volar angulation
Displacement
Radial shortening
Comminution
Ulnar styloid fracture
Associated injuries to the TFCC or carpus
Neurovascular status
Patient's functional status

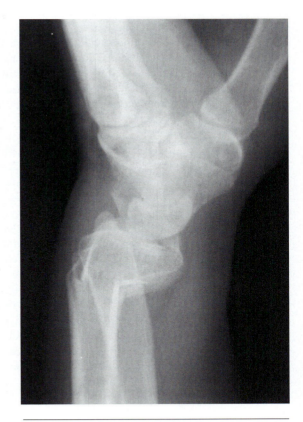

SMITH FRACTURE. A *Smith fracture*, or a reverse Colles fracture, is a volarly displaced fracture of the distal radius (Fig. 4-27).[40,41] The mechanism of injury is either a direct blow to the dorsum of the wrist or a fall onto a supinated wrist. Clinically, there is a "garden-spade" deformity, with the hand and wrist volarly displaced in relation to the forearm. These fractures often require ORIF.

BARTON FRACTURE. A *Barton fracture* involves dorsal or volar subluxation of the hand and wrist secondary to a fracture of the dorsal or volar rim of the distal radial articular surface (Fig. 4-28).[42] A volar Barton fracture is equivalent to a Smith fracture that enters the radiocarpal joint. Volar Barton fractures often need ORIF with volar buttress plating.

FIGURE 4-27. Smith fracture. Fracture through the metaphysis of the distal radius with volar displacement. (Copyright David T. Schwartz, M.D.)

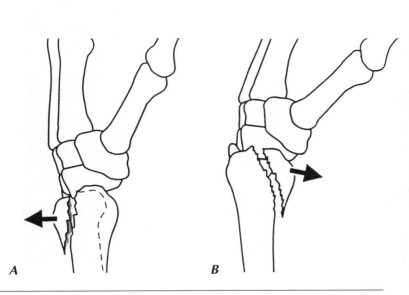

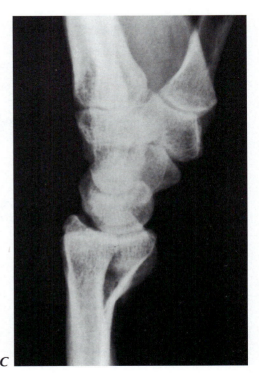

FIGURE 4-28. Dorsal *(A)* and volar *(B)* Barton fracture. Fracture of the dorsal or volar lip of the distal radius articular surface with subluxation of the radiocarpal joint. *C.* Volar Barton fracture. There is slight volar subluxation at the radiocarpal joint. (Copyright David T. Schwartz, M.D.)

CHAUFFEUR'S FRACTURE. The *chauffeur's, backfire,* or *Hutchinson fracture* is an oblique fracture through the radial styloid involving the distal articular surface of the radius (Fig. 4-29).[32] A scapholunate dissociation is commonly associated. Treatment includes closed reduction and percutaneous pinning, with repair of the scapholunate ligament if necessary.

DISTAL RADIOULNAR JOINT DISLOCATION.   Dislocation of the DRUJ is usually seen in association with diplaced distal radius fractures such as Colles, Smith, or Galeazzi fractures (see below). It has significant clinical implications because the radiocarpal joint and the triangular fibrocartilage are usually also disrupted. An isolated DRUJ dislocation is considerably less common (see Chapter 2, Fig. 2-4*B*). The distal ulna may be displaced volarly or dorsally with respect to the radius. On a correctly positioned lateral view, the displacement is readily seen. The dorsal cortices of the distal radius and ulna should lie close together. However, if the lateral view is rotated, the distal ulnar displacement can be difficult to discern. One helpful radiographic landmark is that the ulna styloid normally "points" to the dorsal surface of the triquetrum even when the lateral view is rotated. CT readily detects DRUJ dislocation and subluxation.

Pediatric Injuries

Fractures at the wrist and forearm are common in children. There are two distinct types of pediatric wrist injuries: fractures of the distal radial metaphysis and fractures involving the growth plate. Carpal fractures are distinctly uncommon in children because the carpals are incompletely ossified.

TORUS FRACTURES   In younger children (4 to 10 years of age), because of the pliability of the distal radial metaphysis, fractures tend to be incomplete greenstick fractures or buckle (torus) fractures (Fig. 4-30). These fractures may be minimally displaced and subtle radiographically. Typically, the dorsal cortex of the distal radius is compressed at the site of the buckle fracture. This region must be carefully examined on the lateral radiograph. A slight but abrupt angulation of the cortex may be the only radiographic sign of a fracture (Fig. 4-30*D*). The pronator quadratus fat stripe is often bowed out or partly obliterated.

GROWTH-PLATE FRACTURES.   In older children (8 to 14 years of age), fractures through the growth plate of the distal radius are common (see chap. 22, Fig. 22-9). Salter-Harris type II fractures are the most frequent (Fig. 4-30*E*). Salter-Harris type I fractures are also common.   Nondisplaced injuries are radi-

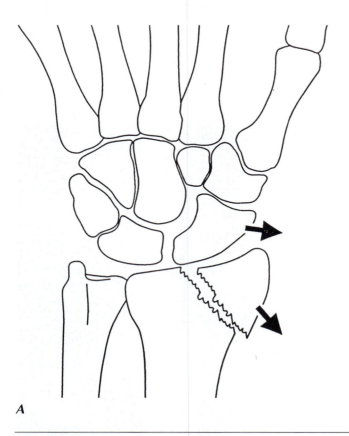

A

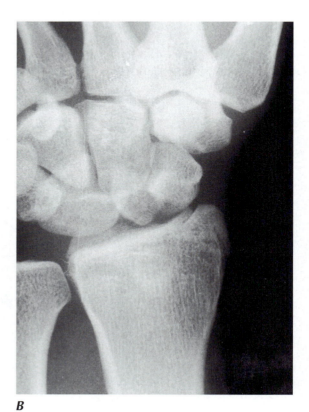

B

FIGURE 4-29.   Chauffeur's or backfire fracture. There is a fracture through the radial styloid. If the fracture is large, there is radial subluxation of the carpus.

ographically subtle. Minimal displacement or widening of the growth plate can be difficult to detect, and comparison views of the uninjured side are helpful in assessing the width or appearance of the growth plate. Bowing or obliteration of the pronator quadratus fat stripe is a clue to the presence of a frac-ture. A nondisplaced grade I Salter-Harris fracture may have no radiographic abnormality. Management of the patient should include appropriate splinting despite negative radiographs. Grades III to V Salter-Harris fractures make up only 5% of all injuries of the distal radius growth plate.

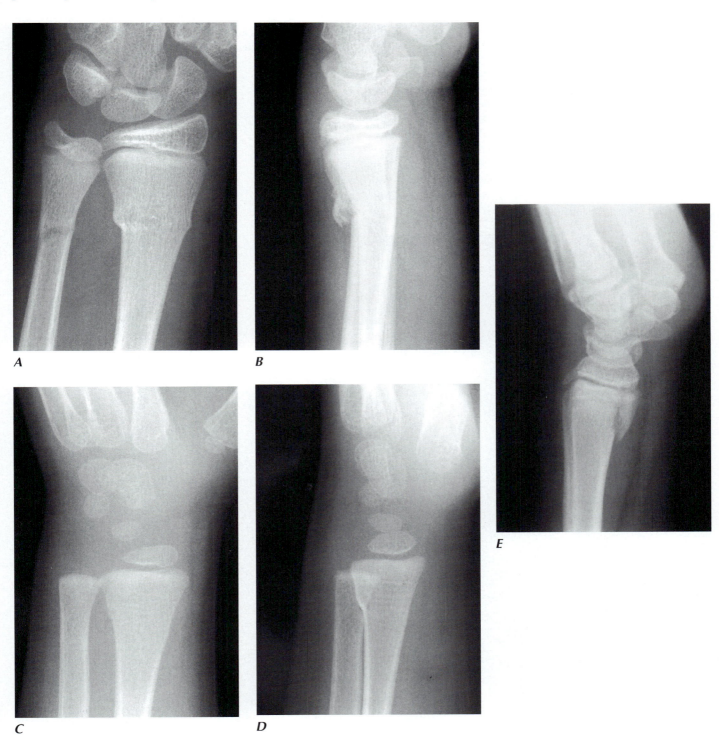

FIGURE 4-30. Pediatric fractures of the metaphysis of the distal radius. *A* and *B*. Greenstick fracture. *C* and *D*. A subtle torus (buckle) fracture of the dorsal cortex is best seen on the lateral view. *E*. Grade II Salter-Harris fracture through the growth plate of the distal radius. The fracture involves the metaphysis. Note that the pronator quadratus fat stripe is bowed forward.

Forearm Fractures

Although the diagnosis of forearm fractures is usually straightforward, the management of displaced forearm fractures and their complications can be difficult. Nonoperative treatment of many forearm fractures yields unsatisfactory results. For maximum functional recovery, anatomic reduction is essential. ORIF with compression plating is usually performed for displaced forearm fractures.

ISOLATED ULNAR SHAFT FRACTURES.   An isolated fracture of the ulnar shaft is known as a *nightstick fracture* (Fig. 4-31). This usually results from a direct blow to the forearm. It is important to assess the joint above and below the fracture, looking especially for dislocation of the radial head at the elbow. If the fracture is angulated more than 10° or offset more than 50% of the bone width, the incidence of nonunion and malunion increases, warranting ORIF. Nondisplaced or minimally displaced fractures are usually treated with a long arm cast.

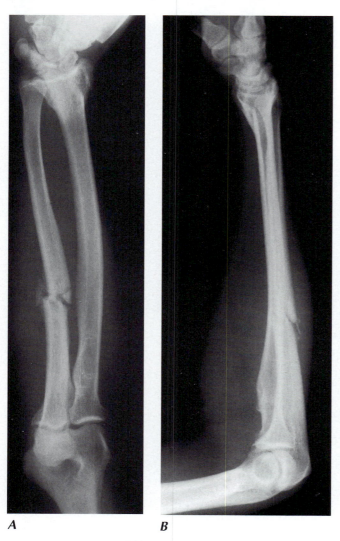

A   *B*

FIGURE 4-31.   Nightstick fracture. A nondisplaced or minimally displaced fracture of the ulnar shaft that is not associated with an injury at the wrist or elbow.

GALEAZZI FRACTURE.   The *Galeazzi fracture,* also known as a *Piedmont fracture,* is a fracture of the distal third of the radius with dislocation of the distal radioulnar joint and ulnar-carpal articulation (Fig. 4-32).[43,44] This fracture results from a fall on an outstretched hand with the forearm hyperpronated. Pain, swelling, ecchymosis, and deformity are seen. Associated injuries of the elbow and wrist as well as neurovascular problems should be anticipated.

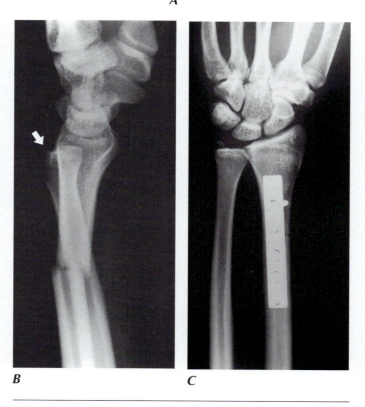

A

B   *C*

FIGURE 4-32.   Galeazzi fracture. Displaced fracture through the distal third of the radial shaft. Dislocation of the distal ulna is evident on the lateral view (*arrow*). ORIF is necessary. (Copyright David T. Schwartz, M.D.)

AP and lateral radiographs of the forearm demonstrate the fracture. Radiography of the joint above and below the forearm fracture (elbow and wrist) must be included to avoid missing associated injuries, such as the distal ulnar dislocation. Radiographic signs of disruption of the DRUJ on the AP view include an ulnar styloid fracture, radial shortening greater than 5 mm, widening of the DRUJ, and malalignment of the distal ulna with the carpus. On the lateral film, subluxation or dislocation of the ulna with respect to the radius is usually obvious: the shaft of the ulna does not overlie the radius and the ulnar styloid does not point to the dorsal surface of the triquetrum. Treatment includes ORIF.

MONTEGGIA FRACTURE. The *Monteggia fracture* is a fracture of the proximal ulnar shaft associated with dislocation of the radial head at the elbow.[45] This injury is usually due to a fall on an outstretched hand with the forearm in maximal pronation. It can also result from a forceful direct blow to the ulnar

surface of the forearm. Clinically, there is deformity of the forearm. The elbow must be examined to detect the dislocation of the radial head. Routine radiographs of the forearm and elbow are adequate to make the diagnosis. The radial head is dislocated when a line drawn through the proximal radial shaft (the radiocapitellar line) does not intersect the capitellum.[46]

Monteggia lesions are classified into four types (Fig. 4-33).[47] In a type I lesion, there is anterior angulation of the ulnar fracture with anterior dislocation of the radial head. This is the most common type, accounting for 60 to 80% of cases (Fig. 4-34).[48]

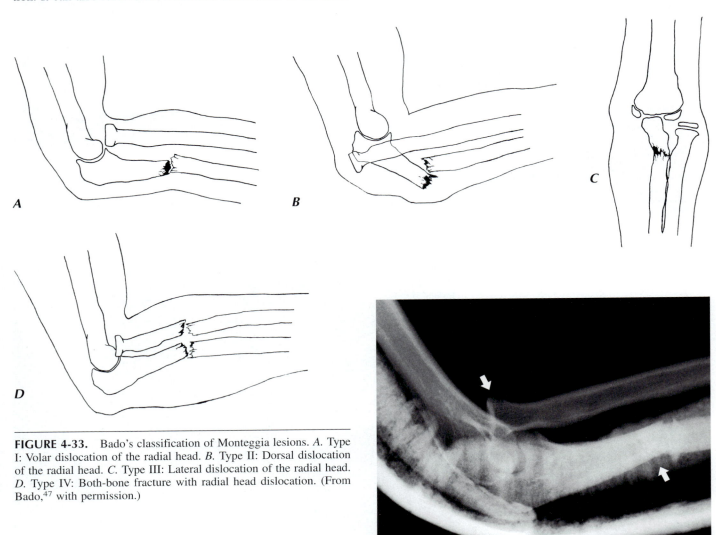

FIGURE 4-33. Bado's classification of Monteggia lesions. *A.* Type I: Volar dislocation of the radial head. *B.* Type II: Dorsal dislocation of the radial head. *C.* Type III: Lateral dislocation of the radial head. *D.* Type IV: Both-bone fracture with radial head dislocation. (From Bado,[47] with permission.)

FIGURE 4-34. Type I Monteggia fracture. Fracture of the proximal ulnar shaft and volar dislocation of the radial head *(arrows)*.

A type II lesion consists of posterior angulation of the ulnar fracture with posterior dislocation of the radial head (Fig. 4-35). A type III lesion consists of a fracture of the proximal ulnar metaphysis with lateral dislocation of the radial head. In type IV, there are fractures of both the radial and ulnar shafts with anterior dislocation of the radial head.

Treatment in adults requires open reduction and internal fixation (Fig. 4-35C). Forearm fractures in children younger than 10 years of age are managed with closed reduction and cast immobilization. In children, continuing growth of the radius and ulna after the fracture has healed corrects residual deformity.[49]

BOTH-BONE FOREARM FRACTURES. Concurrent fractures of the radial and ulnar shafts are the result of a direct blow, motor vehicle collision, or fall (Fig. 4-36). The injury is usually obvious and is accompanied by pain, swelling, and deformity. A careful neurologic examination is essential. Tense swelling can cause a compartment syndrome. Radiographic views of the forearm, wrist, and elbow are needed to demonstrate the full extent of the injury. Low-energy fractures are usually transverse or oblique, whereas high-energy fractures are comminuted. Treatment usually involves open reduction and internal fixation.

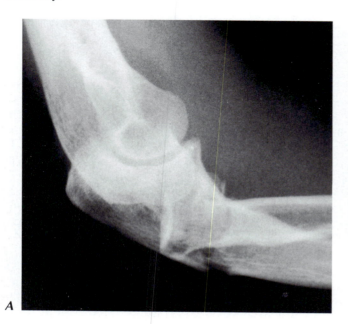

A

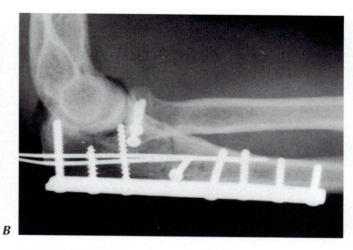

B

FIGURE 4-35. *A.* Type II Monteggia fracture. Fracture of the proximal ulnar shaft and posterior dislocation of the radial head. *B.* ORIF of a type II Monteggia fracture with an associated fracture of the radial head.

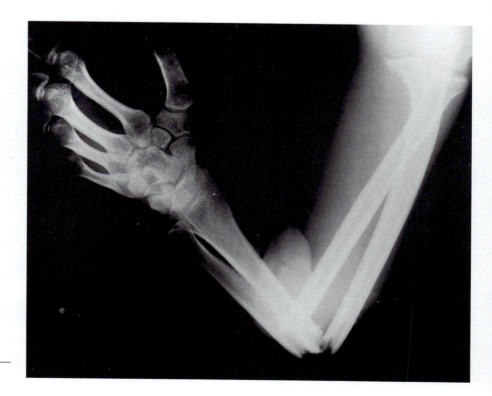

FIGURE 4-36. Both-bone forearm fracture.

ERRORS IN INTERPRETATION

CARPAL FRACTURES.   The most important error in interpreting wrist radiographs is failing to consider the possibility of significant injury even though the radiographs appear normal. This is especially true for scaphoid fractures, because they can be subtle or nondetectable radiographically, and there are significant consequences if they are missed (Fig. 4-10). The standard wrist radiographic series, including a *scaphoid* view, fails to demonstrate the fracture in 10 to 20% of scaphoid fractures. Many other carpal fractures and ligamentous injuries are radiographically subtle. The radiographs must be systematically inspected, concentrating on areas of easily missed injuries such as the proximal metacarpals (Fig. 4-6). Supplementary views are needed to detect certain injuries. For instance, the carpal tunnel view can detect a fracture of the hook of the hamate and the supination oblique view can detect a fracture of the fifth metacarpal base.

Because of the complexity of the radiographic anatomy of the carpals, some shadows can be misinterpreted as fractures. These include normal cortical and trabecular irregularities. The radial articular surface of the scaphoid often ends with a slight "bump" that can look like cortical irregularity due to a fracture

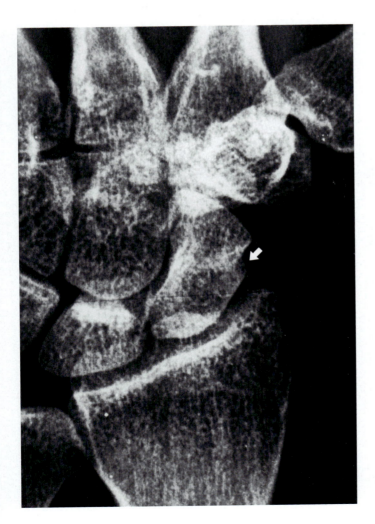

(Fig. 4-37). Foreshortening and overlap of the distal pole of the scaphoid can mimic the increased trabecular density of an impacted fracture (Fig. 4-10*B*). Good-quality films and repeat films with different positioning help clarify questionable findings. Ultimately, reexamination of the patient for tenderness in the area of question usually resolves the problem.

DISTAL RADIUS FRACTURES.   Nondisplaced distal radius fractures can be subtle in both adults and children. Bulging or obliteration of the pronator quadratus fat stripe is a radiographic clue to a fracture (Fig. 4-26). A fine osseous line at the remnant of the distal radius growth plate may persist into adulthood. This should not be misinterpreted as an impaction fracture. In older children at the time that the growth plate is about to fuse, the growth plate creates a small bulge in the cortex of the distal radius that should not be mistaken for a fracture.

FOREARM FRACTURES.   Displaced fractures of the forearm are often associated with dislocations at the elbow or wrist, known as *Monteggia* and *Galeazzi* fractures. These injuries can be missed when the joint above and below the more obvious forearm fracture is not examined clinically or radiographically. In one series of pediatric forearm fractures, 50% of the 12 Monteggia fractures were misdiagnosed at the time of initial presentation.[50] All of these patients had elbow radiographs, but the alignment of the proximal radius and capitellum was incorrectly assessed.

COMMON VARIANTS

Accessory ossicles are much less frequent in the wrist than in the midfoot. They should not be confused with fractures. These small bone fragments are smooth and well corticated and the adjacent bone appears intact (Fig. 2-2*B*). Small fracture fragments have an irregular appearance and do not have a corticated margin; also, the adjacent bone has a cortical gap where the fracture fragment originated.

ADVANCED STUDIES

A *bone scan* is helpful in detecting and excluding occult fractures. However, a bone scan depends on new bone formation to show increased uptake at a fracture. This takes several days to develop. In addition, early after an injury, the increased blood flow to an area of soft tissue injury can show increased uptake, simulating a fracture. Therefore, a bone scan is not useful within the first days after an injury.

MRI can be used to detect fractures unseen by conventional radiography.[15] Unlike bone scans, MRI is positive soon after an

FIGURE 4-37.   A small irregularity of the scaphoid surface should not be misinterpreted as a fracture. It represents the edge of the articular cartilage (*arrow*).

injury. However, MRI is usually unavailable for studying acute wrist injuries. In addition, the cost of MRI is considerable.

CT has limited use in the wrist because of the many planes in which bone surfaces and fractures occur. In certain circumstances, axial CT can be useful. Subluxation of the distal radioulnar joint is difficult to identify with certainty on plain films and is better seen by CT. The bones surrounding the carpal tunnel are readily seen on axial CT, whereas the plain film carpal tunnel view may not give a clear image of these structures.

Three-dimensional CT has also been used in the evaluation of specific carpal bone deformities, fracture displacement, and identification of small bone fragments. CT delineates the amount of fracture displacement as well as the magnitude of carpal bone dislocation. Three-dimensional CT increases the definition and clarity of images of the carpal bones.[51,52]

CONTROVERSIES

Controversies arise primarily in the treatment of patients with "negative" wrist radiographs. It is an error to assume that the patient is suffering from a "wrist sprain" that has limited potential for disability. Negative wrist radiographs do not eliminate the possibility of significant injury. A scaphoid or other carpal fracture, distal radius fracture, DRUJ dislocation, or ligament injury may not be discerned on initial radiographs. The proper approach in managing patients with injuries of the wrist when radiographs fail to demonstrate an injury is to treat the patient as though a significant injury were present. For occult scaphoid fractures and nondisplaced growth-plate injuries, this includes adequate splinting and timely reevaluation.

Because as few as 7% of patients immobilized for a suspected scaphoid fracture actually have such an injury, many patients who do not have a fracture undergo prolonged immobilization and are removed from work for 10 to 14 days.[53] Moreover, there is no definite evidence that immediate immobilization prevents the complications of avascular necrosis and nonunion of the scaphoid. In fact, 1 of the 13 patients with occult scaphoid fractures studied by Murphy developed nonunion despite early and complete immobilization.[15] Other practitioners have suggested that less aggressive splint immobilization is adequate as long as a repeat clinical examination can be assured within 4 to 5 days.[54] The use of a bone scan on the fourth day after the injury is an alternative approach.[15] If the bone scan is negative, it probably excludes a serious injury. This approach has not, however, been validated by long-term study. In any case, it is an error to reassure a patient with a "wrist sprain" that it is an inconsequential injury that needs only minimal supportive dressing and elective follow-up care for persistent symptoms.

ACKNOWLEDGMENTS

With special thanks to those who made this chapter a reality: Steve Getch, our medical artist; Carol Dean, our wonderful secretary; Media Services—Akron City Hospital—SUMMA.

Also, in loving memory of my father, Dr. Mangal Dass Chawla, who taught me the value of hard work, dedication, self-discipline, and honesty.

REFERENCES

1. Larsen CF, Lauritsen J: Epidemiology of acute wrist trauma. *Int J Epidemiol* 22:911, 1993.
2. Waeckerle JF: A prospective study identifying the sensitivity of radiographic findings and the efficacy of clinical findings in carpal navicular fractures. *Ann Emerg Med* 16:733, 1987.
3. Ruby LK, Cooney WP III, An KN, et al: Relative motion of selected carpal bones: A kinematic analysis of the normal wrist. *J Hand Surg Am* 13:1, 1988.
4. Taleisnik J: The ligaments of the wrist. *J Hand Surg Am* 1:110, 1976.
5. Mayfield JK, Johnson RP, Kilcoyne RF: The ligaments of the human wrist and their functional significance. *Anat Rec* 186:417, 1976.
6. Rogers LF: *The Radiology of Skeletal Trauma*, 2d ed. New York: Churchill Livingstone, 1992, pp. 749–759.
7. Kirk M, Orlinsky M, Goldberg R, Brotman P: The validity and reliability of the navicular fat stripe as a screening test in detection of navicular fractures. *Ann Emerg Med* 19:1371, 1990.
8. Sasaki Y, Sugioka Y: The pronator quadratus sign: Its classification and diagnostic usefulness for injury and inflammation of the wrist. *J Hand Surg Br* 14:80, 1989.
9. Botte MJ, Gelberman RH: Fractures of the carpus, excluding the scaphoid. *Hand Clin* 3:149, 1987.
10. Smith DK, Cooney WP III, An KN, et al: The effects of simulated unstable scaphoid fractures on carpal motion. *J Hand Surg Am* 14:283, 1989.
11. Weber ER, Chao EY: An experimental approach to the mechanism of scaphoid waist fractures. *J Hand Surg Am* 3:142, 1978.
12. Gelberman RH, Menon J: The vascularity of the scaphoid bone. *J Hand Surg Am* 5:508, 1980.
13. Freed HA, Shields NN: Most frequently overlooked radiographically apparent fractures in a teaching hospital emergency department. *Ann Emerg Med* 13:900, 1984.
14. Dias JJ, Thompson J, Barton NJ, Gregg PJ: Suspected scaphoid fractures: The value of radiographs. *J Bone Joint Surg Br* 72:98, 1990.
15. Murphy DG, Eisenhauer MA, Powe J, Pavlofsky W: Can a day 4 bone scan accurately determine the presence or absence of scaphoid fracture? *Ann Emerg Med* 26:434, 1995.
16. Imaeda T, Nakamura R, Miura T, Makino N: Magnetic resonance imaging in scaphoid fractures. *J Hand Surg Br* 17:20, 1992.
17. Cooney WP, Dobyns JH, Linscheid RL: Fractures of the scaphoid: A rational approach to management. *Clin Orthop* 149:90, 1980.
18. Langhoff O, Andersen JL: Consequences of late immobilization of scaphoid fractures. *J Hand Surg Br* 13:77, 1988.
19. Ruby L: Fractures and dislocations of the carpus, in Browner BD, Jupiter JB, Levine AM, Trafton PG (eds): *Skeletal Trauma*. Philadelphia: Saunders, 1992, p. 1027.
20. Hocker K, Menschik A: Chip fractures of the triquetrum. Mechanism, classification and results. *J Hand Surg Br* 19:584, 1994.
21. Peltier LF: The classic. Concerning traumatic malacia of the lunate and its consequences: Degeneration and compression fractures. Privatdozent Dr. Robert Kienbock. *Clin Orthop* 149:4, 1980.

22. Ruby L: Fractures and dislocations of the carpus, in Browner BD, Jupiter JB, Levine AM, Trafton PG (eds): *Skeletal Trauma.* Philadelphia: Saunders, 1992, p. 1036.

23. Meldon SW, Hargarten SW: Ligamentous injuries of the wrist. *J Emerg Med* 13:217, 1995.

24. Mayfield JK, Johnson RP, Kilcoyne RK: Carpal dislocations: Pathomechanics and progressive perilunar instability. *J Hand Surg Am* 5:226, 1980.

25. Frankel VH: The Terry-Thomas sign. *Clin Orthop* 129:321, 1977.

26. Cope JR: Rotatory subluxation of the scaphoid. *Clin Radiol* 35:495, 1984.

27. Gilula LA, Weeks PM: Post-traumatic ligamentous instabilities of the wrist. *Radiology* 129:641, 1978.

28. O'Brien ET: Acute fractures and dislocations of the carpus. *Orthop Clin North Am* 15:237, 1984.

29. Alffram PA, Goran CH: Epidemiology of fractures of the forearm. *J Bone Joint Surg Am* 44:105, 1962.

30. Colles A: On the fracture of the carpal extremity of the radius. *Edinburgh Med Surg J* 10:182, 1814.

31. Cooney WP, Linscheid RL, Dobyns JH: Fractures and dislocations of the wrist, in Rockwood CA, Green DP, Bucholz RW, Heckman JD (eds): *Rockwood and Green's Fractures in Adults,* 3d ed. Philadelphia: Lippincott-Raven, 1996, pp. 745–867.

32. Muller ME, Nazarian S, Koch P, Schatzker J: *EDS Classification AO des Fractures: Les Os Longs.* Berlin: Springer-Verlag, 1990.

33. Frykman G: Fracture of the distal radius including sequelae-shoulder hand finger syndrome, disturbance in the distal radioulnar joint and impairment of nerve function: A clinical and experimental study. *Acta Orthop Scand* (Suppl) 108:1, 1967.

34. Friberg S, Lundstrom B: Radiographic measurements of the radiocarpal joint in normal adults. *Acta Radiol Diagn Stockh* 17:249, 1976.

35. Porter M, Stockley I: Fractures of the distal radius: Intermediate and end results in relation to radiologic parameters. *Clin Orthop* 220:241, 1987.

36. van der Linden W, Ericson R: Colles' fracture. How should its displacement be measured and how should it be immobilized? *J Bone Joint Surg Am* 63:1285, 1981.

37. Palmer AK, Werner FW: Biomechanics of the distal radioulnar joint. *Clin Orthop* 187:26, 1984.

38. Edwards H, Clayton EB: Fractures of the lower end of the radius in adults. *BMJ* 1:61, 1929.

39. Doczi J, Springer G, Renner A, Martsa B: Occult distal radial fractures. *J Hand Surg [Br]* 20:614, 1995.

40. Louis DS: Barton's and Smith's fractures. *Hand Clin* 4:399, 1988.

41. Smith RW: *A Treatise on Fractures in the Vicinity of Joints, and on Certain Forms of Accidental and Congenital Dislocations.* Dublin: Hodges and Smith, 1854.

42. Barton JR: Views and treatment of an important injury to the wrist. *Med Exam* 1:365, 1838.

43. Hughston JC: Fracture of the distal radius shaft: Mistakes in management. *J Bone Joint Surg Am* 39:249, 1957.

44. Galeazzi R: Ueber ein besonderes Syndrom bei Verletzungen in Bereich der Unterarmknocken. *Arch Orthop Unfallchir* 35:557, 1934.

45. Monteggia GB: *Instituzione Chirugiche,* Milan: G. Maspero, 1813–1815.

46. McLaughlin, HL: *Trauma.* Philadelphia: Saunders, 1959.

47. Bado JL: The Monteggia lesion. *Clin Orthop* 50:71, 1967.

48. Boyd HB, Boals JC: The Monteggia lesion. A review of 159 cases. *Clin Orthop* 66:94, 1969.

49. Mabrey JD, Fitch RD: Plastic deformation in pediatric fractures: Mechanism and treatment. *J Pediatr Orthop* 9:310, 1989.

50. Gleeson AP, Beattie TF: Monteggia fracture-dislocation in children. *J Accid Emerg Med* 11:192, 1994.

51. Nakamura R, Horii E, Tanaka Y, et al: Three-dimensional CT imaging for wrist disorders. *J Hand Surg Br* 14:53, 1989.

52. James SE, Richards R, McGrouther DA: Three-dimensional CT imaging of the wrist: A practical system. *J Hand Surg Br* 17:504, 1992.

53. Staniforth P: Scaphoid fractures and wrist pain—time for new thinking. *Injury* 22:435, 1991.

CHAPTER 5

THE ELBOW AND DISTAL HUMERUS

David M. Chuirazzi / Ralph J. Riviello

The elbow is an intricate structure of great functional importance. Injuries to the elbow are frequently encountered by emergency physicians, and radiographic findings of elbow injuries can be subtle. This is especially true in children because of the presence of several ossification centers that appear at different ages. To correctly interpret the radiographs, the normal ossification sequence must be understood. If improperly diagnosed, pediatric fractures can result in significant morbidity. Therefore, a separate discussion of the pediatric elbow is provided below.

CLINICAL DECISION MAKING

The decision to obtain radiographs is based on a complete history and physical examination. Two mechanisms of injury are responsible for most elbow fractures—a fall on the outstretched hand and a direct blow to the elbow. The physical examination includes inspection, palpation, and assessment of range of motion and neurovascular integrity. Simple inspection may reveal deformity or dislocation. The olecranon and epicondyles lie close to the skin surface and are therefore readily palpated for evidence of fracture. The radial head and coronoid process lie deeper within the joint and cannot be directly palpated. Fractures in these areas are evident by causing limitation of the elbow's motion.

Limited range of elbow motion to flexion-extension or supination-pronation is a sensitive indicator of elbow injury. In one series, the inability to fully extend the elbow had a sensitivity of 91% in detecting a fracture or joint effusion.[1] Although no prospectively studied guidelines exist for deciding when to order elbow films, it is logical to obtain radiographs in patients who have the appropriate mechanism of trauma, significant pain, localized bone tenderness, or decreased range of motion. On the other hand, radiographs are not indicated in a child with a classic "nursemaid's elbow" (subluxation of the annular ligament) if the symptoms resolve after appropriate reduction maneuvers.

Even when initial radiographs do not show a fracture, patients with significant signs or symptoms or clinical or radiographic evidence of a joint effusion should be immobilized and referred for orthopedic follow-up. In adults, an occult radial head fracture is most likely. In children, an occult supracondylar humeral fracture is common.

Elbow radiographs are helpful in some patients with overuse syndromes who gradually develop pain or joint stiffness. In active children and adolescents, radiographs may reveal osteochondritis dissecans (lateral condyle) or "Little Leaguer's elbow" (medial epicondylar degeneration). However, in simple cases of adult lateral epicondylitis (tennis elbow), radiographs are unnecessary.

When joint pain or stiffness is not caused by trauma, radiography can detect a joint effusion that is difficult to diagnose by physical exam. The finding of an atraumatic joint effusion prompts suspicion of infection, rheumatoid arthritis, gout, and hemarthrosis (e.g., from hemophilia).[2, 3] Extraarticular causes of elbow pain such as olecranon bursitis do not require radiography unless joint space extension is suspected. Isolated olecranon bursitis is usually apparent on physical examination.

ANATOMY AND PHYSIOLOGY

The elbow joint is a complex hinge joint with three articulations located within a single synovial cavity: the humeroulnar joint (between the trochlea and trochlear notch of the ulna), the humeroradial joint (between the capitellum and the radial head), and the proximal radioulnar joint (between the radial head and the radial notch of the ulna) (Fig. 5-1). These articulations allow both stability and free range of motion, including flexion-extension of the elbow and pronation-supination of the forearm.[4]

The distal humerus widens to form the proximal articular components of the elbow joint, the medial and lateral condyles, which are also called the *trochlea* and *capitellum*. The trochlea articulates with the ulna, and the capitellum articulates with the radial head. The distal humerus just proximal to the articular surface has two depressions: the coronoid fossa on the anterior side and the olecranon fossa on the posterior side. Two collections of fat tissue, the anterior and posterior fat pads, are found within these depressions and are important in the radiographic evaluation of the elbow.

The proximal ulna has a crescent-shaped articular surface called the *trochlear notch,* which ends anteriorly in the coro-

77

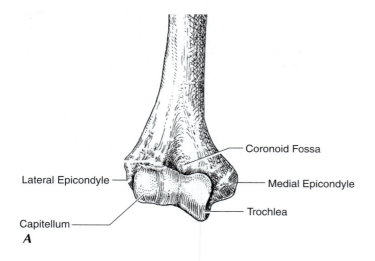

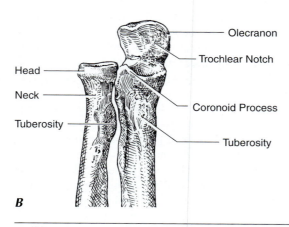

FIGURE 5-1. The skeletal anatomy of the bones forming the elbow—distal humerus, proximal ulna, and proximal radius (anterior view). Three articulations are contained in a single joint capsule—humeroulnar, humeroradial, and proximal radioulnar. (From Pansky B: *Review of Gross Anatomy*, 6th ed. New York: McGraw-Hill, 1996, with permission.)

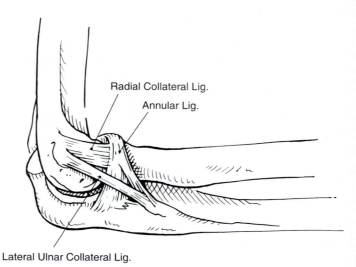

FIGURE 5-2. Ligaments of the elbow—lateral view. The radial head is held in place against the ulna by the annular ligament. The lateral and medial ulnar collateral ligaments attach between the ulna and the humeral epicondyles. The radial collateral ligament stabilizes the annular ligament and the lateral epicondyle of the humerus. (From Dee R, Hurst LC, Gruber MA, Kottmeier SA: *Principles of Orthopedic Practice*, 2d ed. New York: McGraw-Hill, 1997, with permission.)

noid process and posteriorly in the olecranon process. The coronoid process and olecranon lie in their respective fossae during flexion and extension. The proximal surface of the radial head has a central depression to permit rotation as it articulates with the spherical capitellum.

Muscles of the upper arm and forearm insert on the bones of the elbow. The biceps inserts on the radial tuberosity, the brachialis inserts on the ulnar tuberosity and coronoid process, and the triceps inserts on the olecranon. The medial and lateral epicondyles are the origin of the forearm flexor-pronator muscles and the forearm extensor muscles, respectively.

The stability of the elbow is maintained by several ligaments (Fig. 5-2). The annular ligament holds the radial head in place. Both ends of the annular ligament attach to the proximal ulna, and the annular ligament encircles the radial head without a direct osseous attachment. The radial collateral ligament extends from the lateral epicondyle and inserts onto the annular ligament. The ulnar collateral ligament has two fibrous bands that

offer strong ligamentous support for the elbow. The posterior band extends from the medial epicondyle to the medial surface of the olecranon, and the anterior band extends from the medial epicondyle to the coronoid process.[4]

RADIOGRAPHIC TECHNIQUE

Radiographic evaluation of the elbow includes anteroposterior (AP) and lateral projections Table 5-1. Most injuries are identified with these two views. Occasionally, additional views, such as oblique views, are necessary to detect a fracture.

Anteroposterior View. Correct positioning for the AP film is with the elbow extended and the forearm supinated (Fig. 5-3*A* and *B*). If full extension cannot be accomplished because of pain or swelling, the radial head and the capitellum are superimposed and inadequately visualized.

TABLE 5-1

Standard and Supplementary Radiographic Views of the Elbow

	POSITION	EVALUATION OF ADEQUACY	LIKELY FINDINGS
Anteroposterior (AP)	Elbow in full extension Forearm supinated	Elbow fully extended. No overlap of forearm bones.	Most fractures are visible. Radiocapitellar line.
Lateral	Elbow flexed 90° Humeral condyles perpendicular to film Forearm midway between supination and pronation	Elbow flexed 90° Humeral condyles superimposed	Most fractures are visible. Anterior and posterior fat pads Anterior humeral line Radiocapitellar line
SUPPLEMENTARY VIEWS			
Lateral oblique	Position for AP view, then rotate forearm to 45° hypersupination	Radial head projected free of the ulna	Radial head fractures Lateral condyle fractures
Medial oblique	Position for AP view, then pronate forearm 45°	Coronoid process seen without overlap.	Medial condyle fractures.
Capitellum view	Position for lateral, then direct beam 45°	Radial head projected free of coronoid process	Radial head and capitellum fractures
Olecranon view	Flex elbow and supinate forearm X-ray beam tangential to olecranon	Axial view of olecranon	Olecranon fracture in sagittal plane.

Lateral View.   For the lateral radiograph, the elbow is flexed 90°. The humeral condyles are perpendicular to the plane of the film and the forearm is midway between supination and pronation (Fig. 5-3*C* and *D*). In the absence of rotation, the curved articular surfaces of the capitellum and trochlea are superimposed and their respective joint spaces are visible. Correct positioning is necessary to show the joint space and articular relationships. Ninety degrees of elbow flexion is needed to accurately detect a joint effusion by demonstrating displacement of the elbow fat pads.

Oblique Views.   *Medial and lateral oblique projections* provide a better view of their respective condyles. These views are obtained with the elbow extended. For the medial oblique view, the x-ray beam is directed medially at a 45° angle; the lateral condyle and epicondyle are seen without overlap (Fig. 5-4*A*). The lateral oblique view is obtained with the opposite orientation and this view shows the radiocapitellar articulation (Fig.

5-4*B*). In children, lateral condylar fractures are often difficult to see on routine films alone. Therefore, oblique films are obtained on all pediatric patients with a traumatic hemarthrosis and no evidence of fracture on routine AP and lateral films.[5]

Capitellum View.   The *capitellum view* is obtained in the same position as the lateral film but with the x-ray beam angled at 45° cephalad (Fig. 5-4*C*). This exposes the radial head and the radiocapitellar articulation free of overlap by the trochlea and proximal ulna. This view helps to detect some radial head fractures.

Olecranon View.   The *axial olecranon view* is obtained with the elbow flexed at about 50° and the forearm supinated. The x-ray beam is directed perpendicular to the olecranon (Fig. 5-4*D*). The olecranon view is helpful in detecting fractures of the olecranon process that are in an oblique or longitudinal plane.

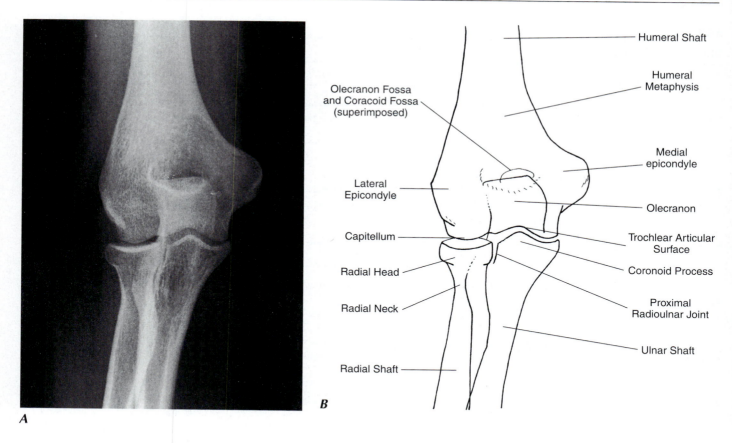

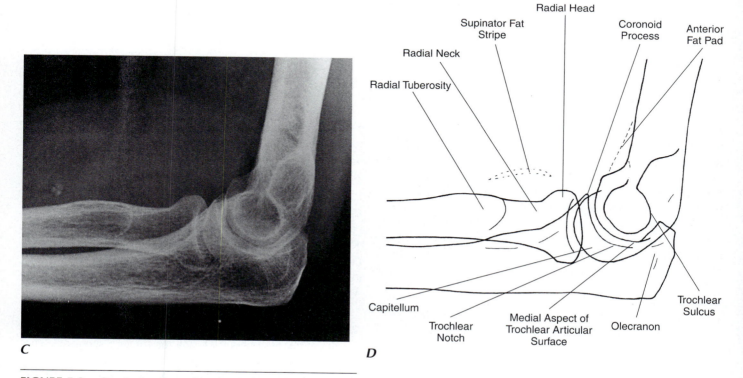

FIGURE 5-3.   Standard radiographic views of elbow. *A* and *B*. AP view. *C* and *D*. Lateral view.

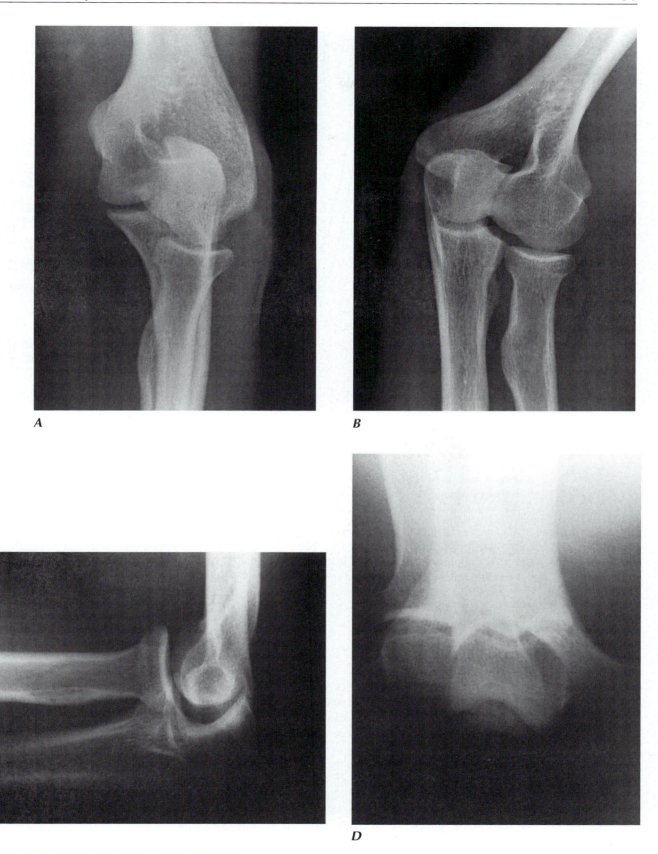

FIGURE 5-4. Supplementary radiographic views of elbow.
A. Medial oblique radiograph. *B.* Lateral oblique radiograph.
C. Capitellar view. *D.* Axial olecranon view.

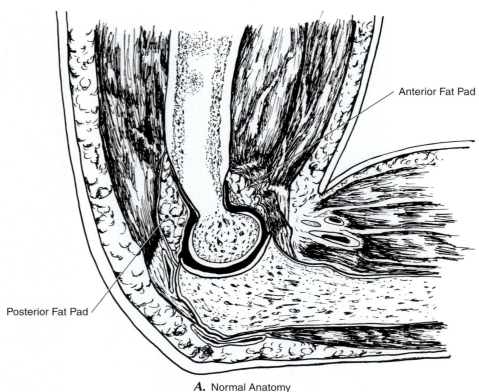

Anterior Fat Pad

Posterior Fat Pad

A. Normal Anatomy

RADIOGRAPHIC ANALYSIS

Many elbow fractures and dislocations are obvious radiographically. In these cases, the radiographs demonstrate the full extent of the injury and permit appropriate treatment. However, a significant number of fractures are subtle. Some nondisplaced fractures can only be inferred by the presence of a joint effusion.

Fat-Pad Sign

Two collections of fat tissue are contained within the outer fibrous layer of the elbow joint capsule (Fig. 5-5A). The anterior fat pad lies within the coronoid fossa, and the posterior fat pad lies within the olecranon fossa. The anterior fat pad is normally visible on the lateral view as a radiolucent stripe lying close to the coronoid fossa. The posterior fat pad is not normally visible because it is entirely contained within the olecranon fossa when the elbow is flexed. In the presence of a joint effusion or hemarthrosis, fluid fills the joint space, lifting the anterior and posterior fat pads (Fig. 5-5B). On the lateral radiograph, elevation of the anterior fat pad or visualization of the posterior fat pad is abnormal (Fig. 5-5D). When the anterior fat pad is displaced and elevated by an effusion, its radiographic appearance is likened to a ship's sail—the "sail sign."[3]

Evidence of a traumatic joint effusion is a sensitive indicator of an intraarticular fracture.[6] However, the absence of a fat-pad sign does not entirely exclude a fracture. Lack of a fat-pad sign can be due to disruption of the joint capsule, insufficient blood collection, or suboptimal radiographic technique (i.e., a lateral view that is rotated or taken without 90° of elbow flexion).[7] It is important to use a "bright light" to search for the fat-pad signs because skeletal radiographs are often overpenetrated with respect to the soft tissues. If the lateral radiograph is taken with the elbow in extension, the olecranon process displaces the fat pad from its resting place, causing a false-positive posterior fat-pad sign (Fig. 5-5E).

In many instances, the joint effusion is easier to detect than the fracture itself. Any intraarticular fracture can cause a fat-pad sign. In adults, traumatic joint effusions are most often caused by a radial head fracture. In children, a supracondylar fracture is most common. Both fractures can be radiographically subtle or undetectable. All patients with positive fat-pad signs are treated empirically for a fracture with appropriate immobilization and referral. In some instances, additional radiographic views, such as oblique views, should be obtained. For example, in a child a posterior fat pad prompts further investigation with oblique views to exclude a lateral condylar fracture. In an adult, oblique views or a capitellum view can reveal a radial head fracture, although documentation of such a fracture does not alter clinical management.

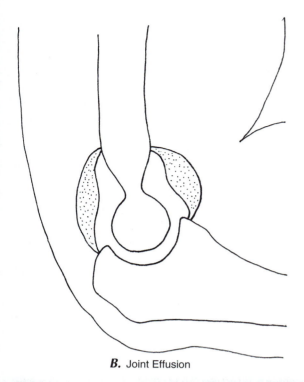

B. Joint Effusion

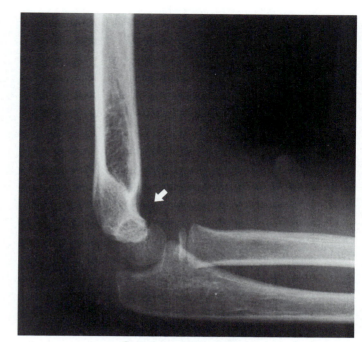

C. Normal Anterior Fat Pad

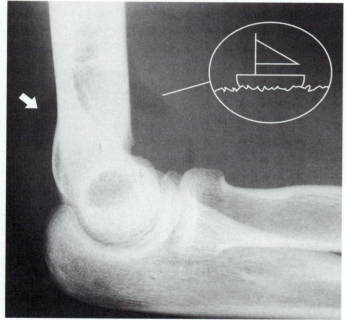

D. Abnormal Fat Pads

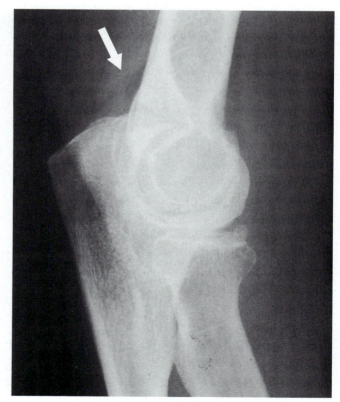

E. False-Positive Fat Pads

FIGURE 5-5.   The fat pads of the elbow joint. *A.* Normal positions of the anterior and posterior fat pads as they lie in their respective fossae. *B.* Displacement of both fat pads by a joint effusion. *C.* Normal anterior fat pad in a child (see Fig. 5-1*C*). *D.* Anterior fat pad "sailing". The posterior fat pad is also seen (*arrow*). *E.* A false-positive posterior fat pad is due to elbow extension.

Systematic Analysis of Adult Elbow Radiographs

A careful and systematic radiograph analysis is necessary to detect elbow injuries. Attention is directed to sites prone to injury and easily missed injuries (Fig. 5-6). The ABC'S mnemonic summarizes the important findings in elbow radiographs: adequacy and alignment, bones, cartilage, and soft tissues (Table 5-2).

Adequacy.   The study must include both the AP and lateral views. On the AP view, the elbow is fully extended and the forearm is supinated so that there is no overlap of the radius and ulna (Fig. 5-3A). A proper lateral view is taken with the joint flexed to 90° and the humeral condyles (trochlea and capitellum) superimposed (Fig. 5-3C). If the positioning is rotated, the condyles will not be superimposed and the joint space will not be visible. Suboptimal technique is acceptable when an extensive fracture precludes proper positioning.

Alignment.   The normal anatomic relationships between the radial head and capitellum and between the trochlea and trochlear notch must be confirmed in every radiographic view. The *radiocapitellar line* is drawn through the mid-shaft of the proximal radius, which should normally intersect with the middle of the capitellum. An intact radiocapitellar line implies normal articulation between the capitellum and radial head.

Bones.   One begins by looking for obvious skeletal injuries involving the distal humerus and proximal radius and ulna. All cortical surfaces are inspected for breaks, flecks of bone, or buckling. The trabeculae are examined for disruption or impaction. If no obvious fractures are seen, the radiograph is reviewed for frequently missed injuries. In adults, subtle fractures occur at the radial head and neck, the olecranon, the coronoid process, and, rarely, the articular surface of the capitellum.

Soft Tissues.   A joint effusion is sought by evaluating the elbow *fat pads*. The presence of an abnormal fat pad prompts evaluation for a subtle fracture, especially at the radial head, although any intraarticular fracture can cause a joint effusion. Supplementary views can disclose a radial head fracture. However, these views are not always necessary because all such patients should be assumed to have a nondisplaced radial head fracture and be treated accordingly. Special olecranon views are obtained to diagnose a nondisplaced, oblique olecranon fracture if there is tenderness or swelling over the olecranon process.

The *supinator fat stripe* can occasionally help detect a subtle radial head fracture. This radiolucent line is visible on the lateral film and represents a fascial plane resting on the supinator muscle. It is located along the volar aspect of the forearm about 1 cm from the radial head and neck. It normally lies parallel to the radial shaft. The supinator fat stripe line is distorted or obliterated by a fracture of the radial head or neck.[8]

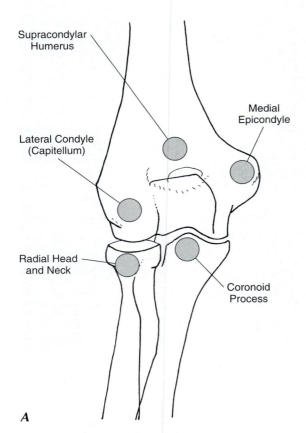

Supracondylar Humerus

Lateral Condyle (Capitellum)

Radial Head and Neck

Medial Epicondyle

Coronoid Process

A

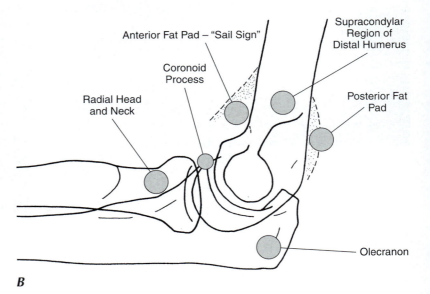

Anterior Fat Pad – "Sail Sign"

Coronoid Process

Radial Head and Neck

Supracondylar Region of Distal Humerus

Posterior Fat Pad

Olecranon

B

FIGURE 5-6.   Sites prone to injury and easily missed injuries—adult. *A.* AP view. *B.* Lateral view.

TABLE 5-2

The ABC'S of Elbow Radiographs

Adequacy	**AP view:** Elbow fully extended. No overlap of radius and ulna. **Lateral view:** Elbow flexed 90°. Humeral condyles superimposed.
Alignment	**Radiocapitellar line:** Aligned in all views. Disruption occurs in radial head dislocations, elbow dislocations, and displaced fractures of the lateral condyle (capitellum). **Anterior humeral line** (children): On lateral view, the line should intersect the middle third of the capitellum. Posterior displacement of the capitellum is seen in supracondylar fractures.
Bones	**Distal humerus:** Supracondylar region, humeral condyles (capitellum and trochlea), intercondylar area, epicondyles **Radius:** Head, neck, and proximal shaft **Ulna:** Olecranon, coronoid process, and proximal shaft **In children**, assess ossification centers for correct order for appearance and position: **CRITOE.**
Cartilage	Examine joint space on AP and lateral views. The pediatric elbow is largely cartilage.
Soft tissues	**Anterior fat pad:** Abnormally elevated with joint effusion ("sail sign") **Posterior fat pad:** Always pathologic If either fat pad is positive, reexamine for subtle fracture: radial head (adult), supracondylar fracture (child), or other intraarticular fracture. **Supinator fat stripe:** Obliterated or distorted in proximal radius or ulna fractures.

ELBOW RADIOGRAPHS IN CHILDREN

The interpretation of pediatric elbow radiographs is challenging because of the many growth plates and secondary ossification centers (Fig. 5-7).

Developmental Considerations

Knowledge of the sequence of appearance of the ossification centers of the elbow is essential for the correct interpretation of pediatric elbow radiographs (Fig. 5-8). There is variation in the age at which each ossification center appears, but the order of ossification is always the same. A mnemonic used to remember this order is CRITOE: *c*apitellum, *r*adial head, *int*ernal (medial) epicondyle, *t*rochlea, *o*lecranon, and *e*xternal (lateral) epicondyle.[9] The age in years at which each ossification center appears is roughly the sequence of odd numbers between 1 and 11: 1, 3, 5, 7, 9, 11 (Table 5-3).[8]

The capitellum is the first center to ossify and is visible by the age of 1 year. The radial head appears next at age 3 years.

The medial epicondyle appears at age 5 years. Early in its development, the medial epicondyle ossification center may appear to be widely displaced from the humerus.[7] The medial epicondyle is the last growth center to fuse; as late as age 18 in boys.[10] The trochlear epiphysis ossifies at about age 7. It arises from multiple centers and has an irregular appearance. Next to appear is the olecranon, at age 9. Finally, at age 11, the lateral epicondyle appears. It does not directly fuse with the humeral shaft but joins the capitellum and trochlea before the entire conglomerate fuses to the humeral shaft in early adolescence.[9]

Systematic Analysis of Pediatric Radiographs

The interpretation of radiographs must be approached systematically (Table 5-2). One searches for common fractures and easily missed injuries (Fig. 5-9). The first step is to assess the quality of the film, as outlined for adult patients.

Bones. The cortical surfaces of each bone are inspected for breaks, flecks of bone, or buckling. The joint space is examined for small bone fragments or entrapment of the medial epicondyle.

The ossification centers are assessed (Fig. 5-8). The proper sequence of ossification centers is correlated with the patient's age using the CRITOE mnemonic. Although the age of appearance varies, the sequence of appearance of the ossification centers is constant. For example, what appears to be a trochlear ossification center when the medial (internal) epicondyle is not present may actually be an avulsed medial epicondyle that is entrapped within the elbow joint.

Soft Tissues. The anterior and posterior fat-pad signs are sought. In the child, a supracondylar fracture is the most common injury.

Alignment. Two anatomic relationships must be confirmed: the anterior humeral line and the radiocapitellar line. These signs help to identify subtle injuries. The *anterior humeral line* is drawn along the anterior surface of the humerus on the lateral view. This line normally intersects the middle third of the capitellum (Fig. 5-10). In a subtle supacondylar fracture, posterior displacement of the capitellum relative to the anterior humeral line may be the only sign of injury.[11]

The *radiocapitellar line* is drawn through the midshaft of the proximal radius and should bisect the capitellum (Fig. 5-11). This relationship should be maintained in all radiographic views. Disruption occurs in dislocations of the radial head, elbow dislocations, and displaced fractures of the lateral condyle (Fig. 5-12). The radiocapitellar line is disrupted in a

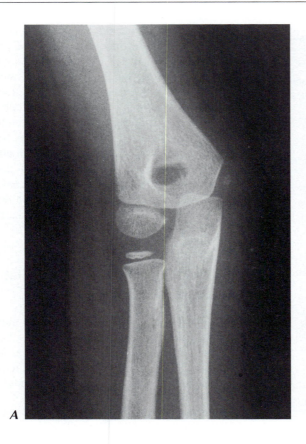

A

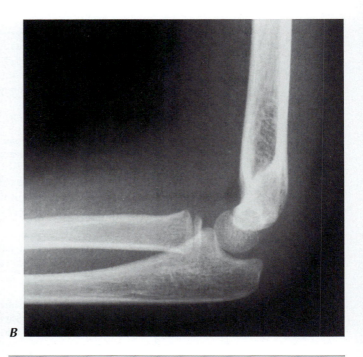

B

FIGURE 5-7.   Standard radiographic views in a child. *A*. AP radiograph of a 6-year-old male with three secondary ossification centers present: the capitellum, radial head, and medial (internal) epicondyle. *B*. Lateral radiograph.

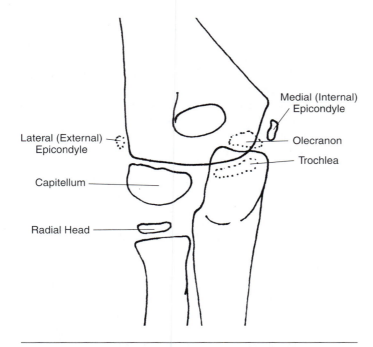

FIGURE 5-8.   Secondary ossification centers of the elbow. The elbow of a 6-year-old showing age-appropriate ossification centers: capitellum, radial head, and medial epicondyle. Future ossification centers are indicated by the broken lines: trochlea, olecranon, and lateral epicondyle. The sequence of appearance of the ossification centers is given by the mnemonic CRITOE—capitellum, radial head, internal (medial) epicondyle, trochlea, olecranon, and external (lateral) epicondyle.

TABLE 5-3

Ossification Centers of the Elbow: CRITOE

OSSIFICATION CENTER	**SEQUENCE AND AGE OF APPEARANCE**	**RANGE OF AGE OF APPEARANCE**
Capitellum	1 year	1–8 months
Radial Head	3 years	3–6 years
Internal (Medial) Epicondyle	5 years	3–7 years
Trochlea	7 years	7–10 years
Olecranon	9 years	8–10 years
External (Lateral) Epicondyle	11 years	11–12 years

Growth plates close at age 14 to 17 years. Medial epicondyle fuses at age 15 to 18 years.

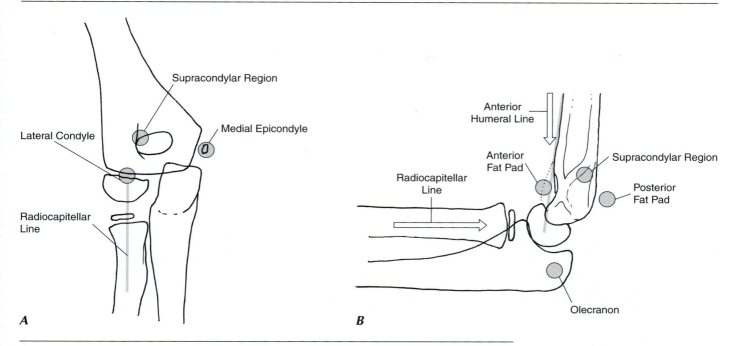

FIGURE 5-9. Sites prone to injury and easily missed injuries—child. *A.* AP view. *B.* Lateral view.

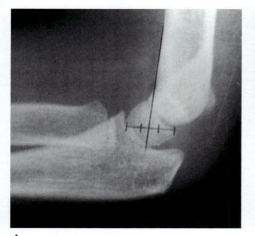

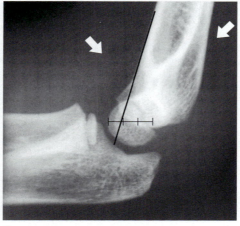

FIGURE 5-10. The anterior humeral line. *A.* Normal radiograph. The anterior humeral line intersects the middle third of the capitellum. *B.* Supracondylar fracture. The capitellum is displaced posteriorly so that the anterior humeral line intersects the anterior third of the capitellum. The fracture line is faintly visible along the volar surface of the distal humerus. There are anterior and posterior fat pad signs (*arrows*).

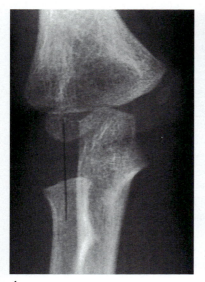

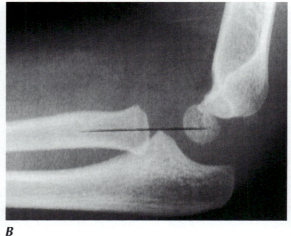

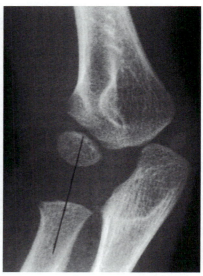

FIGURE 5-11. The radiocapitellar line. The line is normally maintained regardless of the projection.

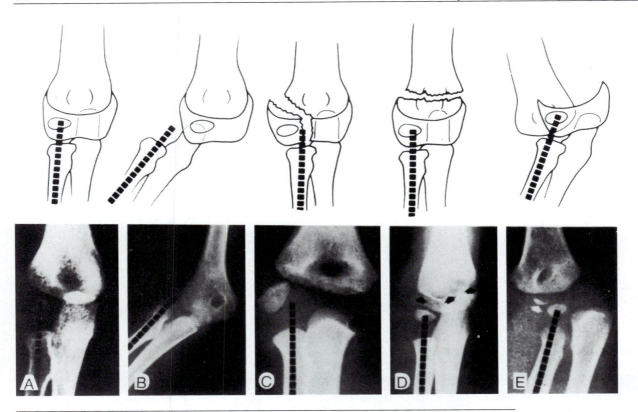

FIGURE 5-12. The radiocapitellar line is helpful in differentiating various fractures and dislocations. *A.* Normal elbow. *B.* Elbow dislocation. *C.* Displaced fracture of the lateral condyle. *D.* Supracondylar fracture. The fracture line is shown with arrows. *E.* Separation of the entire distal humeral epiphysis. A fleck of bone (*arrow*) may be pulled off the lateral condyle, denoting a Salter-Harris type II fracture/separation. (From DeLee JC, Wilkins KE, Rogers LF, Rockwood CA: Fracture-separation of the distal humeral epiphysis. *J Bone Joint Surg* 62A:46, 1980, with permission.)

Monteggia fracture/dislocation and is maintained in a nursemaid's elbow.[5,7]

COMMON ABNORMALITIES—ADULTS

Elbow fractures occur mostly as a result of indirect forces on the elbow due to a fall on an outstretched arm. Other injuries are due to direct blows to the elbow. Assessment of radiographs is guided by knowledge of the common injuries, which vary with the age of the patient (Table 5-4).

Radial Head and Neck Fractures

Fractures involving the proximal radius are the most common elbow injuries in adults and represent 50% of all fractures about the elbow.[12] The usual mechanism involves impaction of the radial head against the capitellum during a fall on the outstretched hand. A fracture of the radial head is clinically suspected when, after an appropriate mechanism, there is difficulty

with elbow range of motion, swelling due to a joint effusion, or tenderness over the lateral aspect of the elbow. Radiographs show disruption of the cortex of the radial head, double lines of cortical bone related to compression of fracture fragments, or a step-off deformity of the concave articular surface (Fig. 5-13). In nondisplaced fractures, these findings can be subtle, requiring oblique or capitellar views for visualization. A joint effusion is often present, as indicated by an anterior or posterior fat-pad sign.

Fractures of the proximal radius are graded using the Mason classification.[13] Type I injuries, the most common form, are displaced less than 2 mm. Type II injuries have ≥2 mm of displacement or depression and involve at least 25% of the radial head. Type III fractures are severely comminuted. A severely comminuted fracture of the radial head may have an associated injury that can be difficult to recognize. The force causing fragmentation of the radial head can also cause subluxation of the distal radioulnar joint at the wrist and disruption of the interosseous membrane. This injury is known as an *Essex-Lopresti fracture.* Although rare, it mandates that evaluation of the wrist be performed in the setting of type III fractures of the radial head.

TABLE 5-4

Common Injuries by Age

Adult	Incidence			Child	Incidence
		Most likely			
Radial head or neck fracture	50%			Supracondylar fracture	60%
Olecranon fracture	20%	↑		Lateral condylar fracture	15%
Elbow dislocation	15%			Medial epicondyla fracture	10%
				Radial neck or head fracture	6–12%
Others:		↓			
Distal humerus fracture				Others:	
Capitellum fracture				Elbow dislocation	
Coronoid fracture		**Least likely**		Olecranon fracture	
Monteggia injury				Monteggia injury	
				Complete epiphyseal	
				separation (rare)	

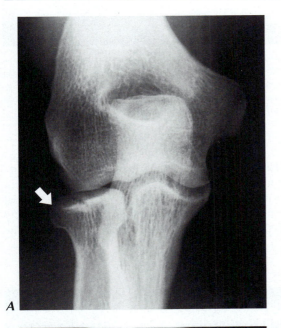

A

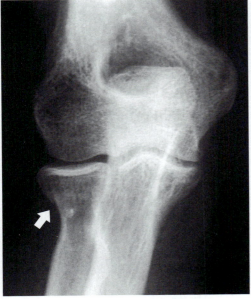

B

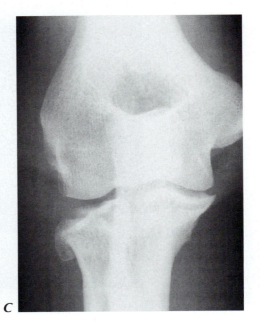

C

FIGURE 5-13. Fractures of the radial head and neck. *A.* A minimally displaced fracture of the radial head (*arrow*). *B.* A minimally depressed fracture of the radial neck (*arrow*). *C.* A grade III severely comminuted and depressed fracture of the radial head.

Olecranon Fractures

Olecranon fractures are more common in adults than in children and adolescents. They represent 20% of adult elbow injuries but only 5% of those in children.[14] These fractures are usually caused by direct trauma to the elbow. The remainder are related to falls on the outstretched hand with the elbow in flexion.[15]

Clinical findings include pain and swelling over the olecranon and inability to extend the elbow. The fracture line is usually perpendicular to the long axis of the ulna. Olecranon fractures are best seen on the lateral radiograph (Fig. 5-14). Traction applied by the triceps muscle can distract the fracture fragments.

Occasionally, the fracture line is oriented along the long axis of the ulna. When nondisplaced, it is difficult to identify on standard radiographs. The axial olecranon view may be helpful in showing the fracture.[5] Clinical signs suggestive of a fracture include local tenderness and swelling at the olecranon. A fat-pad sign may be present.

Elbow Dislocations

In adults, this is the third most common joint dislocation, following dislocations of the shoulder and interphalangeal joints of the hand. In children, the elbow is the most common dislocation. Elbow dislocation most often occurs during hyperextension. The olecranon locks into the olecranon fossa and the coronoid abuts the trochlea. During a fall on an outstretched arm, hyperextension occurs at the elbow, and the olecranon acts as a fulcrum to pry the joint apart.

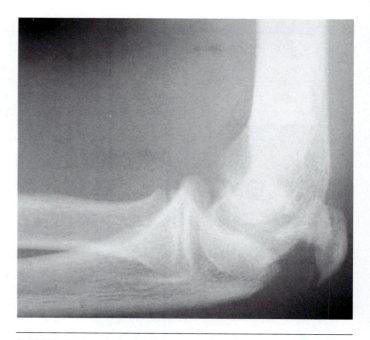

FIGURE 5-14.   A markedly displaced olecranon fracture. Traction by the triceps tendon causes displacement of the fracture. Surgical fixation is necessary both to counteract the pull of the triceps and restore the articular surface of the trochlear notch.

Elbow dislocations are named by the direction of displacement of the ulna relative to the distal humerus. Ninety percent are posterior or posterolateral (Fig. 5-15).[16] Medial and lateral dislocations are much less common (Fig. 5-16). Approximately one-half of elbow dislocations have associated injuries. The

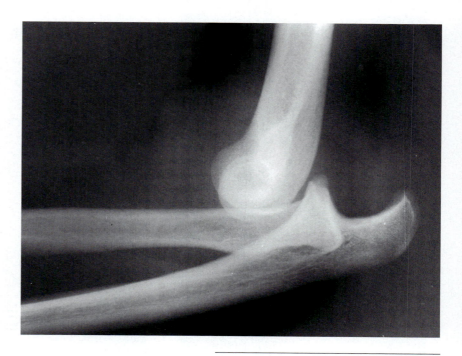

FIGURE 5-15.   Posterior elbow dislocation.

most common is a fracture of the medial epicondyle, followed by a fracture of the proximal radius and coronoid process. Although radio-graphic diagnosis of elbow dislocation is usually straightforward, difficulty arises with detection of subtle associated fractures. These associated injuries, particularly if the fracture fragment becomes entrapped within the joint space, are most often identified on postreduction films (Fig. 5-17).[5] Clinical signs of entrapment include the inability to reduce the dislocation and a limited range of motion after reduction.[17] An entrapped coronoid or medial epicondyle requires surgical correction. Median nerve entrapment can occur during reduction of a posterior dislocation.

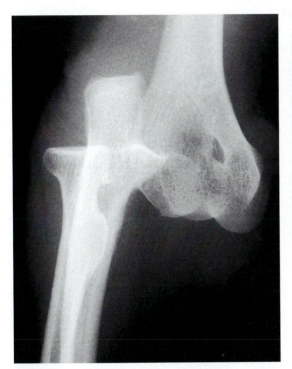

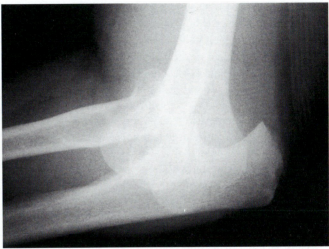

B

FIGURE 5-16. Lateral elbow dislocation.

A

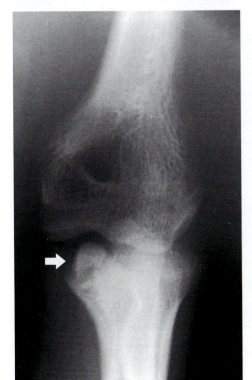

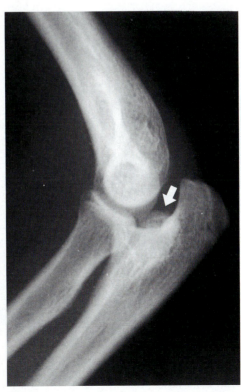

A

B

FIGURE 5-17. Entrapped fracture fragment. Postreduction radiographs of an elbow dislocation reveal entrapment of a bone fragment that was not evident on the initial radiographs. The entrapped fragment prevents complete reduction of the dislocation.

Monteggia Fracture/Dislocations

In 1814, Giovanni Battista Monteggia described difficulties while treating a fracture involving the proximal third of the ulna in association with anterior dislocation of the proximal radius. Four types of injuries are seen.[18] Type I Monteggia injuries involve the proximal third of the ulna with anterior displacement of the distal ulnar fragment and anterior dislocation of the radial head (Figs. 5-18, 5-19, 5-20). This is the most common form, occurring in 65% of cases. Type II injuries have posterior angulation of the ulnar fragment with posterior dislocation of the radial head. Eighteen percent of Monteggia injuries are type II. In type III injuries, the ulna is fractured just distal to the coronoid process, and there is lateral dislocation of the radial head. Type III injuries occur almost exclusively in children 5 to 9 years old.[19] The least common are type IV injuries, which combine the classic Monteggia fracture/dislocation with a fracture of the proximal third of the radius.

Rather than being caused by linear forces transmitted through the bones of the forearm or angular forces with the fulcrum at the elbow, the Monteggia injury results from rotatory forces. As a person falls, the hand may contact the ground and become anchored while the arm and body rotate around the forearm. This results in forceful internal rotation, fracture of the proximal ulna, and dislocation of the radial head.[18]

The Monteggia injury is sometimes confused with an anterior fracture/dislocation of the elbow when a fracture occurs at the trochlear notch of the ulna. One must pay close attention to the proximal radioulnar articulation, which is disrupted in a Monteggia fracture/dislocation yet remains intact during an anterior fracture dislocation.[20] The disrupted radioulnar articulation makes the Monteggia injury more difficult to repair.

Distal Humerus Fractures

Although distal humerus fractures are considerably more common in children, they do occur with moderate frequency in adults, especially older adults with osteoporosis. The mechanism is typically a fall directly on the flexed elbow. Management of these fractures can be difficult. Because of the large

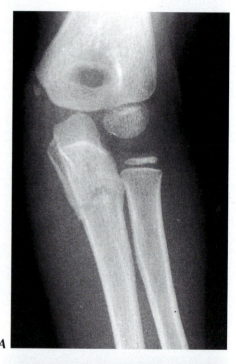

A

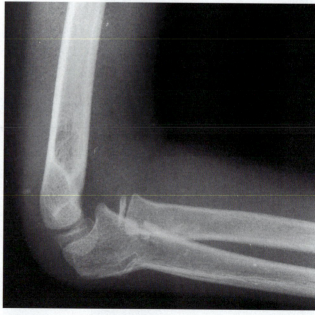

B

FIGURE 5-18.   The Monteggia fracture/dislocation, type I. There is a displaced fracture of the proximal ulnar shaft with anterior dislocation of the articulation between the radius and capitellum.

FIGURE 5-19.   A subtle Monteggia fracture/dislocation in a child. Disruption of the radiocapitellar joint is not evident on the AP radiograph (*A*). Anterior dislocation of the radial head is seen on the lateral view (*B*).

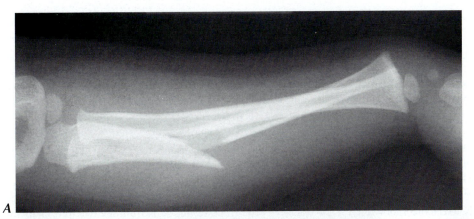

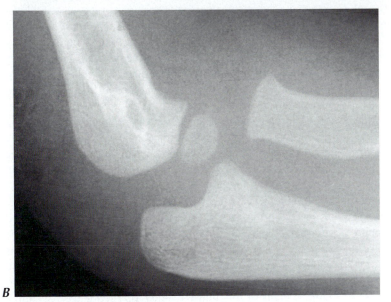

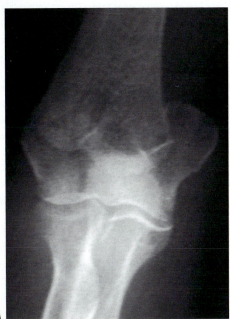

FIGURE 5-20. Subtle Monteggia lesion. The Monteggia injury could be missed in this young child with a markedly displaced mid-shaft ulnar fracture (A). Malalignment of the radiocapitellar articulation is slight on this view and might remain undiscovered without a lateral elbow radiograph (B).

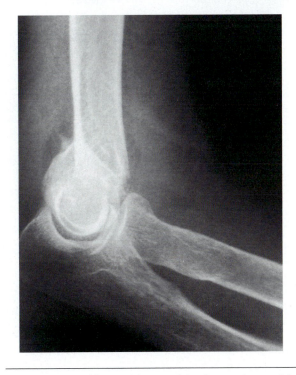

joint surface at the distal humerus, the articular surfaces are often involved and there is risk of subsequent functional impairment.[21,22] About 80% of these fractures are intraarticular and involve both humeral condyles.[23] The most common variety has a Y-shaped fracture line extending through the intercondylar region (Fig. 5-21). About 15% of distal humerus fractures involve only one condyle. Two-thirds of these are isolated fractures of the articular surface of the capitellum, which can be difficult to see on the radiographs. The remaining third are oblique fractures that involve either the medial or lateral humeral condyle. About 5% of distal humeral fractures are extraarticular, most being transverse fractures across the supracondylar region. Rarely, adults will have an avulsion fracture of the medial epicondyle.

FIGURE 5-21. Y-shaped intercondylar fracture in an adult.

COMMON ABNORMALITIES—CHILDREN

Supracondylar Fractures

The supracondylar fracture is the most common elbow fracture in children, accounting for 60% of all pediatric elbow fractures (Table 5-4). The fracture line crosses horizontally across the condyles, the coronoid fossa, and the olecranon fossa. The fracture is actually intraarticular and is therefore more properly called a *transcondylar fracture*. The usual mechanism involves a fall on the outstretched hand.[11] In nearly all cases, the distal fragment is displaced posteriorly. One percent of these fractures are caused by forces applied directly to the olecranon and have anterior displacement.

Supracondylar fractures can be either complete or incomplete. Complete fractures are easily identified (Fig. 5-22). Incomplete fractures can be subtle and may not have a discrete fracture line or break in the cortex (Fig. 5-23).[11] Incomplete injuries include greenstick fractures, cortex buckling (torus fractures), and "plastic bowing." Assessment of the *anterior humeral line* is the best way to detect a subtle supracondylar fracture (Fig. 5-10A). On the lateral film, a line drawn along the anterior surface of the humeral shaft normally intersects with the middle third of the capitellar ossification center. With a supracondylar fracture, the distal portion of the humerus is usually displaced posteriorly, so the anterior humeral line passes anterior to the middle third of the capitellum.[11] A fat-pad sign is another important clue to the presence of this fracture. In a child without a visible fracture, the presence of a fat-pad sign should be presumed to indicate an occult supracondylar fracture.

Loss of the normal valgus carrying angle is the most common complication of a complete supracondylar fracture. Se-verely displaced fractures can injure the brachial artery and median nerve. All complete or displaced supracondylar fractures require orthopedic consultation. Because most displaced supracondylar fractures are now being treated with operative internal fixation and early mobilization, the incidence of Volkmann's ischemic contracture (forearm compartment syndrome) has substantially declined.

Lateral Condylar Fractures

Fractures of the lateral humeral condyle are Salter-Harris type IV fractures. The fracture line runs from the metaphysis of the lateral condyle to the intercondylar region of the unossified epiphysis (Fig. 5-24).[24,25] These injuries account for 10 to 20% of pediatric elbow fractures and tend to occur in infants and young children. Most result from a fall on the outstretched hand with the forearm supinated. Incomplete fractures, which are nondisplaced, can be extremely subtle. Complete fractures are usually displaced posteriorly and inferiorly by the traction forces of the forearm extensor muscles. Any separation is significant because of the high incidence of nonunion. Treatment usually requires internal fixation. Even nondisplaced fractures must be followed closely to detect secondary displacement from the pull of the extensor tendons.

Routine films often underestimate the degree of displacement or can miss a nondisplaced fracture. A posterior fat pad is usually seen with this injury. Oblique radiographs may be necessary to demonstrate the fracture. Therefore, oblique films should be considered on all children with a posterior fat pad and no evidence of fracture on a standard elbow study.[5] Radiographic signs of this injury include a posterior fat-pad sign, a

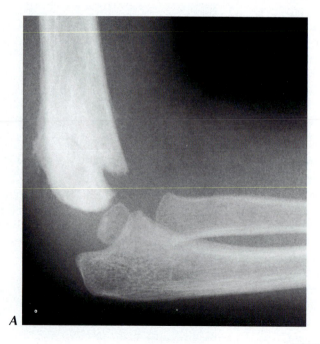

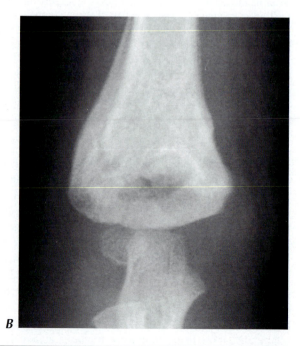

FIGURE 5-22.   A displaced supracondylar fracture. This fracture requires immediate reduction.

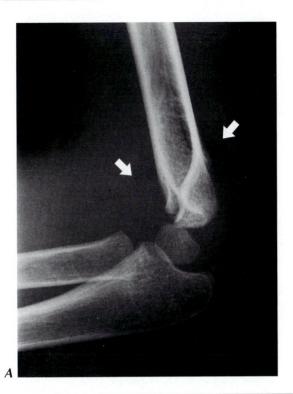
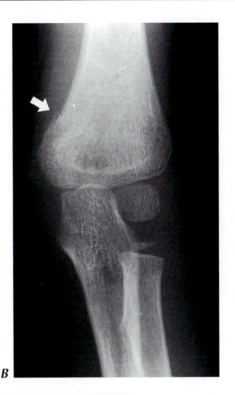

FIGURE 5-23. An incomplete supracondylar fracture. This fracture is akin to a green-stick or buckle fracture. *A.* On the lateral view, anterior and posterior fat-pad signs are seen (*arrows*). The anterior humeral line along the anterior cortex of the humeral shaft intersects the anterior third, rather than the middle third, of the capitellum. *B.* On the AP view, there is slight buckling of the medial surface of the humeral metaphysis (*arrow*).

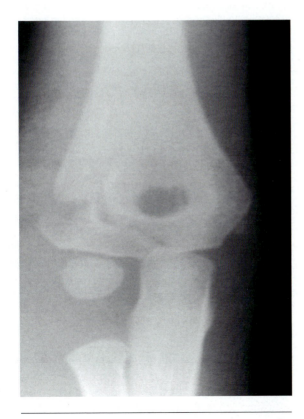

FIGURE 5-24. Fracture of the lateral humeral condyle. The amount of displacement mandates surgical repair.

lateral metaphyseal flake (a thin rim of bone separated from the distal humeral metaphysis), and, if the fracture is displaced, disruption of the radiocapitellar line.

Medial Epicondylar Fractures

Although uncommon in adults, medial epicondylar injuries are common in later childhood and adolescence. The flexor-pronator muscles of the forearm and the ulnar collateral ligament attach to the medial epicondyle. The injury is caused by traction of these structures during valgus stress. Four types of injuries to the medial epicondyle are seen: avulsion, avulsion with entrapment, avulsion associated with elbow dislocation, and, rarely, a Salter-Harris type IV fracture involving the entire medial humeral condyle.

Avulsion. Avulsions of the medial epicondyle result from a fall on the outstretched hand, direct valgus impact, or violent contraction of the flexor-pronator muscle group—"Little Leaguer's elbow" in child baseball pitchers.[26] (The term *Little Leaguer's elbow* is also applied to a chronic overuse syndrome

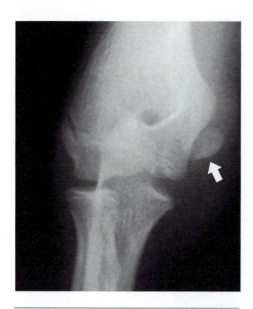

FIGURE 5-25. Medial epicondylar avulsion. The medial epicondyle is displaced inferiorly owing to traction from the flexion-pronator muscles.

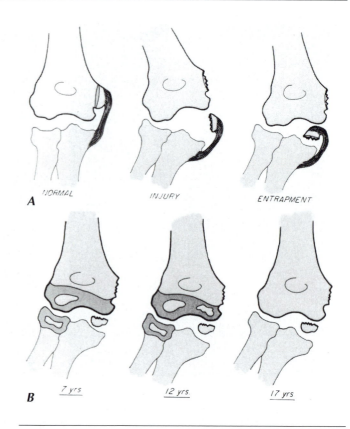

FIGURE 5-26. Avulsion of the medial epicondyle. *A.* Entrapment of the medial epicondyle is possible owing to traction of the ulnar collateral ligament during valgus stress. *B.* The resultant radiographic appearance of entrapment is illustrated before trochlear ossification (7 years), after trochlear ossification (12 years), and at maturity (17 years). Before 9 years of age, the trochlea is not ossified and the entrapped medial epicondyle should not be misinterpreted as a trochlea ossification center. The trochlear ossification center never appears before there is an ossified medial epicondyle. (From Chessare JW, Rogers LF, White H, Tachdjian MO: Injuries of the medial epicondylar ossification center of the humerus. *AJR* 129:49, 1977, with permission.)

characterized by fragmentation and hypertrophy of the medial epicondyle.) The avulsed medial epicondyle is often inferiorly displaced by traction of the flexor-pronator muscles. This injury is best identified on the AP radiograph (Fig. 5-25).[27] Although the lateral film does not directly visualize the injury, it can be of value. Because the medial epicondyle is extraarticular, a simple avulsion fracture does not cause a joint effusion.[28] The presence of a positive fat-pad sign on the lateral film in a patient with medial epicondylar fracture suggests entrapment or a Salter-Harris type IV medial condylar fracture.[29]

Entrapment.   The medial epicondyle can become entrapped within the elbow joint. The valgus stress responsible for the medial epicondyle avulsion fracture transiently opens the joint space allowing the fracture fragment to enter the joint. The radiographic findings must be correlated with the expected age-dependent appearance of the elbow's ossification centers (Fig. 5-26). Before the age of normal trochlear ossification, at 7 to 10 years, the entrapped medial epicondyle must not be mistaken for the trochlear ossification center.[27] After ossification of the trochlea, the entrapped medial epicondyle is located between the trochlea and the coronoid process. Joint effusions are often seen in medial epicondyle entrapment, whereas an effusion is absent with simple medial epicondyle avulsions.

Avulsion with Elbow Dislocation.   Avulsion of the medial epicondyle is often seen with elbow dislocations.[30] As the elbow is dislocated, the ulnar collateral ligament exerts traction on the medial epicondyle, causing an avulsion fracture. The position of the medial epicondyle is variable; it must be clearly identified on postreduction films to exclude joint entrapment. Entrapment is suspected clinically when there is limited range of motion after reduction (Fig. 5-27).[27]

Salter-Harris Type IV Fracture of the Medial Condyle.   The rarest of these injuries is a Salter-Harris type IV fracture involving the medial humeral condyle. This injury should not be misinterpreted as a simple avulsion of the medial epicondyle. The fracture line extends from above the medial condyle to the capitellar-trochlear groove in the epiphysis. The fracture fragment includes the medial portion of the distal humeral metaphysis (including the medial epicondyle) and a portion of the cartilaginous trochlea. If the trochlea has not yet ossified, a "metaphyseal flake" avulsed along with the medial epicondyle provides the only clue to the diagnosis (Fig. 5-28).[29,31] Medial condylar fractures result in significant morbidity because they are unstable and require operative repair. A Salter-Harris type IV medial condylar fracture is suspected when there is a joint effusion, a metaphyseal flake, or joint instability with lack of elbow mobility on physical examination.

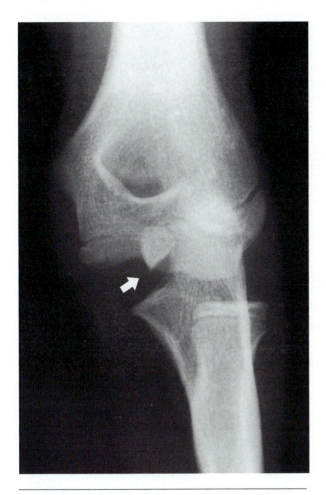

FIGURE 5-27. Entrapment of the medial epicondyle that occurred during an elbow dislocation.

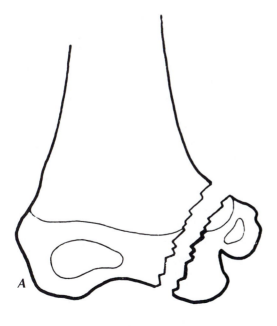

Separation of Entire Distal Humeral Epiphysis

Separation of the entire distal humeral epiphysis is a rare injury. It usually results from a fall on the outstretched hand, from lifting an infant by the forearm, or, in rare cases, by birth injury.[32,33] This injury is a Salter-Harris type I or II fracture at the junction between the distal humeral metaphysis and the epiphysis. It occurs prior to fusion of the epiphysis.[34]

Separation of the humeral epiphysis can be mistakenly diagnosed as an irreducible dislocation of the elbow or a fracture of the lateral condyle.[35] The differentiation is important because these latter lesions require open reduction, whereas epiphyseal separation is treated with closed reduction. The radiocapitellar line is used to distinguish these injuries (Fig. 5-12). With complete epiphyseal separation, the radial head maintains its normal relationship to the capitellum. With dislocation of the elbow or a lateral condylar fracture, the radiocapitellar line is disrupted. Finally, epiphyseal separation causes the radiocapitellar articulation to be displaced medially, whereas in elbow dislocations, the radius and ulna are almost always deviated laterally.[34]

Nursemaid's Elbow

The annular ligament secures the radial head to the ulna. In children below 5 years of age, it is only loosely attached to the radius.[36,37] With extension and forced pronation of the elbow, the annular ligament slips over the radial head and becomes entrapped within the radiocapitellar joint. This common pediatric injury is called a *pulled elbow* or *nursemaid's elbow*. The classic mechanism involves lifting the child by the wrist. The child immediately complains of pain and refuses to use the involved arm.[36] The arm is held at the side with the elbow flexed and the forearm in midpronation. Although this injury is sometimes referred to as "radial head subluxation," that term is incorrect, because it is actually the *annular ligament* that is subluxed. The radial head is neither subluxed nor dislocated.

There is no reason to obtain radiographs if the history and physical examination reveal classic findings for this condition, because the radiographic evaluation would be normal. The radiocapitellar line is always maintained. Radiographs are indicated if the history or physical examination is atypical or if there is failure to reduce the injury.

Two common maneuvers are used to reduce a nursemaid's elbow. The first is elbow supination with flexion. The second involves supination and extension of the elbow. This latter maneuver is often performed when the child is being positioned for radiography and frequently restores the annular ligament to its normal position.

FIGURE 5-28. Fracture of the medial condyle in the immature elbow prior to trochlear ossification. (From Chessare JW, Rogers LF, White H, Tachdjian MO: Injuries of the medial epicondylar ossification center of the humerus. *AJR* 129:49, 1977, with permission.)

ERRORS IN INTERPRETATION

Fracture of the Radial Head.   Fracture of the radial head is the most common adult elbow fracture (Fig. 5-13). Subtle fractures are difficult to see, and a small percentage of fractures are not evident on initial radiographs.[38] Fractures of the radial head are suspected in adults when a joint effusion is present without a visible fracture.

Supracondylar Fracture.   Up to 25% of cases of incomplete supracondylar fractures are inconspicuous greenstick fractures, buckling of a cortex, or plastic bowing.[11] In such instances, it is critical to search for a joint effusion and assess the anterior humeral line (Figs. 5-5, 5-10, and 5-23).

Failure to Recognize a Joint Effusion.   Because of an occasionally indistinct appearance, the sail sign of the anterior fat pad is easier to overlook than a posterior fat pad. A fat pad is missed if the film is overpenetrated and not viewed with a bright light. A joint effusion alerts the physician to either a radial head fracture (in adults) or a supracondylar fracture (in children).

Fracture of the Coronoid Process.   A fractured coronoid process is frequently associated with elbow dislocations. The coronoid fracture can become entrapped in the joint during relocation. This injury should be sought in all elbow dislocations.

Dislocation of the Radial Head.   Dislocation of the radial head is associated with an ulnar shaft fracture in a Monteggia fracture/dislocation. The dislocation of the radial head can be overlooked, especially when the ulnar fracture is located distally. Monteggia fracture/dislocations are uncommon in childhood and can be difficult to detect when the ulna undergoes plastic bowing rather than a discrete fracture.[39] To avoid this error, one should always confirm radiocapitellar alignment.

Osteochondritis Dissecans.   In children 10 to 15 years of age, chronic, repetitive, valgus stress can result in a disruption of the blood supply to a focal area of the capitellar surface. The small lucency that develops in the bone can be overlooked, with eventual progression to fragmentation and the formation of loose bodies in the joint (Fig. 5-29).[40,41]

Failure to Recognize an Entrapped Medial Epicondyle. Knowledge of the normal ossification sequence prevents mistaking an entrapped fragment as a trochlear ossification center (Fig. 5-27). Avulsion of the medial epicondylar ossification center is common during elbow dislocation. Postreduction films must be examined for entrapment of the fragment in the joint space (Fig. 5-28).

Lateral Condylar Fracture in Children.   When they are not displaced, lateral condylar fractures may be evident only on oblique projections. A posterior fat pad is almost always present and should prompt the ordering of oblique films when this injury is suspected (Fig. 5-24).[5]

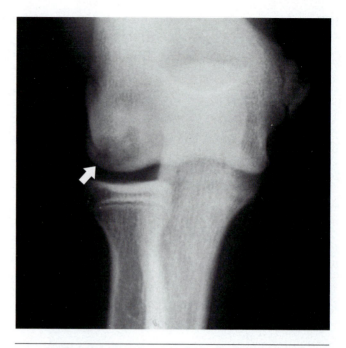

FIGURE 5-29.   Osteochondritis dissecans. Irregular lucency and sclerosis of the capitellum is seen.

Failure to Distinguish Separation of the Entire Distal Humeral Epiphysis from an Elbow Dislocation.   Two observations lead to the correct diagnosis. First, medial displacement is the usual result of separation of the distal humeral epiphysis, whereas medial dislocation of the elbow is extremely rare. Second, the radiocapitellar line is maintained in the distal epiphyseal separation, whereas it is disrupted in an elbow dislocation (Fig. 5-12*E*).

COMMON VARIANTS

In children, there is frequently variation in the appearance of the ossification centers between the two elbows. The olecranon and trochlear ossification centers are notorious for an irregular and fragmented appearance that simulates a fracture. In addition, an ossification center may remain partially nonunited into adult life.[8] Differentiation of these normal variants from fractures is based on clinical findings and the radiographic appearance of the fragment (e.g., rounded, smooth cortex).

In the adult elbow, cortical notches above the medial epicondyle can mimic a fracture (Fig. 5-30). Another variant is the supracondylar process of the distal humerus. This linear, horn-like osseous structure protrudes from the volar surface superior to the medial epicondyle and points toward the joint. Direct blows to the supracondylar process can result in a fracture and damage to the median nerve.[42]

Accessory ossicles are rare at the elbow. The patella cubiti is a sesamoid bone that develops in the triceps tendon.[43] Other ossicles include the antecubital bone, the paratrochlear bone, and the accessory coronoid.

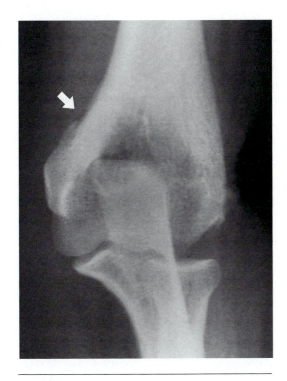

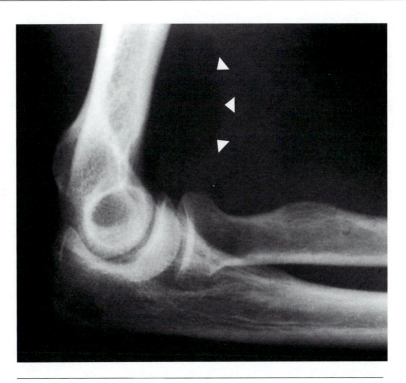

FIGURE 5-30. A cortical notch on the medial surface of the distal humerus simulates a fracture (*arrow*).

FIGURE 5-31. A lipoma mimicking a joint effusion (anterior fat-pad sign).

A lipoma is occasionally located at the distal humerus. The radiographic appearance of the lipoma can mimic a joint effusion (Fig. 5-31).

CONTROVERSIES

Comparison Films

Comparison views are often used to assess ossification centers in children. The comparison film helps to distinguish subtle fractures from normal developmental anatomy. Nevertheless, the value of comparison films is debatable. Rickett and Finlay[44] reviewed the use of comparison radiographs in an emergency department and concluded that no additional information was provided. These films served only to "emphasize the abnormal or normal feature already shown." A similar study showed that the diagnostic accuracy among residents, emergency physicians, and a pediatric radiologist was not improved by the use of comparison films in elbow trauma.[45] However, both of these studies focused on specific situations, such as identifying subtle displacement of the medial epicondyle or gauging alignment in fracture reduction. The usefulness of comparison views is further limited by the developmental asymmetry that often occurs in the pediatric elbow. More important than comparison views is a firm working knowledge of developmental anatomy. Nevertheless, in selected cases, a comparison view of the contralateral elbow can prove useful to the clinician.

Significance of a Positive Fat Pad without an Identified Fracture

The need for repeat radiographic evaluation 1 to 2 weeks after initial presentation has been an area of conflicting opinion. One study of patients with fat-pad signs and no fracture found that 29% had a identifiable fracture on follow-up.[46] Other studies advise against repeat films because of a lower incidence of delayed fracture recognition (6 to 12%); most such fractures are nondisplaced fractures of the radial head.[38] The yield on such films is low and does not change treatment. Management of patients with joint effusions and no identifiable fracture entails informing the patient about the possibility of an undetected fracture, arranging follow-up, and providing conservative treatment (immobilization with a sling or splint) until symptoms subside.

CONCLUSION

Radiographic evaluation of the elbow requires a systematic approach. The clinician must be aware of common injuries and their respective radiographic findings. Subtle injuries can be inferred from abnormal fat pads. Firm knowledge of anatomy is critical, and important anatomic relationships such as the radiocapitellar line and the anterior humeral line should be confirmed on all films. During the review of pediatric films, keeping in mind the correct sequence of ossification centers helps to differentiate an injury from normal development. When a systematic review of elbow radiographs is coupled with a complete history and physical, appropriate injury recognition is ensured.

REFERENCES

1. Hawksworth CR, Freeland P: Inability to fully extend the injured elbow: An indicator of significant injury. *Arch Emerg Med* 8:253, 1991.

2. Hunter RD: Swollen elbow following trauma. *JAMA* 230:1573, 1974.

3. Murphy WA, Siegel MJ: Elbow fat pads with new signs and extended differential diagnosis. *Radiology* 124:659, 1977.

4. Williams PL, Warwick R, Dyson M, Bannister LH: *Gray's Anatomy,* 13th ed. London: Churchill Livingstone, 1989, p. 505.

5. Rogers LF: The elbow and forearm, in Rogers LF (ed): *Radiology of Skeletal Trauma,* 2d ed. New York: Churchill Livingstone, 1992, pp. 749–836.

6. Hall-Craggs MA, Shorvon PJ: Assessment of the radial head–capitellum view and the dorsal fat-pad sign in acute elbow trauma. *AJR* 145:607, 1985.

7. Brodeur AE, Silberstein MJ, Graviss ER, Luisiri A: The basic tenets for appropriate evaluation of the elbow in pediatrics. *Curr Probl Diagn Radiol* 12:1, 1983.

8. Tachdjian MO: Introduction, in Tachdjian MO (ed): *Pediatric Orthopedics,* 2d ed. Philadelphia, Saunders, 1990, pp. 60–61.

9. Silverman FN: The bones: Normals and variants, in Silverman FN, Kuhn JP (eds): *Caffey's Pediatric X-ray Diagnosis: An Integrated Imaging Approach,* 9th ed. St. Louis: Mosby, 1992, pp. 1492–1496.

10. McCarthy SM, Ogden JA: Radiology of postnatal skeletal development. *Skel Radiol* 7:239, 1982.

11. Rogers LF, Malave S, White H, Tachdjian MO: Plastic bowing, torus, and greenstick supracondylar fractures of the humerus: Radiographic clues to obscure fractures of the elbow in children. *Radiology* 128:145, 1978.

12. Conn J, Wade PA: Injuries of the elbow: A ten year review. *J Trauma* 1:248, 1961.

13. Goldberg I, Peylan J, Yosipovitch Z, Tiqva P: Late results of excision of the radial head for isolated closed fracture. *J Bone Joint Surg* 68:675, 1986.

14. Maylahn DJ, Fahey JJ: Fractures of the elbow in children. *JAMA* 166:220, 1958.

15. Horne JG, Tanzer TL: Olecranon fractures: A review of 100 cases. *J Trauma* 21:469, 1981.

16. Neviaser JS, Wickstrom JK: Dislocation of the elbow: A retrospective study of 115 patients. *South Med J* 2:172, 1977.

17. Floyd WE, Gebhardt MC, Emans JB: Intra-articular entrapment of the median nerve after elbow dislocation. *J Hand Surg* 12A:704, 1987.

18. Bado JL: The Monteggia lesion. *Clin Orthop* 50:71, 1967.

19. Bruce HE, Harvey P, Wilson JC: Monteggia fractures. *J Bone Joint Surg* 56A:1563, 1974.

20. Kenn-Cohen BT: Fractures of the elbow. *J Bone Joint Surg* 48:1623, 1966.

21. Aitken GK, Rorabek CH: Distal humeral fractures in the adult. *Clin Orthop* 207:191, 1986.

22. Risenborough EJ, Radin EL: Intercondylar T fractures of the humerus in the adult. *J Bone Joint Surg* 51A:130, 1969.

23. Henley MB: Intra-articular distal humeral fractures in adults. *Orthop Clin North Am* 18:11, 1987.

24. Badelon O, Bensahel H, Mazda K, Vie P: Lateral humeral condylar fractures in children: A report of 47 cases. *J Pediatr Orthop* 8:31, 1988.

25. Fontanetta P, Mackensie DA, Rosman M: Missed, maluniting, and malunited fractures of the lateral condyle. *J Trauma* 18:329, 1978.

26. Brogdon BG, Crow NE: Little Leaguer's elbow. *AJR* 83:671, 1960.

27. Chessare JW, Rogers LF, White H, Tachdjian MO: Injuries of the medial epicondylar ossification center of the humerus. *AJR* 129:49, 1977.

28. Silberstein MJ, Brodeur AE, Graviss ER, Luisiri A: Some vagaries of the medial epicondyle. *J Bone Joint Surg* 63:524, 1981.

29. De Boeck H, Casteleyn PP, Opdecam P: Fracture of the medial humeral epicondyle. *J Bone Joint Surg* 69A:1442, 1987.

30. Smith FM: Medial epicondylar injury. *JAMA* 142:396, 1950.

31. Fahey JJ, O'Brien ET: Fracture-separation of the medial condyle in a child confused with fracture of the medial epicondyle. *J Bone Joint Surg* 53:1102, 1975.

32. DeLee JC, Wilkins KE, Rogers LF, Rockwood CA: Fracture-separation of the distal humeral epiphysis. *J Bone Joint Surg* 62A:46, 1980.

33. McIntyre WM, Wiley JJ, Charette RJ: Fracture-separation of the distal humeral epiphysis. *Clin Orthop* 188:98, 1984.

34. Ruo GY: Radiographic diagnosis of fracture-separation of the entire distal humeral epiphysis. *Clin Radiol* 38:635, 1987.

35. Rogers LF, Rockwood CA: Separation of the entire distal humeral epiphysis. *Radiology* 106:393, 1973.

36. Schunk JE: Radial head subluxation: Epidemiology and treatment of 87 episodes. *Ann Emerg Med* 19:1019, 1990.

37. David ML: Radial head subluxation. *Am Fam Physician* 35:143, 1987.

38. deBeaux AC, Beattie T, Gilbert F: Elbow fat pad sign: Implications for clinical management. *J R Coll Surg Edinb* 37:205, 1992.

39. Gleeson AP, Beattie TF: Monteggia fracture-dislocation in children. *J Accid Emerg Med* 11:192, 1994.

40. Fritz RC, Brody GA: MR imaging of the wrist and elbow. *Clin Sports Med* 14:315, 1995.

41. Jawish R, Rigault P, Padovani JP, et al: Osteochondritis dissecans of the humeral capitellum in children. *Eur J Pediatr Surg* 3:97, 1993.

42. Kolb LW, Moore RD: Fractures of the supracondylar process of the humerus. *J Bone Joint Surg* 49:532, 1967.

43. Schwarz GS: Bilateral antecubital ossicles (fabellae cubiti) and other rare accessory bones of the elbow. *Radiology* 69:730, 1957.

44. Rickett AB, Finlay DB: An audit of comparison views in elbow trauma in children. *Br J Radiol* 66:123, 1993.

45. Chacon D, Kissoon N, Brown T, Galpin R: Use of comparison radiographs in the diagnosis of injuries of the elbow. *Ann Emerg Med* 21:895, 1992.

46. Morewood DJ: Incidence of unsuspected fractures in traumatic effusions of the elbow joint. *BMJ* 295:109, 1987.

CHAPTER 6

THE SHOULDER AND PROXIMAL HUMERUS

WILLIAM MAGUIRE / DAVID T. SCHWARTZ

The shoulder is the most mobile joint in the body. It allows humans to manipulate the environment by positioning their hands. However, this mobility comes with a price; the shoulder is quite vulnerable to instability. The *shoulder girdle* encompasses four articulating regions—glenohumeral, acromioclavicular (AC), sternoclavicular, scapulothoracic. This chapter focuses on the glenohumeral joint and the nearby structures, including the proximal humerus, adjacent portions of the scapula, and the acromioclavicular region.

The shoulder is subject to a wide variety of injuries and nontraumatic conditions. It is also the site of referred pain from thoracic and abdominal disorders. The patterns of shoulder injury vary according to the age of the patient. Elderly patients tend to have fractures of the proximal humerus and the acromion due to osteoporosis. Younger patients, particularly those involved in athletics, are prone to soft tissue injuries such as AC separations, glenohumeral dislocations, and rotator cuff tears. The shoulder is also subject to numerous degenerative conditions and overuse syndromes.[1]

CLINICAL DECISION MAKING

Patients presenting to the emergency department (ED) with pain in the area of the shoulder and upper arm must be evaluated clinically prior to the ordering of radiographs. Certain life-threatening emergencies can cause shoulder pain, including cardiac ischemia, aortic dissection, pneumothorax, and ruptured abdominal viscera (e.g., spleen). Once these life-threatening causes of shoulder pain have been considered, radiographic evaluation of the shoulder can begin.

The decision to order radiographs of the shoulder is guided by the history and physical examination. Important factors to consider include the mechanism of injury and the existence of prior injuries or degenerative conditions. Both shoulders should be exposed to allow visual comparison and palpation of key structures. Palpation of bones follows an orderly pattern, beginning with the suprasternal notch, clavicle, coracoid process, area of the AC joint, greater tuberosity of the humerus, scapular spine, and vertebral border. The soft tissues should likewise be examined, including the muscles of the rotator cuff, subacromion and subdeltoid bursae, axillae, and muscles of the shoulder girdle.[2]

Patients with Shoulder Trauma. In the patient with shoulder trauma, several findings indicate the need for radiographs: obvious deformity, pain on motion of the shoulder, decreased range of motion, and moderate to severe tenderness. If a patient has only minor tenderness and is able to perform full range of motion, then radiographs can be omitted. One must be certain that the adjoining structures—chest, ribs, cervical spine, clavicle, sternum, or scapula—are also nontender. If they are tender, radiographs of these areas should be ordered.

Because most of the shoulder is covered by a thick envelope of muscle, it is difficult to distinguish bone tenderness from soft tissue tenderness. However, the AC region has only a thin cutaneous covering and is easily palpated for deformity and bone tenderness. Radiographs are ordered if there is more than mild tenderness of the AC joint.

Elderly patients with shoulder pain following trauma merit special consideration. Fractures of the distal clavicle and proximal humerus are common in the elderly, so the threshold should be lower for ordering radiographs in older patients.[3] Fractures of the humeral shaft are usually obvious on clinical examination and cause marked pain, deformity, and abnormal motion at the site of the fracture. Any patient with a physical examination indicative of a clavicular or scapular fracture requires specific clavicular or scapular views because fractures can be missed on radiographic views of the shoulder.

Patients with Nontraumatic Shoulder Pain. Many nontraumatic conditions cause shoulder pain and some have characteristic radiographic findings. Moreover, life-threatening intrathoracic and intraabdominal processes can cause referred pain in the shoulder. Intraabdominal disorders that can cause shoulder pain include ruptured ectopic pregnancy, gallbladder disease, liver disease, and intraabdominal blood or pus. Lesions of the lung apex (e.g., Pancoast tumor) or thoracic outlet can also cause shoulder pain.

Certain patients warrant special consideration. Patients with a history of malignancy, sickle cell disease, or steroid use should have radiographs of the shoulder ordered liberally. Patients with osteoarthritis can have significant shoulder pain, and radiographs are helpful in establishing this diagnosis. However, because osteoarthritis is a chronic condition, no ED visit should be attributed to osteoarthritis without consideration of alternative causes of shoulder pain.

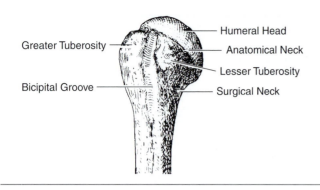

FIGURE 6-1. Anatomy of the proximal humerus. (Modified from Pansky B: *Review of Gross Anatomy,* 6th ed. New York: McGraw-Hill, 1996. With permission.)

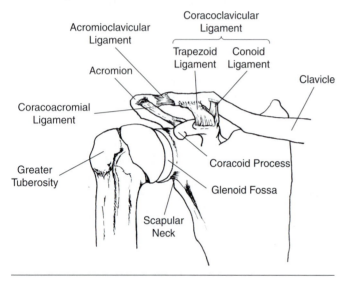

FIGURE 6-2. Ligamentous anatomy of the shoulder.

ANATOMY AND PHYSIOLOGY

The shoulder is composed of three bones (the proximal humerus, scapula, and clavicle). The articular surface of the proximal humerus is the humeral head. The junction between the articular surface and adjacent humerus is the anatomic neck. The "surgical neck" of the humerus is where the humeral shaft begins to widen into the metaphysis. This is the site of most proximal humeral fractures. There are two protuberances on the humeral metaphysis—the greater and lesser tuberosities. Between the tuberosities is a groove for the tendon of the long head of the biceps (Fig. 6-1).

The acromion, coracoid process, and clavicle are held together by ligaments (Fig. 6-2). The strongest ligament is the coracoclavicular ligament. The AC ligament anchors the distal clavicle to the acromion. The coracoacromial ligament spans the region superior to the humeral head.

The glenohumeral joint has a very wide range of motion. The glenoid fossa is a shallow depression serving as the articular surface for the humeral head. The shallowness of the glenoid fossa contributes to both the mobility and instability of the shoulder. The only skeletal component stabilizing the glenohumeral joint is the acromion, which forms a roof over the joint.

The glenohumeral joint is surrounded by a muscular envelope called the rotator cuff. It is composed of four muscles, three of which—the supraspinatus, infraspinatus, and teres minor—insert onto the greater tuberosity of the humerus. The subscapularis muscle inserts on the lesser tuberosity. The humeral head receives its blood supply from the anterior and posterior circumflex arteries, which encircle the humeral neck.

The scapula is a large, flat bone with two prominences (the acromion and the coracoid) that serve as a scaffold for the glenohumeral joint. The clavicle is a strut that attaches the shoulder to the thoracic skeleton. The clavicle has an S shape that extends from the manubrium to the acromion. On the inferior surface, the clavicle has muscular attachments to the chest wall (pectoralis major and deltoid muscles); on its superior and lateral surfaces are insertions of the sternocleidomastoid and trapezius muscles.[4]

Developmental Considerations.   At birth, the acromion, coracoid, and glenoid are cartilaginous and not visible on plain radiographs. The coracoid ossification center appears at 1 to 2 years of age. A subcoracoid and upper glenoid ossification center appears at about 10 years of age. Ossification centers for the glenoid margin, inferior angle, scapular border, and acromion appear at puberty and fuse between 20 and 25 years of age. The humeral shaft is ossified at birth. The main ossification center of the humeral head is present at birth or appears shortly thereafter. Ossification centers for the greater and lesser tuberosities appear in the first year of life. The three ossification centers of the proximal humerus coalesce between the third and seventh years to form a single epiphysis.

RADIOGRAPHIC TECHNIQUE

The standard radiographic series for the shoulder often varies from institution to institution (Table 6-1). Frequently, only anteroposterior (AP) views of the shoulder are obtained. To evaluate patients with trauma, some institutions use an AP view and a scapular Y view. In other institutions, a complete trauma series includes three orthogonal projections of the shoulder: an AP view, a scapular Y view, and an axillary view.[5] This provides complete information about complex fractures and dislocations.

Anteroposterior Shoulder Views

In patients with no history of recent trauma, two AP views are obtained (Fig. 6-3). In one, the arm is in external rotation, while in the other, the arm is in internal rotation. When the arm is externally rotated, the greater tuberosity of the humerus is seen in profile. With the arm in internal rotation, the greater tuberosity of the humerus is seen *en face* over the humeral head and the lesser tuberosity is near the glenohumeral joint.

Although these two views constitute the "standard shoulder series" in some institutions, they may be insufficient in evaluating shoulder trauma. AP shoulder views provide inadequate

TABLE 6-1

Radiographic Views of the Shoulder

VIEW	POSITION	EVALUATION OF ADEQUACY	LIKELY FINDINGS
AP view, external rotation	Patient in frontal plane Humerus externally rotated	Shoulder at 30–40° oblique plane Greater tuberosity of humerus seen laterally *in profile*	Obvious fractures and dislocations Greater tuberosity fracture AC injuries Calcifications of supraspinatus tendon
AP view, internal rotation	Humerus internally rotated	Proximal humerus seen with greater tuberosity *en face* Lesser tuberosity over the glenohumeral joint	Obvious fractures and dislocations Lesser tuberosity fracture Widening of AC space Calcification of infraspinatus, teres minor, or subscapularis tendons
Posterior oblique view (Grashey view)	Patient in 40° posterior oblique position	Lateral view of glenohumeral joint Clear joint space between humeral articular surface and glenoid fossa	Posterior shoulder dislocation (glenohumeral surfaces overlap) Degenerative narrowing of joint space.
Scapular Y view	Patient angled so body of scapula is perpendicular to film	Frontal view of glenohumeral joint Scapula has Y shape Humeral head is visible	Shoulder dislocations Anterior Posterior Scapular fractures
Axillary view	Patient supine with arm abducted X-ray beam directed from apex of axilla to film cassette	Identify glenoid rim and position of humeral head	Shoulder dislocations Anterior Posterior Impaction fractures of humeral head Glenoid rim fractures Acromion fractures

information about the glenohumeral joint because the glenohumeral joint is seen in an oblique orientation. In addition, although the two AP views provide different views of the proximal humerus, the glenohumeral joint and the scapula are seen from only one perspective.

In some cases, a *neutral AP view* is obtained. This view has the advantage of not requiring the patient to rotate the arm, which can be painful. The drawback of this view is that the "neutral position" varies from patient to patient.

Lateral Scapular View (Y View)

The scapular lateral or Y view does not require movement of the injured shoulder (Fig. 6-4). This view is obtained by positioning the patient's body rather than the arm. The view is nearly perpendicular to standard AP views. It identifies glenohumeral dislocations, humeral fractures, and some scapular fractures.[6]

In a normal Y view, the humeral head overlies the center of the glenoid cavity. In most patients, the glenoid itself is not seen; the glenoid fossa is located at the junction of the three arms of the Y. In anterior or posterior dislocations of the gleno-

humeral joint, the humeral head displaces in the corresponding direction with respect to the glenoid fossa.

Posterior Oblique View (Grashey View)

The posterior oblique radiograph provides a view oriented parallel to the glenohumeral joint (Fig. 6-5). This view is obtained with the patient in a 45° posterior oblique orientation. Because the glenoid fossa is seen in profile, it can be examined for narrowing of the joint space (due to loss of articular cartilage or a posterior shoulder dislocation).[7] One difficulty in obtaining the posterior oblique view is that there are no clear anatomic landmarks for the technician to use in positioning the patient. As a result, the view does not always provide a precise view of the glenohumeral joint space.

Axillary View

The axillary view provides an axial view of the shoulder that clearly delineates the glenohumeral joint (Fig. 6-6). The clavicle and coracoid project anteriorly, the acromion and the acromioclavicular joint overlie the humeral head, and the lesser

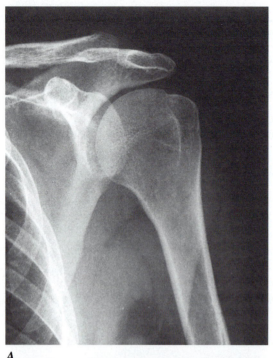

A

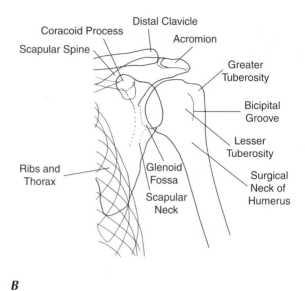

B

FIGURE 6-3. *A* and *B*. AP radiograph with shoulder in external rotation. *C*. AP radiograph with shoulder in internal rotation.

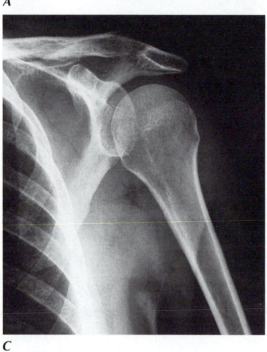

C

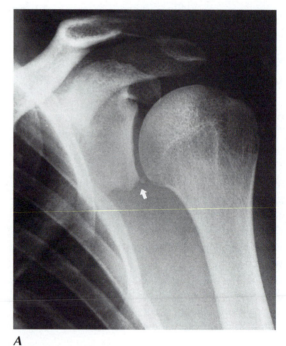

A

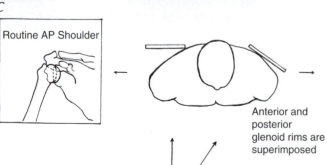

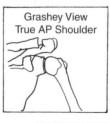

B

FIGURE 6-5. *A*. Grashey view (posterior oblique view). The glenohumeral joint space is seen without overlap. The humerus is in external rotation (the greater tuberosity is lateral). The clavicle is foreshortened. A small fracture is seen at the inferior aspect of the glenoid rim (Bankhart lesion)(*arrow*). *B*. Positioning for the routine AP shoulder radiograph and the Grashey view.

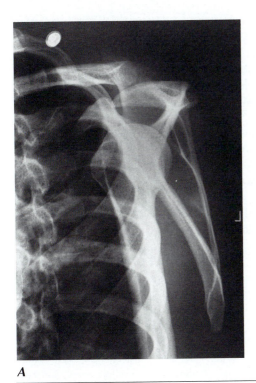

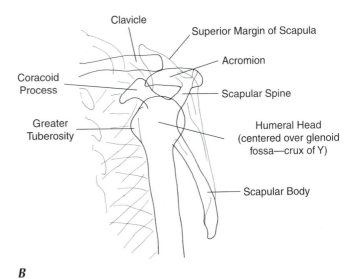

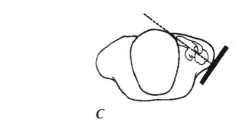

A

FIGURE 6-4. *A, B.* Y view of the shoulder. *C.* Positioning for the Y view of the shoulder. (From Perry CR, Elstrom JA, Pankovich AM: *Handbook of Fractures.* New York: McGraw-Hill: 1995. With permission.)

B

C

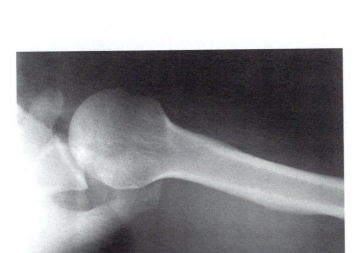

A

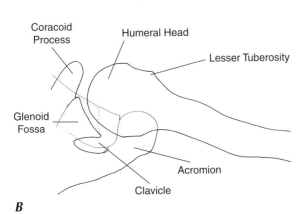

B

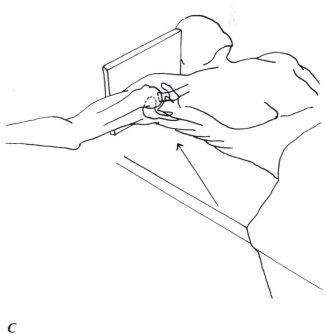

C

FIGURE 6-6. *A, B.* Axillary view of the shoulder. *C.* Positioning for the axillary view.

tuberosity lies anteriorly. In positioning this view, the patient is supine, the film cassette is placed against the superior aspect of the shoulder, and the x-ray beam is directed into the apex of the axilla. This view requires the patient to abduct the injured arm.[8] Ideally, the patient abducts the arm to 90°, but this is frequently impractical in a patient with shoulder trauma. Fifteen degrees of abduction is less painful and reduces the risk of displacing a fractured humeral neck. Displacement of a humeral neck fracture increases the risk of avascular necrosis of the humeral head.[9]

Humeral Views

The two standard views of the humerus are the AP and the lateral. The AP view shows the humeral shaft, humeral head, humeral neck, and distal humerus (epicondyles, olecranon fossa, capitellum, and trochlea). The lateral view shows the dorsal and ventral margins of the humeral shaft and the superimposed medial and lateral epicondyles.

RADIOGRAPHIC ANALYSIS

Anteroposterior View

When examining shoulder radiographs, there are two principal regions to consider: the glenohumeral region and the acromioclavicular region. In addition, peripheral regions—the clavicle, scapula, ribs, and thorax—must be examined (Table 6-2) (Fig. 6-7). First, the technical adequacy of the images is assessed. The orientation of the greater tuberosity is noted. The greater tuberosity is laterally located if the humerus is externally rotated, and seen *en face* if the humerus is internally rotated.

Glenohumeral Region.   One begins with examination of glenohumeral alignment. The humeral head should be seated within the glenoid fossa. The overlap of the humeral head and glenoid fossa should appear normal, although there are no definite measurements for assessing this. The distance between the articular surfaces of the humeral head and anterior glenoid rim should be 6 mm or less.

Next, the bones of the glenohumeral region are examined, beginning with the proximal humerus. The articular surface, trabecular pattern, greater tuberosity, lesser tuberosity, humeral neck, and proximal humeral shaft are evaluated. The glenoid fossa and scapular neck are inspected for fractures such as a small chip fracture from the glenoid rim. Calcifications in soft tissue are noted, especially superior to the humeral head. In chronic tears of the rotator cuff, there is a reduced distance between the humeral head and the acromion.

Acromioclavicular Region.   A bright light is used to view the AC region because it is usually underpenetrated (dark). The alignment of these bones is assessed, beginning with the width of the joint space. The inferior margin of the clavicle should be in line with the inferior margin of the acromion. The supe-

rior margin of the clavicle is normally slightly higher than that of the acromion because the clavicle has a greater cross-sectional diameter. The distance between the coracoid process and the clavicle should be less than 11 mm; wider separation implies a tear in the coracoclavicular ligaments. Internal rotation stresses the AC joint, which can improve the detection AC joint separations.[10]

The AC region should be examined for fractures of the distal clavicle or acromion. Degenerative changes, and calcifications are noted. A bone spur from the acromion is associated with impingement syndrome.

Other Regions.   Finally, other regions of the shoulder are assessed. One should look for midshaft fractures in the clavicle. On the scapula, the coracoid process, acromion, scapular body, and scapular spine are checked. The ribs are inspected for fractures and lytic lesions. The lung is examined for pneumothorax or other lesions.

Additional Views

Other views, such as the Y view or the axillary view, are then examined. The relationship of the humeral head to the glenoid fossa is noted so as to identify an anterior or posterior dislocation. The proximal humerus, glenoid rim, scapula, coracoid process, and acromion are examined for fractures.

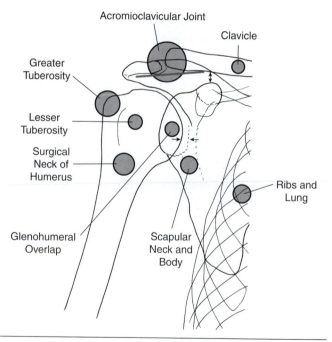

FIGURE 6-7.   Sites of common injury and easily missed injuries. The space between the humeral head and the anterior rim of the glenoid fossa should be 6 mm or less *(facing arrows).* The AC joint space should be 3 to 5 mm wide. The inferior margins of the clavicle and acromion should be aligned *(line).* The space between the coracoid process and clavicle should be less than 11 mm *(double arrow).*

TABLE 6-2

Systematic Analysis of Shoulder Radiographs

Adequacy			At least two views are included and properly performed.
AP view	Glenohumeral region	Alignment	Note orientation of greater tuberosity. It is laterally located if humerus is externally rotated and seen *en face* if humerus is internally rotated. In anterior dislocation, humeral head is markedly displaced medially and inferiorly. Assess amount of overlap of humeral head and glenoid fossa.
		Bones	Proximal humerus (articular surface, trabecular pattern, humeral neck, greater tuberosity, lesser tuberosity, proximal humeral shaft). Glenoid fossa and scapular neck—including small chip fractures from glenoid rim. Note degenerative changes.
		Soft tissues	Calcifications superior to humeral head. Superior migration of humeral head closer to the acromion is seen in chronic tears of the rotator cuff.
	Acromioclavicular region (a bright light may be needed to examine this region)	Alignment	The inferior margin of the clavicle should be aligned with the inferior margin of the acromion. (The superior margin of the clavicle is normally higher than the acromion.) The width of the AC joint space, is normally 3 to 5 mm. The distance between the coracoid process and the clavicle should be less than 11 mm. Wider separation implies a tear of the coracoclavicular ligaments.
		Bones	Distal clavicle fractures. Acromion fractures. Degenerative changes, old injuries, and calcifications.
	Other Regions		Clavicle: Midshaft fractures. Scapula: Coracoid process, acromion, scapular body and spine. Ribs: Fractures or other lesions. Lung: Pneumothorax or lesions in the lung.
Other views—Scapular Y view or Axillary view	Alignment		Note relationship of humeral head to glenoid fossa, looking for anterior or posterior dislocation
	Bones		Fractures of the proximal humerus, glenoid rim, scapular neck, coracoid process, and acromion.

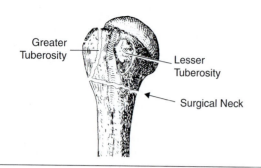

Greater
Tuberosity
Lesser
Tuberosity
Surgical Neck

FIGURE 6-8. Classification of proximal humeral fractures. Fractures are classified by the number of displaced parts, from two to four parts involving the surgical neck, greater tuberosity, or lesser tuberosity. Nondisplaced fractures are considered one-part fractures.

COMMON ABNORMALITIES

Trauma to the shoulder is common. The mechanisms of injury and types of injuries depend on the age of the patient. In younger individuals, injuries are frequently associated with work-related or athletic activities.[11] In elderly patients, falls are a frequent cause of fractures and dislocations.[12]

Proximal Humeral Fractures

Most proximal humeral fractures occur at or just proximal to the surgical neck of the humerus. They usually result from a fall on an outstretched arm or a direct blow. When inspecting the radiographs for fractures, all the margins of the humeral head and neck must be followed: they should appear smooth and contiguous. Some nondisplaced fractures are quite subtle. When humeral neck fractures are displaced, there is danger of avascular necrosis of the humeral head.

The most well-known scheme for classifying proximal humeral fractures was developed by Neer.[13] The Neer classification is based on the number of displaced fracture fragments involving the four principal anatomic components of the proximal humerus: the greater tuberosity, lesser tuberosity, the surgical neck and the humeral shaft (Fig. 6-8). Fractures are classified as one-, two-, three- or four-part, depending on the number of fragments as well as their angulation or displacement (Fig. 6-9). With a proximal humeral fracture, a hemarthrosis can cause widening of the joint space between acromion and humeral head causing it to appear malaligned. This phenomenon is called *pseudodislocation* (Fig. 6-10). A Y view, axillary view or occasionally CT is needed to confirm that the humeral head is not dislocated.

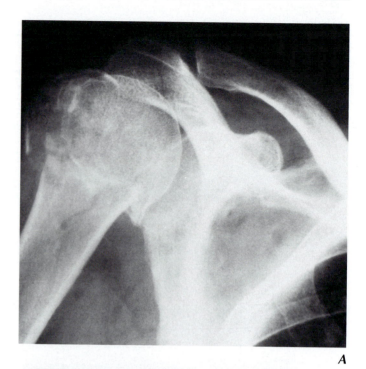

A

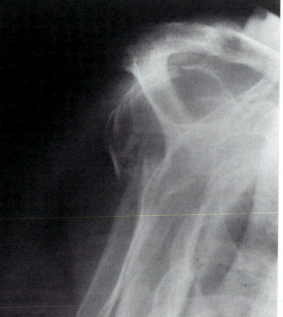

B

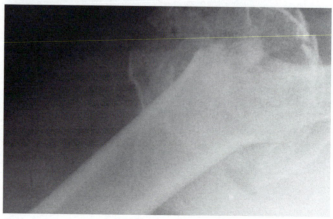

C

FIGURE 6-9. A three-part proximal humeral fracture involving the surgical neck (with impaction and comminution) and the greater tuberosity. There was no dislocation on the Y view or axillary view (*B* and *C*).

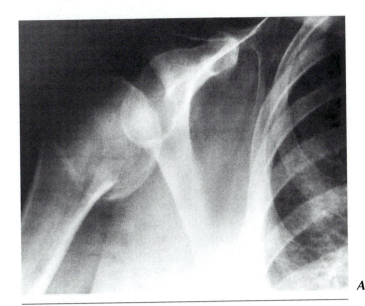

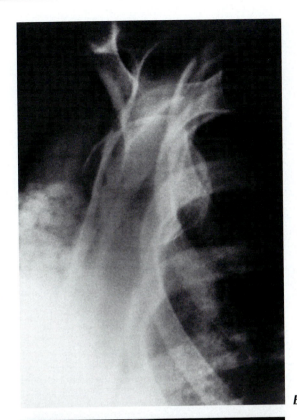

A

B

FIGURE 6-10. Pseudodislocation. On the AP view *(A)*, an impacted fracture of the surgical neck is seen. The humeral head appears dislocated from the glenoid fossa. On the Y view *(B)*, the humeral head is centered on the glenoid fossa (crux of the Y), confirming that no dislocation is present. Inferior displacement of the humeral head is due to distention of the joint capsule by a hemarthrosis. (Copyright David T. Schwartz, M.D.)

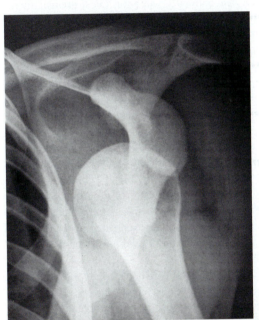

A

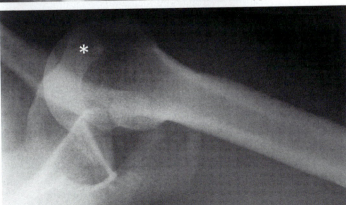

C

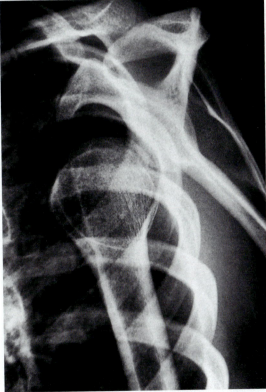

B

FIGURE 6-11. Anterior shoulder dislocation. *A.* On this AP view, the proximal humerus is greatly displaced from the glenoid fossa and lies in a subcoracoid position. The humerus is externally rotated and abducted. *B.* On the Y view, the humeral head is located anterior to the glenoid fossa, overlying the ribs. *C.* On an axillary view, the humeral head is displaced anterior to the glenoid fossa, overlying the coracoid process *(asterisk).*

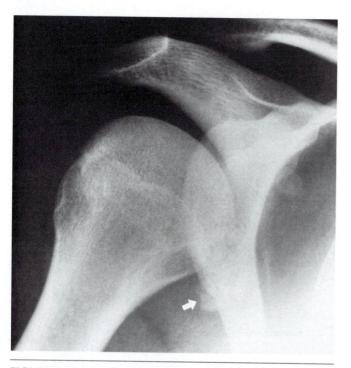

FIGURE 6-12.   Bankart lesion. A fracture of the inferior glenoid rim is seen in a patient with a prior anterior shoulder dislocation. (Also see Fig. 6-4*A*).

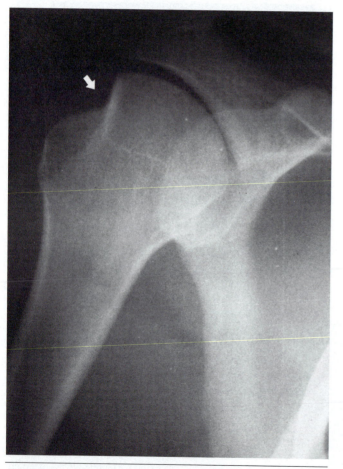

FIGURE 6-13.   Hill-Sachs deformity. A large impaction fracture is present on the lateral surface of the humeral head. This patient had multiple prior anterior shoulder dislocations.

With proximal humeral fractures, an associated dislocation must be diagnosed. This is because a mildly displaced fracture of the proximal humerus is treated with a simple sling or splint, whereas a fracture/dislocation must be reduced. A posterior dislocation can be especially difficult to detect. Because the AP views usually cannot exclude a posterior dislocation, a Y view or axillary view should be obtained. The axillary view must be performed cautiously to avoid causing displacement of the fracture.

Fractures of the Humeral Shaft

Humeral shaft fractures are usually clinically obvious. Radiographically, they are quite apparent. AP and lateral views of the humerus should be obtained if a humeral shaft fracture is suspected. The number of fracture fragments and the degree of angulation of the fragments are important to note. Neurovascular integrity (especially of the redial nerve) must be assessed clinically.

Shoulder Dislocations

The glenohumeral joint is the most frequently dislocated joint in the body because it is so shallow and highly mobile. About 95% of shoulder dislocations are anterior. These are usually obvious clinically and radiographically. Posterior dislocations are infrequent (about 5%). These can be subtle radiographically and are misdiagnosed in as many as 50% of cases at the time of ED presentation. Unfortunately, the consequences of delayed diagnosis are substantial. Nonetheless, by understanding the clinical and radiographic manifestations of this uncommon injury, misdiagnosis can usually be avoided.

ANTERIOR SHOULDER DISLOCATIONS.   Anterior shoulder dislocations are usually due to a fall with the arm abducted, extended, and externally rotated. On clinical examination, there is an obvious step-off deformity with a prominent acromion and an empty glenoid fossa. A visible or palpable fullness is often present anterior to the shoulder, representing the displaced humeral head. The arm is fixed in external rotation and is often abducted.

Radiographically, the findings are equally obvious (Fig. 6-11). The humeral head is completely displaced from the glenoid fossa. In about 90% of cases, the humeral head is in a subcoracoid location. A subglenoid location is seen in most of the remaining cases. Rarely, the humeral head is subclavian or even intrathoracic. Subclavian and intrathoracic shoulder dislocations occur in the setting of severe trauma.

Although it is impossible to tell on the AP radiograph whether the dislocated humeral head is located anterior or posterior to the glenoid fossa, the presence of an anterior dislocation can be deduced from certain findings on the AP radiograph. With an anterior dislocation, the humeral head is greatly displaced out to the glenoid fossa. This cannot occur with a posterior dislocation because the muscles of the rotator cuff prevent such displacement. In addition, with an anterior dislocation, the humeral head is fixed in external rotation with the

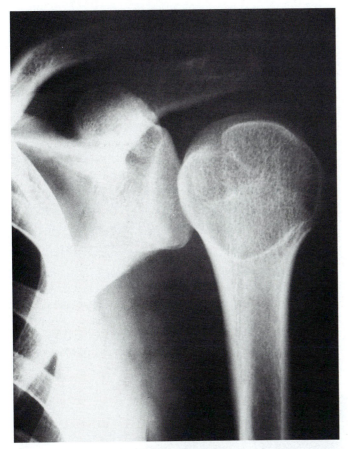

A

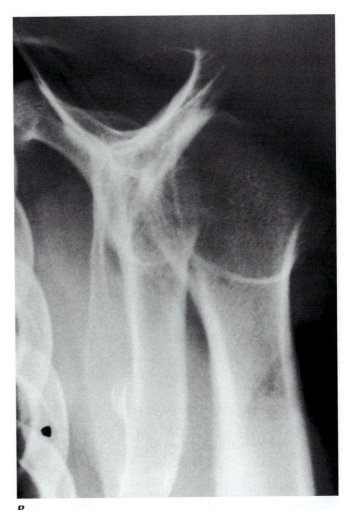

B

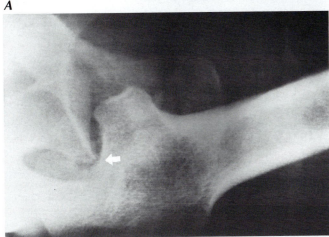

C

FIGURE 6-14. Posterior shoulder dislocation. *A.* On the AP view, the humeral head is displaced lateral to the rim of the glenoid fossa and there is diminished overlap between the humeral head and the glenoid fossa. The proximal humerus is fixed in internal rotation and looks like a "light bulb on a stick." *B.* On the Y view, the humerus is displaced posterior to the glenoid fossa (away from the ribs). *C.* The axillary view in another patient shows the humeral head displaced posterior to the glenoid fossa (opposite the coracoid process). This patient had prior posterior dislocations and has a large impaction fracture on the anterior surface of the humeral head. This is referred to as a "reverse Hill-Sachs" fracture (*arrow*). (Copyright David Schwartz, M.D.).

greater tuberosity located along the lateral aspect of the humeral head. Furthermore, the clinical findings themselves are essentially diagnostic of an anterior dislocation. The Y view and the axillary view directly demonstrate anterior displacement of the humeral head relative to the glenoid fossa, although these views are not usually necessary to establish the correct diagnosis.[14]

Radiographs are necessary before reduction of the dislocation to detect an associated fracture of the proximal humerus, which occurs in 15% of cases (see below). Fractures of the glenoid rim are commonly associated with glenohumeral dislocations. Typically, glenoid rim fractures are small chip fractures associated with a detachment of the glenoid labrum (Fig. 6-12). This rim fracture is known as a *Bankart lesion.*[15] A large frac-

ture may necessitate open reduction if it becomes entrapped. Fifty percent of anterior dislocations are associated with an impaction fracture of the posterolateral surface of the humeral head caused by the anteroinferior rim of the glenoid (Fig. 6-13). This is known as a *Hill-Sachs deformity.*[16] It appears as a vertical line along the humeral head. Anterior glenohumeral dislocations are often recurrent and occur with minimal trauma. In the patient with recurrent shoulder dislocations, the Hill-Sachs deformity can be large because of repeated impaction fractures.

POSTERIOR SHOULDER DISLOCATION. Posterior shoulder dislocations are uncommon because the supporting structures along

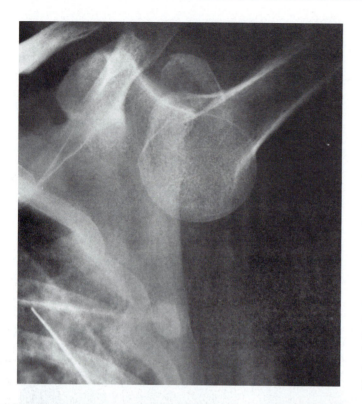

FIGURE 6-15.   Inferior shoulder dislocation. In this patient, who had a fall from a great height, the humeral head is dislocated inferior to the glenoid fossa. This is known as *luxatio erecta,* because the arm is fully abducted and directed superiorly.

the posterior aspect of the glenohumeral joint are strong. The mechanism of injury is typically a direct blow to the anterior shoulder or a fall on an outstretched arm with the shoulder adducted and internally rotated. A posterior shoulder dislocation also can occur during a seizure or electrical shock when the muscles about the shoulder are in tetanic contraction. The muscles causing internal rotation and posterior displacement are stronger than the opposing muscles, and so a posterior dislocation occurs.

The clinical findings of a posterior dislocation are more subtle that those of an anterior dislocation. Nonetheless, when the clinical findings are specifically sought, a posterior dislocation is usually quite evident. The shoulder is held in adduction and internal rotation, and the patient is unable to externally rotate the upper arm. There may be a palpable or visible depression along the anterior aspect of the shoulder and a fullness of the posterior aspect.

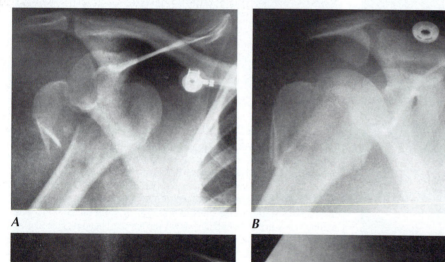

A   *B*

C   *D*

FIGURE 6-16.   Shoulder fracture/dislocations. *A.* Avulsion of the greater tuberosity is seen in this patient with an anterior shoulder dislocation. *B.* With reduction of the dislocation, the greater tuberosity returns to its normal position. *C.* In another patient, there is an anterior dislocation and fracture of the humeral neck. This cannot be reduced using standard closed technique. Open reduction is often necessary. (Copyright David T. Schwartz, M.D.) *D.* In a patient with a humeral neck fracture, a concomitant posterior dislocation is seen on the axillary view. The posterior dislocation could be missed on an AP shoulder radiograph. (*D.* from Pettrone FA: *Athletic Injuries of the Shoulder.* New York: McGraw-Hill, 1995. With permission.)

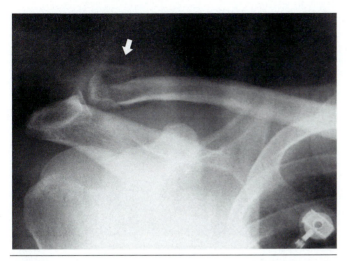

FIGURE 6-17. Distal clavicular fracture. The AC region is a common site of injury during shoulder trauma. This region of the radiograph often must be inspected using a bright light. Distal clavicular fractures are seen in the elderly (*arrow*), whereas injuries of the AC joint are more common in young adults.

The radiographic findings are also subtle, which accounts for the high rate of misdiagnosis (Fig. 6-14). On the AP radiograph, there is a decrease in the overlap of the humeral head and the glenoid fossa. The humeral head is fixed in internal rotation and it is impossible to obtain an external rotation view. Finally, there may be a vertical line representing an impaction fracture on the anteromedial surface of the humeral head. This is known as a *trough line* or a reverse Hill-Sachs deformity.

The posterior displacement of the humeral head is directly seen on the other radiographic views of the shoulder. The Y view reveals that the humeral head is slightly posterior to the crux of the Y, although the displacement can be minimal. The axillary view shows this injury best, the humeral head clearly displaced posterior to the glenoid fossa.

On a posterior oblique view (Grashey view), there is overlap in the normally clear glenohumeral joint space. However, because it is difficult to get absolutely correct positioning of this view, a clear glenohumeral joint space is not always seen, even in a normal shoulder.

OTHER SHOULDER DISLOCATIONS. An inferior shoulder dislocation is known as *luxatio erecta* (Fig. 6-15). The mechanism involves sudden forced abduction and tearing of the floor of the shoulder capsule with protrusion and entrapment of the humeral head inferiorly. *Superior dislocations* are rare. They typically involve a fall that strikes the elbow while the patient's arm is abducted, and the elbow is flexed.

FRACTURE/DISLOCATIONS. With anterior dislocations, avulsion fractures of the greater tuberosity are fairly common (Fig. 6-16). The supraspinatus muscle is attached to the fracture fragment. These fractures do not alter the techniques of reduction and the greater tuberosity fragment is usually brought back in position at the time of the shoulder reduction. On the other hand, fractures of the humeral neck in association with dislo-

cations must not be managed with standard techniques of closed reduction.[17]

When associated with a humeral head fracture, a concomitant posterior dislocation can be difficult to detect. An axillary view is often necessary in the patient with a proximal humeral fracture in order to exclude posterior dislocation. However, when obtaining this view, a humeral neck fracture can become displaced in the process of abducting the arm. The most common fracture associated with a posterior dislocation is a lesser tuberosity avulsion fracture, and so a posterior shoulder dislocation should always be suspected when a lesser tuberosity fracture is present.

Acromioclavicular Injuries

In reviewing radiographs of the shoulder, the AC region must be specifically examined for distal clavicular fractures or separation of the AC joint (Fig. 6-17). A bright light is often necessary because this region of the radiograph is usually dark (underpenetrated). However, injuries to this area are clinically evident by palpation of the shoulder. The distance between the coracoid process and the clavicle should be less than 11 mm. Greater separation implies a tear of coracoclavicular ligaments. The acromion itself is also assessed for fractures.

Clavicular Fractures

The patient with a fractured clavicle may complain of shoulder pain. It is important to palpate the entire length of the clavicle in patients with trauma to the shoulder. There is little soft tissue overlying the clavicle, so the need for specific clavicular views can usually be determined by physical examination. The middle and distal clavicle is visible on AP views of the shoulder and should be inspected for fractures. It is particularly important to review the clavicle in children, because the clavicle is frequently fractured. The middle third is most commonly fractured.

Scapular Fractures

Any fracture of the scapula should prompt a search for injuries to the chest, neck, and brachial plexus. Scapular fractures are classified by location, such as the body, spine, and acromion (Fig. 6-18). Fractures of the scapular neck and glenoid are associated with humeral fractures and dislocations.

Nontraumatic Lesions

A number of nontraumatic conditions are diagnosed by radiography. Certain patients with shoulder pain warrant special consideration. When intravenous drug abusers complain of shoulder pain, an infection of the sternoclavicular joint may be

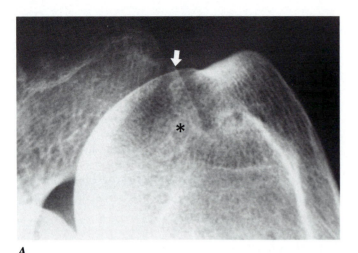

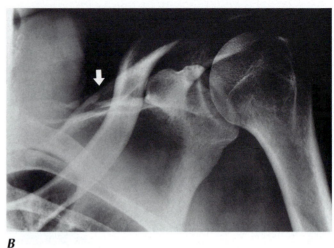

A   *B*

FIGURE 6-18.   Scapular fractures. The scapula should be inspected on any patient with shoulder trauma. *A.* A small fracture of the acromion (*asterisk*) is seen projected through the humeral head. *B.* A fracture of the scapular spine is visible overlapping the clavicle.

present. Patients with sickle cell anemia, particularly children, who complain of pain in the shoulder may have septic arthritis causing widening of the glenohumeral joint spaces.[18] They can also sustain bone infarctions of the proximal humerus.

Patients who chronically use corticosteroids may also present with osteonecrosis of the humeral head. Radiographs show a crescent of subchondral radiolucency representing collapsed necrotic bone.

Primary tumors of the bone and surrounding soft tissues in the shoulder are rare. These are usually evident on plain radiographs of the shoulder, causing an area of hypertrophic bone growth. Metastatic lesions and Paget disease of the shoulder are also seen on plain radiographs. In patients with known malignancies (particularly of the prostate, thyroid, or breast) who have shoulder pain, a radionuclide scan should be obtained if no lesions are found on plain radiographs.

Soft Tissue Abnormalities

In calcific periarthritis (calcific tendonitis), crystals of hydroxyapatite are deposited in the periarticular areas, most commonly in the region of the supraspinatus tendon (Fig. 6-19). Pain in a shoulder may be caused by collagen vascular disorders, such as ankylosing spondylitis and rheumatoid arthritis. There are marginal erosions adjacent to the articular surface of the humeral head and narrowing of the joint space.[19]

Injury to the *rotator cuff* causes soft tissue abnormalities on plain radiographs. Large tears in the rotator cuff cause decreased acromiohumeral space (less than 7 mm) with subacromial and greater tuberosity sclerosis. In addition, the humeral head is superiorly subluxed and lies close to the inferior surface of the acromion. This is characteristic of a chronic rotator cuff tear. Calcified acromial spurs can also be seen.[20]

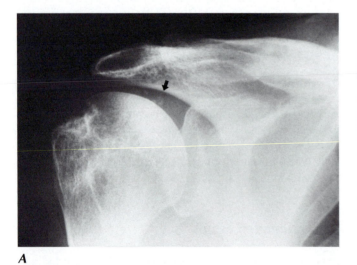

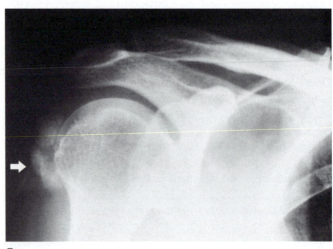

A   *B*

FIGURE 6-19.   Calcific tendinitis. *A.* Calcification is seen in the supraspinatus tendon. *B.* A large deposit of calcium is seen in the subdeltoid bursa. Calcific tendinitis can cause sudden shoulder pain when an acute inflammatory response develops.

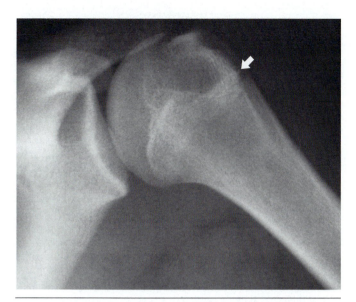

FIGURE 6-20. Epiphyseal growth plate. The proximal humeral growth plate in an older child has an irregular appearance that should not be misinterpreted as a fracture.

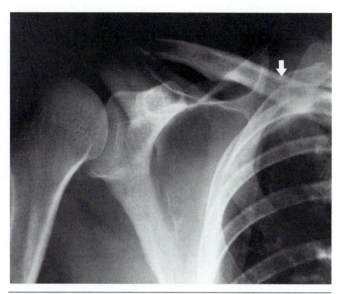

FIGURE 6-21. Rib fracture. A fracture of the second rib is seen at the corner of the radiograph in this patient, who had fallen onto his shoulder *(arrow).*

ERRORS IN INTERPRETATION

Interpretive errors are minimized by following a consistent pattern in reviewing radiographs of the shoulder. The correct views for a suspected abnormality must be obtained. Although most abnormalities are radiographically obvious, some can be subtle and may be misdiagnosed if not specifically sought.

Nondisplaced or impacted fractures of the humeral head and neck in an individual with osteoporosis can be difficult to detect. The cortical margins and trabeculae should be carefully examined, looking for discontinuity, abrupt angulation, or impaction. This is important with a shoulder dislocation, because an unrecognized humeral neck fracture will be displaced during attempted closed reduction. Conversely, the hemarthrosis that accompanies a humeral neck fracture distends the joint capsule and can simulate displacement due to a dislocation (Fig. 6-10). In older children, the growth plate of the humeral head has an irregular appearance that can be mistaken for a fracture (Fig. 6-20). On the other hand, a minimally displaced Salter-Harris I fracture through the physis (growth plate) is subtle. Clinical examination and comparison views can be helpful.

Posterior shoulder dislocations are missed in up to 50% of cases. Additional views such as the Y and axillary views confirm the abnormality.

Injuries at the AC joint can be missed because this area is usually overpenetrated and must be examined using a bright light. In the young adult, AC separation is common; whereas in the elderly, distal clavicular fractures are more common. Since midshaft clavicular fractures can present as shoulder pain, the midclavicle should be examined. If clinical suspicion is high for a scapular fracture, specific scapular AP and Y views should be obtained.

Finally, abnormalities in the adjacent ribs and lung (fracture, pneumothorax) can cause shoulder pain. These "corners" of the radiograph must not be neglected (Fig. 6-21).

COMMON VARIANTS

In adults, several accessory centers of ossification can occur. These include the inferior rim of the glenoid, the inferior angle of the scapula, the coracoid process (infracoracoid bone), and the area near the acromion (os acromiale). In some individuals, the coracoid tubercle may be large and articulate with the clavicle. This is also referred to as the *coracoclavicular joint.* In some individuals, a lucent zone appears at the greater tuberosity of the humerus—this can be quite striking. It should not be confused with a lytic lesion. In addition, areas of periosteal thickening can be seen at the deltoid insertion.

Ossification centers for the glenoid margins, inferior angle, scapular border, and acromion appear at puberty and fuse between the ages of 20 and 25. Unfused ossification centers may be mistaken for fractures. When there is a question, views on the unaffected side can be obtained for comparison. The AC joint and coracoclavicular joint are difficult to evaluate prior to ossification. Fortunately, they are rarely injured in adolescents.

Another variant seen in children is the "vacuum phenomenon." This is a semilunar, radiolucent shadow sometimes seen in the glenohumeral joints of children or young adults. It is a transient phenomenon and clinically insignificant. The glenoid process may also appear irregular in prepubescent children.

ADVANCED IMAGING

For the emergency physician, advanced imaging techniques for shoulder evaluation are generally unnecessary. Ultrasound is used for examination of the rotator cuff. Ultrasound can also be valuable in assessing suspected pyogenic joint effusions. Magnetic resonance imaging (MRI) is widely used by orthopedists in evaluating a variety of shoulder disorders. Computed tomography (CT) of the shoulder can confirm a posterior dislocation if plain films are nondiagnostic. CT is also occasionally needed to differentiate a pseudodislocation caused by a humeral neck fracture from a true dislocation.

CONTROVERSIES

The choice of radiographs of the shoulder is a source of controversy among practitioners. The views required to constitute an adequate screening examination for traumatic and nontraumatic pain in the shoulder are debated. There is no uniformly accepted standard.

Another controversy is the usefulness of postreduction radiographs after anterior dislocations of the shoulder. Most institutions require postreduction films as part of the routine evaluation of dislocation treatment and evaluation. The utility of these radiographs is questionable.[21] Hendley and Knox found that postreduction films rarely revealed any new clinically significant abnormalities.

REFERENCES

1. Pavlov N, Frieberger RH: Fractures and dislocations about the shoulder. *Semin Roentgenol* 13:85, 1978.
2. Hoppenfeld S: *Physical Examination of the Spine and Extremities.* New York: Appleton-Century-Crofts, 1976.
3. Lind T, Kroener K, Jensen J: The epidemiology of fractures of the proximal humerus. *Arch Orthop Trauma Surg* 108:285, 1989.
4. Poppen NK, Walker PS: Normal and abnormal motion of the shoulder. *J Bone Joint Surg* 58A:195, 1976.
5. Rockwood CA Jr, Green DP: *Fractures in Adults,* 3d ed. Philadelphia: Lippincott, 1991, p. 1065.
6. Rubin SA, Gray RL, Green WR: The scapular "Y": A diagnostic aid in shoulder trauma. *Radiology* 110:725, 1974.
7. Slivka J, Resnick D: An improved radiographic view of the glenohumeral joint. *J Can Radiol Assoc* 30:83, 1979.
8. Sartoris DJ, Resnick D: Plain film radiography: Routine and specialized techniques and projections, in Resnick D, Niwayama G (eds): *Diagnosis of Bone and Joint Disorders,* 2d ed. Philadelphia: Saunders, 1988, pp. 2–55.
9. Dingley A, Denham R: Fracture dislocation of the humeral head. *J Bone Joint Surg* 55A: 1973.
10. Vanarthos WJ, Eckman E, Bohrer SB: Radiographic diagnosis of acromioclavicular joint separation without weight bearing: Importance of internal rotation of the arm. *AJR* 162:120, 1994.
11. Rockwood CA: Subluxations and dislocations about the shoulder, in Rockwood CA Jr, Matson FA III (eds): *Fractures in Adults,* 2d ed. Philadelphia: Lippincott, 1984, p. 722.
12. Mann R, Neal EG: Fractures of the shaft of the humerus in adults. *South Med J* 58:264, 1965.
13. Neer CS II: Displaced proximal humerus fractures: I. Classification and evaluation. *J Bone Joint Surg* 52A:1077, 1970.
14. Seeger LL: *Diagnostic Imaging of the Shoulder.* Baltimore: Williams & Wilkins, 1992, pp. 17–19.
15. Pavlov H, Warren RF, Weiss CB Jr, Dines DM: The roentgenographic evaluation of anterior shoulder instability. *Clin Orthop Rel Res* 194:153, 1985.
16. Hill HA, Sachs MD: The grooved defect of the humeral head: A frequently unrecognized complication of the shoulder joint. *Radiology* 35:690, 1940.
17. Hersche O, Gerber C: Iatrogenic displacement of fracture-dislocations of the shoulder: A report of seven cases. *J Bone Joint Surg* 76B:30, 1994.
18. Steinbach HL: Infections of the bones. *Semin Roentgenol* 1:337, 1966.
19. Sharbaro JL: The rheumatoid shoulder. *Orthop Clin North Am* 6:593, 1975.
20. Post M, Silver R, Singh M: Rotator cuff tear: Diagnosis and treatment. *Clin Orthop* 173:78, 1983.
21. Hendley GW, Knox K: Clinically significant abnormalities in postreduction radiographs after anterior shoulder dislocation. *Ann Emerg Med* 28:399, 1996.

CHAPTER 7

THE CLAVICLE AND SCAPULA

RODOLFO QUERIOZ / ANDREW SUCOV

Even though standard radiographic images of the shoulder include portions of the clavicle and scapula, shoulder radiographs are not intended to study the clavicle and the sternoclavicular (SC) joint. They are inadequate for complete evaluation of the scapula. In shoulder radiographs, the lateral portion of the clavicle is overpenetrated (dark) because the radiograph is exposed to show the glenohumeral area. Specific radiographic views of the clavicle and scapula should be requested when an injury to these areas is suspected.

Clavicular fractures are common and account for 4 to 15% of all fractures. They are much more common in children.[1] The majority of these fractures occur in the middle third of the clavicle and are caused by a fall or a direct blow. Acromioclavicular (AC) separation is common in young adults. AC separation usually occurs as result of a direct blow or a fall on the shoulder.

Fractures of the *scapula* are uncommon. Fractures of the scapular body, neck, or spine often result from severe trauma to the shoulder and upper chest. In fact, scapular fractures are typically a marker for high-energy thoracic injury. Injuries to the ribs, lung, and shoulder are commonly found in patients with scapular fractures. In victims of major trauma, scapular fractures may be overlooked on initial evaluation because of the gravity of associated injuries.[2] On the other hand, isolated scapular fractures can occur without associated visceral injuries and an isolated scapular fracture alone is not itself a significant marker for increased mortality. Scapular fractures can also result from electrical shock,[3] seizures,[4] and as a complication of cardiopulmonary resuscitation.[5] In victims of major trauma, the high rate of associated injuries is clinically more significant than the scapular fracture.[6,7]

CLINICAL DECISION MAKING

Pain and a decreased range of motion are the most common reasons for ordering radiographs of the shoulder girdle. Palpation of the entire shoulder region, with an emphasis on the clavicle and scapula, is the basis for ordering radiographs. These superficial bones show tenderness, deformity, or ecchymosis. Injuries to the upper ribs and cervical spine can cause radiation of pain to the shoulder.

For injuries localized to the clavicle, especially of the medial third, clavicular films are recommended. For diffuse, nonlocalized pain, the standard shoulder series is ordered initially. Shoulder views show the majority of the lateral and middle thirds of the clavicle, which are the most common sites of fracture. A shoulder series does not, however, show medial-third clavicular fractures or fractures of the scapular body.[8]

High-yield clinical criteria have not been developed for radiography of the upper extremity, and approximately 80% of radiographs show no fractures.[9] The olecranon-manubrium percussion sign (percussion on the olecranon with auscultation over the manubrium—the audible note is changed with a fracture) may be more specific for the presence of a fracture, but it does not indicate the fracture location and hence does not determine the appropriate radiographic study.[10]

Both the clavicle and scapula lie over neurovascular bundles, the upper ribs, and the pleural cavity. Fractures to the clavicle are rarely associated with injuries to these underlying structures.[11] The body of the scapula is heavily protected by surrounding muscles and usually requires massive energy transfer to produce a fracture. The presence of a scapular fracture indicates the need to exclude an underlying injury to the lungs, ribs, or vascular structures. Fractures of the clavicle generally do not require further study.

Dislocation at the SC junction is demonstrated by swelling and deformity at the proximal aspect of the clavicle. Most dislocations are anterior and present with an obvious disparity between the two sides. Rarely, the dislocation is posterior. Posterior SC dislocations may show only subtle swelling and tenderness at the SC junction without significant deformity. SC dislocations are best evaluated by computed tomography (CT). They are not well demonstrated on plain radiographs. CT also demonstrates mediastinal injuries, which are more likely with posterior dislocation.

In the evaluation of a multiply-injured trauma patient, initial screening films are likely to include radiographs of the cervical spine and chest. The borders of these films do reveal clavicular and scapular injuries. After the patient is stabilized, specific radiographs of the clavicle or scapula are obtained when clinically indicated.[12,13] Neurovascular compromise resulting from a fracture of this area requires earlier investigation.

ANATOMY

The primary function of the upper limb is the positioning of the hand. The upper limb is formed by a number of articulations, including the highly mobile glenohumeral joint. The shoulder in combination with multiple neck and chest muscles forms the pectoral girdle. The clavicle is an important component in providing stability to the pectoral girdle connecting the manubrium of the sternum to the acromion process of the scapula.

The clavicle is S-shaped (Fig. 7-1). The clavicle is divided into thirds: a middle third, a medial (or proximal) third, and a lateral (or distal) third. The medial end of the clavicle is attached to the sternum by SC ligaments and to the first rib by the costoclavicular (rhomboid) ligament (Fig. 7-2). The rhomboid fossa is a depression of the inferior aspect of the medial clavicle and the site of attachment of the rhomboid ligament. The lateral third of the clavicle is firmly bound to the scapula by the coracoclavicular and AC ligaments. The pectoralis major and deltoid muscles attach to the inferior surface of the clavicle. The sternocleidomastoid and trapezius insert on the superior surface of the clavicle. The brachial plexus and great vessels of the upper extremity are located posterior and inferior to the medial and middle thirds of the clavicle and superior to the first rib. Ossification of the clavicle starts by the fifth week of fetal life. The medial epiphysis does not ossify until late in adolescence, between 15 and 19 and possibly as late as 23 years of age.

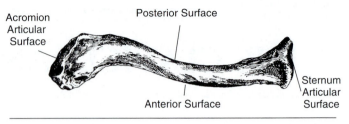

FIGURE 7-1. Skeletal anatomy of the clavicle (superior view). (From Pansky B: *Review of Gross Anatomy*, 6th ed. New York: McGraw-Hill, 1996. With permission.)

The scapula is a triangular flat bone in close contact with the posterior aspect of the upper thorax (Fig. 7-3). Because of its multiple muscle attachments, the scapula helps to stabilize the pectoral girdle. The superior lateral angle bears the glenoid fossa. The scapular neck connects the glenoid fossa with the body of the scapula. The scapular spine is a large ridge that extends to the acromion. The scapular spine divides the body of the scapula into a supraspinous fossa and a larger infraspinous fossa. The acromion articulates with the distal clavicle to form the AC joint. The coracoid process is located slightly medial to the glenoid fossa and projects anteriorly, superiorly, and laterally. The brachial plexus and major vessels of the upper extremity cross anterior to the scapula, just inferior to the base of the coracoid process.

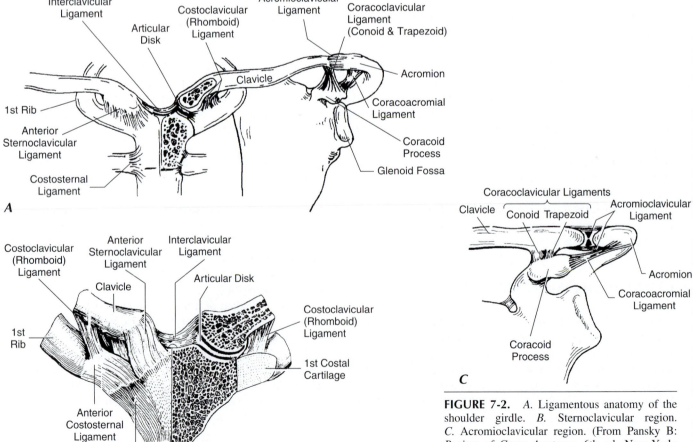

FIGURE 7-2. *A.* Ligamentous anatomy of the shoulder girdle. *B.* Sternoclavicular region. *C.* Acromioclavicular region. (From Pansky B: *Review of Gross Anatomy*, 6th ed. New York: McGraw-Hill, 1996. With permission.)

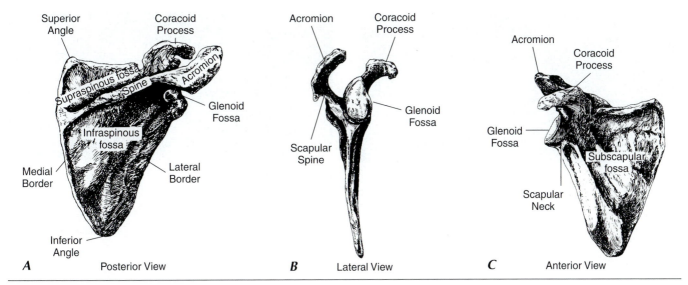

FIGURE 7-3. Skeletal anatomy of the scapula. *A.* Posterior view. *B.* Lateral view. *C.* Anterior view. (From Pansky B: *Review of Gross Anatomy*, 6th ed. New York: McGraw-Hill, 1996. With permission.)

RADIOGRAPHIC TECHNIQUE

Clavicle

The routine radiographic evaluation of the clavicle includes a straight anteroposterior (AP) view and an angled AP view (Table 7-1; Fig. 7-4). Ideally, the two radiographic views should be obtained at 90° to each other. However, because of the anatomic location of the clavicle, this is impossible. The second view is obtained in the AP direction with varying degrees of cephalic angulation of the x-ray beam.

AP View. The AP view is taken with the patient in a supine or upright position. The anterior surface of the clavicle is perpendicular to the x-ray beam. This view identifies most fractures. The lack of overlying soft tissue in the region of the clavicle dictates a radiographic exposure one-half to one-third that used for standard AP views of the shoulder.

TABLE 7-1

Clavicular Radiographic Views

VIEW	TECHNIQUE	ADEQUACY	LIKELY FINDINGS
Anteroposterior view of the clavicle	Supine or upright position. The anterior surface of the clavicle is perpendicular to the x-ray beam.	Correct exposure and positioning allows good visualization of the entire clavicle. The medial end of the clavicle does not overlap the thoracic spine.	In combination with the angled view, identifies most clavicular fractures.
Angled view of the clavicle	The x-ray beam is directed anteroposteriorly and angled 15° cephalad.	There is minimal overlap of the clavicle with the scapula and upper ribs.	Fractures through the middle and medial thirds of the clavicle.
Serendipity view	The x-ray beam is directed anteroposteriorly and angled 40° cephalad. The x-ray beam is centered on the manubrium.	The medial thirds of both clavicles are visualized.	Anterior and posterior sternoclavicular dislocation.
Stress views	Upright position. The x-ray beam is directed anteroposteriorly. 10- to 15-lb weights are suspended from the arms with wrist straps.	Both AC joints should be imaged on a large film cassette to allow comparison with the opposite side.	Confirms nondisplaced AC tear that is not seen on the standard views. Assesses the degree of ligament disruption when mild AC separation is seen on initial views.

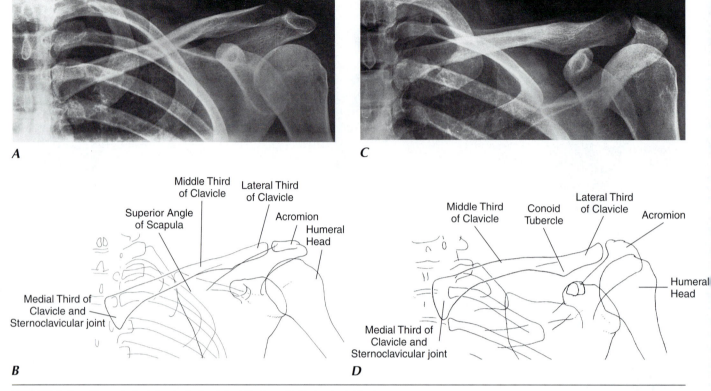

FIGURE 7-4.   Normal clavicle. *A, B.* Straight AP view. *C, D.* Angled AP view.

Angled AP View.   The angled view is taken with the x-ray beam angled cephalad (15°) and tangential to the chest wall. This reduces overlap of the scapula and upper ribs. In some cases, a nondisplaced fracture through the middle third of the clavicle is seen only on this view.

Stress Views.   Stress views are infrequently used in the emergency department (ED). They are obtained when one suspects a nondisplaced tear of the AC ligament that is not seen on the standard view. Stress views are also used to assess the degree of ligamentous disruption when mild AC separation is seen on the initial views. An AP view that includes both shoulders is obtained as 10- to 15-lb weights are suspended from the patient's arms with wrist straps. The weights are suspended from the wrists rather than held by the patient to ensure complete muscle relaxation. Both AC joints are imaged on a single large film to allow comparison. The role of stress views in the ED is debated because a clinical diagnosis of AC injury is made on physical examination and the treatment is not altered by radiographic demonstration of the injury (see "Controversies," below).

Sternoclavicular Views.   On a standard AP radiograph there is considerable overlap of osseous structures at the medial third of the clavicle. The *serendipity view,* an angled AP radiograph obtained with the patient supine, is used to evaluate the SC joint. The x-ray beam is directed 40° in a cephalic direction and is centered on the manubrium. With an anterior SC dislocation, the affected clavicle projects superior to the normal clavicle. In a posterior SC dislocation, the clavicle projects inferior to the normal clavicle. CT is currently the procedure of choice

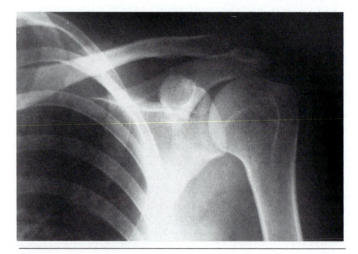

FIGURE 7-5.   Normal AP radiograph of the shoulder. This provides an initial view of the clavicle and scapula, although neither bone is seen in its entirety and only one view of each bone is given.

when SC dislocation is suspected. It provides excellent spatial resolution and defines the degree of displacement of the clavicle. CT is particularly important in a posterior SC dislocation because of the risk of injuring adjacent mediastinal structures (major vessels, esophagus, trachea).

Scapula

Standard radiographs of the shoulder and chest make up the initial screening examination of the scapula. The shoulder AP

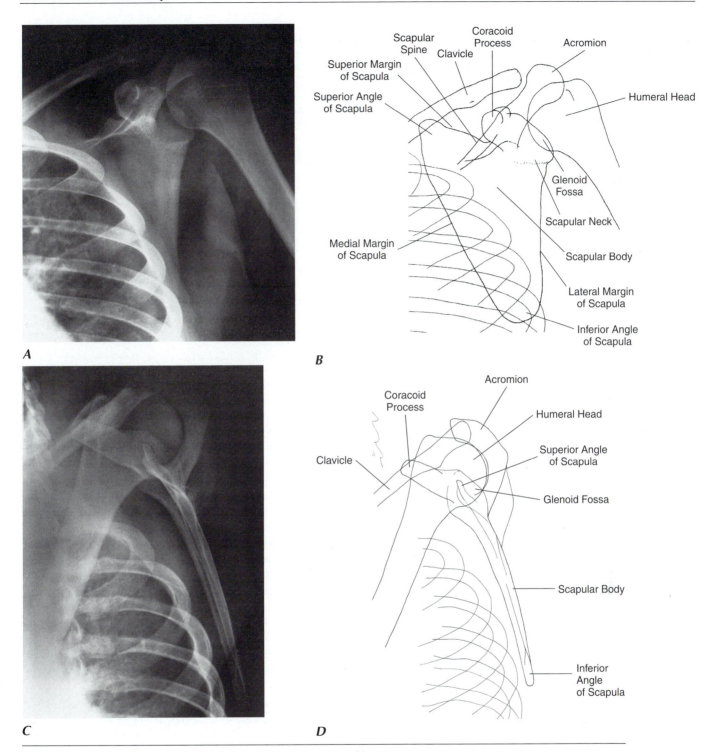

FIGURE 7-6. Normal scapula. *A, B.* AP view. *C, D.* Transscapular (Y) view.

view provides good demonstration of the glenoid fossa, scapula, neck, and acromion. However, most of the body of the scapula is obscured by the lateral aspect of the upper ribs (Fig. 7-5). Dedicated views of the scapula provide better detail when a scapular injury is specifically identified (Table 7-2; Fig. 7-6).

AP View. The AP view of the scapula is obtained by abducting the arm 90°. This moves the scapula laterally, allowing visualization of the lateral border and inferior angle. An alternate view is obtained by having the patient rotate the contralateral

shoulder approximately 45°. This is also called a posterior oblique view. In a modified AP view, the x-ray beam is angled 45° caudally and is centered over the glenoid. This provides an excellent view of the anterior glenoid.

Transscapular Y View. In the transscapular Y view, the coronal plane of the scapula is perpendicular to the film cassette. This is achieved by rotating the ipsilateral shoulder anteriorly. The x-ray beam is directed parallel to the coronal plane of the scapula.

TABLE 7-2

Scapular Radiographic Views

VIEW	TECHNIQUE	ADEQUACY	LIKELY FINDINGS
AP view of the shoulder	Supine or upright position. The x-ray beam is directed anteroposteriorly.	The glenohumeral joint, neck of the scapula, and acromion are seen.	Fractures of the glenoid rim, acromion, and scapular neck.
AP view of the scapula	The upper arm is abducted to minimize overlap of the scapula with the ribs.	The body of the scapula is more completely visualized.	Fractures of the body and neck of the scapula.
Posterior oblique view	The shoulder is rotated by approximately 45°.	Anterior and posterior rims of the glenoid fossa overlap. Glenohumeral joint space seen.	Fractures of the glenoid fossa.
Transscapular Y view	The coronal plane of the scapula is perpendicular to the film cassette.	The scapular body, coracoid process, and scapular spine are clearly defined.	Displaced fractures of the scapular body.

Axillary View.   The axillary view helps evaluate fractures of the acromion and coracoid process. It shows the articulation between the distal clavicle and the acromion. The axillary view also helps evaluate glenohumeral joint dislocations. The patient is supine with the arm slightly abducted. The x-ray beam is directed into the axilla and the film casette is located along the superior aspect of the shoulder.

RADIOGRAPHIC ANALYSIS

Some fractures are best seen on only one view. Therefore, at least two views should be obtained. The first step in interpreting a radiographic series is to evaluate its technical adequacy, including penetration and positioning. A targeted approach is based on knowledge of the most common lesions affecting the clavicle and scapula. This approach is supplemented by the findings on the patient's clinical examination.

Knowledge of normal anatomy, development, and common variants is required. For example, the epiphysis of the coracoid process or acromion in an adolescent patient could be mistaken for a fracture.

Clavicle

A targeted approach is based on recognizing the most common sites of clavicular injuries (Table 7-3). The radiographic evaluation is directed to the middle third of the clavicle, the AC and SC articulations, and surrounding structures (Fig. 7-7).

Middle Third.   The majority of clavicular fractures involve the middle third. Adults usually have significant separation of the bone fragments, making the fracture easy to detect. In younger patients, a greenstick fracture can be subtle. Nondis-

placed fractures may be seen on only one view. If the diagnosis is in doubt, additional views with different angulations are obtained. After the middle third is evaluated, the cortex is followed medially and laterally. The medial aspect of the clavicle is difficult to evaluate because of superimposition of the ribs.

AC Joint and Lateral Third.   The next step is to carefully examine the AC joint space, which should be of uniform width. Dislocation of the AC joint is best evaluated with the angled view of the clavicle. The inferior cortex of the clavicle should align with the inferior cortex of the acromion. The upper margins of the acromion and clavicle often do not align because the clavicle is wider than the acromion. Although the width of the AC joint space varies, it should not exceed 8 mm. The difference between the two sides should not exceed 2 mm. If the AC joint space shows increased width or a step-off between the acromion and clavicle, ligamentous disruption has probably occurred. Weight-bearing (stress) views may be needed for further evaluation.

Injuries to the coracoclavicular ligaments are associated with vertical displacement of the clavicle and an increased coracoclavicular interspace. This distance is measured from the undersurface of the clavicle to the coracoid process. Although the distance varies greatly in individual patients, the normal distance is less than 11 to 13 mm. In addition, this distance depends on the patient-film distance and the angle of the x-ray beam.

Finally, fractures of the lateral third of the clavicle are sought. Lateral clavicular fractures are more common in the elderly.

SC Joint and Medial Third.   Alignment of the medial clavicle with the sternum is checked. The SC joint is evaluated by comparing it with the contralateral side, looking for uniformity in the width of the joint spaces. In the case of SC dislocation,

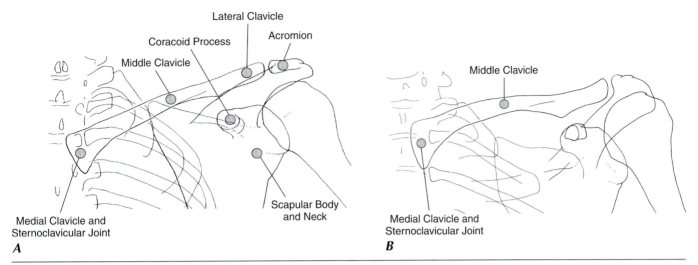

FIGURE 7-7. Sites prone to injury and easily missed injuries—clavicle. *A.* AP view. *B.* Angled view.

the medial ends of the clavicle are at different levels on the AP view. Additional views, such as the serendipity view, may be needed. High suspicion of SC dislocation warrants consideration of CT, especially when a posterior dislocation is suspected.

Examination of Nearby Structures. One should evaluate adjacent bones (ribs, scapula, proximal humerus) and soft tissues. Pneumothoraces or pleural fluid may be seen. The lung apices are checked for pulmonary lesions.

Reexamination. When one fracture is found, attention is given to the other segments of the clavicle as well as surrounding bones and soft tissues. The tendency to end the search when a fracture is found should be avoided because this can lead to other findings being overlooked. The physical exami-

nation is then repeated, with attention to the mechanism of injury and the radiographic findings.

Scapula

A targeted approach for evaluating scapular injuries concentrates on the most commonly injured areas and on injuries that are easily missed (Table 7-4; Fig. 7-8). Scapular fractures are often visible on only one view, so each region must be carefully examined on all views.

Scapular Body, Spine, Neck, and Glenoid. The scapular body, spine, neck, and glenoid rim are the most common sites of injury. The chest film often serves as the starting point in

TABLE 7-3

Systematic Analysis of Clavicular Radiographs

Determine study quality	One or two views are needed. Obtain 15° angled view if no fracture is seen on straight AP view.
Focus on the middle-third	Fractures are most common in the middle-third. Nondisplaced fractures may be seen in only one view. If in doubt, order additional AP views with slightly different angulation.
Evaluate the AC joint and lateral-third of the clavicle	Evaluate the AC and coracoclavicular spaces. The AC joint space should not exceed 8 mm. The coracoclavicular distance is less than 13 mm. The inferior cortex of the clavicle should align with the inferior cortex of the acromion. Elevation of the lateral-third of the clavicle is seen in AC separation.
Evaluate the sternoclavicular (SC) joint and medial-third of the clavicle	The SC joint space should be uniform in width. Look carefully for elevation or depression of the medial-third of the clavicle. Compare with the contralateral side.
Examine nearby structures	Evaluate the lung apex for pneumothoraces or pulmonary lesions. Check the ribs, scapula, and humerus for fractures.
Consider additional studies	If there is suspicion for a fracture of the medial-third of the clavicle or an SC dislocation, AP radiographs with cephalad angulation (35 to 40°) should be obtained (serendipity view). Order further studies as indicated (e.g., CT scan for further evaluation of suspected SC dislocation; comparison or stress views in suspected AC separation).

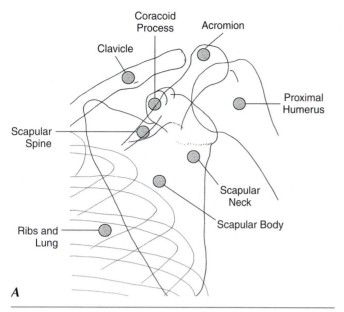

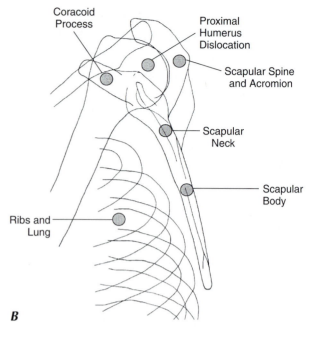

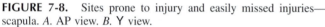

FIGURE 7-8.   Sites prone to injury and easily missed injuries—scapula. *A.* AP view. *B.* Y view.

evaluating scapular injuries. Many fractures are related to high-impact trauma, and associated injuries are frequently seen. In reviewing the initial trauma chest film, one should pay close attention to both scapulae. The use of symmetry is often helpful in assessing abnormalities. By drawing a line through the thoracic spinous processes, one can compare the distance from this line to the medial borders of the scapula. Fracture fragments of flat bones such as the scapula often overlap, so the fracture appears as a bright line on the AP view. Fractures of the scapular body are often visible only on the Y view. The normally smooth curves of the scapula body seen on end in this view are disrupted or angulated. The posterior oblique view can be helpful in evaluating the glenoid fossa.

Acromion and Coracoid Processes.   Isolated fractures of the acromion and coracoid process are rare and usually result from direct trauma. Alignment of the inferior margin of the acromion with the inferior margin of the clavicle is checked. Occasionally, fractures of the coracoid process are not seen on standard views. An AP view of the shoulder with 20 to 45° of cephalic angulation is helpful. The positioning of the humeral head in the glenoid fossa, especially on the Y view, is observed.

Nearby Structures.   Associated injuries in the surrounding bones and soft tissues are sought. Scapular fractures can be associated with other injuries around the shoulder, especially in the setting of severe trauma. The presence of clavicular or high rib fractures increases the possibility of scapular injuries. Unsuspected pneumothorax and indirect signs of thoracic aorta injury (e.g., widening of the upper mediastinum, loss of the right paratracheal stripe, loss of definition of the aortic arch, apical cap) are also considered in reviewing the radiographs.

TABLE 7-4

Systematic Analysis of Scapular Radiographs

Determine study quality	Two views are included (AP and Y view). On the Y view, the body of the scapula should project posterior to the ribs.
Evaluate the scapular body, spine, neck, and glenoid	Examine the scapular body, spine, and neck on the AP and Y views. Fracture fragments of flat bones like the scapula body may overlap and appear as a thin white line.
Focus on the acromion and coracoid processes	Acromion fractures are best evaluated with the AP and axillary views. Coracoid fractures are difficult to see. Follow the outline of the coracoid process on the AP and lateral views as well as the axillary view.
Examine nearby structures	Examine the ribs, clavicle, and humerus for a fracture. Evaluate the lung for pneumothorax or mass lesions.
Consider additional studies	Order further studies as indicated, e.g., CT scan for further evaluation of a scapular fracture with questionable glenoid involvement. Displaced or comminuted intraarticular fractures may require surgical treatment.

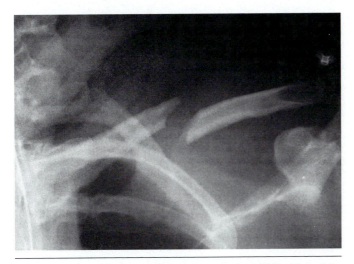

FIGURE 7-9. A displaced fracture through the middle third of the clavicle. The medial part is elevated by the pull of the sternocleidomastoid muscle, and the distal part is depressed by the weight of the arm.

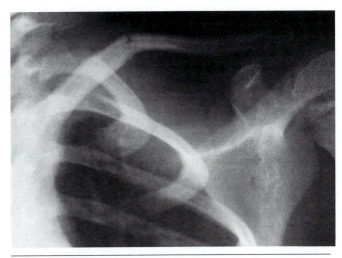

FIGURE 7-10. A greenstick fracture through the middle third of the clavicle in a child.

COMMON ABNORMALITIES

Clavicular Fractures

The clavicle is the most commonly fractured bone in childhood. Some 75 to 82% of clavicular fractures involve the middle third of the clavicle. The lateral third is involved in 12 to 21% of cases, and the medial third in 3 to 6%.[1,8,14] Clavicular fractures in children heal readily with immobilization, even when displaced. In adults, a greater force of injury is needed to fracture the middle portion of the clavicle. Associated injuries are more frequent in adults, and the prognosis for healing is worse.

MID-CLAVICULAR FRACTURES. The clavicle is weakest in its middle third. The mid-clavicle is the attachment of several muscles and ligaments. These attachments create forces in different directions.[15] With a mid-clavicular fracture, the medial segment is elevated, owing to the pull from the sternocleidomastoid muscle, and the lateral fragment is depressed, because of the weight of the upper extremity. Fractures of the mid-clavicle are usually transverse or comminuted (Fig. 7-9). In younger patients, mid-clavicular fractures are frequently greenstick fractures (Fig. 7-10). Nondisplaced fractures can be difficult to see radiographically and may be visible on only one view (Fig. 7-11). The normal S-curve of the middle portion of the clavicle should not be misinterpreted as angulation due to a fracture.

LATERAL CLAVICULAR FRACTURES. Fractures of the lateral third of the clavicle are subdivided according to their position relative to the coracoclavicular ligament.[16,17] If the integrity of the AC and coracoclavicular ligaments is maintained, these fractures are stable and not displaced (Fig. 7-12). With disruption of the ligaments attached to the medial clavicular fragment, the medial segment is displaced superiorly, due to the pull from

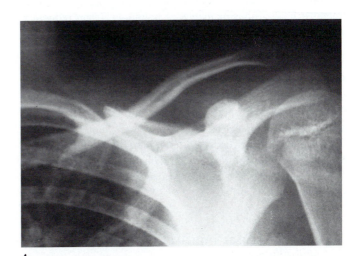

A

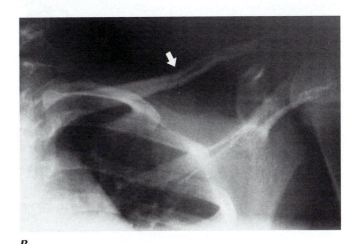

B

FIGURE 7-11. A nondisplaced fracture through the middle third of the clavicle. *A*. The fracture is barely visible on the straight AP view. *B*. The angled view shows the fracture.

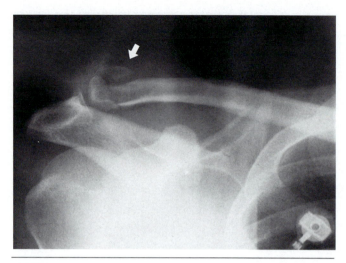

FIGURE 7-12.   A fracture through the lateral third of the clavicle.

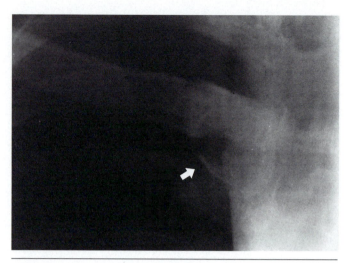

FIGURE 7-13.   A fracture through the medial third of the clavicle.

the sternocleidomastoid muscle. Displaced lateral clavicular fractures have a high incidence of nonunion. Open reduction and internal fixation are often recommended for these fractures.[18]

MEDIAL CLAVICULAR FRACTURES.   Fractures of the medial third of the clavicle are uncommon (Fig. 7-13). Medial clavicular fractures are usually nondisplaced. In adolescents and young adults, medial epiphyseal separation occurs more frequently than fractures of the medial third and require open fixation.[19] Medial clavicular injuries are difficult to detect radiographically and are best evaluated with a steeply angled AP radiograph (the serendipity view) or CT.

Acromioclavicular Injuries

AC separations are common. They usually occur from a fall or direct blow on the acromion or, less commonly, from a fall on an outstretched hand.[20] AC separations are classified as types I, II, and III, according to the degree of injury to the AC and coracoclavicular ligaments. An extended classification adds three types of severe AC disruption (Fig. 7-14).

Type I injuries involve a minor sprain to the fibers of the AC ligaments. The radiographic examination is normal. The joint is stable, and the term *acromioclavicular sprain* is used to describe this injury.

Type II injuries, also called *sublimation of the AC joint,* involve a disruption of the AC ligaments that allows displacement of the clavicle and widening of the AC space (Fig. 7-15). The coracoclavicular ligament remains intact. To detect this injury, the alignment of the inferior margins of the clavicle and acromion are examined. For mildly displaced grade II injuries, comparison views are helpful to detect slight degrees of separation. The clinical examination of patients with type I and II injuries reveals tenderness over the AC joint with no or minimal deformity.

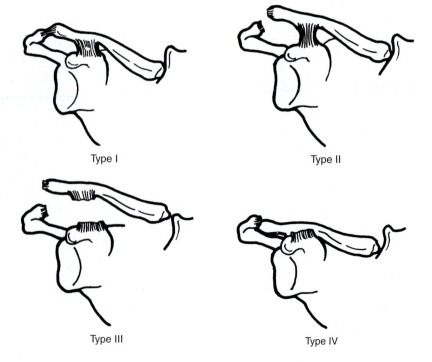

FIGURE 7-14.   Classification of the six types of acromioclavicular dislocations. Types IV, V, and VI are usually associated with major traumatic injuries. Types I, II, III are usually more localized injuries due to moderate degrees of trauma. (From Perry CR, Elstrom JA, Pankovich AM: *Handbook of Fractures.* New York: McGraw-Hill, 1995. With permission.)

Type III injuries involve complete disruption of the AC and coracoclavicular ligaments. The coracoclavicular distance is greater than 13 mm (Fig. 7-16). The elevated distal clavicle tenting the skin above the shoulder is obvious on clinical examination.

The extended classification adds types IV, V, and VI (Fig. 7-14).[21] These involve posterior, superior, and inferior dislocation of the distal clavicle relative to the acromion. These severe dislocations are often associated with neurovascular injuries and major trauma.

Weighted stress views have been advocated for AC injuries. Weighted views can demonstrate greater displacement than seen on the initial view. Theoretically, they can demonstrate a type II injury when no displacement is seen on the nonweighted view. The use of weighted views in the ED remains controversial because treatment is not altered (see "Controversies," below).

The majority of type I and II injuries receive conservative management. Most patients recover fully after shoulder immobilization with a sling or strapping. Management of type III injuries is controversial. Some authors suggest surgical repair of all type III injuries, and others advocate conservative management, similar to that used for type I and II injuries. Surgical repair is attempted only after failure of conservative measures. Types IV, V, and VI are severe injuries that require hospitalization and surgical repair.

Sternoclavicular Dislocations

SC injuries are usually evident on physical examination. Patients have local tenderness, swelling, and deformity. However, SC injuries can be difficult to see radiographically, often requiring supplementary views. The spectrum of SC injuries

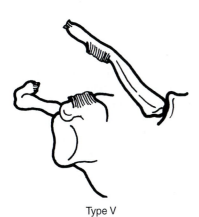

Type V

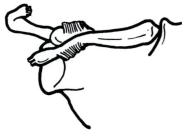

Type VI

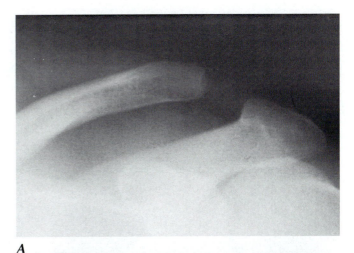

A

B

FIGURE 7-15. Type II AC separation. *A.* The AC joint space is widened and the clavicle is superiorly displaced. *B.* A comparison view of the opposite normal side shows that the inferior margin of the clavicle aligns with the inferior margin of the acromion. The superior margins do not align because the clavicle is thicker than the acromion.

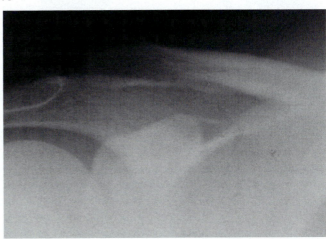

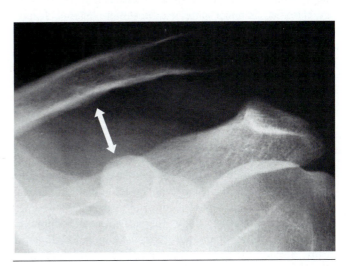

FIGURE 7-16. Type III AC separation. The distal end of the clavicle is widely displaced from the acromion and the distance between the superior surface of the coracoid process and the inferior surface of the clavicle is greater than 13 mm (arrow).

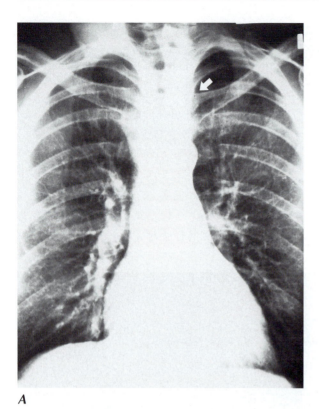

A

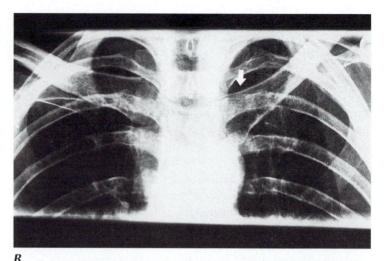

B

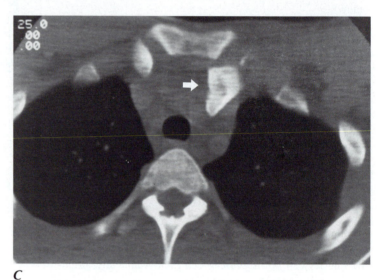

C

FIGURE 7-17. Sternoclavicular dislocation. *A.* On the PA chest radiograph, malalignment of the sternoclavicular joint is difficult to see. The superior margin of the left clavicle is slightly lower than on the right. *B.* On a radiograph of the sternoclavicular region, there is inferior displacement of the medial end of the clavicle, this indicating posterior dislocation (*arrow*). *C.* The diagnosis is confirmed by CT (*arrow*). There is hemorrhage within the nearby mediastinum. (*A* and *B* courtesy of David T. Schwartz, M.D.)

ranges from a nondisplaced sprain to dislocation. Dislocations are classified as either anterior or posterior. Anterior dislocations are characterized by displacement of the clavicle anterior to the sternum. Anterior dislocations account for 90% of cases. Posterior dislocations are associated with a number of serious complications. The great vessels, trachea, esophagus, thoracic duct, and lungs can be injured by the medial end of the clavicle (Fig. 7-17).

An anterior SC dislocation is usually caused by an anterior blow to the shoulder. A posterior dislocation is caused by either a blow to the posterior aspect of the shoulder or direct impact on the medial clavicle. On physical examination, anterior dislocations reveal a palpable lump. Posterior dislocations may be associated with a palpable depression or a lump on the chest wall due to soft tissue swelling. Therefore, it can sometimes be difficult to distinguish anterior from posterior dislocation clinically. Because the clinical implications of anterior and posterior dislocations are quite different, additional views are necessary to confirm the diagnosis. CT is easy to perform and effectively demonstrates the direction and degree of displace-

ment as well as injury to underlying structures. CT is also helpful in detecting fractures of the medial third of the clavicle.

The ossification center of the medial epiphysis appears in adolescence, and the growth plate may not close until age 23 years. In adolescents and younger adults, most SC dislocations occur at the point of least resistance—the growth plate. For this reason, a large number of SC dislocations are actually separations of the clavicular epiphysis.

Scapular Fractures

The positioning of the scapula close to the torso and its surrounding musculature is responsible for the low incidence of scapular body fractures. Scapular fractures represent 3 to 5% of shoulder injuries.[22] High-speed collisions involving cars and motorcycles are responsible for approximately 75% of cases.[20] Isolated scapular fractures also occur from a fall or a direct blow to the shoulder region.

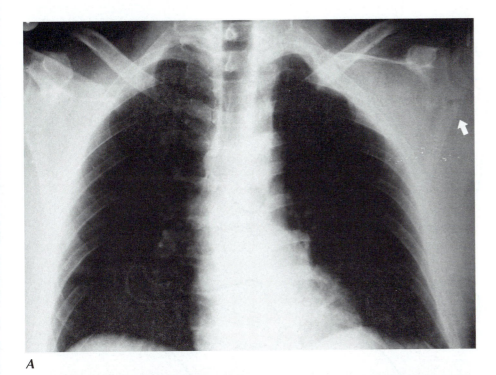

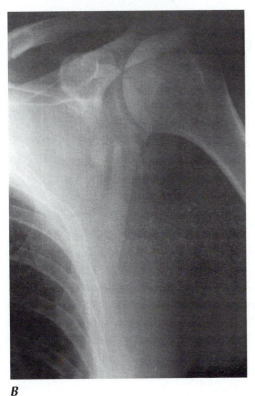

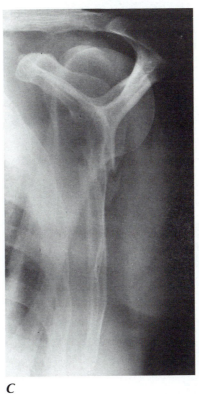

A

B

C

FIGURE 7-18. Scapular fractures seen on the initial trauma chest radiograph. *A.* The portable chest film of a major trauma victim shows a comminuted fracture of the left scapular neck and body. There is also a fracture of the midclavicle. *B* and *C.* The AP and lateral (Y) radiographs provide greater detail of the fracture.

Scapular fractures often result from severe traumatic forces, and life-threatening injuries may be present. The most commonly associated injuries are rib fractures, lung contusions, pneumothoraces, clavicular fractures, brachial plexus, and vascular injuries. The chest film serves as the initial screening examination for trauma involving the shoulder girdle (Fig. 7-18).

Fractures of the scapular body or neck account for approximately 80% of cases (Fig. 7-19).[23–25] Fractures of the scapu-lar body are either horizontal, vertical, or comminuted. Fractures through the scapular neck usually parallel the glenoid fossa (Fig. 7-20). Avulsion fractures involve the coracoid and acromion processes, and the inferior angle of the scapula.

Fractures of the glenoid region are either extensions of fractures of the scapular neck or small chip fractures off the glenoid rim. Fractures of the glenoid rim are usually associated with shoulder dislocations.

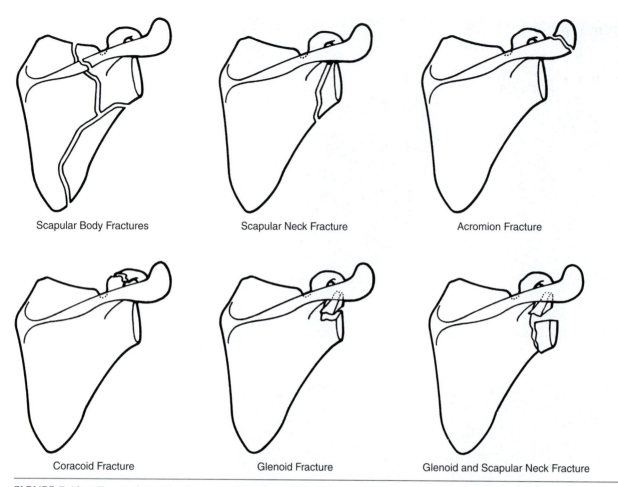

Scapular Body Fractures   Scapular Neck Fracture   Acromion Fracture

Coracoid Fracture   Glenoid Fracture   Glenoid and Scapular Neck Fracture

FIGURE 7-19.   Types of scapular fractures. (From Perry CR, Elstrom JA, Pankovich AM: *Handbook of Fractures*. New York: McGraw-Hill, 1995. With permission.)

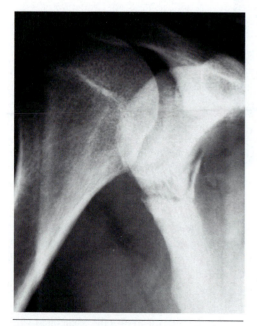

FIGURE 7-20.   Fracture of the scapular neck.

Isolated fractures of the acromion occur from either a direct blow or, less commonly, from superior displacement of the humeral head (Fig. 7-21). Acromion fractures are usually vertically oriented and located at the junction of the acromion and the scapular spine. The presence of an os acromiale (a persistent secondary ossification center) should not be confused with a fracture. Fractures of the coracoid process can occur from a direct blow or in association with an AC dislocation or anterior dislocation of the shoulder. The fracture is usually transverse and located at the base of the coracoid process.

Scapulothoracic Dissociation

Scapulothoracic dissociation represents a closed forequarter amputation of the upper extremity. This injury results from either extreme force applied to the anterolateral portion of the shoulder or severe traction on the shoulder.[26] Patients are usually involved in high-speed motor vehicle collisions and have severe associated injuries. The scapulothoracic anatomy is disrupted, with associated AC joint separation, distracted clavic-

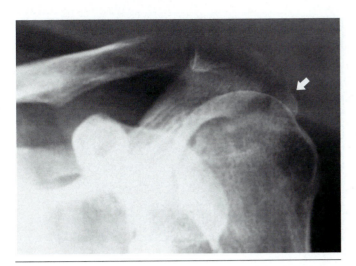

FIGURE 7-21. Fracture of the acromion.

ular fracture, or SC separation. Injury to the subclavian artery and brachial plexus is common. The trauma chest radiograph gives the first indication of this injury by showing a laterally displaced scapula. Concomitant AC separation, SC dislocation, or distracted clavicular fracture are important clues to this injury.[27-29]

ERRORS IN INTERPRETATION

Nondisplaced fractures of the lateral third of the clavicle are occasionally missed in patients with shoulder trauma. On shoulder films, this region is usually overpenetrated because the radiograph is exposed to penetrate the thicker region of the glenohumeral joint. Therefore, in addition to palpation of the AC joint, this portion of the radiograph should be examined using a "bright light." The cortical outline must be carefully examined, especially in elderly or osteopenic patients.

In some standard AP views of the clavicle, the S curve of the middle portion of the clavicle can be misinterpreted as angulation due to a fracture. The angled view is helpful in defining the curved middle third of the clavicle. In difficult cases, a comparison view of the contralateral clavicle may be necessary.

Nondisplaced fractures of the acromion and coracoid process can be overlooked. Careful attention should be paid to the outline of the coracoid process and acromion, especially on the Y and axillary views.

Other injuries that can be overlooked include medial clavicular fractures and dislocations, nondisplaced fractures of the middle third of the clavicle (seen on only one view), and scapular fractures. When high clinical suspicion of an injury exists despite negative radiographs, all available films must be carefully reviewed and additional views be obtained.

Rib fractures and pneumothoraces are often associated with injuries to the shoulder girdle, especially in major trauma. Pneu-

mothorax can occur with an isolated fracture of the clavicle.[11] The visualized areas of the rib cage and lung apices should be carefully inspected.

COMMON VARIANTS

Secondary ossification centers of the coracoid process and acromion can be mistaken for fractures on radiographs of adolescents and young adults (Table 7-5). The secondary ossification centers of the acromion and coracoid process fuse by age 15 years. Two other ossification centers in the scapula occur at the medial (or vertebral) border and the inferior angle. These ossification centers are usually fused by age 25 years.

The acromion is formed by as many as three ossification centers. When one of these centers fails to fuse, an os acromiale is seen. The axillary view of the shoulder provides an image of the acromion and helps exclude a fracture (Fig. 7-22).

Nutrient foramina and vascular channels are usually seen in the upper aspects of the scapular body and adjacent to the scapular neck. Nutrient foramina are usually horizontal, parallel the upper border, have sclerotic margins, and should not be mistaken for fractures. Nutrient channels are also seen in the superior and inferior borders of the clavicle.

The medial epiphysis of the clavicle does not ossify until the late teens and can be confused with a fracture. Many muscles insert on the clavicle, including the sternocleidomastoid, trapezius, deltoid, pectoralis major, and subclavius. These insertions often produce an irregular, ragged appearance of the clavicular cortex and can mimic an inflammatory process.

TABLE 7-5

List of Common Variants

Clavicle
Medial epiphysis: Does not ossify until the late teens and can be confused with a fracture.
Muscle insertions: The insertion of the sternocleidomastoid, trapezius, deltoid, pectoralis major, and subclavius muscles produce an irregular and ragged appearance of clavicle cortex, not to be confused with periosteal reaction or an inflammatory process.
Rhomboid fossa: Defect in the inferior margin of the medial clavicle secondary to insertion of the costoclavicular ligaments.

Scapula
Secondary ossification centers of the acromion and coracoid processes: These secondary ossification centers fuse by age 15 years and can be mistaken for fractures in adolescent and young adults.
Os acromiale: An os acromiale is seen when one of the ossification centers of the acromion fails to unite with the scapular spine.
Nutrient foramina and vascular channels: These are usually seen in the upper aspects of the scapular body and adjacent to the scapular neck.

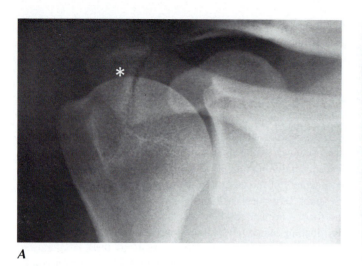
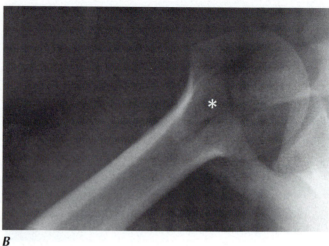

A   *B*

FIGURE 7-22.   Os acromiale. This normal variant is an unfused secondary ossification center. It should not be misinterpreted as a fracture. The axillary view can help define abnormalities of the acromion *(B)*.

The rhomboid fossa is a small defect in the inferior margin of the medial clavicle. It is the insertion of the costoclavicular ligaments that holds the first rib to the medial clavicle (see Fig. 7-2B) and can simulate a lytic lesion (Fig. 7-23).

ADVANCED STUDIES

In most cases, plain radiographs provide all the necessary information for evaluating patients with trauma to the scapula and clavicle.

Although special plain film views have been devised for evaluating injuries to the medial third of the clavicle and SC joint, CT is the imaging study of choice (Fig. 7-17). Axial slices through the medial clavicle clearly demonstrate the intact cortex and the normal anatomy of the SC joint. CT can also demonstrate the great vessels, trachea, esophagus, thoracic duct, and lungs. CT should be ordered when plain films are inconclusive and there is high clinical suspicion for injury.

CT is helpful in evaluating fractures of the glenoid fossa, especially in cases of small avulsion fractures with possible intraarticular fragments. CT with three-dimensional surface rendering shows a clear spatial distribution of bone fragments and is also helpful in evaluating possible glenoid fractures (Fig. 7-24).

Posterior SC dislocations are rare but can be associated with vascular compromise, including compression of the carotid artery and subclavian vessels. If clinical or radiologic suspicion of vascular injury exists, an angiogram should be obtained.[19]

CONTROVERSIES

Obtaining weighted (stress) views has been advocated in injuries to the AC joint to assess the degree of ligamentous disruption. Type I and II injuries may appear the same on nonweighted (nonstress) views, and displacement of type III injuries may be underestimated. Stress views allow improved grading of injuries compared with plain views. However, grading the injury does not appear to have any influence on ED treatment.[30–33] The majority of all injuries, including type III, are treated conservatively with immobilization and pain control. The only difference appears to be when to seek orthopedic referral. Type I and II injuries can be followed up when the condition fails to improve over 1 to 2 weeks, while type III injuries should be assessed for further evaluation within 3 to 7 days.

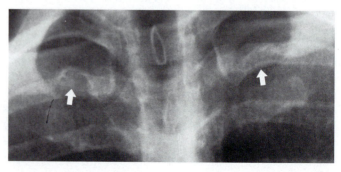
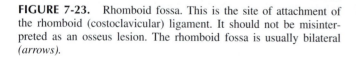

FIGURE 7-23.   Rhomboid fossa. This is the site of attachment of the rhomboid (costoclavicular) ligament. It should not be misinterpreted as an osseus lesion. The rhomboid fossa is usually bilateral *(arrows)*.

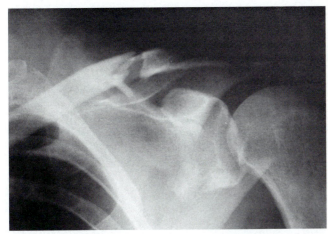

A

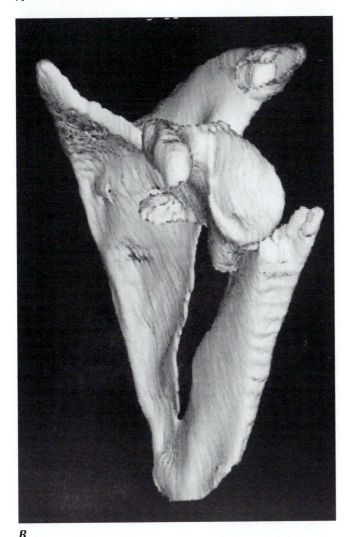

B

FIGURE 7-24. The anatomy of a complex scapular fracture is clearly shown with a surface rendered in three-dimensional CT. *A.* Plain film. *B.* CT.

REFERENCES

1. Nordqvist A, Petersson C: The incidence of fractures of the clavicle. *Clin Orthop* 300:127, 1994.
2. Harris RD, Harris JH Jr: The prevalence and significance of missed scapular fractures in blunt chest trauma. *AJR* 151:747, 1988.
3. Dumas JL, Walker N: Bilateral scapular fractures secondary to electrical shock. *Arch Orthop Trauma Surg* 111:287, 1992.
4. Shaw JL: Bilateral posterior fracture dislocation of the shoulder and other trauma caused by convulsive seizures. *J Bone Joint Surg* 53:1437, 1971.
5. Kam ACA, Kam PCA: Scapular and proximal humeral head fractures: An unusual complication of cardiopulmonary resuscitation. *Anaesthesia* 49:1055, 1994.
6. Buckley SL, Gotschall C, Robertson W Jr, et al: The relationship of skeletal injuries with trauma score, injury severity score, length of hospital stay, hospital charges, and mortality in children admitted to a regional pediatric trauma center. *J Pediatr Orthop* 14:449, 1994.
7. Stephens NG, Morgan AS, Corvo P, Bernstein BA: Significance of scapular fracture in the blunt-trauma patient. *Ann Emerg Med* 26:439, 1995.
8. Neustadter LM, Weiss MJ: Trauma to the shoulder girdle. *Semin Roentgenol* 26:331, 1991.
9. Royal College of Radiologists Working Party: Radiography of injured arms and legs in eight accident and emergency units in England and Wales. *BMJ* 291:1325, 1985.
10. Adams SL, Yarnold PR, Mathews J: Clinical use of the olecranon-manubrium percussion sign in shoulder trauma. *Ann Emerg Med* 17:484, 1988.
11. Meeks RJ, Riebel GD: Isolated clavicle fracture with associated pneumothorax: A case report. *Am J Emerg Med* 9:555, 1991.
12. Ada JR, Miller ME: Scapular fracture. *Clin Orthop* 269:174, 1991.
13. Lange RH, Noel SH: Traumatic lateral scapular displacement: An expanded spectrum of associated neurovascular injury. *J Orthop Trauma* 7:361, 1993.
14. Herscovici D Jr, Sanders R, DiPasquale T, Gregory P: Injuries of the shoulder girdle. *Clin Orthop* 318:54, 1995.
15. Harrington MA Jr, Keller TS, Seiler JG, et al: Geometric properties and the predicted mechanical behavior of adult human clavicles. *J Biomech* 26:417, 1993.
16. Neer CS: Fractures of the distal third of the clavicle. *Clin Orthop* 58:43, 1968.
17. Heppenstall RB: Fractures and dislocations of the distal clavicle. *Orthop Clin North Am* 6:477, 1975.
18. Edwards DJ, Kavanagh TG, Flannery MC: Fractures of the distal clavicle: A case for fixation. *Injury* 23:44, 1992.
19. Lewonowski K, Bassett GS: Complete posterior sternoclavicular epiphyseal separation. *Clin Orthop* 281:84, 1992.
20. Smith MJ, Stewart MJ: Acute acromioclavicular separations. *Am J Sports Med* 7:62, 1979.
21. Williams GR, Nguyen VD, Rockwood CA Jr: Classification and radiographic analysis of acromioclavicular dislocations. *Appl Radiol* 18(2):29, 1989.
22. Hardegger FH, Simpson LA, Weber BG: The operative management of scapular fractures. *J Bone Joint Surg* 66B:725, 1984.
23. Imatani RJ: Fractures of the scapula: A review of 53 fractures. *J Trauma* 15:473, 1975.
24. McGahan JP, Rab GT, Dublin A: Fractures of the scapula. *J Trauma* 20:880, 1980.

25. Wilbur MC, Evans EB: Fractures of the scapula—An analysis of forty cases and review of the literature. *J Bone Joint Surg* 59A:358, 1977.

26. Oreck SL, Burgess A, Levine AM: Traumatic lateral displacement of the scapula: Radiographic sign of neurovascular disruption. *J Bone Joint Surg* 66A:758, 1984.

27. Sampson LN, Britton JC, Eldrup-Jorgensen J, et al: The neurovascular outcome of scapulothoracic dissociation. *J Vasc Surg* 17:1083, 1993.

28. Sheafor DH, Mirvis SE: Scapulothoracic dissociation: Report of five cases and review of the literature. *Emerg Radiol* 2:279, 1995.

29. Lange RH, Noel SH: Traumatic lateral scapular displacement: An expanded spectrum of associated neurovascular injury. *J Orthop Trauma* 7-361, 1993.

30. Bossart PJ, Joyce SM, Manaster BJ, et al: Lack of efficacy of "weighted" radiographs in diagnosing acute acromioclavicular separation. *Ann Emerg Med* 17:20, 1988.

31. Cook, DA, Heiner JP: Acromioclavicular joint injuries. *Orthop Rev* 19:510, 1990

32. Orban DJ: Shoulder injuries, in Harwood-Nuss A, Linden C, Luten RC, et al (eds): *The Clinical Practice of Emergency Medicine.* Philadelphia: JB Lippincott, 1991, pp. 405–407.

33. Bannister GC, Wallace WA, Stableforth PG, et al: The management of acute acromioclavicular dislocation. *J Bone Joint Surg* 71B:848, 1989.

CHAPTER 8

THE FOOT

JOHN WARTELLA / ROSS COHEN / DAVID T. SCHWARTZ

Foot injuries are commonly seen in the emergency department (ED). Over 15% of sports-related injuries are isolated to the foot, and most of these (58%) involve hiking and walking activities. Unusual activities, such as ballet and modern dance, are also responsible for foot injuries. Falls and jumps from significant heights as well as crush mechanisms cause foot injuries that result in considerable disability.

CLINICAL DECISION MAKING

Although there are no specific guidelines for ordering radiographs of the entire foot, midfoot guidelines are included as part of the Ottawa rules for ankle injuries.[1,2] Clinical decision making is largely based on judgment and experience. The mechanism of the traumatic event increases suspicion for certain injuries. For example, forced inversion of the foot is associated with a fracture of the proximal fifth metatarsal. Although a physical examination is essential to determine the need for radiography, such signs as soft tissue swelling and ecchymosis are poor indicators of skeletal injury. Localized bone tenderness over the midfoot and the inability to bear weight are more specific signs of a fracture.

Clinical decision rules for ordering radiographs of the midfoot are a part of the Ottawa ankle rules because midfoot injuries are often caused by the same mechanisms of injury responsible for fractures involving the ankle (see Chap. 9, Fig. 9-1).[1,2] The guidelines suggest that foot radiographs are indicated if there is localized bone tenderness at the navicular and the base of the fifth metatarsal. Inability to bear weight both at the time of injury and in the emergency department (ED) is another indication to obtain a radiographic study. Weight bearing is defined as the ability to take four steps despite the presence of limping.

Fractures of the calcaneus occur after falls, jumps, or other axial compression injuries. The height of a fall may seem minor (e.g., off a stepladder) and still result in a calcaneal fracture. Localized tenderness involving the heel and an appropriate mechanism are sufficient reasons for ordering radiographs of the calcaneus. Minimally displaced fractures of the posterior portion of the calcaneus can be difficult to see on standard foot radiographs. If such a fracture is suspected but not seen on the standard foot views, an axial calcaneal view should be ordered. Fractures of the thoracolumbar spine are associated with calcaneal fractures and are caused by the transmission of axial loading forces from the heel to the spinal column.[3] In the patient with a calcaneal fracture due to axial loading, the spine must be carefully examined for injury.

Metacarpal tenderness following a traumatic event is also an indication for ordering foot radiographs. If a distal phalanx sustains an isolated injury, radiographic evaluation of the toe can be deferred. Nonetheless, most injuries of the great toe should be evaluated radiographically in order to detect a fracture, because these injuries may require more aggressive treatment.

Nontraumatic foot pain may be due to a stress fracture or foreign body. This is especially true in the presence a peripheral neuropathy (e.g., diabetic neuropathy). Some patients may be unaware of a needle embedded in the plantar soft tissue of the foot. Puncture wounds to the sole should be carefully examined to detect any remnant foreign body.

ANATOMY AND PHYSIOLOGY

The three anatomic regions of the foot are the hindfoot, midfoot, and forefoot (Fig. 8-1). The hindfoot consists of the talus and calcaneus; the midfoot consists of the cuneiforms, cuboid, and navicular; and the forefoot consists of the metatarsals and phalanges. The *Chopart joint* (midtarsal joint) separates the hindfoot from the midfoot. The *Lisfranc joint* (tarsometatarsal joint) separates the midfoot from the forefoot.

Hindfoot

The talus articulates with distal tibia and fibula to form the ankle joint. The talus is divided into the body, neck, and head. The superior articular surface of the talus is called the *talar dome* or *trochlea*. The superior surface of the talar dome articulates with the distal tibia. The medial and lateral surfaces of the talar dome articulate with the medial malleolus and lateral malleolus. The inferior surface of the talus articulates with the calcaneus forming the *subtalar joint.* Anteriorly, the talar head articulates with the navicular.

The calcaneus is divided into anterior, middle, and posterior parts. The posterior portion of the calcaneus, the heel bone, is known as the *posterior tuberosity.* It does not articulate with other bones. The most posterior surface of the calcaneus is the

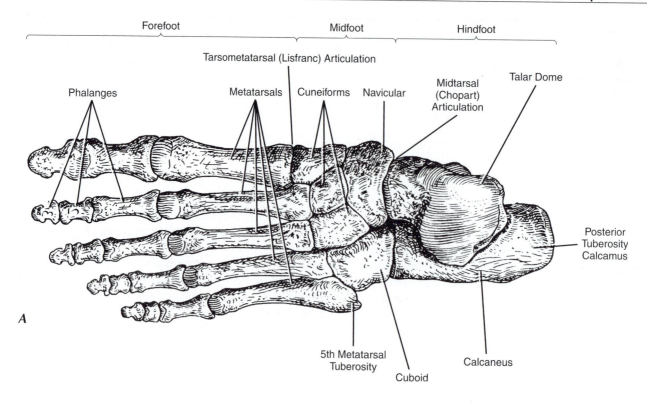

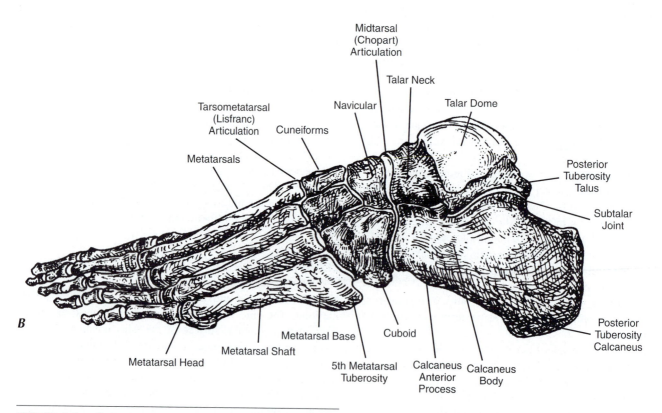

FIGURE 8-1.   Skeletal anatomy of the foot. *A.* Top view. *B.* Side view. (Modified from Pansky B: *Review of Gross Anatomy,* 6th ed. New York: McGraw-Hill, 1996, with permission.)

site of the insertion of the Achilles tendon. The middle part of the superior surface of the calcaneus declines sharply. The anterior part of the superior surface of the calcaneus begins at the deep recess known as the *sinus tarsi* and continues anteriorly and upwardly on the anterior process of the calcaneus. The anterior process of the calcaneus is the site of origin of the bifurcate ligament, which inserts on the navicular and the cuboid. Anteriorly, the calcaneus articulates with the cuboid.

Midfoot

The *navicular* is on the medial side of the midfoot. It has a large posterior concavity that articulates with the talar head. The anterior surface of the navicular articulates with the three cuneiform bones. The lateral surface of the navicular (along with the lateral surface of the third cuneiform) articulates with the cuboid. In about 30% of patients, there is no lateral articulation of the navicular with the cuboid. The cuneiforms are named the first (most medial), second (middle), and third (most lateral). The cuneiforms articulate with their respective metatarsal bones (first, second, and third). The *cuboid* is a square-shaped bone on the lateral aspect of the foot. The posterior border of the cuboid articulates with the calcaneus. Anteriorly, the cuboid articulates with the fourth and fifth metatarsals.

Forefoot

The metatarsals are small long bones. They extend from the tarsals to the phalanges. The second metatarsal is usually 1 cm longer than the first. The developing child has a longitudinal apophysis at the base of the fifth metatarsal that is sometimes mistaken for a fracture.

There are two phalanges in the great toe and three in each of the other toes. The middle and distal phalanges of the fifth (little) toe are commonly fused. Two sesamoid bones are found inferior to the plantar surface of the first metatarsal head.

RADIOGRAPHIC TECHNIQUE

The standard foot series includes the anteroposterior (AP), lateral, and internal (medial) oblique views (Fig. 8-2; Table 8-1). Radiographic technique is important because widely contrasting densities exist between the hindfoot and forefoot areas. The bones and soft tissue margins must both be adequately seen.

Other views are needed in certain situations (Table 8-2). Detecting certain posterior calcaneal fractures can be difficult using standard foot views, and an *axial calcaneal view* is ordered when a calcaneal fracture is suspected but not apparent on plain films (Fig. 8-3). At some institutions, a *lateromedial oblique calcaneal view* is also obtained. Fractures of the talar dome and body are often best seen on ankle radiographs (AP and 45° internal oblique views). Injuries to the extreme medial aspect of the midfoot (first cuneiform and medial tuberosity of the navicular) are sometimes better seen on an *external oblique view*.

TABLE 8-1

Standard Radiographic Views of the Foot

VIEW	POSITION	EVALUATION OF ADEQUACY	LIKELY FINDINGS
AP view	Patient is supine or sitting with knee flexed. Plantar surface of foot in contact with the cassette.	Equal distance between the second through fifth metatarsals. The cuneiforms and cuboid are visible with some superimposition.	Detects most metatarsal fractures. Lisfranc fracture dislocations. Navicular, cuneiform, and sesamoid fractures.
Internal oblique view	The patient is supine or sitting. The medial edge of foot is against the film and lateral edge of foot is raised 30°. X-ray beam perpendicular to the film cassette.	Third through fifth metatarsals are seen without superimposition. Navicular, cuboid, third cuneiform, talar head, and calcaneus are demonstrated.	Metatarsal fractures are seen, especially fourth & fifth. Cuboid fractures.
Lateral view	Patient is recumbent on the affected side. Plantar surface is perpendicular to the cassette.	The entire foot and ankle are demonstrated. There is no rotation.	In combination with the AP view, detects most fractures. Calcaneal fractures are seen. Bohler angle is calculated.

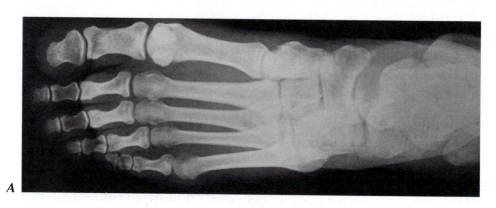

A

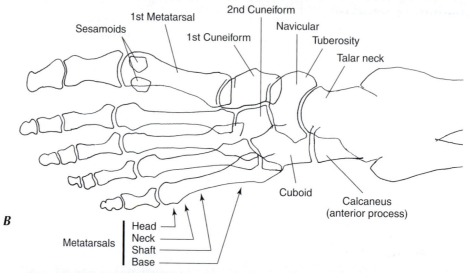

1st Metatarsal

Sesamoids

2nd Cuneiform

1st Cuneiform

Navicular

Tuberosity

Talar neck

Cuboid

Calcaneus
(anterior process)

Metatarsals
Head
Neck
Shaft
Base

B

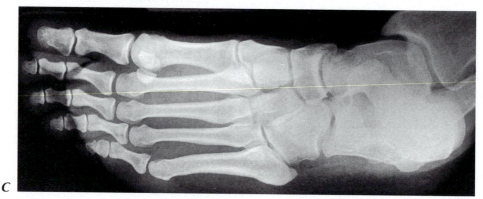

C

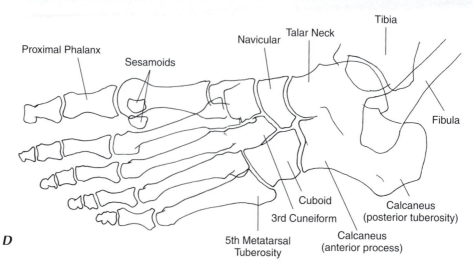

Tibia

Proximal Phalanx

Navicular

Talar Neck

Sesamoids

Fibula

Cuboid

3rd Cuneiform

Calcaneus
(posterior tuberosity)

5th Metatarsal
Tuberosity

Calcaneus
(anterior process)

D

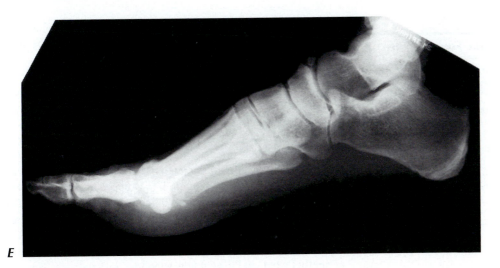

E

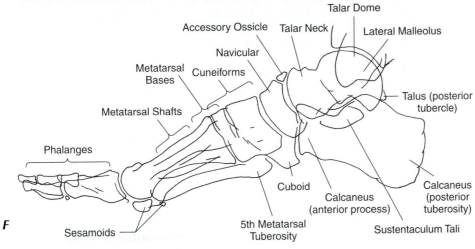

F

FIGURE 8-2. Standard radiographic views of the foot. *A* and *B*. AP view. *C* and *D*. Internal oblique view. *E* and *F*. Lateral view.

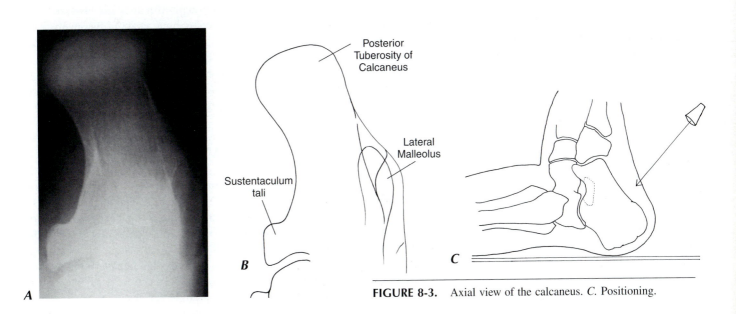

A

B

C

FIGURE 8-3. Axial view of the calcaneus. *C*. Positioning.

TABLE 8-2

Additional Radiographic Views of the Foot and Toes

Calcaneus	Axial view of posterior tuberosity.
Talus	Ankle views (AP and 45° internal oblique) show talar dome and body.
Cuneiform (I) Navicular-medial tuberosity	External oblique foot view.
Toes	Coned-down views (AP and internal oblique).
Great toe	Coned-down views (AP and lateral).

For isolated toe injuries, coned-down AP and internal oblique views of the individual toe are preferred. For the great toe, AP and lateral views are obtained.

Anteroposterior View

The anteroposterior (AP) view demonstrates the structures in the midfoot and forefoot (Fig. 8-2A and B). To obtain the AP image, the patient sits on the table, the knee is flexed, and the foot is placed flat on the cassette. The x-ray beam has a 15° cranial angle away from the long axis of the foot. This view shows the midfoot and forefoot, although there is overlap at the lateral margin of the foot (fourth and fifth metatarsals). The hindfoot is not well seen.

Internal Oblique View

On the internal (medial) oblique view, there is less overlap of the fourth and fifth metatarsals and the cuboid than on the AP view (Fig. 8-2C and D). The first and second metatarsals have more overlap than on the AP view. The internal oblique view is obtained by first placing the sole of the foot flat against the film cassette and then raising the lateral side of the foot to an angle between the foot and the film of 30°. The x-ray beam is perpendicular to the cassette. This view also shows the anterior process of the calcaneus and can detect small avulsion fractures at the site of the insertion of the bifurcate ligament.

Lateral View

The hindfoot is best seen on the lateral view of the foot (Fig. 8-2E and F). This view is obtained with the patient either in a frog-leg position or lying on the affected side. The lateral edge of the injured foot is placed on the cassette with the foot perpendicular to the cassette and the x-ray beam is directed straight to the midpoint of the foot. The lateral view demonstrates the calcaneus and talus. This view can also show avulsion fractures

of the dorsal surface of the talar neck and navicular. The metatarsals are not well seen on the lateral projection because of overlap.

Calcaneus—Axial Projection

The axial calcaneal view is obtained with either a plantodorsal or a dorsoplantar orientation (Fig. 8-3). The *plantodorsal projection* is obtained with the patient lying or sitting supine with the leg extended. A strip of cloth is wrapped around the ball of the foot and the foot is held in dorsiflexion at a 90° angle. The cassette is flat and the x-ray beam is directed at a cranial angle 40° away from the long axis of the foot (Fig. 8-3C). For the *dorsoplantar projection,* the patient is prone, the knee is gently flexed, and the ankle is supported on sandbags. The film is perpendicular to the x-ray table and placed against the sole of the foot. The x-ray beam is directed at a 40° caudal angle to the long axis of the foot.

The axial projection is used to detect fractures oriented along the longitudinal axis of the posterior tuberosity of the calcaneus. The sustentaculum tali is also shown on this view.

Calcaneus—Lateromedial Oblique

The lateromedial oblique provides an unobstructed image of the anterior aspect of the subtalar joint. This view is obtained with the patient sitting or lying with the hip and knee flexed. The ankle is in a right-angle position and the medial edge of the foot is placed against the cassette. The leg is rotated, coming to rest against a foam wedge, so that a 45° angle is formed. The x-ray beam is perpendicular to the cassette. In addition to providing greater detail of the subtalar joint, this view also shows the cuboid and navicular.

Toe Views

Injuries to the second through fifth toes are assessed with coned-down AP and internal oblique views of the involved toe. Because the x-ray beam is not centered on the toes, standard foot views can miss a subtle injury to the toes because of insufficient detail and distortion. In addition, the toes are poorly seen on the standard foot lateral view due to overlap. Injuries to the great toe are imaged with an AP and lateral view.

RADIOGRAPHIC ANALYSIS

Analysis of foot radiographs begins by focusing on sites of common injury (Fig. 8-4).[4] The site of maximal tenderness is carefully inspected. A systematic analysis then includes a step-wise review of the hindfoot, midfoot, and forefoot in each radiograph (Table 8-3). The AP and internal oblique views show the forefoot and midfoot best, whereas the lateral view shows the hindfoot and midfoot best. Finally, those areas where subtle injuries can be missed are carefully reviewed again.

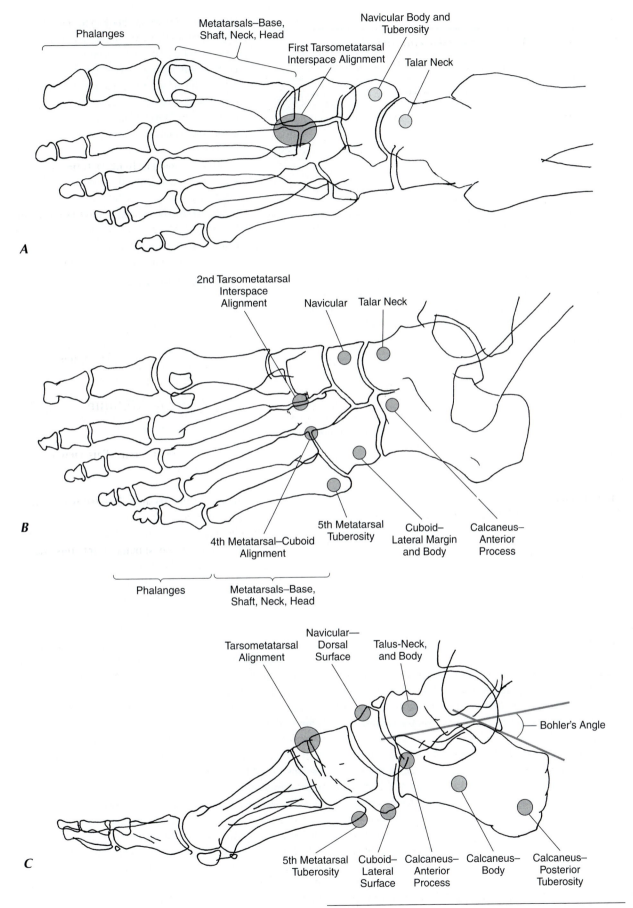

FIGURE 8-4.   Sites prone to injury and easily missed injuries.
A. AP view. *B.* Internal oblique view. *C.* Lateral view.

TABLE 8-3

Systematic Analysis of Foot Radiographs

AP view	Forefoot	Metatarsal shafts, heads, MTP joints, phalanges
	Midfoot	Metatarsal bases (I, II, III). The medial side of the second metatarsal base should align with the medial edge of the second cuneiform. Navicular (body and medial tuberosity). Cuneiforms (I, II).
	Hindfoot	Talonavicular and calcaneocuboid articulations (midtarsal joint).
Internal oblique view	Forefoot	Metatarsal shafts, heads, metatarsophalangeal joints, phalanges.
	Midfoot	Metatarsal bases (III, IV, V). Fifth metatarsal base—a common site of fracture Fourth metatarsal base (medial edge) aligns with the medial border of the cuboid and the third metatarsal base (lateral border) aligns with the lateral edge of the third (lateral) cuneiform. Cuboid. Cuneiform (III).
	Hindfoot	Talus: head and neck. Calcaneus: anterior process and body. Talonavicular and calcaneocuneiform articulations.
Lateral view	Hindfoot	Calcaneus: tuberosity, body, and anterior process. Bohler's angle (20° to 40°). Talus: body, dome, posterior tuberosity (os trigonum), neck, and head. Subtalar articulation.
	Midfoot	Superior border of midfoot: Malalignment due to dislocation. Avulsion fractures of superior border of talar neck. Cuboid and fifth metatarsal tuberosity.
	Forefoot	Metatarsals and phalanges not well seen due to overlap.

Anteroposterior View

The AP view provides most information about the forefoot. Sequential inspection of the metatarsals begins with the first metatarsal. Each metatarsal is reviewed from the base to the shaft and finally the head. The metatarsal shafts should be roughly parallel.

The alignment of the metatarsal bases with the cuneiforms and cuboid is carefully examined. The lateral edge of the second metatarsal base should be aligned with the lateral edge of the second cuneiform. Abnormal alignment here prompts closer inspection for a Lisfranc (tarsometatarsal) fracture/dislocation.

The phalanges are inspected for fracture and dislocation. Each proximal phalanx should be aligned with the corresponding metatarsal.

Next, the midfoot tarsal bones are examined. The anterior navicular surface should be smooth. The three cuneiforms are inspected for fracture and their articular relationships with the navicular are examined. Fracture of the midfoot tarsals or in-

terruption of their normal articular relationships should prompt a careful review of the Lisfranc (tarsometatarsal) joint. Disruption of the Lisfranc joint appears as medial or lateral displacement of the first metatarsal and lateral displacement of the second through fifth metatarsals. When dislocation occurs at the Lisfranc joint, metatarsal and tarsal fractures are often seen.

Finally, the hindfoot is inspected. The AP view provides limited information about the talus and calcaneus. Portions of the midtarsal (Chopart) joint are seen and should have smooth articular surfaces and a uniform joint space. Rarely, an avulsion fracture is seen.

Internal Oblique View

The internal (medial) oblique projection is examined in the same manner as the AP view. The lateral metatarsals and cuboid are seen without overlap and should be carefully reviewed. The base of the fifth metatarsal is a common site of fracture. The anterior process of the calcaneus is also well seen. This site is carefully checked for an avulsion fracture.

Lateral View

In examining the lateral view, one should inspect the hindfoot first, then the midfoot, and finally the forefoot. The distal elements of the tibia and fibula are also inspected for a fracture.

When evaluating the *talus*, the relationship of the talar dome with the articular surface of the tibia is noted. The articular surfaces and joint space should appear as a smooth arc. The rest of the talus is then examined from posterior to anterior, starting with the body, proceeding to the neck, and finishing with the talar head. One should look for tiny avulsion fractures at the anterosuperior border of the talus. An accessory ossicle, the *os trigonum,* is often seen posterior to the articular surface. The subtalar joint is inspected for its proper relationship with the calcaneus. Likewise, the articular relationship between the navicular and the talar head is noted.

Next, the *calcaneus* is examined. The cortex and trabeculae are inspected for disruption. *Bohler's angle* is assessed if a calcaneal fracture is suspected (Fig. 8-5).[5] Bohler's angle is measured at the intersection of two lines drawn on the superior surface of the calcaneus. The first line connects the superior margin of the posterior tuberosity with the posterior facet; the second line connects the posterior facet with the anterior process of the calcaneus. The normal value of the Bohler's angle is 20 to 40°. An angle of less than 20° suggests a depressed calcaneal fracture; however, a normal Bohler's angle does not exclude a calcaneal fracture.

The bones of the midfoot are then inspected. On the lateral

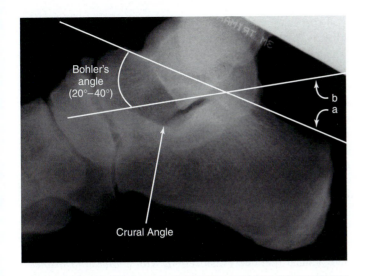

FIGURE 8-5. Bohler's angle. Bohler's angle is formed between a line drawn along the superior surface of the posterior tuberosity *(a)* and a line connecting the superior tip of the subtalar articular surface and the superior tip of the anterior process *(b)*. Bohler's angle is normally between 20 and 40°. A diminished Bohler's angle is seen with most compression fractures of the calcaneal body. The angle between the subtalar articular surface and the superior surface of the anterior process is known as the *crural angle.*

view, parts of the navicular, cuboid, and first cuneiform are seen. The superior margin of the navicular is checked for small avulsion fractures.

The metatarsals usually have so much overlap that detection of abnormalities is difficult. If the metatarsal bases are superiorly displaced relative to the tarsals, an injury to the Lisfranc joint is likely. The base of the fifth metatarsal is inspected for a fracture.

COMMON ABNORMALITIES

Talar Fractures

The talus is the second most frequently fractured tarsal bone after the calcaneus. Many of these injuries are minor avulsion fractures associated with ankle injuries, most often of the dorsal or lateral surfaces of the talus. Osteochondral fractures of the talar dome articular surface occur with ankle injuries and are described in Chap. 9. Other common and more serious injuries are fractures through the talar head, neck, body, or posterior process. Talar neck fractures are the most common. Talar dislocations are seen with severe trauma, most often involving the subtalar joint. In about half of talar dislocations, there is an associated fracture of the talar neck. The blood supply to the talus is tenuous. Most of the blood supply to the talar body arrives via the talar neck. Therefore, fractures of the talar neck are often complicated by avascular necrosis of the talus.

FRACTURES OF THE TALAR NECK. Talar neck fractures occur when the foot is forcibly dorsiflexed. The neck of the talus is compressed against the anterior tibial plafond. This injury was first described in World War I aviators who, in crash landing,

had jammed a foot against the rudder bar. These fractures are therefore sometimes referred to as "aviator's astragalus." Nowadays, a common mechanism of injury is a front-end automobile crash in which the driver's foot hits the brake pedal.

Owing to the tenuous blood supply of the talus, fractures involving the talar neck can lead to avascular necrosis. The more severe the fracture, the greater the risk of avascular necrosis. Important elements to note in describing fractures of the talar neck are displacement as well as malalignment of the subtalar and talonavicular joints (Fig. 8-6). About half of the fractures of the talar neck and body are associated with subtalar dislocation or posterior dislocation of the talar body (Fig. 8-7).

Fractures involving the talar neck are best seen on the lateral and AP views of the foot. Because of overlap of the sustentaculum tali with the inferior aspect of the talus, evaluation

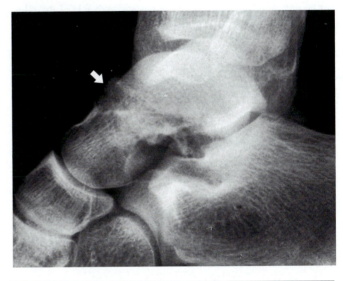

FIGURE 8-6. Talar neck fracture. A fracture through the talar neck with dorsal displacement.

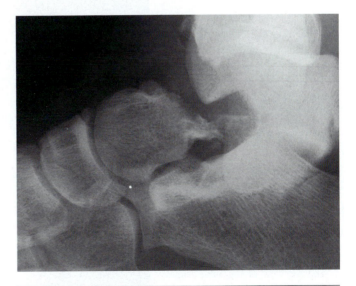

FIGURE 8-7. Fracture/dislocation of the talar neck. In this severe injury, the talar body fragment is dislocated posteriorly with respect to the subtalar joint and ankle mortise. There is substantial risk of avascular necrosis of the talus.

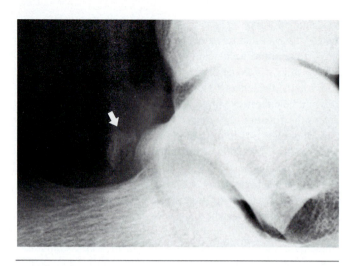

FIGURE 8-8. Os trigonum. This common accessory ossicle should not be mistaken for a fracture of the posterior tubercle of the talus.

of the subtalar joint can be difficult on plain films. CT may be needed for complete evaluation of a fracture of the talar neck.

FRACTURES OF THE TALAR BODY. Talar body fractures are usually associated with high-velocity, high-energy injuries (e.g., a fall from a great height or a motor vehicle accident). Nondisplaced fractures of the talar body can be difficult to see. Ankle radiographs (AP and lateral views) are used to evaluate the talar body. A 45° internal oblique view of the ankle can also help delineate a talar body fracture.

OS TRIGONUM. The *os trigonum* is a common accessory ossicle that can mimic a fracture of the posterior talus (Fig. 8-8). An os trigonum is seen in 8% of the population. It has smooth,

well-corticated margins. However, pain elicited with foot dorsiflexion suggests a fracture of the posterolateral tubercle of the talus or a fracture through its cartilaginous attachment, resulting in displacement of the os trigonum.

FRACTURES OF THE TALAR HEAD. Talar head fractures often occur during a fall in which the force is transmitted through the forefoot to the talus. The standard foot views usually show the fracture. However, a 45° internal oblique view of the ankle or CT may be required.

Talar Dislocations

There are two types of talar dislocation: total talar dislocation and subtalar (peritalar) dislocation. With a *total talar dislocation,* the talus is completely disarticulated from both the ankle and calcaneus. This is often an open injury and is often accompanied by a talar neck fracture (Fig. 8-7). Clinically, there is obvious deformity of the hindfoot.

SUBTALAR DISLOCATION. In a *subtalar dislocation,* the talocalcaneal (subtalar) and talonavicular joints are disrupted (Fig. 8-9). With medial subtalar dislocations, the foot is angled medially and the head of the talus is palpable laterally. In the rare lateral dislocation, the talar head is palpated medially. With closed dislocations, emergent reduction is performed prior to radiographic study if there is risk of skin necrosis. Postreduction films are essential to detect associated fractures.

Ankle views should be obtained when a total talar or subtalar dislocation is suspected. The ankle AP view best shows the disarticulation. The lateral view is helpful in identifying associated fractures to the talus, tibia, and navicular.

FIGURE 8-9. Subtalar dislocation. *A.* The AP view of the ankle shows medial displacement of the calcaneus at the subtalar joint. The talus is normally situated in the ankle mortise. *B.* The lateral view shows dislocation between the talus and calcaneus.

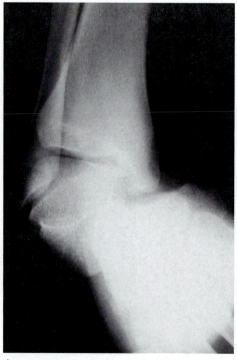

A

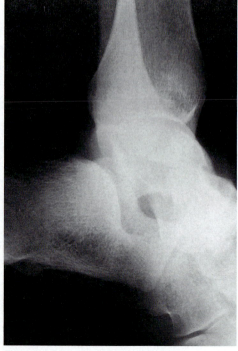

B

Calcaneal Fractures

The calcaneus is the most commonly fractured tarsal bone. Common sites of calcaneal fractures include the body, the anterior process, and the posterior tuberosity. Comminuted compression fractures of the body of the calcaneus are the most frequent and are associated with considerable posttraumatic morbidity.

The lateral view is essential in evaluating the calcaneus. Both cortical and trabecular bone must be examined closely for disruption. Curvilinear radiodense areas within the calcaneus indicate overlap of fracture fragments and may be the only evidence of fracture. The *Bohler's angle* is measured to assess the magnitude of compression of a fractured calcaneus (Fig. 8-5). Nevertheless, some calcaneal fractures have a normal Bohler angle.

COMPRESSION FRACTURES OF THE CALCANEAL BODY.   Fractures of the body of the calcaneus often demonstrate some degree of compression. Compression fractures result from a fall or jump landing on the feet. The injury is suggested by an ecchymotic and tender heel. Calcaneal body fractures (especially with compression) are usually detected on standard foot views. However,

axial and oblique calcaneal views are needed to detect more subtle injuries. With compression, the Bohler's angle is almost always less than 20° (Fig. 8-10). Computed tomography (CT) is used to fully define complex calcaneal fractures.

Because most calcaneal compression fractures result from a high fall, vertebral body fractures are common. In fact, vertebral fractures occur in over 20% of calcaneal fractures.[6] The thoracolumbar junction (T12-L2) is most often involved. Therefore, in evaluating a patient with a calcaneus fracture, one must examine the axial skeleton carefully. In addition, there is a significant risk of concomitant fractures in other skeletal regions, such as the knees and hips.

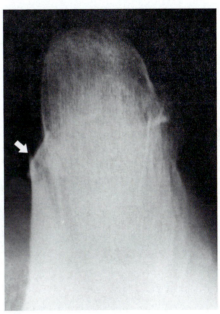

B

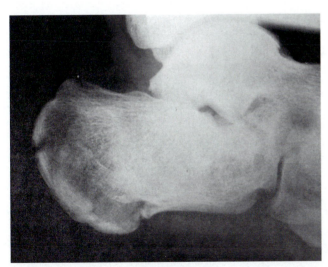

A

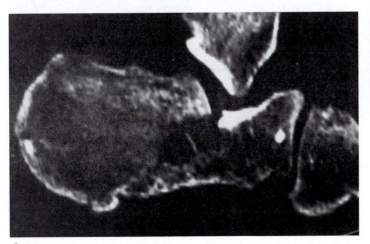

C

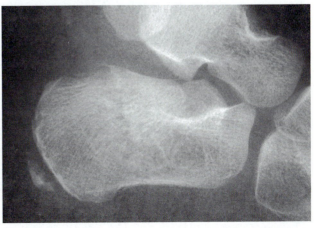

D

FIGURE 8-10.   Calcaneal compression fractures. *A.* There is a comminuted compressed fracture of the calcaneal body and posterior tuberosity. Bohler's angle is flat (0°). *B.* The axial view shows a fracture across the posterior tuberosity. *C.* CT sagittal reconstruction image shows the anatomy of the fracture. *D.* A compression fracture in a child. The fracture line is difficult to see, whereas the flattening of Bohler's angle reveals the magnitude of the injury.

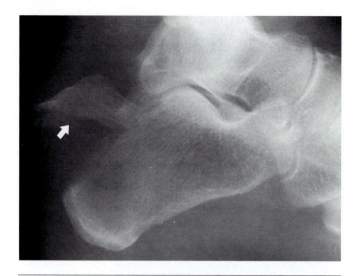

FIGURE 8-11.   Avulsion fracture of the posterior tuberosity. The superior surface of the posterior tuberosity is avulsed off by the pull of the Achilles tendon. Because of its radiographic appearance, this fracture is sometimes called a "beak" fracture.

FRACTURES OF THE POSTERIOR TUBEROSITY.   A fracture of the posterior tuberosity of the calcaneus usually results from a jump or fall. The patient is unable to walk and plantarflexion is difficult. The lateral radiograph best identifies this injury. When it is displaced, the injury is obvious. If a nondisplaced longitudinal or oblique fracture of the posterior calcaneal tuberosity is suspected and is not visible on the lateral view, an axial view of the posterior calcaneus should be performed (see Fig. 2-1). Avulsion fractures of the superior surface of the posterior tuberosity are due to the pull of the Achilles tendon (Fig. 8-11).

FRACTURES OF THE ANTERIOR PROCESS.   A fracture of the anterior process of the calcaneus occurs at the insertion of the bifurcate ligament (Fig. 8-12). This is best seen on the lateral or internal oblique views of the foot.

FRACTURES OF THE SUSTENTACULUM TALI.   Fracture of the sustentaculum tali results from axial loading applied to an inverted foot. The sustentaculum tali is a medial structure; therefore the patient with this fracture has tenderness and swelling just distal to the medial malleolus. Sustentaculum tali fractures are often best seen on the axial calcaneal view. CT provides the best images of this injury.

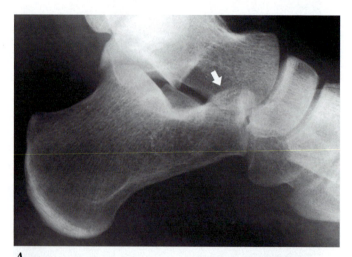

A

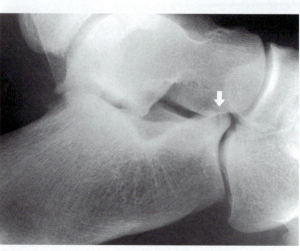

B

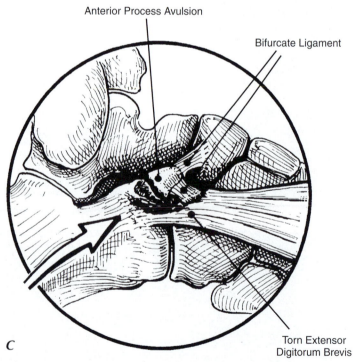

C

FIGURE 8-12.   Fracture of the anterior process of the calcaneus. *A.* The superior corner of the anterior process of the calcaneus is a frequent site of fracture. The injury is due to avulsion from the pull of the bifurcate ligament that attaches to the navicular and cuboid. *B.* The fracture can be small and is occasionally missed. *C.* Line drawing (From Martise JR, Lerinsohn EM: *Imaging of Athletic Injuries,* McGraw-Hill, 1992, with permission.)

Midtarsal Dislocations

Chopart joint is the articulation between the hindfoot and midfoot. Dislocation at the Chopart joint is rare. When it does occur, fractures of the adjacent bones are frequent. On the lateral view, talonavicular dislocation is usually obvious.

Midfoot Fractures

Fractures of the cuboid, cuneiforms, and navicular are usually due to either axial loading or crush injuries. Avulsion fractures occur as a result of inversion and eversion of the ankle and foot.

Isolated midfoot fractures are uncommon. For example, a cuboid fracture is often associated with a calcaneal fracture, and a cuneiform fracture is frequently seen in association with a metatarsal fracture.

NAVICULAR FRACTURES. Dorsal chip fractures result from foot inversion and are thus associated with ankle sprains. Fractures through the body of the navicular are usually vertical and sometimes horizontal. Crush-compression injuries usually involve the anterior surface of the navicular. Medial fractures involve the navicular tuberosity and may be visible only on an external oblique view. Navicular fractures can be complicated by avascular necrosis and nonunion (Fig. 8-13).

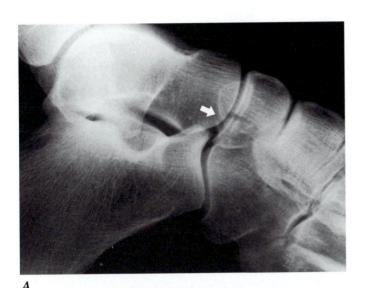

A

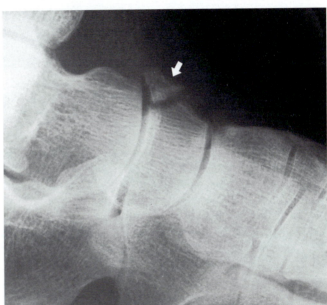

B

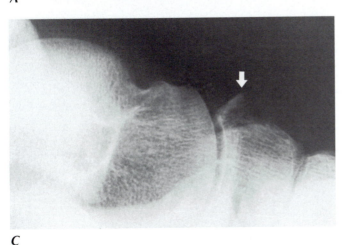

C

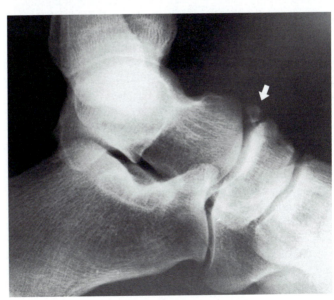

D

FIGURE 8-13. Navicular fractures. *A.* Transverse fracture through the body of the navicular. *B.* An avulsion fracture from the dorsal surface of the navicular is occasionally seen with ankle sprains. *C.* A small avulsion fracture can be subtle. *D.* This accessory ossicle (os supranaviculare) has a well-corticated, smooth margin. It should be recognized as a normal variant and not mistaken for an acute fracture.

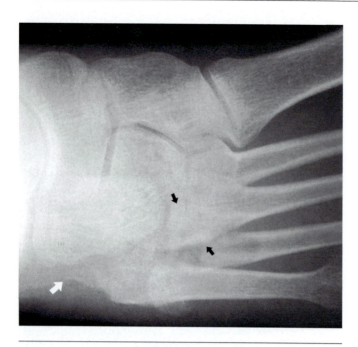

FIGURE 8-14.   This cuboid fracture is associated with fractures of the fourth and fifth metatarsal bases.

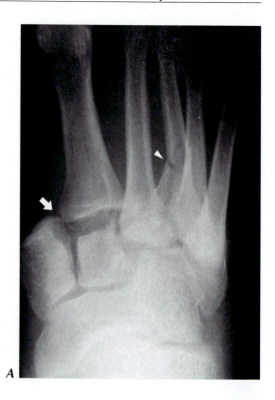

A

FRACTURES OF THE CUBOID AND CUNEIFORMS.   Fractures of the cuboid and cuneiforms are usually visible on the standard foot series, although the radiographic findings can be subtle. Cuboid fractures are often associated with fractures of the calcaneus and navicular. Fractures of the cuneiforms are usually associated with a Lisfranc (tarsometatarsal) fracture/dislocation. In fact, an apparently isolated cuneiform fracture is often actually a Lisfranc fracture/dislocation that has spontaneously reduced. Severe compression forces result in a cuboid fracture called a "nutcracker" fracture. Cuboid avulsion fractures occur at both the lateral margin and the inferior pole (Fig. 8-14). CT may be needed to fully characterize cuboid and cuneiform injuries.

Tarsometatarsal (Lisfranc) Fracture/Dislocation

Tarsometatarsal dislocations are referred to as *Lisfranc fracture/dislocations,* or Lisfranc fractures.[7,8] Unlike most orthopedic eponyms, this eponym does not honor the person who first described the injury; rather, Lisfranc described the anatomy of the tarsometatarsal articulation. Usually, high-energy trauma causes this injury such as a frontal-impact auto collision or a fall.[9] Diabetic neuropathy resulting in Charcot disease (neuropathic arthropathy) is also associated with Lisfranc fracture/dislocations due to repetitive stress. Although Lisfranc fracture/dislocations represent severe derangement of the foot, the radiographic findings can be subtle.

The tarsometatarsal joint has strong ligamentous connections between the metatarsals and the adjacent cuneiforms and cuboid. The second metatarsal in particular has strong connections to the cuneiforms. It is difficult for the second metatarsal to dislocate without sustaining a transverse fracture through its base. Therefore, a fracture through the proximal second metatarsal is indicative of an injury to the Lisfranc joint.

Radiographic detection of the Lisfranc fracture/dislocation is based on the observation that the medial edge of the second metatarsal does not align with the medial edge of the second cuneiform.[10] This is seen on the AP and internal oblique projections of the foot. In addition, the medial aspect of the base of the fourth metatarsal is normally aligned with the medial edge of the cuboid, the fifth metatarsal notch (end of the articular surface) is normally aligned with the lateral surface of the cuboid, and the lateral aspect of the first metatarsal is nor-

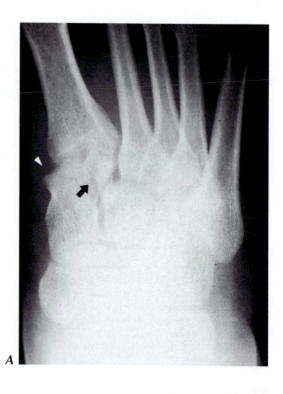

A

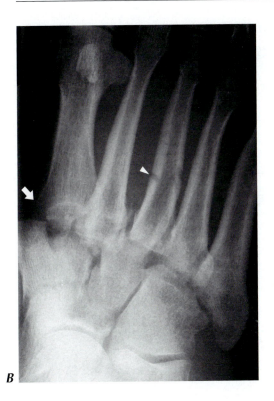

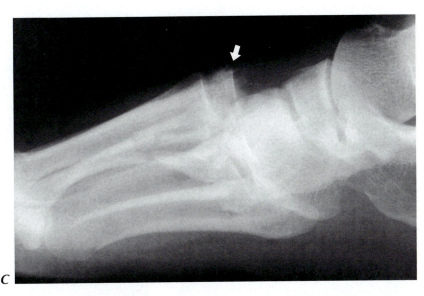

B

C

FIGURE 8-15. Lisfranc fracture/dislocation, homolateral type. In this severely displaced injury, the first metatarsal is dislocated from the first cuneiform (*arrow*) *(A* and *B)*. A fracture of the third metacarpal shaft is also present (*arrowhead*). On the lateral view *(C)*, the metatarsals are dorsally displaced relative to the midfoot.

mally aligned with the lateral edge of the medial cuneiform. Any alteration in these alignments suggests a dislocation. On the lateral view, there may be malalignment of the dorsal surfaces of the cuneiforms and metatarsal bases—the metatarsal bases are displaced dorsally with respect to the cuneiforms.

Displacement of a Lisfranc dislocation is described as either homolateral or divergent. The *homolateral type* has lateral displacement of the first metatarsal, along with lateral displacement of the second through fifth metatarsals (Figs. 8-15 and 8-16).

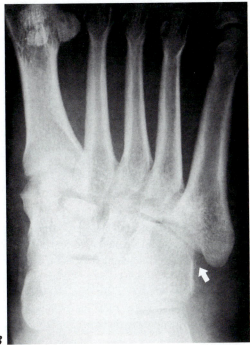

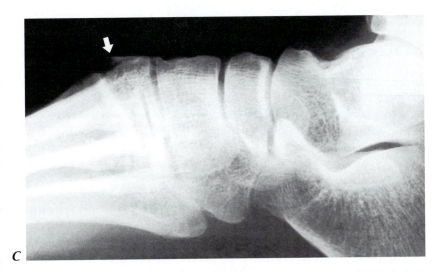

B

C

FIGURE 8-16. Lisfranc fracture/dislocation, homolateral type. In this patient, the radiographic findings are more subtle. On the AP view *(A)*, there is a fracture of the first cuneiform (*arrow*) and malalignment of the base of the first metatarsal and first cuneiform (*arrowhead*). On the internal oblique view *(B)*, the base of the fifth metatarsal is slightly displaced laterally relative to the cuboid (*arrow*). On the lateral view *(C)*, a small avulsion fracture from the dorsal surface of the metatarsal bases is seen (*arrow*).

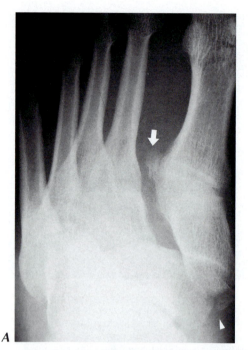

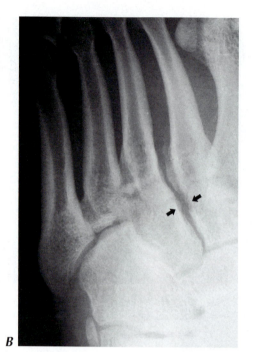

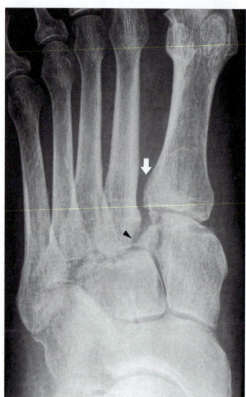

In the *divergent type,* the first metatarsal (and occasionally the second metatarsal) dislocates medially or stays fixed and the more lateral metatarsals are displaced laterally (Fig. 8-17). With a Lisfranc injury, there are frequently fractures of the cuneiforms, metatarsal shafts, and bases of the metatarsals.

Metatarsal Fractures

Metatarsal fractures may involve the base, shaft, neck, or head of the metatarsal. Standard radiographic projections are adequate for the diagnosis of metatarsal fractures. The AP projection usually offers the most information (Fig. 8-18). The oblique view occasionally provides better visualization, especially of the lateral metatarsals. The lateral projection is less useful because of metatarsal overlap. Nonetheless, the lateral projection can show displacement of the fracture and dislocation at the metatarsophalangeal joints. Sometimes, a metatarsal fracture is visible on only one view.

FIGURE 8-17.   Lisfranc fracture/dislocation, divergent type. *A.* On the AP view, there is marked widening of the space between the first and second cuneiforms and metatarsal bases (*arrow*). A small fracture is present at the medial surface of the navicular (*arrowhead*). *B.* In the oblique view, widening between the second and third cuneiforms and metatarsal bases is seen (*arrows*). *C.* A subtle divergent Lisfranc dislocation/fracture is indicated by the slight widening of the space between the first cuneiform and base of the second metatarsal (*arrow*). A small fracture of the second metatarsal base is present (*arrowhead*). Although the fracture and displacement appears slight, the derangement of the foot at the tarsometatarsal joint is severe. (*C.* Copyright David Schwartz, M.D.)

Fractures of the Fifth Metatarsal

The base (tuberosity) of the fifth metatarsal is a common site of fracture, usually due to inversion of the ankle and foot. Inversion creates tension on the peroneus brevis tendon and the lateral fibers of the plantar fascia, which causes avulsion at their insertion sites on the tuberosity of the fifth metatarsal (Fig. 8-19). This tuberosity avulsion fracture must be distinguished from a fracture of the fifth metatarsal shaft, which is usually

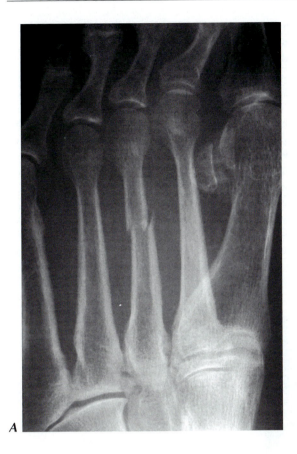

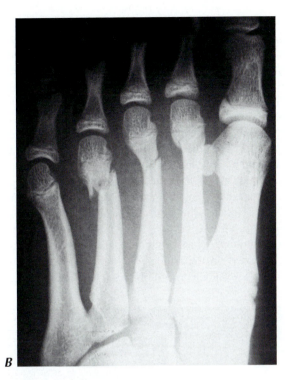

FIGURE 8-18. Metatarsal fractures. *A.* An isolated fracture through the shaft of the third metatarsal. *B.* Fractures of the neck of the second, third, and fourth metatarsals.

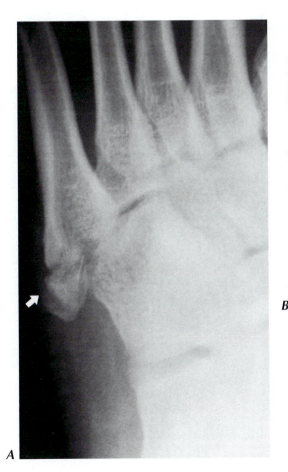

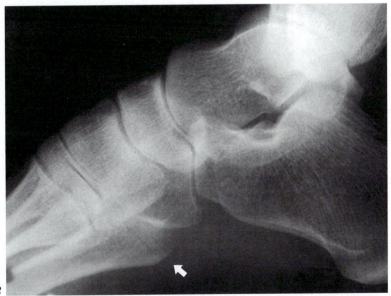

FIGURE 8-19. "Pseudo-Jones" fractures. *A.* An avulsion fracture of the fifth metatarsal tuberosity is seen on this oblique view. *B.* A subtle fracture is seen on this lateral view.

due to a direct blow or repeated stress on the lateral margin of the foot (Fig. 8-20). Robert Jones described a transverse fracture through the proximal fifth metatarsal shaft in 1902 after he sustained the injury while dancing.[11] Both fractures of the fifth metatarsal shaft and of the tuberosity are often referred to as a *Jones fracture*, although the term is properly applied only to the fracture of the proximal portion of the metatarsal shaft. The tuberosity avulsion fracture is therefore sometimes called a *pseudo-Jones fracture*.[12,13] The tuberosity fracture is considerably more common than the metatarsal shaft fracture.

Occasionally, a tuberosity avulsion fracture is missed. This occurs because the mechanism of injury is the same as that causing a common ankle sprain—inversion of the ankle. If only ankle radiographs are ordered, the fracture of the fifth metatarsal base is at the bottom corner of the radiograph—or it may not even be included on the radiograph. The lateral margin of the foot must be examined in all patients with an "ankle sprain" and foot radiographs should be ordered if there is tenderness in this area.

An unfused apophysis of the fifth metatarsal base is seen in children and adolescents and should not be misinterpreted as a fracture (Fig. 8-21). The unfused apophysis is oriented along the long axis of the foot, whereas a tuberosity avulsion fracture is transverse. The *os vesalianum* is an accessory bone located near the base of the fifth metatarsal. This accessory bone can be mistaken for a fracture. Smooth cortical margins are consistent with an accessory ossicle than a fracture. Irregular margins imply fracture.

Fractures of the tuberosity of the fifth metatarsal usually heal quickly, without sequelae. On the other hand, the true Jones fracture at the proximal metaphyseal shaft has a high incidence of nonunion because it involves the weight-bearing lateral margin of the foot. The true Jones fracture must be treated with a full cast.

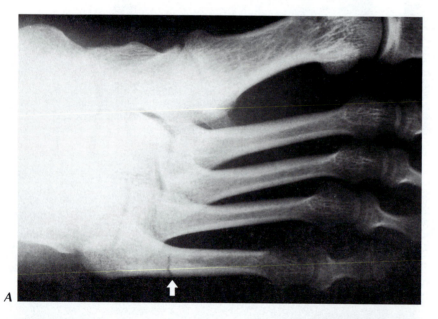

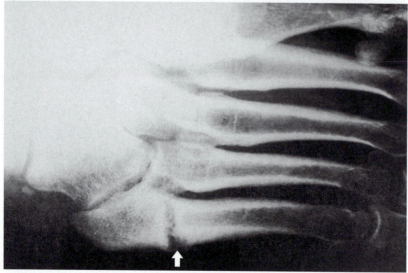

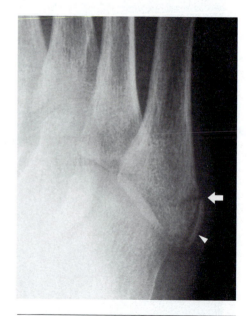

FIGURE 8-21. A normal unfused apophysis of the fifth metatarsal tuberosity is seen in this adolescent *(arrowhead)*. This should not be mistaken for a fracture. In this patient, there is also a fracture across the base of the metatarsal *(arrow)*.

FIGURE 8-20. Jones fracture. *A.* A transverse fracture through the proximal shaft of the fifth metatarsal. *B.* This fracture is often complicated by nonunion.

Phalangeal Fractures

Toe fractures are common. The most frequently involved toe is the fifth, because of its vulnerable position. Although phalangeal fractures are often trivialized, they are quite painful.

Standard radiographic views of the involved toe usually show the fracture (Fig. 8-22). Foot radiographs may fail to show the fracture because the toe is far from the central ray of the x-ray beam and is therefore not well visualized. Phalangeal fractures are described as transverse, oblique, spiral, comminuted, intraarticular, and extraarticular. Chronic digital deformities such as hammertoes, claw toes, mallet toes, and hallux abductovalgus distort radiographic imaging, making evaluation more difficult. When a fracture is suspected, one should place the toes as parallel to the x-ray plate as possible during imaging.

Sesamoid Fractures

Sesamoid fractures are rare. When they do occur, they are frequently misdiagnosed. Patients often relate no history of trauma. Compounding this difficulty is the fact that bipartite sesamoids are common (they are found in about 30% of persons) (Fig. 8-23). A smooth margin suggests a bipartite bone, and a rough or irregular margin is probably a fracture.

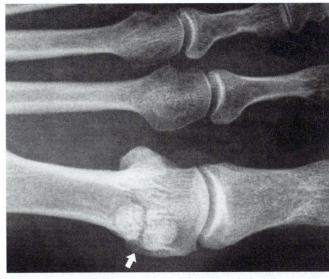

A

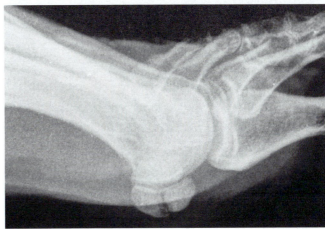

B

FIGURE 8-23. A bipartite sesamoid was found incidentally on this radiograph of the foot. The margins are well-corticated, suggesting that this is not an acute injury.

Stress Fractures

Stress fractures often involve the metatarsals, occasionally the navicular, and rarely the calcaneus.[14] The most common location for a stress fracture is the diaphyseal region of the metatarsals. There is no radiographic evidence of stress fracture until about 14 days following the fracture, when periosteal changes are seen (Fig. 8-24). The bone callus has a fluffy radiographic appearance. The clinical presentation is similar to that of inflammatory processes such as tendinitis or capsulitis. An earlier diagnosis can be made using a technetium-99 bone scan.

Freiberg Infraction

Freiberg infraction is an osteochondrosis (avascular necrosis) that most often involves the head of the second metatarsal[15,16] (Fig. 8-25). The third metatarsal is less often involved, and the

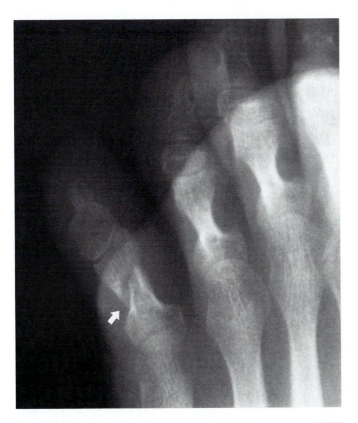

FIGURE 8-22. A fracture through the proximal phalanx of the little toe is seen on this AP view.

fourth metatarsal rarely. This disorder is seen most often in females during childhood. The etiology is uncertain. On radiography, there is fragmentation of the cortical surface of the second metatarsal. Eventually, the metatarsal head becomes flattened. *Köhler disease,* also seen in children, is osteochondrosis of the navicular bone.

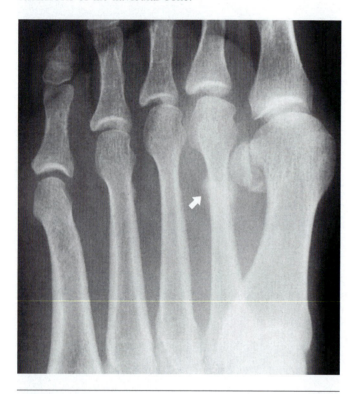

FIGURE 8-24. A "fuzzy" periosteal reaction due to a stress fracture *(arrow)* is seen around the distal second metatarsal shaft. The patient presented with nontraumatic foot pain that had been present for several weeks.

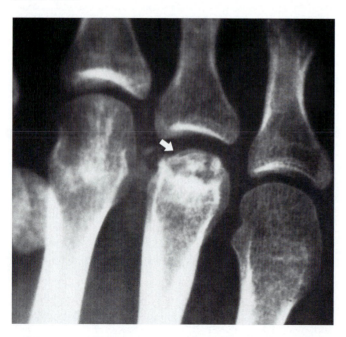

FIGURE 8-25. There is collapse of the second metatarsal head due to idiopathic avascular necrosis. The patient presented with foot pain not due to trauma. This is known as a Freiberg infraction.

Plantar Puncture Wounds

The decision to image a patient with a puncture wound to the foot can be difficult.[17–19] A thorough history gives the clinician an idea about the depth of penetration and whether the penetrating object remained intact. Punctures in the area of the metatarsal heads are common.[20] If the history suggests a retained foreign body, plain radiography should be performed.[21–23]

If the wounding agent is radiolucent, then CT or ultrasonography is a preferable imaging technique.[24] CT is superior in detecting soft tissue foreign bodies.[25] CT also helps localize the object in three dimensions, which can assist in its removal. Real-time *ultrasonography* with a high-frequency (15 MHz) transducer can localize soft tissue foreign bodies. However, complex echo shadows caused by fascial planes, tendons, and muscles can make identification difficult.

In some patients, a foreign body will be present without a good history of stepping on a sharp object. For this reason, radiographs should be obtained in patients with unexplained localized foot cellulitis or cellulitis unresponsive to antibiotics (Fig. 8-26).

ERRORS IN INTERPRETATION

Lisfranc Fracture/Dislocation

Although the Lisfranc tarsometatarsal fracture/dislocation causes severe derangement of the foot, the radiographic findings can be subtle if the amount of displacement is minimal (Fig. 8-16).[10] The key radiographic observation is loss of the normal alignment between the medial border of the base of the second metatarsal and the medial border of the second cuneiform. Small fractures of the metatarsal bases and cuneiforms also suggest this injury.

Jones Fractures

A fracture of the tuberosity at the base of the fifth metatarsal occasionally occurs in the patient with a "sprained ankle." The lateral margin of the foot must be examined clinically; when it is tender, foot radiographs should be obtained. On ankle radiographs, the fracture is easily missed because it lies outside or near the edge of the x-ray film (Fig. 8-19). Treatment of this fracture is symptomatic, with a compressive dressing and limited weight bearing.

Proximal fifth metatarsal fractures must be described accurately, and the eponym *Jones fracture* should be avoided. This eponym has been applied to both fractures of the tuberosity and those of the metatarsal shaft. Because the management and prognosis of these two injuries are significantly different, the fracture should be described anatomically rather than with the eponym (Fig. 8-20). Finally, an unfused apophysis at the fifth metatarsal base is normal in children and adolescents, although it can look much like a fracture (Fig. 8-21).

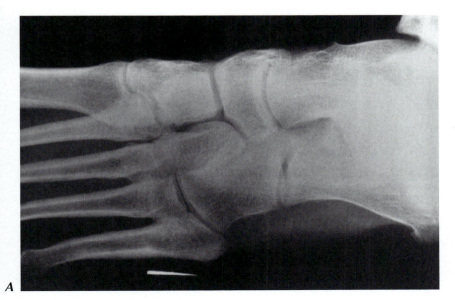

A

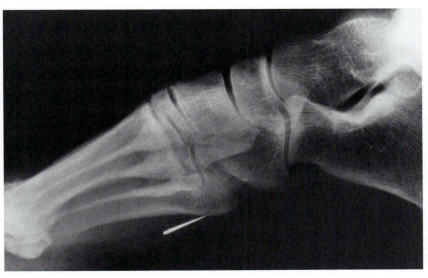

B

FIGURE 8-26. A metallic foreign body is seen along the lateral margin of the foot. The patient had localized cellulitis of the foot that was unresponsive to antibiotics. The patient was unaware of having stepped on a sharp object.

Avulsion Fractures of the Midfoot

Small avulsion fractures of the midfoot can occur in patients who have ankle "sprains." The midfoot should be carefully examined clinically and the radiographs should be closely inspected for fractures. Common sites of avulsion fractures are the dorsal surface of the navicular, the anterior process of the talus, and the lateral margin of the cuboid (Fig. 8-13*D*).

Calcaneal Fractures

Fractures of the *posterior tuberosity* of the calcaneus (heel bone) that are oriented in the long axis or oblique plane may not be visible on the lateral foot film. Because this region is not shown on AP or oblique foot radiographs, an axial view of the calcaneus should be obtained when this injury is suspected (Fig. 2-1).

A small avulsion fracture is common at the superior corner of the *anterior process* of the calcaneus, the site of origin of the bifurcate ligament. This region should be examined on lateral and internal oblique radiographs in all patients with midfoot injuries (Fig. 8-12*B*).

Stress Fractures

Stress fractures of the foot are common. They occur after excessive walking or athletic activity. There is either an acute event or chronic repetitive activity. Some patients develop stress fractures without a definite inciting event. Plain radiographs are negative up to 2 weeks after the injury. After that period, bone sclerosis develops. In the tarsals, a band of sclerosis is seen within the trabecular portion of the bone. Along the metatarsal shaft, a subtle zone of periosteal elevation and callus formation develops (Fig. 8-24).

COMMON VARIANTS

Accessory ossicles of the foot are common (Fig. 8-27). Some of these are located at the same sites as avulsion fractures. They are distinguished from fractures by their characteristic location; smooth, well-corticated margins; and the lack of pain or tenderness. The *os trigonum* is at the posterior process of the talus and is the most common accessory ossicle (Fig. 8-8). Secondary ossicles that occur at sites of avulsion fracture include the *os supratalare, os supranaviculare, os peroneum* at the cuboid, *os vesalianum* at the fifth metatarsal tuberosity, and the *os calcaneus secondarius* at the anterior process of the calcaneus (Fig. 8-13*D*). Two sesamoids bones at the base of the great toe invariably present. In up to 30% of persons, one of the sesamoids is bipartite (Fig. 8-23).

ADVANCED STUDIES

Although not required in the ED, CT is used to completely define the anatomy of complex calcaneal and talar fractures. Thin CT slices are obtained in both the axial (plantar) and coronal planes. CT is also used in patients with a possible retained foreign body from a plantar puncture wound if it is not visible with plain radiography. In patients suspected of having a stress fracture of the foot but with negative plain radiographs, *bone scintigraphy* can provide earlier diagnosis.

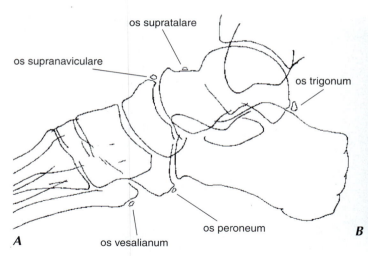

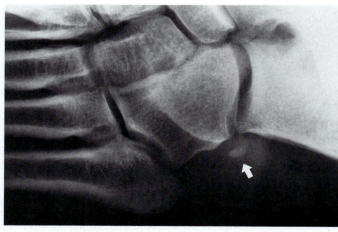

FIGURE 8-27. *A.* Accessory ossicles of the tarsals are common. *B.* The os peroneum is seen adjacent to the cuboid.

CONCLUSION

Fractures of the foot are common and some injuries are easily misdiagnosed. A thorough history and physical examination are essential prior to radiographic study. A description of the mechanism of injury and localization of pain helps in interpreting the radiographs. When doubt exists as to the presence of a fracture, supplementary views and special studies such as CT and bone scans may be required. Since most foot fractures do not require immediate surgical intervention, there is usually time for a complete outpatient evaluation after initial provisional treatment. If further studies are needed, immobilization and avoidance of weight bearing are prescribed and the patient is referred for consultation.

REFERENCES

1. Steill IG, Greenberg GA, et al: Decision rules for the use of radiography in acute ankle injuries. *JAMA* 269:1129, 1993.
2. Steill IG, McKnight, et al: Implementation of the Ottawa ankle rules. *JAMA* 271:828, 1994.
3. Edward CP: Fractured os calcis and lumbar vertebra. *Can Med Assoc J* 103:177–179, 1970.
4. Karasick D: Fractures and dislocations of the foot. *Semin Roentgenol* 29:152, 1994.
5. Chen MY, Bohrer SP, Kelley TF: Boehler's angle: A reappraisal. *Ann Emerg Med* 20:122, 1991.
6. Wilson DW: Functional capacity following fractures of the os calcis. *Can Med Assoc J* 95:908, 1966.
7. Arntz CT, Hansen ST: Dislocations and fracture/dislocations of the tarsometatarsal joints. *Orthop Clin North Am* 18:105, 1987.
8. Foster SC, Foster RR: Lisfranc's tarsometatarsal fracture/dislocation. *Radiology* 120:79, 1976.
9. Vuori A: Lisfranc joint injuries: trauma mechanisms and associated injuries. *J Trauma* 35:40, 1993.
10. Englanoff G, Anglin D, Hutson HR: Lisfranc fracture/dislocation: A frequently missed diagnosis in the emergency department. *Ann Emerg Med* 26:229, 1995.
11. Jones R: Fractures of the base of the fifth metatarsal bone by indirect violence. *Ann Surg* 35:697, 1902.
12. Kavanaugh JH, Brower TD, Mann RV: The Jones fracture revisited. *J Bone Joint Surg (Am)* 60-A:776, 1978.
13. Munro TG: Fractures of the base of the fifth metatarsal. *J Can Assoc Radiol* 4:260, 1989.
14. Meyer SA, Saltman CL, Albright JP: Stress fractures of the foot and leg. *Clin Sports Med* 12:395, 1993.
15. Helal B, Gibb MB: Freiberg's disease: A suggested pattern of management. *Foot Ankle* 8:94, 1987.
16. Freiberg AH: Infraction of the second metatarsal: A typical injury. *Surg Gynecol Obstet* 19:191, 1914.
17. Schwab RA, Powers RD: Conservative therapy of plantar puncture wounds. *J Emerg Med* 13:291, 1995.
18. Chisholm CD, Schlesser JF: Plantar puncture wounds: Controversies and treatment recommendations. *Ann Emerg Med* 18:1352, 1989.
19. Verdile VP, Freed HA, Gerard J: Puncture wounds to the foot. *J Emerg Med* 7:193, 1989.
20. Patzakis MJ, Wilkins J, Brein WW, et al: Wound sites as a predictor of complications following deep nail punctures of the foot. *West J Med* 150:545, 1989.
21. Lammers RL, Magill T: Detection and management of foreign bodies in soft tissue. *Emerg Med Clin North Am* 10:767, 1992.
22. Flom LL, Ellis GL: Radiologic evaluation of foreign bodies. *Emerg Med Clin North Am* 10:163, 1992.
23. Chanley DP, Manz JA: Non-metallic foreign bodies in the foot: Radiography versus xeroradiography. *J Foot Surg* 25:45, 1986.
24. Chudnofsky CR, Sebastion S: Special wounds: Nail bed, plantar puncture and cartilage. *Emerg Med Clin North Am* 10:813, 1992.
25. Kuhns LR, Borlazats, Seigel RF, et al: An in vitro comparison of CAT scan, xerography, and radiography in the detection of soft tissue foreign body. *Radiology* 132:218, 1979.

CHAPTER 9

THE ANKLE AND LEG

BRANDT WILLIAMSON / DAVID T. SCHWARTZ

Ankle injuries make up 3% or more of emergency department (ED) visits, and radiographs of the ankle account for 10% of all radiographs ordered in the ED.[1–4] In fact, ankle sprains are the most frequent sports-related orthopedic injury, especially in competitive athletics.[5,6] Although many ankle injuries initially appear minor, up to 44% of patients have persistent symptoms 1 year after injury.[7] Even though people at age extremes are at greater individual risk for sustaining an ankle fracture, most fractures are seen in patients who are 21 to 30 years of age.[1]

The ankle is a complex joint that possesses an extraordinary amount of mobility while under extreme mechanical stress. The body of the talus and the subtalar joint are important for the mechanical functioning of the ankle. The anatomy and mechanics of the midshaft tibia and fibula are less complex than that of the ankle. Some ankle injuries result in midfoot fractures or in fractures of the proximal tibia or fibula. Fractures of the tibial shaft are often severe injuries that pose the risk of neurovascular compromise and compartment syndrome.

CLINICAL DECISION MAKING

Although most patients with acute ankle injuries are evaluated radiographically, only about 15% of ankle radiographs obtained in the ED demonstrate a fracture. The decision to obtain radiographs depends on clinical findings that can discriminate between a fracture and a purely ligamentous injury. In North America in 1993, about $500 million was spent annually on ankle radiographs. Therefore, about $425 million was spent on radiography in patients without a fracture. Guidelines have been developed to increase the efficiency of radiologic evaluation while not missing any significant fractures. These criteria were developed in Canada by Stiell et al., and have become known as the *Ottawa ankle rules.*[8] The Ottawa ankle rules are clinical decision guidelines that help determine when to obtain radiographs on a patient with an ankle injury (Fig. 9-1).

The Ottawa rules are used to evaluate both the ankle and the midfoot because midfoot fractures are often associated with ankle injuries. The Ottawa rules entail a simple stepwise evaluation. First, if there is bone tenderness at the posterior edge of the distal 6 cm or tip of either the fibula or tibia, radiographs of the ankle are obtained. Tenderness at the anterior aspect of the distal fibula is not an indication to obtain radiographs because that is the common region of tenderness with ankle sprains. If there is tenderness over the base of the fifth metatarsal or over the navicular, foot radiographs are ordered. If there is no bone tenderness in these regions of the foot or ankle, the ability to bear weight on the injured ankle is assessed.

Radiographs should be ordered if the patient is unable to bear weight both at the time of the injury and in the ED. Weight bearing is defined as the ability to take four steps (two steps on the injured ankle). The rules consider the patient able to bear weight even if there is a marked limp.

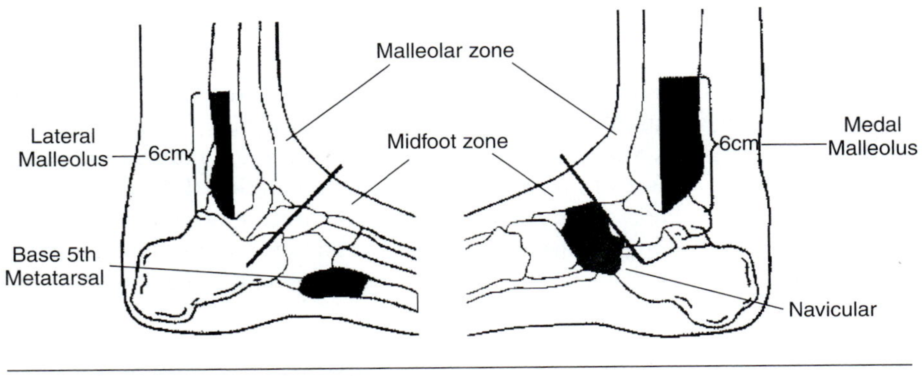

These criteria apply only to patients above 18 years of age, although a small study has demonstrated their applicability in children.[9] Patients who were excluded during the development of these rules were pregnant patients, patients with isolated skin injuries, those with injuries that occurred 10 days or more prior to evaluation, and patients returning for repeat evaluations. Also excluded were patients with altered mentation due to intoxication or head trauma and those with other painful, distracting injuries.

The use of the Ottawa rules remains

FIGURE 9-1. The Ottawa ankle rules. 1. Bone tenderness: *Ankle*—posterior surface (distal 6 cm) or tip of lateral or medial malleolus. *Midfoot*—navicular or base of the fifth metatarsal. 2. Inability to bear weight (four steps) *both* immediately at the time of injury and in the ED. Avulsion fractures of the malleolar tip less than 3 mm in breadth are excluded because they are not considered clinically significant. These rules remain secondary to the clinical judgment and common sense of the physician. Altered sensorium, other distracting injuries, and underlying bone disorders must be considered. Patients under the age of 18 were not studied. (From Stiell IG, Greenberg GH, McKnight RD, et al: Decision rules for the use of radiography in acute ankle injuries: Refinement and prospective validation. *JAMA* 269:1127–1132, 1993. With permission.)

somewhat controversial. A large multicenter study confirmed their accuracy.[10] Other authors have occasionally found missed fractures when the Ottawa rules were used.[11,12] However, those studies have been criticized because the Ottawa rules were not correctly applied.[13] An analysis of the cost-effectiveness of these rules supports their efficiency and contribution toward cost containment.[14]

Indications for obtaining radiographs of the tibia and fibula are less controversial. Midshaft tibial and fibular fractures are usually obvious clinically. Occasionally, they can be subtle, especially in children with greenstick or torus fractures. With a nondisplaced fracture of the tibial or fibular shaft, edema and ecchymosis can be minimal if the periosteum is intact.

ANATOMY AND PHYSIOLOGY

Proper radiographic interpretation and clinical evaluation require an understanding of ankle anatomy and biomechanics. The ankle is a hinge joint, made up of three bones—the tibia, fibula, and talus (Fig. 9-2). The tibia contributes to the medial and superior aspect of the joint. On the medial side, the tibia forms the medial malleolus. Superiorly, the tibia forms the *plafond* (French for *ceiling*). The fibula contributes to the lateral aspect of the ankle and forms the lateral malleolus. The posterior lip of the distal tibia is sometimes referred to as the *posterior malleolus.*

The distal tibia and fibula are held together by three ligaments: the anterior inferior tibiofibular ligament, the posterior inferior tibiofibular ligament, and the interosseous membrane (Fig. 9-3). The resulting fibrous joint between the tibia and fibula is called the *syndesmosis.*

The ligaments that provide lateral and medial ankle stability are grouped into the lateral and medial collateral ligament complexes (Fig. 9-3). The lateral collateral ligaments include the anterior talofibular, calcaneofibular, and posterior talofibular ligaments. These ligaments originate from the fibula and insert on the talus and calcaneus. On the medial side of the ankle, the deltoid ligament inserts mostly on the talus, but also has insertions on the navicular.

The inferior component of the ankle joint is the talus. The superior part of the talus is the talar *dome* or *trochlea*. The articulation of the talus with the tibia and fibula resembles a hinged joint similar to a mortise-and-tenon. The tibiofibular surface that articulates with the talar dome is the *mortise*. The primary weight-bearing element of the mortise is the tibial plafond. The entire weight of the body is borne by the talus, and so minimal changes in the surface of the talar dome result in chronic pain and joint dysfunction.

The three bones and three ligament groups of the ankle can be viewed as forming a ring. This ring must be intact for the ankle to remain stable. These structural components include the lateral malleolus, lateral collateral ligaments, deltoid ligament, medial malleolus, tibiofibular syndesmosis, and talar dome. If a break occurs in only one of those components, the injury is stable. If two components of the ring are broken, the ankle loses

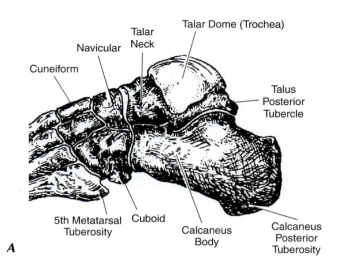

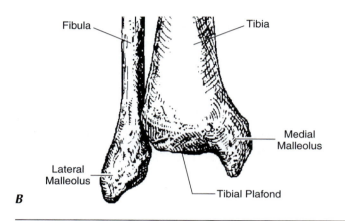

FIGURE 9-2.   Bones of the ankle. *A.* Lateral view of the foot. *B.* Anterior view of the distal tibia and fibula. (From Pansky B: *Review of Gross Anatomy,* 6th ed. New York: McGraw-Hill, 1996. With permission.)

its stability. If the entire width of the mortise joint space is not uniform, the injury is likely to be unstable.

Ankle mechanics are closely related to injury patterns. Because of the transverse-wedge shape of the talar dome, the ankle is more stable in dorsiflexion than in plantar flexion. The wedge-shape of the talus also allows for inversion of the ankle in plantar flexion and slight eversion in dorsiflexion.

Ankle Positions and Motions—Terminology

The terminology used to describe the motions causing injury of the ankle is confusing because some of the terms are used inconsistently by various authors (Fig. 9-4). Rotation of the foot relative to the long axis of the lower leg is termed *internal rotation* and *external rotation* depending on the direction of motion of the foot relative to the leg. In the original Lauge-Hansen terminology, *inversion* and *eversion* were used to describe the mo-

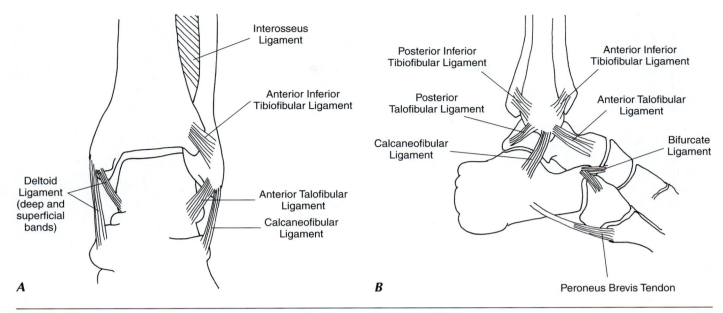

FIGURE 9-3. Ligamentous anatomy of the ankle. *A.* Anterior view. *B.* Lateral view.

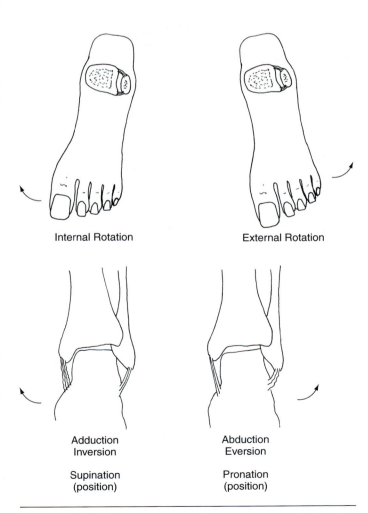

FIGURE 9-4. Terminology of motion causing injury at the ankle.

tions of internal and external rotation. Nowadays, the terms inversion and eversion are used differently, as stated below. External rotation is the most common mechanism causing ankle fractures.

Adduction and *abduction* describe motion of the talar dome within the ankle mortise—rotated inward and outward around the long axis of this foot. *Supination* and *pronation* describe the position of the foot relative to the ankle. The ankle is supinated when the foot is rotated inward along the long axis of the foot—i.e., the same motion as the force of adduction. The ankle is pronated when the foot is rotated externally along its long axis—i.e., the same motion as the force of abduction. *Inversion* is a motion similar to adduction and supination, although some authors distinguish inversion as involving the subtalar joint as well as the ankle joint. From a practical standpoint, *inversion* and *adduction* could be used interchangeably. Inversion (or adduction) is the most common mechanism of an ankle sprain. *Eversion* is the opposite motion to inversion and is similar to abduction and pronation.

RADIOGRAPHIC TECHNIQUE

Radiographic evaluation of the ankle includes three views—*lateral, anteroposterior* (AP), and *mortise* views (Fig. 9-5). Although the AP and lateral views show most fractures, the integrity of the joint is best assessed on the mortise view (Table 9-1).

The Anteroposterior View

The AP view shows the distal tibia and fibula, and the talar dome (Fig. 9-5*A* and *B*). The joint space is not entirely visible

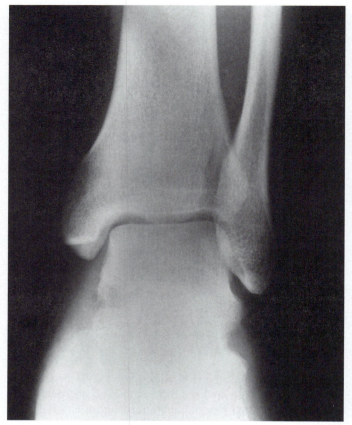

A

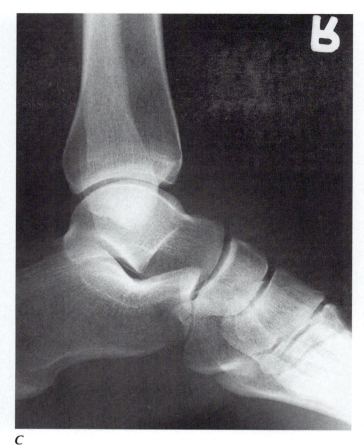

C

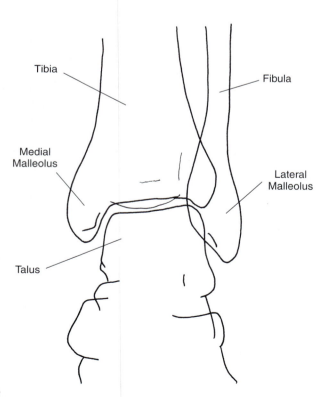

Tibia

Fibula

Medial
Malleolus

Lateral
Malleolus

Talus

B

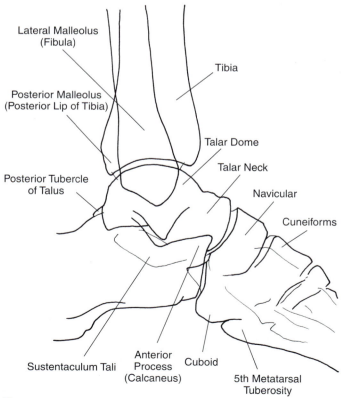

Lateral Malleolus
(Fibula)

Tibia

Posterior Malleolus
(Posterior Lip of Tibia)

Talar Dome

Talar Neck

Posterior Tubercle
of Talus

Navicular

Cuneiforms

Sustentaculum Tali

Anterior
Process
(Calcaneus)

Cuboid

5th Metatarsal
Tuberosity

D

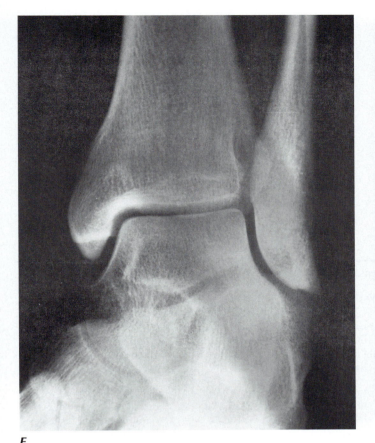

E

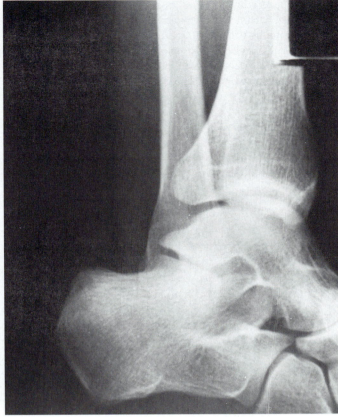

G

FIGURE 9-5. Normal ankle radiographs. *A* and *B*. AP view. *C* and *D*. Lateral view. *E* and *F*. Mortise view. *G*. "Poor" lateral view, showing "posterior malleolus" and distal fibula.

Medial
Clear Space

Distal Tibiofibular
Joint
(Lateral
Clear Space)

Tibiofibular
Overlap

Talar Dome

F

because of overlap of the lateral malleolus on the tibia and talus. The distal tibiofibular joint space is usually visible. The distal tibia and fibula overlap by at least 6 mm.

The Lateral View

On a correctly positioned lateral view, the medial and lateral margins of the talar dome are superimposed and the joint space appears as a semicircular arc of uniform width. The lateral view is useful for seeing the anterior and posterior margins of the distal tibia. The distal fibula projects through the distal tibia (Fig. 9-5C and D). The base of the fifth metatarsal should be visible.

The Mortise View

The mortise view is an AP view with the ankle internally rotated 15° to 20°. This view depicts the entire joint space without overlap, and therefore permits assessment of subtle disruptions of the ankle joint (Fig. 9-5D and E). The entire joint space should be uniform in width. The area between the medial malleolus and talus is called the *medial clear space*. The area between the lateral malleolus and the talus, which extends into the distal tibiofibular joint space, is called the *lateral clear space*. The distal tibia and fibula should overlap slightly (about 1 mm). If there is no overlap, the tibiofibular syndesmosis is abnormally widened and the integrity of the ankle joint may be compromised.

Additional Views

Additional radiographic views include the external oblique, the internal oblique, the "poor" lateral, and stress views.

These views have a limited role in the emergency evaluation of ankle injuries. The *external oblique* is obtained with 45° of external rotation. It is useful for posterior tibial fractures and distal fibular fractures that are not seen on the standard views. The *internal oblique view* is obtained with 45° of internal rotation and provides another view of the joint. The *"poor" lateral* is similar to the lateral view but with the foot rotated externally 15°. It can provide better definition of the posterior tibial lip. *Stress views* are used to demonstrate ligamentous injuries and do not, in general, play a role in the acute setting.

TABLE 9-1

Standard and Supplementary Radiographic Views of the Ankle

VIEW	POSITION	EVALUATION OF ADEQUACY	LIKELY FINDINGS
AP	Supine position, leg extended. Foot dorsiflexed with plantar surface perpendicular to x-ray cassette.	Absence of rotation confirmed by open medial clear space. Slight superimposition of lateral malleolus on talus.	In combination with lateral will identify most fractures: lateral and medial malleolus, and distal tibia and fibula.
Lateral	Recumbent on affected side. Leg in lateral position. Plantar surface of the foot is perpendicular to the x-ray cassette.	Distal tibia, distal fibula, tibiotalar joint, and tarsals shown in lateral position. Fibula should be superimposed over posterior tibia. Medial and lateral margins of the talar dome are superimposed, so the joint space appears as a clear arc.	In combination with AP view, identifies most fractures. Spiral fracture of distal fibula. Posterior lip of distal tibia. Ankle effusion. Base of fifth metatarsal.
Mortise	Supine or sitting, leg extended. Foot dorsiflexed, plantar surface perpendicular to x-ray cassette. Ankle rotated internally with the malleoli parallel to plane of the film cassette (15–20° internal rotation).	Talotibial joint space is well demonstrated. Medial and lateral malleolar joint spaces are open.	True anteroposterior view of tibiotalar articulating surface. Assess integrity of the ankle mortise. Unobstructed view of the medial and lateral clear space.
SUPPLEMENTARY VIEWS			
External oblique	Supine or sitting, leg extended. Foot dorsiflexed with plantar surface perpendicular to x-ray cassette. Ankle rotated externally 45°.	Malleoli superimposed on talus. Fibula superimposed on anterior tibia. Talus and calcaneus visible with articulations obscured.	Posterior tibial fractures. Helpful in defining Salter-Harris type I and II distal fibular fractures.
Internal oblique	Supine or sitting, leg extended. Foot dorsiflexed with the plantar surface perpendicular to the x-ray cassette. Ankle rotated internally 45°.	Lateral malleolus and tibiofibular articulation well visualized.	Unobstructed view of medial and lateral clear space. Talar body and neck.
"Poor" lateral	Similar to routine lateral, but the long axis of the foot is tilted 15°, toes pointed down, with heel elevated on a towel or sponge.	Posterior lip of the tibia superimposed on fibula.	Fracture of the posterior tibial lip ("posterior malleolus").

RADIOGRAPHIC ANALYSIS

A systematic approach should be applied to ankle radiographs so as to avoid missing a subtle fracture as well as to determine the full extent of the injury. An *ABC'S* approach prompts one to examine each film for *ad*equacy and alignment and injuries to the *b*ones, *c*artilage, and *s*oft tissue. A *targeted approach* is based on knowledge of ankle injury patterns and directs attention to specific sites of common injury and areas of frequently missed injuries.

Adequacy. The first step is to determine the *adequacy* of the study. A complete set of three standard views must be obtained. The films must be properly exposed and positioned and must include all relevant structures—e.g., the distal tibial and fibular shafts, the proximal fifth metatarsal, and the body of the calcaneus (Table 9-1).

Targeted Approach

A targeted approach is based on a knowledge of ankle injury patterns (Table 9-2). The radiographic evaluation is directed to sites prone to injury and sites of frequently missed injury (Fig. 9-6).

Examine the Malleoli. Approximately 90% of fractures about the ankle involve the malleoli—lateral, medial, and posterior (posterior lip of the distal tibia). Therefore, the review of the films begins with these areas. The distal fibula (lateral malleolus) is the most common site of injury. Although most fractures are easily detected, nondisplaced oblique fractures and small avulsion fragments are often difficult to see or are visible on only one view. One should note the level of the injury relative to the mortise as well as the amount of displacement and angulation. The medial malleolus and, on the lateral view, the posterior lip of the distal tibia (posterior malleolus) should also be inspected for signs of fracture.

Small avulsion fractures usually occur at the distal tip of the lateral malleolus. It is often necessary to examine the films with a "bright light" in order to detect these small bone fragments. A nondisplaced oblique fracture of the lateral malleolus is often only visible on the lateral view. Oblique views or a "poor" lateral view can occasionally demonstrate the fracture more clearly.

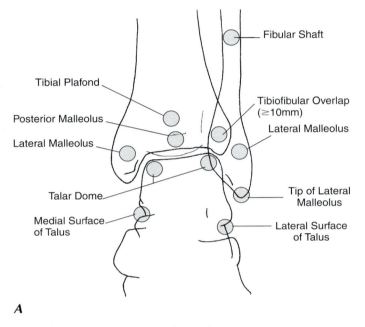

A

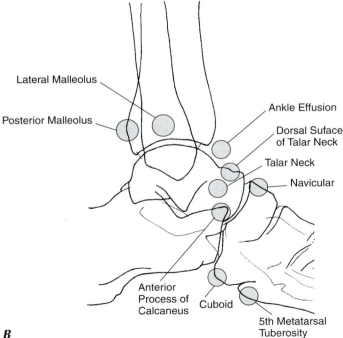

B

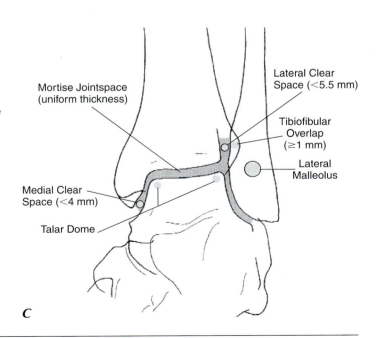

C

FIGURE 9-6. Sites prone to injury and easily missed injuries. *A.* AP view. *B.* Lateral view. *C.* Mortise view.

TABLE 9-2

Systematic Analysis of Ankle Radiographs

Determine study quality	All three views are included. On the lateral view, the malleoli should be superimposed. On the AP, the fibula and tibial plafond are above the talus. On the mortise view, the entire talar dome and joint space are seen without overlap. The proximal aspect of the fifth metatarsal is included on the lateral and mortise views.
Focus on the lateral, medial and posterior malleolus	Obvious fractures are readily detected. The lateral malleolus is most commonly injured, but the medial and posterior malleoli must also be inspected. Note the relationship of the level of the fracture to the mortise. Nondisplaced fractures may only be seen on one view (e.g., spiral fracture of lateral malleolus seen only on lateral view). Carefully check for tiny avulsions off the tips of the malleoli or talus.
Evaluate the mortise	On the mortise view, the entire joint space should be uniform in width. Look for widening of the medial clear space and distal tibiofibular clear space as well as shifting of the talus within the mortise. Scrutinize the joint space for small osteochondral fracture fragments from the talar dome.
Reexamine	If a fracture or joint space deformity is found, reexamine the other areas of the ankle for subtle injuries.
Examine the bones outside of the ankle joint—tarsals and peripheral areas	On the lateral view, look for small avulsion fractures involving the *tarsal bones,* particularly the navicular, talus, and anterior calcaneus. Check the proximal aspect of the *fifth metatarsal* for an avulsion fracture. Check the most proximal element of the *fibula* seen on the film. An abnormality may suggest a more proximal fracture and the need for a complete study of the tibia and fibula.
Reevaluate	Order further studies as indicated (e.g., complete tibiofibular radiographs, oblique views, foot films, comparison views in children).

Examine the Mortise. The next step is to examine the joint space of the ankle mortise. This is important for assessing the structural integrity of the ankle. The articular surfaces are best visualized on the mortise view. The spaces between the articular surfaces should be of uniform width on all sides of the ankle mortise.

Although various measurements are applied to the width of the joint space, the uniformity of the joint space is the key observation (Fig. 9-5C). The medial clear space is located between the medial surface of the talar dome and the medial malleolus. It should be about 4.0 mm wide. The width of the space between the distal tibiofibular joint should be about 5.5 mm. Widening of these joint spaces implies ligamentous disruption. A slight amount of widening (up to 2.0 mm) of the medial clear space can occur with an isolated lateral malleolar fracture, but greater widening indicates disruption of the deltoid ligament.

When the joint space of the mortise is inspected, attention should be directed to any small bone fragment within the joint that may represent an osteochondral fracture of the talar dome. On the lateral view, there should be a uniform clear space between the talar dome and the tibial plafond.

Reexamine. If a *fracture* of one malleolus is found or there is distortion of the ankle mortise, the other malleoli should be carefully reexamined for evidence of a subtle fracture or ligamentous disruption. This provides a complete assessment of the

extent of the injury and the integrity of the ankle joint.

In some instances, radiographs of the entire length of the tibia and fibula should be obtained to detect a more proximal fibular fracture (e.g., Maisonneuve and Dupuytren fractures; see below). Proximal fractures should be suspected when no fibular fracture is seen on the ankle radiographs despite the presence of a medial malleolar fracture or widening of the mortise joint space. Because of the difficulty in predicting proximal fibular fractures, some clinicians order complete tibiofibular radiographs in all patients with displaced ankle fractures. It is important to check for such proximal injuries by physical examination. All patients with ankle injuries should be examined for tenderness over the leg and knee.

Examine Peripheral Areas. Sites that are not the primary focus of ankle radiographs are next inspected. The most proximal portion of the fibula seen on the AP and mortise views should be examined for evidence of a fracture. The proximal portion of the fifth metatarsal should be examined on the lateral and mortise radiographs because an avulsion fracture of the tuberosity (base) of the fifth metatarsal is frequently seen with ankle inversion injuries.

Midfoot fractures are often associated with ankle injuries, and the tarsal bones should be examined on ankle radiographs. Injuries include avulsion fractures from the navicular, the cuboid, the talar neck, and the anterior process of the calcaneus.

ABC'S Approach

Alignment and Bones.   Proper *alignment* dictates that, on all three views, the talar dome should lie within the ankle mortise and beneath the tibial plafond. In analyzing the *bones,* all cortical margins are traced for disruption. The trabecular network is scrutinized for impaction, deformity, or lucency. One must be particularly careful when examining areas of overlap. For example, on the lateral view, the fibula must be traced throughout the area where it is superimposed on the tibia. If there is question of an abnormality in an area of overlap, oblique films better reveal the abnormality.

Cartilage.   *Cartilage* occupies the articular spaces of the ankle, and the radiographic assessment of the joint space is key to determining the stability of the ankle. On the mortise view, the entire joint space should be of uniform thickness (Fig. 9-5C). Widening of the lateral clear space between the distal fibula and tibia suggests disruption of the syndesmosis, with resultant instability of the joint. Widening of the medial clear space between the medial side of the talar dome and the medial malleolus suggests tearing of the deltoid ligament.

Soft Tissues.   *Soft tissue swelling* is frequently seen with ankle injuries because the overlying soft tissues are normally so thin that swelling is easily detected. However, the value of this finding in determining the nature or severity of an injury is limited. Soft tissue swelling is seen in the region of the lateral or medial malleolus on the AP and mortise views using a "bright light." Although soft tissue swelling increases the suspicion of a fracture, there is little relation between the extent of soft tissue swelling and the presence of a fracture.

On the lateral view, a *joint effusion* appears as a soft tissue "teardrop" (a bulge) anterior to the distal end of the talus (Fig. 9-7). An effusion should prompt one to look carefully for subtle avulsion injuries and nondisplaced fractures. One recently published study found that a large ankle effusion correlates well with the presence of a fracture.[15]

The *Achilles fat triangle* is seen on the lateral view and is formed by the Achilles tendon, the posterior tuberosity of the calcaneus, and the deep muscle layer. With a calcaneal fracture, distal tibial fracture, fibular fracture, or Achilles tendon rupture, the well-defined triangular borders are lost or distorted. Of these injuries, a rupture of the Achilles tendon is primarily a clinical rather than a radiographic diagnosis.

COMMON ABNORMALITIES

A precise description of the manner in which the ankle was injured suggests the most likely pattern of injury. Knowledge of the position of the ankle and the direction of the forces causing the injury helps to predict the fracture and the resulting radiographic findings. Unfortunately, the injury usually occurs so quickly that the patient is unable to describe the position of the ankle and the direction of the injuring forces. However, know-

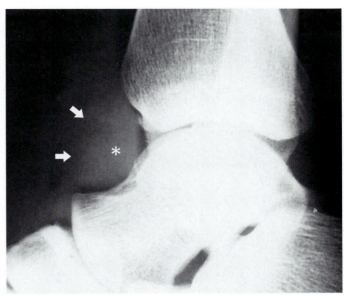

A

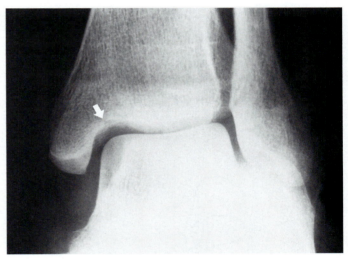

B

FIGURE 9-7.   Ankle joint effusion. A prominent round soft tissue bulge is seen anterior to the ankle joint on the lateral view (*A*). This represents a joint effusion, which, in the setting of trauma, is a hemarthrosis. The radiographs should be closely re-examined for a fracture. On the AP view (*B*), a subtle fracture of the medial malleolus is seen (*arrow*). (Copyright David T. Schwartz, M.D.)

ing the typical patterns of ankle injuries enables the physician to search for specific associated injuries when one fracture is found.

Mechanisms of Injury

The most common mechanism of injury to the ankle is *inversion,* also termed *supination-adduction* (Fig. 9-8). In adults, this usually does not cause a fracture but rather a sprain of the lateral ankle ligaments. When a fracture occurs, it is a transverse fracture of the lateral malleolus below the level of the ankle

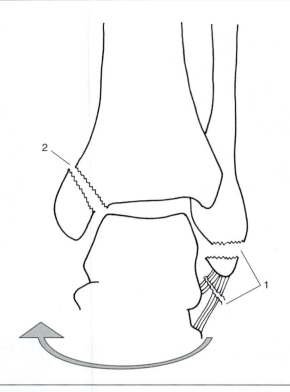

FIGURE 9-8.　Injuries produced by inversion (supination-adduction) of the ankle. 1. The most common ankle injury is a tear of the lateral collateral ligaments. Alternatively, there is a transverse fracture of the lateral malleolus. 2. Greater traumatic force also produces an oblique fracture of the medial malleolus extending up from the mortise (2).

mortise. The fracture is due to tensile forces of the lateral ankle ligaments. With more severe injuries, the medial malleolus is fractured in an oblique orientation.

The most common mechanism responsible for ankle fractures is *external rotation* (Fig. 9-9). The convention for describing displacement is to refer to the motion of the distal part relative to the proximal part. Therefore, in external rotation, the foot rotates externally with respect to the leg. Clinically, the patient's foot is usually planted on the ground and the patient's body rotates *internally* relative to the foot. This produces a sequence of fractures and ligamentous tears that encircle the ankle mortise. The site of the first injury that occurs is dependent on the position of the foot at the time of injury (i.e., whether the foot is supinated or pronated).

Ligament Mechanics

Differences in the strength of ligaments and bones have implications for injury patterns. With inversion injuries in adults, a ligamentous sprain is more common than a fracture. At the syndesmosis, the posterior tibiofibular ligament is stronger than the anterior tibiofibular ligament. Therefore, an avulsion fracture is more likely to occur at the posterior aspect of the syndesmosis than at the anterior region.

In children, the ligaments of the ankle are stronger than the epiphyseal growth plate. Therefore, a fracture through the growth plate (Salter-Harris fracture) is more likely than an ankle sprain.

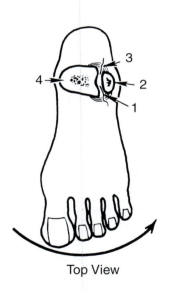
Top View

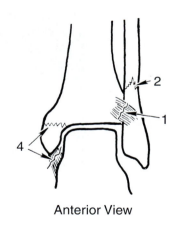
Anterior View

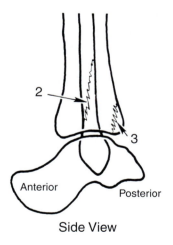
Side View

FIGURE 9-9.　Injuries produced by external rotation of the ankle. As the talus rotates within the ankle mortise, a series of injuries is produced. The sequence of injuries depends on the position of the foot at the time of injury. The sequence illustrated here occurs when the foot is supinated. This causes tension on the lateral collateral ligaments and anterior joint capsule and relaxes the medial collateral (deltoid) ligament. 1. Tear of the anteroinferior tibiofibular ligament. 2. Spiral fracture of the lateral malleolus beginning at the level of the mortise. 3. Tear of the posteroinferior tibiofibular ligament or avulsion fracture of the posterior malleolus. 4. Transverse fracture of the medial malleolus or tear of the deltoid ligament. This injury corresponds to Lauge-Hansen SER-4 (supination-external rotation, grade 4). When the foot is pronated at the time of injury, the deltoid ligament is pulled tight and the medial malleolus is injured first. This is followed by a fracture of the lateral malleolus, typically above the level of the mortise. (From Rogers LF: *The Radiology of Skeletal Trauma*, 2d ed. New York: Churchill-Livingstone, 1992. With permission.)

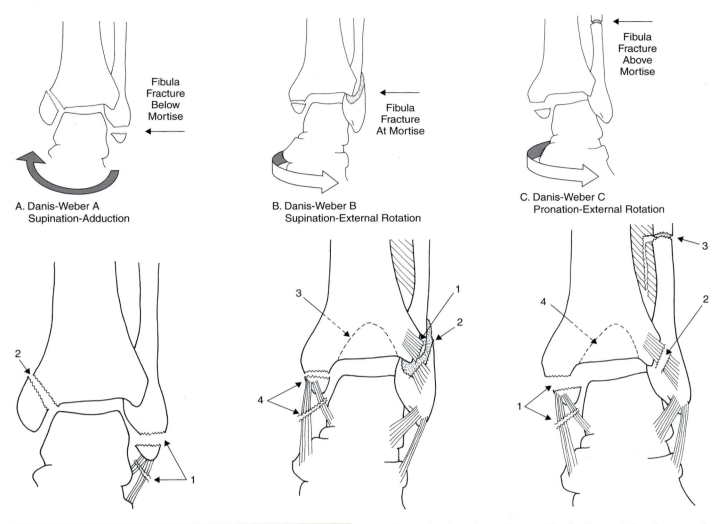

FIGURE 9-10. The Danis-Weber and Lauge-Hansen classification schemes of ankle injuries. The relationship between these two classification systems is illustrated. The numbers refer to the sequence (staging) of injury (see Table 9-3). *A.* A transverse fracture below the mortise (Danis-Weber A) is due to inversion (supination-adduction). *B.* A spiral fracture at the level of the mortise (Danis-Weber B) is due to external rotation of a supinated ankle. *C.* A fracture above the mortise (Danis-Weber C) is due to external rotation of a pronated ankle.

Lauge-Hansen Classification

The Lauge-Hansen classification scheme is based on the pattern of injury caused by the traumatic force. It is useful in understanding complex injury patterns by relating the mechanism of injury to the anatomic pathology seen on the radiograph (Fig. 9-10). There are 17 different injuries grouped into five major categories (Table 9-3).[16]

A two-part name is used to describe the injury (e.g., supination–external rotation). The first part defines the position of the foot at the onset of trauma. The second part describes the motion of the talus within the mortise, which predicts the stresses on the bones and ligaments during injury.

By reviewing the radiographic findings, it is often possible to determine the injury mechanics based on the Lauge-Hansen classification. Avulsion injuries normally produce horizontal (transverse) fractures; impaction forces typically produce oblique fractures; and torsional forces produce spiral fractures.

Danis-Weber Classification

The Danis-Weber system is based on the level of the fracture of the distal fibula (Fig. 9-10).[16] It is simpler than the Lauge-Hansen system and is more directly related to operative treatment decisions (Table 9-4). The type A fracture occurs below (distal to) the mortise. This tends to be a stable fracture, treated with closed reduction and casting unless there is a medial malleolus fracture. The type B fracture is a spiral fracture that starts at the level of the mortise. Type B may be stable or unstable depending on the presence of other injuries aside from the lateral malleolus fracture. The type C fracture is above the level of the mortise and disrupts the ligamentous connections between the tibia and fibula (the tibiofibular ligaments and interosseous membrane) below the fracture. The type C injury is extremely unstable, requiring surgical fixation.

TABLE 9-3

Lauge-Hansen Classification—Based on Mechanism of Injury

Supination-external rotation 60% of ankle fractures	SER 1	Tear of the anteroinferior tibiofibular ligament (AITFL)
	SER 2	Spiral fracture of lateral malleolus at mortise
	SER 3	Fracture of the posterior malleolus or tear PITFL
	SER 4	Low fracture of the medial malleolus or deltoid ligament tear
Pronation-external rotation 20% of ankle fractures	PER 1	Low fracture of the medial malleolus or deltoid ligament tear
	PER 2	Tear of the anteroinferior tibiofibular ligament (AITFL)
	PER 3	High fracture of the lateral malleolus (above mortise)
	PER 4	Fracture of the posterior malleolus or tear PITFL
Supination-adduction (inversion) 20% of ankle fractures	SAD 1	Low fracture of the lateral malleolus or tear of lateral ligaments
	SAD 2	Oblique fracture of the medial malleolus at mortise
Pronation-abduction (eversion) <0.5% of ankle fractures	PAB 1	Low fracture of the medial malleolus or tear of deltoid ligament
	PAB 2	Tear of the inferior tibiofibular ligaments
	PAB 3	Oblique fracture of the lateral malleolus at mortise
Pronation-dorsiflexion Pilon fracture (axial loading) <0.5% of ankle fractures	PDF 1	Transverse fracture of the medial malleolus
	PDF 2	Fracture of the anterior lip of the tibia with displacement
	PDF 3	Supramalleolar fracture of the fibula
	PDF 4	Transverse fracture of the tibia, often with comminution

NOTE: SAD 1 is the most common ankle injury, usually resulting in a sprain of the lateral ligaments. PAB 1 and PER 1 have a similar radiographic appearance. PAB 2 and PER 2 have a similar radiographic appearance.

TABLE 9-4

Danis-Weber Classification of Ankle Injuries

TYPE	DESCRIPTION	TREATMENT
A	Horizontal fibular avulsion below the mortise with associated oblique fracture of the medial malleolus.	Conservative, except if medial malleolus fracture is present
B	Spiral fracture of the lateral malleolus with horizontal avulsion fracture of the medial malleolus and a tear of the inferior tibiofibular ligaments.	Surgery likely unless only lateral malleolus fracture is present
C	High fibular fracture with rupture of the inferior tibiofibular ligaments, and a horizontal avulsion fracture of the medial malleolus.	Surgery necessary

Naming Fractures

Certain fractures are referred to by descriptive names and eponyms (Table 9-5). Although they concisely describe common and characteristic injury patterns and are of some histor-ical interest, eponyms are often misapplied and should usually be avoided. Proper radiographic, anatomic, and orthopedic terms should always be used to describe the radiologic find-ings and injury.

COMMON FRACTURE PATTERNS

Malleolar fractures are by far the most common fractures of the bones forming the ankle. They can occur as single injuries or in combination with other fractures. Lateral malleolar frac-tures are the most frequent, followed by medial and "posterior" malleolus fractures. Occasionally, the fibular shaft rather than the distal fibula is fractured. Fractures to the distal tibial meta-physis (plafond) are distinct from malleolar fractures. They are caused by a different mechanism of injury (axial compression).

Malleolar Fractures

SINGLE MALLEOLAR FRACTURES.   Lateral malleolar fractures are by far the most common fracture involving the ankle. They are most often caused by external rotation or inversion (ad-duction). Inversion is the most frequent cause of ankle injury and usually results in an isolated sprain of the anterior talofibu-lar ligament. Occasionally, a small avulsion fracture is seen at the tip of the lateral malleolus (Fig. 9-11). Such a fracture may be barely visible as a faint osseous chip. The presence of such a small fracture does not alter the management of an ankle sprain.

Forceful inversion (adduction) results on a horizontal lateral malleolar fracture below the level of the mortise (Fig. 9-12).

External rotation results in a spiral fracture of the lateral malleolus at or above the level of the mortise (Fig. 9-13). When it is not displaced, a spiral lateral malleolar fracture may not be visible on the AP view and is only seen with difficulty on the lateral view owing to overlap by the tibia. Distal fibular fractures also occur at the fibular shaft 4 to 10 cm above the mortise (Fig. 9-14). When the fibular fracture is above the mortise, the syndesmosis is disrupted and the lateral malleolus and talus are laterally displaced.

Isolated *medial malleolar fractures* are uncommon and are caused by external rotation

TABLE 9-5

Descriptive Names and Eponyms for Fractures of the Leg and Ankle

Aviator's astragalus	All fractures and fracture dislocations to the talus.
Dupuytren fracture	Fracture of the fibular shaft above the mortise with rupture of the interosseous membrane and the distal tibiofibular ligaments. There is lateral talar shift and a fracture of the medial malleolus and/or deltoid ligament tear.
Jones fracture	A transverse fracture of the proximal shaft of the fifth metatarsal. Not an avulsion fracture of the fifth metatarsal base (tuberosity)—a "pseudo-Jones" fracture.
Maisonneuve fracture	Fracture to the proximal fibula with rupture of the tibiofibular syndesmosis. Commonly associated with rupture of the deltoid ligament or medial malleolar fracture.
Pilon fracture	Fracture with comminution of the tibial plafond.
Tillaux fracture	Fracture to the distal lateral tibia at articulating surface.

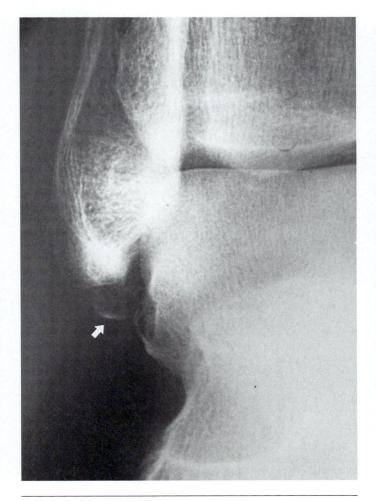

FIGURE 9-11. Avulsion fracture of the lateral malleolus. A tiny bone fragment is seen at the tip of the distal fibula in this patient with a sprained ankle (*arrow*). The presence of a small avulsion fracture does not alter the management of the patient.

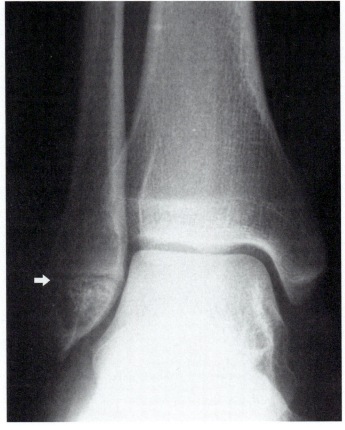

FIGURE 9-12. An isolated transverse fracture of the lateral malleolus in an adolescent male. This injury was caused by forceful inversion (adduction) of the ankle. It is classified as a supination-adduction grade I injury (SAD I). These fractures are below the level of the mortise (Danis-Weber type A). The fracture should not be mistaken for a residual open growth plate. The fibular growth plate closes before that of the distal tibia.

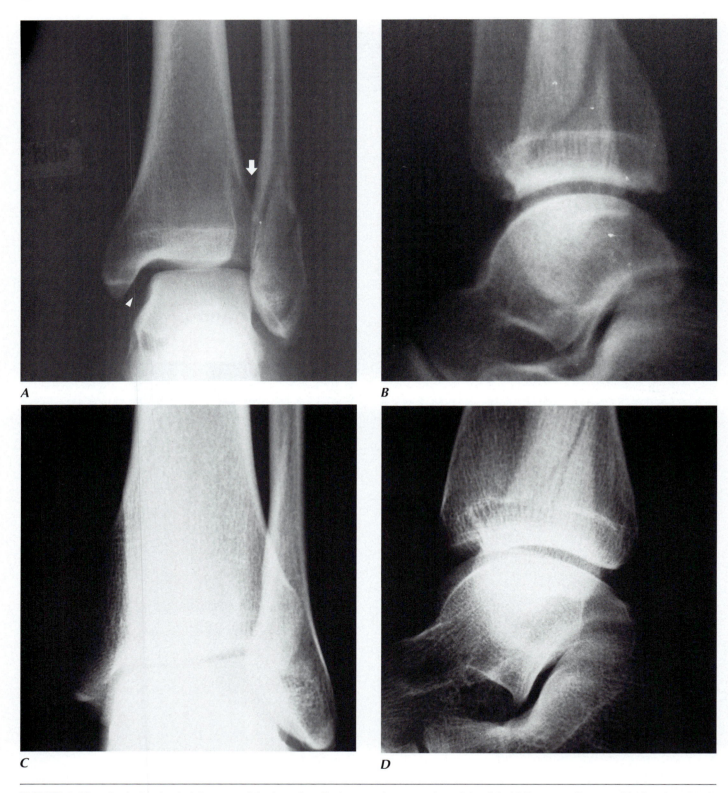

A

B

C

D

FIGURE 9-13. An isolated spiral fracture of the lateral malleolus. The injury is caused by external rotation and is classified as a supination-external rotation grade 2 injury (SER-2). The injury occurs at the level of the mortise (Danis-Weber B). On the mortise view (*A*), there is mild widening of the distal tibiofibular joint space, suggesting injury to the syndesmosis (*arrow*). There is also mild widening of the medial joint space (*arrowhead*). Slight widening of up to 2 mm is common with such lateral malleolar fractures and is not necessarily due to tearing of the deltoid ligament. Greater widening does imply disruption of the deltoid ligament. On the lateral view (*A*), the fracture is seen through the distal tibia.

An isolated nondisplaced lateral malleolus fracture may be seen only on the lateral view. In another patient, the AP view (*C*) shows no sign of the fracture because it lies oblique to the x-ray beam. On the lateral view (*D*), the fracture is seen projected through the distal tibia.

or abduction. They are usually associated with a lateral malleolar fracture or lateral ligamentous injury that disrupts the ankle mortise (Fig. 9-15). The fracture may be a tiny chip pulled off the tip of the medial malleolus (Fig. 9-16).

BIMALLEOLAR FRACTURES.   Bimalleolar fractures involve both the lateral and the medial malleoli. If a single malleolar fracture is discovered, a second fracture or ligament tear may exist at the opposite malleolus. While a single malleolar fracture is considered stable, two fractures are unstable and require operative repair.

With forceful inversion (adduction), there is a horizontal fracture of the lateral malleolus below the level of the mortise

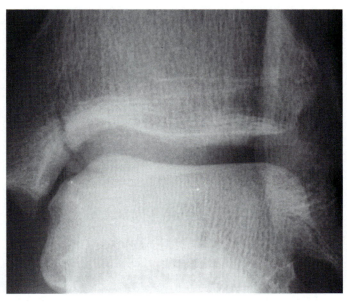

FIGURE 9-15.   An oblique fracture of the medial malleolus. This is caused by forceful inversion (adduction) of the ankle. It is associated with injury to the lateral collateral ligaments or a transverse fracture of the lateral malleolus. It is classified as supination-adduction grade 2 (SAD2).

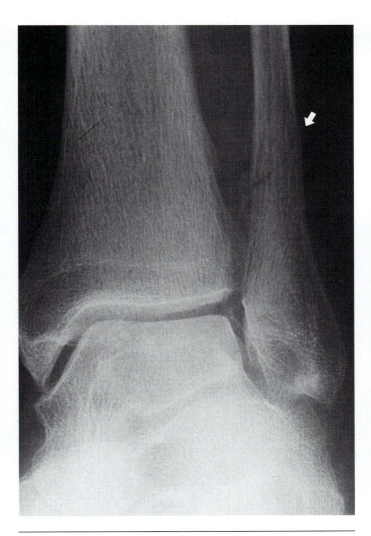

FIGURE 9-14.   An isolated fracture of the lateral malleolus above the mortise. The injury is caused by external rotation and is classified as a pronation–external rotation grade 3 injury (PER 3), which typically occurs above the level of the mortise (Danis-Weber C). These injuries generally require internal fixation owing to associated injury of the syndesmosis. However, in this nondisplaced facture, the syndesmosis may be intact. Stress views are needed to determine ligament stability.

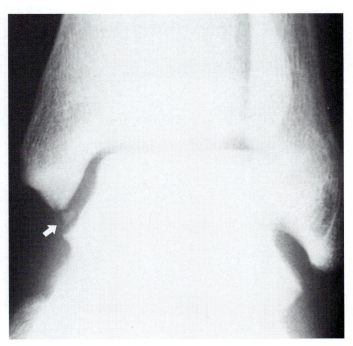

FIGURE 9-16.   A tiny avulsion fracture of the medial malleolus. This is due to traction on the deltoid ligament during external rotation of a pronated ankle (pronation–external rotation grade 1, or PER 1). It is unusual for this to occur as an isolated injury; therefore other fractures or ligamentous injuries must be carefully sought.

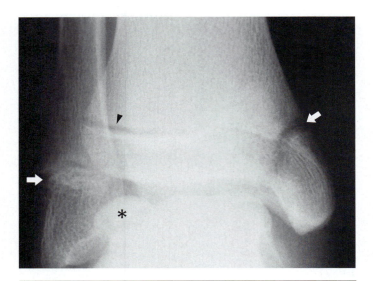

FIGURE 9-17.   A bimalleolar fracture due to forceful inversion in an adolescent. There is a transverse fracture through the lateral malleolus and an oblique fracture through the medial malleolus. The lateral portion of the distal tibial growth plate is open (*arrowhead*). This is classified as supination–adduction grade 2 (SAD 2). There is also a fracture through the lateral aspect of the talar dome (*asterisk*).

and an oblique fracture of the medial malleolus at the level of the mortise (Fig. 9-17). With forceful external rotation, there is a spiral fracture of the lateral malleolus and a horizontal fracture of the medial malleolus below the level of the mortise (Fig. 9-18). According to Lauge-Hansen, when the foot is supinated at the time of external rotation, the lateral malleolus fracture occurs at the level of the mortise (Danis-Weber B). When the foot is pronated at the time of external rotation, the fibular fracture occurs above the mortise (Danis-Weber C).

TRIMALLEOLAR FRACTURES.   Trimalleolar fractures are caused by external rotation, and are extremely unstable. The ankle mortise is disrupted and posterolateral subluxation of the talus is frequently seen (Fig. 9-19). The posterior portion of the distal tibia (posterior malleolus) is fractured due to tension on the posteroinferior tibiofibular ligament. Large fractures of the posterior malleolus are caused by axial compression when the foot is plantar flexed. When a significant portion of the articular surface is involved, operative fixation of the posterior malleolus is necessary (Fig. 9-20).

DUPUYTREN FRACTURE.   The Dupuytren fracture is a fracture of the fibular shaft 4 to 10 cm above the mortise. The in-

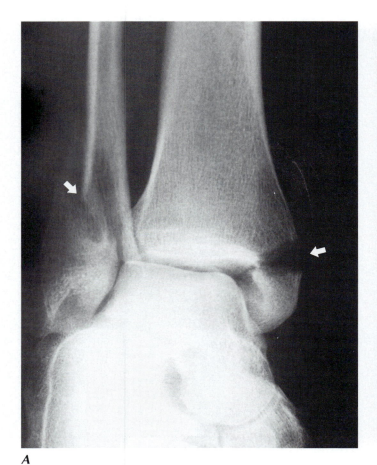

A

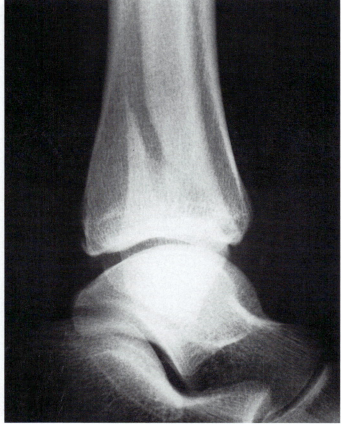

B

FIGURE 9-18.   A bimalleolar fracture due to forceful external rotation. There is a spiral fracture of the lateral malleolus originating at the level of the mortise and a horizontal fracture of the medial malleolus. This is classified as supination–external rotation grade 4 (SER 4) or Danis-Weber B. It is an unstable injury.

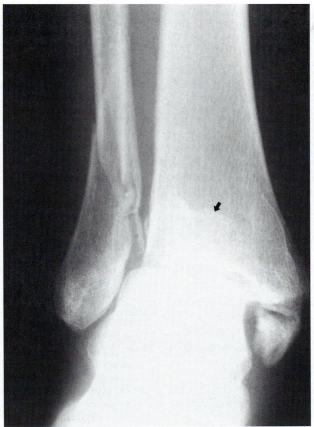

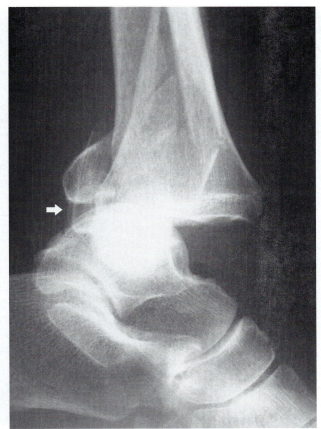

A

B

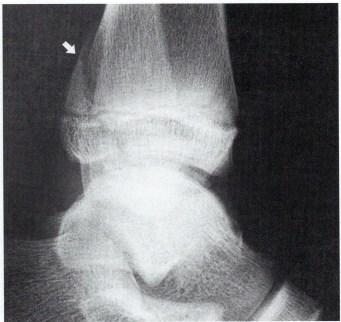

FIGURE 9-20. A large fracture of the posterior malleolus involving one-quarter of the articular surface. This fracture is due to axial compression on the plantar flexed ankle. Smaller posterior malleolar fractures are due to avulsion of the posteroinferior tibiofibular ligament.

FIGURE 9-19. A trimalleolar fracture due to forceful external rotation. There is a spiral fracture of the distal fibular shaft just above the level of the mortise and a horizontal fracture of the medial malleolus. Displacement of the distal fibula implies rupture of the tibiofibular syndesmosis. The small posterior malleolar fracture is seen on the AP, view projected through the distal tibia, and on the lateral view (*arrow*). The talus is dislocated posterior to the tibia. This is classified as pronation–external rotation grade 4 (PER 4) or Danis-Weber C.

terosseous membrane is torn distal to the level of the fracture and the mortise is severely disrupted (Fig. 9-21). The talus is often laterally displaced due to rupture of the deltoid ligament. Fractures of the medial malleolus, posterior malleolus, and anterior tibial tubercle usually accompany a Dupuytren fracture. The Dupuytren fracture is equivalent to a severe pronation–external rotation injury (Lauge-Hansen), and Danis-Weber C.

The fibular fracture may be seen at the superior margin of the film or may even lie beyond the edge of the film. If the talus is shifted laterally on the AP view or the tibia is separated from the talus, a fracture of the fibular shaft should be suspected. If a fibular fracture is not seen on routine views, additional views that show more of the proximal fibula should be obtained.

MAISONNEUVE FRACTURE. A Maisonneuve fracture is a fracture of the proximal fibular shaft that results from external rotation. Although an isolated fracture of the proximal fibular

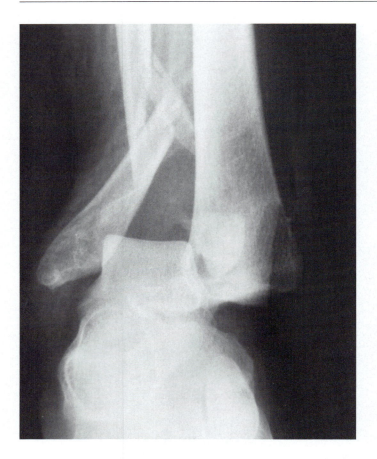

shaft usually warrants little concern regarding the ankle joint, with a Maisonneuve fracture the tibiofibular syndesmosis is disrupted and the ankle is unstable (Figs. 9-22 and 9-23). This injury is usually associated with a medial malleolar fracture (or deltoid ligament rupture) and often a posterior malleolar fracture.

Radiographic clues to a Maisonneuve fracture can be subtle. If there is a medial or posterior malleolar fracture and no lateral malleolar fracture, complete clinical and radiologic evaluation of the leg is indicated. Another sign of a Maisonneuve fracture is widening of the medial joint space between the medial malleolus and the talus in the absence of a distal fibular fracture. In all patients with ankle injuries, the knee and lower leg must be examined for tenderness indicative of a syndesmosis injury.

Tibial Plafond Fractures—Pilon Fractures

Tibial plafond fractures result from axial loading. They frequently extend up the tibial metaphysis in an oblique or spiral manner. They are also termed *pilon (pylon) fractures*. Pilon fractures are intraarticular fractures of the distal tibia (Fig. 9-24). About 20% of these injuries are open. They can be severely comminuted and are often associated with a distal fibular fracture.

FIGURE 9-21.　A Dupuytren fracture of the distal fibula occurs 4 to 10 cm above the mortise (PER 4). There is marked disruption of the mortise.

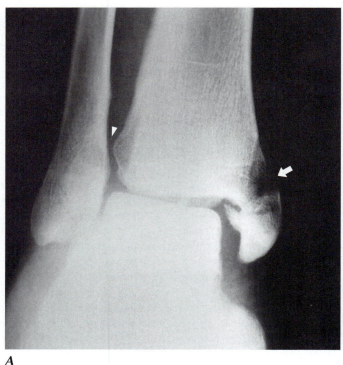

A

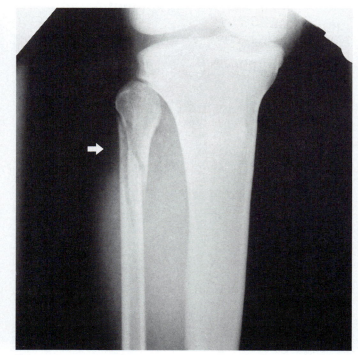

B

FIGURE 9-22.　A Maisonneuve fracture. On the AP view of the ankle (*A*), there is an oblique fracture of the medial malleolus (*arrow*). There is no fracture of the lateral malleolus. The distal tibiofibular articulation is widened (no overlap of the distal tibia and fibula) (*arrowhead*). This pattern is suggestive of a Maisonneuve fracture. A subsequent radiograph of the proximal fibula revealed a spiral fracture (*B*). The patient did not complain of knee or leg pain. (Copyright David T. Schwartz, M.D.)

FIGURE 9-23. Maisonneuve fracture—mechanism of injury. External rotation of the talus within the ankle mortise causes diastasis of the distal tibiofibular articulation. The torsional force is transmitted up the fibular shaft, resulting in a fracture of the proximal fibula. The proximal fibular fracture is indicative of disruption of the ankle mortise. In Maisonneuve's original analogy (1840) of external rotation injury, rotation of the measuring stick (or talus) wedges apart two books (the ankle mortise), causing diastasis and fractures at the ankle. (From Rockwood CA, Green DP: *Fractures in Adults,* 2d ed. Philadelphia: Lippincott, 1984. With permission.)

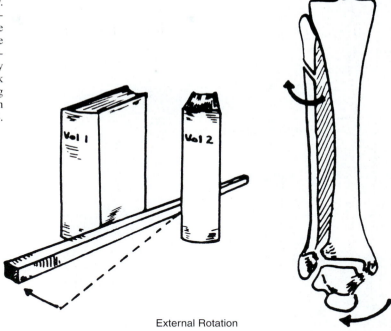

External Rotation

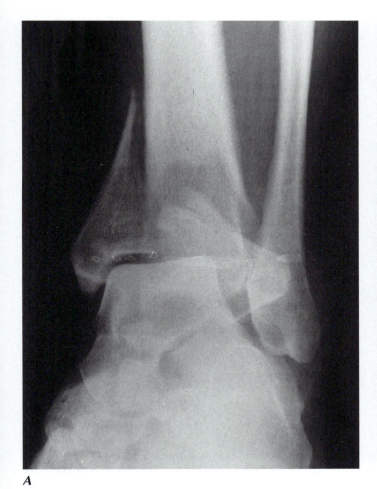

A

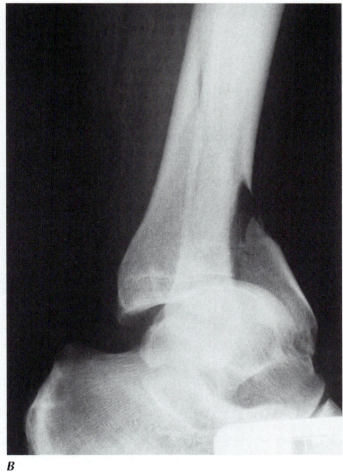

B

FIGURE 9-24. Pilon fracture. Forceful axial loading causes a comminuted fracture of the tibial plafond.

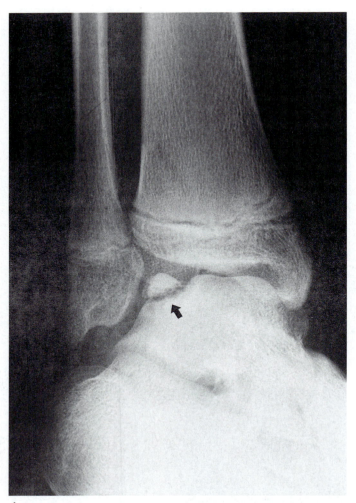

Typical mechanisms of injury would be a jump from a great height or a head-on car crash with the foot on the brake pedal, in which the talus is driven into the tibia. Pilon fractures are usually easily detected, but a complete radiographic examination of the leg is necessary to define the proximal extent of the tibial fracture. Pilon fractures are frequently associated with injuries to the calcaneus, tibial plateau, hip, pelvis, and spine. They may resemble bimalleolar or trimalleolar fractures, although a fracture of the tibial plafond is characteristic of the pilon fracture.

Fractures of the Talar Dome

Fractures involving the talar dome have significant clinical implications. These injuries can cause long-term problems if managed incorrectly because of the weight-bearing requirements of the articular surface of the talus. Chronic arthritic problems can persist if a bone fragment remains within the joint space for a prolonged period of time. The AP view is best for revealing these fractures (Fig. 9-25).

Fractures of the talar dome occur when an inverted foot (either dorsiflexed or plantar flexed) sustains a vertical (axial) force through the talus. Most fractures of the talar dome occur either

FIGURE 9-25. Fracture of the talar dome. *A.* A large talar dome fracture is seen in this child with ankle trauma. *B.* A subtle fracture is seen on the medial side of the talar dome. Although the fracture is small and nondisplaced, it can have significant long-term consequences.

A

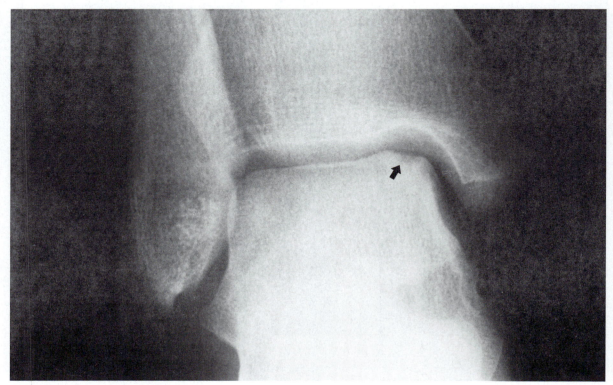

B

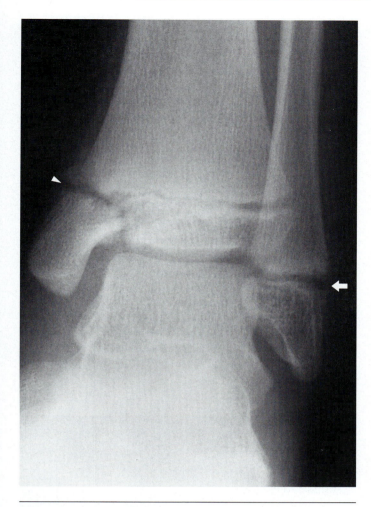

FIGURE 9-26. Fracture of the growth plate at the ankle. There is a minimally displaced fracture through the distal fibular growth plate (*arrow*). In children, such growth plate fractures are more common than ligament sprains. A fracture through the medial malleolus is also present (*arrowhead*).

on its anterolateral or posteromedial surface. Occasionally, an osteochondral fracture is radiographically occult on initial examination. Later, the typical appearance of osteochondritis dissecans develops.

The position of the foot on the radiograph is important in the identification of talar dome fractures. A plantar flexed foot better demonstrates posteromedial lesions; dorsiflexion better shows anterolateral lesions. Because the ankle is most often in neutral position (or slightly plantar flexed), posterior and posteromedial talar dome fractures are better seen. Moreover, posteromedial fractures tend to be larger and more "scooped out" than are anterolateral lesions. Anterolateral lesions of the trochlea are often wafer-thin and difficult to see on plain films. An ankle effusion seen on the lateral radiograph should heighten the suspicion of a subtle fracture about the ankle, including a talar dome fracture. Sometimes these lesions are seen only on computed tomography (CT) or magnetic resonance imaging (MRI).

Fractures in Children

In children, fractures frequently involve the *epiphyseal growth plate*. The pattern of injury can be complex. The most common ankle fracture in children involves avulsion of the tip of the lateral malleolus.[18] The next most common is a fracture of the *fibular epiphyseal plate* (Fig. 9-26). Epiphyseal plate fractures of the distal tibia and fibula account for 15 to 25% of all growth-plate injuries, second only to injuries involving the distal radius.[19] Epiphyseal plate fractures are common because of the weakness of the growth plate relative to the ligaments. Ligamentous disruption is extremely unusual in children. It is far more likely for a child below 10 years of age to sustain a fracture of the distal fibular growth plate than a ligament sprain.

A nondisplaced Salter-Harris type I fracture of the distal fibula can be difficult to detect. Although radiographs may appear "normal," the patient must be treated empirically as though a fracture were present. Periosteal reaction is seen 14 days after the injury, confirming the fracture. With a minimally displaced fibular epiphysis, a supplementary external oblique view may reveal the displacement. Similar difficulties exist for a nondisplaced fracture through the epiphyseal plate of the distal tibia, although most fractures involving the distal tibial epiphyseal plate are Salter-Harris types II to IV. These are more easily seen because there is an attached bony fragment. However, the fracture fragment can be quite small.

Closure of the distal fibular growth plate and the distal tibial growth plate is usually complete at 14 years for females and 16 years for males.[20] Since the physes of the fibula and tibia close at about the same time, a fracture should be suspected if there is a fused epiphysis to one bone and an open epiphyseal plate to the other.

JUVENILE TILLAUX FRACTURE. The juvenile Tillaux fracture is a consequence of the gradual closure of the tibial epiphyseal growth plate (Figs. 9-27 and 9-28). Closure of the tibial growth plate begins at its medial aspect and proceeds laterally. Once initiated, fusion of the tibial epiphysis takes 2 to 3 years. When the medial margin of the epiphysis is fused and the lateral margin is open, external rotation causes a Salter-Harris type III fracture of the lateral tibial epiphysis (the tibial plafond). The immature lateral regions of the distal tibial growth plate are fractured while the nearly fused medial portion of the growth plate is intact.

This fracture can be difficult to visualize with standard radiographic views and is often missed on initial evaluation. Anterior displacement of the tibial epiphysis is often obscured by the overlapping fibula on the lateral view. CT (preferably with three-dimensional reconstruction) is frequently required to make a definitive diagnosis.

TRIPLANE FRACTURE. The triplane fracture is an unusual fracture of the distal tibia that occurs prior to closure of the epiphyseal plate. It accounts for 5 to 10% of pediatric intraarticular fractures.[21] This complex fracture involves three different fracture elements—the metaphysis, the epiphyseal plate, and

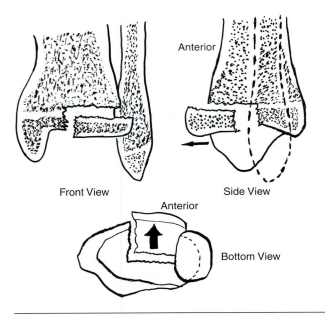

Front View   Side View

Anterior

Bottom View

FIGURE 9-27.   Juvenile Tillaux fracture. The lateral aspect of the distal tibial epiphysis is pulled off by the anteroinferior tibiofibular ligament. The medial aspect of the distal tibia, including the medial malleolus, is not involved because the medial portion of the growth plate has closed.

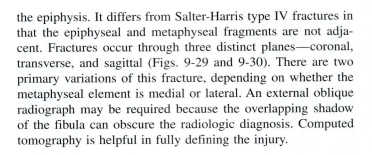

the epiphysis. It differs from Salter-Harris type IV fractures in that the epiphyseal and metaphyseal fragments are not adjacent. Fractures occur through three distinct planes—coronal, transverse, and sagittal (Figs. 9-29 and 9-30). There are two primary variations of this fracture, depending on whether the metaphyseal element is medial or lateral. An external oblique radiograph may be required because the overlapping shadow of the fibula can obscure the radiologic diagnosis. Computed tomography is helpful in fully defining the injury.

Fractures Involving the Leg

The proper anatomic term for the area between the knee and ankle is the *leg*—the "lower leg" is a misnomer. Fractures of the leg involve the tibial or fibular shaft.

TIBIAL SHAFT.   In the adult, tibial shaft fractures are due both to direct impact and rotational injury. In young children, fractures due to torsion are common. In children, fractures may cause minimal clinical findings. If the mechanism suggests a possibility of fracture, a radiograph should be ordered.

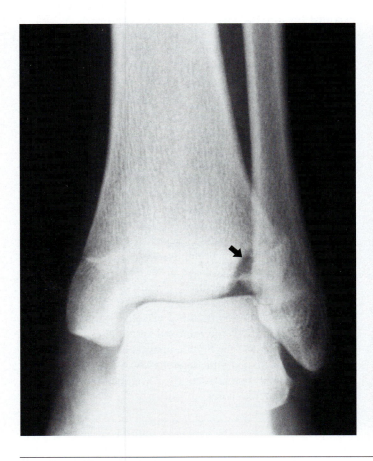

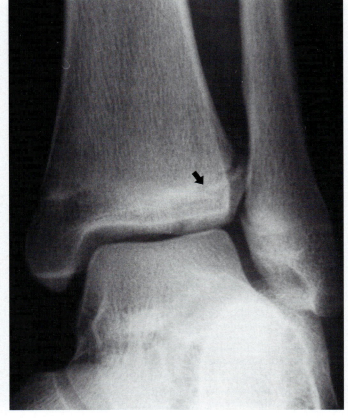

FIGURE 9-28.   A juvenile Tillaux fracture in a 12-year-old girl. The AP view (*A*) shows a vertical fracture through the lateral portion of the tibial epiphysis. This is partly hidden by the overlapping lateral malleolus. The mortise view (*B*) shows the extent of the fracture. Note that the medial portion of the distal tibial growth plate is closed.

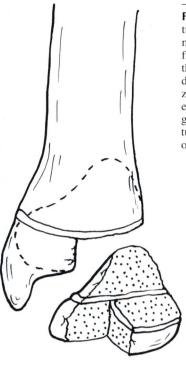

FIGURE 9-29. Triplane fracture. Schematic diagram of the most common type of triplane fracture. There is a fracture in the sagittal plane through the distal tibial epiphysis, a horizontal fracture through the lateral portion of the distal tibial growth plate, and a coronal fracture through the posterior malleolus.

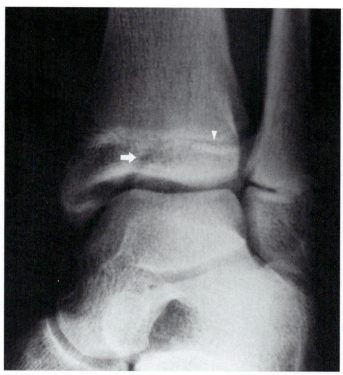

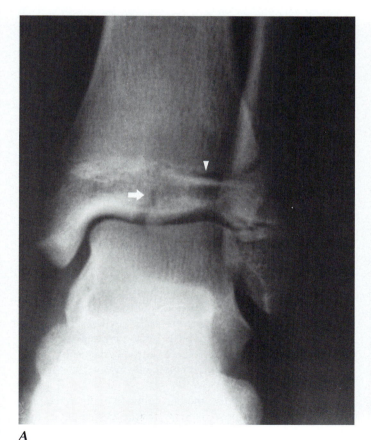

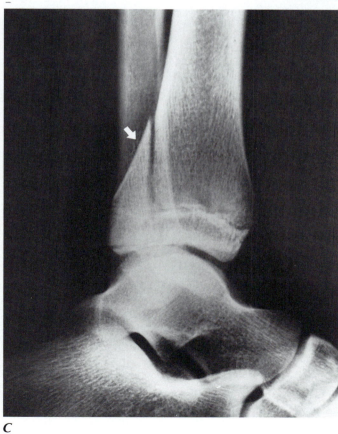

A

C

FIGURE 9-30. A triplane fracture in a 14-year-old boy. On the AP and mortise views (*A* and *B*), there is a vertical fracture through the tibial epiphysis (*arrow*) and a horizontal fracture through the lateral portion of the growth plate (*arrowhead*). The medial portion of the growth plate is closed. The fibular growth plate is also slightly widened. On the lateral view (*C*), a posterior malleolar fracture is seen (*arrow*). This third fracture in the coronal plane distinguishes a triplane from a Tillaux fracture.

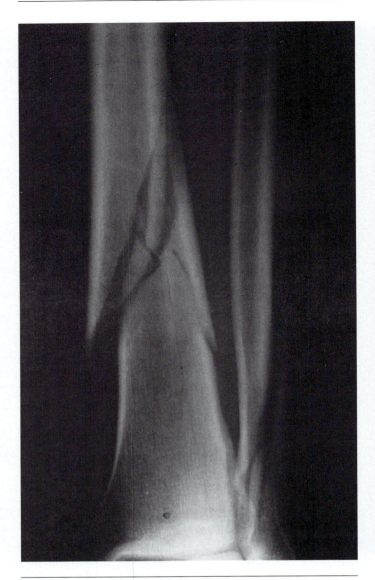

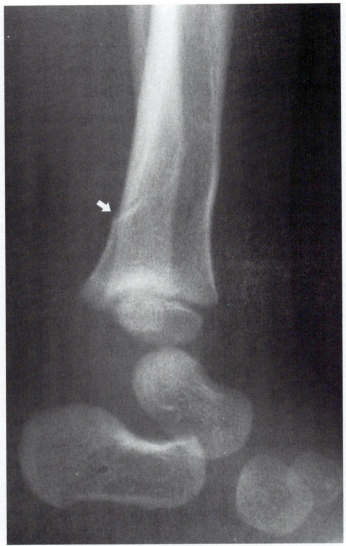

FIGURE 9-31.   A comminuted spiral fracture of both the tibia and distal fibula. The fracture is due to torsional forces.

FIGURE 9-32.   A torus (buckle) fracture of the distal tibia in a young child.

FIBULAR SHAFT.   The fibular shaft is a non-weight-bearing bone. Therefore, the ability to ambulate does not exclude the possibility of a fracture to the shaft of the fibula. This is particularly true in the elderly. If trabecular detail is well visualized, it is unlikely that fractures of the fibula or the tibia will be missed. If a fracture is present, the neurovascular status of the limb must be carefully assessed.

BOTH BONE FRACTURES.   Fractures of both the tibia and fibula are more commonly encountered than single bone injuries. Close attention must be paid to a possible neurovascular injury or compartment syndrome (Fig. 9-31).

PEDIATRIC LEG INJURIES.   In the pediatric population, torus fractures of the leg bones are common (Fig. 9-32). The *toddler's fracture* is a spiral fracture of the tibial shaft in children ages 12

to 24 months (Fig. 9-33). It is due to aggressive attempts at taking the first steps. It usually is minimally displaced. The radiographs can have only subtle abnormalities or may be negative. A presumptive diagnosis is therefore made based on clinical findings. In such cases, repeat studies at 10 days are necessary to reveal callus formation at an otherwise radiographically occult fracture. Toddler's fractures less commonly involve the distal tibial metaphysis.

Up to age 40 months, another common tibial fracture is termed the *CAST* fracture (*c*hildren's *a*ccidental *s*piral *t*ibial fracture). This is an isolated fracture of the diaphysis and is caused by a twisting mechanism. The possibility of an associated and less apparent greenstick fracture of the fibula must be considered.

Up to age 5 years, most fractures to the tibia are spiral and are due to a twisting mechanism of injury. Between the ages of 5 and 10 years, children more commonly have transverse fractures of the tibia that result from direct lateral impact.

ERRORS IN INTERPRETATION

Fractures of the Fifth Metatarsal

Ankle sprains commonly result from an inversion injury. The same forces that cause ankle sprains can also cause a fracture of the proximal fifth metatarsal. With inversion, the peroneus brevis tendon is stretched as it courses beneath the lateral malleolus and avulses its osseous attachment at the base of the fifth metatarsal (Fig. 9-3B). Tension on the plantar aponeurosis also contributes to the avulsion injury.

This fracture can be missed when only ankle radiographs are ordered (Fig. 9-34). All ankle radiographs should include the base of the fifth metatarsal. Moreover, clinicians should always palpate the base of the fifth metatarsal prior to ordering radiographs so as to assess the likelihood of a fifth metatarsal fracture. If there is tenderness, foot radiographs should be ordered.

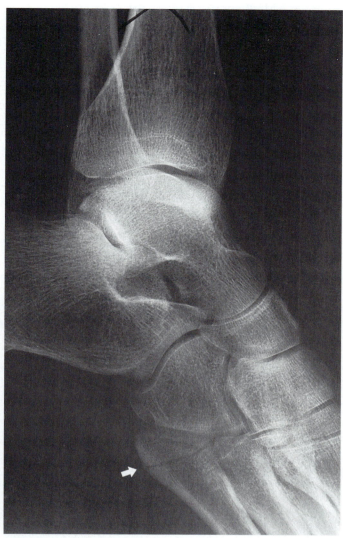

FIGURE 9-34. An avulsion fracture through the tuberosity at the base of the fifth metatarsal is visible at the corner of the ankle film obtained in a patient with a "sprained ankle." This region should be examined in all ankle radiographs.

On the other hand, in older children, the physician should not mistake the *apophysis of the fifth metatarsal* for a fracture (see Chap. 8, Fig. 8-21). Fractures are transverse to the long axis of the metatarsal; whereas the apophyseal plate follows the long axis. Moreover, fractures are tender on clinical examination.

Maisonneuve Fractures

A Maisonneuve fracture can be difficult to detect if there are no ankle fractures and only minimal displacement of the mortise. The proximal fibular fracture is not seen if only the standard ankle radiographs are obtained. Widening of the space between the talus and the medial malleolus or separation of the distal tibiofibular joint should alert the physician to obtain radiographs of the entire tibia and fibula. The knee and leg must be examined for tenderness in all patients with ankle injuries.

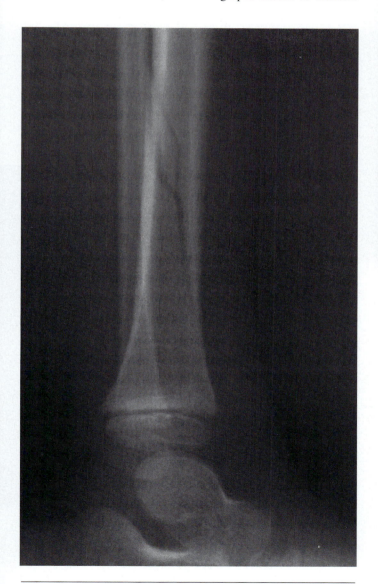

FIGURE 9-33. A toddler's fracture in a young child is a spiral fracture of the tibial shaft.

Fractures of the Talar Dome

Osteochondral fractures of the talar dome are often missed initially because the fracture fragment can be minute (Fig. 9-25*B*). Fractures of the talar dome are diagnosed on films repeated 6 to 8 weeks after the injury, when the patient complains of con-

tinued pain and joint stiffness.[24] If the small fragment separates from the talus, this isolated piece of bone usually requires surgical removal.

Fractures of the Lateral Malleolus

Nondisplaced lateral malleolar fractures can be difficult to see on the standard radiographs (Figs. 9-11 to 9-13). The lateral view can show a spiral fracture projected through the tibia.

Tarsal Fractures

Other fractures that are associated with ankle injuries include avulsion of the calcaneus, navicular, and talus (Fig. 9-35; see chap. 8, Fig. 8-12). These tiny fractures can be difficult to detect.

Stress Fractures

Stress fractures are typically seen in the older, osteopenic patient or in the young athlete. Radiographically, they appear as a sclerotic band extending across the distal tibial or fibular shaft. Curiously, with tibial stress fractures, a history of overuse is often absent. These fractures can occur in less active older peo-

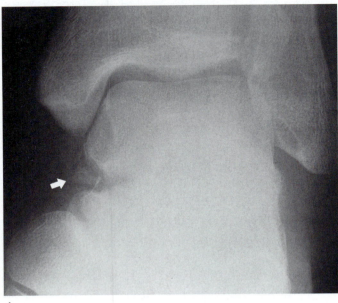

A

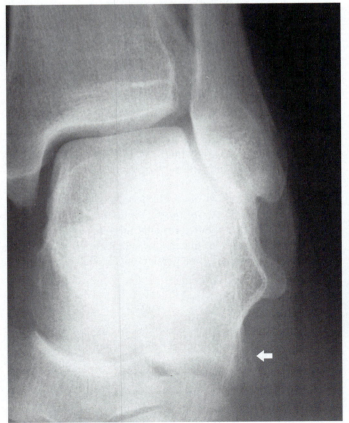

B

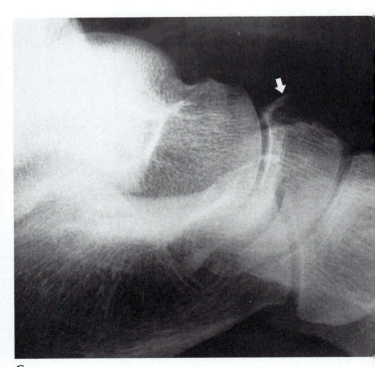

C

FIGURE 9-35.   Midfoot avulsion fractures. *A.* A small bone fragment is seen at the medial aspect of the talus at the insertion of the deltoid ligament (*arrow*). *B.* A tiny fragment is avulsed off the lateral aspect of the talus (*arrow*). *C.* An avulsion fracture from the dorsal surface of the navicular.

ple. Stress fractures also occur in young patients with osteopenia due to disuse following an ankle injury. The stress fracture results from ill-advised attempts to bear weight on the weakened bone. Female distance runners often have stress fractures of the distal fibula.

COMMON VARIANTS

Accessory ossicles are common at the ankle. These bones can be mistaken for a fracture. The most common is the os trigonum, which results from failure of the posterior talar process to fuse with the talus (Fig. 9-36). A well-rounded surface with uniform cortex is more consistent with an accessory bone than with a fracture. An osseous fragment is sometimes found at the distal fibula. A well-rounded, smooth cortex suggests a secondary ossification site or an old fracture fragment (Fig. 9-37).

ADVANCED STUDIES

Stress Radiographs

Stress radiographs are used to determine the extent of ligamentous injury. Stress views are not a routine part of the ED evaluation. At the initial presentation, pain and swelling usually preclude obtaining stress views. Stress views are generally obtained by the orthopedist and often require local

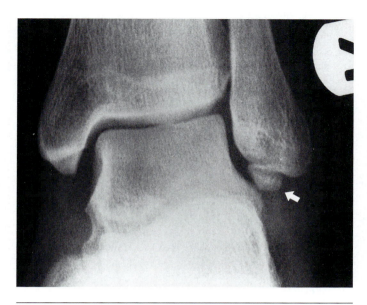

FIGURE 9-37. Nonunion of an old distal fibular fracture. There are smooth, well-corticated margins.

anesthesia to provide sufficient pain control and relaxation to perform the study. The adequacy of stress radiographs is technique-dependent—they are only 38% sensitive as compared with arthrography.[23] Both eversion and inversion stress views should be taken. A 10° shift in the joint space suggests rupture of the anterior talofibular ligament and the calcaneofibular ligament. If comparison views are used, a difference of 2 to 3 mm at the joint space is abnormal. Additional studies such as MRI or arthrography are often necessary to define the injury fully. These studies are directed by an orthopedic consultant.

Advanced Imaging

Fractures requiring CT include complex fractures involving the distal tibia, such as pilon and triplane fractures. This is decided by the orthopedic consultant because of the complexity of these injuries.

The use of MRI and arthrography for sprains, joint capsule injuries, and injuries to the syndesmosis is best directed by the orthopedist. These studies are rarely available to the emergency physician, and add little to the provisional acute treatment of most injuries.

REFERENCES

1. Varnish T, Clark WRY, Young RA, et al: The ankle injury—indications for selective use of x-rays. *Injury* 14:507, 1983.
2. Dunlop MG, Beattie TF, White GK, et al: Guidelines for selective radiological assessment of inversion ankle injuries. *BMJ* 293:603, 1986.

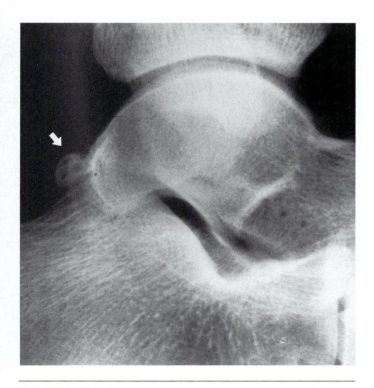

FIGURE 9-36. Os trigonum. A common accessory ossicle of the posterior tubercle of the talus.

3. Cockshott WP, Jenkin JK, Pui M: Limiting the use of routine radiography for acute ankle injuries. *Can Med Assoc J* 15:129, 1983.

4. Sujitkumar P, Hadfield JM, Yates DW: Sprain or fracture? An analysis of 2000 ankle injuries. *Arch Emerg Med* 3:101, 1986.

5. Garrick JG, Requa RK: The epidemiology of foot and ankle injuries in sports. *Clin Sports Med* 7:29, 1988.

6. Garrick JG: The frequency of injury, mechanism of injury and epidemiology of ankle sprains. *Am J Sports Med* 5:241, 1977.

7. Dettori JR, Basmania CJ: Early ankle mobilization: Part II. A one-year follow-up of acute, lateral ankle sprains (a randomized clinical trial). *Mil Med* 159:20, 1994.

8. Stiell IG, McKnight RD, Greenburg GH, et al: Decision rules for use of radiography in acute ankle injuries: Refinement and prospective validation. *JAMA* 269:1127, 1993.

9. Chande VT: Decision rules for roentgenology of children with acute ankle injuries. *Arch Pediatr Adolesc Med* 149:255, 1995.

10. Stiell I, Wells G, Laupacis A, et al: A multicenter trial to introduce clinical decision rules for the use of radiography in acute ankle injuries. *BMJ* 311:594, 1995.

11. Pigman EC, Klug RK, Sanford S, et al: Evaluation of the Ottawa clinical decision rules for the use of radiography in acute ankle and midfoot injuries in the emergency department: An independent site assessment. *Ann Emerg Med* 24:41, 1994.

12. Lucchesi GM, Jackson RE, Peacock WF, et al: Sensitivity of the Ottawa rules. *Ann Emerg Med* 26:1, 1995.

13. Stiell IG, Greenberg GH, McKnight RD, Wells GA: The "real" Ottawa ankle rules. *Ann Emerg Med* 27:103, 1996.

14. Anis AH et al: Cost-effective analysis of the Ottawa ankle rules. *Ann Emerg Med* 26:422, 1995.

15. Clark WCT, Janzen DL, Ho K, et al: Detection of radiographically occult ankle fractures following acute trauma: Positive predictive value of an anle effusion. *AJR* 164:1185, 1995.

16. Lauge-Hansen N: Fractures of the ankle: II. Combined experimental-surgical and experimental-roentgenologic investigation. *Ann Surg* 60:957, 1950.

17. Weber BGI: Die *Verletzungen des Oberen Sprunggeleukes.* Bern: Hans Huber, 1966.

18. Landin LA, Danielsson LG: Children's ankle fractures: Classification and epidemiology. *Acta Orthop Scand* 54:634, 1983.

19. Sloan EP, Rittenberry TJ: Ankle and foot injuries. In: Reisdorff EJ, Roberts MR, Wiegenstein JG (eds): *Pediatric Emergency Medicine.* Philadelphia: Saunders, 1993, p. 978.

20. Sarrafian SK: *Anatomy of the Foot and Ankle,* 2d ed. Philadelphia: Lippincott, 1993, p. 34.

21. Whipple TL, Martin DR, McIntyre LF, et al: Arthroscopic treatmet of triplane fractures of the ankle. *J Arthroscop Rel Surg* 9:456, 1993.

22. O'Donoghue D: *Treatment of Injuries in Athletes,* 3d ed. Philadelphia: Saunders; 1976, pp. 698–746.

23. Sauser DD, Nelson RC, Lavine MH, Wu CW: Acute injuries of the lateral ligaments of the ankle: Comparison of stress radiography and arthrography. *Radiology* 148:653, 1983.

CHAPTER 10

THE KNEE

TERRY KOWALENKO / DAVID T. SCHWARTZ

The knee is the largest joint in the body. It is particularly vulnerable to injury because of its location and the magnitude of the deforming forces it must resist. The knee sustains skeletal or soft tissue injuries by several mechanisms, including rotatory, compressive, and transverse (lateral) forces. Severe traumatic forces, such as automobile or motorcycle accidents and falls from great heights, produce major fractures and joint disruption. Young adults (especially athletes) are vulnerable to ligamentous and soft tissue injuries because of the relative strength of the bones at that age. In the elderly, relatively minor trauma can lead to fractures because the bones become weaker than the supporting soft tissue structures. In children, the growth plate (physis) and sites of ligamentous attachment are the areas of relative weakness and are the most common areas of injury.

Most knee radiographs are obtained in the emergency department (ED) to exclude fractures following trauma. More than a million studies are ordered annually in the ED; of these, most plain films are normal and less than 15% have clinically significant findings.[1] Nevertheless, significant soft tissue injuries can exist in the absence of radiographic findings.[2,3] Several imaging adjuncts are available, including computed tomography (CT), musculoskeletal ultrasound (MSUS), and magnetic resonance imaging (MRI). MRI is currently the modality of choice in diagnosing acute and chronic soft tissue injuries and occult fractures about the knee.[4]

CLINICAL DECISION MAKING

It is important to obtain an accurate history of a knee injury. A thorough physical examination is essential to detect fractures and soft tissue injuries. The physical examination involves inspection, assessment of range of motion, palpation for soft tissue and bone tenderness or joint effusion and neurovascular testing. Valgus (medially directed) and varus (laterally directed) stresses are applied to the knee to detect laxity of the medial collateral ligament (MCL) and lateral collateral ligament (LCL). Anterior and posterior drawer tests detect femorotibial translation, indicating rupture of the anterior cruciate ligament (ACL) or posterior cruciate ligament (PCL).

Despite these efforts, the initial physical examination may miss significant injuries; for example, within 1 to 2 hours after an injury, muscle spasm can develop that masks ligamentous injury. Even after a thorough history, physical examina-

tion, and radiographic evaluation, the diagnosis is incomplete in 31% of cases and is incorrect in 13%.[5]

Only 6 to 11% of all knee radiographs obtained are positive for fracture.[6-8] Several investigators are developing guidelines to help assist clinicians on the decision to order knee radiographs (Table 10-1).[9-14] The goal is to reduce the number of radiographic studies ordered without missing any significant injuries. Stiell et al. recommend knee radiographs for acute knee injuries with one or more of the following conditions: (1) patient's age 55 years or older, (2) tenderness at the head of the fibula, (3) isolated tenderness of the patella, (4) inability to flex to 90°, and (5) inability to bear weight for four steps both immediately and in the ED.[10,12] In a prospective study of 1096 adults with acute knee injuries, 63 (5.7%) were determined to have clinically important fractures, and 5 (0.5%) had clinically unimportant fractures. All 63 clinically important fractures were identified by the decision rules.[12]

Two other groups of investigators have derived decision rules for knee radiography. Weber et al. studied 242 patients, 28 (11.6%) of whom had fractures.[13] These investigators suggested that radiography was not necessary if the patient was under 50 years old, able to walk without a limp, and had a twisting mechanism of injury without an effusion. In two-thirds of these patients, blunt impact was the mechanism of injury, and this group had a higher incidence of fractures. Application of the decision rules would reduce the need to obtain radiographs in 29% of ED patients with knee trauma.

Bauer et al. studied 213 injuries in 209 patients, of whom 18 (8%) had fractures.[14] They suggested that patients should have radiographs only if they were unable to walk or had effusion or ecchymosis. These criteria would eliminate the need to obtain radiographs in 39% of ED patients with knee trauma.

The exact methodology in these studies must be considered before attempting to apply the associated decision rules. In addition, the latter two rules have not been validated with a prospective trial. Furthermore, the existence of three sets of decision rules for knee radiography adds to the difficulty in deciding which guidelines to apply. The proposed decision rules are useful only as preliminary guidelines when one is attempting to determine which patients need radiographs; they should not replace clinical judgment.

In patients with nontraumatic knee pain, the indications for plain radiographs are unclear. Plain radiographs may show evidence of old or occult injuries, loose bodies, osteoarthritis, tumors, infection, avascular necrosis, gout, or pseudogout.

TABLE 10-1

Decision Rules for Knee Radiography

STIELL ET AL.[10,12] RADIOGRAPHS SHOULD BE OBTAINED IF ONE OR MORE OF THE FOLLOWING IS PRESENT:	WEBER ET AL.[13] RADIOGRAPHS ARE *NOT* NECESSARY IF THE PATIENT:	BAUER ET AL.[14] RADIOGRAPHS SHOULD BE OBTAINED IF ONE OR MORE OF THE FOLLOWING IS PRESENT:
1. Inability to bear weight for four steps both at the time of injury and in the ED	1. Can walk without a limp	1. Unable to bear weight
2. Inability to flex the knee 90°	2. Twisted the knee and does not have an effusion	2. Effusion present
3. Tenderness over the patella	3. Is younger than 50 years old	3. Ecchymosis about the knee
4. Tenderness over the fibular head		
5. Age 55 years or older		

ANATOMY AND PHYSIOLOGY

The knee is made up of three articulations involving four bones: (1) a ginglymus joint (a complex hinge in which the center of rotation changes with the angle of flexion) between the femur and tibia, (2) an arthrodial (gliding) joint between the femur and patella, and (3) a diarthrodial joint between the head of the fibula and the proximal tibia (Fig. 10-1).

The superior extent of the knee is the supracondylar portion of the distal femur. The medial and lateral femoral condyles are separated by the *intercondylar notch.* The intercondylar notch extends anteriorly to form the *patellofemoral groove,* which is the articulating surface for the patella.

The femoral condyles articulate with the medial and lateral tibial plateaus, which are the flattened, smooth articulating surfaces on the superior aspect of the tibial condyles. The surface of the tibial plateau is angled posteriorly approximately 15° below the horizontal plane. The tibial plateaus are separated by a ridge of bone called the *intercondylar eminence.* The intercondylar eminence has two projections, the medial and lateral tibial spines. The *anterior tibial tubercle* is a protuberance on the anterior surface of the proximal tibia, which serves as the insertion site of the patellar tendon.

The head of the fibula articulates with the proximal tibia inferior and posterior to the lateral tibial condyle. The proximal tibiofibular joint allows minimal gliding of the fibula along the tibia. The plane of the joint varies among individuals from almost horizontal to vertical.

The *patella,* the largest sesamoid bone in the body, lies within the fibers of the quadriceps tendon. A thin sheet of the quadriceps tendon extends over the anterior surface of the patella and joins the *patellar tendon,* which extends from the apex (inferior aspect) of the patella and inserts into the anterior tibial tuberosity. The posterior surface of the patella has a medial and lateral articulating facet separated by a ridge. These facets articulate with the femoral condyles at the patellofemoral groove.

The two main intraarticular ligaments are the cruciate ligaments (Fig. 10-2). The *anterior cruciate ligament* (ACL) orig-

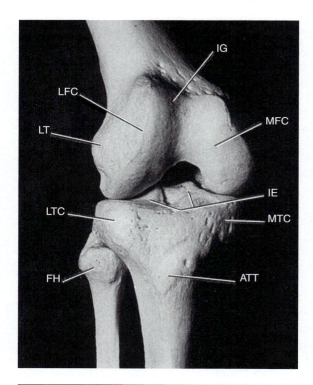

FIGURE 10-1. Bones of the knee: LT, lateral tubercle; MFC, medial femoral condyle; LFC, lateral femoral condyle; IG, intercondylar groove (articular surface for patella); MTC, medial tibial condyle; LTC, lateral tibial condyle; IE, intercondylar eminence (tibial spines); ATT, anterior tibial tubercle; FH, fibular head (patella not shown). (From Pansky B: *Review of Gross Anatomy,* 6th ed. New York: McGraw-Hill, 1996. With permission.)

inates from the posterior medial surface of the lateral femoral condyle within the intercondylar notch, and inserts on the intercondylar eminence just anterior and lateral to the medial tibial spine. The ACL prevents anterior slippage of the tibia and limits extension and medial rotation of the knee. The *posterior cruciate ligament* (PCL) originates from the middle of the medial femoral condyle within the intercondylar notch. It inserts on the midposterior aspect of the tibia, just below the joint line. The PCL prevents posterior slippage of the tibia and limits extension.

The collateral ligaments provide medial and lateral support for the knee. The *medial collateral ligament* (MCL) originates on the medial surface of the medial femoral condyle and inserts onto the tibial metaphysis. The MCL is important in resisting a valgus (medially directed) force on the knee.

The *lateral collateral ligament* (LCL) is complex, consisting of intra- and extracapsular ligaments.[15–18] The deepest layer is the lateral capsular ligament. Superficial to this is the iliotibial band, an extracapsular structure that inserts on the anterolateral surface of the tibia. The biceps femoris tendon adds lateral support and inserts on the fibular head. The MCL is stronger than the LCL.

Both the medial and lateral *menisci* cushion, lubricate, and stabilize the knee. The menisci are crescent-shaped and are attached to the intercondylar eminence of the tibia. In cross section, both menisci are wedge-shaped, with the broader surface at the periphery.

The knee has the largest synovial membrane in the body. Multiple bursae adjacent to the tendons and muscles aid in smooth knee movement. Some bursae, such as the suprapatellar bursa, communicate with the knee joint itself.

The popliteal artery courses through the popliteal fossa and is fixed both proximally and distally. This fixation allows little displacement, which makes the popliteal artery vulnerable to injury following tibiofemoral knee dislocation and fractures of the proximal tibia.[19]

The sciatic nerve bifurcates at the proximal popliteal fossa into the common peroneal nerve (lateral) and the tibial nerve (medial), which continues directly into the calf. The common peroneal nerve courses over the head and around the neck of the fibula. Injury to the proximal fibular neck is associated with a common peroneal nerve injury. This results in an inability to dorsiflex the foot (foot drop) and decreased sensation to the posterior and lateral surfaces of the leg and dorsum of the foot.

In children, the distal femoral and proximal tibial epiphyses are present from birth to the age of approximately 18 years. The patella begins to ossify between the ages of 3 and 6 years. In children, growth plates and tendon insertions are more commonly injured than bone.

RADIOGRAPHIC TECHNIQUE

Two to four standard radiographic views are used to evaluate the knee: anteroposterior (AP), lateral, and, depending on the institution, internal and external oblique views.[20] Supplementary radiographic views include the axial ("sunrise") patellar view, the intercondylar notch view, and oblique views (if not in-

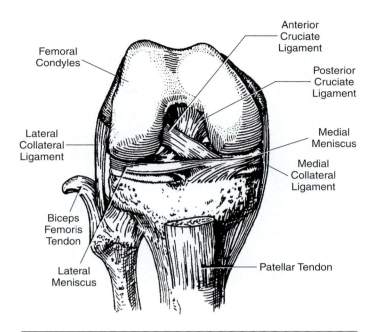

FIGURE 10-2. Soft tissues of the knee. Anterior view. The knee is flexed and the patella has been removed. The cruciate ligaments are seen within the intercondylar notch of the distal femur. (From Pansky B: *Review of Gross Anatomy,* 6th ed. New York: McGraw-Hill, 1996. With permission.)

cluded in the standard knee series). The clinical examination and initial plain-film findings determine whether supplemental radiographs are needed (Table 10-2).

Anteroposterior (AP) View

The AP radiograph is obtained with the cassette centered under the fully extended knee. The x-ray beam is directed perpendicular to the joint (Fig. 10-3).

Lateral View

The lateral radiograph is obtained with the cassette adjacent to the lateral aspect of the knee while the patient lies on the affected side (Fig. 10-3). The knee is flexed 20 to 30°. The x-ray beam is directed 5° cephalad to prevent the joint space from being obscured by the magnified image of the longer medial femoral condyle. The lateral view can also be obtained in a cross-table fashion. This technique can reveal a fat-blood level within the joint (lipohemarthrosis). A lipohemarthrosis is caused by leakage of blood and fat from an intraarticular fracture or a torn ACL or PCL. The cross-table technique is especially helpful in evaluating trauma patients because it requires less movement of the patient.

Oblique Views

The oblique views are the external (anterolateral) and internal (anteromedial) views (Fig. 10-4). The patient lies supine and

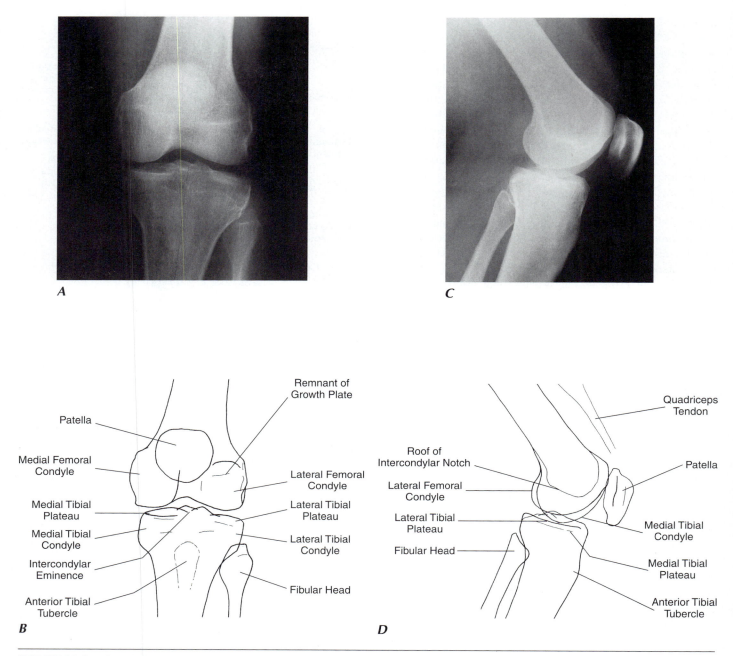

A

C

Remnant of Growth Plate

Patella

Medial Femoral Condyle

Medial Tibial Plateau

Medial Tibial Condyle

Intercondylar Eminence

Anterior Tibial Tubercle

Lateral Femoral Condyle

Lateral Tibial Plateau

Lateral Tibial Condyle

Fibular Head

B

Quadriceps Tendon

Roof of Intercondylar Notch

Lateral Femoral Condyle

Lateral Tibial Plateau

Fibular Head

Patella

Medial Tibial Condyle

Medial Tibial Plateau

Anterior Tibial Tubercle

D

FIGURE 10-3.   Standard radiographs of the knee. *A* and *B*. AP view. *C* and *D*. Lateral view.

the film cassette is posterior to the knee. The external oblique view is obtained with the affected extremity rotated 45° laterally. The internal oblique view is obtained with the extremity rotated 45° medially. The x-ray beam is directed perpendicular to the knee joint. The external oblique view demonstrates the medial tibial plateau, medial femoral condyle, and lateral margins of the patella. The internal oblique view shows the lateral tibial condyle, lateral femoral condyle, and medial margins of the patella. Oblique views are useful in detecting subtle fractures of the tibial plateau and vertical patellar fractures near the margins of the patella. In addition, the internal oblique view shows the proximal tibiofibular joint space.[21]

Supplementary Views

Additional radiographs include the axial ("sunrise") patellar view, tunnel ("notch") view, tibial plateau view, and stress views. The *sunrise view* is a tangential view of the patella (Fig. 10-5).[22,23] The knee is flexed 50 to 60° while the patient is supine or prone and the x-ray beam is directed tangentially across the patellofemoral joint. The patella is seen within the notch of the patellofemoral groove of the femur. The sunrise view is used to detect vertical fractures of the patella and osteochondral fractures of the patella after reduction of a patellar dislocation.

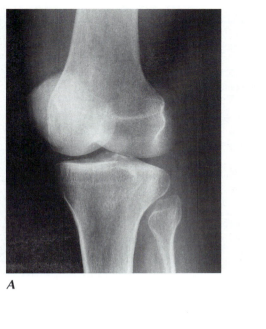

A

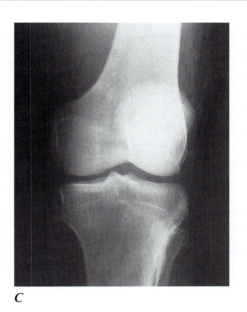

C

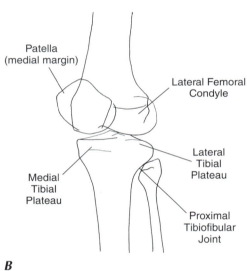

Patella
(medial margin)

Lateral Femoral
Condyle

Medial
Tibial
Plateau

Lateral
Tibial
Plateau

Proximal
Tibiofibular
Joint

B

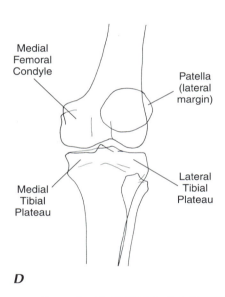

Medial
Femoral
Condyle

Patella
(lateral
margin)

Medial
Tibial
Plateau

Lateral
Tibial
Plateau

D

FIGURE 10-4.   Oblique radiographs of the knee. *A, B.* Internal oblique view. *C, D.* External oblique view.

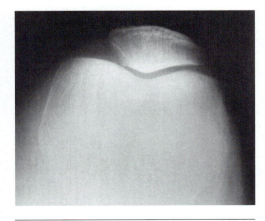

FIGURE 10-5.   Sunrise patellar view.

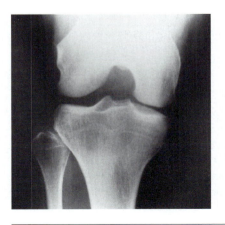

FIGURE 10-6.   Intercondylar notch view.

TABLE 10-2

Standard and Supplementary Radiographic Views of the Knee

VIEW	POSITION	EVALUATION OF ADEQUACY	LIKELY FINDINGS
AP	Supine position, leg extended. Cassette centered under knee. X-ray beam directed perpendicular to joint.	Tibial spines and tibial eminence located in middle of tibial plateaus. Horizontal dimensions of the medial and lateral joint spaces are equal. Patella lies near the midline overlying the patellofemoral groove. Lateral tibia and fibular head overlap slightly.	In combination with lateral, will identify most fractures. Patella is seen projected through the distal femur, so nondisplaced patella fractures may not be visible.
Lateral	Recumbent on affected side. Cassette on lateral side of knee. Knee flexed 20 to 30°.	Minimal rotation. Femoral condyles nearly superimposed. Medial condyle slightly larger and more posterior due to magnification. Medial and lateral tibial plateaus appear as well-defined cortical lines.	In combination with AP view, will identify most fractures. Knee effusion (suprapatellar bursa). Horizontal patellar fractures. Patellar location. Anterior tibial tuberosity.
Cross-table lateral	Supine position. Knee flexed 20 to 30°. Cassette on medial side. Horizontal x-ray beam.	Same as lateral view except lateral femoral condyle is more magnified.	Lipohemarthrosis.
External oblique	Supine position. Leg extended. Extremity rotated 45° laterally. X-ray beam directed perpendicular to joint.	Medial femoral condyle and medial tibial plateau. Tibial plateaus appear elongated in horizontal plane. Lateral margin of patella.	Fractures of the medial femoral condyle, medial tibial plateau, and lateral margin of patella.
Internal oblique	Supine position. Leg extended. Extremity rotated 45° medially. X-ray beam directed perpendicular to joint.	Lateral femoral condyle and lateral tibial plateau. Medial patellar margin. Fibula and tibiofibular joint well visualized.	Fractures of the lateral femoral condyle, lateral tibial plateau, and medial margin of patella. Proximal fibular fractures and disruptions of tibiofibular joint.
Axial patellar view ("Sunrise")	Supine or prone position. Knee flexed 50 to 60°. Edge of patella centered on cassette. X-ray directed tangentially through patellofemoral joint.	Patella lies atop femoral condyles and the patellofemoral groove. Patellofemoral joint space and posterior surface of patella well delineated.	Vertically oriented patellar fractures. Osteochondral fracture fragments within patellofemoral joint space.
Intercondylar notch view (Tunnel view)	Prone position. Knee flexed 40°. X-ray beam directed perpendicular to long axis of leg at center of popliteal fossa.	Optimal visualization of intercondylar notch and intercondylar eminence.	Loose bodies within joint. Avulsions at intercondylar notch—cruciate ligament insertions. Osteochondritis dissecans.

The *notch view* is a posteroanterior (PA) view obtained by placing the patient in a prone position, flexing the knee approximately 40° (resting the foot on a support). The x-ray beam is directed perpendicular to and centered on the popliteal depression. This "open joint" view is designed to optimize visualization of the intercondylar eminence and intercondylar notch. It is obtained for a suspected avulsion of the ACL or PCL (Fig. 10-6).

To better visualize the tibial plateau, an angled beam or *tibial plateau view* is used. This AP view is obtained by directing the x-ray beam 15° caudad, providing a tangential view of the tibial plateau.[24] This view is useful in assessing the depth of depression of a tibial plateau fracture, although it has now been largely supplanted by CT.

Although seldom necessary in the ED, *stress views* can confirm or exclude ligamentous injuries.[25–27] Radiographs are taken with valgus stress to evaluate the MCL and varus stress to evaluate the LCL. In children, stress views are used to differentiate growth plate fractures from ligamentous injuries.

RADIOGRAPHIC ANALYSIS

The skeletal anatomy of the knee is fairly straightforward, and many fractures are radiographically obvious. However, minimally displaced fractures are often radiographically subtle, and a systematic approach is necessary to avoid missing such injuries (Table 10-3).

Systematic analysis of knee radiographs focuses on sites of common injury and sites of easily missed fractures (Fig. 10-7). After an initial review and assessment of the technical adequacy of each view, each bone is carefully examined for subtle fractures, cortical deformity, or trabecular impaction. The joint space and surrounding soft tissues are inspected for small bone fragments due to ligamentous avulsion fractures and osteochondral fractures. Although small, such fractures cause significant articular derangement. In each view, the following regions are examined successively:

Proximal tibia—tibial plateaus (especially lateral), tibial condyles, and intercondylar eminence
Distal femur—femoral condyles, intercondylar notch, and supracondylar region
Joint space—look for asymmetry, fracture fragments
Patella—look for fractures, displacement, and effusion (suprapatellar bursa seen on the lateral view)
Proximal fibula, proximal tibiofibular articulation, and anterior tibial tuberosity

Anteroposterior (AP) View

A properly positioned AP view is centered on the articular surfaces so that both the medial and lateral joint spaces are open. The horizontal dimensions of the medial and lateral tibial plateaus are roughly equal. The intercondylar spines are located near the midline within the intercondylar notch of the femur. The patella is superimposed on the distal femur, near the midline. The inferior pole (apex) of the patella is at the level of the intercondylar notch. The fibular head overlaps the lateral tibial condyle (Fig. 10-3).

In studying the AP radiograph, the tibia is examined first. The cortex and trabeculae of the tibia are inspected, paying close attention to the tibial plateaus (looking for discontinuity or impaction), tibial condyles, tibial spines (looking for avulsion fractures), and the proximal tibiofibular articulation. The trabeculae of the medial tibial condyle are normally more dense than those of the medial side because the medial side carries more body weight. Increased trabecular density on the lateral side is abnormal and indicates a fracture of the lateral tibial plateau. The joint spaces are examined, looking for intraarticular osteochondral fractures and avulsions. Next, the femoral condyles and supracondylar area are examined. The inter-

condylar notch is examined for fracture fragments. Finally, the superimposed outline of the patella is traced for fractures or subluxation.

Lateral View

On a lateral view, the medial and lateral femoral condyles should be almost completely superimposed. However, exact superimposition is not possible and a small amount of rotation is often present. Standard positioning of the lateral view places the film cassette against the lateral aspect of the knee so that the medial femoral condyle is farther from the x-ray film and is therefore more magnified. The medial condyle therefore appears slightly larger than the lateral condyle (Fig. 10-3).

The medial and lateral tibial plateaus appear as sharp, well-defined cortical lines. Each tibial plateau is equidistant to and articulates with its respective femoral condyle.

The surface of the cortical bone at the roof of the intercondylar notch projects through the femoral condyles. The origin of the ACL is located at the intersection of this intercondylar roof line and a line drawn down the posterior cortex of the femoral shaft. The fibular head partly overlaps the lateral tibial condyle.

The patella has a quadrilateral shape and lies anterior to the femoral condyles. The quadriceps and infrapatellar tendons can be seen because they are highlighted by adjacent radiolucent fat tissue. The quadriceps tendon attaches to the superior border of the patella and is separated from the anterior surface of the femur by the prefemoral (suprapatellar) fat pad. The infrapatellar joint space is occupied by the infrapatellar fat pad, which appears as a triangular area of relative radiolucency.

Systematic review of the lateral view begins with the femoral condyles. These are inspected for breaks or deformity of the cortex or trabeculae. The articular surfaces should be smooth. The lateral femoral articular surface is somewhat flattened on its anteroinferior aspect, while the medial condylar surface is continuously curved. The slight flattening of the lateral condyle is known as the lateral femoral condylar sulcus.

Next, the proximal tibia is examined. Each tibial plateau surface is inspected for cortical breaks, angulation, or trabecular impaction. The intercondylar eminence is examined for fractures or avulsions. Then, the anterior tibial tuberosity and proximal fibula are examined.

Next, the patella is examined. Horizontally oriented patellar fractures are readily seen on the lateral view. The position of the patella is assessed. The patella position cannot be accurately determined by using the location of the patella relative to the tibiofemoral joint space, because this varies depending on the amount of flexion or extension of the knee. Instead, the *Insall-Salvati ratio* (infrapatellar tendon ratio) is used.[28] Optimally, a lateral radiograph is obtained with the knee in 30° of flexion to place the patellar tendon under tension. The length of the infrapatellar tendon (inferior pole of the patella to the tibial tuberosity) and the length of the patella are measured. The ratio of the length of the infrapatellar tendon to the patella is normally 0.8 to 1.0; a ratio greater than 1.2 means that the

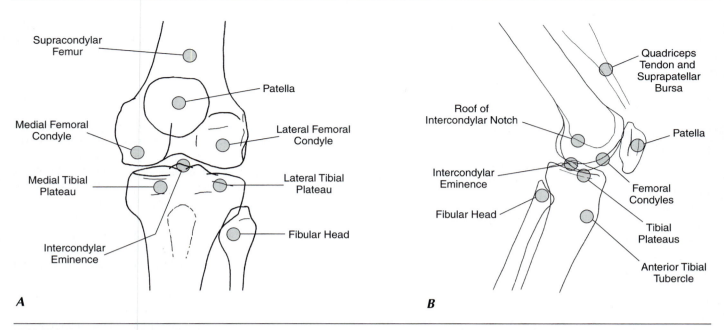

FIGURE 10-7.   Sites prone to injury and easily missed injuries. *A.* AP view *B.* Lateral view *C.* Internal oblique view *D.* External oblique view.

patella is high-riding (*patella alta*). Patella alta is associated with an infrapatellar tendon rupture. A low-riding patella (*patella baja*) is present when the Insall-Salvati ratio is less than 0.8. Patella baja is seen with quadriceps tendon rupture, neuromuscular disease, and achondroplasia.

Finally, the lateral radiograph is inspected for signs of a knee joint effusion. The suprapatellar bursa extends superiorly from the posterosuperior margin of the patella and divides the prefemoral fat pad into anterior and posterior components. The bursa is normally less than 5 mm wide and is sometimes visible as a thin, slightly opaque stripe within the prefemoral fat pad. The suprapatellar bursa is continuous with the knee joint and becomes distended if the patient has knee effusion.

Knee Effusion.   In an acutely traumatized patient, knee effusion is a sign of a fracture or serious soft tissue injury.[29–32] An effusion that develops immediately after injury is due to hemorrhage within the joint. A hemarthrosis is seen in partial and complete ACL tears, meniscal injuries, PCL tears, and osteochondral fractures. Effusions that develop later after injury do not have the same significance.

Small effusions can be difficult to detect radiographically and are better diagnosed by physical examination. A small effusion is detected by manually compressing the suprapatellar region and palpating the medial and lateral sides of the patella for a fluid bulge. Larger effusions are detected on the lateral radiograph because of distension of the suprapatellar bursa (Fig. 10-8).[33,34]

Knee effusions distend the suprapatellar bursa, which is continuous with the knee joint. The suprapatellar bursa is occasionally visible on the lateral radiograph as a thin soft tissue stripe that extends proximally from the posterosuperior margin of the patella. It lies posterior to the quadriceps tendon and anterior to the prefemoral fat pad. The suprapatellar bursa is normally less than 5 mm wide in adults. With a small effusion, the suprapatellar bursa is 5 to 10 mm wide. With larger effusions, the quadriceps tendon is displaced anteriorly and the suprapatellar bursa is distended. A very large effusion displaces the patella anteriorly, causing it to rotate forward. The soft tissue layers of the suprapatellar region are obliterated, and the quadriceps tendon appears thickened (Fig. 10-9).[35] Incorrect positioning of the lateral radiograph with excessive knee flexion or rotation can obscure findings of an effusion. Occasionally, a large effusion can be identified on the AP radiograph. It appears as abnormal soft tissue density adjacent to the patella.

Lipohemarthrosis may be the only radiographic sign of an occult fracture of the distal femur or proximal tibia. The cross-table lateral view shows a distinct layer in the suprapatellar bursa between the blood below and more radiolucent fat above (Fig. 10-10).[36] Differentiating a simple suprapatellar effusion and lipohemarthrosis can be difficult. Both have a fusiform shape. A lipohemarthrosis has an anterior lucent layer of fat and an opaque posterior layer. The position of the prefemoral fat pad anterior to the suprapatellar bursa can also appear as a triangular lucency superior to the patella and may be misinterpreted as a radiolucent fat layer of a lipohemarthrosis. However, the fat pad does not extend behind the patella, while a lipohemarthrosis does.

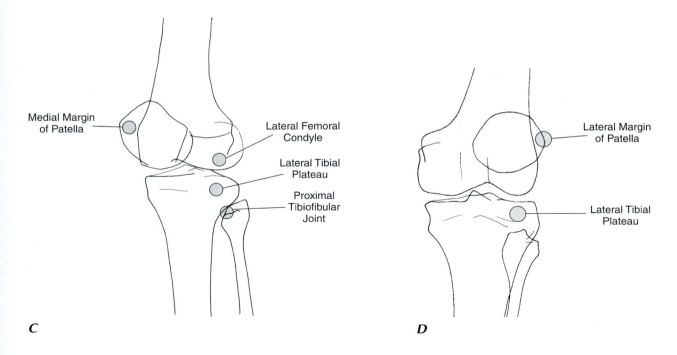

C   D

TABLE 10-3

Systematic Analysis of Knee Radiographs

Determine study quality	At least two views are included—AP and lateral. In some centers, internal and external oblique views are routine. On an AP view without rotation, the intercondylar spines and patella are near the midline. On the lateral view, the knee is flexed 30° and the femoral condyles are nearly superimposed. The medial and lateral tibial plateaus appear sharp. The patella is anterior to the femoral condyles with a clear patellofemoral joint space.
Look for skeletal abnormalities	Examine the cortical margins and trabecular architecture. Tibial plateaus (especially lateral tibial plateau) Tibial condyles (especially lateral avulsion—Segond fracture) Femoral condyles Joint space—avulsion of intercondylar eminence Patella—fracture, elevation, or inferior displacement Proximal fibula
Examine the lateral view for an effusion	An effusion causes increased density in the suprapatellar region and obliterates the fat deep to the quadriceps tendon. A cross-table view can reveal a fat-fluid level (lipohemarthrosis) due to an intraarticular fracture.
Reexamine	If a fracture or joint space deformity is found, reexamine other areas of the knee for subtle injuries. If there are questionable abnormalities on the AP and lateral views or if an effusion is present and standard views do not demonstrate a fracture, consider supplementary views such as oblique views or a tunnel view to better evaluate the tibial plateaus, femoral condyles, and intercondylar eminence. Obtain a sunrise patellar view and/or oblique views if the patient is especially tender over the patella (a vertical patellar fracture may not be seen on other views).

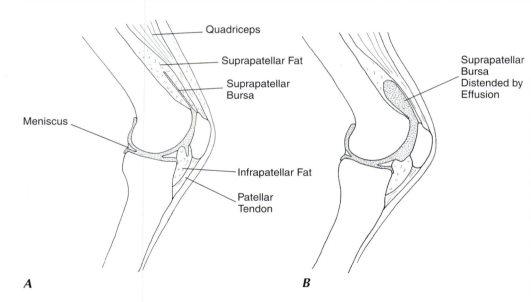

FIGURE 10-8. Radiographic detection of a knee effusion. *A*. The suprapatellar bursa normally contains a minimal amount of joint fluid and is not usually radiographically visible or is less than 5 mm in thickness. The quadriceps tendon is visible in the suprapatellar region because it is adjacent to radiolucent fat (subcutaneous and suprapatellar fat). *B*. A knee effusion distends the suprapatellar bursa. The effusion is seen as an oblong fluid collection in the suprapatellar region. The normally well-defined margins of the quadriceps tendon are obliterated. With a large effusion, the patella is displaced anteriorly.

Oblique Views

The internal and external oblique views demonstrate the femoral condyles, tibial plateaus, and patella from a different orientation than seen on the AP and lateral radiographs (Fig. 10-4). Some fractures may be seen only on an oblique view. The articular surfaces are particularly well demonstrated on the oblique views and should be carefully inspected for subtle fractures. The tibial plateau appears elongated in the horizontal plane. In addition, the margins of the patella are seen projected

beyond the femur. The fibular head and tibiofibular joint space are seen on the internal oblique view.

If not routinely included in the knee series, oblique views should be obtained if a fracture of the tibial plateau, or, less commonly, the femoral condyle, is suspected but not seen on the AP or lateral views. These fractures are suspected if the mechanism of injury is severe, if the patient has considerable pain on weight bearing, or if a lipohemarthrosis is seen. Vertically oriented fractures of the medial or lateral margins of the patella are also seen on oblique views. Such fractures are

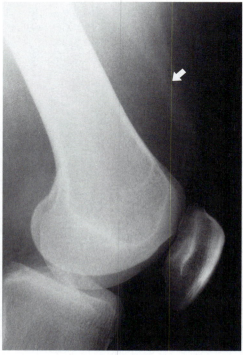

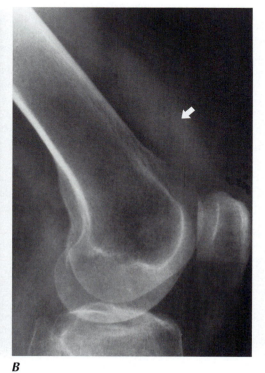

FIGURE 10-9. Knee effusion. *A*. Normally, a slender quadriceps tendon is outlined by subcutaneous and suprapatellar fat. *B*. With a knee effusion, the suprapatellar fat is displaced by fluid in the suprapatellar bursa. Definition of the quadriceps tendon is lost. There is swelling in the suprapatellar region and anterior displacement of the patella.

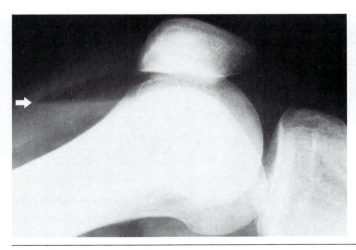 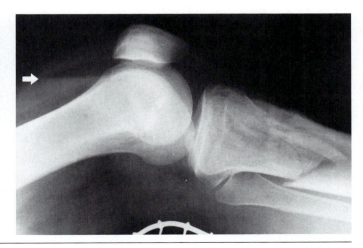

FIGURE 10-10. Lipohemarthrosis. A fat-blood level is seen in this patient with a proximal tibial fracture. A lipohemarthrosis implies that there is an intraarticular fracture. When no obvious fracture is seen in a patient with a hemarthrosis, a subtle fracture should be carefully sought, such as a tibial plateau fracture, tibial spine fracture, or osteochondral fracture. A proximal tibia fracture was present in this patient.

suspected clinically if the patient has tenderness over the patella.

Axial (Sunrise) Patellar View

The sunrise view gives an excellent view of the patella lying in the patellofemoral groove (Fig. 10-5). This view is used to see vertically oriented patellar fractures, which are not visible on the lateral view and are difficult to see on the AP view because of overlap by the distal femur. Osteochondral fractures within the patellofemoral joint can also be seen on this view. Vertically oriented grooves on the anterior surface of the patella are normal and should not be mistaken for fractures.

Tunnel (Notch) View

The tunnel view provides optimal visualization of the intercondylar notch and intercondylar eminence (Fig. 10-6). It is used to detect avulsions of the insertion sites of the cruciate ligaments, loose bodies within the joint (osteochondromatosis), and erosion of the articular surface (osteochondritis dissecans). Small avulsion fractures off the medial or lateral margins of the tibial condyles and tibial plateau fractures are occasionally better seen on this view.

Common Abnormalities

The type of knee injury depends on the magnitude and direction of the injuring forces, the position of the knee (flexed or extended) at the time of the trauma, and the age of the patient. In older adults, osteoporosis weakens the bone and fractures can occur following minor trauma. In young adults, the bones are stronger, and soft tissue injury without fracture is common. The frequency of various fractures about the knee seen in the

ED has been established by several recently published clinical studies (Table 10-4).

Medially directed forces (valgus) are common and result in medial ligament tears, with or without lateral bone injury. Laterally directed forces (varus) are less common and cause lateral soft tissue injuries. Direct anterior impact with the knee extended causes ACL injury. Anterior forces with the knee flexed causes injury to the patella and possibly the PCL. A direct axial load, as with jumping injuries, results in tibial plateau injuries. Twisting injuries result in various soft tissue injuries and avulsion fractures. Forced flexion of the knee while the knee extensors are contracted results in extensor mechanism injuries. Combined injuries are common.

Patellar Fractures

Patellar fractures are the most common fracture involving the knee. They are classified as vertical, transverse, proximal/distal pole, marginal, stellate, or osteochondral (Fig. 10-11).

TABLE 10-4

Frequency of Fractures in Patients Presenting to the Emergency Department*

Patella	40%	77
Tibial plateau	32%	62
Fibular head	9%	17
Distal femur	8%	16
Tibial spine	7%	13
Tibial tuberosity	2%	3
Loose body	1%	2
Segond	0.5%	1
Medial tibial	0.5%	1
Total		192

*Data from four papers.[10,12–14]

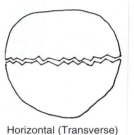
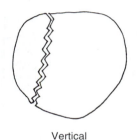
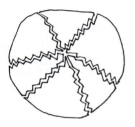
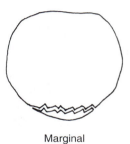

Horizontal (Transverse)   Vertical   Stellate   Marginal

FIGURE 10-11.   Types of patellar fractures.

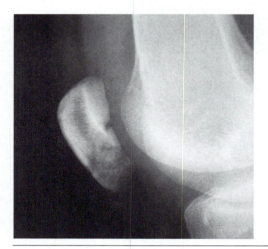

FIGURE 10-12.   A nondisplaced transverse (horizontal) fracture is best seen on the lateral view. A mild suprapatellar effusion is present. This is the most common patellar fracture. The extensor mechanism is intact.

Most patellar fractures result from a direct blow. Other fractures are due to forced flexion. Transverse fractures account for about half of all patellar fractures. The fracture usually involves the midportion of the patella. The fragment is either nondisplaced or widely displaced. They are easy to identify on a lateral radiograph (Figs. 10-12 and 10-13). The next most common patellar fractures are stellate (burst) fractures, which account for about one-third of patellar fractures. These are usually the result of direct blows. Stellate fractures are easy to visualize on AP and lateral radiographs (Fig. 10-14).

Vertical or marginal fractures account for approximately 15% of patellar fractures. They are the result of patellar dislocation or direct blows to the edges of the patella. Longitudinal (vertical) fractures are often nondisplaced and may not be visible on routine views. This fracture can be difficult to see on the AP view because the distal femur overlaps the patella. Oblique and sunrise patellar views help to identify these fractures (Figs. 10-15 and 10-16).

Proximal or distal pole avulsion fractures are less common.

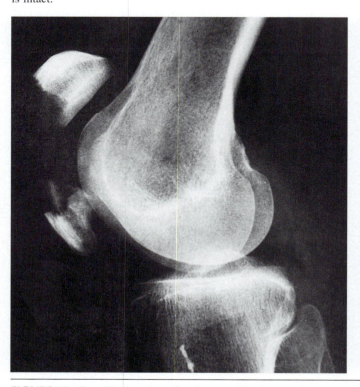
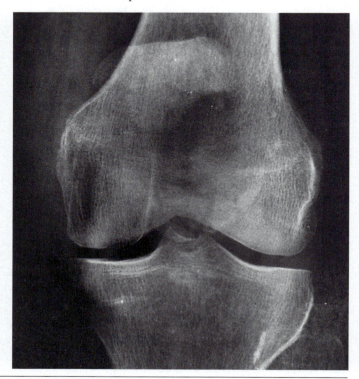

FIGURE 10-13.   Displaced patellar fracture. The fracture fragments are widely displaced and the extensor mechanism of the knee is disrupted. The distal fragment has migrated inferiorly closer to the anterior tubercle of the tibia. The proximal fragment is pulled superiorly by the quadriceps. The fracture can also be seen on the AP radiograph. Treatment consists of excision of the distal fragment and wire suturing.

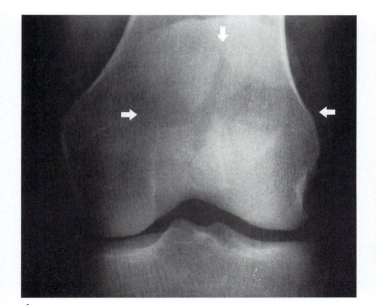

A

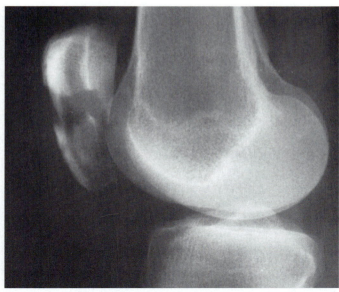

B

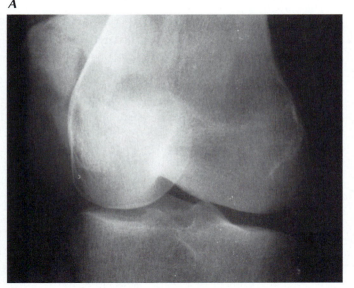

C

FIGURE 10-14. Stellate patellar fracture (*A–C*). These fractures are usually due to direct trauma and are usually nondisplaced because the extensor retinaculum is intact.

The fracture may consist of a large or small fracture fragment. Disruption of the infrapatellar region may result in a high-riding patella (patella alta) (Fig. 10-17).

Tibial Plateau Fractures

Tibial plateau fractures are the second most common type of knee fractures (after patellar fractures). More than half of the patients who sustain a tibial plateau fracture are 50 years of age or above.[37–39] Plateau fractures are important because they affect knee alignment, stability, and motion. They range in severity from minimally displaced fractures to severely dis-

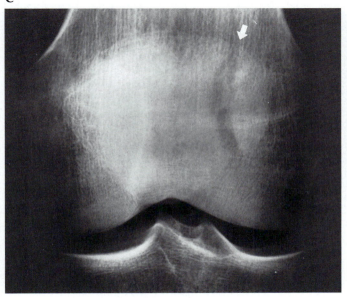

A

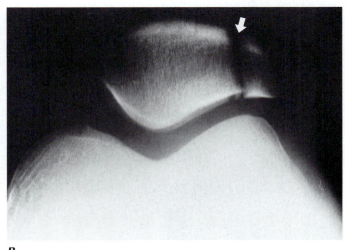

B

FIGURE 10-15. Vertical patellar fracture (*A* and *B*). These fractures are usually nondisplaced. They may be visible on the AP view but are most easily seen on the "sunrise" patellar view.

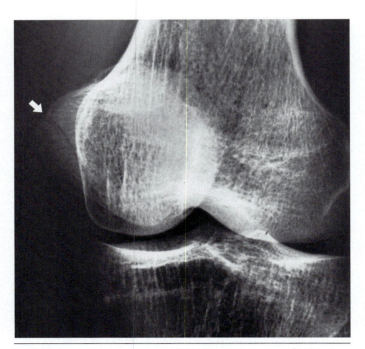

FIGURE 10-16. A vertical patellar fracture seen only on an oblique radiograph. The fracture runs in a slightly oblique plane and was not seen on a sunrise patellar view. (Copyright David T. Schwartz, M.D.)

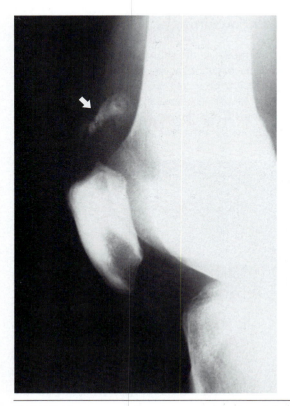

FIGURE 10-17. Avulsion of the superior pole of the patella. Note that the patella is low-riding, which indicates that the extensor mechanism is disrupted.

placed and comminuted injuries disrupting the entire proximal tibia.

The most common mechanism of injury causing a tibial plateau fracture is a valgus force combined with axial loading. The typical clinical scenario, responsible for 25 to 50% of tibial plateau fractures, is the "bumper" or "fender" injury from a vehicle-pedestrian collision. Tibial plateau fractures are also caused by axial loading, such as that which occurs when a person falls or jumps and lands on the feet. Postmenopausal women with osteoporosis are at increased risk of sustaining a tibial plateau fracture. These can occur with minimal trauma during normal daily activities, such as going down stairs or stepping off a curb.[40]

The lateral tibial plateau is involved in 75 to 90% of cases. An isolated lateral tibial plateau fracture is seen in 55 to 70% of cases. An isolated medial tibial plateau fracture occurs in 10 to 23% of cases, and combined medial and lateral fractures occur in 11 to 31% of cases. Many tibial plateau fractures have associated ligamentous and meniscal injuries.

The classification of tibial plateau fractures depends on the site of the fracture and displacement of major fragments (Fig. 10-18). Tibial plateau fractures are divided into six types. *Compression fractures* of the joint surface make up 26% of fractures. These almost always involve the lateral plateau. *Vertical split fractures* near the joint margin make up 24%. *Combined vertical split and compression fractures* make up 26%. *Oblique fractures of the medial condyle,* in which the fracture extends from near the intercondylar eminence to the cortex of the medial metaphysis and involves nearly the entire condyle, make up 13%. *Posterior split fractures* involving a fragment from the posterior portion of the tibial plateau make up 3%. *Bicondylar fractures* account for approximately 10% of cases. These are caused by severe trauma to the proximal tibia that creates a separation of the tibial condyles and drives them inferiorly with respect to the shaft. These fractures, which have an inverted-Y configuration, are associated with a high incidence of ligamentous and neurovascular injuries, and more than 50% are associated with subcondylar fractures or fractures of the proximal tibial shaft. Retropulsed fragments from a comminuted tibial plateau fracture can damage the popliteal artery.

Tibial plateau fractures that are separated more than 4 mm or have articular surface depression of more than 8 to 10 mm generally need open reduction and internal fixation. The depth of plateau surface depression is difficult to determine on the AP view because the plateau surface slopes 15° from the horizontal plane. A 15° caudad-angled AP view (tibial plateau view) can provide a more accurate assessment of the depth of plateau surface depression. However, CT, especially with coronal and sagittal reconstructions, has supplanted the plain-film tibial plateau view.

Most tibial plateau fractures are easy to identify on the standard AP and lateral views (Figs. 10-19 through 10-22). However, about 22% of tibial plateau fractures are minimally displaced and can be subtle (Figs. 10-23 and 10-24). With minimally displaced vertical split fractures, the fracture line often lies in an oblique plane and is therefore not visible on an AP or lateral radiograph. If not routinely obtained, oblique

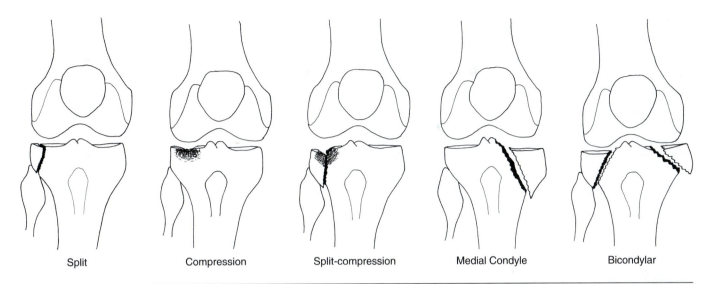

FIGURE 10-18. Classification of tibial plateau fractures.

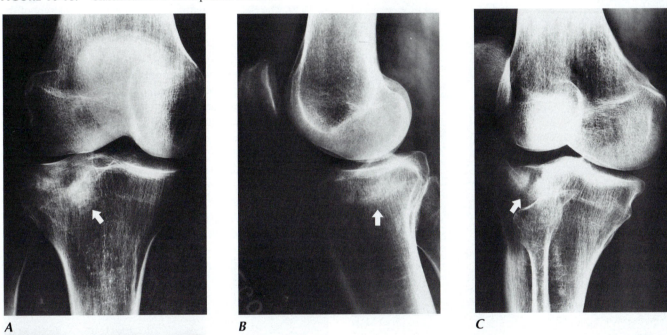

FIGURE 10-19. A split-compression tibial plateau fracture. Impaction causes increased bone density below the lateral tibial plateau on the AP and lateral radiographs (*A* and *B*). The cortical surface of the tibial plateau appears intact. The split-compression nature of the fracture is evident on the oblique view showing a vertical fracture line (*C*). This amount of depression of the tibial plateau mandates surgical elevation and fixation with a contoured side-plate and screws (*D*). (Copyright David T. Schwartz, M.D.)

views should be added if a nondisplaced tibial plateau fracture is suspected but not seen on the standard radiographs. Suspicion of a tibial plateau fracture is based on clinical signs (effusion, inability to bear weight) or radiographic findings (lipohemarthrosis or irregularity of the tibial plateau surface).

A minimally displaced compression fracture can also be difficult to see on standard radiographs because the tibial plateau surface slopes 15° from the horizontal plane and is not seen tangentially on the AP view. Increased trabecular density beneath the lateral tibial plateau surface is a subtle radiographic sign of a depressed

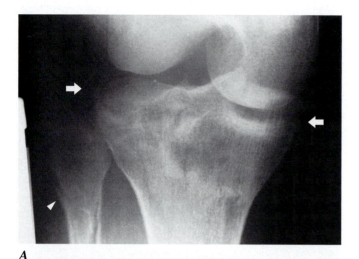

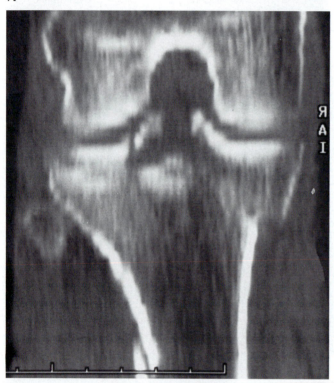

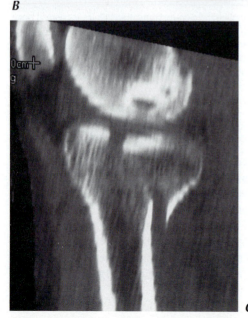

FIGURE 10-20. A bicondylar fracture is seen on the AP view (*A*). There is also a fibular neck fracture (*arrowhead*). The magnitude of displacement of the fracture fragments is revealed by CT-reconstructed images in the coronal and sagittal planes (*B* and *C*).

tibial plateau fracture on the AP film. Normally, the medial tibial condyle has greater trabecular density because it bears more body weight. On the lateral view, both tibial plateau surfaces should be identified and closely examined for depression or cortical interruption, indicative of a fracture. Oblique views should be obtained to confirm the fracture if any of these radiographic signs are present.

Segond Fractures

This type of fracture was first described by Paul Segond in 1879 in cadaveric experiments. It was first recognized on radiographs in 1936. The Segond fracture is a small avulsion fracture of the lateral margin of the lateral tibial condyle at the site of attachment of the lateral capsular ligament (Fig. 10-25). It is generally 2 to 10 mm below the surface of the tibial plateau. The fracture fragment is a 10- by 3-mm elliptical fragment and is displaced several millimeters from the tibial condyle. A Segond fracture, caused by internal rotation and varus stress, often occurs during sports injuries.[41,42] This fracture should be distinguished from an avulsion of the fibular styloid, although both injuries can coexist.

The Segond fracture is significant because 75 to 100% of patients have an associated ACL injury.[43,44] Meniscal injuries are also commonly associated with the Segond fracture. The Segond fracture is best seen on the AP view. Associated soft tissue injuries are seen on MRI.[45,46]

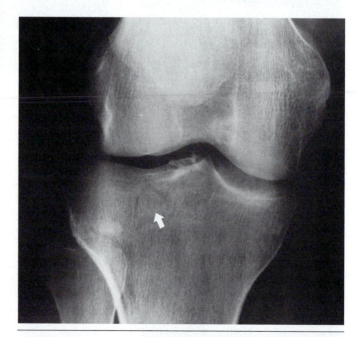

FIGURE 10-21. A subtle split-compression tibial plateau fracture. There is slight impaction of the trabecular pattern of the lateral tibial condyle and minimal cortical interruption near the intercondylar eminence.

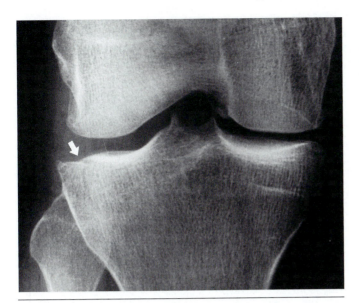

FIGURE 10-22. A subtle split fracture is seen at the lateral aspect of the lateral tibial plateau. (Copyright David T. Schwartz, M.D.)

FIGURE 10-23. A tibial plateau compression fracture in an elderly female with osteoporosis. There is a thin line of cortical bone with subjacent trabecular impaction below the lateral tibial plateau. (Copyright David T. Schwartz, M.D.)

Intercondylar Eminence Fractures (Fractures of the Tibial Spine)

Three types of fractures of the intercondylar eminence are described.[47] Type I is an intercondylar avulsion fracture that is minimally elevated. Type II is an intercondylar avulsion fracture that is incompletely detached and "hinged" to the tibia posteriorly. In type III-A, the tibial eminence is completely ele-

vated off the tibia. In type III-B, the tibial eminence is completely separated and rotated as much as 90°, such that the articulating surface of the fragment is directed posteriorly. Type III injuries are often associated with collateral ligamentous injuries and peripheral meniscal detachments. A fracture at the base of the intercondylar eminence or of the medial tibial spine may indicate ACL disruption. Isolated fractures of the lateral intercondylar spine do not involve the cruciate ligaments. Frac-

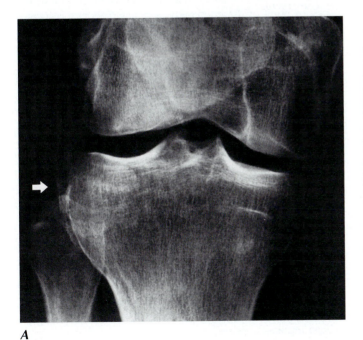

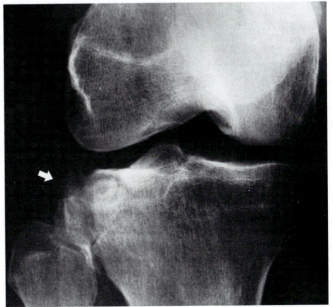

A   *B*

FIGURE 10-24. A tibial plateau fracture is seen clearly only on an oblique view. On the AP view, there is slight irregularity and increased density of the trabeculae below the lateral tibial plateau (*A*). The fracture is clearly seen on the oblique view (*B*). This is because the fracture line lies in an oblique plane. (Copyright David T. Schwartz, M.D.)

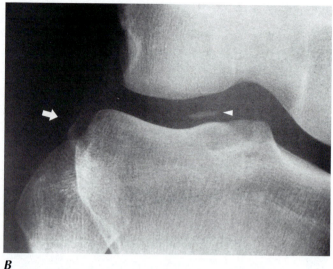

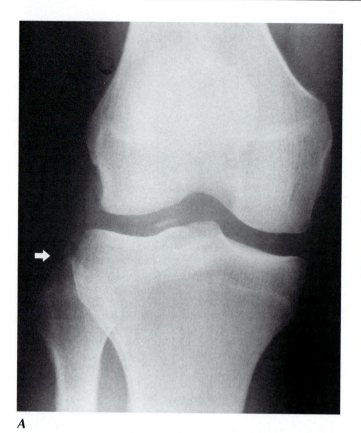

A

B

FIGURE 10-25.   Segond fracture. Forceful internal rotation of the tibia when the knee is flexed causes avulsion at the insertion of the lateral capsular ligament (the Segond fracture) (*arrow*) and tearing of the anterior cruciate ligament. In this patient, there is also a small avulsion fracture of the anterior tibial spine at the insertion of the anterior cruciate ligament (*arrowhead*). The Segond fracture is a subtle but important clue to the presence of an ACL tear. (Courtesy of Thomas Akre, D.O., Ingham Region Medical Center, Lansing, Michigan.)

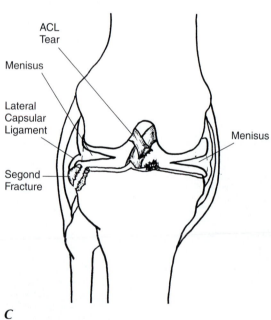

C

Avulsion Fractures of the Anterior Cruciate Ligament

The ACL originates from the lateral femoral condyle at the most posterior point of the intercondylar notch. This site is located on the lateral film at the intersection of the posterior femoral shaft and the intercondylar notch line. It is more clearly seen using a tunnel view. A fracture here is rare.

An avulsion fracture at the tibial insertion is more common and is easier to see. On both the AP and lateral views, the fracture appears as a bone fragment along the anterior slope of the intercondylar eminence. In children, the anterior aspect of the tibial epiphysis may be avulsed. Avulsion of the anterior tibial spine is more common in children than in adults because of weakness of the epiphyseal plates in the immature skeleton.

TABLE 10-5

Radiographic Findings of Anterior Cruciate Ligament Injury

Anterior displacement >5 mm of the tibia relative to the
    femur on lateral projection (tibial anterotranslation)
Segond fracture
Fracture of the fibular head or styloid process
Nondisplaced fracture of the posterior tibial plateau
Lipohemarthrosis
Deepened lateral femoral condylar notch

tures of the intercondylar eminence are often diagnosed on standard radiographs but may be better seen on a tunnel view. Fractures at the base of the intercondylar eminence occur frequently in children and adolescents (Fig. 10-26).

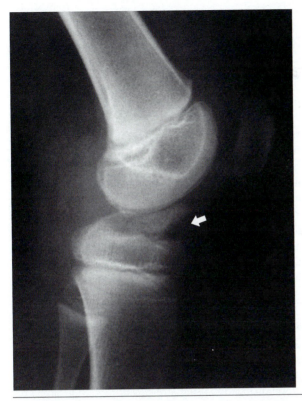

and is known as *tibial anterotranslation.* This reflects extensive damage to the ACL, collateral ligaments, joint capsule, and menisci. Other radiographic findings suggesting an ACL tear include Segond fracture, fibular head avulsion fracture, nondisplaced fracture of the posterior tibial plateau hemarthrosis, and a deepened lateral femoral condylar notch. Clinical indicators of an ACL tear are a sudden "pop" and an acute hemarthrosis (Table 10-5).

Osteochondral Fractures

Osteochondral fractures most often occur at the medial articular surface of the patella and the anterior part of the lateral femoral condyle (Fig. 10-27). These are thin, curved fragments of cortical bone and covering cartilage. The small, radiographically visible bone fragment is much smaller than the entire cartilaginous portion. Osteochondral fractures often result from lateral patellar dislocation. These fragments are best seen on a sunrise or internal oblique radiograph. An osteochondral fragment acts as a loose foreign body in the joint, causing impaired movement, locking, and degenerative disease. The fragments are usually located in the anterior portion of the joint space. The site of origin is seldom seen on routine radiographs. Osteochondral fractures generally require MRI or arthroscopic evaluation.

FIGURE 10-26. Intercondylar eminence fracture in a 9-year-old boy. There is a hinged-type elevation of the intercondylar eminence at the site of insertion of the anterior cruciate ligament. These injuries are more common in children. In adults, tear of the ACL is the usual injury.

Rupture of the Anterior Cruciate Ligament

Anterior displacement of greater than 5 mm of the tibia relative to the femur on a lateral view indicates an ACL rupture. This is the radiographic equivalent of the anterior drawer sign

Fractures of the Femoral Condyle

Femoral condyle fractures are intraarticular fractures caused by valgus or varus stress with axial loading. They can affect one or both condyles, and can occur in multiple planes. Fractures of the femoral condyle are often associated with fractures of the tibial plateau. They also occur in forced hyperextension,

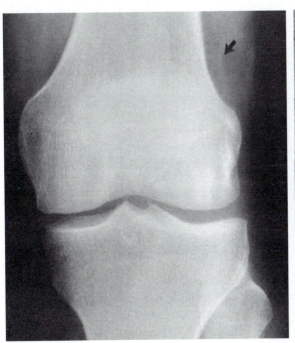

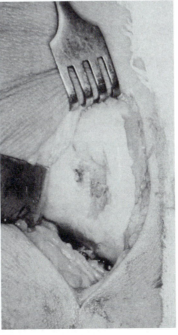

FIGURE 10-27. Osteochondral fracture. *A.* A thin sliver of bone is adjacent to the lateral femoral condyle in a 16-year-old youth who injured his knee during a long jump in track. These injuries typically occur when the patella impacts against the lateral femoral condyle, as during a patellar dislocation. The small sliver of bone reflects a large defect in the articular cartilage. *B.* The operative view demonstrates the large defect in the articular surface of the lateral femoral condyle. (From Larson RL, Jones DC: Dislocations and ligamentous injuries of the knee, in Rockwood CA, Green DP (eds): *Fractures in Adults,* 2d ed. Philadelphia: Lippincott, 1984. With permission.)

A   *B*

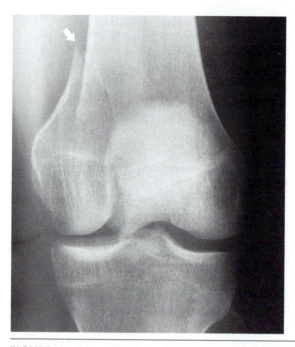

FIGURE 10-28. Femoral condyle fracture. The medial femoral condyle is sheared off the distal femur in this patient who was thrown off of a motorcycle.

when the tibial eminence is driven against the inner portion of the intercondylar notch. Severely comminuted condylar fractures are often associated with a spiral fracture of the distal femur.

When one condyle is involved, the fracture is oriented in a vertical, oblique, coronal, or coronal-oblique plane. When both condyles are involved, these fractures have a T or Y shape. Standard views detect most of these fractures, but tunnel views may be helpful in revealing subtle condylar fractures (Fig. 10-28). CT is performed to evaluate fractures of the femoral condyle fully.

Supracondylar Femoral Fractures

Supracondylar femoral fractures usually result from considerable force. They may be comminuted, transverse, or oblique. The distal fragment is often angulated posteriorly or rotated. These fractures also occur in patients with severely demineralized or otherwise weakened bone. In children, the weakest area is the epiphyseal-metaphyseal junction, where most fractures occur.

Supracondylar fractures can be associated with significant blood loss, and the fragment can injure the popliteal artery. These fractures are also associated with fractures or dislocations about the hip.

Floating Knee

Floating knee is a term used to describe combined fractures of the distal femur and tibial shaft.[48] This injury isolates the knee

from the limb above and below, leaving it "floating." It usually results from a high-impact force (e.g., motor vehicle accidents, vehicle-pedestrian collisions).

Knee (Tibiofemoral) Dislocation

Tibiofemoral knee dislocations require a high-energy impact. The incidence of knee dislocations is low. The dislocation is named by the direction of displacement of the tibia relative to the femur. Anterior dislocation is the most common, followed by posterior dislocation. Anterior dislocations usually result from a hyperextension injury, and posterior dislocations result from direct anterior impact to a flexed knee. Lateral, medial, and rotary dislocations occur less frequently.

Both clinically and radiographically, tibiofemoral dislocations are easy to see; although, some dislocations have reduced spontaneously at the scene of the injury.[42] The tibia is displaced relative to the femur (Fig. 10-29). Tibiofemoral dislocations are associated with other skeletal, soft tissue, neurologic, and vascular injuries. In one study, 53% of patients had fractures involving the tibial plateau (20%), distal femur (12%), tibia and fibula (10%), isolated fibula (6%), and isolated tibia (4%).[49] Tibiofemoral dislocation usually results in rupture of both cruciate ligaments, the joint capsule, and extracapsular ligaments.[50] The peroneal nerve is injured in approximately one-third of tibiofemoral dislocations; the prognosis for improvement is poor if complete palsy occurs at the time of the injury.

The most devastating complication of a tibiofemoral knee dislocation is an injury to the popliteal artery. The popliteal artery is fixed both proximally and distally to the popliteal fossa. Popliteal artery injury occurs in 23 to 60% of tibiofemoral dislocations.[51–53] Therefore, in all patients with a tibiofemoral dislocation, an arteriogram is recommended. Patients with comminuted distal femoral or proximal tibial fractures are also at high risk of arterial injury. Clinical signs of popliteal artery injury include pallor, coolness, cyanosis, or delayed capillary refill. Other physical signs of popliteal artery injury include a bruit or pulsatile hematoma. However, a patient can have a significant popliteal artery injury despite normal pulses and normal capillary refill.[54,55]

For patients with obvious limb ischemia, emergency arteriography is mandatory. This can be performed in the operating room, which avoids the delay of obtaining a formal arteriogram in the radiology department. Irreversible ischemia occurs within 6 to 8 hours. Further delay results in an 86% amputation rate.[56] Even without signs of limb ischemia, arteriography is recommended following tibiofemoral dislocation.[53,57]

Stress Fractures and Insufficiency Fractures

Stress fractures are caused by abnormal or excessive forces acting on normal bone, whereas *insufficiency fractures* are caused by physiologic forces acting on abnormal or weakened bone. The proximal tibia is the most common site of stress and in-

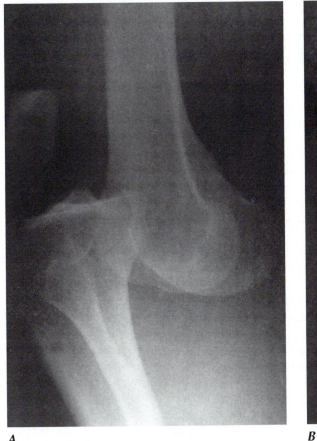

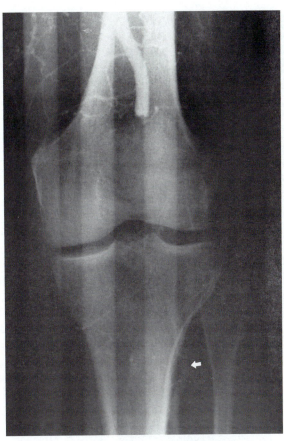

A   *B*

FIGURE 10-29.   Knee dislocation (tibiofemoral dislocation). *A.* The tibia is displaced far anterior to the femoral condyles. This is the most common form of knee dislocation and results from forceful hyperextension. There is great risk of popliteal artery injury. *B.* Despite immediate reduction of the dislocation, the popliteal artery was torn and completely thrombosed. There is faint filling of the proximal tibial artery by collateral flow through the geniculate arteries (*arrow*).

sufficiency fractures around the knee. Patients have pain anterior to the proximal tibia, below the joint line. The initial radiograph may be normal. A vague band of sclerosis or endosteal callus appears within 3 to 7 weeks. Stress and insufficiency fractures can be difficult to diagnose on plain films and often require bone scintigraphy and MRI for identification.

Elderly patients sustain insufficiency fractures of the proximal tibia and supracondylar portion of the femur; these appear similar to stress fractures. Osteopenic bone "hides" insufficiency fractures.

Anterior Tibial Tubercle Fractures

Acute fractures of the anterior tibial tubercle occur most often in adolescents involved in jumping activities and soccer. They are avulsion injuries at the site of attachment of the patellar tendon.[58,59] Fractures of the anterior tibial tubercle are classified into three types. Type I is a fracture of the distal portion of the anterior tibial tubercle; type II is a fracture of the entire tubercle; and type III is a fracture of the entire tubercle that extends proximally to separate off a contiguous portion of the anterior tibial epiphysis. These fractures are easy to detect be-

cause the fracture fragments are sharp and lack cortical bone on one or more surfaces (Fig. 10-30). These features distinguish it from Osgood-Schlatter disease.

Fractures of the Fibular Head and Neck

Fibular head and neck fractures are usually visible on standard radiographs (Fig. 10-31). These fractures occur with either valgus or varus forces. A direct blow to the lateral aspect of the knee fractures the fibular neck. There is often an associated fracture of the lateral tibial condyle. Excessive varus forces cause a fibular head avulsion fracture. This is often associated with fractures of the proximal tibia and disruption of the biceps femoris tendon and LCL. The peroneal nerve and anterior tibial artery may be injured.

Fractures of the proximal third of the fibula can also be associated with fractures of the tibial shaft or rupture of the distal tibiofibular ligament and interosseous membrane. A fracture of the proximal fibula that occurs in association with injury of the tibiofibular syndesmosis is known as a *Maisonneuve fracture*. The Maisonneuve fracture usually presents as an ankle injury, with the proximal fibular fracture being relatively less

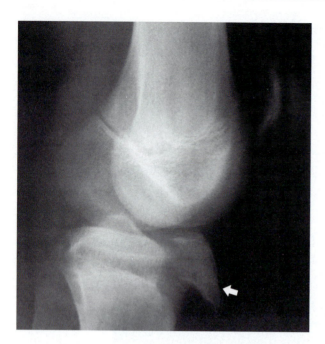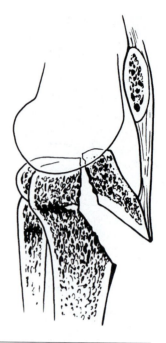

FIGURE 10-30.   Fracture of the anterior tibial tubercle. There is a type III avulsion fracture of the anterior tibial tubercle in this adolescent boy. The fracture extends through the anterior portion of the proximal tibial epiphysis. (From Kling TF: Avulsion of the tibial tubercle, in Pizzutillo PD (ed): *Pediatric Orthopaedics in Primary Practice.* New York: McGraw-Hill, 1997. With permission.)

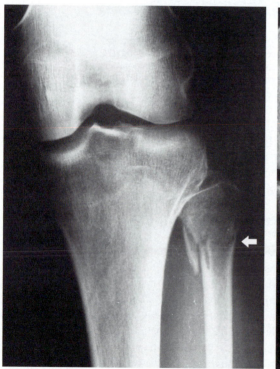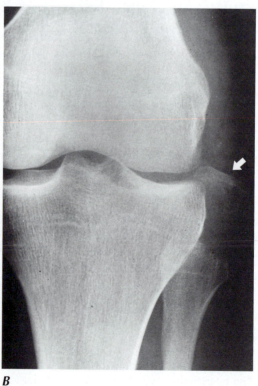

A   *B*

FIGURE 10-31.   Proximal fibular fractures. *A.* Direct impact to the lateral aspect of the knee can result in simple or comminuted fractures of the fibular head or neck. These may be associated with fractures of the lateral tibial plateau.

   B. A varus (medially directed) force results in avulsion of the tip of the fibular head at the insertion of the biceps femoris tendon or lateral collateral ligament. Lateral peroneal nerve injuries are associated with these fractures.

   Fractures of the proximal fibular shaft are due to torsion forces of the lower leg or ankle. (Maisonneuve fracture; see Chapter 9). Examination of the ankle should be performed when such injuries are encountered.

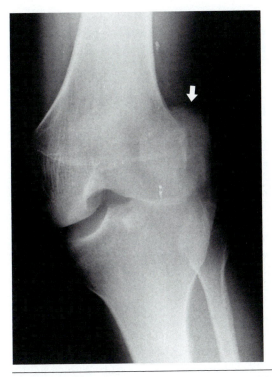

FIGURE 10-32. Lateral patellar dislocation. Radiographs are not needed to make the diagnosis. However, postreduction radiographs should be obtained to search for associated osteochondral fractures, usually involving the articular surface of the lateral femoral condyle.

symptomatic. Occasionally, a Maisonneuve fracture presents primarily as a knee injury and a less prominent ankle injury. In either case, these injuries must not be missed because this is an unstable injury of the ankle and tibiofibular syndesmosis.

Proximal Tibiofibular Joint Dislocation

Proximal tibiofibular joint dislocations and subluxations are rare. The diagnosis can be difficult to confirm on plain radiographs because the findings are subtle and are affected by rotary positional changes in the limb.[60] Knee effusions are generally absent. These injuries often occur with fractures near or within the joint and are therefore often overlooked. About 60% of proximal tibiofibular joint dislocations are unrecognized at initial presentation.[61,62] Most can be diagnosed with well-positioned AP and lateral views. In one study, the AP and lateral radiographs identified 72.5% of cases. Identification of tibiofibular joint dislocation is aided by the use of an internal oblique view or CT.[60]

Anterolateral dislocations are most common. The lateral view shows the fibular head displaced anteriorly so that it almost entirely overlaps the tibial condyle. Normally, only a portion of the overlying head of the fibula is anterior to the posterior cortex of the lateral tibial condyle. On the AP view, the fibular head is displaced laterally and the interosseous space is widened.

Posteromedial dislocations occur less frequently. They result from a direct blow and are often associated with peroneal nerve injury. The lateral view shows the fibula posterior to the tibial condyle. On the AP view, the fibular head lies behind the tibial condyle.[63]

Patellar Dislocations

The patella is usually dislocated laterally. Patellar dislocations frequently occur in sports activities that require abrupt changes

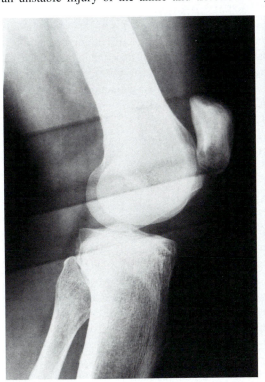

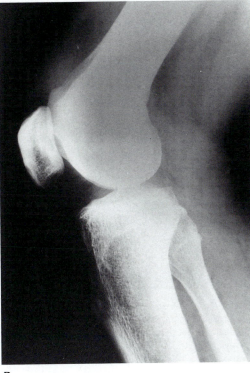

FIGURE 10-33. Patella alta. This older man fell when his legs buckled, causing bilateral disruption of the knee extensor mechanisms. On the left, he has a high-riding patella due to patellar tendon rupture (*A*). On the right, there is a quadriceps tear. The patella is low-riding and there is a soft tissue defect in the suprapatellar region (*B*). (Copyright David T. Schwartz, M.D.)

A   *B*

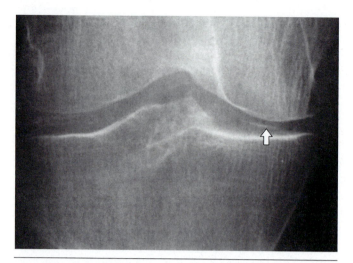

FIGURE 10-34. Chondrocalcinosis. Degenerative calcification of the articular cartilage and meniscus occurs in older individuals with osteoarthritis. The patient may develop an acute crystal-induced arthritis due to calcium pyrophosphate ("pseudogout").

in direction while running. A blow to the medial patella can also cause this injury. In complete lateral dislocation, the patella lies lateral to the lateral femoral condyle. Infrequently, minor degrees of subluxation are seen. Patellar dislocations are often associated with osteochondral fractures; such a fracture is seen on the sunrise view as a small fragment within the joint space.

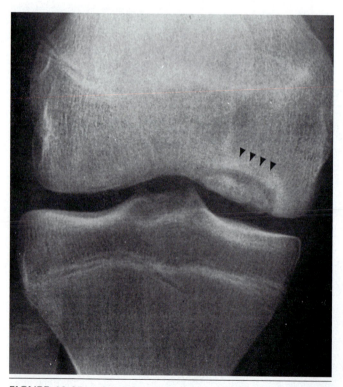

FIGURE 10-35. Osteochondritis dissecans in an adolescent youth involving the articular surface of the medial femoral condyle. There is a focal area of avascular necrosis due to repetitive minor trauma. (From Martire JR, Levinsohn EM: *Imaging of Athletic Injuries.* New York: McGraw-Hill, 1992. With permission.)

Although the diagnosis is obvious on clinical examination and prereduction radiographs are not mandatory, postreduction radiographs should be obtained to search for associated fractures (Fig. 10-32).[64]

Patellar Tendon Injuries

Patellar tendon injury and rupture are usually clinically obvious. The patient feels a "pop." With complete rupture, the patient is unable to extend the knee and has swelling with tenderness in the infrapatellar region. The tear usually occurs where the infrapatellar tendon inserts on the patella.[65]

The lateral radiograph shows a soft tissue opacity due to hemorrhage in the region of the patellar tendon, and the normally sharp interface between the patellar tendon and the underlying fat pad is obliterated. Occasionally, an avulsion fracture fragment off the inferior pole of the patella is present. With complete rupture, a high-riding patella is seen (Fig. 10-33). The Insall-Salvati ratio is used to assess the position of the patella. The ratio of the length of the infrapatellar tendon (inferior pole of patella to the tibial tuberosity) and the length of the patella are measured. The normal value is 0.8 to 1.0. With an infrapatellar tendon ratio of greater than 1.2, a high-riding patella (patella alta) is present.

Quadriceps Tendon Rupture

Quadriceps tendon rupture usually occurs in the elderly and is associated with gout and diabetes mellitus.[66] The hallmark clinical finding is the inability to extend the knee, and a palpable suprapatellar defect.

The lateral radiograph can show signs of this injury. Obliteration of the quadriceps tendon and surrounding hematoma is seen in all patients. The sharp fat planes and suprapatellar fat pad are obliterated by hematoma. In 67% of cases, a suprapatellar mass (representing proximal retraction of torn tendon) and suprapatellar calcific densities (representing avulsed bone fragments of the patella) are seen.[66–68] A low-riding patella (patella baja) is seen in 56% of cases (Insall-Salvati ratio of less than 0.8).[69]

Nontraumatic Disorders

Osteoarthritis. Osteoarthritis or degenerative joint disease is a common cause of knee pain, especially in the elderly. It can occur in younger patients following traumatic injuries. Radiographically, osteoarthritis is characterized by joint space narrowing, irregular articular surfaces, subchondral sclerosis, and marginal osteophytes. Moderately advanced osteoarthritis can mask a nondisplaced fracture. Loose intraarticular bodies are common and can mimic fractures.

Chondrocalcinosis. Chondrocalcinosis is characterized by

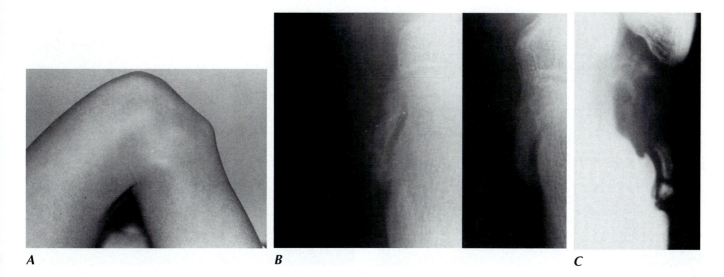

A   *B*   *C*

FIGURE 10-36. Osgood-Schlatter disease. *A.* This patient has a tender and prominent anterior tibial tubercle. There are usually no distinctive radiographic findings. Radiographs are indicated to exclude other disorders, such as a neoplasm. *B.* The anterior tibial tubercle has a variable radiographic appearance. *C.* In this patient, the anterior tubercle is fragmented because of repetitive stress. Symptoms resolved after excision of the ossicle. (From Stanitski CL: Osgood Schlatter's disease, in Pizzutillo PD (ed): *Pediatric Orthopaedics in Primary Practice.* New York: McGraw-Hill, 1997. With permission.)

calcification of the articular cartilage. It is associated with osteoarthritis and is caused by calcium pyrophosphate dihydrate deposition (pseudogout). Patients present with acute pain and effusion that mimics gout. The radiograph demonstrates a thin line of calcification parallel to the tibial condyles (Fig. 10-34).

Osteochondritis Dissecans. Osteochondritis dissecans causes knee pain in older children and adolescents. The knee is the most common site of osteochondritis dissecans, especially affecting the medial femoral condyle. Radiographically, there is a shallow, concave defect along the articular surface of the femoral condyle. Osteochondritis dissecans is a focal area of posttraumatic subarticular avascular necrosis following a subchondral fracture. The margins of the defect are smooth and sclerotic. A separate piece of bone may be found within the concave defect or within the joint space (Fig. 10-35).

Osgood-Schlatter Disease. Osgood-Schlatter disease is believed to result from repeated contraction of the quadriceps muscle resulting in, subclinical avulsions of the anterior tibial tubercle.[70] It occurs most frequently in boys between the ages of 10 and 15 years. Patients have pain, swelling, and tenderness over the tibial tuberosity. The radiograph may show elevation of the tubercle away from the shaft, with accompanying soft tissue swelling anterior to the tubercle. The tubercle may be fragmented, and the separate ossicles are rounded with complete margins of cortical bone. Osgood-Schlatter disease is a clinical and not a radiographic diagnosis. It must be distinguished from an acute fracture of the anterior tibial tubercle (Fig. 10-36).

ERRORS IN INTERPRETATION

The knee is a site of frequent radiographic misinterpretation, occurring in 3% of ED radiographs (Table 10-6). Some common knee injuries are often misdiagnosed; in fact, proximal tibial fractures were the most frequently missed injury in one series in which 15.8% (3 of 19) were misdiagnosed. Also commonly missed are distal femur fractures (9.5%, or 2 of 21) and patellar fractures (5.7%, or 3 of 53). Knee fractures are also missed in the setting of multiple trauma because of the need to attend to life-threatening injuries. Careful examination of the radiographs for these sites of injury minimizes the chances of misdiagnosis (Fig. 10-7).

TABLE 10-6

Easily Missed Fractures about the Knee

Tibial plateau fractures
Femoral condyle fractures
Ligament avulsions:
    Segond fractures
    Tibial eminence fractures
    Intercondylar notch avulsions
Osteochondral fractures (patella, femoral condyle)
Patellar fractures (vertical or oblique)
Extensor mechanism injuries
    Patellar tendon, quadriceps tendon—patella alta and patella baja
Stress fractures and insufficiency fractures
Proximal tibiofibular dislocations and subluxations
Salter-Harris growth plate injuries in children

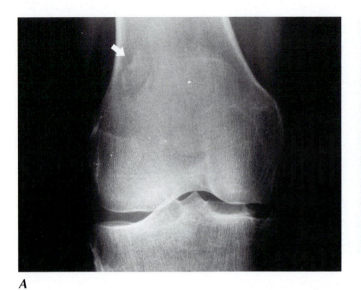

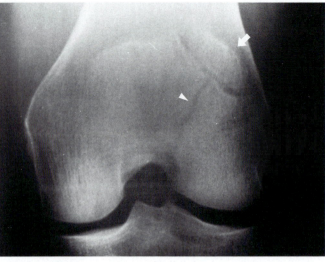

A　　　　　　　　　　　　　　　　　　　　　　　　　　　　*B*

FIGURE 10-37.　Bipartite patella. An unfused accessory ossification center is a common variant and is known as a *bipartite patella*. It typically occurs on the superior lateral margin of the patella (*A*) (*arrow*). It can be distinguished from a fracture by its irregular sclerotic margins. It is nontender and generally bilateral. The accessory ossification center may be split into two or more parts, resulting in a tripartite or multipartite patella. This patient has a bipartite patella as well as an oblique patellar fracture (*arrowhead*) that was initially misinterpreted as a "tripartite" patella (*B*). (Copyright David T. Schwartz, M.D.)

Bipartite Patella

The bipartite and multipartite patellae are normal variants that can be mistaken for fractures. Normally, the patella develops from one ossification center but occasionally from more. The additional ossification center is usually in the upper outer quad-

rant of the patella. It has smooth, rounded cortical margins and may not correspond accurately in size or shape to the adjacent fossa. Often, bipartite and multipartite patellae are bilateral (Fig. 10-37).

COMMON VARIANTS

Fabella

The fabella is an accessory calcification located in the lateral head of the gastrocnemius muscle. It is seen posterior and lateral to the knee. The fabella can be bifid or irregular (Fig. 10-38).

Pellegrini-Stieda Disease

Pellegrini-Stieda disease is relatively common. Calcification is present in and around the MCL at its insertion on the medial femoral epicondyle. It is thought to be caused by an old avulsion injury of the MCL with subsequent calcification within the subperiosteal hematoma. Pellegrini-Stieda disease must be distinguished from an acute avulsion injury (Fig. 10-39).

ADVANCED STUDIES

Computed Tomography (CT)

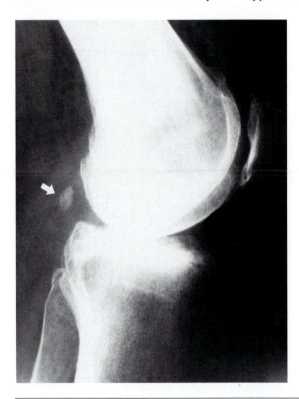

FIGURE 10-38.　The fabella is a common sesamoid that develops within the tendon of the lateral head of the gastrocnemius muscle (*arrow*).

CT is an excellent radiographic adjunct for evaluating certain knee injuries, especially tibial plateau fractures (Fig. 10-20). CT with multiplanar reconstruction is effective for evaluating

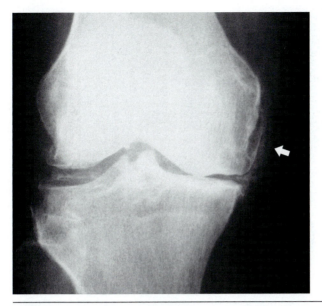

FIGURE 10-39. Pellegrini-Stieda disease. Calcification at the site of attachment of the MCL on the medial femoral epicondyle. Chondrocalcinosis is also present in this patient.

the anterior and posterior borders of the tibial plateau, establishing the location of fracture fragments in comminuted fractures, determining the extent of articular involvement and the amount of depression of the fractures. CT is also useful in evaluating the femoral condyles, osteochondral fractures, the patellofemoral joint, proximal tibiofibular stress fractures, proximal tibiofibular joint dislocations, and quadriceps tendon rupture.

Magnetic Resonance Imaging (MRI)

The multiplanar and soft tissue imaging capabilities of MRI accurately localize and characterize many knee lesions.

Cruciate Ligament Tears. One of the principal roles for MRI is to diagnose a cruciate ligament tear, especially a tear of the ACL. An ACL tear appears as a disruption of the fibers, increased signal intensity, and indistinct delineation of the fibers. Other associated findings include an effusion, hemarthrosis, and nondisplaced fractures. Less specific signs are a buckled PCL and tibial anterotranslation (the MRI equivalent of a positive anterior drawer test) (Figs. 10-40 and 10-41).

Menisci. MRI is the best noninvasive technique for evaluating the menisci. Meniscal tears cause defects with increased signal intensity within the normally hypointense meniscal substance. MRI can correctly characterize the orientation and extent of the tear (Fig. 10-42).

Other Structures. Other soft tissue structures demonstrated by MRI include the collateral ligaments, bursae, extensor mechanism, articular cartilage, intramedullary bone (bone bruises and occult fractures), biceps femoris tendon, and pes anserinus complex.

Articular cartilage defects can be evaluated with a special MRI protocol for cartilage. Normal articular cartilage has a uniformly high signal intensity. Loose cartilage is seen as hypointense fragments within the knee joint or a distended bursa.

Nondisplaced fractures and stress fractures that are radi-

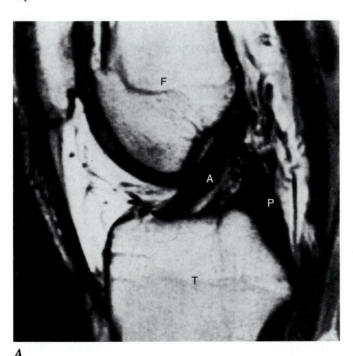

A

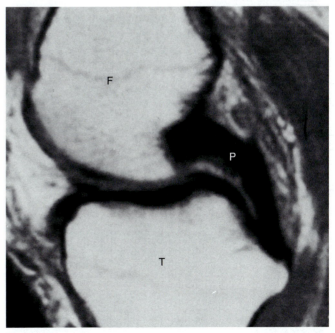

B

FIGURE 10-40. Normal MRI appearance of the cruciate ligaments. (T1-weighted images). *A*. The normal anterior cruciate ligament has fibers of intermediate signal running through the mostly low-signal (dark) ligament. *B*. The normal posterior cruciate ligament has a uniform dark appearance. Its shape is like that of a hockey stick. (From Martire JR, Levinsohn EM: *Imaging of Athletic Injuries.* New York: McGraw-Hill, 1992. With permission.)

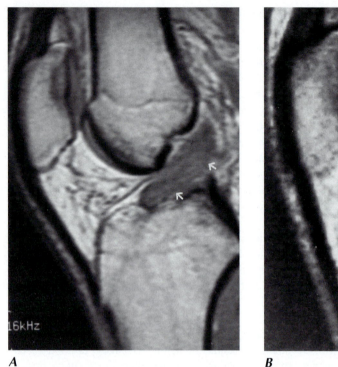 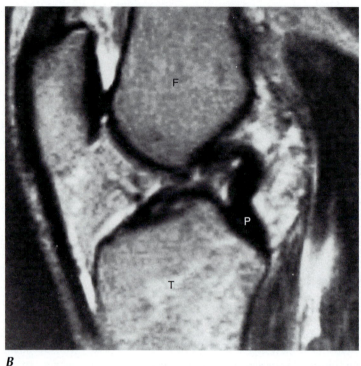

A   *B*

FIGURE 10-41.   MRI of an anterior cruciate ligament tear. *A.* A torn and edematous anterior cruciate ligament. The ACL has an increased signal with an inhomogeneous appearance and blurring of fibers (*arrows*). (From Dee R, Hurst LC, Gruber MA, Kottmeier SA: *Principles of Orthopaedic Practice,* 2d ed. New York: McGraw-Hill, 1997. With permission.) *B.* In another patient with a complete ACL tear, there is buckling of the posterior cruciate ligament due to anterior slippage of the tibia. This is the MRI equivalent of an abnormal anterior drawer sign. (From Martire JR, Levinsohn EM: *Imaging of Athletic Injuries.* New York: McGraw-Hill, 1992. With permission.)

ographically occult appear on MRI as linear, hypointense signals extending from the cortex through the intramedullary bone. MRI, in contrast to bone scan, detects abnormalities immediately after the injury.

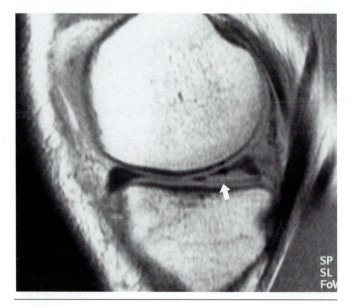

FIGURE 10-42.   MRI of a meniscus tear (T1-weighted image). The normal, uniformly dark appearance of the posterior horn of the medial meniscus is interrupted by a high-signal-intensity tear.

Musculoskeletal Ultrasonography (MSUS)

In the hands of a trained ultrasonographer, MSUS has a wide range of applications in diagnosing acute knee pathology. Ultrasonography is an ideal modality for imaging tendons. The hyperreflective interfaces between the fascicles and septa are well demonstrated by MSUS. The interface between the different intratendinous structures is also clearly demarcated. Its lower cost compared with MRI makes MSUS appropriate for repeat and follow-up examinations.

Tendons.   Tendon tears are discrete hypoechoic gaps between the separated ends of the disrupted tendon. Quadriceps tendon tears are either complete or incomplete. The tears are usually located 1 to 2 cm above the patella. Transection of the quadriceps tendon is associated with slackening of the patellar tendon. Patellar tendon tears commonly occur immediately below the patella.

Tears of the semimembranosus and biceps femoris tendons are rare. They appear as anechoic gaps in the tendons. The semimembranosus tendon usually tears near its tibial insertion. The torn biceps femoris tendon usually retracts from its fibular insertion and is found above the level of the femoral condyles.

Tendinitis is more common than tendon tears. Tendinitis causes focal or generalized enlargement and hypoechogenicity of the tendon, with increased interfibrillar distances between the fascicles. "Sonographic palpation" elicits tenderness when the transducer is directly over the area of tendinitis. Patellar tendinitis ("jumper's knee") is common, usually involving the proximal tendon. Tendinitis of the biceps femoris and semimembranosus tendons appears as focal enlargement and hypoechogenicity, usually at the level of the femorotibial joint.

Bursae. The suprapatellar, prepatellar, superficial and deep infrapatellar, and semimembranosus-gastrocnemius bursae are sacs of synovial fluid. When they are distended with fluid, sonography can characterize location, size, synovial thickening, internal debris, and rupture. In addition, MSUS can guide needle aspiration.

Inflammatory disease, such as rheumatoid arthritis or gout, show a typical irregular synovial reaction with floating internal particulate-crystalline debris within the fluid-distended bursa. Panni and tophi are seen as coalescing echoes within the bursa.

Baker Cyst. A Baker cyst represents abnormal distension of the semimembranosus-gastrocnemius bursa. This bursa communicates with the femorotibial joint in 50% of individuals. As fluid accumulates in the semimembranosus-gastrocnemius bursa, a large "horseshoe-shaped" Baker cyst is seen by ultrasonography. Baker cyst rupture causes subcutaneous and intramuscular edema of the gastrocnemius.

Ligaments. Intraarticular ligaments are best demonstrated by MRI. However, the MCL, LCL, and iliotibial band are readily accessible to MSUS, which can detect tears of these ligaments. The PCL is also seen without difficulty. The ACL is indirectly demonstrated on MSUS, and an ACL tear appears as an anechoic cyst representing a hematoma adjacent to the inner margin of the lateral femoral condyle.

Osteochondral Defects. Most focal irregularities of the articular cartilage occur in the surface of the femoral condyle. The articular cartilage is examined sonographically with the knee in flexion (exposing the anterior femoral condyles) and extension (allowing visualization of the posterior femoral condyles). Articular cartilage defects appear as focal clefts or step-off deformities. Acutely, the cartilage is focally thickened because of edema. A loose body is sought when an articular surface defect is detected. A loose fragment of cartilage appears as a high-level echo within the joint capsule. The ability to visualize a radiolucent cartilage fragment is an important feature of MSUS.

Nondisplaced Fractures and Stress Fractures. The normal cortical surface appears as an uninterrupted linear acoustic interface. A fracture is seen as an anechoic cleft or step-off deformity along the normally smooth linear cortex. A subperiosteal hematoma appears as a lenticular hypoechoic cystlike lesion immediately above the interrupted cortex. Callus formation in nondisplaced or stress fractures appears as a mixed hypo- and hyperechoic nodule over the interrupted cortex.

Infection. MSUS can be used to determine the site of suspected infection about the knee. Cellulitis is seen as widening of the superficial subcutaneous tissue with hypoechoic pools of lymphangitic fluid. Abscesses are focal, walled-off lesions with abnormal central hypoechoic fluid usually containing internal echogenic speckles, which represents either debris or gas. Septic or inflammatory arthritis presents as complex fluid distending the joint capsule and bursa, with irregular thickening of the synovium associated with adhesions, septations, and mobile debris of varying sizes.

Menisci. The menisci are intraarticular and best evaluated with MRI. However, both lateral and medial menisci can be seen on MSUS. Tears appear as discrete linear anechoic clefts across the hyperechoic, triangular-appearing meniscus. Nonvisualization of the meniscus suggests a tear and displacement of the entire meniscus.

ACKNOWLEDGMENT

Thanks are given to Dr. Antonio Bouffard for his assistance on the Advanced Studies section.

REFERENCES

1. Kannus P, Jarvinen M: Routine radiographs in acute knee distortions. *Orthopedics* 11:1591, 1988.
2. Fishwick NG, Learmonth DJA, Finlay DBL: Knee effusions, radiology and acute knee trauma. *Br J Radiol* 67:934, 1994.
3. Sanville P, Nicholson DA, Driscoll DA: The knee. *BMJ* 308:121, 1994.
4. Yao L, Lee JK: Occult intraosseous fracture: Detection with magnetic resonance imaging. *Radiology* 167:749, 1988.
5. Oberlander MA, Shalvoy RM, Hughston JC: The accuracy of the clinical knee examination by arthroscopy (abstr). *Am J Sports Med* 21:773, 1993.
6. Gleadhill DNS, Thomson JY, Simms P: Can more effective use be made of x-ray examinations in the accident and emergency department? *BMJ* 294:943, 1987.
7. Pennycook AG, Rai A: Knee radiographs: A substitute for proper clinical examination within the accident and emergency department. *Injury* 24:383, 1993.
8. Stiell IG, Wells GA, McDowell I, et al: Use of radiography in acute knee injuries: Need for clinical decision rules. *Acad Emerg Med* 2:966, 1995.
9. Seaberg DC, Jackson R: Clinical decision rule for knee radiographs. *Am J Emerg Med* 12:541, 1994.
10. Stiell IG, Greenberg GH, Wells GA, et al: Derivation of a decision rule for use of radiography in acute knee injuries. *Ann Emerg Med* 26:405, 1995.
11. Saxena AC, Norris RL, Rinstuen K, et al: The role of knee radiographs in the emergency department: A prospective study (abstr). *Ann Emerg Med* 21:658, 1992.
12. Stiell IG, Greenberg GH, Wells GA: Prospective validation of a decision rule for the use of radiography in acute knee injuries. *JAMA* 275:611, 1996.
13. Weber JE, Peacock WF, Jackson RE, et al: Clinical decision rules

discriminate between fractures and nonfractures in acute isolated knee trauma. *Ann Emerg Med* 26:429, 1995.

14. Bauer SJ, Hollander JE, Thode HC, et al: A clinical decision rule in the evaluation of acute knee injuries. *J Emerg Med* 13:611, 1995.

15. Siebacher JR, Inglis AF, Marshall DVM, Warren RS: The structure of the posterolateral aspect of the knee. *J Bone Joint Surg* 64(A):467, 1986.

16. Johnson LL: Lateral capsular ligament complex: Anatomical and surgical considerations. *Am J Sports Med* 7:156, 1979.

17. Hughston JC, Andrews JR, Cross MJ, Moschi A: Classification of knee ligament instabilities: Part II. The lateral compartment. *J Bone Joint Surg* 58(A)173, 1976.

18. DeLee JC, Riley MB, Rockwood CA Jr: Acute straight lateral instability of the knee. *J Sports Med Phys Fit* 11:404, 1983.

19. Hall Jr RF, Gonzales M: Fracture of the proximal part of the tibia and fibula associated with an entrapped popliteal artery. *J Bone Joint Surg* 68(A):941, 1986.

20. Cockshott WP, Racoveanu NT, Burrows DA: Use of radiographic projections of the knee. *Skel Radiol* 13:131, 1985.

21. Daffner RH, Tabas JH: Trauma oblique radiographs of the knee. *J Bone Joint Surg* 69(A):568, 1987.

22. Hughston JC: Subluxation of the patella. *J Bone Joint Surg* 50(A):1003, 1968.

23. Kimberlin GE: Radiological assessment of the patelofemoral articulation and subluxation of the patella. *Radiol Technol* 45:129, 1973.

24. Moore TM, Harvey JP: Roentgenographic measurement of tibial plateau depression due to fracture. *J Bone Joint Surg (A)* 56:155, 1974.

25. Stäubli HU, Jakob RP: Anterior knee motion analysis measurement and simultaneous radiography. *Am J Sports Med* 19:172, 1991.

26. McPhee IB, Fraser JG: Stress radiography in acute ligamentous injuries of the knee. *Injury* 12:383, 1981.

27. Rijke AM, Gortz HT, McCue FC III, et al: Graded stress radiography of injured anterior cruciate ligaments. *Invest Radiol* 26:926, 1991.

28. Insall J, Salvate E: Patella position in the normal knee joint. *Radiology* 101:101, 1971.

29. Maskell TW, Finlay DB: The prognostic significance of radiologically detected knee joint effusions in the absence of associated fracture. *Br J Radiol* 63:940, 1990.

30. Casteleyn PP, Handelberg F, Opdecam P: Traumatic haemarthrosis of the knee. *J Bone Joint Surg* 70(B):404, 1988.

31. Holmgren BS: Flüssiges Fett im Kniegelenk nach Trauma. *Acta Radiol* 23:131, 1942.

32. Noyes FR, Bassett RW, Grood ES, et al: Arthroscopy in acute traumatic hemarthrosis of the knee. *J Bone Joint Surg* 62(A):687, 1980.

33. Hall FM: Radiographic diagnosis and accuracy in knee joint effusions. *Radiology* 115:49, 1975.

34. Butt P, Lederman H, Chuang S: Radiology of the suprapatellar regron. *Clin Radiol* 34:511, 1983.

35. Swischuk LE: *Emergency Radiology of the Acutely Ill or Injured Child.* Baltimore: Williams & Wilkins, 1994, pp. 331–355.

36. Nelson SW: Some important diagnostic and technical fundamentals in the radiology of trauma with particular emphasis on skeletal trauma. *Radiol Clin North Am* 4:251, 1966.

37. Dovey H, Heerfordt J: Tibial condyle fractures. *Acta Chir Scand* 137:521, 1971.

38. Reibel DB, Wade PA: Fractures of the tibial plateau. *J Trauma* 2:337, 1962.

39. Ottolenghi CE: Vascular complications in injuries about the knee joint. *Clin Orthop* 165:148, 1982.

40. Rogers LF: The knee and shafts of the tibia and fibula, in *Radiology of Skeletal Trauma,* 2d ed. New York: Churchill Livingstone, 1992, pp. 1199–1317.

41. Goldman AB, Pavlov H, Rubenstein D: The Segond fracture of the proximal tibia: a small avulsion that reflects major ligamentous damage. *AJR* 151:1163, 1988.

42. Norwood LA Jr, Andrews JR, Meisierling RC, Clancy GL: Acute anterolateral rotatory instability of the knee. *J Bone Joint Surg* 61(A):704, 1979.

43. Manaster BJ, Andrews CL: Fractures and dislocations of the knee and proximal tibia and fibular. *Semin Roentgenol* 29:113, 1994.

44. Dietz GW, Wilcox DM, Montgomery JB: Segond tibial condyle fracture: Lateral capsular ligament avulsion. *Radiology* 159:467, 1986.

45. Capps GW, Hayes CW: Easily missed injuries around the knee. *Radiographics* 14:1191, 1994.

46. Weber WN, Neumann CH, Barakos JA, et al: Lateral tibial rim (Segond) fractures: MR imaging characteristics. *Radiology* 180:731, 1991.

47. Kimbrough EE: Concomitant unilateral hip and femeral shaft fractures—a too frequently unrecognized syndrome: Report of five cases. *J Bone Joint Surg* 43(A):443, 1961.

48. Blake R, McBryde A: The floating knee: Ipsilateral fractures of the tibia and femur. *South Med J* 68:13, 1975.

49. Treiman GS, Yellin AE, Weaver FA, et al: Examination of the patient with a knee dislocation: The case for selective arteriography. *Arch Surg* 127:1056, 1992.

50. Bratt HD, Newman AP: Complete dislocations of the knee without disruption of both cruciate ligaments. *J Trauma* 34:383, 1993.

51. Varnell RM, Coldwell DM, Sangeorzan BJ, Johansen KH: Arterial injury complicating knee disruption. *Am Surg* 55:699, 1989.

52. Green NE, Allen BL: Vascular injuries associated with dislocation of the knee. *J Bone Joint Surg* 59(A):236, 1979.

53. Bunt TJ, Malone JM, Moody M, et al: Frequency of vascular injury with blunt trauma–induced extremity injury. *Am J Surg* 160;226, 1990.

54. Peck JJ, Eastman AB, Bergan JJ, et al: Popliteal vascular trauma: A community experience. *Arch Surg* 125:1339, 1990.

55. McCoy GF, Hannon DG, Bair RJ, Templeton J: Vascular injury associated with low-velocity dislocations of the knee. *J Bone Joint Surg* 69(B):285, 1987.

56. Green NE, Allen BL: Vascular injuries associated with dislocations of the knee. *J Bone Joint Surg* 59(A):236, 1977.

57. Montgomery JB: Dislocation of the knee. *Arthrop Clin North Am* 18:149, 1987.

58. Hand WL, Hand CR, Dunn AW: Avulsion fractures of the tibial tubercle. *J Bone Joint Surg* 53(A):1579, 1971.

59. Ogden JA, Tross RB, Murphy MJ: Fracture of the tibial tuberosity in adolescents. *J Bone Joint Surg* 62(A):205, 1980.

60. Keogh P, Masterson E, Murphy B, et al: The role of radiography and computed tomography in the diagnosis of acute dislocation of the proximal tibiofibular joint. *Br J Radiol* 66:108, 1993.

61. Turco VJ, Spinella AJ: Anterolateral dislocation of the head of the fibula in sports. *Am J Sports Med* 13:209, 1985.

62. Ogden JA: Subluxation and dislocation of the proximal tibiofibular joint. *J Bone Joint Surg* 56(A):145, 1974.

63. Ogden JA: Dislocation of the proximal fibula. *Radiology* 105:547, 1972.

64. Ahstrom JP Jr: Osteochondral fracture in the knee joint associated with hypermobility and dislocation of the patella. *J Bone Joint Surg* 47(A):1491, 1965.

65. Nichols CF: Patellar tendon injuries. *Clin Sports Med* 11:807, 1992.

66. Kaneko K, Demouy EH, Brunet ME, Bezian J: Radiographic diagnosis of quadriceps tendon rupture: Analysis of diagnostic failure. *J Emerg Med* 12:225, 1994.

67. Ramsey RH, Miller GE: Quadriceps tendon ruptures: A diagnostic trap. *Clin Orthop* 70:161, 1970.

68. Newberg A, Wales L: Radiographic diagnosis of quadriceps tendon rupture. *Radiology* 125:367, 1977.

69. Barasch E, Lombardi LJ, Arene L, Epstein E: MRI visualization of bilateral quadriceps tendon rupture in a patient with secondary hyperparathyroidism: Implications for diagnosis and therapy. *Comput Med Imag Graph* 13:407, 1989.

70. Cohen B, Wilkinson RW: The Osgood-Schlatter lesion: A radiological and histological study. *Am J Surg* 95:731, 1958.

CHAPTER 11

THE HIP AND PROXIMAL FEMUR

DENNIS HANLON / TIM EVANS

Fractures about the hip are the most common type of lower extremity fracture in the elderly.[1–4] The incidence of these fractures has increased dramatically over the past several decades and will continue to increase as the population ages. Fractures of the proximal femur are complicated by prolonged rehabilitation and significant mortality. The financial cost of the 250,000 fractures about the hip that occur annually exceeds $1.25 billion[3]. In children, in contrast to the elderly, such fractures account for less than 1% of fractures. However, proximal femoral fractures can be devastating if the growth plate is injured or if the tenuous blood supply to the femoral head is disrupted.[5]

Hip radiographs are usually obtained to evaluate traumatic injuries. Most of these injuries are demonstrated on routine radiographs. However, a nondisplaced fracture about the hip in the elderly can be extremely difficult to detect and additional views or adjunctive imaging studies may be needed. Radiographs are also used to evaluate chronic hip pain, acute infections, inflammatory processes, or disorders of development.

Most radiographs of the femoral shaft are obtained to evaluate a fracture. The femoral shaft is extremely strong and requires a large force to fracture. Fractures of the femoral shaft are associated with significant morbidity because of hemorrhage, fat emboli, or associated injuries. Femoral shaft fractures are an indicator of major trauma and potentially life-threatening visceral injuries.

CLINICAL DECISION MAKING

Radiographic evaluation is performed in individuals with obvious evidence of a fracture or dislocation such as deformity, rotation, or shortening of the lower extremity. Patients with pain in the hip, thigh, or groin after direct trauma or transmitted forces (e.g., a blow to the knee with the hip flexed) require evaluation. Elderly patients who complain of pain in the hip, thigh, or groin after minor trauma need radiographs. The elderly can sustain fractures even in the absence of trauma because of osteoporosis or metastatic disease. Such patients may have minimal physical findings and can even be able to walk. A patient may present with knee pain rather than hip pain. Chronic corticosteroid users are predisposed to osteoporosis and avascular necrosis (AVN). Individuals with hip pain and fever require radiographs to check for the widened joint space associated with a septic joint. Children who complain of hip pain need a radiographic study of the hip, even in the absence of trauma, to investigate the possibility of a slipped capital femoral epiphysis (SCFE) and Legg-Calvé-Perthes (LCP) disease (AVN of the femoral head). Children complaining of knee pain may require imaging studies of their hips to look for SCFE and LCP disease if the knee examination is normal.

ANATOMY

The femur is the longest, largest, and strongest bone in the body and consists of a head and neck, the body or shaft, and distal condyles (Fig. 11-1). The hemispherical femoral head articulates in a ball-in-socket fashion with the acetabulum to form the hip joint. The superior aspect of the femoral shaft has two prominent tubercles, the *greater* and *lesser trochanters*. The *intertrochanteric line* connects the trochanters anteriorly; the *intertrochanteric crest* connects them posteriorly. The gluteus medius and minimus muscles attach to the greater trochanter. The iliopsoas muscle inserts on the lesser trochanter. The bones

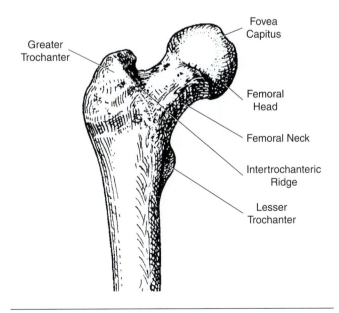

FIGURE 11-1. Anatomy of the proximal femur. (Modified from Pansky B: *Review of Gross Anatomy*, 6th ed. New York: McGraw-Hill, 1996, with permission.)

217

of the hip joint are held in place by these and other muscles and ligaments. The articular capsule attaches above the intertrochanteric line anteriorly. Posteriorly, the capsule attaches to the base of the femoral neck. The trochanters are therefore extracapsular.

The blood supply to the femoral head has three sources (Fig. 11-2). The largest contribution is from the circumflex arterial ring that encircles the base of the femoral neck and lies outside the joint capsule. Branches from the circumflex ring course along the femoral neck. These are subject to disruption from displaced fractures of the femoral neck. An additional blood supply is through the medullary cavity of the femoral neck. A third, smaller portion is the foveal artery within the ligamentum teres. The ligamentum teres originates in the centrum of the acetabulum and inserts on the fovea centralis. The fovea centralis is a depression in the center of the femoral head's articular surface. Disruption of the blood supply to the femoral head by a fracture of the femoral neck can result in a vascular necrosis of the femoral head.

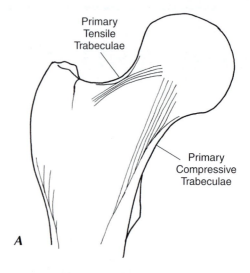

A

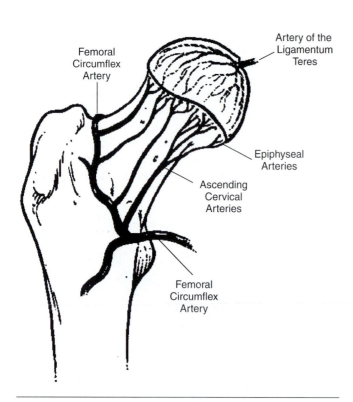

FIGURE 11-2. Blood supply to femoral head. Most of the blood supply to the femoral head comes from the circumflex arterial ring, which is located outside the joint capsule at the base of the femoral neck, along the intertrochanteric ridge. The circumflex ring is derived from the deep femoral artery. Ascending cervical arteries branch from the circumflex ring and traverse along the femoral neck to supply the femoral head. The cervical arteries are susceptible to disruption by a femoral neck fracture. A smaller contribution to the blood supply of the femoral head is from the artery in the ligamentum teres, which traverses the acetabular joint space and enters the fovea of the femoral head. (From Dee R, Hurst LC, Gruber MA, Kottmeier, SA. *Principles of Orthopedic Practice*, 2d ed. New York: McGraw-Hill, 1997, with permission.)

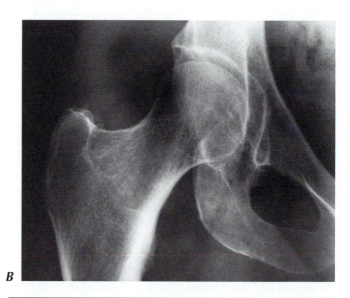

B

FIGURE 11-3. Trabecular pattern of the proximal femur. There are two main sets of structural trabeculae that support the weight of the body across the proximal femur: the primary compressive and primary tensile trabeculae. Radiograph of an elderly female with osteoporosis (*B*). The primary trabeculae are accentuated in osteoporosis owing to loss of secondary and interconnecting trabeculae.

The femoral nerve arises from the second through fourth lumbar nerve roots and provides sensory innervation to the hip and the skin of the medial and anterior thigh. The posterior division of the obturator nerve arises from the same lumbar nerve roots and supplies both the hip and the knee joints. Therefore, pain arising from the hip joint may be referred to the thigh and knee.

The proximal femur is strengthened by two main groups of trabeculae (Fig. 11-3). Compressive trabeculae extend vertically from the femoral head toward the medial aspect of the femoral neck. Tensile trabeculae arch from the femoral head past the superior cortex of the femoral neck toward the greater trochanter. Disruption of the trabecular lines is a radiographic sign of a proximal femur fracture.

TABLE 11-1

Radiographic Views of the Hip

VIEW	POSITION	EVALUATION OF ADEQUACY	LIKELY FINDINGS
AP view of pelvis*	Supine position. Legs extended. Hips internally rotated 15° (great toes touching). X-ray beam centered on pelvis.	Entire pelvis and proximal femur included. Femoral neck elongated. Greater trochanter in profile. Lesser trochanter less prominent. No rotation—left and right sides of pelvis symmetrical.	Most fractures and dislocations. Allows comparison with opposite hip.
Frog-leg view	Supine position. Hip and knee of affected side flexed, hip abducted and rotated externally. In children, include both sides of pelvis.	Axial projection of femoral neck. Greater trochanter projected over neck of femur.	Femoral neck and intertrochanteric fractures. SCFE, in children.
Cross-table lateral (groin lateral) view	Supine position. Unaffected hip flexed 90° with ankle supported. Beam directed perpendicular to femoral neck. Injured hip is not moved.	View includes acetabulum, ischial tuberosity, and proximal femur. Greater and lesser trochanters overlap. Femoral neck anteverted 30° to femoral shaft.	Femoral neck and intertrochanteric fractures. Hip dislocation.
Posterior oblique view	Involved side of pelvis rotated posteriorly 45°. (Opposite side of pelvis elevated 45°.) Hip and knee flexed.	Iliac wing and proximal femur. Anterior rim of acetabulum. Posterior column of acetabulum.	Proximal femur fractures. Fractures of acetabulum.
Anterior oblique view	Involved side of pelvis rotated anteriorly (elevated) 45°.	Obturator foramen. Posterior rim of acetabulum. Anterior column of acetabulum.	Fractures of acetabulum.

SCFE, slipped capital femoral epiphysis

*An AP view centered on involved hip can provide better visualization of femoral neck, but does not permit complete evaluation of nearby pelvis.

RADIOGRAPHIC TECHNIQUE

Conventional radiography is the best and least expensive way to evaluate hip disorders (Table 11-1)[6,7]. When the patient is severely injured or there is a markedly displaced fracture about the hip, only a single anteroposterior (AP) view is performed. In other cases, at least two views at right angles to each other are needed to define the anatomy of a skeletal injury. Although the AP view is readily obtained, a direct lateral projection of the hip is not possible because of overlap by the soft tissues and skeleton of the pelvis. Two techniques are used to provide a second view of the proximal femur that is nearly perpendicular to the AP view: the frog-leg view and the cross-table lateral view. A posterior oblique view is an alternative when positioning is difficult. The second view is important for demonstrating such common injuries as femoral neck fractures, intertrochanteric fractures, and SCFE. Nondisplaced fractures may not be visible on the AP view.

AP View. The routine radiographic examination of the hip begins with an AP view of the pelvis (Fig. 11-4). Although an AP view centered on the hip provides slightly better visualization of the hip than does an AP view of the pelvis, a hip radiograph does not provide a complete view of the adjacent pelvis (i.e., the pubic rami and iliac wing). Because injuries to the pelvis are common following hip trauma, it is generally recommended that physicians obtain an AP view of the entire pelvis rather than an AP view of the affected hip only.

When the patient lies supine in a relaxed, neutral position, the femoral neck is slightly rotated externally and therefore appears foreshortened on the radiograph (Fig. 11-5). This foreshortening can obscure subtle injuries to the femoral neck. The presence of such external rotation can be recognized because the lesser trochanter appears prominent. Visualization of the femoral neck is improved by having the patient rotate the hips internally about 15° until the great toes touch. While this may be impossible for a severely injured patient, this technique optimizes visualization of the femoral neck on the AP view. On a correctly performed AP view, the femoral neck is elongated and the lesser trochanter is less prominent. Although standard positioning of an AP hip radiograph specifies slight internal rotation of the leg, a standard AP view of the pelvis view is often taken with the legs in a neutral position. However, when an AP

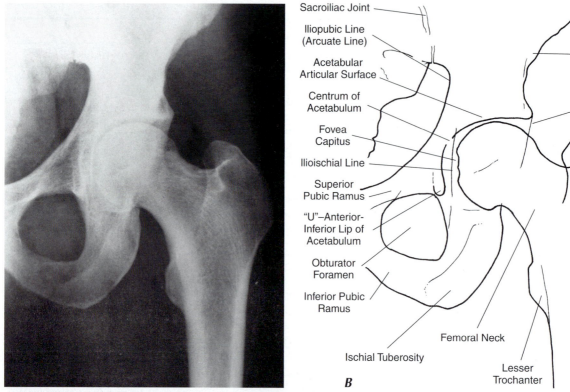

A

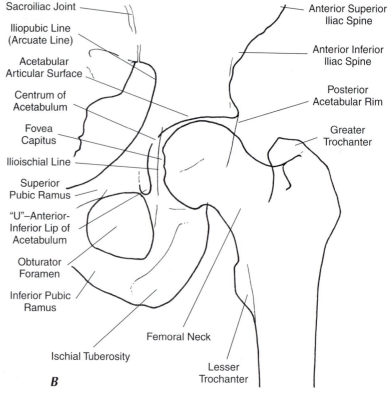

Sacroiliac Joint

Iliopubic Line
(Arcuate Line)

Acetabular
Articular Surface

Centrum of
Acetabulum

Fovea
Capitus

Ilioischial Line

Superior
Pubic Ramus

"U"–Anterior-
Inferior Lip of
Acetabulum

Obturator
Foramen

Inferior Pubic
Ramus

Ischial Tuberosity

Anterior Superior
Iliac Spine

Anterior Inferior
Iliac Spine

Posterior
Acetabular Rim

Greater
Trochanter

Femoral Neck

Lesser
Trochanter

B

FIGURE 11-4. The standard AP radiograph of the hip. Although the AP radiograph of the hip (*A*) provides closer detail of the involved hip, the AP pelvis radiograph (*C*) is usually preferred in the emergency department because it encompasses the entire pelvis adjacent to the hip and shows the opposite side, which is useful for comparison.

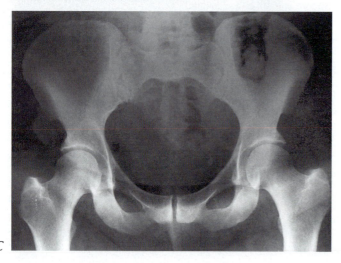

C

pelvis view is being used to evaluate the hips, the 15° internal rotation technique should be used.

Frog-Leg View. The frog-leg view visualizes the femoral head and neck in a plane nearly perpendicular to that of the AP view (Fig. 11-6). This is actually an AP view taken with the hip flexed, abducted, and externally rotated. It is useful in demonstrating pathology of the proximal femur. However, because this view requires movement of the injured hip, it can be painful and can cause displacement of a fracture. In addition, the view of the femoral neck is not entirely perpendicular to the view seen on the AP view. Nevertheless, positioning for the frog-leg lateral view is simple and it should be obtained when the patient can be positioned without undue pain. A frog-leg view of the entire pelvis is useful in children suspected of having SCFE because the opposite femoral head is seen for comparison.

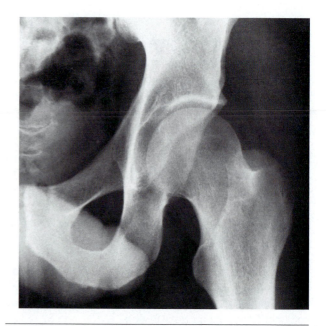

FIGURE 11-5. Suboptimal positioning of a hip radiograph. At rest, the legs tend to rotate externally. This causes foreshortening of the femoral neck on the radiograph. (On a properly performed hip radiograph, the legs are slightly rotated internally, which fully elongates the femoral neck.)

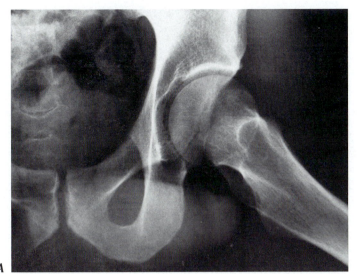

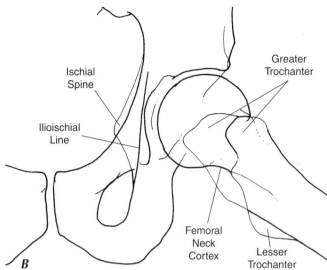

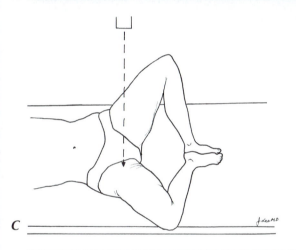

FIGURE 11-6. *A, B.* Frog-leg view of the hip. *C.* Positioning.

Cross-Table Lateral View. In the cross-table lateral or *groin lateral view,* the film is placed lateral to the involved hip and the contralateral leg is raised. The x-ray beam is directed horizontally from the medial groin laterally toward the film (Fig. 11-7). This view has the advantage of not requiring the patient to move the injured leg when there is a femoral fracture or hip dislocation.

Oblique Views. Oblique views of the hip are useful in demonstrating fractures of the acetabulum. The posterior oblique view can also reveal nondisplaced fractures of the femoral neck and lesser trochanter that are not seen on the AP view. The posterior oblique view is used as a substitute for the frog-leg or lateral view when positioning for these views is difficult.

Femoral Shaft Radiography. The radiographic examination of the femoral shaft consists of an AP and a lateral projection. Because of the length of the adult femur, it is usually impossible to see the entire bone on a single film plate. Midshaft fractures of the femur are often associated with injuries to the knee and hip. Therefore, in patients with suspected fractures of the femoral shaft, it is critical that radiographs be obtained to adequately see the joints above and below the injury.

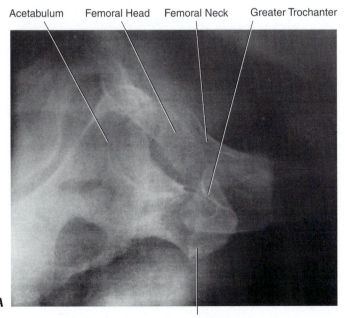

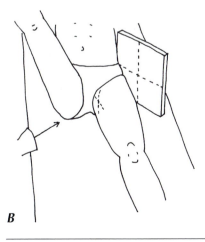

FIGURE 11-7. *A.* Cross-table lateral view of the hip. *B.* Positioning. (*A.* From Ballinger PW: *Merrill's Atlas of Radiographic Positions and Radiologic Procedures,* 7th ed. St. Louis: Mosby, 1995. With permission.)

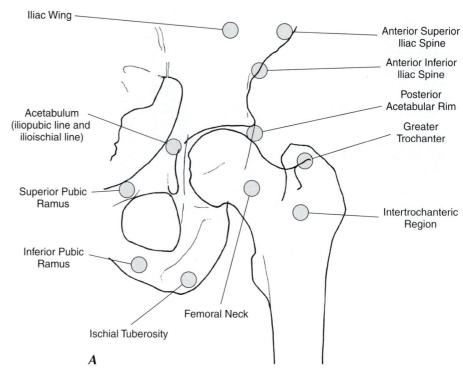

A

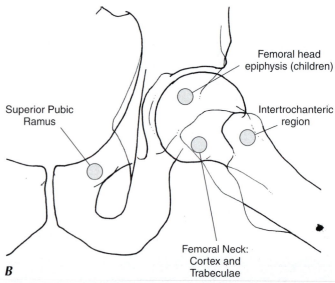

B

FIGURE 11-8.   Site prone to injury and easily missed injuries.

RADIOGRAPHIC ANALYSIS

Interpretation of radiographs begins with an initial quick review to look for obvious deformities. Often, these abnormalities are so dramatic that they draw one's attention away from less striking but significant, injuries. Therefore, a systematic review of the radiographs must be performed with a focus on both common (Fig. 11-8) and subtle injuries (Table 11-2).

Adequacy.   A systematic review begins with an assessment of the adequacy of the films. Two projections should be included: an AP view of the pelvis and a lateral hip projection (either frog-leg or cross-table). A correctly positioned AP view has the patient's hip rotated internally about 15°, elongating the femoral neck.

Alignment.   The overall alignment is then assessed. The symmetry of the entire pelvis is noted. The femoral head must lie within the acetabulum, and the medial half of the femoral head should overlap the posterior acetabular rim. A line connecting the inferior margin of the superior pubic ramus should curve smoothly to connect with the medial margin of the femoral neck. This is known as *Shenton's line* (Fig. 11-9). Disruption of Shenton's line indicates hip pathology (usually a femoral neck fracture).

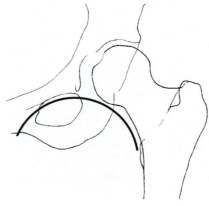

FIGURE 11-9.   Shenton's line. A line drawn along the inferior aspect of the femoral neck forms a continuous, smooth arc with the lower border of the superior pubic ramus.

TABLE 11-2

Systematic Analysis of Hip Radiographs

Initial review	Look for obvious abnormalities—fractures or dislocations	
Adequacy	An AP and lateral views are included unless patient is too ill to obtain a lateral view. AP of the entire pelvis is preferred. AP of hip must include the ipsilateral pubic rami and iliac bone. Hip is slightly rotated internally so that femoral neck is elongated. Lesser trochanter appears small, mostly hidden by femoral shaft.	
Check overall alignment	*Symmetry*—left and right sides have similar appearance. *Femoral head*—located within acetabulum. *Shenton's line*—inferior margin of superior pubic ramus makes smooth curve with medial margin of femoral neck.	
Proximal femur	Femoral neck Femoral head Intertrochanteric region Greater trochanter Lesser trochanter	Cortex—breaks or discontinuity. Trabeculae—disrupted, impacted (sclerosis), or distracted. Abnormal alignment of the femoral head and neck.
Articular surfaces	Femoral head surface	Smooth except central depression—fovea centralis.
	Acetabular joint surface	Smooth except central discontinuity—centrum.
	Joint space	Superior portion 4 to 5 mm wide. Medial portion 8 to 9 mm wide. No more that 2 mm difference between sides.
Acetabulum	Ilioischial line Iliopubic line (arcuate line) U (anteroinferior rim)	The "radiographic teardrop". All lines smooth, continuous, and symmetrical.
	Anterior and posterior rims	Look for fracture fragments.
Pelvis (peripheral areas)	Pubic rami Ischial ramus Ischial tuberosity Iliac body (acetabular dome) Iliac wing and crest	Look for fractures, discontinuity, impaction, or distortion of contour indicative of a fracture.
Lateral view	Femoral neck Trochanteric region	Cortical or trabecular discontinuity, impaction, or disruption.

Proximal Femur. Examination of the bones concentrates first on the proximal femur. This includes the femoral head, femoral neck, intertrochanteric region, and the greater and lesser trochanters. The cortex should be smooth and without breaks or abrupt angulations. Both the compressive and tensile trabeculae are examined for evidence of discontinuity or dis-

ruption. A band of increased trabecular density (sclerosis) is seen where fracture fragments are impacted. A band of decreased density (rarefaction) is seen when the fracture is distracted.

Articular Surfaces. Next, the articular surfaces are examined. The surface of the femoral head should be smooth and continuous except for the depression of the fovea centralis. The acetabular articular surface should likewise be smooth and continuous except for a central discontinuity due to the centrum of the acetabulum.

The joint space is then examined. It should be smooth and slightly wider medially than along its superior portion. The joint space of both hips should be the same width (within 2 mm). In the adult, the medial joint space is 8 to 9 mm wide and the superior joint space is 4 to 5 mm wide.[7]

Hip disorders are categorized by whether the joint space is narrowed, widened, or normal.[6,7] A narrowed joint space indicates loss of cartilage due to mechanical stress on the joint (osteoarthritis) or inflammation, such as rheumatoid arthritis. A widened space (2 mm larger than the unaffected side) usually indicates fluid (blood, infection, or inflamed synovial fluid) within the joint.

Acetabulum. The radiographic lines of the acetabulum are reviewed: the ilioischial line, the iliopubic line (continuous with the arcuate line), and the radiographic U (inferoanterior rim of the acetabulum). These lines converge with the articular surface of the acetabulum to form the *radiographic teardrop* (Fig. 11-4) (see chapter 12, Fig. 12-6). The anterior and posterior rims of the acetabulum are seen projecting through the femoral head.

Pelvis. The adjacent pelvis is then examined. This includes the pubic rami; the ischial tuberosity; the dome of the acetabulum; and the iliac spines, wing, and crest. Fractures to these areas are common following hip trauma.

Lateral View. Finally, the lateral view is examined. This view is useful in defining the anatomy of the subcapital region of the femoral head, particularly the anterior and posterior cortices. The trochanteric region and acetabulum are examined for evidence of fractures. Cortical discontinuity, medullary impaction, and distortion are sought. In suspected dislocations of the hip, the alignment of the bones on the cross-table lateral view reveals whether the dislocation is anterior or posterior. SCFE is often poorly seen on an AP view of the hip, yet may be clearly shown on a frog-leg lateral view.

COMMON ABNORMALITIES

Fractures of the Proximal Femur

Fractures of the proximal femur are classified on the basis of their location and relationship to the joint capsule (Table 11-3) (Fig. 11-10). *Intracapsular fractures*, particularly femoral neck fractures with displacement, have a significant incidence of avascular necrosis (AVN) of the femoral head. The more proximal an intracapsular fracture, the greater the risk of AVN. *Extracapsular fractures* do not disrupt the blood supply and therefore are not complicated by AVN.

FEMORAL HEAD FRACTURES.   Femoral head fractures are usually associated with hip dislocations. The clinical findings depend on the associated dislocation. The incidence of femoral head fractures associated with posterior dislocations is 10 to 16%, while the incidence reported with anterior dislocations is 22 to 77%. Femoral head fractures are usually best seen on radiographs obtained following the reduction of the dislocation.

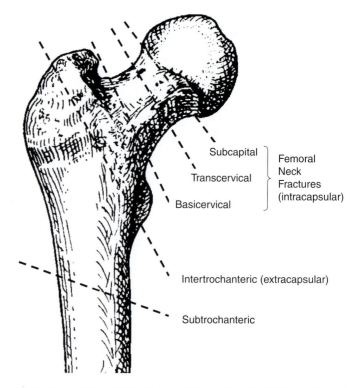

FIGURE 11-10.   Classification of proximal femoral fractures. Fractures of the femoral neck are intracapsular. Subcapital fractures are the most frequent. Intertrochanteric and subtrochanteric fractures are extracapsular.

Femoral head fractures include depressions, flattening, or transchondral fractures. The radiographic findings are often quite subtle (Fig. 11-11). Some authorities recommend computed tomography (CT) following all hip dislocations to look for femoral head fractures and fracture fragments within the joint space.

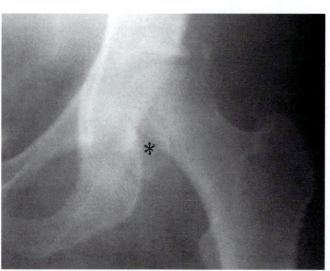

A

FIGURE 11-11.   Femoral head fracture. *A*. AP view. Note abnormal contour of the femoral head inferiorly (asterisk). *B*. CT scan clearly demonstrates a fracture fragment of the left femoral head that is completely rotated.

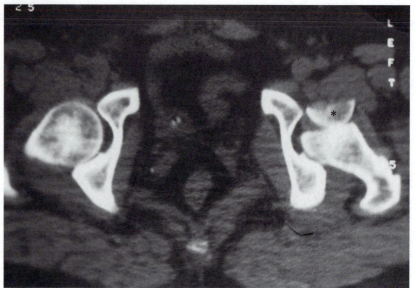

B

FEMORAL NECK FRACTURES.   Femoral neck fractures are unusual in healthy young persons and require high-energy forces such as falls from great heights or motor vehicle accidents. However, femoral neck fractures are common in the elderly (particularly women) because of osteoporosis. These patients often have minimal or no trauma. The fracture is often the result of multiple microfractures sustained over time.

The clinical presentation depends on the degree of displacement and extent of the fracture (Fig. 11-12). Elderly patients with minimally displaced fractures complain of pain in the groin, hip, or knee and may be able to walk (although usually with a limp). Physical examination may reveal tenderness of the hip or mild pain on range of motion. The leg is shortened if the fracture is impacted. As the degree of displacement and impaction increases, the leg becomes increasingly shortened and externally rotated. Many nondisplaced or impacted fractures are difficult to see on plain films. If a femoral neck fracture is suspected from the physical examination and the plain films are nondiagnostic, further imaging studies, e.g. magnetic resonance imaging (MRI), are indicated.

TABLE 11-3

Classification of Proximal Femur Fractures

Intracapsular
    Femoral head
    Femoral neck
        Subcapital (most common)
        Transcervical
        Basicervical
Extracapsular
    Intertrochanteric
    Greater trochanter
    Lesser trochanter
    Subtrochanteric

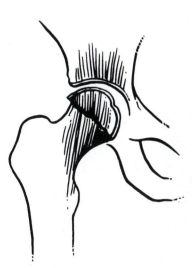

I Incomplete impacted

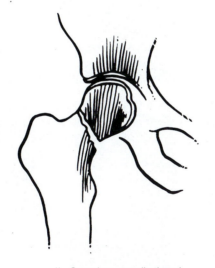

II Complete non-displaced

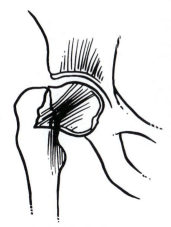

III Partially displaced

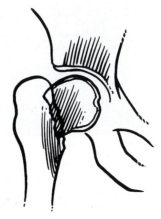

IV Fully displaced

FIGURE 11-12.   The Garden classification of femoral neck fractures. I. Incomplete impacted fracture, usually valgus angulation. II. Complete, nondisplaced fracture, usually valgus angulation. III. Complete, partially displaced fracture, usually varus angulation. IV. Completely displaced fracture with no engagement of the fracture parts. (From Dee R, Hurst LC, Gruber MA, Kottmeier SA: *Principles of Orthopedic Practice*, 2d ed. New York: McGraw-Hill, 1997, with permission.)

Subcapital fractures occur at the junction of the femoral head and neck. These are the most common femoral neck fractures. A displaced subcapital fracture is usually obvious on the AP radiograph (Fig. 11-13). However, nondisplaced fractures can be radiographically inapparent (Fig. 11-14). Femoral neck fractures are the most commonly missed fracture about the hip.[8] Subtle radiographic findings must be sought in the elderly pa-

tient presenting with hip pain (Table 11-4). These include superimposition of the base of the femoral head on the superior cortex of the femoral neck, disruption or angulation of the trabecular lines, abnormal angulation between the femoral head and femoral neck, and foreshortening of the femoral neck. An impacted fracture results in a transverse band of increased density in the subcapital region.

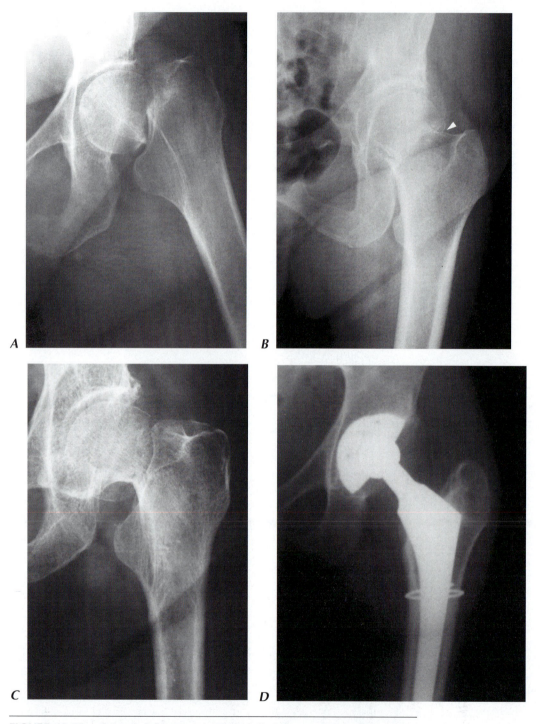

FIGURE 11-13.   Subcapital fractures. *A*. Marked displacement, Garden class IV. *B*. Complete fracture with valgus angulation, Garden class II. *C*. Complete, partially displaced fracture with varus angulation, Garden class III. *D*. Postoperative total arthroplasty after a femoral neck fracture. The acetabulum is replaced when there is preexisting degeneration of the articular surface.

TABLE 11-4

Radiographic Signs of Nondisplaced Subcapital Fractures

1. Disruption of the normally smooth line of the cortex.
   Superimposition of the base of the femoral head on the cortex of the femoral neck.

2. Disruption of the normal trabecular architecture.

3. Foreshortening of the femoral neck.
   Can also be caused by improper patient positioning.

4. Abnormal angle between the femoral neck and femoral head.
   Normally, 120–135°.

5. Transverse band of increased density across femoral neck.
   Impacted fracture.

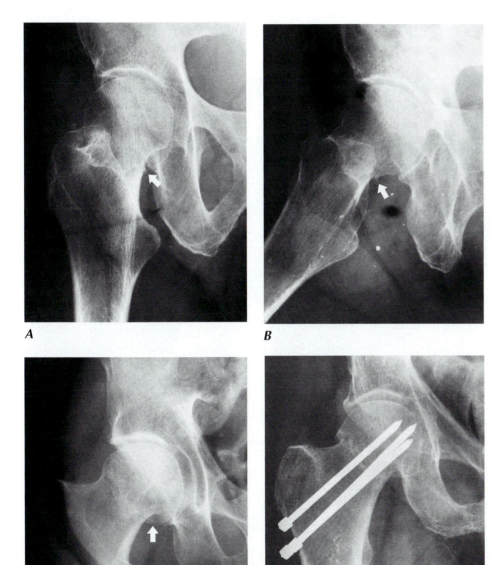

A

B

C

D

FIGURE 11-14. Nondisplaced subcapital fractures in two elderly patients with osteoporosis. *A.* On the AP view, the compressive trabeculae are interrupted and the medial cortex is slightly buckled. *B.* On the frog-leg lateral view, minimal irregularity of the medial cortex is seen. *C.* In another patient, impaction of the femoral head is seen. *D.* Postoperative radiograph. Stabilization of the femoral neck with cancellous screws. (*A* and *B* courtesy of Evan Schwartz, MD, Assistant Professor of Orthopedics, Catholic Medical Center, New York.)

When standard radiographs are nondiagnostic, several management strategies are used to ensure an appropriate diagnosis. Options include bed rest at home with repeat radiographs in 10 to 14 days or hospital admission for further imaging studies. Advanced studies such as bone scan, tomography, CT, or MRI play an important role in the diagnosis of occult fractures of the proximal femur. The bone scan was formerly the most commonly used. However, the bone scan is nonspecific and does not become positive until 3 to 5 days (or longer) after the injury. CT can identify fractures poorly seen on plain films; however, MRI is more sensitive. Although MRI is expensive, the overall cost is decreased because of the earlier diagnosis[9-11] (Fig. 11-15).

Transcervical fractures cross the midportion of the femoral neck. *Basicervical* fractures involve the junction of the base of the neck and the trochanters. Both of these are uncommon and are readily diagnosed on the AP view because of their displacement. Children are more likely than adults to have basicervical fractures. In adults, basicervical fractures are often due to underlying bone lesions, such as metastasis.

INTERTROCHANTERIC FRACTURES. Intertrochanteric fractures are the most common extracapsular fractures. These injuries usually result from falls in the elderly. Osteoporosis is the main predisposing factor. The patient with an intertrochanteric fracture is usually unable to walk. The affected leg is shortened and externally rotated to a much greater extent than with femoral neck fractures. This is the result of the powerful rotary force exerted by the iliopsoas muscle at its insertion on the distal fragment.

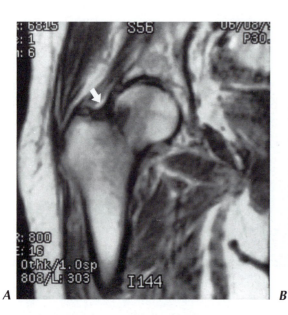

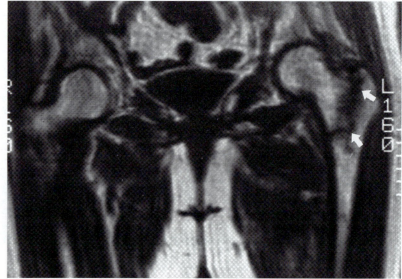

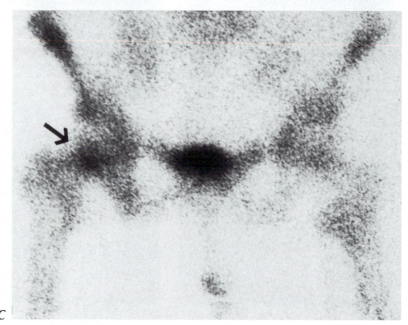

FIGURE 11-15. Imaging of occult fractures of the proximal femur. The initial plain radiographs were negative in these elderly patients with hip pain after minor trauma. Although MRI does not directly visualize bone, the fracture is evident owing to the decreased signal intensity where there is hemorrhage and edema within the marrow along the line of the fracture (T1-weighted images). *A.* Femoral neck fracture. *B.* Intertrochanteric fracture. *C.* Bone scan showing uptake at the site of an occult femoral neck fracture. (*A* and *B.* From Dee R, Hurst LC, Gruber MA, Kottmeier, SA: *Principles of Orthopedic Practice,* 2d ed. New York, McGraw-Hill, 1997, with permission.) (*C.* From Martire JR, Levinsohn EM: *Imaging of Athletic Injuries.* McGraw-Hill, 1992, with permission.)

A   *B*

C

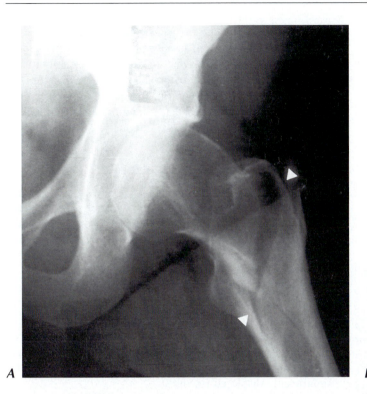
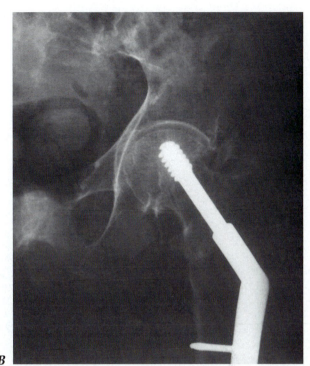

FIGURE 11-16.   Intertrochanteric fracture. *A.* A three-part fracture involving the lesser trochanter. *B.* Postoperative radiograph showing a sliding-screw device. The screw in the femoral neck slides into the collar at the base of the femoral neck. The apparatus is fixed by a plate and screws along the proximal femoral shaft.

Intertrochanteric fractures are classified by the number of fragments (Fig. 11-16). In a two-part fracture, the fracture line extends between the greater and lesser trochanters. The addition of a fracture involving either the greater or lesser trochanter is a three-part fracture. The addition of fractures involving both the greater and lesser trochanters is a four-part fracture. The stability of the fracture decreases as the number of parts increases. Because of the rich blood supply of the extracapsular region, these fractures have the potential for healing rapidly and well. Intertrochanteric fractures do not pose the same risk of AVN of the femoral head as do femoral neck fractures.

Intertrochanteric fractures are usually easy to diagnose radiographically. Two views of the area must be obtained to assess the number of fragments adequately and determine the degree of angulation. Occasionally, the fracture is visible only on the lateral view.

GREATER TROCHANTER FRACTURES.   Isolated fractures of the greater trochanter occur in two distinct age groups. The most common is an avulsion fracture in adolescent athletes. The second most common type of greater trochanter fracture occurs in elderly patients who fall and land directly on the greater trochanter. These patients are able to walk and have tenderness over the greater trochanter without evidence of shortening, rotation, or limited range of motion.

These injuries can be difficult to detect radiographically for two reasons. First, because the patient is ambulatory with minimal clinical findings, the injury may not be suspected. Second, the radiographic technique used to penetrate the entire hip overexposes the greater trochanter. Therefore, adequate visualization of the greater trochanter requires "bright lighting" the film (i.e., by using a high-intensity viewer) or obtaining other views (usually an oblique projection). With aging, the margin of the greater trochanter develops an irregular appearance that obscures or mimics a fracture.

LESSER TROCHANTER FRACTURES.   Fractures of the lesser trochanter almost always occur in young athletes. They are caused by forceful contraction of the iliopsoas muscle. In adults, this injury occurs in the presence of metastatic disease of the lesser trochanter.

SUBTROCHANTERIC FRACTURES.   Subtrochanteric fractures occur up to 5 cm below the inferior margin of the lesser trochanter. These fractures are due to major trauma and occur in a younger age group. When these injuries occur in the absence of significant trauma, usually in older patients, a pathologic fracture due to metastasis, Paget's disease, or other bone disease must be considered.

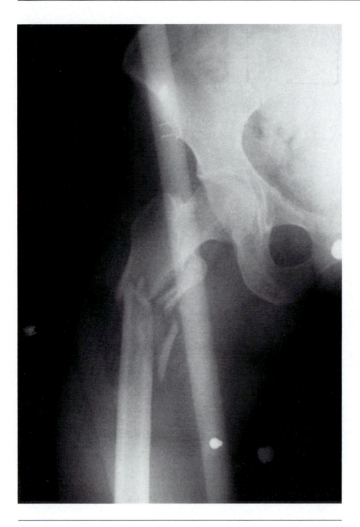

The proximal fracture fragment is flexed, abducted, and externally rotated, producing an outward protrusion of the greater trochanter. If the fragments are overriding, the leg is shortened.

These injuries are easy to diagnose radiographically (Fig. 11-17). Because of the strong forces required to produce these injuries, there are often associated injuries, such as acetabular fractures and hip dislocations.

Avulsion Fractures about the Hip

Avulsion fractures occur primarily in adolescent athletes. Forceful contraction of the involved muscle group causes these injuries (Table 11-5). Patients complain of pain and difficulty walking. They have localized tenderness and limitation of movement of the involved muscle group.

Radiographically, these injuries can be difficult to diagnose (Fig. 11-18). Findings depend on the patient's age, the degree of apophyseal ossification, and the age of apophyseal closure. These injuries may be undetectable in younger patients. Treatment is symptomatic and includes ice, analgesia, no weight bearing, and orthopedic referral. Surgery may be necessary for significantly displaced fractures.

FIGURE 11-17.   Subtrochanteric fracture. There is a separate fragment of the lesser trochanter.

TABLE 11-5

Avulsion Fractures About the Hip

FRACTURE SITE	MUSCLE GROUP	MECHANISM
Anterior superior iliac spine	Sartorius	Hip flexion
Anterior inferior iliac spine	Rectus femoris	Hip flexion
Ischial tuberosity	Hamstrings	Knee flexion
Greater trochanter	Gluteus medius and minimus	Abduction, external rotation
Lesser trochanter	Iliopsoas	Flexion with leg extended, internal rotation

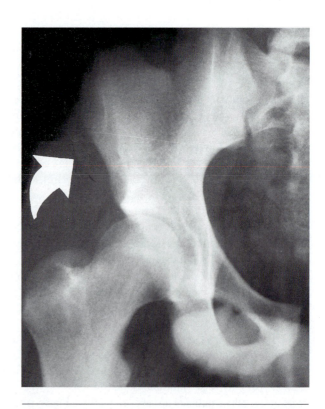

FIGURE 11-18.   Avulsion fracture of the anterior superior iliac spine.

Hip Dislocations

The characteristics of hip dislocations depend on the age of the patient. In adults, it requires great force, such as a motor vehicle accident, to dislodge the femoral head from the acetabulum. In a patient who has had a total hip replacement, the prosthesis can dislocate spontaneously or after minimal trauma. Young children are more likely to dislocate their hips than to sustain a fracture of the femoral neck. These dislocations may occur following minimal trauma, from falls, or from doing splits. In older children, increased force is necessary to dislocate the hip. The incidence of AVN of the femoral head increases with delayed reduction of the dislocation.

POSTERIOR DISLOCATIONS.   Posterior dislocations of the hip are the most common. The usual mechanism is a motor vehicle crash in which the knee strikes the dashboard. If the thigh is adducted at the time of impact, the forces transmitted along the femoral shaft displace the femoral head posteriorly and laterally with respect to the acetabulum. Depending on the degree of flexion of the hip at the time of impact, the hip will also be directed superiorly. Fractures of the acetabulum, patella, tibia, and the femoral head, neck, and shaft are associated with posterior hip dislocations.

The clinical findings can be predicted from the mechanism of injury. The affected leg is shortened, flexed, adducted, and internally rotated. Because great force is required to produce a posterior hip dislocation, patients with this injury are generally victims of multiple trauma. Therefore, the first radiograph obtained is the AP pelvis. In this projection, the dislocated femoral head is usually located superior to the acetabulum (Fig. 11-19).

Less commonly, the femoral head lies directly posterior to the acetabulum. In these cases, the dislocation is diagnosed radiographically by noting that the affected femoral head appears smaller than the opposite normal femoral head because the posteriorly dislocated femoral head lies closer to the radiographic film cassette. In addition, the lesser trochanter of the affected hip appears smaller or is not visible because the posteriorly dislocated hip is internally rotated and adducted.

While the AP pelvis film generally demonstrates the dislocation adequately and provides sufficient information to characterize its position, this radiograph is inadequate for evaluating associated injuries. Other views, such as a lateral or oblique view, must be obtained. Some authors recommend CT scanning of the hip following reduction of posterior dislocations to search for acetabular fractures, femoral head fractures, and fracture fragments within the joint. Others suggest CT scanning only if an acetabular fracture is identified on the plain films or if the reduction is not anatomic.

ANTERIOR DISLOCATIONS.   Anterior dislocations are less common than posterior dislocations, accounting for only 10 to 15% of all hip dislocations. Anterior dislocations result from forced abduction and external rotation of the leg. Anterior dislocations are associated with femoral head fractures. Acetabular and femoral neck fractures are less likely than with anterior hip dislocations than posterior dislocations.

On examination, the patient's hip is abducted and externally rotated. The hip is flexed if the femoral head lies adjacent to the obturator foramen. If the femoral head lies superiorly (adjacent to the pubic or iliac bones), the hip may be either slightly flexed or extended.

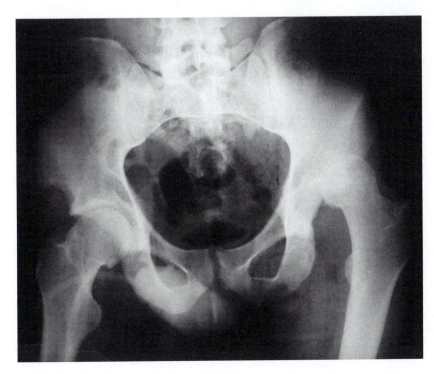

FIGURE 11-19.   Posterior hip dislocation. The left femoral head lies superior to the acetabulum and the hip is adducted and internally rotated.

On the AP radiograph, the femoral head is usually located medial to the acetabulum, in contrast to the superolateral position of a posterior hip dislocation. The lesser trochanter is prominent because the proximal femur is in external rotation. The affected femoral head appears larger than the contralateral femoral head because of the magnification that results from its being farther away from the film cassette. The anterior location of the femoral head is confirmed on the cross-table lateral radiograph (Fig. 11-20).

CENTRAL DISLOCATIONS.   The traumatic impact that produces a posterior dislocation generally displaces the femoral head in a superior and lateral direction. This occurs when the hip is adducted at the time of impact. However, if the thigh is abducted at the time of impact, the forces direct the femoral head through the acetabulum (Fig. 11-21). The resulting medial displacement of the femoral head into the pelvis is termed a *central hip*

dislocation. It can also result from a direct blow to the lateral aspect of the hip.

PROSTHESIS DISLOCATIONS.   A hip prosthesis can dislocate anteriorly or posteriorly following minimal trauma. Prosthesis dislocation is more likely if the hip is subjected to unusual forces, unusual positions, or if malalignment of the components occurred during surgery. The clinical presentation depends on the direction of the dislocation. Two radiographs taken perpendicular to each other diagnose the type of dislocation (Fig. 11-22).

Arthropathies

Arthropathies result from one of three processes: inflammation, deposition, or degeneration (Table 11-6). Inflammatory arthropathies affecting the hip include rheumatoid arthritis and ankylosing spondylitis. Degenerative arthritis (osteoarthritis) can affect the hip primarily (by abnormal mechanical stress placed on the joint) or secondarily (by deposition of a foreign substance into the cartilage).[12,13]

Radiographically, the assessment of a hip arthropathy begins by observing the direction that the femoral head has moved within the acetabulum. It can move in one of three directions: medially, superomedially, or superolaterally. Uniform loss of cartilage results in movement in a superomedial direction. This indicates a primary cartilage problem due to an inflammatory or deposition arthropathy. Medial or superolateral movement indicates nonuniform loss of cartilage due to abnormal mechanical stress.

INFLAMMATORY ARTHROPATHIES.   Inflammatory arthropathies are characterized by aggressive destruction of cartilage by erosion. *Rheumatoid arthritis* is a bilaterally symmetrical polyarthropathy. It produces a uniform loss of cartilage and superomedial migration of the femoral head. Generalized osteoporosis and bone erosion without evidence of new bone formation are also seen.

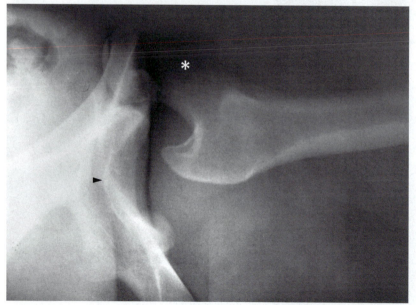

A

B

FIGURE 11-20.   Anterior hip dislocation. *A.* On the AP view, the left femoral head appears to be within the acetabulum. However, the anterior direction of the dislocation can be surmised by the fact that the femur is externally rotated (the femoral head overlies the femoral neck). *B.* On a cross-table groin lateral, the femoral head (*asterisk*) is seen dislocated anterior to the acetabulum (*arrowhead*). (Copyright David T. Schwartz, MD, New York.)

TABLE 11-6

Radiographic Features of Arthropathies

Type	Joint space narrowing	Migration of femoral head	Bone changes	Osteophyte production	Other features
Osteoarthritis	Nonuniform, localized, irregular	Medially, superiorly, or superolaterally	Subchondral cysts, subchondral sclerosis (eburnation)	Prominent, particularly on acetabulum and medial aspect of femoral head	Deformity, malalignment
Rheumatoid arthritis	Uniform, symmetrical	Superomedially or centrally	Generalized osteopenia, bone erosion	Minimal or absent	Associated systemic symptoms
Ankylosing spondylitis	Symmetrical	Superomedially	No change in mineralization, minimal erosions	Mild to moderate	Ossification of ligaments, bilateral associated sacroilitis
Pseudogout	Variable, gradual loss of joint space	Superomedially	Bone density variable, cysts	Moderate	Cartilaginous calcifications
Gout	Minimal	Superomedially (slight)	Initially normal, later, "punched out"	Mild to moderate	Rarely affects hips

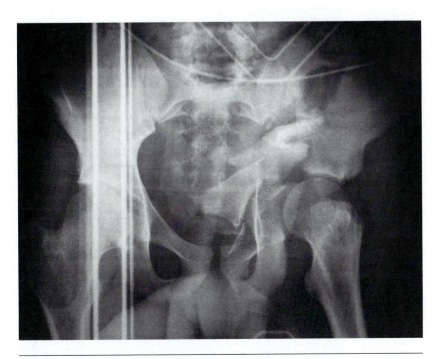

FIGURE 11-21. Central hip dislocation with acetabular fracture. (Courtesy of Dr. Jeffery L. Bleazzard, Sparrow Hospital, Lansing, MI.)

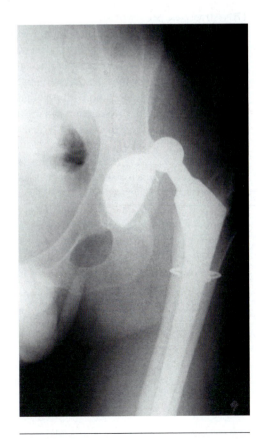

FIGURE 11-22. Posterior dislocation of a hip prothesis.

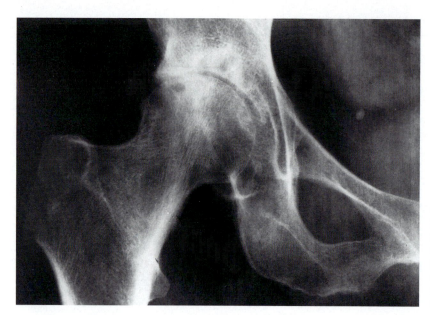

FIGURE 11-23.   Osteoarthritis. There is marked joint space narrowing, subchondral sclerosis, and cyst formation of both the femoral and acetabular articular surfaces. There is asymmetrical joint space narrowing with superior migration of the femoral head. Osteophyte formation at the margins of the joint are also frequently seen.

The hip is the most common appendicular joint affected by *ankylosing spondylitis*.[6,12] The femoral head migrates in a superomedial direction. With ankylosing spondylitis, the mineralization of the bones is maintained and erosions are minimal. Ligamentous ossification is also observed. Ankylosis occurs early in the disease. The hip is not usually affected by psoriatic arthritis or Reiter's syndrome.

DEPOSITION ARTHROPATHIES.   The most common deposition arthropathy affecting the hip is *calcium pyrophosphate disease (pseudogout)*. True gout rarely affects the hip. In pseudogout, uniform loss of cartilage and superomedial migration of the femoral head occur within the acetabulum. The destruction of cartilage is slower in deposition arthropathies than with the inflammatory types. Bone production and repair are marked. This results in the formation of bone cysts and osteophytes at the femoral head and acetabulum.

DEGENERATIVE ARTHROPATHIES.   Degenerative arthropathy (osteoarthritis) is characterized by abnormal weight bearing across the hip and resultant abnormal mechanical stresses. A nonuniform loss of cartilage and superolateral migration of the femoral head occur within the acetabulum. Osteophyte formation is prominent, particularly at the medial aspect of the femoral head. Bone deposition occurs along the inner aspect of the femoral neck and in the articular surfaces of the acetabulum (Fig. 11-23).

Avascular Necrosis

AVN is also known as *aseptic necrosis, osteonecrosis,* and *ischemic necrosis*.[14,15] It frequently complicates femoral neck frac-

tures and hip dislocations. AVN may be idiopathic or secondary to various conditions, including exogenous steroid therapy, alcohol abuse, gout, sickle cell disease, dysbarism, and renal osteodystrophy. Patients complain of hip or groin pain that increases with weight bearing. The pain may radiate to the medial thigh or knee.

Radiographic findings lag behind clinical symptoms by several months. There are several radiographic stages (Table 11-7 and Fig. 11-24). Early AVN is often difficult to distinguish from degenerative arthritis. The major differentiating feature of AVN

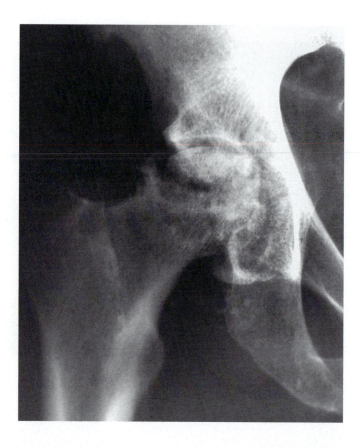

FIGURE 11-24.   Avascular necrosis of femoral head. The femoral head shows characteristic mottling, sclerosis, and deformity. There is also joint space narrowing, which is a late finding.

TABLE 11-7

Avascular Necrosis of the Femoral Head

STAGE	SYMPTOMS	RADIOGRAPHIC FINDINGS	TREATMENT
I	None to mild. Hip or groin pain.	Plain films normal. MRI or bone scan abnormal.	No weight bearing, core decompression
II	Pain increases with weight bearing. Decreased range of motion (ROM).	Femoral head maintains normal contour but mottled with densities and lucencies.	Same as I
III	Progressively increasing pain and decreased ROM.	Loss of femoral head contour. "Crescent sign."	Osteotomy or THR*
IV	Further worsening of symptoms.	Severe collapse of femoral head with cystic changes. Osteophytes. Narrowed joint space.	THR

*THR, total hip replacement.

TABLE 11-8

Radiographic Comparison of AVN and Osteoarthritis*

	AVASCULAR NECROSIS	OSTEOARTHRITIS
Joint space	Well preserved until late	Early, nonuniform loss
Bony change of femoral head	Mottled with increased densities and lucencies	Subchondral Sclerosis (eburnation)
	Loss of contour Subchondral arc-like lucency ("crescent sign") Collapse (late)	Subchondral cysts Flattened femoral head (late) Collapse (very late)
Osteophytes	Not prominent until late	Prominent

*These entities may be indistinguishable after loss of joint space in AVN.

is the preservation of the joint space until the most advanced stages (Table 11-8).

Nonoperative therapy fails to halt the progression of AVN. It is beneficial to achieve an early diagnosis. Although both bone scan and MRI can make this diagnosis early, MRI is more specific and accurate.[14,16] Treatment depends on the extent of the disease and is determined primarily by the orthopedic consultant. Early diagnosis before collapse of the femoral head allows core decompression rather than total hip replacement. After collapse of the femoral head, total hip replacement is the only treatment option.

Pathologic Fractures

Pathologic fractures are defined as fractures of abnormal bone. They may be caused by minor trauma or may occur in the absence of any trauma. The abnormal bone is caused by disuse, infection, maldevelopment, metabolic disease, or metastatic disease. The hip is the third most common site, following the spine and pelvis, for osseous metastasis. If a patient with a known cancer (especially of the breast, lung, thyroid, kidney, or prostate) has a fracture, close radiographic examination for evidence of metastasis is mandatory. Radiographic findings suggestive of a pathologic fracture include calcification, periosteal reaction, generalized osteopenia, thinned or destroyed cortical bone, and a sclerotic rim. Pathologic fractures resulting from metastasis are rarely located in the subcapital area; most are intertrochanteric or subtrochanteric (see chapter 2, Fig. 2-8). Fracture management is made complicated by the poor bone quality.

Fractures in Children

Fractures of the proximal femur are uncommon in children. Fractures of the developing hip usually involve the physis (growth plate) and are often complicated by subsequent growth disturbance.[5,17–19] Pediatric hip fractures are often nondisplaced because of the relatively strong periosteum. The amount of displacement determines the incidence of AVN. Management of proximal femoral fractures in children differs from that in adults. Because children tolerate immobility better, and no current prosthesis allows for growth, internal fixation is used much less often than in adults, except for screw fixation of SCFE.

In evaluating children with hip injuries, it is important to know the radiographic appearance of the growth plates, the ages at which the secondary ossification centers first became visible, and the ages at which the growth plates close (Table 11-9 and Fig. 11-25). With this anatomic knowledge and an understanding of the types of pediatric hip injuries, most fractures are easy to identify.

Disorders of the Developing Hip

SLIPPED CAPITAL FEMORAL EPIPHYSIS.   SCFE is a progressive posteromedial displacement of the proximal femoral epiphysis.[17,20,21] The onset is often insidious. The patient presents with a limp and hip pain. However, the patient may complain only of knee, thigh, or groin pain. SCFE occurs in late childhood or early adolescence. It usually is seen in overweight children, although it can occur in tall, thin persons. SCFE is bilateral in 20 to 30% of cases. The second slip usually occurs within 1 year of the initial presentation. On physical examination there is limited internal rotation. When the patient attempts to flex the affected hip, it rotates externally and abducts (Whitman's sign).

Both AP and frog-leg lateral views of the pelvis and hips are necessary. In mild cases, the radiographic diagnosis can be difficult. Asymmetry of the position of the femoral head epiphysis is typical. A line drawn along the superior aspect of the femoral neck does not intersect the femoral head epiphysis. On the AP view, Shenton's line is disrupted. In mild cases, the slippage is seen only on the frog-leg view (Fig. 11-26).

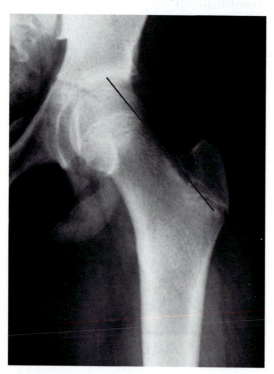

FIGURE 11-25.   Normal hip of an older child. The unfused growth plates of the femoral head and greater trochanter should not be misinterpreted as fractures. A line drawn along the margin of the femoral neck normally intersects the edge of the femoral head epiphysis.

TABLE 11-9

Secondary Ossification Centers of the Hip

LOCATION	APPEARANCE (AGE)	CLOSURE (AGE/YEARS)	COMMENT
Capital femoral epiphysis	First year of life (3 months)	18–20	15% of femoral length
Greater trochanter	1.5–4.5 years	16–20	
Lesser trochanter	13 months	16–20	
Anterior superior iliac spine	Puberty	20–25	
Anterior inferior iliac spine	Puberty	20–25	
Ischial tuberosity	Puberty	20–25	
Posterior acetabulum	14–18 years	20–25	May persist as os acetabuli

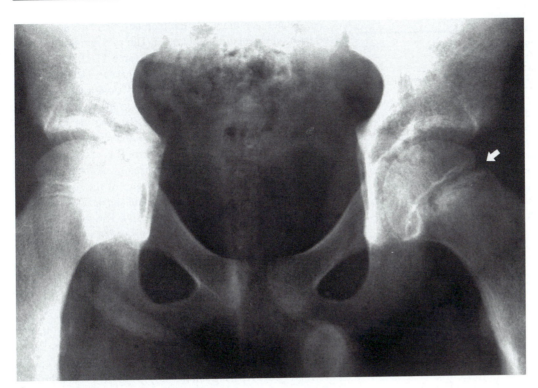

A

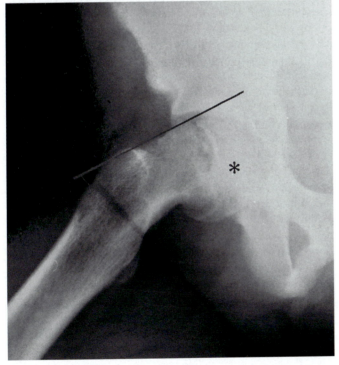

B

FIGURE 11-26. Two examples of subtle slipped capital epiphysis (SCFE). *A.* On the AP view, there is slight widening of the growth plate in comparison to the opposite side. There is medial slippage of the femoral head, i.e., no part of the femoral head intersects a line drawn along the superior margin of the femoral neck. *B.* In another patient, the frog-leg view shows medial slippage of the femoral head. The AP view was normal.

Unilateral widening of the physis may be the only finding. The frog-leg view should include both hips so that the opposite normal hip can be used for comparison. SCFE is graded by the amount of slippage of the femoral head epiphysis seen on the AP radiograph. In mild SCFE, the slippage is less than one-third the diameter of the femoral head, moderate SCFE is between one-third and one-half, and severe SCFE is greater than one-half.

Initial management includes no weight bearing, orthopedic referral and subsequent surgical fixation. Complications of SCFE include AVN and chondrolysis.

LEGG-CALVÉ-PERTHES (LCP) DISEASE. LCP disease is idiopathic AVN of the proximal femoral epiphysis.[22] It occurs primarily in boys between 3 and 10 years of age. The patient presents with a limp and complain of hip, groin, or knee pain. The onset is insidious. This disorder is bilateral in 10 to 20% of cases. Physical examination reveals limited internal rotation and abduction.

TABLE 11-10

Stages of Legg-Calvé-Perthes (LCP) Disease

STAGE	RADIOGRAPHIC FINDINGS
Necrotic	Bulging hip capsule.
	Crescent sign.
	Increased density of femoral epiphysis.
Fragmentation	Epiphysis deforms.
	Femoral neck widens.
Reossification	Increased density at margins of epiphysis.
	Continued widening of femoral neck.
Remodeling	Coxa magna, coxa brevis, coxa irregularis.
	Osteochondritis dissecans.

An AP pelvis radiograph that includes both hips and a frog-leg lateral view should be obtained. The radiographic findings depend on the stage of the disorder (Table 11-10). Initially, a bulging hip joint capsule is caused by synovitis. A subchondral lucency, known as the *crescent sign of Caffey*, may be seen (Fig. 11-27). The crescent sign is caused by a fracture of the necrotic bone, and it is best seen on the frog-leg view. With progression to the fragmentation stage, the necrotic bone is replaced with fibrocartilage (Fig. 11-28). This results in a mottled radiographic appearance. Formation of new bone then occurs, which can cause premature closure of the growth plate. Permanent deformity of the femoral head can develop, although some remodeling continues until maturity. The four patterns of deformity are coxa magna, coxa brevis, coxa irregularis, and osteochondritis dissecans. The prognosis depends on the age of the patient at the time of presentation, which correlates with the stage of disease. LCP disease must be recognized early and referred to an orthopedist.

SEPTIC ARTHRITIS. The hip is the most common site of joint infection in children younger than age 5 years of age. Septic arthritis is an orthopedic emergency; delay in diagnosis can result in permanent joint damage. In younger children, the clinical presentation is often nonspecific. Infants present with fever, irritability, and refusal to move the leg. Older children present with pain, limp, and inability to bear weight.

An AP pelvis radiograph that includes both hips is necessary. When the joint is infected, an increased distance between the medial aspect of the epiphysis and the inferomedial acetabulum is seen.[23] This radiographic finding is most sensitive in the neonate. The majority of radiographs in children older than 1 year of age are normal. Ultrasound can detect an effusion not seen on plain film. In addition to imaging studies, a complete blood count, blood cultures, and a sedimentation rate are needed. Arthrocentesis under fluoroscopy is mandatory whenever this diagnosis is highly suspected regardless of radiographic and laboratory findings. Management consists of early recognition, orthopedic consultation, aspiration, intravenous antibiotics, and arthrotomy to relieve joint pressure.

OSTEOMYELITIS. Acute osteomyelitis of the proximal femur occurs more commonly in children than in adults.[17,24] The clinical presentation of osteomyelitis is similar to that of septic arthritis except that gentle, passive range of motion is possible with osteomyelitis. Initially, radiographs are normal or show soft tissue swelling and obliteration of muscle fascial planes. Periosteal elevation and lytic lesions are seen after 10 to 14 days. Because a radionuclide bone scan is positive earlier than plain radiographs (within 3 days), bone scan is the mainstay of early diagnosis. CT and MRI can reveal early destructive changes. Intravenous antibiotics, orthopedic consultation, and hospital admission are necessary.

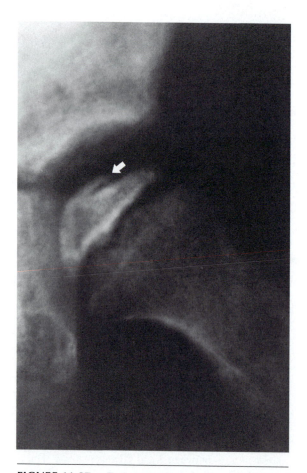

FIGURE 11-27. Early avascular necrosis of the femoral head (Legg-Calvé-Perthes disease). The "crescent sign" of Caffey is a subchondral lucency, resulting from a collapse of necrotic bone (*arrow*).

TOXIC SYNOVITIS. Toxic synovitis, also known as *transient synovitis*, is the most common cause of hip pain in children between age 3 and 10 years.[17,20] It is a self-limited disease of unclear etiology that must be differentiated from serious causes

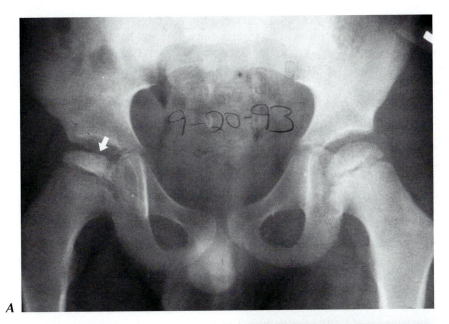

A

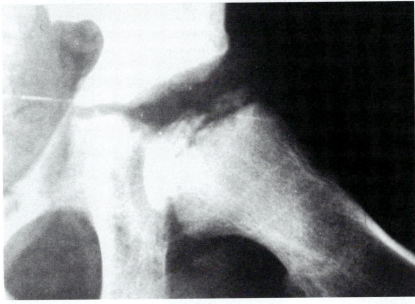

B

FIGURE 11-28. Avascular necrosis of the femoral head (Legg-Calvé-Perthes disease). There is progressive loss of volume and fragmentation of the femoral head in moderate (*A*) and severe (*B*) cases. (Courtesy Ellen Cavanaugh, MD, Sparrow Hospital, Lansing, Michigan.)

of hip pain such as septic arthritis and osteomyelitis. Although the etiology is unknown, many patients have had preceding viral infections. The patient presents with a limp or hip pain, and physical examination reveals limited internal rotation. Radiographs are usually normal but may show bulging of the joint capsule. The white blood cell count and sedimentation rate are normal or slightly elevated. Joint aspiration is mandatory if a septic joint is suspected. Management includes analgesia, limitation of activities, and orthopedic consultation and follow-up.

ERRORS IN INTERPRETATION

Subtle and Occult Fractures of the Femoral Neck. Although displaced fractures of the femoral neck are obvious, nondisplaced or impacted femoral neck fractures can be extremely difficult to see on plain films (Fig. 11-14).[10] Subtle radiographic findings of nondisplaced subcapital fractures include discontinuity of the normally smooth line of cortical bone, disruption of the normal trabecular pattern, a transverse band of increased density, foreshortening of the femoral neck, and abnormal angulation between the femoral neck and the femoral head (Table 11-4).[7]

In an occult fracture, the radiographs are negative, and adjunctive imaging studies such as bone scan, conventional tomography, CT, or MRI are necessary.[9–11] There is variation in the choice of adjunctive study. Bone scan has been the most commonly employed, but it is nonspecific and is not expected to be positive for three to five days after the injury.[11] Although CT may identify some fractures not easily seen on plain films, MRI is more sensitive for truly occult fractures.[9–11] Although MRI is expensive, overall cost is lower thanks to earlier diagnosis (Fig. 11-15).[9]

Stress Fractures and Insufficiency Fractures of the Femoral Neck.   These fractures are often difficult to detect radiographically. Stress fractures are caused by excessive, repetitive impact on normal bone. They are primarily seen in athletes (especially long-distance runners) and military recruits. Insufficiency fractures occur in abnormal bone subjected to routine stress. They occur in the elderly with osteoporosis. Bone scan is the preferred test in suspected stress fractures.[25] These fractures are classified into two types: tension (involving the superior aspect of the femoral neck) and compression (involving the inferior aspect of the femoral neck). Tension-type stress fractures may require operative repair, whereas compression-type stress fractures respond to conservative management.

Fractures of the Pubic Rami and Other Pelvic Fractures.   Pelvic fractures are often present in patients with hip trauma. Pubic ramus fractures are the most common (Fig. 11-29). Patients complain of groin pain that increases with walking. As isolated fracture of the iliac wing causes lateral hip pain that increases with abduction. The pelvis must be closely examined in all patients with a suspected hip fracture.

Avulsion Fractures.   An avulsion fracture is often misdiagnosed as a "muscle pull" because these injuries are subtle radiographically. Knowledge of the radiographic appearance of the apophysis and the expected age of closure is essential (Fig. 11-18).

Septic Hip.   Septic arthritis is a true orthopedic emergency. This diagnosis is not excluded by a normal radiograph. In fact, the majority of patients above 1 year of age have a normal radiograph rather than one showing an increased joint space.[23]

Arthrocentesis is mandatory when this diagnosis is suspected. Overreliance on plain radiographs must be avoided.

Fractures of the Posterior Acetabular Rim.   Although technically a pelvic fracture, a posterior acetabular rim fracture injury is commonly associated with posterior hip dislocations. These fractures can be subtle on plain films. CT easily demonstrates the fragment. When a posterior hip dislocation is difficult to reduce, the cause may be an entrapped bone fragment (Fig. 11-30).

Fracture Mimics.   Osteophytes of the femoral head and gluteal skin folds that project over the femoral neck can mimic a fracture line (Fig. 11-31). On the other hand, a gluteal skin fold or osteophyte can lie over and obscure a fracture.

The os acetabuli is an accessory ossicle that can mimic an acetabular fracture or a fracture of the femoral neck, depending on its location.[26] The cortex of an accessory ossicle is well rounded and sclerotic, differentiating it from a fracture fragment.

The femoral shaft often has a prominent vascular channel for its nutrient artery. This can be distinguished from a fracture because the vascular channel has sclerotic margins, involves only one cortex of the femoral shaft and has an oblique orientation directed away from the knee. The clinical findings are of course different for a vascular channel than for a fracture.

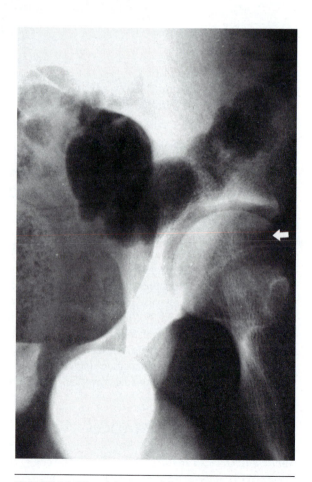

FIGURE 11-30.   A fracture of the posterior acetabular rim.

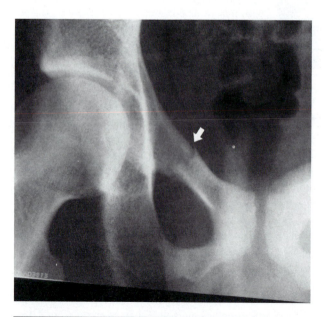

FIGURE 11-29.   A superior pubic ramus fracture was found in this elderly patient, who complained of hip pain after minor trauma.

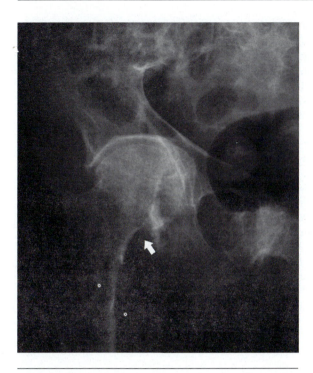

FIGURE 11-31.   The acetabular rim overlies the femoral neck. The overlapping shadow should not be misinterpreted as a fracture.

ADVANCED IMAGING

Supplementary imaging modalities are used when plain radiographs are negative or equivocal. The choice of imaging study is determined by the specific clinical problem, patient characteristics, consultant preference, availability and cost.

Bone Scan.   Radionuclide studies are used to evaluate suspected fractures, infections, or other diseases when there are no radiographic abnormalities. Occult fractures of the femoral neck, osteomyelitis, and neoplasms can be detected by bone scan.[10] The advantages of bone scan include its widespread availability, relatively low cost, and ability to demonstrate disease activity. However, with an occult fracture, abnormal uptake is not seen for 3 to 5 days after the injury. Even more time may be required in elderly patients with osteoporosis. In addition, both arthritis and synovitis cause abnormal tracer uptake.[6] The increasing availability of MRI has reduced the role of bone scan.

Computed Tomography.   CT provides highly detailed cross-sectional images of the hip region. CT can detect nondisplaced fractures, periosteal reactions, calcifications, and neoplasms.[7] It can demonstrate some fractures not seen on plain radiography and is used to determine the nature of an abnormality seen on bone scan. Specific indications for CT include acetabular fractures, fractures of the femoral head, irreducible hip dislocations (due to an intraarticular bone fragment), and differentiation tumors from stress fractures.[13] Compared with MRI, CT is less expensive, more readily available, and provides better bone resolution. However, CT does not demonstrate soft tissues as well as MRI. The disadvantages of CT include cost, radiation exposure, and inability to visualize cartilage.[7]

Magnetic Resonance Imaging.   MRI is now widely used to evaluate the acutely injured or painful hip.[7,9,11,14] Its advantages include direct multiplanar imaging, soft tissue detail, great sensitivity, and lack of ionizing radiation. It is the test of choice for AVN and is used to follow LCP.[22] In many institutions, MRI has replaced bone scan in the diagnosis of an occult fracture. The disadvantages of MRI include lack of availability, cost, time, and inferior display of small osseous abnormalities. One study reported a reduced cost of evaluating occult fractures of the femoral neck because of earlier diagnosis and decreased length of hospital stay.[9] In patients with suspected hip injuries, MRI often finds other fractures or soft tissue injuries, such as occult fractures of the pubic rami (Fig. 11-15).[27]

CONTROVERSIES

Because elderly patients with osteoporosis may sustain fractures with minimal or no trauma, the threshold for ordering radiographs should be low. The evaluation and management of the patient suspected of having an occult fracture of the femoral neck is a matter of controversy. The goal is to confirm the diagnosis and prevent a nondisplaced fracture from becoming displaced. Admission to the hospital for further diagnostic studies is not cost-effective but may be necessary in some patients with preexisting medical problems or who are in difficult social situations. If discharged to home, patients should not bear weight and should return for repeat radiographs in 7 to 10 days. However, elderly patients often have difficulty using crutches to eliminate weight bearing and thus risk displacement if a fracture is present. Use of adjunctive studies (CT, MRI, bone scan) is becoming a preferred strategy. MRI, although expensive, can make an earlier diagnosis.

REFERENCES

1. Levy DB, Hanlon DP, Townsend RN: Geriatric trauma. *Clin Geriatr Med* 9:601, 1993.
2. Pierron RL, Perry HM, Grossberg F, et al: The aging hip. *J Am Geriatr Soc* 38:1331, 1990.
3. Hay EK: That old hip: The osteoporosis process. *Nurs Clin North Am* 26:43, 1991.
4. Zuckerman JD: Hip fracture. *N Engl J Med* 334:1519, 1996.
5. Stewart C: The clinical spectrum of adult and pediatric hip injuries: Predisposing factors, evaluation, and definitive management. *Emerg Med Rep* 15:91, 1994.
6. Brower AC, Kransdorf MJ: Imaging of hip disorders. *Radiol Clin North Am* 28:955, 1990.
7. Pitt MJ, Lund PJ, Speer DP: Imaging of the pelvis and hip. *Orthop Clin North Am* 21:545, 1990.
8. Miller MD: Commonly missed orthopedic problems. *Emerg Med Clin North Am* 10:151, 1992.

9. Deutsch AL, Mink JH, Waxman AD: Occult fractures of the proximal femur: MR imaging. *Radiology* 170:113, 1989.

10. Alba E, Youngberg R: Occult fractures of the femoral neck. *Am J Emerg Med* 10:64, 1992.

11. Evans PD, Wilson C, Lyons K: Comparison of MRI with bone scanning for suspected hip fracture in elderly patients. *J Bone Joint Surg* 76B:158, 1994.

12. Brower AC: Appendicular arthropathy. *Orthop Clin North Am* 21:405, 1990.

13. Schon L, Zuckerman JD: Hip pain in the elderly: Evaluation and diagnosis. *Geriatrics* 43:48, 1988.

14. Lang P, Genant HK, Jergesen HE, et al: Imaging of the hip joint. *Clin Orthop* 274:135, 1992.

15. Resnick D, Niwayama G: Osteonecrosis: diagnostic techniques, specific situations, and complications, in Resnick D (ed): *Diagnosis of Bone and Joint Disease,* 3d ed. Philadelphia: Saunders, 1995, pp. 3495–3515.

16. Basset LW, Gold RH, Reicher M, et al: MRI in the early diagnosis of ischemic necrosis of the femoral head: Preliminary results. *Clin Orthop* 214:237, 1987.

17. Urbanski LF, Hanlon DP: Pediatric orthopedics. *Top Emerg Med* 18:73, 1996.

18. Canale ST: Fractures of the hip in children and adolescents. *Orthop Clin North Am* 21:341, 1990.

19. Colona PC: Fractures of the hip and femur in children. *Am J Surg* 6:793, 1992.

20. Spatz DK: Hip pain in children. *Res Staff Phys* 33:57, 1987.

21. Lehman WB: Slipped capital femoral epiphysis, in Dee R, Mango E, Hurst LC, (eds): *Principles of Orthopaedic Practice.* New York: McGraw-Hill, 1989, pp. 1101–1109.

22. Bowen JR: Legg-Calvé-Perthes, in Dee R, Mango E, Hurst LC, (eds): *Principles of Orthopaedic Practice.* New York: McGraw-Hill, 1989, pp. 1110–1122.

23. Volberg FM, Sumner TE, Abramson JS, et al: Unreliability of radiographic diagnosis of septic hip in children. *Pediatrics* 74:118, 1984.

24. Mercier LR, Pettid FJ, Tamisiea DG, et al: Infections of bone and joint, in Mercier LR (ed): *Practical Orthopedics,* 4th ed. Philadelphia: Mosby–Year Book, 1995, pp. 262–277.

25. Kupke MJ, Kahler DM, Lorenzoni MH, et al: Stress fracture of the femoral neck in a long distance runner: Biomechanical aspects. *J Emerg Med* 11:587, 1993.

26. Daffner RH: Skeletal pseudofractures. *Emerg Radiol* 2:96, 1995.

27. Bogost GA, Lizerbraum EK, Crues JV: MR imaging in evaluation of suspected hip fracture: Frequency of unsuspected bone and soft-tissue injury. *Radiology* 197:263, 1995.

CHAPTER 12

THE PELVIS

FRED HUSTEY / LAILA MOETTUS WILBER

Traumatic injuries to the pelvis range from minor isolated pubic ramus fractures to lethal disruptions of the pelvic ring. When major pelvis fractures are seen, it is important to rapidly identify and treat associated complications. These patients often have multiorgan system injuries.[1] Morbidity and mortality rates are high, ranging from 5 to 20%, and mortality is as high as 60% in open fractures.[2–4] Pelvic fractures themselves are a source of significant blood loss, leading to hemorrhagic shock. A retroperitoneal hematoma due to a pelvic fracture can contain several liters of blood. In addition, there is a high rate of visceral injuries, such as urethral tears (up to 14%), bladder rupture (up to 15%),[5] rectal or colonic perforation, gynecologic injuries, and involvement of the lumbosacral plexus.

CLINICAL DECISION MAKING

With regard to the radiography of the pelvis, there are four important decisions to be made: (1) when to obtain an anteroposterior (AP) pelvis film; (2) when to suspect pelvic hemorrhage and obtain angiography; (3) when to suspect visceral injuries, especially involving the urinary tract; and (4) when supplementary radiographic studies are needed for more complete orthopedic assessment.

Anteroposterior Pelvis Radiography

In deciding when to obtain an AP radiograph of the pelvis, it is useful to categorize traumatic injuries as minor, moderate, or severe. The distinction between these groups ultimately depends on the physician's clinical judgment. One must consider the mechanism of injury, physical findings, and associated injuries (Table 12-1). Using the guidelines of the *Advanced Trauma Life Support* (ATLS) *Manual*, which are primarily concerned with severe multiorgan system trauma, an AP pelvis film is obtained in all trauma victims once they are stabilized. This recommendation is based on the frequency of significant pelvic injuries in victims of major trauma and the grave consequences that result from overlooking such a pelvic injury. By routinely obtaining a pelvic radiograph in the initial "trauma series" (cervical spine, chest, and pelvis), one minimizes the chance of missing a pelvic injury. A pelvic injury can be missed in a multitrauma victim not because of a lack of clinical findings but rather because the presence of other grave injuries distracts the clinician from noticing the pelvic injury.

With victims of "moderate" or minor trauma, the ATLS policy of routine pelvic study should not be applied indiscriminately; pelvic radiographs are ordered selectively. There are several studies suggesting that patients without pelvic pain or tenderness who are alert, not intoxicated, without significant head injury, and without other distracting injuries do not need pelvic radiographs.[2,6] There are no clinical decision rules for the pelvis that have been prospectively studied and validated. Therefore, clinical judgment is necessary to decide how much pain or tenderness should prompt the ordering of radiographs. Certain groups are at high risk. The elderly woman who falls and complains of hip pain should have a pelvic film because fractures of the pubic rami (and of the proximal femur) are common. In younger patients, a greater force of injury and degree of pain are expected with skeletal injury.

Pelvic Angiography

Pelvic hemorrhage can be life-threatening, requiring rapid identification and treatment. Pelvic bleeding can be arterial, venous, or osseous. In the hemodynamically unstable patient with a significant pelvic fracture and a negative diagnostic peritoneal lavage, pelvic angiography and embolization of arterial hemorrhage can be lifesaving. To control significant venous bleeding, external fixation may be performed prior to angiography in order to decrease blood loss resulting from pelvic venous disruption.[7,8]

Visceral Injuries

The incidence of visceral injuries associated with pelvic fractures is high. Blood at the urethral meatus, gross hematuria, a high-riding prostate, and perineal ecchymosis suggest a urethral or bladder disruption. If a urethral tear is suspected in a male patient, a Foley catheter should not be inserted until a retrograde urethrogram is performed. Attempts at catheter insertion in the male may convert a partial urethral tear to a complete tear, which is difficult to repair surgically. Gross hematuria may also be due to a bladder rupture, which can be diagnosed by cystography. However, if pelvic angiography is being con-

TABLE 12-1

Indications for Pelvic Radiography

PHYSICAL EXAMINATION	UNRELIABLE EXAMINATION
Gross deformities, including rotation of the hip and shortening of the extremity	Head injury
	Inability to assess pain and neurologic status accurately (including patients with spinal cord injury)
Ecchymosis, swelling, or laceration over the pelvis, perineum, lower lumbar and medial thigh	Drug and/or alcohol intoxication
Blood at the urethral meatus	
Gross hematuria	
Instability on pelvic compression*	
Tenderness to palpation	
Rectal examination with abnormal tone, high-riding prostate, bony protuberances	

*A controversial maneuver. Hemostasis may be disrupted by movement of an unstable pelvis.

sidered, cystography must be deferred because radiographic contrast material that has extravasated from a ruptured bladder interferes with angiographic imaging. In addition, if abdominal computed tomography (CT) is to be performed, cystography should also be deferred because extravasated contrast from an intraperitoneal bladder rupture interferes with the identification of intraperitoneal hemorrhage on CT. Vaginal or rectal bleeding in the setting of a pelvic fracture is indicative of an open fracture with bone fragments penetrating these tissues.

Supplementary Skeletal Radiographs

Only after the patient has been adequately stabilized should further skeletal radiologic evaluation of the pelvis be considered. Additional studies aid in determining orthopedic management. This is usually deferred until after the patient is admitted to the hospital.

Patients in whom disruption of the pelvic ring is noted on the initial AP radiograph need further radiographic investigation to fully define the skeletal injury. Traditionally, this was accomplished with inlet and outlet views, which are AP views of the pelvis with the beam angled caudad and cranially. However, CT provides better anatomic delineation of the extent of the pelvic fracture and has therefore become the primary imaging modality in pelvic ring disruptions. Acetabular fractures also warrant further imaging, and CT has largely replaced supplementary oblique (Judet) views. CT reveals the anatomy and extent of acetabular fractures in great detail. CT can also identify intraarticular bone fragments that would otherwise go undetected.[9] Judet views should be used in conjunction with CT to identify fractures in the axial plane that are poorly seen on CT.

Occasionally, supplementary plain-film views are used in the emergency department (ED) to clarify a questionable abnormality on the routine AP film. However, clinical findings often resolve the issue. For example, if there is a question of a subtle, nondisplaced acetabular fracture on the AP film and the

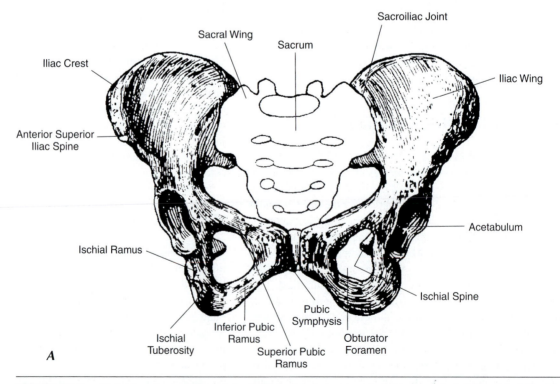

A

FIGURE 12-1. Skeletal anatomy of the pelvis. *A.* The pelvis is composed of two innominate bones (shaded) and the sacrum. There are three articulations–two sacroiliac joints and the pubic symphysis. *B.* Innominate bone (lateral view). *C.* Innominate bone (medial view) The quadrilateral plate is the medial surface of the acetabulum, which forms the radiographic ilioischial line. (From Pansky B: *Review of Gross Anatomy*, 6th ed. New York: McGraw-Hill, 1996. With permission.)

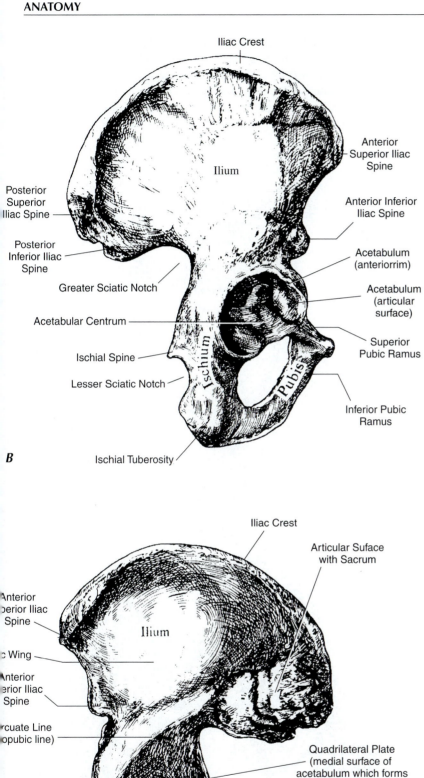

Figure B (top):
- Iliac Crest
- Ilium
- Anterior Superior Iliac Spine
- Anterior Inferior Iliac Spine
- Acetabulum (anterior rim)
- Acetabulum (articular surface)
- Superior Pubic Ramus
- Inferior Pubic Ramus
- Posterior Superior Iliac Spine
- Posterior Inferior Iliac Spine
- Greater Sciatic Notch
- Acetabular Centrum
- Ischial Spine
- Lesser Sciatic Notch
- Ischium
- Pubis
- Ischial Tuberosity

B

Figure (bottom):
- Iliac Crest
- Articular Suface with Sacrum
- Ilium
- Anterior Superior Iliac Spine
- Iliac Wing
- Anterior Inferior Iliac Spine
- Arcuate Line (iliopubic line)
- Superior Pubic Ramus
- Quadrilateral Plate (medial surface of acetabulum which forms the radiographic ilioischial line)
- Ischial Spine
- Ischial Ramus
- Pubis
- Ischium
- Pubic Symphysis (articular surface)
- Obturator Foramen
- Ischial Tuberosity
- Inferior Pubic Ramus

patient has minimal pain, it is unlikely that the questionable radiographic abnormality represents a fracture. If there is significant pain of the hip, oblique (Judet) views can demonstrate the fracture and confirm the diagnosis. Supplementary plain radiographs can also be helpful when CT images are compromised by scatterings from metallic implants.

ANATOMY

The pelvis is a relatively rigid ring with minimal flexibility. It is composed of three bones and three joints (the symphysis pubis and two sacroiliac [SI] joints) (Fig. 12-1). The ilium, the ischium, and the pubis are collectively known as the *innominate bone.* They merge to create the acetabulum. The two innominate bones form the anterior and lateral parts of the pelvic ring. The major component of the posterior pelvis is the sacrum. A ridge runs along the inner surface of the innominate bone that makes up the inner circumference of the pelvis and is known as the *arcuate line.*

The anterior portion of the innominate bone is formed by the superior and inferior pubic rami and the body of the pubic bone. The pubic rami together with the ischial ramus form the obturator ring. The body or midportion of the innominate bone makes up the acetabulum. The acetabular articular surface is crescent-shaped and is open inferiorly. The nonarticular center of the acetabulum is called the *centrum.* The innominate bone is thin in this region. Both anterior and posterior to the thin central region are stronger sections of bone forming the anterior and posterior columns of the acetabulum. Superior to the acetabulum is the strong, weight-bearing portion of the ileum known as the acetabular dome. The flat, medial surface of the body of the innominate bone is called the *quadrilateral plate.* The posterior and superior portion of the innominate bone is made up of the iliac wing, bordered by the iliac crest and the articular surface of the SI joint.

The stability of the posterior pelvis is maintained by the SI joints (Table 12-2). The iliolumbar ligaments link the ilium and the transverse process of the fifth lumbar vertebra, providing additional posterior support. The innominate bones are also joined to the sacrum by the sacrotuberous and sacrospinous ligaments, which form a strong sling across the base of the pelvis (Fig. 12-2). The fibrocartilaginous pubic symphysis and its supporting ligaments provide stability to the anterior portion of the ring. The anterior elements are weaker and more easily

TABLE 12-2

Major Ligaments of the Pelvis

Anterior and posterior sacroiliac ligaments	Support SI joints
Iliolumbar ligament	From transverse process of L5 to posterior iliac crest
Sacrotuberous ligament	From inferior sacrum to ischial tuberosity
Sacrospinous ligament	From inferior sacrum to ischial spine
Pubic symphysis and associated ligaments	Stabilize pelvis anteriorly

disrupted than the posterior elements. The anterior pelvis is important in shielding the urethra and bladder from blunt forces.

The visceral compartments of the pelvis are divided by the arcuate line into the false pelvis above and the true pelvis below. The false pelvis, or major pelvis, lies above the arcuate line and contains the lower portion of the abdominal viscera.

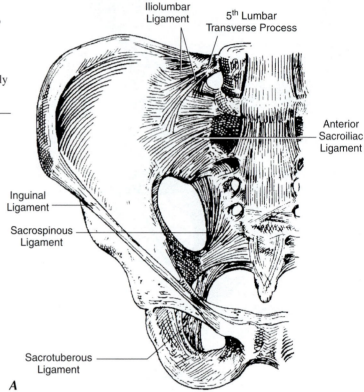

A

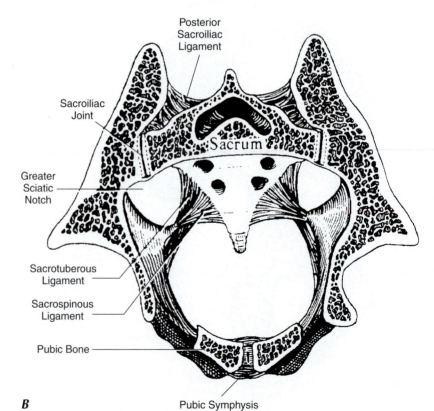

B

FIGURE 12-2. Ligamentous anatomy of the pelvis. *A.* Anterior view of the pelvis. *B.* Coronal section showing the ligamentous support of the pelvis. (From Pansky B: *Review of Gross Anatomy*, 6th ed. New York: McGraw-Hill, 1996. With permission.)

The true pelvis, or minor pelvis, lies below the arcuate line and contains the pelvic organs and neurovascular structures.

The major arteries of the pelvis include the common iliac, internal iliac, and external iliac arteries (Fig. 12-3). Branches of the internal iliac artery are especially susceptible to injury. Trauma to the anterolateral pelvis may tear the pudendal and vesical arteries. The superior gluteal artery passes through the sciatic notch and is often injured during shearing of the SI joint. Involvement of the median sacral, lateral sacral, and iliolumbar arteries can occur with sacral fractures. Pelvic veins accompany the arteries and sustain similar injuries.

Skeletal Development

In children, separate ossification centers of the innominate bone are present (Fig. 12-4). The triradiate cartilage (Y-shaped cartilage) is formed by the merger of the ilium, ischium, and pubis at the acetabulum. There are separate ossification centers for the ischial and pubic rami, the iliac crests, the iliac and ischial spines, and the ischial tuberosities. The femoral capital epiphysis is another ossification center.

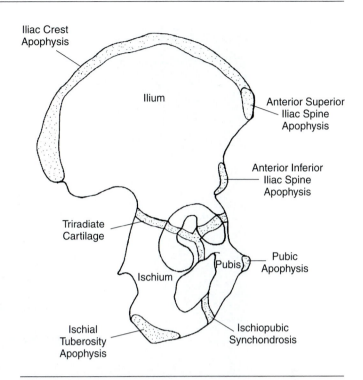

FIGURE 12-4. Growth plates and ossification centers in the developing pelvis, including the triradiate cartilage. (Adapted from Rogers LF: *The Radiology of Skeletal Trauma*, 2d ed. New York: Churchill-Livingstone, 1992. With permission.) (Adapted from *Gray's Anatomy: The Anatomical Basis of Medicine and Surgery.* PL Williams, LH Bannister, MM Berry. Harcourt Brace, London, 1995.)

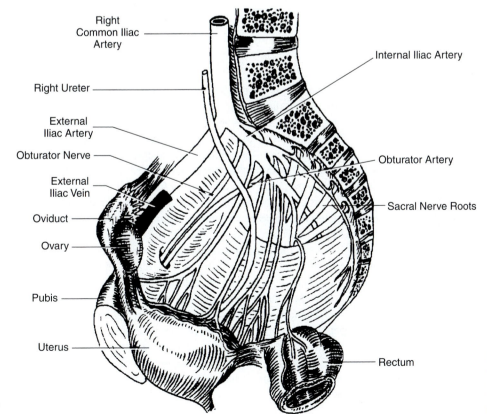

FIGURE 12-3. Visceral anatomy of the pelvis. The major arteries and sacral nerve roots are shown. (From Pansky B: *Review of Gross Anatomy*, 6th ed. New York: McGraw-Hill, 1996. With permission.)

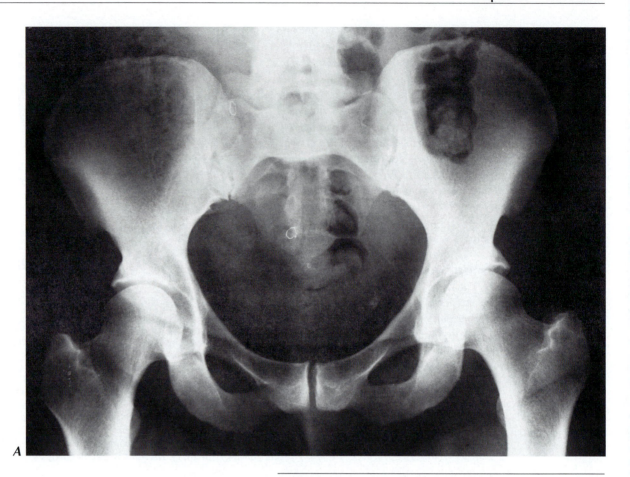

FIGURE 12-5.   *A, B.* Radiographic anatomy of the AP pelvis view.

RADIOGRAPHIC TECHNIQUE AND RADIOGRAPHIC ANATOMY

Standard AP Pelvis View

The radiographic assessment of pelvic trauma is unique in skeletal radiography because only one view is obtained—an AP radiograph (Fig. 12-5). On the AP view, most injuries to the sacral wings, iliac bones, ischium, pubis, and femoral neck are identified. While easily and rapidly obtained in the acute trauma setting, the AP view can miss injuries to the acetabulum, sacroiliac joints, and sacrum. In addition, even when a fracture is identified on the AP view, this single view may not define the extent of the injury completely.

Radiographic Anatomy

There are several anatomic landmarks to identify on a plain AP radiograph of the pelvis (Fig. 12-5). The *arcuate line* makes up the inner circumference of the pelvic skeleton. Posteriorly, the arcuate line is continuous with the sacral neuroforaminal lines. Anteriorly, the arcuate line is also known as the *iliopubic line* or the iliopectineal line. The *ilioischial line* is a radiographic line representing the surface of the quadrilateral plate of the innominate bone (the medial wall of the acetabulum). The anteroinferior rim of the acetabular surface forms a radiographic U. The *radiographic teardrop* is formed by the confluence of the articular surface of the acetabulum, the anteroinferior rim of the acetabulum, and the ilioischial line (Fig. 12-6). The articular surface of the acetabulum often has a gap or irregularity in its midportion due the interruption of the articular surface by the *centrum*. There is a corresponding irregularity in the articular surface of the femoral head, known as the *fovea*, where the ligamentum teres inserts.

Depending on the exact angle of the x-ray beam through this region of the pelvis, the three components of the radiographic teardrop might not align to give the teardrop appearance. In a nonrotated pelvic radiograph, asymmetry is due either to a fracture through the acetabulum or a displaced disruption of the pelvic ring.

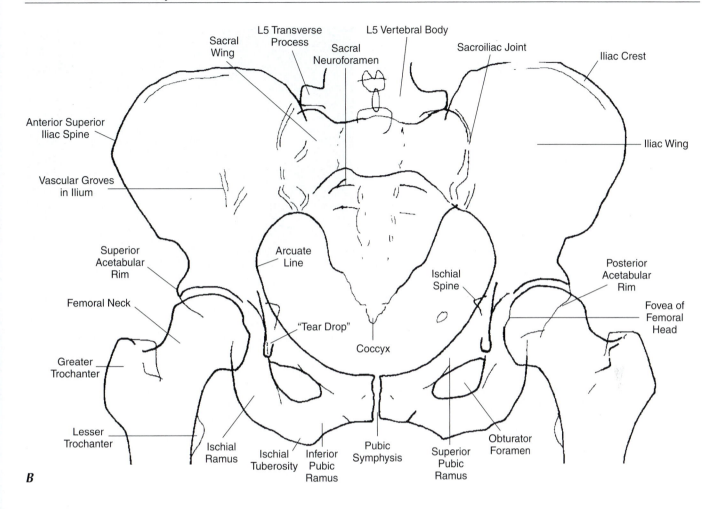

B

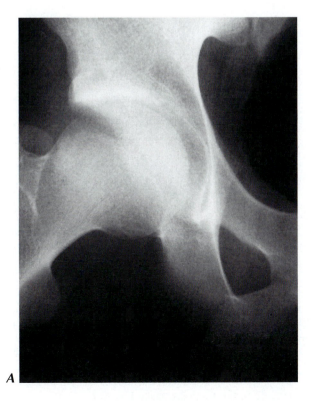

A

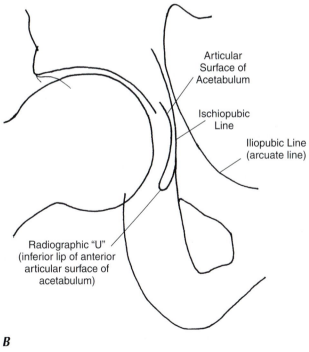

B

FIGURE 12-6. The "radiographic teardrop" of the acetabulum. The alignment of the ischiopubic line with the radiographic U depends on the positioning of the patient. The complete teardrop is not always seen.

Pediatric Anatomy

Incomplete ossification results in radiographically open growth plates and secondary ossification centers (Figs. 12-4 and 12-7). Complete closure does not occur until late adolescence or early adulthood.

Supplementary Radiographic Views

There are several supplementary methods by which pelvic injuries are further evaluated (Table 12-3). However, CT has largely supplanted these supplementary plain-film views in most circumstances.

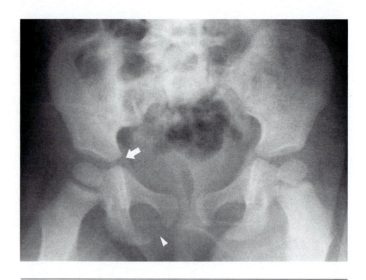

FIGURE 12-7.   Growth plates and ossification centers in a 2-year-old child. The triradiate cartilage (*arrow*), ischiopubic synchondrosis (*arrowhead*), and femoral head growth plate are open. None of the apophyseal ossification centers of the pelvis are seen at this age.

TABLE 12-3

Radiographic Views of the Pelvis

VIEW	POSITION	FINDINGS
Anteroposterior (AP)	Supine position. Pubic symphysis is aligned with the sacral spinous processes. Entire iliac crest, lower lumbar spine, and proximal femurs included. Position with hips in neutral position with slight external rotation is acceptable. If a nondisplaced femoral neck fracture is suspected, 15° of internal rotation of the hips is preferred.	Most injuries to the pubic rami, sacral wings, iliac bones, acetabulum, ischium, and proximal femur.
Anterior Judet view (internal oblique) (obturator oblique)	Supine position with patient anteriorly rotated with affected hip elevated 45°.	Acetabular fractures: anterior column (iliopubic line) and posterior rim.
Posterior Judet view (external oblique) (iliac oblique)	Supine position with patient anteriorly rotated with unaffected hip elevated 45°.	Acetabular fractures: posterior column (ilioischial line) and anterior rim.
Inlet	40 to 50° of caudal angulation perpendicular to the plane of the pelvic inlet.	Inward displacement of the pelvic rim and acetabulum. Displacement of the ilium at the sacroiliac joint.
Outlet	35 to 40° of cephalad angulation.	Fractures of the sacrum, sacroiliac disruption, fractures of the anterior pubic region, and obturator ring.
Lateral sacral view		Transverse fracture of sacral body.
Computed tomography	Axial slices through the iliac and sacal wings, the acetabular dome, and the acetabulum. Thin slices through the acetabulum are preferred (1.5 to 5 mm).	Fracture anatomy and complexity including articular involvement and intra-articular bone fragments. Best for acetabular and sacral fractures. May miss injuries that lie in the axial plane. Three-dimensional reconstructions are helpful for complex acetabular fractures.

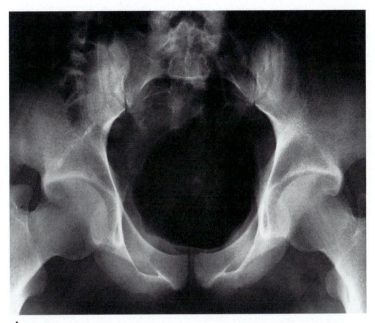

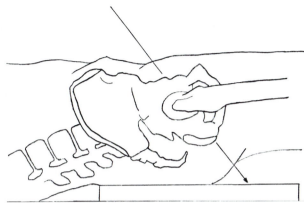

A

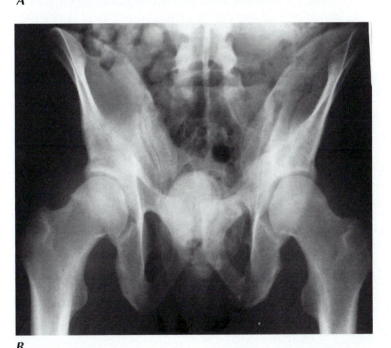

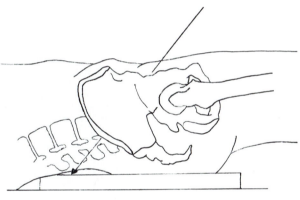

B

FIGURE 12-8. *A.* Inlet view of the pelvis. X-ray beam is angled 25° to 45° caudad. *B.* Outlet view of the pelvis. X-ray beam is angled 35° to 45° cephalad.

INLET AND OUTLET VIEWS. Angled views of the pelvis provide additional information in assessing pelvic ring disruptions (Fig. 12-8). The *inlet view* is obtained by directing the beam 35° to 60° caudad into the midpelvis. This provides better visualization of displacement of the pelvic ring and acetabulum. It is also the best view to demonstrate malalignment at the SI joint, especially posterior displacement of the ilium. The *outlet view* is useful in the evaluation of fractures of the sacrum or SI disruption. This view is obtained by directing the x-ray beam 25°

to 40° cephalad and centered on the pubic symphysis, giving a frontal view of the sacroiliac joints, sacrum, pubic symphysis, and pubic rami.

These angled AP views could potentially be used in the ED if there is a questionable abnormality on the straight AP view (e.g., pubic ramus). Because these views are taken at a different angle than the AP view, they may reveal the injury. With more severe injuries, CT is preferable once the patient has been stabilized.

OBLIQUE (JUDET) VIEWS.   *Oblique (Judet) views* are used to visualize acetabular anatomy (Fig. 12-9). To be positioned for the *anterior Judet view,* the supine patient's affected side is raised 45°. The x-ray beam is directed vertically through the affected hip. Thus the x-ray beam effectively passes medially through the patient at a 45° angle; therefore this view is also called an *internal oblique.* On this view, the obturator ring is seen *en face,* so this view is also called an *obturator oblique* (Fig. 12-9*B*). The anterior column of the acetabulum (the iliopubic line) and posterior lip of the acetabulum are seen. The *posterior Judet view* is obtained with the unaffected hip elevated 45° and the x-ray beam is directed through the affected hip (Fig. 12-9*C*). The view is also called an *external oblique* or *iliac oblique* (since the iliac wing is seen *en face*). The posterior column of the acetabulum (ilioischial line) and anterior rim of the acetabulum are seen.

Judet views are poorly tolerated by injured patients because of the manipulation required for positioning. In such cases, supine oblique views are an alternative, although these views are more difficult to interpret because there is greater distortion.

Currently, CT is the preferred study of acetabular fractures because of its great anatomic definition. Judet views play a secondary role. Occasionally, an injured patient will have a questionable abnormality in the region of the acetabulum on the AP view. In such a circumstance, an oblique (Judet) view might prove useful in the ED.

LATERAL SACRAL VIEW.   The *lateral sacral view* can assess sacral fractures in the transverse plane. Although most sacral fractures are difficult to evaluate fully on plain radiographs and are better defined by CT, fractures that lie in the transverse plane might not appear on CT and be better visualized by plain films.

Computed Tomography

CT provides greater detail for complex pelvic and intraarticular fractures of the hip. CT has largely supplanted the supplementary plain radiographic views of the pelvis mentioned above. CT reconstructions with three-dimensional surface rendering provide excellent anatomical depiction of complex acetabular fractures.

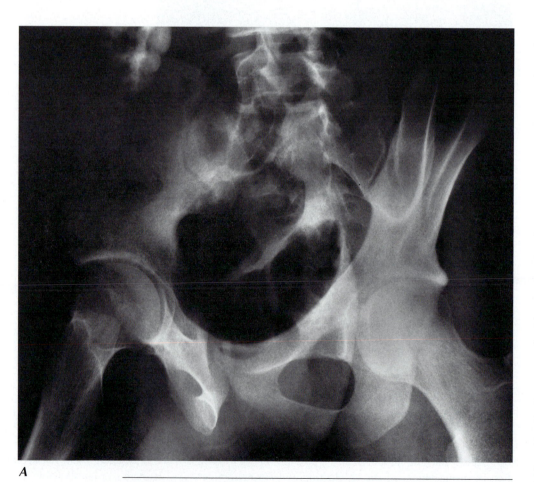

A

FIGURE 12-9.   Oblique (Judet) views of the pelvis. *A.* Oblique view showing both sides of pelvis (anterior oblique view of left side of pelvis; posterior oblique view of right side of pelvis). *B.* Anterior oblique view (obturator oblique or internal oblique view). The injured side of pelvis is raised 45° off table. *C.* Posterior oblique view (iliac oblique or external oblique view). The opposite side of pelvis is raised 45° off table.

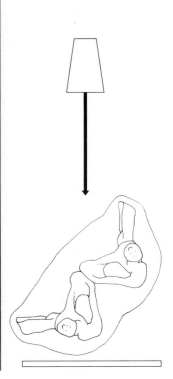

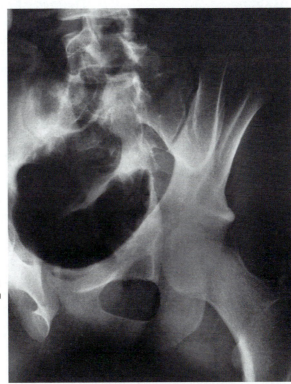

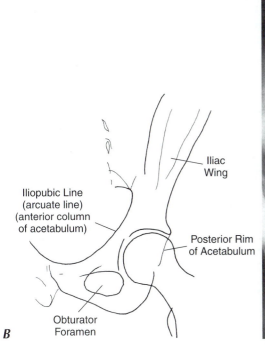

Iliac
Wing

Iliopubic Line
(arcuate line)
(anterior column
of acetabulum)

Posterior Rim
of Acetabulum

Obturator
Foramen

B

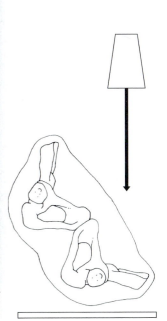

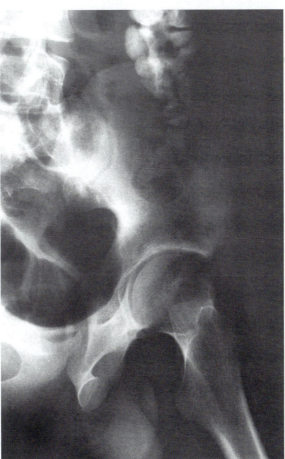

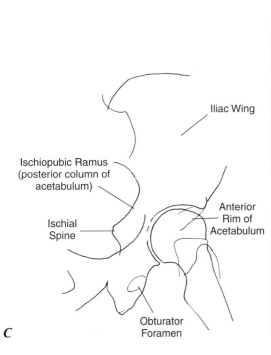

Iliac Wing

Ischiopubic Ramus
(posterior column of
acetabulum)

Ischial
Spine

Anterior
Rim of
Acetabulum

Obturator
Foramen

C

RADIOGRAPHIC ANALYSIS

It is important to use a systematic approach in analyzing the AP pelvis radiograph (Fig. 12-10). The pelvis radiograph can be reviewed as three concentric circles (Table 12-4 and Fig. 12-11), starting with the inner circumference of the pelvis (the arcuate line). Next, the bones of the pelvic ring itself are examined. The third concentric circle is the peripheral zone of structures outside the pelvic ring. If one break is noted in the pelvic ring, a second fracture should be sought.

The *first step* is an initial *overall screening* of the radiograph, looking for obvious fractures. The technical adequacy of the film is assessed, making certain that the pelvis is not rotated and ensuring that the entire pelvis is included.

Inner Circle

The inner circumference of the pelvis is made up of the *arcuate line,* which should be smooth, continuous, and symmetrical. Posteriorly, the arcuate line is continuous with the sacral neuroforaminal lines.

Middle Circle

Next, the middle concentric circle, consisting of the bones of the pelvis itself, is examined. The anterior structures are first reviewed, followed by the lateral structures and finally the posterior structures. Fracture lines, distortion or malalignment, or a lack of symmetry suggests injury.

Anterior. The *anterior structures* are the pubic bone and obturator ring. The pubic symphysis, body of the pubis, and superior and inferior pubic rami are examined bilaterally. Then, the circumference of the obturator foramen is traced. Last, the ischial ramus is inspected. If there is one break in the obturator ring, a second fracture elsewhere is sought, including a fracture of the acetabulum.

Lateral. Next, the *lateral portions* of the pelvis are examined. The integrity of the acetabulum is evaluated. Both sides are compared and should be symmetrical. The anterior and posterior columns of the acetabulum (the ilioischial and iliopubic lines) and the radiographic teardrop are traced (Fig. 12-6). Disruption of the teardrop suggests an injury to the acetabulum. Next, the articular surface of the acetabulum is traced. There is a normal gap in its midportion, at the *acetabular centrum.* The articular surface of the femoral head should nearly parallel the acetabular surface (the superior joint space is slightly narrower than the medial joint space). Last, the dome of the acetabulum (body of the iliac bone) is examined.

Posterior. Next, the *posterior portion* of the pelvis, the sacrum, is examined. The SI joints are inspected for discontinuity and asymmetry. The sacral wings (alae) are checked for fracture. These are the weakest portions of the sacrum because they are pierced by the sacral neuroforamina. The sacral neuroforaminal lines are examined for smoothness or discontinuity, comparing the left to the right. The body of the sacrum, sacral spines, and coccyx are examined.

Outer Circle

The third, outer concentric circle is made up of the *peripheral regions* outside of the pelvic ring—the iliac wings, anterior superior and anterior inferior iliac spines, proximal femurs, ischial tuberosities, and lumbar spine. Fractures in this region do not involve the pelvic ring.

TABLE 12-4

Systematic Analysis of the Pelvis Radiograph

Adequacy	Both iliac crests, proximal femurs, and lower lumbar spine No rotation–The symphysis pubis aligns in the midline with the sacralspinous processes
Initial overview	Anatomic structures are *symmetrical,* smooth in contour, and lack discontinuity or fracture lines
THREE CONCENTRIC CIRCLES	
Inner circle	Arcuate line Sacral neuroforaminal lines
Middle circle Anterior	Superior and inferior pubic rami Obturator ring—if one break is noted, search for a second break Pubic symphysis—no wider than 5 mm
Lateral	Acetabulum—"radiographic teardrop" Iliopubic line, ilioischial line, and radiographic U Articular surface of acetabulum and femoral head Acetabular rims (anterior and posterior) Acetabular dome and body of the ilium
Posterior	Sacrum Sacral neuroforaminal lines and sacral wings SI joints Body of sacrum, coccyx L5 transverse process
Outer circle Anterior	Ischial tuberosity Proximal femur—femoral neck, intertrochanteric region
Lateral	Iliac wing Anterior superior and inferior iliac spines
Posterior	Lumbar vertebrae L5 transverse process fracture (indicates SI joint disruption)
Reevaluate	If there is one break in the pelvic ring or obturator ring, search for a second break If there is a questionable abnormality, additional views may be helpful—inlet, outlet, oblique (Judet) views, or CT

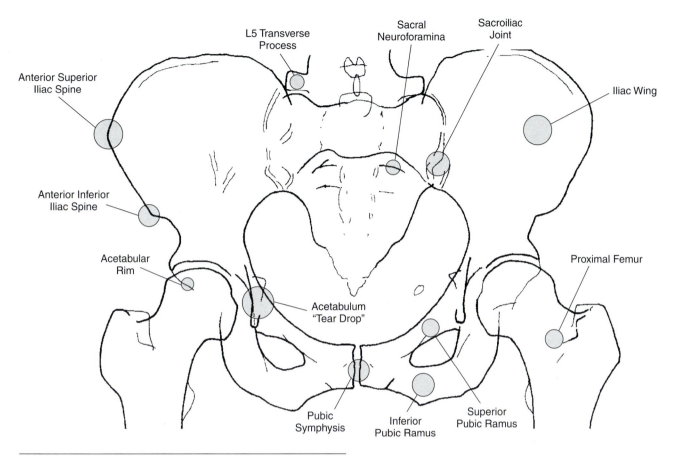

FIGURE 12-10. Sites prone to injury and easily missed injuries.

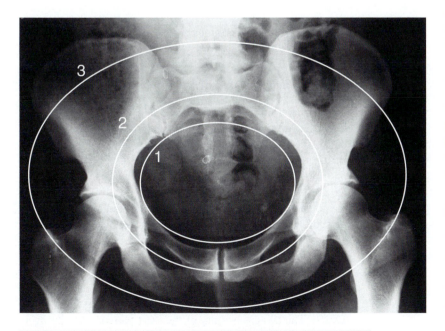

FIGURE 12-11. Three concentric circles—systematic analysis of the AP pelvis radiograph. 1. Inner circle—the arcuate line and sacral neuroforamina. 2. Middle circle—the pelvic bones. 3. Outer circle—peripheral areas outside the pelvic ring.

Fractures of the iliac wing appear as dark fracture lines or bright white lines if the fracture fragments are overlapping. A normal vascular groove must be distinguished from a fracture line. The iliac crest and iliac spines are sites of avulsion fractures. The femoral head, femoral neck, and intertrochanteric region are examined for fractures. Then, the ischial tuberosities are inspected.

Last, the lower lumbar vertebrae are inspected, checking the vertebral bodies, spinous processes, and transverse processes. A fracture through the fifth lumbar transverse process is caused by the pull of the iliolumbar ligament. An L5 transverse process fracture may be the only indication of nondisplaced fracture through the sacroiliac joint (part of a pelvic ring disruption).

Reexamine

If one break in the pelvic ring is found, a second break must be carefully sought. If there is a questionable abnormality, supplementary views (inlet views, outlet views, oblique views, or CT) can be obtained.

The *obturator internus muscle* is often seen on both sides of the pelvis as a dark gray crescent on the inner surface of the acetabulum. Bulging or loss of this line can signify an occult acetabular fracture.[10]

TABLE 12-5

Kane Classification of Pelvic Fractures

I. Fractures of individual bones without disruption of the
pelvic ring
   A. Avulsion fractures
      1. Anterior superior iliac spine
      2. Anterior inferior iliac spine
      3. Ischial tuberosity
   B. Single fracture of pubic ramus
   C. Fracture of the iliac wing (Duverney fracture)
   D. Transverse fracture of the sacrum
   E. Coccygeal fracture
II. Single breaks in the pelvic ring
   A. Fracture of two ipsilateral rami
   B. Fracture near, or slight separation of, the symphysis pubis
   C. Fracture near, or subluxation of, the sacroiliac joint
III. Two or more breaks in the pelvic ring
   A. Double vertical fractures of the pubis (straddle fracture)
   B. Double vertical fractures or dislocation of the pelvis
      (Malgaigne or bucket-handle fracture)
   C. Severe multiple fractures
IV. Acetabular fractures
   A. Nondisplaced
   B. Displaced

TABLE 12-6

Eponyms and Descriptive Names for Pelvic Fractures

Duverney fracture	Iliac wing fracture without disruption of the pelvic ring.
Straddle fracture	Fractures of all four pubic rami (both obturator rings) due to direct anterior impact to pubic region.
Malgaigne fracture	Pelvic ring disruption with unilateral fractures of the pubic rami and ipsilateral posterior injury. Vertical shear mechanism of injury.
Bucket-handle fracture	Pelvic ring disruption with unilateral fractures of the pubic rami and contralateral posterior injury.
Open-book pelvis	Separation of the pubic symphysis with bilateral disruption of the anterior sacroiliac, sacrospinous, and sacrotuberous ligaments.
Closed-book pelvis	Lateral compression injury causing inward displacement of one side of pelvis.

COMMON ABNORMALITIES

Several classification systems of pelvic fractures exist, including those based on location of the fracture (ilium, ischium, pubis, sacrum), the integrity of the weight-bearing arches of the pelvis, and the number of breaks in the pelvic ring. The injury pattern determines mechanical stability, which is important in deciding on definitive management (operative versus nonoperative). In the Kane classification system (Table 12-5), fractures are graded according to increasing complexity and severity: (1) fractures without disruption of the pelvic ring, (2) single breaks in the pelvic ring, (3) double breaks in the pelvic ring, and (4) acetabular fractures. Finally, there are also eponyms and descriptive names applied to various injury patterns. However, these often fail to clarify the nature of the injury (Table 12-6).

Disruptions of the Pelvic Ring

The classification system developed by Young and Burgess (Table 12-7) is based on the observation that the direction of the force of injury determines the fracture pattern. Fractures are grouped into those caused by lateral compression, anteroposterior compression, vertical shear, or a combination of forces.

LATERAL COMPRESSION INJURIES.   Lateral compression injuries are the most common major traumatic injuries (Fig. 12-12). Clinical settings that cause lateral compression injuries include those where a pedestrian has been struck laterally by a moving car or a passenger is injured in a vehicle that has been struck on the side. The lateral compression force creates fractures in the coronal plane across the pubic rami, usually on the side of the impact. Contralateral fractures of the pubic rami may be present. Posteriorly, there is an impaction fracture of the sacrum at the sacral neuroforamina. The sacrospinous and sacrotuberous ligaments are compressed. There are three grades of lateral compression (LC) injury.

LC-I.   The most commonly seen fracture pattern is LC-I (Fig. 12-13). The posterior injury of the LC-I pattern is easily overlooked; it is best detected by careful examination of the margins of the sacral neuroforamina for discontinuity. LC-I injuries are relatively stable.

TABLE 12-7

Young Classification of Pelvic Ring Disruptions

Lateral compression	Fracture of at least one set of pubic rami. Compressive posterior injury
LC-I	Compression of SI region on the side of impact
LC-II	Compression of SI region with either a tear of the posterior SI ligament, or an iliac wing fracture
LC-III	LC-II on side of impact with contralateral external rotation injury—"wind-swept pelvis"
AP compression	Widening of symphysis pubis or pubic rami fractures. Widening of posterior elements (unilateral or bilateral)
APC-I	Minimal widening of pubic symphysis. Posterior elements intact
APC-II	Anterior SI, sacrotuberous, and sacrospinous ligaments disrupted. Posterior SI ligaments intact
APC-III	Posterior SI ligaments disruption as well as anterior SI sacrotuberous, and sacrospinous ligaments
Vertical shear (VS)	Vertical displacement at anterior and posterior pelvis
Mixed injury	Combination of above injury patterns

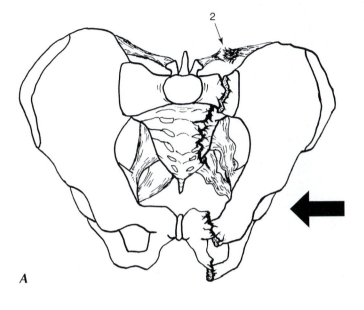

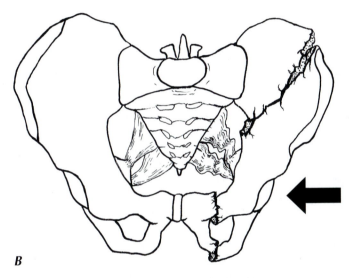

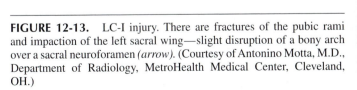

FIGURE 12-12. Lateral compression injuries (LC). A laterally directed force causes inward rotation of the hemipelvis and oblique or coronal fractures of the pubic rami. Posteriorly, there is an impaction fracture of the ipsilateral sacral wing. With grade II injuries, the sacral fracture is more severe and the posterior SI ligaments are torn (*arrow 2*). *B.* Alternatively in a grade II injury, there is a fracture through the iliac wing. These lateral compression injuries are referred to as "closed-book" pelvis.

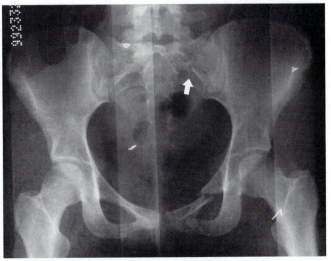

FIGURE 12-13. LC-I injury. There are fractures of the pubic rami and impaction of the left sacral wing—slight disruption of a bony arch over a sacral neuroforamen *(arrow).* (Courtesy of Antonino Motta, M.D., Department of Radiology, MetroHealth Medical Center, Cleveland, OH.)

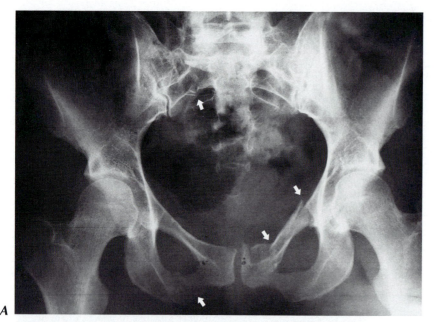

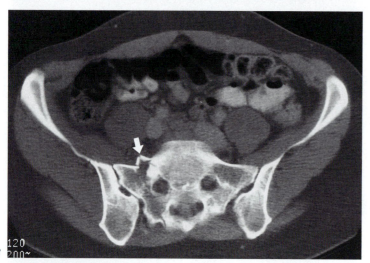

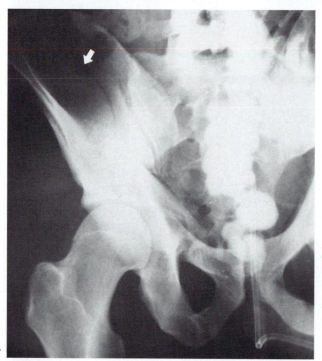

LC-II. A greater lateral compression force produces the LC-II injury (Fig. 12-14). In addition to the fractures of the pubic rami, a displaced fracture of the ipsilateral iliac or sacral wing is present. This fracture usually starts from the inferior portion of the SI joint and extends in a cephalad direction through the posterior iliac wing. Although more mobile to internal rotation than an LC-I, this injury is still relatively stable to external rotation and vertical movement because the sacrotuberous and sacrospinous ligaments are intact. LC-I and LC-II fractures are sometimes called "closed-book" pelvic injuries. They are associated with a lower risk of vascular injury because the volume of the pelvis is essentially reduced by the fracture. Extraperitoneal bladder rupture is associated with LC-II injuries, possibly as a result of impalement with sharp fragments of the pubic rami.

LC-III. LC-III injuries (Fig. 12-15) usually result when a victim is trapped between an unyielding object on one side and an injurious force is applied in a rolling fashion, as when a pedestrian is run over by a motor vehicle. This produces a LC injury on the side of the impact, with external rotational forces on the contralateral side producing tears in the anterior sacrospinous, sacrotuberous, and SI ligaments. This injury produces what is known as the "windswept pelvis." The forces disrupting the contralateral SI joint can also damage the nearby neurovascular structures. These fractures are highly unstable on the side of external rotation.

ANTEROPOSTERIOR COMPRESSION INJURIES. Anteroposterior compression (APC) injuries result from anteriorly or posteriorly directed forces on the pelvis. These injuries can be either directly (a pedestrian struck anteriorly by an oncoming vehicle) or indirectly transmitted through the extremities or the ischial tuberosities (as when a passenger in a motor vehicle is thrown against the dashboard with a flexed hip). There are three grades of APC injuries depending on the degree of ligamentous disruption (Table 12-7) (Fig. 12-16).

FIGURE 12-14. Lateral Compression Injuries. *A.* On the AP radiograph, there are bilateral pubic rami fractures and an impaction fracture through the right sacral wing. *B.* The CT shows the impaction fracture of the sacral wing (*arrow*). *C.* In another patient with lateral compression injury, there are fractures through the iliac wing (*arrow*) and pubic rami. (*A* and *B.* Copyright David T. Schwartz, M.D.)

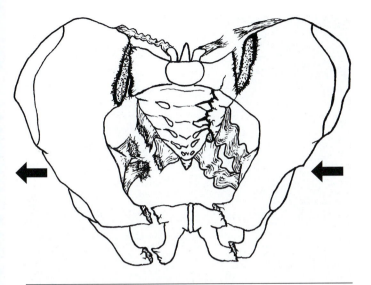

APC-I injuries stretch but do not tear the ligamentous supports of the pelvic ring. Radiographic findings include mild pubic diastasis (less than 3.5 cm) and imperceptible to mild widening of the SI joints (Fig. 12-17).

APC-II injuries tear the anterior SI ligaments as well as the sacrotuberous and sacrospinous ligaments. Radiographic findings include a widened anterior SI joint and an anterior pelvic ring injury. APC-II injuries can produce either unilateral or bilateral findings. Intact posterior ligamentous structures in an APC-II injury serve as a hinge, producing what has been described as the "open-book pelvis" (Fig. 12-18). There is often associated injury to the neurovascular structures, leading to hemorrhage, urethral injury, and neurologic deficits.

APC-III injuries result in complete disruption of the posterior SI ligaments, producing what is sometimes referred to as a "sprung pelvis" (Fig. 12-19). These mechanically unstable injuries are associated with a high rate of neurovascular injury.

FIGURE 12-15. LC-III injury. The forces of injury cause impaction of one side of the pelvis and widening (external rotation) of the contralateral side, with opening of the SI joint and tearing of the sacrospinous and sacrotuberous ligaments. This injury is referred to as a "windswept pelvis."

VERTICAL SHEAR INJURIES. Vertical shear injuries are the least common type of injury to the pelvis. They result from a vertical force, as in a patient who falls from a height and lands on the lower extremities. The pelvis is disrupted in a vertical plane, with cephalad or cephaloposterior displacement of the fracture segment. These are also referred to as *Malgaigne fractures* (Fig. 12-20). Vertical shear injuries are grossly unstable and are associated with a high incidence of neurovascular injury.

MIXED INJURIES. Many injuries represent a combination of the lateral compression, anteroposterior compression, and vertical shear mechanisms. These injuries are classified as having a complex or mixed pattern.

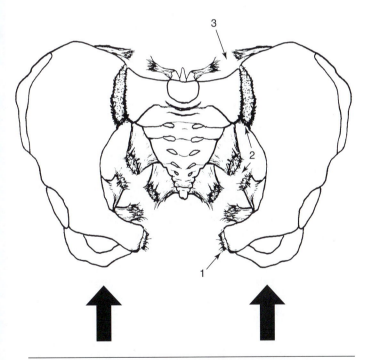

FIGURE 12-16. AP compression injury—open-book pelvis. An anteriorly directed force causes widening of the anterior pelvis, usually separation of the pubic symphysis (1). With grade II injuries, there is widening of one or both of the sacroiliac joints, with tearing of the sacrospinous and sacrotuberous ligaments (2). In grade III injuries, the SI joints are totally disrupted, with tearing of the posterior SI ligaments.

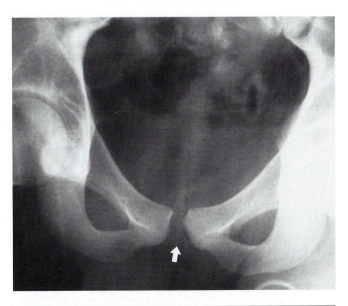

FIGURE 12-17. APC-I injury. There is slight widening of the pubic symphysis >3.5 cm (*arrow*) without widening of the SI joints.

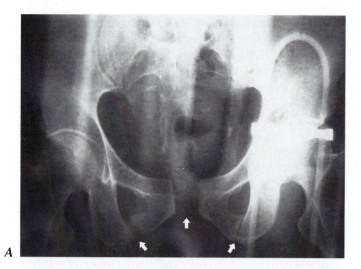

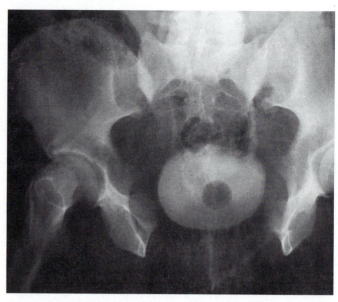

FIGURE 12-19.   APC-III injury. There is marked widening of the pubic symphysis and complete separation of both SI joints. This injury is sometimes referred to as a "sprung pelvis." The bladder is intact as shown by this contrast cystogram. (Foley catheter balloon inflated.) (Courtesy of Antonino Motta, M.D., Department of Radiology, MetroHealth Medical Center, Cleveland, OH.)

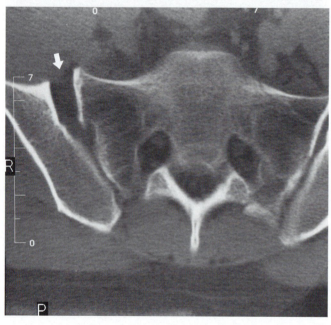

FIGURE 12-18.   APC-II injury. *A.* There is moderate widening of the pubic symphysis as well as bilateral fractures of the pubic rami. Slight widening of the right sacroiliac joint is difficult to detect on the AP view. *B.* CT shows widening of the anterior portion of the right sacroiliac joint. The posterior ligaments are intact. (Courtesy of Antonino Motta, M.D., Department of Radiology, MetroHealth Medical Center, Cleveland, OH.)

Other single breaks in the pelvic ring are less common. Subluxation of the symphysis pubis is rare. Nonetheless, subluxation can occur from direct AP forces. Subluxation of the symphysis pubis is more common in an already lax joint (as in pregnancy approaching parturition). Isolated fractures near the SI joint or subluxation of this joint are exceedingly rare. They usually result from blunt direct trauma to the posterolateral pelvis. Typically, the ilium is displaced posteriorly and toward the midline, overlapping the sacral shadow. Again, if a single break of the pelvic ring is identified, a second break must be carefully sought.

Fractures Not Involving the Pelvic Ring

Fractures without disruption in the pelvic ring also occur (Fig. 12-21). Single fractures of a pubic ramus are the most common type of pelvic fracture (Fig. 12-22). They are often seen in elderly patients and occasionally missed. They are of limited clinical consequence, though they can be painful and limit an older person's ability to live independently. These fractures can account for hip pain in elderly patients who have fallen and do not have a proximal femoral fracture. Fractures of the ischial ramus are rare. They may occur from falls in the sitting position or other direct blunt trauma to the ischial tuberosity.

Single Breaks in the Pelvic Ring

Ipsilateral fractures of the superior and inferior pubic rami are among the most common pelvic fractures. Many of these, however, may actually be mild LC-I injuries. When these injuries are studied with bone scan or MRI, a slight impaction fracture is frequently found in the sacral wing or SI joint. This posterior fracture is usually not of clinical consequence. Ipsilateral fractures of the rami are especially common in the elderly after minor trauma.

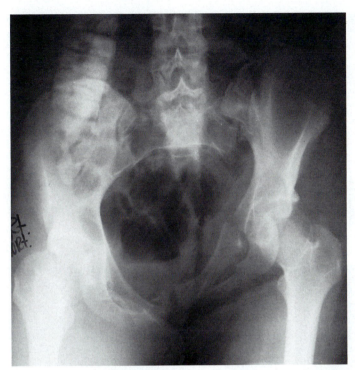

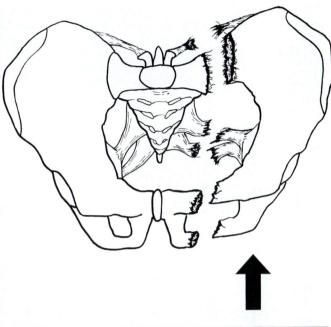

FIGURE 12-20. Vertical shear injury (VS). The left hemipelvis is displaced superiorly and multiple fractures are present. (Courtesy of Antonino Motta, M.D., Department of Radiology, MetroHealth Medical Center, Cleveland, OH.)

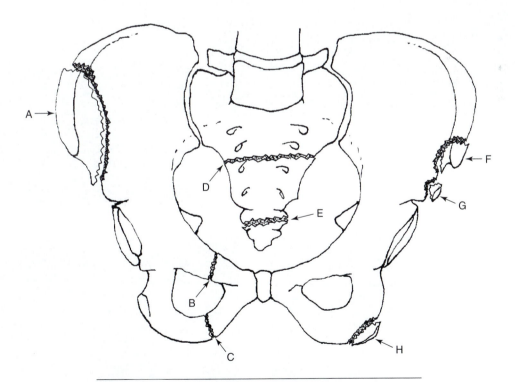

FIGURE 12-21. Isolated fractures that do not disrupt the pelvic ring. *A.* Iliac wing fracture (Duverney). *B.* Superior pubic ramus. *C.* Inferior pubic ramus. *D.* Transverse sacral fracture. *E.* Coccyx fracture. *F.* Anterior superior iliac spine avulsion. *G.* Anterior inferior iliac spine avulsion. *H.* Ischial tuberosity avulsion.

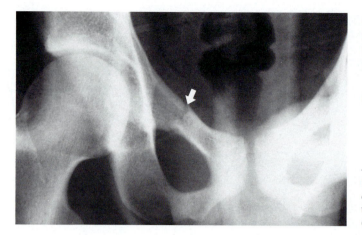

Fractures of the iliac wing result from direct lateral impact to the ilium (Fig. 12-23). These are usually minimally displaced because muscular forces retain the normal position of the ilium. Most are detected on routine AP views of the pelvis.

Avulsion fractures secondary to sudden and forceful muscular contractions are common in young persons with immature

FIGURE 12-22.   Isolated fracture of the pubic ramus. A minimally displaced fracture of the right superior pubic ramus is present. With this injury, a second fracture should be sought in the obturator ring (inferior pubic ramus) and the posterior pelvis (sacral wing).

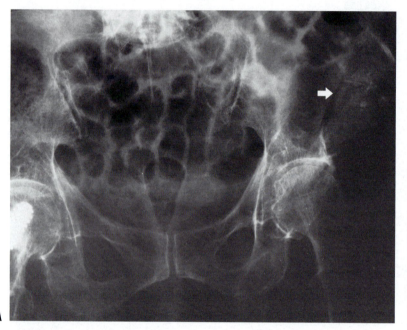

A

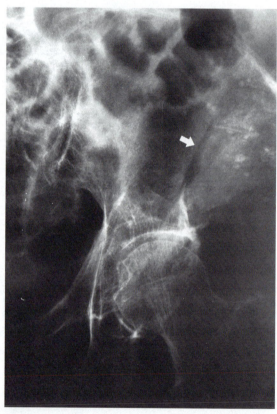

B

FIGURE 12-23.   Fractures of the iliac wing. *A.* A fracture of the iliac wing was missed on the initial radiograph interpretation in this elderly woman who had fallen on her hip. *B.* Examination of the film using a bright light reveals the fracture. *C.* In another patient, a fracture of the anterior iliac wing is faintly visible on the AP pelvic view. *D.* The fracture is readily apparent on CT. (*A* and *B* copyright David T. Schwartz, M.D.)

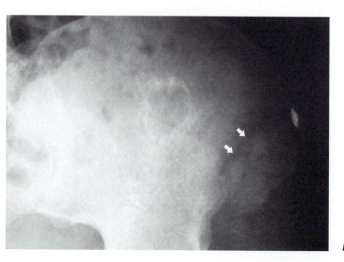

C

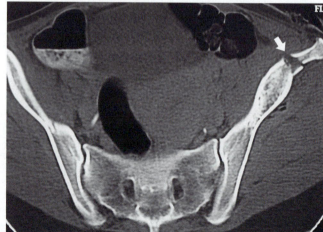

D

bone (e.g., teenage athletes). A sudden pull from the rectus femoris muscle (hip flexor) can result in an avulsion of the anterior inferior iliac spine (Fig. 12-24). Similar force involving the sartorius muscle produces the more common avulsion of the anterior superior iliac spine. Activities that forcefully contract the hamstrings (e.g., hurdling) cause avulsion of the ischial tuberosity.

Isolated fractures of the *sacrum* result from trauma to the posterior pelvis. Sacral fractures are commonly transverse and can be difficult to detect on plain AP radiographs. Since outlet views show the sacral alae and SI joints better, they can be use-

ful in detecting a sacral fracture (Fig. 12-25). A lateral view of the sacrum may be necessary to detect this injury. These injuries are characterized by ecchymosis, edema, pain over the sacrum, and abnormal mobility of the sacrum on rectal examination when bimanual alternating pressure is applied. They are associated with a high incidence of neurologic injury, usually involving higher sacral roots and sparing bowel and bladder function.

Fractures of the *coccyx* are caused by falls in the sitting position. Symptoms include pain on sitting and on defecation. Rising from a sitting position is quite painful. The diagnosis is

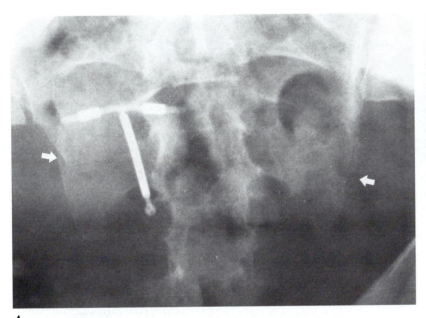

A

FIGURE 12-24. Transverse sacral fracture. *A.* The fracture is difficult to see on the AP view *(arrows). B.* A lateral sacral film reveals the fracture. (A T-shaped intrauterine contraceptive device is present.)

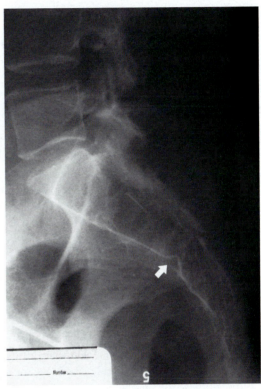

B

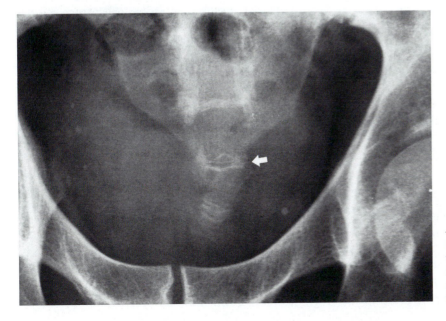

FIGURE 12-25. Fracture of the coccyx. These fractures are diagnosed clinically, by palpation during digital rectal examination. Radiographs are generally not necessary. Normal deformity of the coccyx can be difficult to distinguish from a fracture by radiographs.

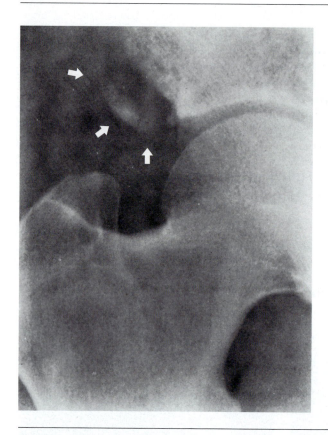

FIGURE 12-26.   An avulsion fracture of the anteroinferior iliac spine is due to the pull of the rectus femoris muscle. This is seen here in an adolescent athlete. (From Martire JR, Levinsohn EM: *Imaging of Athletic Injuries*. New York: McGraw-Hill, 1992. With permission.)

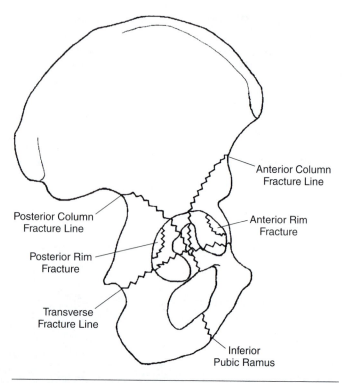

FIGURE 12-27.   Acetabular fractures. The three main fracture lines are shown: anterior column, posterior column, and transverse. Fractures of the anterior and posterior columns extend through the inferior pubic ramus. The Y-shaped fracture involves both the anterior and posterior columns. An anterior wall fracture involves the upper part of the anterior column fracture line and the anterior part of the transverse fracture line. A posterior wall fracture involves the corresponding portions of the posterior column and transverse fracture lines. Fractures of the acetabular rim are usually associated with hip dislocations.

made by rectal examination, showing an exquisitely tender and abnormally mobile coccyx. Radiographs are unnecessary (Fig. 12-26). Because the normal coccyx often has an irregular, deformed appearance, the radiographic signs of a coccygeal fracture are difficult to distinguish from the normal appearance.

Acetabular Fractures

The classification system for acetabular fractures is based on the division of the innominate bone into anterior and posterior columns. Fractures of the posterior (ilioischial) column are more common than fractures of the anterior (iliopubic) column. Posterior column fractures are frequently associated with posterior hip dislocations. Transverse fractures across both acetabular columns are also common. The remaining category includes Y-shaped fractures, in which the acetabulum is broken into three or more fragments. This is the most common type of acetabular fracture (Figs. 12-27 and 12-28).

Comminuted fractures due to direct impact on the hip can actually displace the femoral head through the acetabulum and quadrilateral plate. This injury is known as a *central hip dislo-

cation. Some acetabular fractures are limited to the rim of the articular surface. Posterior rim fractures are more common and are often associated with posterior hip dislocations.

Most acetabular fractures are visible on the standard AP pelvic film. Minimally displaced fractures can be subtle, and there may only be mild distortion or asymmetry of the acetabular contour lines that make up the *radiographic teardrop*. Oblique views (Judet views) can demonstrate a fracture that is not well seen on the AP view (Fig. 12-29).

Fractures of the posterior column disrupt the ilioischial line and may be better seen on the posterior oblique view (external oblique or iliac oblique). Fractures of the anterior column disrupt the iliopubic line and may be better seen on the anterior (internal or obturator) oblique view. Although the acetabular rims are difficult to see because of overlap by the femoral head, they should be scrutinized for evidence of a fracture. CT best defines the extent of an acetabular fracture and helps with operative planning. Judet views are helpful to the orthopedist by visualizing a fracture that lies in the horizontal plane and poorly seen by axial CT. CT is especially helpful because it can detect intraarticular bone fragments that are otherwise undetectable.

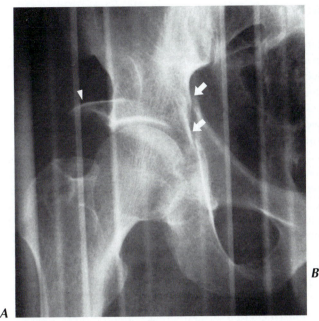

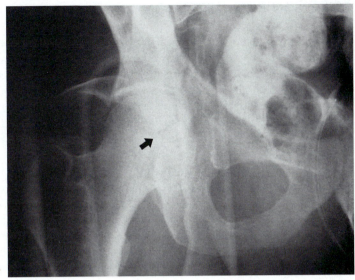

B

A

FIGURE 12-28. Acetabular fracture. *A.* On the AP view, an acetabular fracture involving both the iliopubic (arcuate) and ilioischial lines is seen (*arrows*). A fracture of the posterior acetabular rim is also present (*arrowhead*). *B.* On the obturator (internal) oblique view, the fracture is seen to traverse the entire acetabulum (*arrow*).

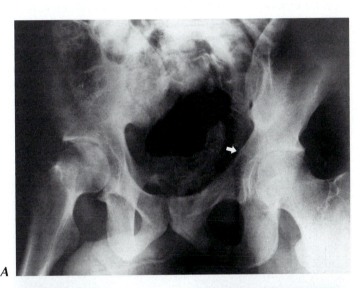

A

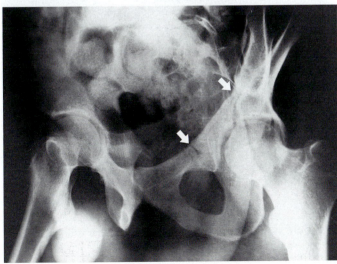

B

FIGURE 12-29. An acetabular fracture revealed by Judet views. *A.* On a slightly rotated AP view, there is only slight buckling of the arcuate line. *B.* On the internal (obturator) oblique view, the fractures are easily seen. *C.* CT shows the fracture clearly. (Copyright David T. Schwartz, M.D.)

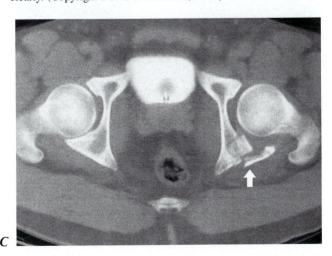

C

ERRORS IN INTERPRETATION

Fractures of the pubic ramus, especially those that are minimally displaced, are occasionally overlooked. Additional AP views at different angles, such as inlet or outlet views, can help clarify questionable abnormalities (Fig. 12-22). Fractures of the iliac crest can be difficult to see in slender elderly patients. Overpenetration of the radiograph in that region is common because there is relatively little soft tissue density compared with the midportion of the pelvis. The films should be viewed with a "bright light" to detect this injury (Fig. 12-23). Minimally displaced acetabular fractures can be difficult to see and must be carefully sought. Oblique (Judet) views may be warranted in questionable cases (Fig. 12-29). A fracture of the L5 transverse process may be the only indication of a nondisplaced injury of the SI joint.

COMMON VARIANTS

Several normal variants can be mistaken for pelvic pathology. Nutrient arteries cause grooves of the iliac wing or acetabular dome that should not be mistaken for fractures. In the child, cartilaginous growth plates such as the triradiate cartilage (of the acetabulum) and apophyses such as in the iliac crest and ischial tuberosity are occasionally misinterpreted as fractures (Figs. 12-30 and 12-31). There may be variation in the closure of the iliopubic and ischiopubic synchondroses, producing an irregular appearance or impression of displacement of the bone along these growth plates. The symphysis pubis may appear to be abnormally widened in the adolescent and may exhibit some malalignment and irregularity in the adult. In adolescents, the ischial tuberosity apophysis can mimic an avulsion fracture.

ADVANCED STUDIES

Computed Tomography.   CT is widely used in the evaluation of pelvic fractures. It is useful in the evaluation of sacral and acetabular fractures, which are frequently missed or poorly delineated on plain radiographs. CT is also helpful when plain radiographs have equivocal findings. Three-dimensional CT is useful in imaging complex skeletal surfaces, especially fractures of the acetabulum.

Most often, CT is used to assess the complete extent of a fracture, the degree of displacement, the presence of intraarticular debris, and the disruption of the articular surface.[11] While not applicable to the initial management by the emergency physician, these CT views are helpful in operative planning by the orthopedic surgeon. CT has also been proposed as an accurate and noninvasive modality for determining ongoing pelvic hemorrhage in the hemodynamically stable patient with pelvic fractures.[12] Extravasation of intravenous contrast is seen.

Cystourethrograms.   *Retrograde urethrograms* and *cystograms* are indicated in some patients with pelvic disruption (see Clinical Decision Making—Visceral Injuries) (Figs. 12-32 and 12-33). These are easily done in the trauma suite to diagnose a urethral or bladder injury. To instill contrast for a retrograde urethrogram in a male patient, a Foley catheter inserted no further than the fossa navicularis or a 50-mL beveled syringe placed in the urethral meatus may be used. For a cystogram, the bladder must be distended with at least 350 mL of contrast (or until the patient complains of discomfort). A scout film, a filled film, and a postvoid film are obtained. Contrast accumulating around loops of bowel or in the dependent por-

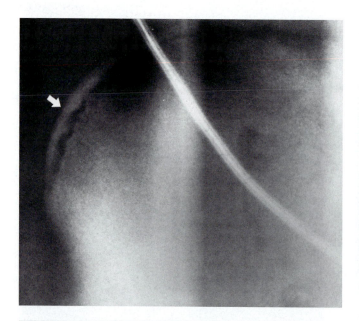

FIGURE 12-30.   Persistent ossification center of the iliac crest in a young adult should not be misinterpreted as an avulsion injury.

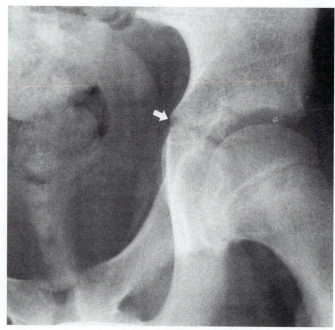

FIGURE 12-31.   Interruption of the arcuate line is due to residual triradiate cartilage in an adolescent. This should not be misinterpreted as a fracture.

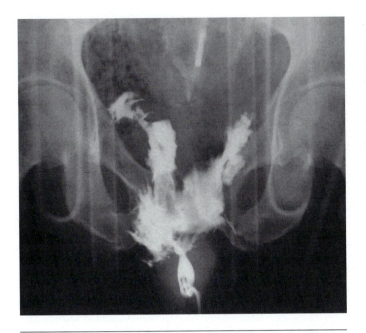

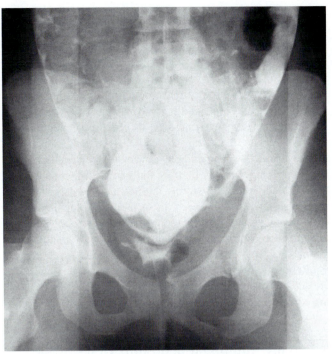

FIGURE 12-32. Retrograde urethrogram demonstrates extensive extravasation of contrast due to urethral disruption in a patient with anterior pelvic fractures. (Courtesy of Antonino Motta, M.D., Department of Radiology, MetroHealth Medical Center, Cleveland, OH.)

FIGURE 12-33. Retrograde cystogram in a patient with pelvic fractures shows intraperitoneal bladder disruption. Contrast is seen throughout the peritoneal cavity. (Courtesy of Antonino Motta, M.D., Department of Radiology, MetroHealth Medical Center, Cleveland, OH.)

tions of the peritoneal cavity is indicative of intraperitoneal tears. Extraperitoneal tears show contrast leaking around the base of the bladder or in the prevesical space. A cystogram should *not* be performed if pelvic angiography or abdominal CT is contemplated for the patient because extravasated contrast will interfere with those studies.

Angiography. Pelvic angiography is indicated when arterial bleeding into the pelvis is suspected (Fig. 12-34). Embolization of the internal iliac arteries can be lifesaving.

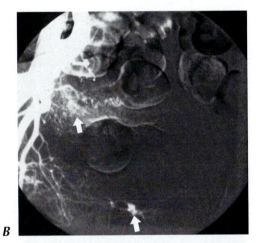

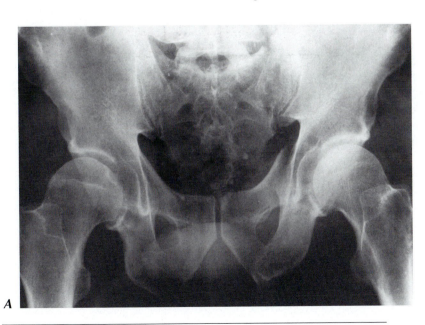

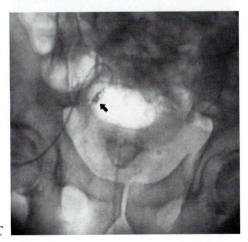

FIGURE 12-34. *A.* A patient with anterior pelvic fractures had persistent blood loss. *B.* An angiogram revealed extravasation from the right internal iliac artery. *C.* Embolization with coils stopped the hemorrhage.

CONTROVERSIES

Do all blunt trauma victims require pelvic radiographs?

The current ATLS protocol is to obtain an AP radiograph of the pelvis on all blunt multitrauma patients.[1] Several studies suggest that a selective approach to ordering radiographs is appropriate for detecting clinically significant pelvic injuries.[2,6,13,14] Pelvic radiography can be omitted in patients with no physical examination findings for a pelvic injury so long as there are no painful distracting injuries and the patient's neurologic status is not impaired. In such cases, foregoing pelvic radiographs saves time and resources and reduces the patient's radiation exposure. However, in the victim of major blunt trauma, routine pelvic radiography is warranted, since pelvic injuries are common and serious in such patients. If pelvic films are always ordered in victims of major trauma, the risk of missing a pelvic injury in these multiply injured patients is reduced.

When are additional plain-film views of the pelvis useful?

With the ready availability of CT, the role of supplementary plain-film views, such as Judet views and inlet-outlet views, has diminished substantially. CT provides greater overall detail than plain imaging. CT can miss injuries that occur in the axial plane. An acetabular fracture that lies in the axial plane may be visible only on the Judet view, and a nondisplaced transverse sacral fracture may be detected only by an outlet view or lateral sacral view. One approach is to obtain CT for all pelvic ring disruptions and to obtain supplementary plain films if there is a specific issue not resolved by CT. In the ED, inlet, outlet, or Judet views could be used to clarify a questionable finding on the AP view.

Another controversy involves obtaining views of the coccyx. Most clinicians agree that a fracture of the coccyx should be diagnosed by a rectal examination that reveals a tender and abnormally mobile coccyx. Furthermore, nondisplaced fractures can be difficult to detect radiographically. A simple coccygeal fracture not involving the sacrum is of little clinical consequence and is managed conservatively and symptomatically. Roentgenography adds little to the disposition and management of such patients.

REFERENCES

1. Alexander RH, Ali J, Aprahamian C, et al: *Advanced Trauma Life Support Student Manual.* Chicago: American College of Surgeons, 1993.
2. Koury HI, Peschiera JL, Welling RE: Selective use of pelvic roentgenograms in blunt trauma patients. *J Trauma* 34:236, 1993.
3. Naam NH, Brown WH, Hurd R, et al: Major pelvic fractures. *Arch Surg* 118:610, 1983.
4. Rothenberger DA, Fischer RP, Strate RG, et al: The mortality associated with pelvic fractures. *Surgery* 84:356, 1978.
5. Heare MM, Heare TC, Gillespy T: Diagnostic imaging of pelvic and chest wall trauma. *Musculoskel Trauma* 27:873, 1989.
6. Salvino CK, Esposito TJ, Smith D, et al: Routine pelvic x-ray studies in awake blunt trauma patients: A sensible policy? *J Trauma* 33:413, 1992.
7. Panetta T, Sclafani SJ, Goldstein AS, et al: Percutaneous transcatheter embolization for massive bleeding from pelvic fractures. *J Trauma* 25:1021, 1985.
8. Ben-Menachem Y, Coldwell DM, Young JW, Burgess AR: Hemorrhage associated with pelvic fractures: Causes, diagnosis, and emergent management. *AJR* 157:1005, 1991.
9. Harley JD, Mack LA, Winquist RA: CT of acetabular fractures: Comparison with conventional radiography. *AJR* 138:413, 1982.
10. Driscoll PA, Ross R, Nicholson DA: The pelvis. *BMJ* 307:927, 1993.
11. Magid D, Fishman EK: Imaging of musculoskeletal trauma in three dimensions. *Radiol Clin North Am* 27:948, 1989.
12. Cerva DS, Mirvis SE, Shanmuganathan K, et al: Detection of bleeding in patients with major pelvic fractures: Value of contrast-enhanced CT. *AJR* 166:131, 1996.
13. Civil ID, Rose SE, Botchlo G, Schwab CW: Routine pelvic radiography in severe blunt trauma: Is it necessary? *Ann Emerg Med* 17:488, 1988.
14. Yugueros P, Sarmiento JM, Garcia AF, Ferrada R: Unnecessary use of pelvic x-ray in blunt trauma. *J Trauma* 39:722, 1995.

CHAPTER 13

THE CERVICAL SPINE

BRENT RUOFF / O. CLARK WEST

Of the 12,000 to 13,000 injuries of the cervical spine sustained in the United States each year, about 30% are associated with spinal cord injury. Of concern, 5 to 10% of spinal cord injuries are sustained or worsened during initial emergency management.[1,2] The majority of cervical spine injuries result from motor vehicle collisions.

The medicolegal aspects of cervical spine injury add to the expense of medical practice.[3] Reduced ordering of cervical spine radiographs in the emergency department (ED) could save as much as $45 million nationwide annually.[4] Nonetheless, the occurrence of a spinal cord injury resulting from a missed diagnosis is a great concern. Balancing patient care against the risk of adverse outcome and the need to conserve resources is a challenge.

The task of interpreting cervical spine radiographs is not a simple one. The cervical vertebrae and their articular relationships are anatomically intricate and the radiographic images of the cervical spine are extremely complex. The emergency physician must be familiar with cervical spine biomechanics and radiographic anatomy and apply that knowledge to the interpretation of radiographs.

CLINICAL DECISION MAKING

The primary role for radiography of the cervical spine in the ED patient is to evaluate blunt cervical trauma. Nonetheless, radiographs are limited in their ability to exclude spinal injury. Initial radiographs may be normal in up to 7% of patients with a cervical injury.[5,6] Moreover, plain radiographs do not evaluate neural structures and cannot exclude neurologic injury. This is especially true in children, where significant spinal cord injuries occur without any plain-film evidence of vertebral column injury.[7–9] This pattern is called SCIWORA—*spinal cord injury without radiographic abnormality*. Assessing the neurologic integrity is done by physical examination and advanced neurologic imaging (i.e., magnetic resonance imaging). In the patient with an altered mental status, the determination of a neurologic deficit is difficult.

In the multisystem trauma patient, management of airway, breathing, and circulation takes priority over radiographic studies. Properly performed, orotracheal intubation is safe even in the patient with an unstable cervical spine injury.[10,11] The task of obtaining images of the cervical spine should not delay life-saving measures during trauma resuscitation. One should maintain cervical spine immobilization and proceed with other interventions until the patient is stable. Only then should a complete cervical spine series be obtained.

The Cervical Spine Trauma Series

In the evaluation of trauma, a three-view series (anteroposterior, lateral, and open-mouth views) is satisfactory for initially identifying injuries. Oblique views do not increase the yield of cervical spine radiographs. Flexion-extension views should be used in carefully selected patients to detect ligamentous injuries. The AP view makes only a limited contribution to the detection of cervical spine fractures. One study suggests that the lateral and open-mouth odontoid views are the only studies required for initial plain-film evaluation of blunt trauma.[12] Additional views or repeated views are often required to assess the cervical spine adequately. In one study, the initial three views were adequate to evaluate the cervical spine in only 41.3% of cases.[13] Commonly, improved visualization of C1 is needed as well as a swimmer's view to inspect the cervicothoracic junction adequately.

Indications for Radiographic Evaluation

Not every patient who presents to the ED in cervical spine immobilization placed by a prehospital provider requires radiography. The emergency physician must consider the mechanism of injury, the patient's mental status, and the presence of other painful "distracting" injuries (Table 13-1).[14] Of these, the mechanism of injury by itself is not an indication for radiographic evaluation. The need for radiographic evaluation and the manner in which the evaluation should proceed is determined by placing patients into various risk-pattern groups (Fig. 13-1). These groups include patients who are (1) asymptomatic, (2) symptomatic *without* neurologic abnormality, and (3) symptomatic *with* neurologic abnormality.

ASYMPTOMATIC PATIENTS. In the alert, nonintoxicated patient without distracting painful injuries who is asymptomatic, radiologic evaluation of the cervical spine can be deferred. The patient must have no pain or tenderness through the entire cervi-

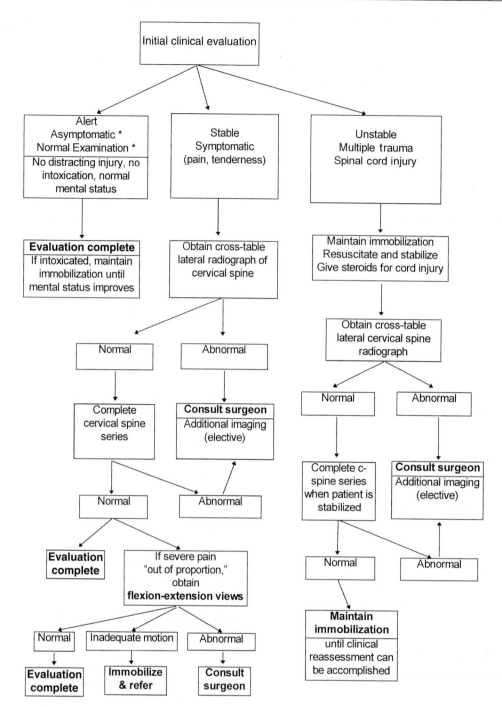

* - No neck pain, no tenderness, full range of motion without pain. CT is indicated in the ED if there is a questionable abnormality on the plain films or if the cervicothoracic junction or cervicocranium is not adequately visualized on the plain films in a patient with clinical suspicion of an injury to those regions.

FIGURE 13-1. Algorithm for evaluating the cervical spine.

cal area during a complete range of motion examination. The patient's mental status must be completely normal. Finally, there can be no painful distracting injury. A distracting injury is typically regarded as a long bone fracture. However, significant posttraumatic cephalgia or shoulder pain can obscure the detection of a cervical injury.

In several large prospective studies, there were no fractures of the cervical spine in asymptomatic patients.[15–17] When cervical fractures occur, patients have tenderness. Hoffman et al. studied 974 victims of blunt trauma for whom cervical spine films were obtained. There were 27 patients with cervical spine fractures. All patients with fractures had at least one of the fol-

TABLE 13-1

Which Patients Require Radiographs?

Sufficient mechanism of injury plus one or more of the following:
- Neck pain or dorsal neck tenderness
- Altered sensorium
- Intoxication
- Other distracting painful injury
- Abnormal neurologic exam

Mechanisms of Injury:
- Deceleration (motor vehicle collision)
- Direct blow to head:
  - Fall from above standing height
  - Diving into shallow water
  - Recreational/sports accidents

lowing findings: midline neck tenderness; evidence of intoxication, altered level of alertness, or a severely painful injury elsewhere. The complaint of neck pain was not, by itself, a discriminating finding, but the presence of cervical tenderness was. Of the 974 patients, 353 (37.3%) were without cervical fracture and had none of the four study characteristics. If radiographs had been obtained only for patients who had at least one of the four study characteristics, all fractures would have been detected, and the number of films ordered would have decreased by more than one-third.[17] In a subsequent study, Hoffman et al. found that only 5 of the total 954 cervical fractures did not meet criteria for obtaining radiographs. Of these, two were suspected of being chronic and three were spinous process fractures. None of these required intervention.[18]

The Nontender Cervical Fracture. The existence of a non-tender cervical spine fracture has been disputed and characterized as a medical myth. The suggestion of a "painless" cervical fracture was made in 1972 by Thambyrajah in the *Medical Journal of Malaysia*.[21] Since then, assertions regarding nontender cervical spine fractures continue to surface. When carefully analyzed, reports of painless cervical spine fractures have failed to meet the strict exclusion criteria outlined above.[22–24]

SYMPTOMATIC PATIENTS WITHOUT NEUROLOGIC ABNORMALITY. Symptomatic patients without neurologic abnormality are those who have some degree of pain or tenderness to the head, neck, or shoulders but have no neurologic deficit. Likewise, patients with blunt head injuries require cervical spine evaluation, especially those with a decreased level of consciousness.[25–28] In symptomatic patients without neurologic abnormality, radiographic evaluation of the cervical spine proceeds by first acquiring a cross-table lateral view. In most settings, if this view is normal, a complete cervical spine series is obtained.

If the lateral radiograph of the cervical spine is abnormal, spinal immobilization is maintained and a spinal surgeon is notified. Additional imaging is obtained only after the patient is fully stabilized. Further imaging may include an open-mouth odontoid view and an AP view as well as computed tomography (CT) evaluation of the abnormal site.

Flexion-Extension Views. If the standard cervical spine series is normal and one suspects ligamentous injury (i.e., there is disproportionate or excessive pain), extension and flexion views are considered. If these radiographs are normal, the examination is finished. If the study is inadequate due to the patient's inability to fully flex or extend the neck, the patient is placed in a rigid cervical collar and referred to a spine surgeon for further evaluation. With ligamentous injury, the flexion-extension views show subluxation of the vertebral bodies or widening of the spinous processes. These views can also demonstrate an otherwise occult spinous process fracture.[29] If the flexion-extension views are abnormal, a spine surgeon is notified.

PATIENTS WITH NEUROLOGIC ABNORMALITY. When a neurologic abnormality is present, spinal immobilization is maintained throughout the resuscitation. Intravenous steroid therapy is promptly initiated for a spinal cord injury (methylprednisolone 30 mg/kg IV bolus, then 5.4 mg/kg/h IV).[30] A cross-table lateral cervical view is obtained. Once this has been done and other life-threatening processes are addressed, the cervical spine series is completed. If the cross-table view is abnormal, the injury must be addressed by a spine surgeon. If the lateral view shows no osseous injury in the presence of a spinal cord injury, the spine surgeon is consulted and additional imaging is performed (usually CT or MRI).

Limitations of the Cross-Table Lateral View

A cross-table lateral view of the cervical spine is, by itself, insufficient to "clear" the neck. If the cross-table view is normal in a mildly symptomatic patient who is not the victim of high-velocity injury, the cervical collar is removed and the three-view trauma series, including an AP and an open-mouth (odontoid) view, is completed. Shaffer found that 6 of 35 (17%) cases of cervical fracture had lateral films interpreted as normal.[31] The sensitivity of the cross-table lateral view for excluding fracture is 85%.[32] The frequency of missed cervical spine injury on lateral film can be as high as 26%.[33] Even when the three-view series is obtained, the fracture miss rate for cervical spine injury can be as high as 20%.[34] This false-negative rate mandates that the multisystem trauma victim be maintained in spinal immobilization in the ED even with "normal" radiographs.

Many cases of false-negative cervical spine radiographs are due to inadequate films, especially failure to visualize the cervicothoracic junction and cervicocranium. False-positive radiographic interpretations also occur. False-positive rates range from 14 to 40%.[34,35]

Computed Tomography

A CT scan is indicated any time a bony abnormality is found on cervical spine films that suggests an unstable injury. The timing of CT is decided by the emergency physician in consultation with the trauma surgeon. Although the radiologic evaluation of blunt cervical trauma begins with plain film study, 2.0 to 4.7% of plain films will fail to show a fracture that is detectable by conventional or computed tomography.[36,37]

ANATOMY AND PHYSIOLOGY

The cervical spine can be divided into two anatomically and functionally distinct regions: the cervicocranium and the lower cervical spine (C_3-C_7). The occiput, atlas, and axis are the *cervicocranium*. The cervicocranium and the lower cervical spine are subject to different patterns of injury. At the cervicocranium, the vertebral canal is large relative to the diameter of the spinal cord. This contributes to the lower incidence of spinal cord injury in patients with cervicocranial fractures who survive to hospital arrival. At the mid- and lower cervical spine, the spinal cord occupies nearly the entire vertebral canal and is therefore frequently injured during spinal column trauma.

The Cervicocranium

The atlas (C1) is a ring of bone with thick lateral masses and no vertebral body (Fig. 13-2). The articulation between C1 and the occipital condyles permits about 13° of flexion and extension.[38]

The axis (C2) is anatomically complex. The dens projects cranially from the C2 vertebral body. The *superior articular facets* of C2 form the "shoulders" of the vertebral body lateral to the dens. The *pars interarticularis* extends posteriorly from the lateral aspect of the axis body and is bounded inferiorly by the *inferior articular facet*. C2 does not have lateral masses or pedicles. Posteriorly, the laminae of C2 form the neural arch and fuse in the posterior midline with the bifid *spinous process*. The atlas (C1) and axis (C2) articulate in such a way as to allow rotation with a small degree of flexion, extension, and lateral tilt.

The stability of the cervicocranium is dependent on several strong ligaments—the anterior longitudinal ligament, the posterior longitudinal ligament, the transverse atlantal ligament, the alar ligaments and the accessory ligaments. In the cervicocranium, the anterior longitudinal ligament is called the *anterior atlantoaxial ligament*, connecting C1 and C2, and the *anterior atlantooccipital ligament*, between C1 and anterior rim of the foramen magnum. The thick *transverse atlantal ligament* (TAL) extends across the ring of C1 and hold the dens against the anterior arch of C1. The transverse ligament also includes small longitudinal slips extending superiorly and inferiorly. The transverse ligament is also called the *cruciform ligament* (or cruciate ligament). The *alar ligaments*, which limit rotation, extend from the dorsolateral surface of the dens upward and laterally to the occipital condyles. The cranial extension of the *posterior longitudinal ligament* (PLL) lies posterior to the cru-

ciform ligament and attaches to the anterior rim foramen magnum. It is also known as the *tectorial membrane*. This tough membrane limits flexion and extension.

The Lower Cervical Spine (C3 – C7)

The lower five cervical vertebrae are all similar in configuration (Fig. 13-3). Each has a cylindrical vertebral body with upturned superolateral borders called the *uncinate processes*. Paired *pedicles* extend laterally from the vertebral body to join the articular masses (lateral masses). The superior and inferior articular facets make up the superior and inferior surfaces of the lateral masses. The articular facet surfaces are tilted 35° forward from the frontal plane. The transverse processes project laterally from the vertebral body and lateral masses. Each transverse process is perforated by a *transverse foramen*. The paired flat *laminae* project posteromedially from the lateral masses and join in the midline. The spinous process projects posteriorly from the midline at the site of fusion of the laminae.

Several ligaments ensure the mechanical stability of the lower cervical spine (Fig. 13-4). The superior and inferior vertebral body endplates are connected by the *annulus fibrosus* of the intervertebral disks. The anterior longitudinal ligament (ALL) extends along the anterior aspect of the vertebral bodies. It is securely attached to the anterior intervertebral disk margins. The posterior longitudinal ligament (PLL) extends along the posterior vertebral bodies. It forms the anterior boundary of the vertebral canal.

The *ligamentum flavum* (yellow ligament) connects the laminae of adjacent vertebrae. The laminae and ligamentum flavum form the posterior boundary of the vertebral canal. The *interspinous ligaments* join the spinous processes in the midsagittal plane. The *supraspinous ligament* is the strong, continuous band linking the tips of the spinous processes.

The motion of the lower cervical spine is the sum of incremental movements that occur at each intersegmental articulation. The segments C3 to C7 allow about 45° of neck rotation. Rotation is limited by the inclination of the apposed facet surfaces and by tightening of the capsular ligaments.

Cervical Spine Stability

Stability of the cervical spine depends on the integrity of skeletal and ligamentous structures. In a *two-column model*, the spine is divided into anterior and posterior columns (Fig. 13-4). The anterior column consists of the vertebral body, the ALL, and the PLL. The posterior column is formed by the neural arch and its supporting ligaments. Stability is dependent on an intact posterior ligament complex that includes the ligamentum flavum, interfacetal capsules, interspinous ligament, and supraspinous ligament.[39] In a *three-column system*, the middle column consists of the PLL, the posterior aspect of the disk annulus, and the posterior aspect of the vertebral body.[40] The middle column plus either the anterior or posterior column must fail for instability to occur.

Biomechanical experiments demonstrate that stability is dependent on intact anterior or posterior elements plus at least

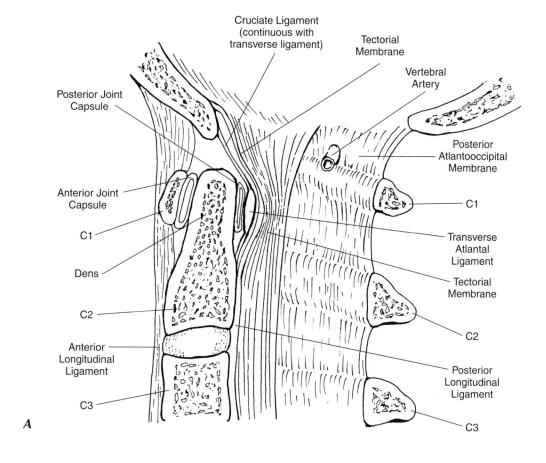

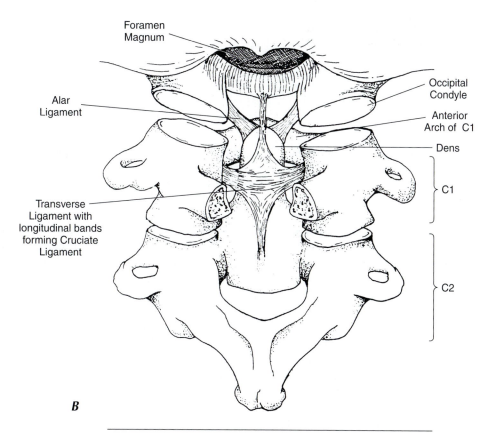

FIGURE 13-2. Anatomy of the cervicocranium. *A.* Sagittal section. *B.* Posterior view (C1 posterior arch is cut away).

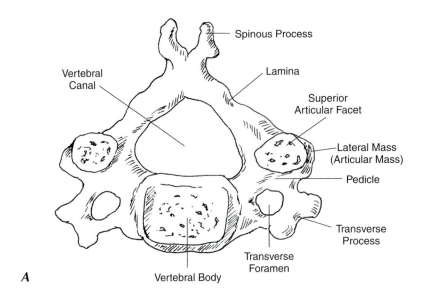

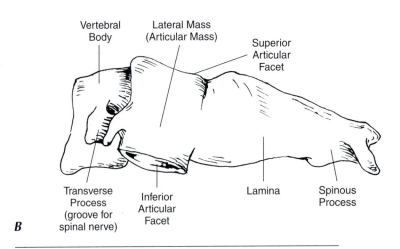

FIGURE 13-3.   A typical lower cervical vertebra (C5). *A.* Top view.
B. Side view.

one ligament of the other column.[41] The upper limit of physiologic motion between adjacent vertebral bodies is 3.5 mm in the horizontal plane and 11° of angulation.

Cervical stability is defined differently by various medical disciplines. From the neurologic standpoint, the cervical spine's stability is defined by its ability to preserve normal neurologic function. The radiologic definition of cervical spine stability derives from a number of radiographic measurements and relationships. Another scheme stratifies instability into three stages based on mechanical and neurologic function. First-degree instability is the loss of mechanical integrity without neurologic damage. Second-degree instability is a neurologic deficit despite mechanical stability. Third-degree instability is both a neurologic deficit and mechanical instability.

In general, the determination of spine stability guides definitive neurosurgical therapy. It is less critical for the emergency physician to assess the degree of spine stability than it is for the surgeon, who must determine definitive treatment. Most patients with cervical spine injury are admitted to the hospital. An occasional patient with a simple fracture (e.g., mild

wedge compression fracture or isolated fracture of the C7 spinous process) may be sent home with close follow-up if adjunctive studies (CT and flexion-extension views) confirm that the injury is mechanically stable.

Delayed (Hidden) Instability.   Mechanical instability can be overlooked at the time of initial evaluation. The instability may be "delayed," causing progressive degeneration of the vertebral column over many months. This occurs with flexion-type injuries that disrupt the posterior ligamentous support of the cervical spine. Up to 3% of spine-injured patients have "hidden" ligamentous injuries without any identifiable radiographic abnormalities in the ED. Pain and muscle spasm accompanying ligamentous injury can prevent patients from having a full range of motion on flexion-extension radiographs. This will mask instability in the ED.[42] Some patients have been reported to develop subacute clinical instability and worsened symptoms within weeks of initial evaluation despite initially normal static and dynamic plain radiographs.[43]

Delayed instability occurs late after the injury due to in-

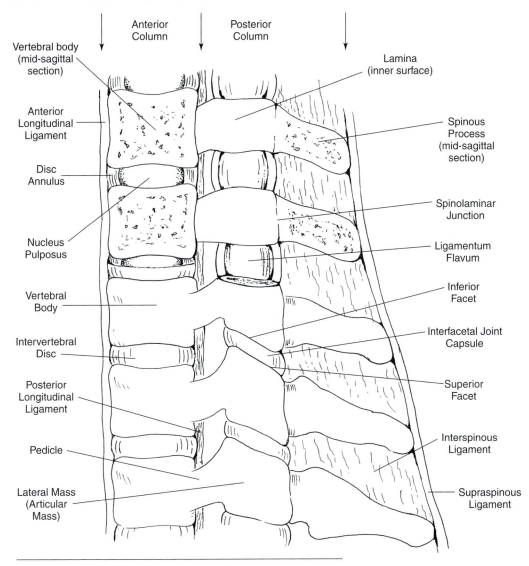

FIGURE 13-4.   Anatomy of the lower cervical spine. The superior two vertebrae are shown cut away in sagittal section.

complete healing and deforming degenerative changes. It occurs in up to 30 to 50% of cases of mild flexion injuries (e.g., hyperflexion sprain or anterior wedge compression fracture) that are treated nonoperatively.

RADIOGRAPHIC TECHNIQUE

Although in the non-trauma patient radiographs of the cervical spine are exposed with the patient in an upright posture, the trauma patient requires radiographic evaluation while immobilized in the supine position. The three principal views in the injured patient are the lateral, anteroposterior (AP), and open-mouth views (OMV) (Table 13-2). In the trauma victim, the initial view is the cross-table lateral. The AP and open-mouth (odontoid) views are then taken with the cervical collar removed, so long as the patient's clinical condition permits.

Supplementary views that are added depending on the clinical circumstances include the swimmer's view, oblique views, pillar views, and flexion-extension studies. CT is used to precisely define injuries identified on plain radiographs,

and to image areas that are difficult to see on the plain films (e.g., cervicocranium, cervicothoracic junction). (See section: *Controversies,* at end of chapter.)

Lateral View

The standard lateral radiograph is performed with the patient upright. The beam is directed perpendicular to the sagittal plane with a 72-in. focal-point-to-film distance (FFD). Most trauma patients are immobilized and receive a supine cross-table lateral view using portable equipment and a shorter FFD (about 40 in.). The film cassette is positioned vertically with its inferior edge touching the patient's shoulder. Gentle caudad traction on the patient's arms improves visualization of the lower cervical vertebrae.

The lateral view shows the cervicocranium, vertebral alignment, the vertebral bodies, intervertebral disk spaces, spinous processes, and the articular facets (Fig. 13-5A and B). To be technically adequate, the film must include the entire cervical spine from the base of the skull to the C7-T1 interface. Extraneous objects (e.g., earrings, necklaces) must be removed. The projection must be a true lateral view with minimal rotation and head tilt. The left and right diamond-shaped articular masses should be superimposed on a correctly performed lateral projection.

Anteroposterior View

The AP projection is performed with the patient's head and neck straight and the cassette centered behind the neck at C4. The beam is centered on the thyroid cartilage and is angled cephalad 20° to avoid overlap by the mandible. This view shows the vertebral bodies of C3 to C7, the intervertebral disk spaces, and the spinous processes (Fig. 13-5C and D).

Open-Mouth View

The open-mouth view (odontoid view) is an anteroposterior projection of C1 and C2 (Fig. 13-5E and F). This view shows the lateral masses of C1, the dens, the C2 vertebral body, the lateral atlantoaxial joints, and the spinous process of C2. The patient is usually supine with the cassette placed behind the neck and centered at C2. The head is positioned so that a line connecting the tip of the upper incisors and the occiput is perpendicular to the cassette.[44] The x-ray beam is directed vertically through the open mouth and the patient is instructed to say "ah."

In a technically adequate open-mouth view, several important structures are seen without interference. The lateral masses of C1, the atlantoaxial articulations, and the dens (except for its tip) are not obscured by overlapping teeth or the skull base. The head and neck are not tilted or rotated. In the absence of rotation, the C2 spinous process is in the midline and aligned with the dens.

If details of the spine are obscured by overlapping structures, the film is repeated with slightly different positioning of the patient. Other techniques can be tried. The "chewing" technique is performed with the same beam and cassette orientation. The patient is instructed to rapidly and repeatedly open and close the mouth (moving the lower jaw only) while a prolonged exposure is performed.[38]

The *Fuch's method* is used to visualize the dens (Fig. 13-6). It is especially useful in young children who do not cooperate with positioning for an open-mouth projection.[45] The cassette is positioned as previously described. The patient's neck is extended so that a line connecting the chin and the tip of the mastoid is perpendicular to the cassette. The beam is directed just caudad to the chin tip. The image of the dens is projected through the foramen magnum. The lateral masses of C1 and C2 are poorly seen on this view. If the patient is suspected to have an injury of the cervicocranium, this view should be avoided because of the requisite neck extension.

If there is a high clinical suspicion of a cervicocranial injury, a CT of C1 and C2 is obtained instead of an open-mouth view. This is especially useful if the patient has a severe head injury and an emergency head CT scan is being performed.

Swimmer's View

The swimmer's view (Twining view) is performed when the cervicothoracic junction is inadequately demonstrated on the standard supine lateral view (Fig. 13-7). The arm on one side is fully abducted over the patient's head, and the opposite shoulder is depressed slightly by traction on the arm. The cassette is placed in a vertical position next to the axilla of the abducted arm and centered just below the cervicothoracic junction.[44] The x-ray beam is directed through the base of the neck. Ideally, the vertebral bodies of the lower cervical segments and cervicothoracic junction are seen.

Patient movement during positioning for this view can cause displacement of an unstable spine.[46] Therefore, a swimmer's view is avoided if there is significant suspicion of cervical injury, and CT of this region is obtained instead. Supine oblique views are an alternative means to see the cervicothoracic junction, although their ability to reliably exclude a cervical injury is uncertain.

The posterior elements of C7 are not well seen on the swimmer's view. Therefore, if the patient has had severe trauma and has significant pain in this area, a swimmer's view may not be adequate to exclude injury. Conversely, if there is low suspicion for injury, a swimmer's view is usually sufficient for evaluation of this region.

Oblique Views

Oblique views can be performed with the patient upright, prone, or supine. Standard upright oblique views are performed by rotating the patient 45° from the posteriorly placed cassette and centering the beam at C4 (Fig. 13-8). Oblique views can be done on supine patients in full spinal immobilization by elevating one side of the spine board on blocks, producing 45° of patient rotation. Alternatively, supine "trauma" oblique views require no patient movement other than placing the x-ray film cassette under the patient. The beam is directed 45° from vertical.[47] To avoid any patient movement, the beam may be angled even further (60°) and the film cassette placed alongside the patient's neck. The main disadvantage of the supine trauma oblique view is that the x-ray beam is not perpendicular to the x-ray film, causing distortion of the structures located farthest from the film. Oblique views requiring head and neck rotation are avoided in the trauma setting. Oblique views demonstrate the pedicles, laminae, intervertebral foramina, and articular facets.

Oblique views are useful in some patients with suspected injuries to the posterior column that are poorly seen on the standard three-view study. Such injuries include unilateral interfacetal dislocation, lateral mass fractures, and lamina fractures.

In many cases, CT will supplant supplementary oblique views. In some institutions, oblique views are included with the standard cervical spine series.

Pillar Views

Pillar views are oblique views with the x-ray beam angled to show the lateral masses. These views require significant head rotation. These views have been largely supplanted by CT.

TABLE 13-2

Radiographic Views of the Cervical Spine

	TECHNIQUE	ADEQUACY	LIKELY FINDINGS
Lateral	Patient supine and immobilized. Cross-table projection. Gentle traction on shoulders.	Entire cervical spine from skull base to superior end-plate of T1. Jewelry and other extraneous objects removed. Minimal rotation—left and right lateral masses superimposed.	Most fractures and dislocations are seen.
AP	Patient supine, head and neck straight.	Neck straight. No rotation—spinous processes in midline.	Vertebral body and uncinate process fractures. Lateral mass fractures. Spinous process fractures.
Open-mouth view	Patient supine. Head and neck straight (no tilt or rotation)	Teeth and skull base do not overlap dens or lateral masses of C1 and C2. Dens and C2 spinous process aligned in the midline. Slight head tilt or rotation causes the lateral masses of C1 to slip laterally with respect to C2.	Jefferson burst fracture of C1. Dens fracture. Avulsion of lateral masses of C1.
SUPPLEMENTARY VIEWS			
Swimmer's view	Patient supine. One arm fully abducted above the head. Caudal traction on opposite arm.	Vertebral bodies of C7 and T1 seen with minimal overlap by the shoulders and clavicles. C2 or C1 should be visible to be able to correctly orient the radiograph.	Vertebral body fractures. Malalignment at the cervicothoracic junction.
Oblique views	Patient upright or supine and rotated 45° to film cassette. Trauma obliques performed with patient supine and x-ray beam angled.	Entire cervical spine visible. Clear view of neuroforamina, pedicles, laminae and lateral masses of ipsilateral side of vertebral column.	Laminar and pedicle fractures. Unilateral interfacetal dislocation.
Flexion-extension views	Patient upright. Patient performs active flexion and extension. Movement stopped if significant pain or neurological deficit develops.	Entire cervical spine visible. Flexion—inferior margin of mandible is vertical. Extension—spinous processes close together.	Flexion—Posterior ligament tears (instability). Fracture displacement may increase. Extension—Anterior ligament injury. Fracture displacement.

Flexion and Extension Views

Dynamic lateral projections (flexion-extension views) are performed only on alert, stable patients (Fig. 13-9). At some institutions, flexion-extension views are performed with physician supervision. When used correctly, the technique successfully and safely demonstrates cervical spine instability in trauma patients with otherwise negative radiographs.[42] The views are done with the patient sitting or standing upright. All movement is performed by the patient. Motion is limited by the patient's discomfort or the onset of neurologic symptoms. First, the patient performs neck flexion (forward flexion), attempting to touch the chin as low on the chest as possible without opening the mouth. Next, the patient performs extension, elevating the chin as far as possible.

These views are used in the ED to reveal instability in carefully selected patients with significant pain and otherwise normal or equivocal radiographs. Flexion and extension views can be helpful in differentiating acute injury from chronic degenerative changes (spondylosis), which cause

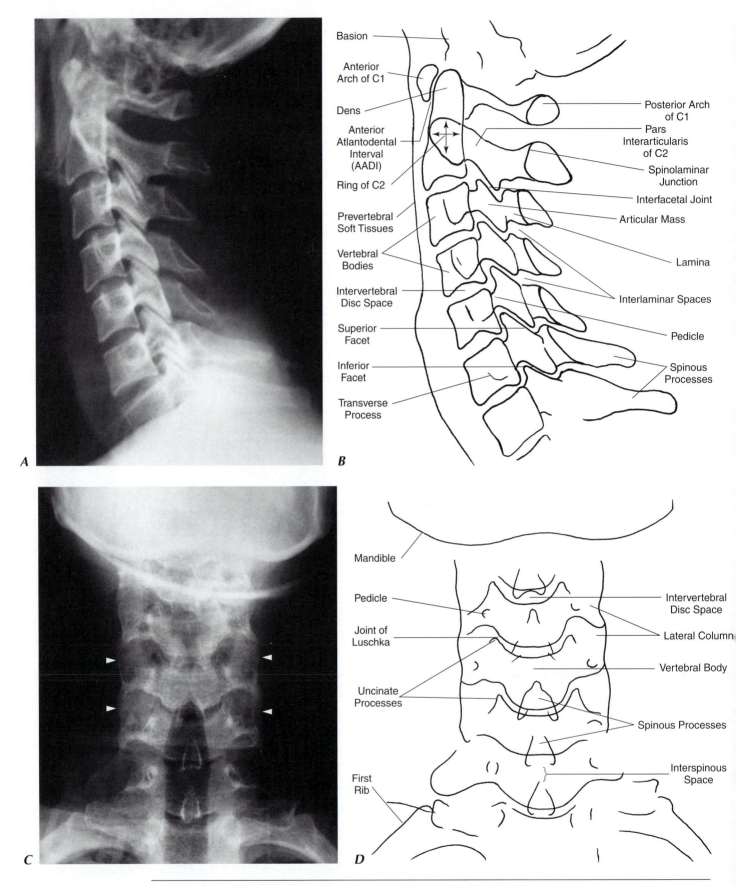

FIGURE 13-5. Normal cervical spine radiographs. *A.* and *B.* Lateral view. The spine is seen from the skull base to C7. The T1 vertebral body is not seen. *C.* and *D.* AP view. This AP view shows the vertebral bodies of C4-C7. C3 is not optimally seen because of the overlying immobilization device and mandible. Note the smooth undulating contour of the lateral columns (*arrowheads*).

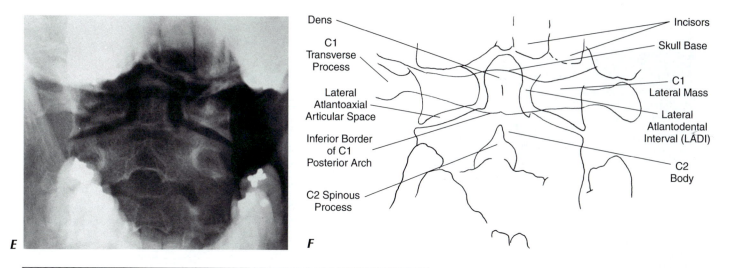

E

F

FIGURE 13-5. (*continued*)   E. and F. Open-mouth view. The head is slightly rotated to the left so that there is slight asymmetry of the dens between the lateral masses of C1. The lateral margins of C1 and C2 are aligned. (© Washington University, used by permission.)

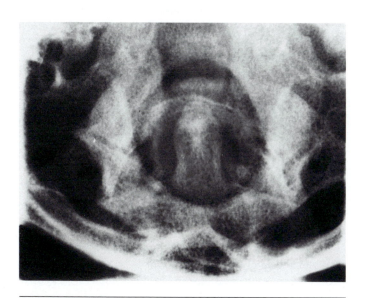

FIGURE 13-6.   Fuchs view. An alternative view of the dens shows the dens projected through the foramen magnum. The lateral masses of C1 and C2 are not seen.

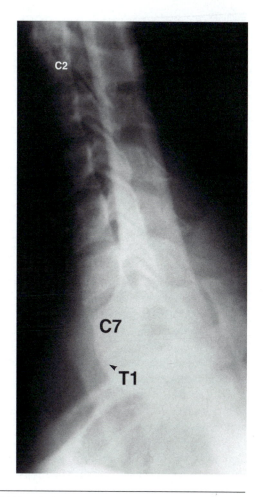

FIGURE 13-7.   Swimmer's view. The swimmer's view shows alignment at the cervicothoracic junction. For orientation, the C2 vertebra at the top of the radiograph can be used as the starting point to count down the vertebrae. The superior cortex of T1 (*arrowhead*) is partially hidden by the overlying humeral head and clavicle. Sufficient detail of the C7-T1 articulation is seen to exclude malalignment. C7 can be traced once the overlying margins of the humerus, clavicle, and scapular spine are identified. (© Washington University, used by permission.)

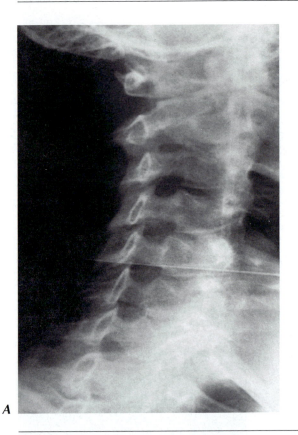

A

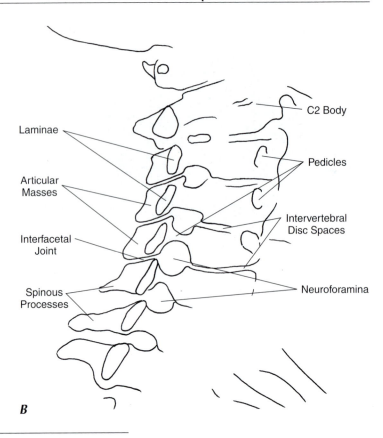

B

C2 Body

Laminae

Pedicles

Articular
Masses

Interfacetal
Joint

Intervertebral
Disc Spaces

Spinous
Processes

Neuroforamina

FIGURE 13-8. Oblique view. The shingle-shaped laminae overlie the articular masses. The laminae are normally aligned to look like "shingles on a roof." The neuroforamina are seen throughout the cervical spine. (© Washington University, used by permission.)

vertebral malalignment. For patients with chronic neck pain syndromes, stress views produced by passively flexing the neck have been advocated.[48] The use of flexion-extension views in the ED is restricted to alert, neurologically intact patients with otherwise normal radiographs who can sit or stand upright and perform active range of motion.

The examination is not "normal" unless adequate range of motion is demonstrated. In full flexion, the upright patient's mandible should be vertical (parallel to the patient's body) with jaws closed. In full extension, adjacent spinous processes should nearly touch. If an adequate range of motion is not demonstrated, cervical immobilization and a repeat examination in several days are required.

Standard criteria for stability, such as measurements of subluxation or angulation, cannot always be applied to radiographs of patients with degenerative changes. These patients can have chronic malalignment that would be classified as mechanically unstable in the acute trauma setting. Flexion-extension views can prove stability. Range of motion may appear to be suboptimal because of the degenerative changes, and it must be assumed that the limitation is due to injury until repeat examination. Immobilization and repeat examination are used liberally for patients with degenerative changes and significant neck pain when range of motion is limited.

COMPUTED TOMOGRAPHY.   Axial slices are obtained through areas of abnormality to define their anatomy more precisely. CT is performed to assess areas of questionable abnormality. CT is also used to visualize areas that may be difficult to see on conventional radiographs, especially the cervicocranium and cervicothoracic junction. The use of CT should be limited to patients with a sufficient clinical suspicion of injury in these areas.

CT can miss fractures that lie in the axial plane (e.g., a fracture across the base of the dens) as well as malalignment in the axial plane (vertebral body displacement). Plain film correlation or CT images reconstructed in the sagittal and coronal planes help to detect these injuries. Helical CT is especially advantageous for producing accurate reconstructed images.

NORMAL RADIOGRAPHIC ANATOMY

Lateral View

A complete lateral view extends from the skull base to the superior margin of the first thoracic vertebra (Fig. 13-5A and B).

CERVICOCRANIUM.   The *basion* is the anterior rim of the foramen magnum cephalad to the tip of the dens. The interval

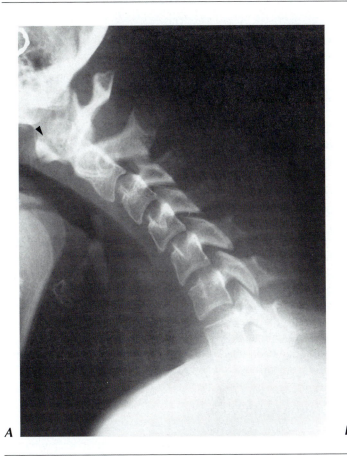

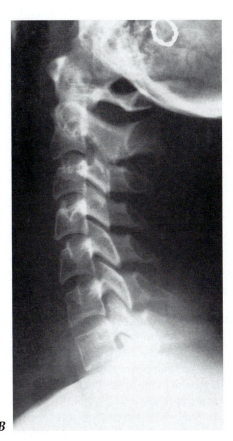

A

B

FIGURE 13-9.   Flexion-Extension Views. *A.* Flexion view. The presence of several unfused vertebral body endplates implies that the patient has not yet reached skeletal maturity. The AADI (predental space) has a slight V shape (normal for this young patient), but the interval is normal in size (*arrowhead*). There is a normal amount of mild anterior slippage of the vertebral bodies at several levels. The intervertebral disk spaces are uniform in size, and the interfacetal articulations are normal. There is no focal increase in an interlaminar or interspinous space. *B.* Extension view. The occiput abuts against C1 posteriorly and there is close approximation of the spinous processes. Alignment of the vertebral bodies is normal and the anterior disk spaces are uniform in size. (© Washington University, used by permission.)

between the basion and the tip of the dens, the *basion-dental interval* (BDI), is normally less than 12 mm in adults[49] (Fig. 13-10). The occipitoatlantal articulation appears as a confluence of bone rather than as a distinct joint.

The anterior arch of C1 is separated from the dens by the *anterior atlantodental interval* (AADI) or *predental space.* The predental space is normally less than 3 mm wide. The slender posterior arches of C1 form the neural arch and posterior tubercle.

The vertebral body of C2 has a characteristic shape. Its anterior and posterior cortical margins are continuous with the anterior and posterior surfaces of the odontoid process. A distinctive confluence of radiographic shadows is formed by the lateral extension of the C2 vertebral body; this is known as the *ring of C2* (Fig. 13-5*A* and *B*).[50] A ring of C2 is formed on each side of the C2 vertebral body. When there is slight rotation, the two C2 rings are not superimposed, and each individual ring is difficult to discern. The inferior articular facets, laminae, and spinous process extend dorsally from the C2 vertebral body.

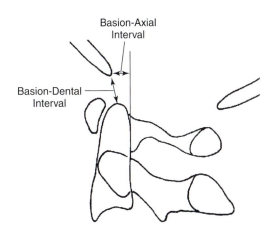

FIGURE 13-10.   The basion-dental interval (BDI) is normally less than 12 mm. The basion-axial interval (BAI) is used in children when the tip of the dens is not ossified. It is normally less than 12 mm.

LOWER CERVICAL SPINE.   From C3 to C7, the anterior and posterior surfaces of the nearly rectangular vertebral bodies assume a mildly lordotic curvature. The posterior surfaces of the vertebral bodies form the anterior surface of the spinal canal. The transverse processes are projected over each vertebral body and appear as small curvilinear densities. The paired diamond-shaped left and right lateral masses and articular facets extend posteriorly. The left and right lateral masses should be superimposed. The superior and inferior articular facets of adjacent vertebrae form the parallel surfaces at the interfacetal joints. Posterior to the lateral masses are the paired laminae. These intersect in the posterior midline with the base of the spinous process. At this location, there is a bright crescent called the *spinolaminar junction*. This forms the dorsal boundary of the spinal canal. The spinous processes gradually increase in size from C3 to C7. The intervertebral disk spaces each have uniform width and are all of similar height.

PREVERTEBRAL SOFT TISSUES.   A distinct soft tissue shadow is formed by the prevertebral soft tissues anterior to the vertebral column (Fig. 13-5A and B). An increase in thickness occurs at C4 due to the interposed esophagus below that level. Maximum "normal" values of prevertebral soft tissue thickness for different levels of the spine are as follows: C1, 10 mm; C2, 5 mm; C3, 7 mm; and C7, 20 mm.[51] The prevertebral soft tissue is wider at C1 due to interposed nasopharyngeal adenoidal tissue. These measurements are unreliable when the pharynx is poorly aerated or when a nasogastric or endotracheal tube obscures the soft tissue boundary. A thin layer of fatty tissue (the *prevertebral fat stripe*) is often visible within the prevertebral soft tissues. The prevertebral fat stripe is obliterated by hemorrhage or edema due to an adjacent injury.

Prevertebral soft tissue swelling can indicate an otherwise occult or subtle cervical spine injury especially of the cervicocranium. However in two large series, the sensitivity and specificity of soft tissue abnormalities was limited.[52,53] Soft tissue thickening is found in only about 60% of patients with injury to the cervicocranium.[54] The specificity of cervicocranial soft tissue swelling is only 84%. In the lower cervical spine, soft tissue swelling is very insensitive and is found in only 5% of cases.

Other authors suggest that changes in the contour of the prevertebral soft tissues, rather than measured thickness, especially in the cervicocranium, is an important indicator of cervical spine injury.[55] The normal contour of the cervicocranial soft tissues closely follows the contour of the anterior aspect of the vertebrae. There is a slight convexity (bulge) anterior to the C2 vertebral body and the anterior tubercle of C1. There is normally a slight concavity (depression) or straightening anterior to the base of the dens and atlantooccipital articulation. Swelling at C1 and the occiput must be distinguished from the nasopharyngeal adenopathy that is often seen in children and young adults. Adenopathy causes a rounded, lumpy contour in the upper cervicocranium.

Due to the interposed esophagus, the prevertebral soft tissues are thicker in the lower cervical spine and are less able to reveal posttraumatic swelling. The contour of the soft tissues in that area normally often becomes narrow or "tucks in" at the cervicothoracic junction. Loss of this narrowing is a sign of swelling due to injury of the lower cervical spine.

Anteroposterior View

The anteroposterior (AP) view shows the vertebral bodies, intervertebral disk spaces, spinous processes, and lateral masses (Fig. 13-5C and D). The upper two cervical segments are obscured by the mandible. The wedge-shaped *uncinate processes* of the vertebral bodies project upward from the lateral borders of the superior end plates, forming the *joints of Luschka*. This gives the vertebral bodies the appearance of interlocking horned structures. The intervertebral disk spaces are of fairly uniform height. The tracheal air shadow tapers at the level of the glottis, where the finely calcified thyroid cartilage may be seen overlying the lateral cervical bony masses. The bifid or chevron-shaped spinous processes project through the vertebral bodies in the midline and are evenly spaced. The facet joints are at an oblique orientation to the x-ray beam and are not visible. The lateral masses therefore appear to be continuous and have a smooth, wavy lateral border.

Open-Mouth View

The open-mouth view is an AP view of the cervicocranium projected through the patient's open mouth (Fig. 13-5E and F). The lateral masses of C1 sit atop the lateral articular surfaces of C2. The lateral borders of the lateral masses of C1 align with the subjacent lateral borders of C2. The atlantoaxial articular surfaces are parallel and symmetrical. The dens is centered between the lateral masses of C1, and the *lateral atlantodental intervals* (LADI) are roughly equal. The transverse processes of C1 are faintly visible. The posterior arch of C1 often overlies the base of the dens and can create an overlapping shadow (Mach band) across the base of the dens. The central incisor teeth at the base of the skull often overlie the tip or body of the dens.

Rotation or lateral tilt of the head causes changes in the alignment of C1 and C2. Lateral tilt causes the lateral border of C1 to move laterally with respect to the subjacent lateral articular surface of C2 and widens the LADI on that side. On the contralateral side, the lateral mass of C1 moves medially in relation to C2, and narrowing the contralateral LADI. Head rotation causes the lateral mass of C1 ipsilateral to the direction of rotation to appear smaller and triangular, and the LADI increases. The opposite lateral mass broadens and becomes more rectangular, while the corresponding LADI decreases.

Oblique Views

The oblique views show the vertebral bodies, pedicles, articular masses, and laminae (Fig. 13-8). The neuroforamina on one side appear as open ovals. The pedicles on the opposite side overlie the vertebral bodies and appear as radiodense ovals. The laminae are teardrop- or disk-shaped densities overlying the articular masses. The laminae are oriented so that each is angled with its inferior edge overlapping the subjacent superior laminar edge posteriorly, appearing like "shingles on a roof." The spinous processes are seen projecting beyond the articular masses.

RADIOGRAPHIC ANALYSIS

A systematic approach to the interpretation of radiographs of the cervical spine is essential. An ABC'S approach to interpretation has been advocated for lateral cervical spine radiographs.[56] Examination of the radiographs should concentrate on sites of common injury and areas of easily missed injuries (Fig. 13-11).

The ABC'S approach to radiographic interpretation examines first adequacy and alignment, and then bones, cartilage, and soft tissues. Adequacy mandates that the entire cervical spine ultimately be included. Alignment, bones, and cartilage (joint spaces) are inspected on all radiographic views. Examination of the prevertebral soft tissues is especially important on the lateral view.

The lateral view is most important because 85% of cervical spine injuries are detected on this image.[57] It must be systematically analyzed before other views are obtained. Next, the open-mouth view is obtained and examined, since most of the remaining injuries are seen on this view. Finally, the AP view is reviewed, usually to corroborate abnormalities seen on the lateral view.

Lateral Cervical Spine

A modification of the ABC'S approach, the (ABC'S)^3 method, provides valuable reminders for lateral view interpretation (Table 13-3) (Fig. 13-5A and B).

Adequacy, Alignment, Atlantodental Interval (A^3)

ADEQUACY. The radiograph must be of sufficient quality to demonstrate skeletal detail and interfaces between air, soft tissue, and bone. The entire cervical spine must be visible from the occiput to the C7-T1 interspace. When the C7-T1 interspace is not completely seen, additional imaging such as a swimmer's view, supine oblique, or CT is necessary. Overlapping jewelry must be removed. The radiograph should have no rotation. Rotation is evident when the left and right diamond-shaped lateral masses of each vertebra are not superimposed.

ALIGNMENT. Four smooth lordotic lines are observed: (1) the anterior vertebral body line (ABL); (2) the posterior vertebral body line (PBL); (3) the posterior border of the spinal canal (the spinolaminar line or SLL); and (4) the tips of the spinous processes (spinous process line or SPL) (Fig. 13-12). These lines are relatively parallel throughout physiologic motion. The distance between the PBL and SLL (the boundaries of the

spinal canal) should be at least 13 mm. Straightening is often seen on the supine cross-table lateral view. With the patient upright, straightening may represent muscle spasm due to an injury.

Displacement or angulation of a vertebral body implies injury. An offset of adjacent vertebral bodies of greater than 3.5 mm suggests instability. The angle formed by the superior surfaces of adjacent vertebral borders should be less than 11°. Although these measurements represent the upper limits of physiologic motion, lesser amounts of malalignment must be viewed with suspicion in the acutely traumatized patient.

Alignment of the articular masses should also be assessed. Gradual loss of superimposition of the paired articular masses and facet joints may represent physiologic rotation, but a sudden or isolated change in superimposition is abnormal.

ANTERIOR ATLANTODENTAL INTERVAL. The AADI, or *predental space*, should be 3 mm or less throughout physiologic motion in adults (up to 5 mm in children). An increase implies disruption and instability of the transverse atlantal ligament (TAL). The anterior arch of C1 and the dens are examined at this time.

Basion-Dental Interval, Base of Dens, Bones (B^3)

THE BASION-DENTAL INTERVAL. In an adult, a distance between the basion and tip of the dens greater than 12 mm implies occipitoatlantal dissociation. In children up to age 13 years, the basion-axial interval (BAI) is used.[49] The distance between the basion and a line extending rostrad along the posterior border of the axis body and dens should be less than 12 mm.

BASE OF THE DENS. Fractures at the base of the dens, if nondisplaced, are difficult to identify on the lateral view. These are better seen on the open-mouth view. Although a cortical break through the base of the dens may be seen, this region is often poorly visualized because of overlap by the lateral masses of C1. Slight displacement is best assessed by observing whether the posterior cortex of the dens is aligned with the posterior surface of the C2 vertebral body.

Inspection of the *ring of C2* aids in detecting a fracture through the upper portion of the vertebral body of C2.

BONES. Systematic inspection of the bones of the cervical spine proceeds from top to bottom. For each vertebra, one begins from the same point (for example, the anteroinferior aspect of each vertebral body) and sequentially examines the vertebral body, articular masses, laminae, and spinous process of that vertebra. Particular attention is given to the upper and lower cervical segments, where the majority of missed fractures occur. Despite the unique shape of the vertebral body of C2, the base of C2 has a similar AP diameter to that of the body of C3. The vertebral bodies of C3 through C7 are essentially rectangular, with smoothly corticated borders. Any abrupt angulation or buckling of the cortex is abnormal. A height disparity of more than 2 mm between the anterior and posterior aspects of any individual vertebral body suggests compression. The cortical

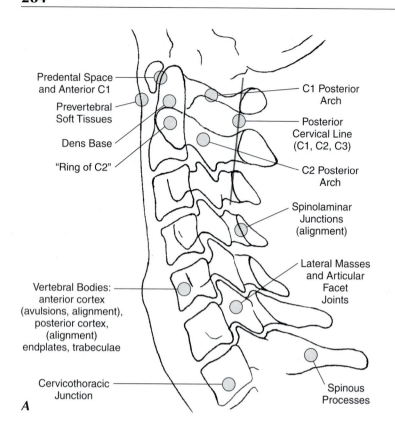

Predental Space and Anterior C1

Prevertebral Soft Tissues

Dens Base

"Ring of C2"

Vertebral Bodies: anterior cortex (avulsions, alignment), posterior cortex, (alignment) endplates, trabeculae

Cervicothoracic Junction

C1 Posterior Arch

Posterior Cervical Line (C1, C2, C3)

C2 Posterior Arch

Spinolaminar Junctions (alignment)

Lateral Masses and Articular Facet Joints

Spinous Processes

A

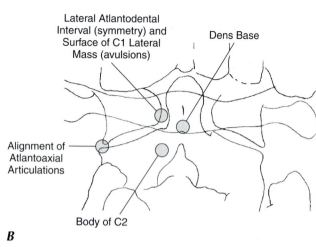

Lateral Atlantodental Interval (symmetry) and Surface of C1 Lateral Mass (avulsions)

Dens Base

Alignment of Atlantoaxial Articulations

Body of C2

B

FIGURE 13-11.   Sites prone to injury and easily missed injuries. *A.* Lateral view. *B.* Open-mouth view. *C.* AP view. *D.* Oblique view.

TABLE 13-3

Systematic Analysis of the Lateral Cervical Spine Radiograph (ABC'S)[3]

A[3]	**Adequacy**: Skull base to the cervicothoracic junction seen.
	  No rotation—left and right lateral masses superimposed.
	Alignment: Four gently lordotic parallel curves (anterior vertebral bodies, posterior vertebral bodies, spinolaminar junctions and tips of spinous processes).
	AADI: Anterior atlantodental interval (predental space) <3 mm (<5 mm in children).
	  Anterior tubercle of C1 intact.

B[3]	**Basion-Dental Interval**: BDI is normally <12 mm.
	  In children, use the basion-axial interval (<12 mm.)
	Base of Dens: Fracture or displacement.
	  Posterior cortex of dens aligned with posterior cortex of C2 vertebral body.
	  Check the "ring of C2."
	Bones: Examine each vertebra in its entirety.
	  Cervicocranium and C5–C7 are most commonly fractured.

C[3]	**Cartilage (disks)**: Intervertebral disk spaces uniform. **Cartilage (facets)**: Interfacetal joint widening or displacement. **Connective tissues (posterior)**: Spinous process or laminar "fanning."
S[3]	**Soft tissues**: Abnormal width or contour of prevertebral soft tissues, especially cervicocranium. **Scan the periphery**: Examine structures outside the spine: skull, mandible, sphenoid sinus, clavicles. **Selective reexamination**: Any area of abnormality is selectively reexamined, including adjacent vertebral segments.

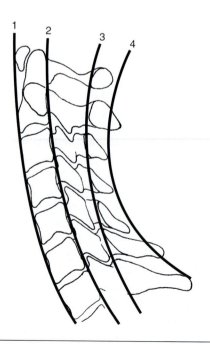

FIGURE 13-12.   Vertebral alignment in the lateral cervical spine radiograph. The four curves of alignment are shown: (1) anterior vertebral body line, (2) posterior vertebral body line, (3) spinolaminar line, and (4) tips of spinous processes.

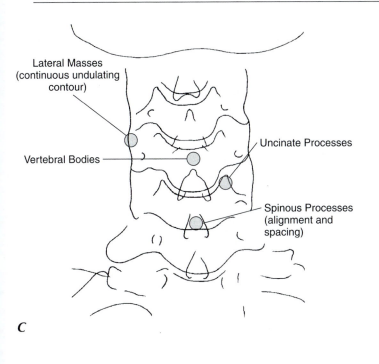

Lateral Masses (continuous undulating contour)

Vertebral Bodies

Uncinate Processes

Spinous Processes (alignment and spacing)

C

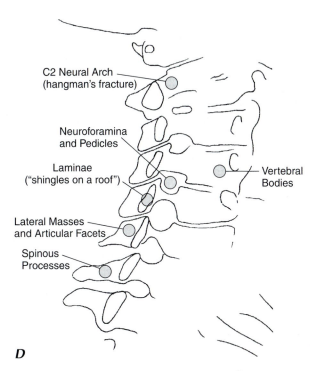

C2 Neural Arch (hangman's fracture)

Neuroforamina and Pedicles

Laminae ("shingles on a roof")

Vertebral Bodies

Lateral Masses and Articular Facets

Spinous Processes

D

margins of the articular masses, laminae, and spinous processes should be free from defect or angulation. The posterior arch of C1 and spinous processes of the lower segments should be carefully examined for fracture.

Cartilaginous Disks, Cartilage of Interfacetal Joints, Connective Tissues (C^3)

DISK SPACES. Adjacent vertebral body end plates are parallel. The intervertebral disk height is uniform throughout the cervical spine. Disk space widening suggests a subjacent compression fracture or ligamentous injury. Disk space narrowing may indicate disk rupture. Diffusely narrowed disk spaces accompany chronic degeneration.

FACET JOINTS. The articular surfaces of opposing facets are parallel and form joint spaces of uniform size at all levels. Widening of the interfacetal space, lack of parallelism, or unmasking of any facet surface indicates pathology, as does rotation of any facet surface from its normal 35° inclination.

POSTERIOR CONNECTIVE TISSUES. The interspaces between the laminae and spinous processes are maintained by the interspinous and supraspinous ligaments. Although the atlantoaxial interspinous space is often larger, the other interspinous spaces

remain fairly consistent at all levels throughout motion. Any focal widening or "fanning" is abnormal. Below C2, adjacent interspinous and interlaminar spaces should not differ by more than 2 mm.

Soft Tissues, Scan the Periphery, Selective Reexamination (S^3)

PREVERTEBRAL SOFT TISSUES. Prevertebral soft tissues normally follow the contour of the anterior surfaces of the vertebral bodies. At the level of C1, its thickness may be up to 10 mm. Between C1 and the top of C4, the soft tissues are fairly narrow (5 to 7 mm). Of greater importance than these measurements is that at C1 and C2, the contour should follow the anterior surfaces of the vertebrae. Any focal bulge, even if the measured thickness is not greater than 5 to 7 mm, may indicate an injury. However, the absence of swelling does not exclude an injury. Below C4, the prevertebral soft tissues approximately triple in thickness, to up to 22 mm, because of the interposed esophagus. Swelling in this area is rarely seen.[58,61]

PERIPHERY OF THE RADIOGRAPH. To ensure complete interpretation, the base of the skull, the mandibles, and the structures of the anterior neck are examined briefly. Fluid in the sphenoid sinus and occipital fractures should be noted. Mandibular fractures may be visible. The contour of the epiglottis, the cortical integrity of the hyoid bone, and the tracheal air shadow require inspection. Foreign bodies in the soft tissues should be identified.

REEXAMINE AREAS OF ABNORMALITY. The discovery of one abnormality should not prevent completion of the systematic analysis. The areas of suspicion detected previously are reexamined as a final step. Adjacent segments are re-inspected and the spine is reviewed for associated abnormalities.

Open-Mouth View

Following interpretation of the lateral cervical spine radiograph, attention is turned to the open-mouth view (Fig. 13-5E and F). This view is systematically analyzed and inspected for signs to corroborate abnormal findings on the lateral film. An ABC'S approach can guide interpretation (Table 13-4).

ADEQUACY. The dens and lateral masses of C1 and C2 should be seen without overlapping teeth, mandible, or skull base. Rotation should be minimal with the dens and the spinous process of C2 aligned in the midline.

ALIGNMENT. The dens is symmetrically located between the lateral masses of C1. Both lateral atlantodental intervals (LADI) are equal. The lateral margins of the articular surfaces of C1 and C2 are aligned. Widening of the lateral masses of C1 in relation to C2 is seen in a Jefferson burst fracture of C1. Slight displacement of both lateral masses of C1 in the same direction and slight asymmetry of the dens is due to tilting or rotation of the head.

BONES. Particular attention is given to the base of the dens. Other fracture sites are the medial aspect of the articular masses of C1 and the body of C2. Overlapping shadows (Mach bands) across the base of the dens must be differentiated from fractures.

CARTILAGE. The lateral articulations of C1 and C2 form parallel joint surfaces.

Anteroposterior View

ALIGNMENT. The spinous processes are normally in the midline. They may gradually deviate to one side if the patient is rotated. Sudden deviation suggests a rotational injury. The articular masses form a smooth, undulating, continuous lateral margin (Fig. 13-5C and D) (Table 13-4).

BONES. The vertebral bodies are of uniform height and width, and their margins should be smooth. Loss of height or increased width prompts a search for cortical lucencies. The uncinate processes extend superiorly from the lateral upper borders of the vertebral bodies, forming the joints of Luschka with the supradjacent vertebra. Disruption of the continuous wavy cortical margin of the lateral columns suggests injury to the articular mass.

CARTILAGE. The intervertebral disk spaces should be consistent in width. The spinous processes are approximately equidistant. Focal widening implies fracture or posterior ligamentous injury.

Swimmer's View

An adequate swimmer's view allows the lower cervical spine and cervicothoracic junction to be seen (Fig. 13-7). The vertebrae are identified by counting down from the distinctive C2 vertebral body. Alignment of the vertebral bodies is the principal observation. Examination of the bones and inspection of the joint and connective tissue relationships is performed in the usual fashion; however, the vertebral structures must be differentiated from overlying bones. One should identify the humerus, clavicle, and ribs, which commonly overlie the vertebrae. If

---

TABLE 13-4

Systematic Analysis of Open-Mouth and AP Radiographs (ABC)

	OPEN-MOUTH VIEW	AP VIEW
Adequacy	No overlap by teeth or skull base. Dens and spinous process of C2 are midline.	No tilt or rotation of neck.
Alignment	Lateral articular surfaces of C1 and C2 aligned. Dens positioned symmetrically between lateral masses of C1.	Spinous processes aligned in midline and evenly spaced. Lateral margin of the lateral masses appears as a continuous, undulating surface.
Bones	Base of the dens. Body of C2. Small avulsions of medial aspects of C1 lateral masses.	Vertebral bodies, uncinate processes, lateral masses, spinous processes.
Cartilage (joint spaces)	Articular spaces between C1 and C2 are even and symmetrical.	Disk spaces of uniform height.

there is high clinical suspicion of a C7 injury, a CT scan should be performed before the region is "cleared."

Oblique Views

Oblique views are optional in many centers. They are most useful for detecting a unilateral facet dislocation (UFD) or fracture of the neural arch (Fig. 13-8).

ALIGNMENT. The anterior and posterior boundaries of the vertebral bodies are aligned. Depending on the angle at which the film is exposed, the laminae, articular masses, or both will be visible. The laminae and/or articular masses should be stacked like "shingles on a roof." Loss of the "shingled" relationship between adjacent laminae or articular masses is seen with a facet dislocation or fracture of the posterior column.

BONES. The pedicles, articular masses, and laminae are inspected for fractures. The examination is focused on an area of abnormal alignment. The neuroforaminal openings are seen.

CARTILAGE. The articular facets and apophyseal joints are examined. Uncovered facet surfaces, widened apophyseal joints, or facets displaced into the subjacent neural groove are indicative of rotational or posterior column injury.

Flexion-Extension Views

Important observations on the flexion-extension views are the adequacy of range of motion and the preservation of normal intervertebral relationships (Fig. 13-9). Adequate flexion is demonstrated when the inferior border of the patient's mandible (with the mouth closed) is vertical—i.e., parallel to the patient's torso. Extension is adequate when adjacent spinous processes are close together and nearly touching. Radiographs that fall short of these parameters are nondiagnostic. Indicators of posterior ligamentous instability include slippage of adjacent vertebral bodies greater than 3 mm, loss of parallelism of adjacent articular facets, unmasking of an articular facet, widening of an interlaminar space, and widening of an interspinous distance more than 2 mm greater than adjacent spaces ("fanning"). Anterior ligamentous injury is present when there is widening of the anterior disk space on the extension view.[58,60]

PEDIATRIC CONSIDERATIONS

Developmental Anatomy

There are several distinctive anatomic characteristics of the cervical spine in children.[1,2] Some of these developmental features result in radiographic findings that could appear pathologic in the adult, mimicking fractures, malalignment, and soft tissue abnormalities. The two principal aspects of the developing spinal column that are responsible for these radiographic findings are (1) incomplete vertebral ossification and open cartilaginous growth plates, and (2) laxity of supporting ligaments

and surrounding soft tissues.

In the child, the supportive ligaments between adjacent vertebrae are relatively lax. This has a protective effect such that the pediatric cervical spine is able to withstand traumatic distortions without fracture or dislocation. Ligamentous laxity accounts, in part, for the low incidence of cervical spine fractures in children. On the other hand, increased mobility of the spinal column allows the spinal cord to be traumatized when there are no radiographically detectable injuries.

Growth plates in developing vertebrae differ from the epiphyseal growth plates in long bones. In long bones, growth occurs only on the metaphyseal side of the growth plate whereas in the spine, the growth plate lays down bone along both of its surfaces. Growth plates in the spinal skeleton are termed *synchondroses* (Figure 13-13).

Cervicocranium. The atlas (C1) has three ossification centers (Fig. 13-13*A*). The anterior arch of the atlas is not ossified at birth and in the young infant. It begins to ossify in the first year of life and becomes fused to the lateral masses by the age 9 years. The posterior arch of C1 is formed from two lateral ossification centers, which fuse in the dorsal midline by 5 years of age.[59]

The ossification centers of the axis (C2) include the vertebral body centrum, two lateral neural arch ossification centers, and three ossification centers for the dens (Fig. 13-13*B*). The body of the dens is formed from two ossification centers, which fuse before birth. The tip of the dens has a notched appearance in early childhood. A separate ossification for the tip of the dens, the *ossiculum terminale*, appears in early childhood and unites with the dens by age 12 years. Between the base of the dens and the centrum of C2 is the subdental synchondrosis. The synchondroses between the neural arches, vertebral body and the dens form an H when C2 is viewed from the front. These growth plates usually fuse by age 6. Occasionally, the subdental synchondrosis persists to about age 11, leaving a transverse lucency at the base of the dens. Any of these radiolucent growth plates could be misinterpreted as a fracture.

Lower Cervical Spine. At birth, each lower cervical vertebra consists of three main ossification centers—the vertebral body *centrum* and the two sides of the neural arch (Fig. 13-13*C*). During childhood, the neural arch fuses posteriorly before fusing with the centrum. The vertebral body is formed from the large central ossification center and the superior and inferior end plates. The end plates do not begin to ossify until adolescence. Therefore, throughout childhood, the vertebral bodies appear shortened and rounded. From adolescence until early adulthood, the end plates appear as thin layers of bone adjacent to the superior and inferior surfaces of the vertebral body centrum.

Radiographic Anatomy

The Lateral View in Children. In *infancy,* the occipitoatlantal articulation is clearly visible (Fig. 13-14*A* and *B*). The anterior arch of C1 is not present at birth, becoming ossified during the

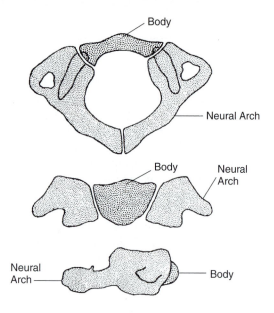

Developmental Anatomy of C-1

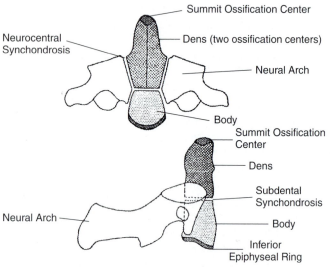

Developmental Anatomy of C-2

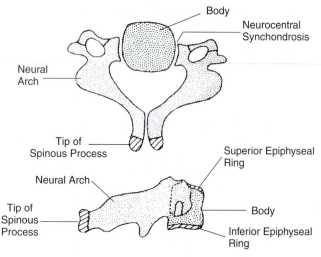

**Developmental Anatomy of the
Lower Cervical Vertebrae (C3-C7)**

FIGURE 13-13. Developmental anatomy of the cervical spine. (From Bailey DK: The normal cervical spine in infants and children. Radiology 59:712, 1952, with permission.)

first year of life. When ossified, it may be located near the superior tip of the dens. This apparent displacement is due in part to the fact that the ossification center of the tip of the dens is not yet visible. The posterior arch of C1 is seen posterior to the dens. The subdental synchrondrosis (growth plate) separates the dens from the body of C2.

Because the tip of the dens is not ossified, determination of the basion dental interval is unreliable in children up to 13 years of age. An alternate measurement is used: the *basion-axial interval* (BAI).[49] The BAI is the distance between the basion and a line extending rostrad along the posterior border of the axis body and dens. The BAI should be less than 12 mm (Fig. 13-10).

The vertebral bodies from C3 to C7 appear rounded anteriorly. The articular facets are indistinct and nearly horizontal. The articular masses and laminae extend posteriorly from the vertebral bodies.

At *age 3 years*, the anterior arch of C1 is completely ossified (Fig. 13–14C). The subdental synchondrosis remains visible. The vertebral bodies are more completely ossified, but the anterior surfaces retain a curved or wedged shape. The articular masses and facets are more distinct but remain horizontal.

In an *8-year-old* child, the lateral cervical radiograph often resembles more closely that of an adult (Fig. 13–14D). The synchondroses of C2 have mostly fused. The anterior curvature of the vertebral bodies has diminished. Separate ossification centers for the superior and inferior end plates of the vertebral bodies have begun to appear. They do not fuse to the vertebral bodies until early adulthood. Articular facets have the normal adult inclination. The neural arches have fused, forming the spinous processes.

FIGURE 13-14. Radiographic anatomy of the cervical spine in children of different ages. *A.* Lateral view, 8-day-old infant. The alignment is normal. Note the subdental synchondrosis *(small arrow)*. The anterior arch of C1 is not yet ossified. The posterior arch of C1 lies posterior to the dens *(curved arrow)*. The vertebral bodies appear rounded anteriorly. The articular facets are indistinct and nearly horizontal. The prevertebral soft tissues are normal in width and contour, measuring 5 mm at C2 and 10 mm anterior to C5. *B.* Lateral view, 8-week-old infant. The large occiput makes the upper cervical segments appear to be flexed in this supine radiograph. The atlantooccipital junction is visible. The anterior arch of C1 is now ossified *(arrow)* and in a normal position somewhat cephalad to the dens. The subdental synchondrosis is visible *(arrowhead)*. The vertebral bodies are rounded. *C.* Lateral view, 3-year-old child. The spine is seen from the occiput to T1. The atlantooccipital joint remains partially visible. The anterior arch of C1 is ossified *(arrow)*. The subdental synchondrosis has nearly disappeared *(arrowhead)*. The vertebral bodies are shortened anteriorly. The facets are more distinct and steeply inclined *(asterisk)*. The posterior neural arches have fused, as indicated by the presence of the spinolaminar junction *(curved arrow)*. *D.* Lateral view, 8-year-old child. The atlantooccipital joint and the subdental synchondrosis are no longer visible. The end plates have not ossified, leaving the anterior vertebral bodies shortened and rounded. The remaining structures have attained their adult configuration. The soft tissues anterior to the occiput and C1 are thickened and lobulated due to enlarged adenoidal tissue *(asterisk)*.

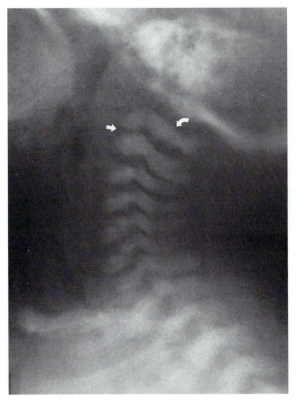

A. Eight-day-old

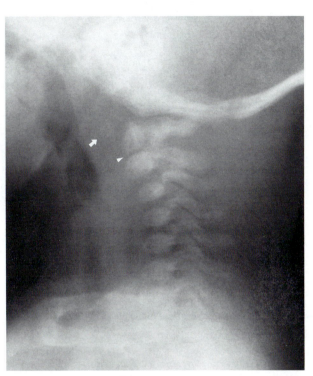

B. Eight-week-old

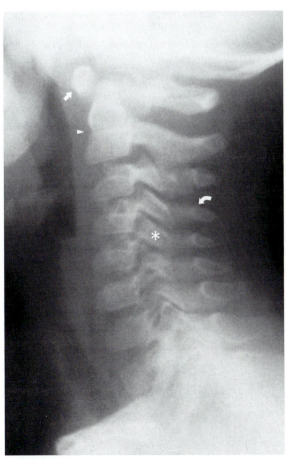

C. Three-year-old

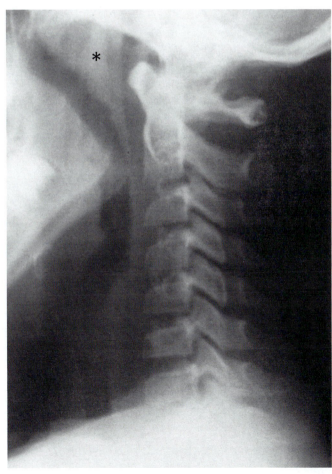

D. Eight-year-old

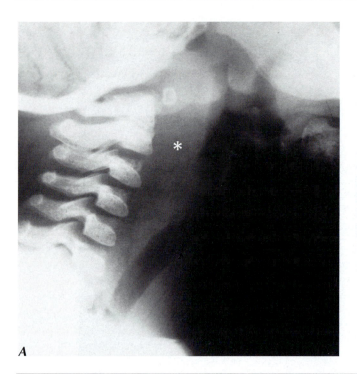

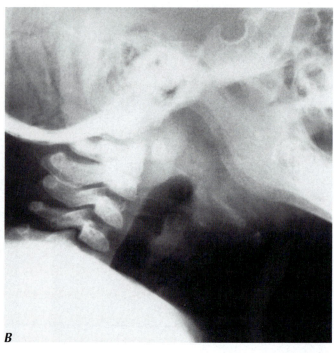

A   *B*

FIGURE 13-15.   Apparent soft tissue swelling in a young child due to poor positioning. Prevertebral soft tissue laxity in a young child can cause marked thickening when the child is crying, flexed forward or swallowing (*A*). A second film with better positioning shows normal prevertebral soft tissues (*B*).

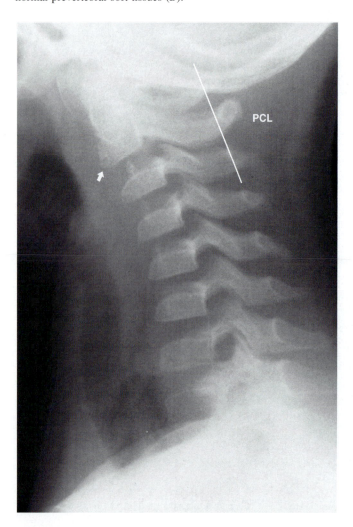

SOFT TISSUE LAXITY.   Ligamentous laxity creates three distinctive radiographic findings in young children. First, the prevertebral soft tissues can appear thickened if the patient's neck is flexed or the patient is swallowing or crying at the time of exposure. This "physiologic pseudomass" of infancy disappears when the radiograph is repeated during inspiration and with the neck extended (Fig. 13-15).

Second, the predental space (*anterior atlantodental interval* or AADI) between the anterior arch of C1 and the dens, can be up to 5 mm wide in children up to about age 8 to 10 years (it is <3 mm in adults) (Fig. 13-14*D*). This is due to laxity of the transverse atlantal ligament. In addition, the cortical surfaces of the predental space are often not parallel especially during neck flexion.[60]

Third, ligamentous laxity allows the vertebral body to slip anteriorly at the C2-C3 and C3-C4 intervertebral disks in children up to age 8 (Fig. 13-16).[43,61] This is termed *pseudosubluxation*. The limit of physiologic vertebral body slippage is gauged by the *posterior cervical line* (PCL). The PCL connects the spinolaminar junctions of C1, C2, and C3. These three points should form a straight line. With C2-C3 pseudosubluxation, the spinolaminar junction of C2 remains within 2 mm of the posterior cervical line.

FIGURE 13-16.   Pseudosubluxation and the posterior cervical line. Lateral view of a 5-year-old boy demonstrates generous anterior movement of C2 relative to C3 (*arrow*). The posterior cervical line (PCL) drawn between the spinolaminar junction of C1 and C3 verifies that this is physiologic. In pseudosubluxation, the spinolaminar junction of C2 is within 2 mm of the PCL.

The AP and Open-Mouth View in Children

The open-mouth view can be difficult or impossible to obtain in young children.[45] When clinical suspicion of an injury to this region is high, a CT scan is often obtained instead. The lateral masses of C1 are ossified at birth. In early childhood, the occipitoatlantal articulation may be visible. Until about age 3, the dens appears shortened and has a notched tip. Between ages of 3 and 6 years, the *ossiculum terminale* appears at the tip of the dens. It fuses with the dens at about age 12 years.

Because the lateral masses of C1 ossify before the lateral articular surfaces of C2, the lateral masses of C1 can appear widened in relation to C2. This normal finding in the young child simulates a Jefferson burst fracture of C1. When doubt exists, a CT scan should be performed.

Up to age 6, the synchondroses of the dens and the body of C2 form a radiolucent H on the open-mouth view. The subdental synchondrosis may remain open until age 11. Open neurocentral synchondroses of the lower cervical vertebrae are seen on the AP radiograph (Fig. 13-17).

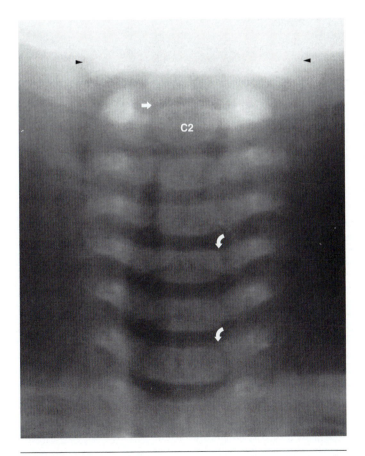

FIGURE 13-17. AP view—2-year-old child. An AP view obtained using the modified Fuchs technique (head slightly extended) demonstrates the cervical spine from the atlantoaxial articulation to C7. The lateral masses of C1 are faintly visible through overlying skull (*black arrowheads*). The subdental synchondrosis separates the dens from the body of C2 (*arrow*). Synchondroses separate the vertebral bodies from the lateral masses at lower levels (*curved arrows*).

COMMON ABNORMALITIES

Injuries of the cervical spine are divided between those of the cervicocranium and those of the lower cervical spine. Injuries of the cervical spine in adults are most common at C2, C5, and C6.[62] Older adults sustain relatively more injuries to the cervicocranium. The preponderance of cervical spine injuries that occur in childhood are at the cervicocranium, although the overall incidence among children is low.

Most cervical spine fractures are readily recognized. Occasionally, the cervical spine injury is difficult to identify, putting the patient at risk for further injury. Most missed injuries are at the cervicocranium and cervicothoracic junction. Injuries at the cervicothoracic junction are missed because the region can be obscured on the lateral radiograph by overlying shoulder musculature. Cervicocranial injuries are missed because of three factors: (1) the anatomy of the region is complex, making the radiographic findings difficult to appreciate; (2) pain and tenderness are poorly localized with high cervical injuries; and (3) neurologic deficits are relatively uncommon in survivors of high cervical injury. The incidence of spinal cord injury in survivors with cervicocranial injuries is relatively low for three reasons: (1) the spinal canal is widest in relation to the size of the spinal cord at the cervicocranium; (2) some cervicocranial fractures actually widen the spinal canal because the neural arch has burst outward; and (3) patients with cord injuries at C1 and C2 generally do not survive to hospital presentation.

Injuries of the lower cervical spine are classified on the basis of the mechanism of injury and the associated forces. Cervicocranial injuries are classified on an anatomic basis.

To better understand lower cervical injuries, the terms used to describe mechanical stresses or motions must be understood. *Flexion* is the forward bending of the head and neck in the midsagittal plane. *Extension* is bending of the head and neck posteriorly in the midsagittal plane. *Lateral bending* is movement of the head in the coronal plane. *Rotation* is turning or pivoting of the head and spinal segments on the vertical axis extending through the torso, neck, and head. *Compression* (axial load) is a force exerted down the vertical axis through the head and spine. *Distraction* is a force vector directed up the vertical axis, creating tension on supporting structures. Most injuries are the result of combined forces such as compressive-extension, compressive-flexion, or distractive-flexion.

Cervical Spine Injuries in Children

Cervical injury is rare in children younger than 16 years of age, accounting for only 2 to 10% of all cervical spine injuries. Furthermore, only 10 to 15% of pediatric spine injuries occur in children younger than 8 years. In young children, the upper cervical spine is the site of most injuries. This is because the child has a relatively heavy head and the neck has a high mechanical fulcrum at C2-C3. The anatomic distribution of injuries in children older than 8 to 12 years is similar to that of adults.[1,2,63]

Spinal cord injury occurs in 10 to 36% of children with cervical fractures or dislocations, and about 10% of cord injuries result in quadriplegia. *Spinal cord injury without radiographic abnormality* (SCIWORA) accounts for about 20% of all spinal cord injuries in children.[7-9] The onset can be delayed up to 4 days after trauma. This late onset is due to delayed compromise of blood supply to the cord. Most patients with SCIWORA are younger than 8 years of age. Prognosis is poor for patients who are younger than age 3 or those who have complete cord lesions. Patients with incomplete lesions tend to improve.[64]

Certain cervical spine injuries are unique to children. Odontoid synchondral fracture-separation (epiphysiolysis dentis) with atlantoaxial dislocation occurs exclusively in young children. Rotary atlantoaxial subluxation or dislocation seldom occurs in patients beyond adolescence. Injuries of the lower cervical spine in children are usually subluxations, dislocations, or compression injuries.[63,65]

Cervicocranial Injuries

Injuries to the cervicocranium are classified anatomically based on the vertebra involved (Table 13-5). Atlas (C1) fractures constitute about 10% of all cervical fractures and 25% of fractures of the cervicocranium. They are associated with other cervical fractures about 50% of the time, especially fractures of C2.[66] The axis (C2) is one of the more commonly fractured cervical vertebrae. Odontoid fractures and neural arch (hangman's) fractures each account for about 35% of fractures of the cervicocranium.[56,67]

OCCIPITOATLANTAL DISLOCATION.   Occipitoatlantal dislocation (OAD) is typically found in patients with severe head trauma. It is a grave and often fatal injury and is frequently discovered postmortem. Damage to the ligaments of the occipitoatlantal joints results in subluxation or complete dislocation. The occiput can be distracted or translocated anteriorly (most common) or posteriorly relative to the atlas.[49] The injury occurs more commonly in children. The victim is usually dead or neurologically devastated, although occasionally a patient survives.

The diagnosis is made on the lateral cervical radiograph (Fig. 13-18). The relationship of the skull base to the atlas is disrupted, as demonstrated by an increased basion-dental interval (BDI) and basion-axial interval (BAI). More severe cases are displaced anteriorly with obvious dislocation of the atlas from the occipital condyles. Severe retropharyngeal swelling can compromise the airway.

OCCIPITAL CONDYLE FRACTURE.   Occipital condyle fractures are being recognized more frequently as more patients receive cervicocranial CT during trauma evaluation. These fractures are caused by impaction from an axial load, extension of a basilar skull fracture, or avulsion by the attachment of the alar ligament following excessive rotation.[6] Patients complain of pain in the upper neck and skull base and may have lower cranial nerve deficits.

TABLE 13-5

Injuries of the Cervicocranium

	LATERAL VIEW	OPEN-MOUTH VIEW
Occipitoatlantal dislocation	Increased BDI and BAI Visible occipitoatlantal joints	
Atlantoaxial dislocation	Increased AADI	Avulsion off medial aspect of C1 lateral mass
Jefferson burst fracture	Increased AADI (occasional) Posterior arch C1 fracture (occasional)	Laterally displaced C1 lateral masses Dens asymmetrical between C1
C1 posterior arch fracture	Posterior arch C1 fracture	
Dens fracture—High (Type II)	Fracture at the dens base Dens displacement (anterior or posterior)	Fracture at base of dens
Dens fracture—Low (Type III)	Disruption of "ring of C2"	Fracture through upper body of C2
Hangman's fracture—Type I	Minimally displaced C2 posterior arch fractures Slight anterolisthesis of C2 vertebral body C2 spinolaminar junction minimally displaced posteriorly	
Hangman's fracture—Type II	Fractured C2 posterior arch Anteriorly displaced C2 vertebral body, +/− angulation C2 spinolaminar junction minimally displaced posteriorly	
Hangman's fracture—Type III	Fractured C2 posterior arch Anteriorly displaced and angulated C2 vertebral body Dislocation of C2–C3 articular facets and displaced posterior arch	
C2 vertebral body fracture	Increased C2 body width ("fat" C2)	

Key: BDI, basion-dental interval; BAI, basion-axial interval; AADI, anterior atlantoaxial interval

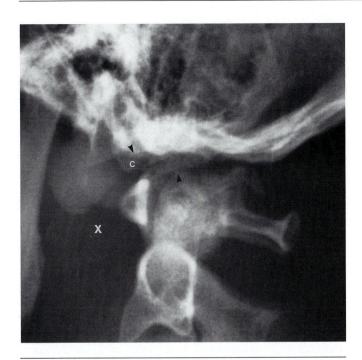

FIGURE 13-18. Occipitoatlantal dislocation. Lateral radiograph demonstrates anterior and cephalad movement of the skull base with respect to C1. The distance between the basion and dens (*small black arrowheads*), the BDI, is greater than 12 mm. The occipital condyles are displaced anteriorly out of the articular facets of C1 (*white C*). There is marked prevertebral soft tissue swelling (white X). This was a fatal injury. (© Washington University, used by permission.)

Plain radiographs seldom offer evidence of injury other than prevertebral soft tissue swelling. In fact, soft tissue swelling should prompt further investigation. The abnormality is demonstrated by axial CT through the occipitoatlantal articulation. Fractures of the avulsion type are unstable, requiring immobilization.

ATLANTOAXIAL DISLOCATIONS. These injuries are uncommon. There are two distinct types: rupture of the transverse ligament and rotary subluxation or dislocation. Most cases of rotatory subluxation or dislocation occur in children.[45]

Isolated Transverse Ligament Disruption. Isolated tearing of the transverse atlantal ligament (TAL) with or without trauma to the dens causes disruption of the atlantodental articulation. Systemic conditions (rheumatoid arthritis, ankylosing spondylitis) or local inflammatory disorders (tuberculosis) weaken the transverse ligament and erode the dens, causing dislocation following even trivial trauma. Traumatic TAL rupture without predisposing systemic illness is unusual and typically occurs in older adults with blunt occipital trauma. Patients usually have minimal neurologic compromise.

A TAL rupture is extremely unstable. The diagnosis is usually made on the lateral plain radiograph by a widened AADI (>3 mm) (Fig. 13-19). However, the diagnosis can be missed when the patient is supine, the neck is slightly flexed, and the dislocation is reduced. In some cases, the BDI may be abnormal. The open-mouth view may reveal a small avulsion fracture from the medial surface of either lateral mass of C1. In

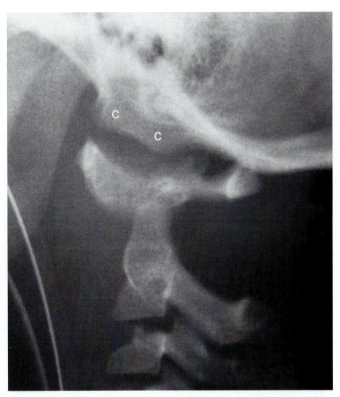

FIGURE 13-19. Atlantoaxial and occipitoatlantal dislocation. Lateral radiograph in a 3-year-old child showing cephalad dislocation of the skull base with respect to C1 and anterior dislocation of C1 with respect to C2. The occipitoatlantal articulation is widened. The occipital condyles (*white C*), are translocated from their fossae in C1. Anterior motion of C1 with respect to C2 is demonstrated by the position of the dens in the central portion of the C1 ring. The AADI is 19 mm. (© Washington University, used by permission.)

cases of spontaneous reduction, retropharyngeal swelling may be the only radiographic clue. The patient's severe neck pain and muscle spasm suggest a serious injury and the need for further study. Careful physician-guided flexion and extension views are advocated in the absence of neurologic injury to detect this ligamentous injury.[67]

Atlantoaxial Rotary Subluxation. In the absence of trauma, atlantoaxial rotary subluxation is called *torticollis* or *wry neck*. It represents physiologic motion that is temporarily fixed because of an inflammatory process or muscle spasm. On the other hand, traumatic subluxation is associated with incomplete ligamentous damage (Fig. 13-20). In the mildest form of traumatic subluxation, it has the same radiographic appearance as that of nontraumatic rotary subluxation. In more severe cases, translocation of the atlantoaxial rotational axis and asymmetrical articulation of the lateral masses of C1 and C2 are present.

The lateral radiograph demonstrates rotation of the atlas, while the paired structures of the remainder of the spine are perfectly superimposed. One lateral mass of C1 projects over the dens, making the predental space indistinct. Traumatic subluxation frequently has retropharyngeal soft tissue swelling. On the open-mouth view, although it is often difficult to obtain, there is asymmetry of the lateral atlantodental intervals and the lateral masses of the atlas.

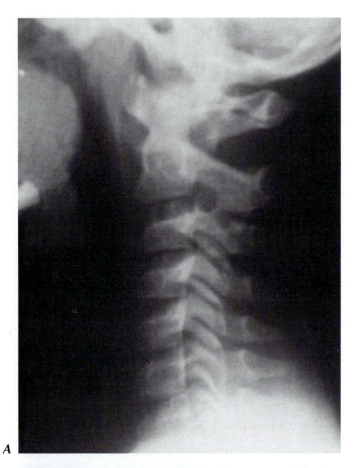

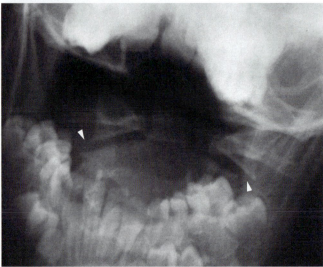

Nontraumatic subluxation is of limited clinical significance and usually resolves spontaneously. Traumatic subluxation is painful and usually requires intervention. These patients are immobilized and require urgent consultation.

Atlantoaxial Rotary Dislocation.   Atlantoaxial rotary dislocation results from severe rotary stress. The patient has considerable pain and distinct posturing. The radiographic appearance is the same as that of severe subluxation. The fixed rotation prevents positioning for an open-mouth radiograph. The diagnosis is made by CT, showing total displacement of the apposed articular surfaces (Fig. 13-21). Immediate consultation is required for treatment.

JEFFERSON BURST FRACTURE OF C1.   Jefferson burst fracture is an axial compression injury involving C1. Because of the slope on the C1 articular surfaces, axial compression causes lateral expulsion of the lateral masses of C1. It was originally described as a four-part fracture, although two- or three-part injuries often occur. In all cases, one fracture involves the anterior arch of C1 and the other the posterior arch. The transverse ligament can be ruptured. Patients may have neck pain, odynophagia, and pain or hypesthesia in the greater occipital nerve distribution. In as many as 53% of patients,[67] Jefferson fractures are associated with fractures of C2.

The lateral radiograph may demonstrate a fracture of the posterior arch (Fig. 13-22). Retropharyngeal swelling is often seen. An increased predental space suggests rupture of the transverse ligament. On the open-mouth view, the lateral masses of C1 are usually displaced off the lateral borders of the C2 superior articular facets. Displacement of greater than 6.9 mm indicates transverse ligamentous disruption, although less displacement does not prove that the traverse ligament is intact.[68] If an open-mouth view is unobtainable, the diagnosis is confirmed by CT, which readily identifies the C1 ring fractures. CT can also identify lateral mass avulsion fractures at the insertion sites of the transverse ligament. In the absence of transverse ligament disruption or other fractures, Jefferson fracture is mechanically stable. Patients are admitted for neck immobilization and advanced imaging.

FIGURE 13-20.   Atlantoaxial rotary subluxation. *A.* Lateral cervical radiograph of an 8-year-old boy with neck pain and rotated head posture after a collision in a soccer game. The lower cervical spine is slightly rotated. Rotation and lateral tilt at the cervicocranium result in an indistinct AADI and lack of superimposition of the lateral masses of C1. The prevertebral soft tissues at C1 are normal. *B.* An open-mouth odontoid projection was obtained despite the patient's fixed head tilt and rotation. The lateral margins of the articular masses of C1 and C2 are malaligned (*arrowheads*), which, in combination with the marked asymmetry of the left and right LADI, indicate lateral tilt to the left. Two findings indicate rightward rotation of the occiput and C1 relative to C2: the left lateral mass of C1 is greater in transverse dimension than the right, and the middle incisors are displaced to the right of the dens. This combination of rotation opposite the direction of extreme lateral tilt represent torticollis or rotatory subluxation. CT was performed to rule-out rotatory dislocation. The patient's symptoms resolved following conservative treatment with cervical support and analgesia.

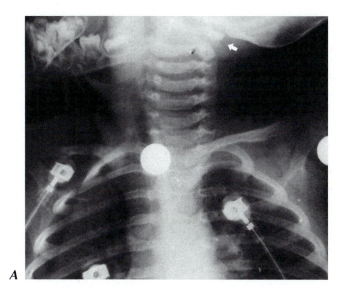

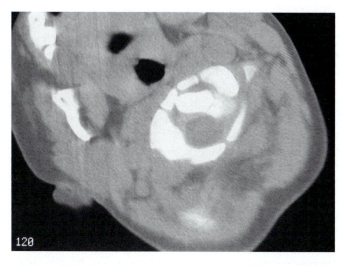

FIGURE 13-21. Atlantoaxial rotary dislocation. *A.* On the AP radiograph, the child's head is fixed in rotation to the right. C1 is rotated with respect to C2 (*arrow*). *B.* CT of C1 shows the dens dislocated with respect to the anterior arch of C1. (Courtesy Ellen Cavenagh, MD, Sparrow Hospital, Lansing, Michigan)

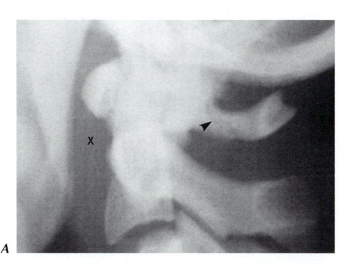

FIGURE 13-22. Jefferson burst fracture. *A.* Lateral radiograph shows a fracture through the posterior arch of C1 (*arrowhead*). Convexity of the retropharyngeal soft tissues indicates swelling (X). *B.* Open-mouth odontoid view shows bilateral widening of the LADI (X) and lateral displacement of the lateral masses of C1 with respect to C2 (*arrows*). A horizontal linear band through the center of the image is due to an overlying spine immobilization backboard. The central incisor teeth project over the dens. (© Washington University, used by permission.)

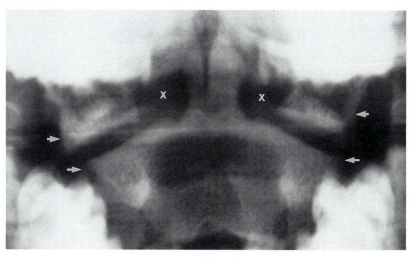

ISOLATED FRACTURE OF THE POSTERIOR ARCH OF C1.   Forceful hyperextension compresses the posterior arch of C1 between the occiput and posterior structures of C2. Patients have occipital pain or pain at the base of the neck.

The fracture is often apparent on the lateral radiograph (Fig. 13-23A and B). The fracture line is usually immediately posterior to the articular masses. The absence of retropharyngeal soft tissue swelling helps to distinguish this injury from a Jefferson burst fracture. Normal alignment of the lateral masses of C1 on the open-mouth view also reduces the likelihood of a Jefferson fracture. An isolated fracture of the posterior arch is considered stable; however, a fracture of C2 accompanies about half of all C1 posterior arch fractures.[65,66] CT is performed in all cases to detect a Jefferson burst fracture or associated C2 fracture. Congenital defects in the abnormalities of the posterior arch of C1 are common and must be differentiated from an acute fracture.

AXIS (C2) BODY FRACTURES.   The mechanism of injury for fractures of the body of C2 is poorly understood. The fracture is vertical and usually oblique, making it difficult to see on the lateral or open-mouth views. Prevertebral soft tissue swelling occurs. The "fat C2" sign (increase in the anteroposterior dimension of the C2 body relative to C3 on the lateral radiograph) is indicative of this fracture.[69] The diagnosis frequently requires CT. Fractures of the body of C2 are potentially unstable.

HANGMAN'S FRACTURE.   The "hangman's fracture," also called *traumatic spondylolisthesis of the axis*, is a bilateral fracture of the neural arch of C2. The mechanism of injury is hyperextension. The fracture is similar to that occurring in judicial hanging. In such a hanging, the distraction force severs the spinal cord. Today, however, most hangman's fractures are produced by hyperextension and compression. This occurs in a motor vehicle head-on collision when the patient's head strikes

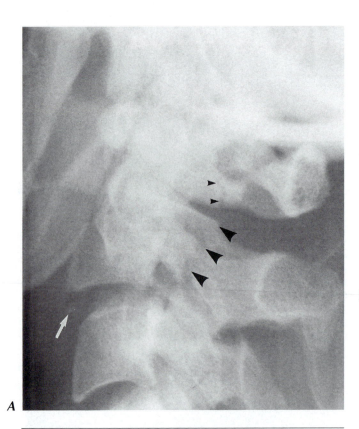

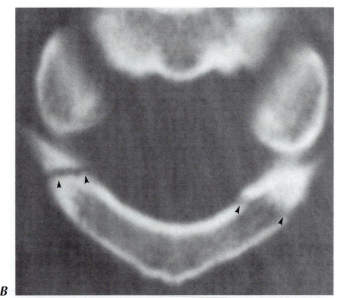

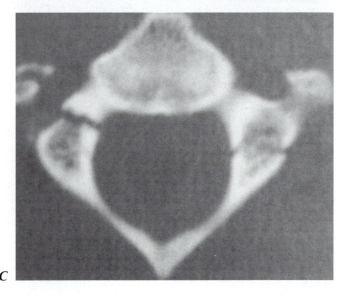

FIGURE 13-23.   Hangman's fracture and fracture of the posterior arch of C1. *A.* Vertically oriented fractures are seen in the posterior arch of C1 (*small black arrowheads*). There are also fractures of the posterior elements of C2 (*large black arrowheads*)—a hangman's fracture. There is mild anterolisthesis of C2 with respect to C3, approximately 3 mm, and avulsion of a small fragment at the anteroinferior corner of C2 (*small white arrow*). The C2-3 disk space is widened anteriorly. *B.* CT at the level of C1 shows bilateral fractures of the posterior arch of C1 (*arrowheads*). There were no fractures of the anterior arch of C1, which excludes a Jefferson burst fracture. *C.* CT at the level of C2 shows bilateral fractures of the lateral masses of C2—a hangman's fracture. (© Washington University, used by permission.)

the windshield while the neck is extended. The compressive nature of the injury results in a lower incidence of spinal cord injury than with a judicial hanging.

The lateral radiograph is diagnostic in most cases (Fig. 13-23A and C).[70] However, when there is minimal displacement, the injury is radiographically subtle.

The Effendi classification subdivides hangman's fractures into three types.[47] Type I fractures, the most common, are minimally displaced.[71] The body of C2 is not displaced, and the anterior longitudinal ligament (ALL) and C2-C3 disk are intact. Type I fractures are considered mechanically stable. Because displacement of the anterior and posterior fragments is minimal, it can be difficult to identify the injury on the radiographs. There may be a slight cortical irregularity of the neural arch of C2 or slight malalignment of the spinolaminar line (posterior cervical line) with posterior displacement of C2. Slight anterior displacement of the C2 vertebral body relative to C3 may also be present. These patients are immobilized and admitted to the hospital.

In type II fractures, the C2-C3 disk is disrupted and the C2 vertebral body is displaced anteriorly. The interfacet articulations are intact. Patients with these injuries are more likely to have neurologic deficits than those with type I fractures. All must be considered unstable.

The rare type III fracture is the result of flexion and compression with subsequent rebound extension. This causes greater displacement of the vertebral body than in a type II fracture. In addition, there is displacement of one or both of the articular facet joints. Associated fractures and neurologic injuries are common. The supporting structures of both the anterior and posterior columns are disrupted and the spine is unstable.

DENS FRACTURES.   Odontoid fractures are often seen in younger patients following motor vehicle accidents (MVAs). They also occur in older adults after falls. They may be associated with fractures of C1. Neurologic injury occurs in up to 25% of cases, ranging from minimal nerve root deficits to quadriplegia.

Dens fractures are classified into three groups depending on the location of the fracture. Type I fractures are caused by avulsion of the dens tip by the alar ligament. These are rarely encountered and are mechanically stable. Some authors doubt the existence of type I injury and classify dens fractures into "high" and "low" categories. Type II or high fractures occur at the base of the dens. These are the most common. Type III or low fractures are oblique fractures through the upper part of the C2 vertebral body.

FIGURE 13-24. Dens fracture, type II. *A.* Lateral radiograph shows discontinuity of the posterior cortex at the base of the dens and a 2-mm-wide fracture (*arrowheads*). The "ring of C2" is intact. *B.* Open-mouth view shows the fracture through the base of the dens (*arrows*). The fracture is partially hidden by a Mach band caused by the overlying posterior arch of C1. Cortical disruption and the jagged fracture line indicate pathology. (© Washington University, used by permission.)

Nondisplaced type II dens fractures can be extremely subtle on plain radiographs (Fig. 13-24). Discontinuity of the dens cortex is usually seen on the open-mouth view. The fracture through the base of the dens is occasionally seen on the lateral view. Displacement makes the injury obvious. Retropharyngeal swelling is expected but not uniformly present. If no abnormality other than soft tissue swelling is evident, CT should be performed and sagittal and coronal reconstructions must be included.

Type II fractures are unstable. Associated fractures are found in about 25% of cases. CT evaluation for an associated C1 injury is necessary. Neurologic injury is more likely when there is displacement or angulation.[65] Nonunion occurs in 26 to 36% of cases regardless of the degree of displacement.[70]

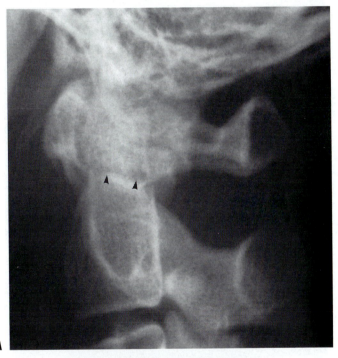

A

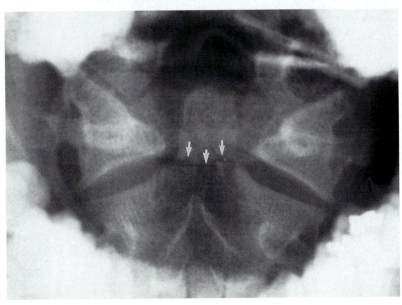

B

Type III or "low" dens fractures are actually fractures of the body of C2. The fracture extends through the superior part of the vertebral body, creating a crater-like defect. The superior fragment consists of the dens attached to a convex C2 body segment (Fig. 13-25). The most easily recognizable abnormalities on the lateral radiograph are prevertebral soft tissue swelling and the disruption of the axis "ring." The open-mouth view often demonstrates the V-shaped fracture through the superior aspect of the axis body. This injury is unstable, but the

prognosis for complete healing is much better than in high dens fractures.

Odontoid synchondral fracture-separation is an injury of the axis in young children. It resembles a dens fracture (Fig. 13-26). The dens is separated from the C2 vertebral body at the subdental synchondrosis. The amount of displacement is variable.[62,64] On the lateral radiograph, the anterior and posterior cortex of the dens and C2 vertebral body are malaligned and sometimes angulated. The injury is mechanically unstable.

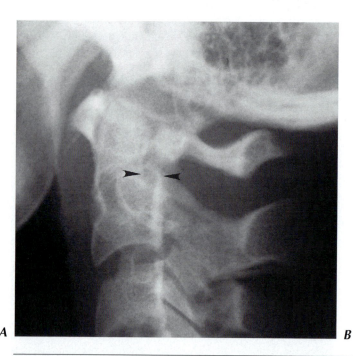

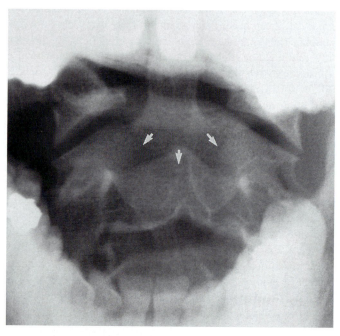

A   *B*

FIGURE 13-25.   Dens fracture, type III. *A.* Lateral view demonstrates 5-mm anterior displacement of the dens with respect to the body of C2. There is discontinuity at the posterosuperior aspect of the "ring of C2" (*arrowheads*). *B.* The open-mouth view shows a subtle linear lucency across the body of C2 just below to the dens (*arrows*).

FIGURE 13-26.   Odontoid synchondral fracture/separation with atlantoaxial dislocation. The basion-dental interval and AADI (predental space) are normal. This implies that the occipitoatlantal joints, altantodental articulation, and TAL are intact. The dens is separated from the body of C2 at the subdental synchondrosis (*arrow*). Anterior displacement of C1 results in narrowing of the vertebral canal. The child had no spinal cord injury.

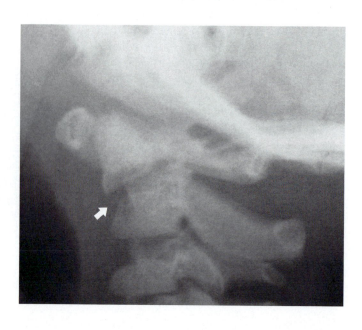

INJURIES OF THE LOWER CERVICAL SPINE

Injuries of the lower cervical spine occur predominately in the segments C5 through C7.[65] About 80% result from flexion mechanisms.[72] The injuries are classified into six categories, according to the forces causing the injury: (1) compressive-flexion, (2) axial-compression, (3) distractive-flexion (and distractive-flexion with rotation), (4) compressive-extension, (5) distractive-extension, and (6) lateral bending (Table 13–6). Patients can have multiple injuries combining two or more of these injury mechanisms.

Compressive-Flexion Injuries

WEDGE COMPRESSION FRACTURE.   Compressive forces come to bear primarily on the anterior aspect of the vertebral body owing to the flexion component of the injury. The superior end plate of the affected vertebra becomes impacted and the anterior cortex buckles. Posterior ligamentous structures are injured to a varying extent depending on the amount they are distracted.

The lateral radiograph shows loss of anterior vertebral body height, impaction of the superior portion of the vertebral body, and discontinuity and angulation of the anterior superior endplate. (Fig. 13-27) Increase in the interspinous or interlaminar distance suggests posterior ligament tearing. Because the interfacetal capsules and posterior column generally remain intact, the compression fracture is stable even if there is partial posterior ligament damage. However, "delayed instability" with progressive loss of vertebral body height and kyphotic angulation can occur when the injury is inadequately treated or not diagnosed.[48]

FLEXION TEARDROP FRACTURE.   Extreme flexion and compression forces result in complete disruption of the vertebral body and the stabilizing elements of all columns. The anterior aspect of the vertebral body is severely comminuted. The anteroinferior portion breaks into a triangular fragment, the "teardrop." The posterior aspect of the vertebral body is retropulsed into the vertebral canal causing spinal cord injury (Fig. 13-28). The posterior ligamentous structures and the articular facets are distracted. Patients experience immediate anterior spinal cord injury, typically maintaining dorsal column function.

The lateral radiograph establishes the diagnosis. The cervical spine has a kyphotic angulation. The anterior portion of the vertebral body is compressed and fractured, forming a distinctive triangular fragment ("teardrop") split from its anteroinferior aspect. The retropulsed posterior body segment encroaches on the vertebral canal. The interfacetal joint spaces, interlaminar space, and interspinous distance are widened at or adjacent to the level of the fracture. The injury is mechanically unstable and the prognosis for neurologic improvement is poor.

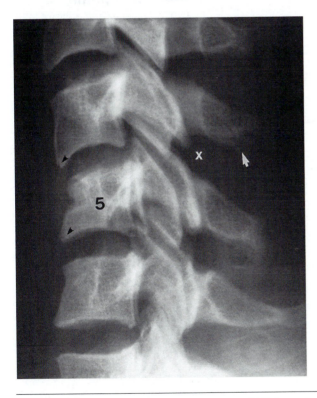

FIGURE 13-27.   Wedge compression fracture of C5. Lateral view of C5 shows buckling of the anterior cortex with vertebral body wedging. There is an avulsion fracture of the spinous process of C4 (*small white arrow*) and a mild increase in the C4-5 interlaminar space (X), which indicate posterior distraction injury. The ring apophyses along the anteroinferior margins of C4 and C5 are nearly completely fused (*small black arrowheads*), indicating that this young individual is near skeletal maturity. The artifacts overlying the posterior elements of C5 and C6 are caused by plastic rings in the cervical collar that can hide or simulate pathology. (© Washington University, used by permission.)

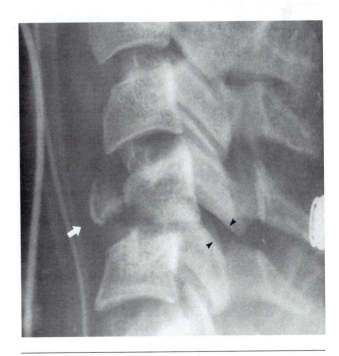

FIGURE 13-28.   Flexion teardrop fracture. A large teardrop fragment has been fractured from the anteroinferior cortex of the C4 vertebral body (*arrow*). There is 5-mm retrolisthesis of the posterior aspect of the C4 vertebral body into the spinal canal. The C4-5 interfacetal joints are widened (*arrowheads*). This patient had complete and permanent neurologic paralysis below the clavicles. (© Washington University, used by permission.)

TABLE 13-6

Injuries of the Lower Cervical Spine Grouped by Mechanism of Injury

	LATERAL VIEW	AP VIEW AND OTHER VIEWS
Compressive-Flexion		
Wedge compression fracture	Loss of anterior vertebral body height Possible spinolaminar widening	
Flexion teardrop fracture	Complex vertebral body fracture, anteroinferior "teardrop" Vertebral body fragment retropulsed Focal kyphosis Spinolaminar widening	
Axial Compression		
Burst fracture	Disruption of anterior and posterior vertebral body lines Increased AP diameter Loss of vertebral body height Vertebral body fracture	Vertebral body fracture Loss of vertebral body height Increased vertebral body width
Distractive-Flexion		

Hyperflexion sprain	Spinolaminar widening
	Focal kyphosis
	Anterolisthesis of vertebral body
	Widened posterior disc space
		Flexion view:
		    Posterior element "fanning"
		    Further vertebral body slippage
		    and interfacetal widening

Bilateral interfacetal dislocation	Anterolisthesis of vertebral body >50% Disk space widening Interfacetal widening or dislocation Spinolaminar widening	
Clay shoveler's fracture	Isolated spinous process fracture (C7)	Spinous process fracture
Distractive-Flexion with Rotation		

Unilateral interfacetal dislocation	Anterolisthesis of vertebral body,
	    up to 25%
	Abrupt loss of facet superimposition
	    ("bowtie" sign)
	Narrow "laminar space"
	Spinolaminar widening
		Spinous processes displaced off midline
		Oblique view:
		    Loss of normal laminar alignment
		    ("shingles on a roof")

Compressive-Extension		
Laminar fracture	Fractured lamina	

Pillar fracture	Displaced articular mass with
	    horizontal facet
	    Articular mass fracture
		Lateral column disruption
		Oblique view:

Pedicolaminar fracture	Fractured lamina Displaced articular mass	Lateral column disruption Oblique view: Articular mass fracture
Distractive-Extension		
Extension teardrop fracture	Triangular anteroinferior body avulsion (C2 most common)	

Hyperextension sprain	Widened anterior disk space
	Occasional small anteroinferior
	    vertebral body avulsion
		Extension view:
		    Abnormal lordosis
		    Anterior disk space widening

Axial Compression Injury ("Burst" Fracture)

Isolated compression along the vertical axis of the spine causes this "explosive" injury. It usually occurs at C4, C5, or C6. The force of injury causes intrusion of the nucleus pulposus into the vertebral body, resulting in vertebral body rupture with centrifugal displacement of the fracture fragments. The extent of anatomic disruption and neurologic damage varies depending on the amount of vertebral body comminution and associated posterior column destruction. Mild burst fractures are difficult to identify with plain radiographs. Severe burst fractures with retropulsion of fracture fragments into the vertebral canal can result in permanent quadriplegia.

Radiographic findings vary depending on the severity of the fracture (Fig. 13-29). The lateral view demonstrates disruption of the superior and inferior end plates with loss of vertebral body height. Fracture fragments are displaced outward, disrupting the anterior alignment of the vertebral bodies and intruding into the vertebral canal posteriorly. In contrast to the kyphotic deformity seen with flexion-teardrop injury, vertebral alignment is maintained in burst fractures. On the AP view, there is loss of vertebral body height. The joints of Luschka below the fracture may appear narrowed and those above may appear widened because of expansion of the vertebral body's transverse diameter. A vertical lucency representing the fracture through the vertebral body may be seen.

Burst fractures require hospital admission. CT imaging defines the full extent of the injury. Although some compression injuries are mechanically stable, severe comminution, neurologic deficits, and posterior element fractures characterize unstable burst fractures.

Distractive-Flexion Injuries (with or without Rotation)

HYPERFLEXION SPRAIN. Hyperflexion sprain results from sudden torso deceleration with unrestricted head and neck movement. The severity of ligament injury is variable, ranging from minor interspinous ligament sprain to complete disruption of the posterior longitudinal ligament and posterior disk annulus. The mechanical stability of the spinal column is variable. Delayed kyphotic deformity from poor ligamentous healing can occur over time.

Radiographic findings correlate with severity of injury and degree of displacement (Fig. 13-30). More severe injuries show an increase in the interspinous and interlaminar spaces ("fanning"), dissociation of the apposed interfacetal joint surfaces, widening of the posterior disk space, and anterior slippage of the vertebral body. Lesser injuries have radiographic findings limited to the posterior column. When the injury is nondisplaced, the initial lateral radiograph appears normal. In this case, a flexion view is needed to establish this diagnosis.[70] The clinical clue to this injury is pain out of proportion to that expected in a patient with normal or equivocal initial radiographs. Emergent consultation is required. Equivocal flexion studies require cervical immobilization and referral.

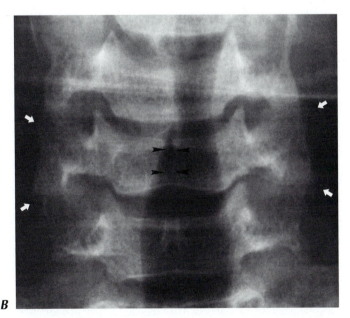

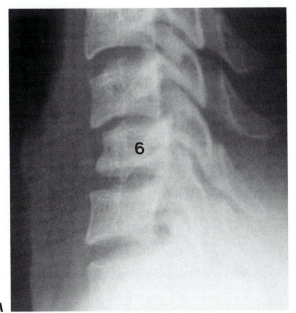

FIGURE 13-29. Burst fracture. *A.* There is loss of height of the C6 vertebral body with retropulsion of a posterior fragment into the vertebral canal. Overall vertebral alignment is maintained. This distinguishes this burst fracture from a hyperflexion teardrop, which produces hyperkyphosis at the level of injury. *B.* AP radiograph shows a mid-sagittal fracture of the C6 vertebral body projecting over the tracheal air column (*arrowheads*). Note slight lateral displacement of the lateral masses of this vertebra (*arrows*). Widening in both the AP and transverse planes indicates a burst fracture. (© Washington University, used by permission.)

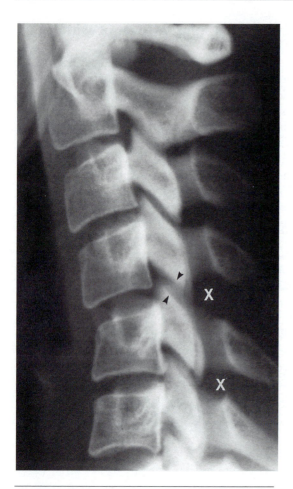

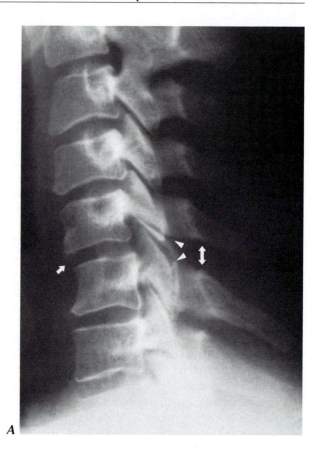

A

FIGURE 13-30. Hyperflexion sprain. Injury to the posterior ligaments is evident by the slight widening of the interspinous and interlaminar spaces at C4-C5 (*X*). The articular facet of C5 is subluxed forward (*arrowheads*). There is a kyphotic angulation at this level.

UNILATERAL INTERFACETAL DISLOCATION.   Unilateral interfacetal dislocation (UID) is caused by distractive-flexion with rotation. The rotational component of the force results in dislocation of the articular facet on one side of the vertebra. The involved articular facet is displaced up and over the subjacent articular facet so that it lies anterior to the subjacent articular mass. The vertebral column is rotated at the level of injury. Patients have severe pain, resist neck movement, and often have nerve root compression. The pure unilateral dislocation is usually mechanically stable and the term *unilateral locked facet* is therefore appropriate. However, if the articular mass is fractured or if the contralateral facet joint is injured, the injury is unstable. Despite mechanical stability, UID requires urgent consultation for reduction. CT is necessary to confirm the injury and to detect associated lateral mass or posterior element fractures.

CT has revealed that facet fractures are more common than previously believed.[73] The fractured facet encroaches on the intervetebral foramen, causing nerve root compression. Any such facet fracture renders UID unstable.

The radiographic signs of UID are usually obvious, although in some cases they are subtle. On the lateral radiograph, there is anterior displacement of the upper vertebral body that is less than 50% of the vertebral body AP-diameter (Figs. 13-31 and 13-32). The left and right diamond-shaped lateral masses, which are normally superimposed on the lateral film, become abruptly offset at the level of injury. This lack of superimposition of the left and right lateral masses creates a characteristic *double-diamond* or *bowtie* configuration. The bowtie appearance is also seen on an incorrectly positioned lateral radiograph in which the patient's head is rotated so that the right and left articular masses are not superimposed. Incorrect patient positioning appears different from UID because malpositioning results in a gradual transition to the bowtie appearance, whereas UID causes an abrupt change from normal superimposition to the rotated bowtie configuration.

Other signs of UID on the lateral radiograph include widening of the spinous processes ("fanning") and displacement of the dislocated facet into the neuroforamen. Finally, the distance between the posterior cortex of the lateral mass and the spinolaminar junction of the dislocated vertebra (the "laminar space") is narrowed.[74]

The AP view shows displacement of the spinous processes out of the midline. The spinous processes above the injury are rotated, and those below the injury remain in the midline.

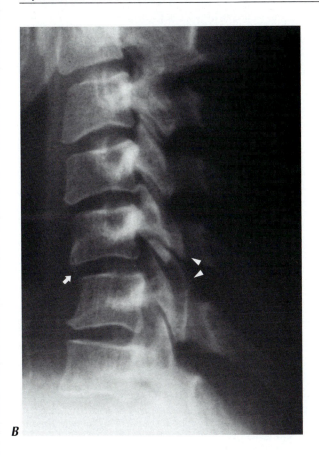

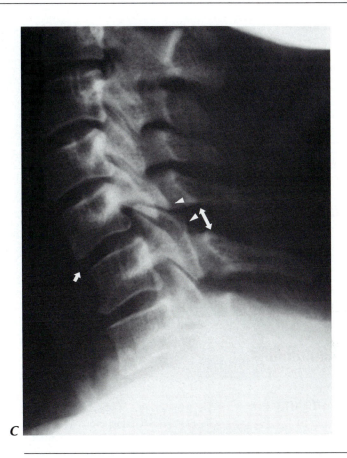

B

C

FIGURE 13-31. Hyperflexion sprain. *A.* A neutral lateral radiograph demonstrates minimal anterolisthesis of C5 with respect to C6, associated with mild kyphosis (*arrow*). There is subluxation of the C5-C6 interfacetal joints (*arrowheads*) compared with adjacent levels and a subtle increase in the interlaminar distance (*double arrow*). *B.* The flexion radiograph shows a slight increase in interfacetal subluxation at C5-C6 (*arrowheads*) and normal interfacetal movement at all other levels. Slight anterolisthesis of C5 on C6 is again seen (*arrow*). The positioning is slightly rotated so that the articular masses gradually lose their parallelism in the lower segments and appear to be doubled at C5 and C6. Flexion is suboptimal because the patient experienced significant pain on movement. *C.* An extension view completes the dynamic evaluation. Adequate extension is demonstrated by exaggeration of the lordosis and reduction in the interlaminar distances from C2 through C5. Note persistence at C5-C6 of mild anterolisthesis (*arrow*), interfacetal subluxation (*arrowheads*), and increased interlaminar distance (*double arrow*). The findings on flexion-extension views confirm the presence of hyperflexion sprain.

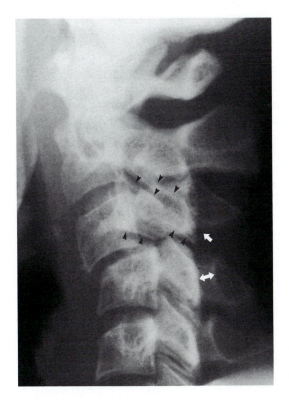

FIGURE 13-32. Unilateral interfacetal dislocation. A unilateral interfacetal dislocation of C3-C4. There is angulation and anterolisthesis of C3 on C4. There is an abrupt rotational malalignment at C3 compared with C4 such that the lateral masses of C3 are not superimposed. This creates a "double diamond" or "bowtie" appearance at C3 (*arrowheads*). The left and right articular masses of each vertebra below this level are normally superimposed. There is slight widening ("fanning") of the spinous processes at C3-C4. The "laminar space" between the posterior cortex of the articular mass and the spinolaminar junction is abruptly narrowed at C3 (*arrow*) compared with lower levels (*double arrow*).

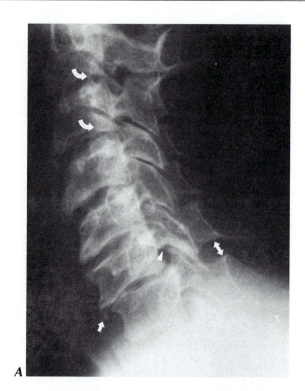

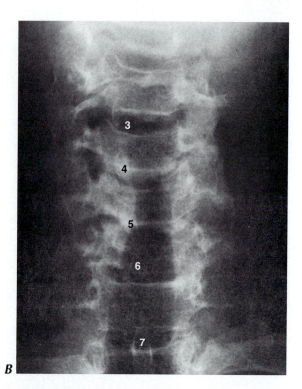

FIGURE 13-33.   Unilateral interfacetal dislocation. *A.* In a patient with considerable degenerative changes, the radiographic findings of a C6-C7 unilateral interfacetal dislocation are subtle. The lateral radiograph demonstrates 4-mm anterolisthesis of C6 on C7 (*arrow*) and narrowing of the spinal canal. One inferior articular facet at C6 is partly uncovered (*arrowhead*). Rotation of the vertebrae above the dislocation results in the appearance of the articular masses in a doubled "bowtie" configuration (*curved arrows*). This is seen more easily at the upper levels. The interlaminar space at C6-C7 is widened (*double arrows*). Findings indicative of degenerative changes include anterior osteophytes at C4-C5 and C5-C6, ALL calcification at C3-C4 and C6-C7, and loss of disk height at C4 through C7. *B.* AP radiograph shows rotation above C7. The spinous processes (numbered) are rotated off the midline above C7. The C6-C7 interspinous distance is increased. The left lateral column appears continuous (normal), but the right lateral column is interrupted by lucencies at C6-C7 and every interspace above (*arrow*). *C.* Right posterior oblique projection demonstrates increased interlaminar distance at C6-C7 (*arrow*), suggesting subluxation of the left C6-C7 interfacetal joint. *D.* Left posterior oblique projection shows dislocation of the right C6 inferior facet into the neuroforamen (*asterisk*). Anterolisthesis of the C6 vertebral body on C7 (*arrow*) and osteophytes from C4 to C7 are seen.

The oblique radiograph is helpful in identifying UID if the lateral and AP views are inconclusive (Fig. 13-33). On the side of the dislocation, the oblique view shows the dislocated articular mass anterior to the subjacent facet resting within the intervertebral neuroforamen. The adjoining lamina projects through the articular mass and lies anterior to the subjacent lamina, disrupting the normal "shingles on a roof" configuration of the lamina.

CT readily demonstrates the facet dislocation, and detects other posterior element fractures that are difficult to see on plain film. On CT, normal facet articulations look like the cross-section of a *hamburger bun*. With a facet dislocation, the hamburger bun is inverted—the facet surfaces do not face one another. This has been termed a *naked facet*.

BILATERAL INTERFACETAL DISLOCATION.   Extreme distractive-flexion causes disruption of all posterior ligamentous structures and transposition of both lateral masses of one vertebra anterior to the subjacent lateral masses. The inferior articular facets above the injury are seated anterior to the subjacent articular

facets and lie within the neuroformina, creating the appearance of a tooth locked in a notch. The destruction of the ligamentous supporting structures creates instability. Therefore, the term *bilateral locked facets* is incorrect and misleading because it implies that the facets are "locked" together and stable. The spinal cord is wedged between the laminae of the segment above and the vertebral body below the disruption, and extensive neurologic injury is common. Occasionally, the facet joints are only partially displaced, a condition called *bilateral perched facets.* The superior vertebral facets are subluxed superiorly and anteriorly, coming to rest above the subadjacent facets.

Bilateral interfacetal dislocation (BID) usually occurs at the lower cervical interspaces. The abnormality is easy to identify on the lateral radiograph (Fig. 13-34). The vertebral body above the dislocation is displaced anterior to the subadjacent vertebra by at least 50% of the vertebral body diameter. With bilateral perched facets, the displacement is less than 50%. Also with BID, the articular surfaces of the facets are exposed, and the inferior tip of the upper articular mass rests in the gutter of the intervertebral foramen.

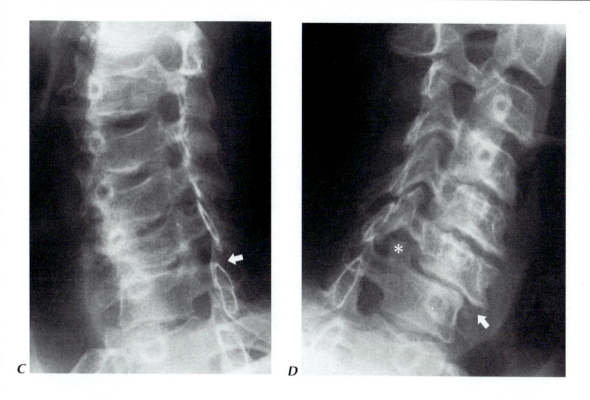

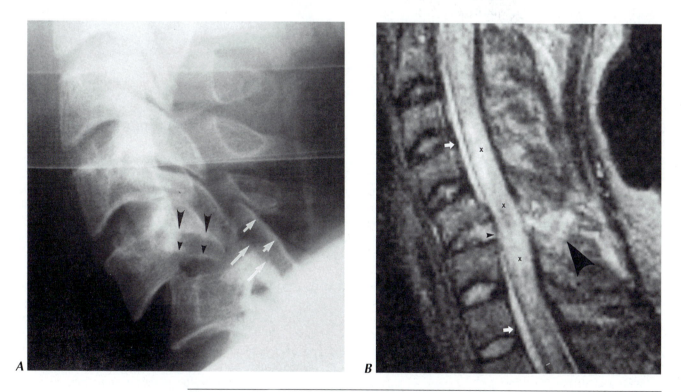

FIGURE 13-34.   Bilateral interfacetal dislocation. *A.* This lateral radiograph shows severe 20-mm anterior slippage of C5 with respect to C6. The facets of C5 (*black arrowheads*) are dislocated anterior to the facets of C6 (*white arrows*). This victim of a water skiing accident presented with flaccid quadriplegia. *B.* A postreduction MRI demonstrates spinal cord hematoma at C5-6 (*small x's*). The posterior longitudinal ligament is disrupted (*small arrowhead*). High signal intensity in the anterior epidural space is due to epidural hematoma (*white arrows*). The C5-6 intervertebral disk is widened posteriorly. High signal in the ligaments of the posterior elements (*large arrowhead*) indicates the posterior distraction injury. (© Washington University, used by permission.)

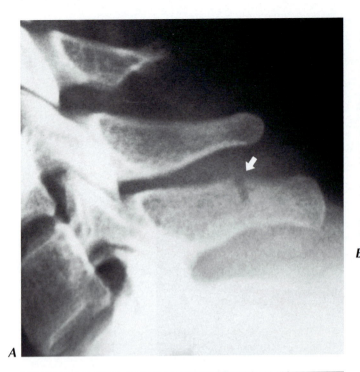

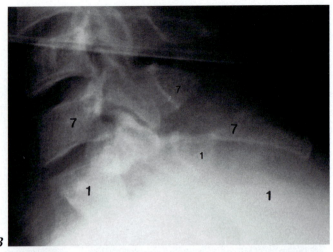

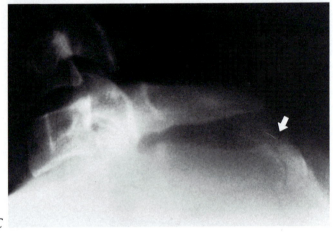

FIGURE 13-35. C7 spinous process fractures. *A.* An isolated fracture of the C7 spinous process. If there are no other skeletal or ligament injuries, this is biomechanically stable. This is a clay shoveler's fracture. The patient sustained a direct blow to the back of the neck. (© David Schwartz, MD, New York University.) *B.* Lateral view of C7 demonstrates a fracture of the spinous process of C7. Partially hidden by the shoulders is a similar fracture of T1. Horizontal lines at the top of the image are due to cervical spine immobilization blocks. These fractures may extend into the posterior neural arch and should not be considered stable. (© Washington University, used by permission.) *C.* An unfused accessory ossification center of the tip of the C7 spinous process is a common anomaly (*arrow*). (© David Schwartz, MD, New York University.)

CLAY SHOVELER'S FRACTURE. A clay shoveler's fracture is an isolated fracture through the spinous process of C7. The fracture can also occur at C6 or T1. The classic mechanism of injury is downward traction on the spinous processes by the muscular attachments to the scapulae during forceful lifting by the arms. The injury also results from forced flexion of the neck while the muscular and ligamentous structures of the posterior neck are under tension. A third mechanism of injury is a direct blow to the spinous process. It should be noted that spinous process fractures can also be caused by hyperextension, in which case the fracture may extend into the adjacent laminae or pedicles. This "compressive-extension" injury is not a true clay shoveler's fracture and is potentially unstable.

With a clay shoveler's fracture, the posterior ligamentous structures are intact, and the injury is stable. Patients complain of pain over the fractured spinous process. A clay shoveler's fracture is well demonstrated on the lateral radiograph when the posterior elements of C7 and T1 are visible (Fig. 13-35). The fracture is typically horizontal or oblique. This injury must be distinguished from an unfused apophysis, which has smooth, well-corticated margins and vertical orientation.

Compressive-Extension Injuries

Compressive-extension causes fractures of the posterior arch, including the pedicles, articular facets, laminae, and spinous processes. Posterior arch fractures are frequently complex and comminuted, involving several spinal levels. These injuries were formerly referred to collectively as *hyperextension fracture-dislocation.*[75] Unilateral posterior element fractures are included in this category.

LAMINAR FRACTURE. Laminar fractures result from compression between adjacent laminae. They can occur at any level, tend to be bilateral, and are often associated with other fractures. The fracture is considered stable if the injury is isolated to one segment and the neurologic examination is normal. When visible on the lateral radiograph, a laminar fracture appears as a lucency in the posterior arch (Fig. 13-36). Occasionally, the fracture is seen on the AP view, projected through the vertebral body. Nondisplaced isolated laminar fractures are often only seen on CT. Neurologic abnormalities suggest associated injuries or comminution of the laminae with impingement by fracture fragments. This requires further imaging. An isolated laminar fracture is usually of limited clinical significance.

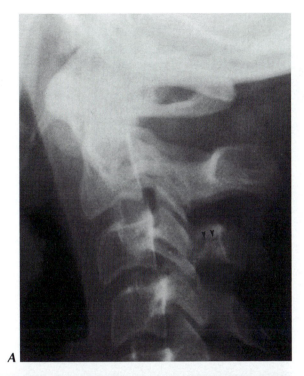

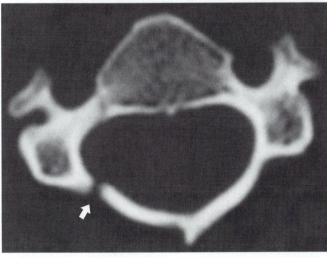

FIGURE 13-36. Laminar fracture. *A.* Lateral radiograph illustrates a horizontally oriented fracture along the right lamina of C3 (*arrowheads*). *B.* Axial CT through C3 demonstrates a right-sided laminar fracture. (© Washington University, used by permission.)

PILLAR FRACTURE. Extension and compression forces that are concentrated on one side produce unilateral articular mass (pillar) fractures. These are also referred to as *extension-rotation injuries.* If isolated to the facet, the injury involves the inferior facet surface more often than the superior facet surface. However, these injuries are often comminuted and occasionally involve other structures of the posterior arch.[70] Articular facet and pillar fractures are probably more common than their reported incidence of 3 to 11%. They usually occur in the lower cervical spine and are associated with radiculopathy in about one-third of patients.[73] If neurologic damage is absent, the injury is considered stable.

The radiographic findings are often very subtle (Fig. 13-37). Fractured inferior facets are often upwardly displaced, altering the usual superimposition of the paired joints on the lateral radiograph. Pillar fractures can be minimally displaced or translocated posteriorly and laterally. When the pillar fracture is nondisplaced, the lateral view may be normal or only a faint vertical lucency may be detectable through the articular mass. If the fracture is displaced, the articular mass is shifted posteriorly relative to the contralateral side and appears as a duplicated lateral mass at the level of fracture. The detached fragment frequently tilts anteriorly, causing the articular surfaces to approach horizontal.

On the AP radiograph, the normally uninterrupted wavy contour of the lateral masses is disrupted by the horizontal articular surface. The fracture fragment can be laterally displaced. Oblique views are helpful if the lateral and AP views are inconclusive. On the oblique projection, the fracture line may be visible in the affected articular mass. CT is required to diagnose the injury fully.

Occasionally, the extension force causes the vertebral body to translocate anteriorly, particularly on the side of the pillar fracture, with a resultant intervertebral disk injury. Disk space narrowing and mild anterolisthesis of the vertebral body are seen. These findings can appear similar to a UID. This fracture is potentially unstable.

PEDICOLAMINAR FRACTURE. A pedicolaminar fracture is caused by compressive-extension with rotation or lateral bending. The posterior arch is compressed asymmetrically between the vertebrae above and below, resulting in fractures through both the pedicle and lamina on the same side. This creates a freely separated lateral mass. For this reason, the injury is also called a *pedicolaminar fracture-separation.* With greater force, the anterior ligaments are disrupted and there is anterolisthesis of the vertebral body. The degree of neurologic damage varies.

The extent of instability depends on the degree to which the anterior longitudinal ligament (ALL) and adjacent disks are injured. In its mildest form, the fracture is nondisplaced and anterior support structures are intact. In a more severe injury, the ALL and one or both of the adjacent disks are disrupted, with resultant anterior slippage of the vertebra. In the most severe injury, the articular mass contralateral to the fracture is dislocated. This is an unstable UID.

The radiographic findings are variable (Fig. 13-38). The findings on the lateral view can be similar to those of a laminar or pillar fracture, including discontinuity of the posterior arch with displacement of the articular mass. With more severe injury, the articular mass is increasingly displaced or comminuted. Anterior slippage of the involved vertebral body signifies disruption of the ALL and intervertebral disk. Anterolisthesis of the vertebral body is most pronounced when the contralateral facet joint is dislocated, and the radiographic findings are those of a UID.

On the AP view, the continuous wavy border of the lateral masses is disrupted. In mild cases, a subtle vertical lucency in the lateral mass corresponding to the pedicle fracture may be the sole radiographic finding. Comminution of the lateral mass may be visible. The anteriorly tilted articular mass can appear

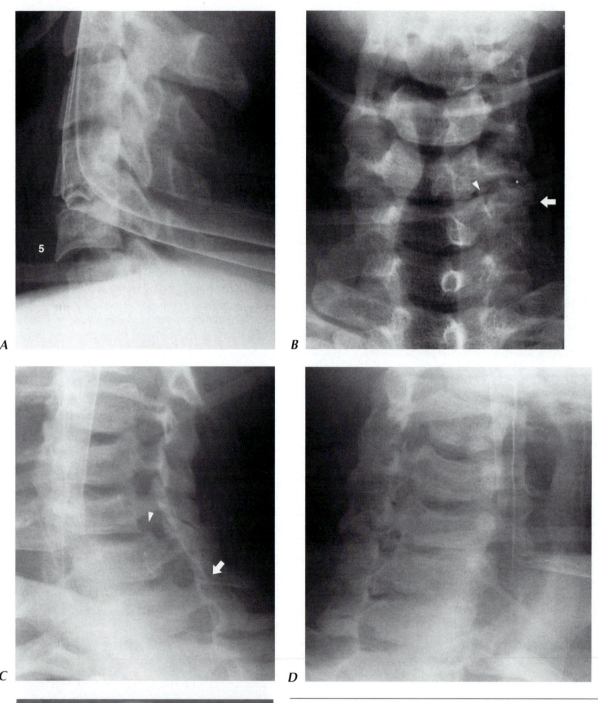

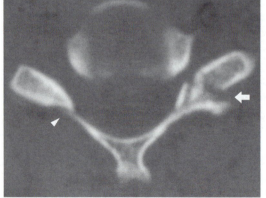

FIGURE 13-37. Pillar fracture. *A.* A supine cross-table lateral cervical view provides inadequate visualization of the spine below C5. Detail is obscured by immobilization blocks. Anterolisthesis of 2 to 3 mm is present at C5-C6, but no other abnormalities are visible. *B.* The AP radiograph demonstrates a C6 "pillar sign" in the left lateral column. The left lateral column is interrupted by a visible C5-C6 interfacetal joint and abnormal lucencies at the C6 level (*arrow*). A small fracture fragment is visible cephalad to the left C6 uncinate process (*arrowhead*). Slight displacement of the C6 spinous process off the midline suggests mild rotation of that segment. *C.* The right oblique view shows anterolisthesis of C5 on C6 (*arrowhead*). The C6 articular pillar is shortened and a lucency crosses its upper portion. The normal "shingled" configuration of the laminae is interrupted at C5-C6, suggesting fracture of the C6 articular pillar with displacement (*arrow*). *D.* The left oblique view, despite overlapping shadows from immobilization and resuscitation apparatus, is normal. *E.* CT demonstrates abnormalities of C6. The left articular pillar and lamina are fractured (*arrow*). Note abrupt and irregular interruption in the cortex and trabeculae. The smooth, faint lucency in the right lamina (*arrowhead*) represents volume-averaging artifact and should not be misinterpreted as a fracture. This was confirmed by finding that adjacent CT slices were normal.

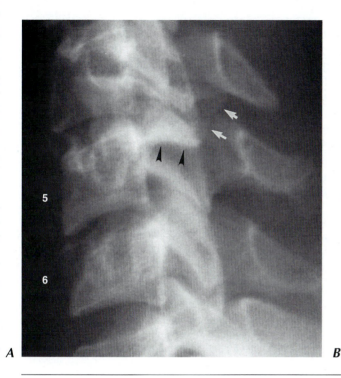

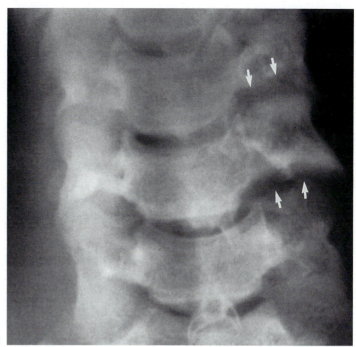

A   *B*

FIGURE 13-38. Pedicolaminar fracture at C5, and wedge compression fracture at C6. *A.* Lateral radiograph demonstrates rotation of the left lateral mass of C5 anteriorly, creating a "horizontal facet" at C5 (*black arrowheads*). The attached laminar fragment projects posteriorly from the horizontal facet (*white arrows*). A wedge fracture of C6 is present, with a separate anterosuperior fracture fragment. *B.* AP radiograph shows rotation of the left lateral mass. Loss of the normal articulation between the lateral masses of C5 and C6 appears as an abnormal lucency in the normally continuous lateral column (*arrows*). The fracture has the typical trapezoidal shape expected with this injury. The vertebral body fracture of C6 is not evident on this view. (© Washington University, used by permission.)

as a trapezoidal structure with horizontal lucent intervals above and below. Although oblique views can further characterize the fracture, CT defines the injury best.

Distractive-Extension Injuries

EXTENSION TEARDROP FRACTURE. Distraction and extension causes the ALL to avulse a triangular bone fragment from the anteroinferior corner of the vertebral body. The fracture occurs most commonly at C2, especially in older adults with degenerative disease. Younger patients occasionally sustain this fracture at lower cervical levels.

The diagnosis is made on the lateral radiograph (Fig. 13-39). A triangular fragment is displaced from the anteroinferior segment of the involved vertebral body. Its vertical dimension tends to be greater than its width. This is because the ALL attaches to the anterior surface of the vertebral body. The fibers of the intervertebral disk are intact, so that the height of the disk space is uniform and vertebral body alignment is maintained. An isolated extension teardrop fracture is mechanically stable and is usually without neurologic compromise.

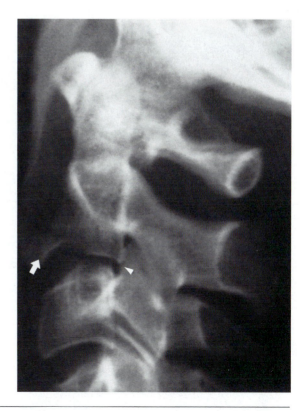

FIGURE 13-39. Hyperextension teardrop of C2. Lateral radiograph demonstrates a large triangular fragment at the anteroinferior corner of C2. The C2-3 disk space is widened and there is slight retrolisthesis of C2 with respect to C3 (*arrowhead*). (© Washington University, used by permission.)

HYPEREXTENSION DISLOCATION (HYPEREXTENSION SPRAIN). Hyperextension causes varying degrees of disruption of the ALL, intervertebral disk, and PLL. Spontaneous reduction can result in fairly normal alignment after the insult. The injury tends to occur in the lower cervical segments and typically results from "whiplash" or a blow to the forehead. The spinal cord is often pinched between the posterior aspect of the vertebral body and the buckled ligamentum flavum.[76] Patients typically have an acute central cord syndrome. Damage to the supporting ligamentous structures leads to mechanical and neurologic instability.

Radiographic findings can be subtle or even normal in contrast to the neurologic deficits that accompany this injury. On the lateral view, a prevertebral hematoma is often seen and appears as diffuse prevertebral soft tissue thickening (Figs. 13-40 and 13-41). There is anterior widening of the intervertebral disk space that is frequently multilevel. A small avulsion fragment from the anteroinferior aspect of the vertebral body may be seen.[77] The fragment tends to have a greater horizontal than vertical dimension, differentiating it from a hyperextension teardrop fracture.[6] Hyperextension teardrop fractures are avulsed by the ALL. The firm attachment of the ALL to the anterior surface of the vertebral body results in a relatively greater vertical dimension of the avulsion fragment. In hyperextension dislocation, distraction occurs at the interface between the vertebral body and intervertebral disk, which causes the inferior end plate of the body to be avulsed by the dense, inelastic Sharpey's fibers of the disk annulus. The resultant fragment is greater in width than in height. In preadolescents, the injury can cause avulsion of an unfused inferior vetebral body endplate ossification center.

Because this is a potentially unstable injury, all patients are hospitalized. Once they have been admitted, elective flexion-extension views are used to assess ligamentous stability. MRI can directly visualize the spinal cord injury and ligament disruption.

Lateral Bending

Lateral bending is the least common type of injury (6%). It is responsible for unilateral posterior element or lateral mass fractures. It also causes compression fractures of one side of the vertebral body. A unilateral fracture of the uncinate process can be seen on the AP view.

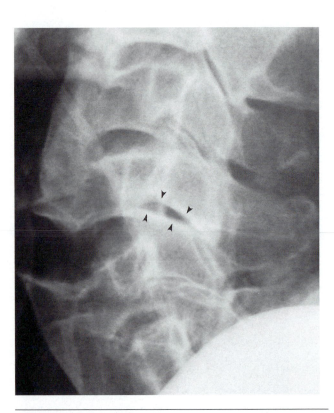

FIGURE 13-40. Hyperextension dislocation. In this patient with diffuse idiopathic skeletal hyperostosis (DISH), there is a 5-mm retrolisthesis of C4 with respect to C5. The anterior osteophytes at this level are fractured and the disk spaces have widened markedly. The C4-5 facet joints are also widened and posteriorly subluxed (*arrowheads*). (© Washington University, used by permission.)

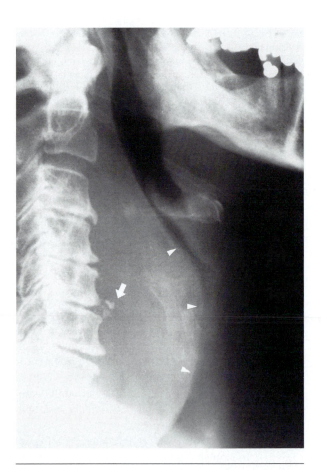

FIGURE 13-41. Hyperextension sprain with avulsion fracture. There is a small osteophyte avulsion fracture off the anterior-inferior corner of the C5 vertebral body (*arrow*). This was due to hyperextension sprain causing traction on the ALL. This small fracture is potentially unstable. There is enormous soft tissue swelling in this patient who was taking coumadin. The airway is critically narrowed (*arrowheads*) and the patient required endotracheal intubation.

ERRORS IN INTERPRETATION

A missed injury of the cervical spine can be particularly devastating. On the other hand, false-positive errors are costly, inconvenient, and irritating to patients (Fig. 13-42). Many false-positives are due to developmental and degenerative variants.

Missed injury is most often the result of suboptimal or inadequate radiographic technique rather than actual errors in the interpretation of good-quality radiographs.[78] The entire cervical spine must be visualized.

Nevertheless, physician error is responsible for some missed injuries, making it important to understand and identify common errors. Some injuries are missed because visible radiographic abnormalities are overlooked by the physician. Other errors result when negative plain films are not followed by additional studies in patients whose clinical findings mandate further evaluation (e.g., pain out of proportion to radiographic findings). Most missed cervical spine fractures occur in patients with other more evident spinal injuries. The additional fracture is missed because it is less radiographically apparent or not carefully considered. These missed injuries are less important to the emergency physician because such patients are generally hospitalized for detailed evaluation. Of greater immediate significance are spinal injuries that are missed because the radiographs are misinterpreted as normal.

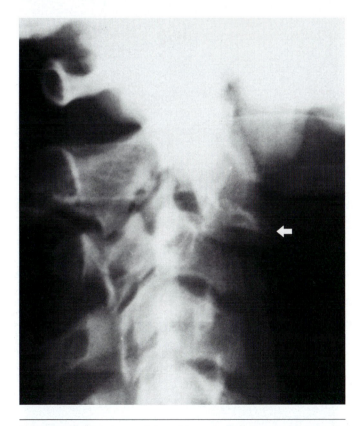

FIGURE 13-42. An overlying object mimics a fracture. A bony abnormality at the C2 vertebral body is seen in the intoxicated lethargic victim of a motor vehicle collision. The patient was immobilized in Gardner-Wells tongs before it was determined that the apparent fracture was actually the overlying finger tip of the physician holding the patient's head. Overreading radiographs can contribute to patient morbidity.

The Cervicocranium. The anatomic complexity and frequent lack of neurologic symptoms make missing an injury common in the cervicocranium.[78] The nondisplaced dens fracture is the most frequently missed significant cervical spine injury.[79] Meticulous attention to image interpretation and liberal use of advanced techniques for suspicious cases decreases the likelihood of error. These advanced techniques include CT with coronal and sagittal reconstructions.

The Cervicothoracic Junction. The cervicothoracic junction is also a region in which injuries are occasionally missed. This usually occurs because radiographic visualization is obscured by the overlapping shoulders and soft tissues. The posterior elements of C7 and T1 are especially difficult to see. The vertebral body, lateral masses, posterior arch, and spinous process of C7 must be seen clearly. The C7-T1 articulation must be visible. Additional studies such as a swimmer's view or CT are needed when the lateral view is incomplete. When the clinical suspicion for injury is high, CT is warranted.

Unilateral Interfacetal Dislocation. The radiographic signs of UID can be subtle, especially if there is no anterolisthesis of the vertebral body or fanning of the spinous processes. The bowtie sign is difficult to appreciate if the displaced lateral mass overlies the vertebral body. The most reliable sign is an abruptly diminished "laminar space" (distance between the posterior cortex of the lateral mass and the spinolaminar junction).[74] Nevertheless, this injury usually causes marked symptoms. Oblique views are frequently helpful. CT should be ordered if subtle abnormalities are not clarified by plain radiographs.

The Posterior Column. Fractures of the spinous process are usually easily seen on plain radiographs except when the C7 and T1 spinous process is obscured by overlapping shoulders. Injuries to the other portions of the neural arch and posterior column are less reliably identified. The frequency of missed fractures of the pedicles, articular facets, and laminae is 33 to 73% when plain films are used alone.[36,79,80] The clinical significance of these fractures is unclear because isolated posterior element fractures are usually mechanically stable. Comminuted fractures are most clinically significant but are generally associated with neurologic injury and are more readily detected radiographically. It is prudent for the clinician to pursue an anatomic diagnosis with CT, oblique, or flexion-extension views whenever plain radiogaphs are inconclusive or nerve root findings are present.

Distinguish Wedge Compression from Burst Fracture. The importance of differentiating a wedge compression fracture from a burst fracture lies in the potential for neurologic injury due to impingement by a bone fragment in burst fractures. In addition, burst fractures are mechanically unstable. Careful examination of the lateral view for violation of the posterior vertebral body line and of the AP view for a vertical fracture lucency distinguishes a burst fracture from a simple wedge compression. In some cases, CT is needed to make the distinction. In addition, the posterior ligamentous structures may be distracted by the flexion injury in wedge compression fractures.[48] In burst fractures, alignment of the posterior neural arch and the interlaminar spaces usually remains normal.

Ligamentous Injury.   Purely ligamentous injury without associated fractures can occur in patients with normal radiographs. These patients are at risk for both immediate and delayed cervical instability.[42] Patients with neuropathy require advanced studies, but some patients have no clinical findings other than pain. The radiographic findings in hyperflexion and hyperextension strain can be quite subtle. In patients at risk, even subtle changes consistent with ligamentous injury should prompt adjunctive imaging. The dictum that 3.5 mm of malalignment or 11° of angulation is permissible does not apply to the patient with acute trauma. Patients with pain out of proportion to that expected with normal or equivocal radiographs should have flexion and extension views unless they are found to be at high risk of cervical injury on clinical examination (e.g., neurologic injury, multiple trauma). Patients with normal standard radiographs but inadequate range of motion on flexion-extension views are managed with cervical immobilization and repeat examination in several days.

COMMON VARIANTS

Numerous anatomic variants are important to recognize. These are grouped into two categories: developmental anomalies and degenerative changes.

Developmental Anomalies.   Incomplete fusion of the posterior arch of C1 occurs in 3 to 4% of patients.[81] It is usually a simple posterior cleft (spina bifida occulta). This anomaly is seen on the open-mouth view. Unilateral or bilateral absence of the posterior arch is seen on the lateral radiograph.[38] An enlarged anterior arch of C1 or hypertrophy of the spinous process of C2 is commonly associated with C1 posterior arch defects (Fig. 13-43). These anomalies generally have no clinical significance.[81]

Anomalous fusion of the ossification centers of the dens causes several findings.[38] The *ossiculum terminale persistens* results from incomplete fusion between the tip and the body of the dens. This appears as a small ossicle resting in a V-shaped dens tip. In other cases, the dens is shortened or absent because of ossification failure. The *os odontoideum* is a well-corticated fragment sitting cephalad to the body of C2 (Fig. 13-44). Whether the os odontoideum is developmental or posttraumatic nonunion of a dens fracture is unclear. The vertebral body typically has a hump representing the remnant of the base of the dens. The os odontoideum can cause mechanical instability and require operative fixation.

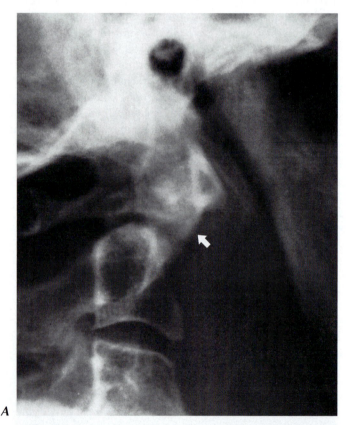

A

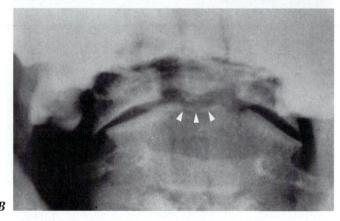

B

FIGURE 13-44.   Os odontoideum. *A.* Lateral view showing anterior slippage of the dens fragment relative to the body of C2 (*arrow*). The margins are smooth and well corticated indicating that this is not an acute injury. *B.* Open-mouth view shows the os odontoideum separated from the body of C2 (*arrowheads*). (Copyright David Schwartz, M.D.)

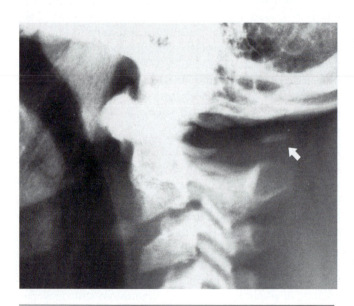

FIGURE 13-43.   Congenital incomplete posterior arch of C1. There is only faint ossification of the posterior tubercle of C1. The anterior arch of C1 shows compensatory hypertrophy.

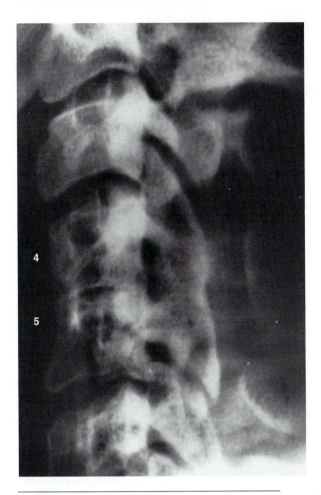

FIGURE 13-45. Congenital block vertebrae. Vertebral bodies of C4 and C5 are fused. A vestigial disk space remains. There is a compensatory reduction in the size of each of the fused vertebral bodies.

Congenital fusion (*block vertebrae*) can occur in any part of the cervical spine from the occipitoatlantal articulation to the lower cervical bodies or posterior arches (Fig. 13-45). Subluxation may appear to be present between the fused segments and adjacent vertebrae.[35] This is usually caused by the decreased anteroposterior diameter of the fused bodies.

Degenerative Changes. Degenerative changes are common in older individuals and include vertebral body malalignment, osteophyte formation, loss of vertebral body height, and calcification of the ALL (Fig. 13-46). Anterolisthesis (anterior slippage of one vertebra relative to the subjacent vertebra) of up to 6 mm can occur when degenerative narrowing of the facet joint is present. Retrolisthesis is due to intervertebral disk space narrowing. Posterior displacement of the superior body occurs as its articular facet slips down the subjacent facet. Calcification of the ALL typically occurs at the inferior edge of the vertebral body and can be mistaken for an avulsion fracture. Disk space widening and prevertebral soft tissue swelling typical of an acute avulsion injury are absent. Degenerative flattening of the vertebral bodies (platyspondylia) can mimic compression fracture. The presence of sclerotic margins and other degenerative changes differentiate the chronic condition from an acute injury.

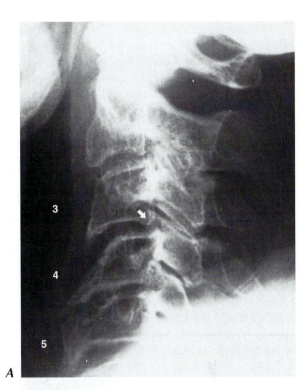

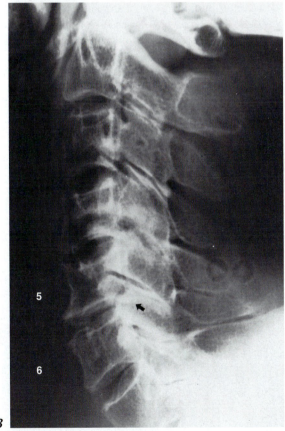

FIGURE 13-46. Degenerative spondylosis. *A.* Anterolisthesis of C3 is due to degenerative narrowing of the C3-C4 facet joints. There is also degenerative loss of anterior vertebral body height of C4 and C5 with marked osteophyte formation. The posterior vertebral body line should be used to assess malalignment in patients with degenerative changes because the anterior surfaces of the vertebral bodies have degenerative deformities. *B.* Retrolisthesis of C5 is due to degenerative disk disease causing disk space narrowing at C5-C6.

Anatomic variants that cannot be differentiated from acute injuries can be further evaluated with CT. In the absence of a fracture, flexion and extension views can be performed to demonstrate stability. However, decreased range of motion is common in degenerative disease, and it can be difficult to differentiate between the expected loss of motion from chronic degenerative changes and the loss of motion caused by acute pain and muscle spasm. When the results are equivocal, patients require cervical immobilization and repeat examination in several days. When signs of instability are found in dynamic studies, immediate surgical consultation is necessary.

Mach Bands.   The shadow of a line of cortical bone superimposed across another bone can create the illusion that a fracture exits in the region of overlap (Fig. 13-47). This optical effect is called a *Mach band.* These bands are distinguished by tracing the line created by the overlapping structure beyond the borders of the involved bone. A Mach band is often seen overlying the base of the dens on the open-mouth view. When doubt exists, a repeat open-mouth view with a slightly different orientation causes the Mach band to move.

Positioning Errors.   Incorrect positioning of the patient can cause confusing findings on plain radiographs. Rotation of the patient on the lateral view causes loss of superimposition of the articular facets. A rotated lateral view can cause the ramus and angle of the mandible to overlap the cervicocranium. On the supine cross-table lateral projection, the cervical spine commonly appears straightened. On the open-mouth view, head tilt and rotation cause asymmetry of the lateral masses of C1 in relation to the body of C2.

ADVANCED STUDIES

Definitive evaluation of a cervical spine injury frequently requires advanced radiographic techniques. The combination of screening plain films and adjunctive CT provides diagnostic accuracy approaching 100%.[36,82] MRI has replaced CT myelography as the principal diagnostic tool in patients with ligamentous or neurologic injuries.

Computed Tomography.   CT has excellent sensitivity in identifying most types of cervical injuries.[36,79,82] Multiple fractures are common in the cervical spine, especially in the cervicocranium, and are usually found in contiguous segments. CT can be used to further evaluate fractures that may have violated the integrity of the spinal canal, posterior element fractures, fractures with neurologic injury, and dislocations. The scan should include the level of interest and the superior and inferior adjacent segments. CT is also used to better define areas that are often poorly seen on plain film, such as the cervicocranium and cervicothoracic junction. Finally, CT is useful to clarify suspicious, but nondiagnostic findings on plain radiographs (Table 13-7).

Despite its excellent ability to detect most fractures, CT can miss fractures that are oriented in the axial plane (e.g., fracture through the base of the dens or a mild wedge compression fracture of a vertebral body). CT can also miss malalignment along the longitudinal axis.[80] Reconstructed images in the cornal and sagittal plane are used to diagnose these injuries. CT has limited ability to assess the integrity of soft tissue structures. Ligamentous injuries without fracture are better assessed using flexion-extension views or MRI.

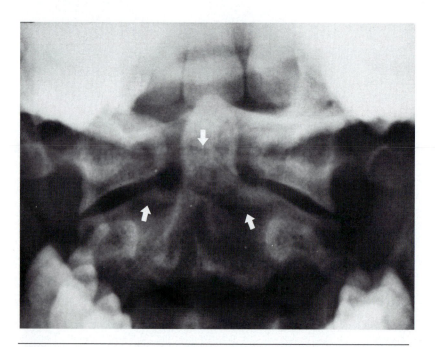

FIGURE 13-47.   Mach bands. An open-mouth view illustrates two Mach bands projecting over the dens. The more cephalad and most prominent is due to the inferior margin of the occipital bone. The more caudad one projects just below the base of the dens, and is due to the posterior arch of C1. (© Washington University, used by permission.)

TABLE 13-7

Indications for CT of the Cervical Spine

Inadequate plain radiographs*
    especially cervicocranium and cervicothoracic junction
Suspicious but nondiagnostic plain radiographs*
Fractures with neuropathy†
Specific injury identified or suspected on plain radiograph†
    Jefferson burst fracture of C1
    Burst fracture of vertebral body
    Posterior element fracture: lateral mass, lamina
    Unilateral facet dislocation
Injuries potentially missed by axial CT
    Dens type II fracture
    Wedge compression fracture
    Hyperflexion sprain
    Hyperextension sprain

*Appropriate for ED evaluation
†Usually performed after ED evaluation

Although some investigators have questioned the association of cervical injury in patients with facial and head trauma,[25,27,28,83] others have found that patients with clinical evidence of severe head injury are at high risk for cervical spine injuries.[26,28] Postmortem studies have shown a significant frequency of injuries to the cervicocranium in severely head-injured patients.[84] The additional CT slices required for the evaluation of C1 and C2 add only a few additional seconds. In a prospective study of 202 patients with "substantial" head trauma (GCS scores of 3 to 6), CT demonstrated 37 fractures of the cervicocranium, of which 19 were missed on standard radiographs.[109] Another study showed a greater incidence (6.7% vs 3.9%) of cervical injury in patients with GCS scores below 14 regardless of the presence or absence of head injury.[28] The cervicocranium is an area where missed injuries commonly occur, and including images of the cervicocranium with CT evaluation of the head is reasonable for trauma patients with a depressed level of consciousness.

CT Myelography.   The inability to identify anatomic detail within the vertebral canal has prompted the use of cervical myelography with CT in cases of clinical spinal cord injury. This procedure is currently used only for patients with contraindications to MRI.

Magnetic Resonance Imaging.   MRI has been reserved primarily for patients who require subacute evaluation. Long scanning times and incompatibility with monitoring and life-support devices, as well as the availability of other imaging modalities, have limited its use in seriously ill patients. Nevertheless, certain injuries are best identified by MRI such as damage to the supporting ligaments of the spine (particularly the ALL and PLL), defining cord integrity, traumatic disk herniation, and vertebral artery occlusion.[6] MRI is useful in evaluating hyperextension injuries; patients with neurologic deficits that are progressing or are unexplained by other radiographic tests; fractures involving the transverse foramen; and traumatic spondylolisthesis requiring reduction. MRI is significantly less sensitive than plain radiographs or CT in identifying bone abnormalities.

Proponents of MRI in the emergency setting argue that it is necessary to differentiate extrinsic compression from intrinsic cord injury in patients with neurologic findings.[77] Because MRI can accurately define the presence and location of acute spinal cord injury, some authorities believe that MRI should be performed as the next adjunctive examination for patients with abnormal plain radiographs or neurologic deficits.[86] In this diagnostic algorithm, CT is performed only if MRI identifies a spinal injury and further definition of skeletal anatomy is necessary to guide clinical decision making.

MRI has replaced CT myelography in defining spinal cord injury (Fig. 13-31*B*). Its use in the emergency evaluation of cervical injury is restricted by limited availability and technical difficulties in unstable patients. Emergency indications may include progressive neurologic deficits or preoperative evaluation of patients requiring emergent cervical decompressive surgery. MRI can help delineate the anatomy of the cervicocranium of young children in whom bones are poorly ossified and ligamentous injury is common.

CONTROVERSIES

The Screening Examination: The Role of CT.   Because CT is superior to plain radiography in defining the specific anatomy of cervical fractures, it has been suggested that it be used to screen all patients suspected of having cervical injury.[36,79,80,82,85,87,88] The diagnostic capabilities of the three-view plain radiographic series were challenged when one study found that 53% of fractures identified by CT were missed by plain radiographs.[36] However, most fractures were found in patients whose plain views identified another fracture or an area of suspicion leading to the CT (only 1 of 49 patients with fractures on CT had normal plain films). Therefore, plain radiographs should be used for initial screening and CT should remain adjunctive.[87] When using CT for areas considered to be abnormal, suspicious, or poorly visualized on a three-view plain radiographic screening examination, the combination yields sensitivity approaching 100%.[82]

Which Plain Film Views?   It is universally agreed that the standard screening examination should include at least the lateral, AP, and open-mouth views. These three views have acceptable sensitivity as a screening tool.[89,90] In some institutions, oblique views are included with the standard series,[91] and others add pillar views.[92] Studies using three views (lateral, AP, and open-mouth) with adjunctive CT have demonstrated excellent sensitivity.

Additional screening views assist in visualizing the lateral structures and allow for clear evaluation of the cervicothoracic junction. A comparison study of three views versus three views plus supine oblique views suggested that oblique views provide additional information useful in making specific anatomic diagnoses; however, the study failed to demonstrate any difference in actual injury detection.[93] An expert panel of the American College of Radiology was unable to reach a consensus regarding the use of oblique views as an initial screening tool but agreed that three views constitute a minimal screening examination.[94] Although the oblique view allows the clinician to identify the anatomic detail of the lateral masses and provides safe viewing of the cervicothoracic junction, its use as a standard screening tool remains a matter of institutional and physician preference.

Is Prevertebral Soft Tissue Swelling a Useful Radiographic Sign? In individual cases, prevertebral soft tissue swelling may be the most radiographically evident sign of a subtle nondisplaced fracture. It is therefore emphasized that this is an important observation to make in all lateral cervical spine films.[95–99] However, when studied in a controlled fashion, the usefulness of thickening of the prevertebral soft tissue shadow seems questionable. In one study of 58 patients (41 of whom had fractures), only 49% of the injured patients had increased soft tissue dimensions. Futhermore, 24% of the noninjured patients (4 of 17) also had thickening.[52] Another study of 318 patients (58 with fractures), also revealed considerable overlap in soft tissue measurements in injured and noninjured patients, with a large number of false-negative and false-positive soft tissue findings.[53] In one of the largest series with 199 patients (106 injured and 93 controls), the upper and lower cervical regions were analyzed separately. The sensitivity of soft tissue swelling in the upper cervical spine (C1 to C4) was only 59% (and specificity 84%) and the number of cases with soft tissue swelling in the region of C4 to C7 was very low, only 5%.[54,99] Although the presence of soft tissue swelling should prompt a search for subtle injuries, the absence of swelling does not exclude an injury.

On the other hand, Harris points out that when carefully examined, changes in the *contour* of the cervicocranial soft tissues are a sensitive indicator of an occult cervicocranial injury. The contour is more useful than measurement of soft tissue thickness at discrete points.[55] The normal prevertebral soft tissue contour closely follows the anterior surfaces of the vertebrae in that region. There is a slight convexity at the C2 vertebral body and anterior tubercle of C1. Anterior to the dens and the atlantooccipital articulation, there is normally a slight concavity or straightening of the soft tissues. Abnormal soft tissue contour near C1 and C2 should prompt further imaging to search for such injuries as atlantooccipital subluxation, occipital condylar fractures, Jefferson burst fracture, fractures of the lateral mass of C1, or hangman fractures. Other pathologic entities and anatomic variants can cause swelling, such as facial fractures, retropharyngeal abscesses, nasopharyngeal adenopathy, or poor pharyngeal aeration due to swallowing or pooling of saliva at the time of exposure.

SUMMARY

Emergency physicians should use clinical criteria to eliminate unnecessary radiographs. Patients with multiple injuries cannot have their cervical spines "cleared" despite normal initial radiographs. A systematic approach to the interpretation of plain radiographs improves diagnostic accuracy. Liberal use of adjunctive imaging improves the sensitivity of plain radiographs.

ACKNOWLEDGMENTS

Thanks for special assistance to Carol B. Nestor and Dr. Martin Pusic.

REFERENCES

1. Bonadio WA: Cervical spine trauma in children: Part I. General concepts, normal anatomy, radiographic evaluation. *Am J Emerg Med* 11:158, 1993.
2. Bonadio WA: Cervical spine trauma in children: Part II. Mechanisms and manifestations of injury, therapeutic considerations. *Am J Emerg Med* 11:256, 1993.
3. McNamara RM, O'Brien MC, Davidheiser S: Post-traumatic neck pain: A prospective and follow-up study. *Ann Emerg Med* 17:906, 1988.
4. Hoffman JR, Schriger DL, Mower W, et al: Low-risk criteria for cervical-spine radiography in blunt trauma: A prospective study. *Ann Emerg Med* 21:1454, 1992.
5. Ringenberg BJ, Fisher AK, Urdaneta UF, et al: Rational ordering of cervical spine radiographs following trauma. *Ann Emerg Med* 17:792, 1988.
6. El-Khoury GY, Kathol MH, Daniel WW: Imaging of acute injuries of the cervical spine: Value of plain radiography, CT, and MR imaging. *AJR* 164:43, 1995.
7. Pang D, Wilberger JE: Spinal cord injury without radiographic abnormalities in children. *J Neurosurg* 57:114, 1982.
8. Farley FA, Hensinger RN, Herzenberg JE: Cervical spinal cord injury in children. *J Spinal Disord* 5:410, 1992.
9. Pang D, Pollack IF: Spinal cord injury without radiographic abnormality in children—The SCIWORA syndrome. *J Trauma* 29:654, 1989.
10. Shatney, CH, Brunner RD, Nguyen TQ: The safety of orotracheal intubation in patients with unstable cervical spine fracture or high spinal cord injury. *Am J Surg* 170:676, 1995.
11. Wright SW, Robinson GG II, Wright MB: Cervical spine injuries in blunt trauma patients requiring emergent endotracheal intubation. *Am J Emerg Med* 10:104, 1992.
12. Holliman CJ, Mayer JS, Cook RT Jr, Smith JS Jr: Is the anteroposterior cervical spine radiograph necessary in initial trauma screening? *Am J Emerg Med* 9:421, 1991.
13. Velmahos GC, Theodorou D, Tatevossian R, et al: Radiographic cervical spine evaluation in the alert asymptomatic blunt trauma victim: much ado about nothing? *J Trauma Injury* 40:768, 1996.
14. Ringenberg BJ, Fisher AK, Urdaneta LF, Midthun MA: Rational ordering of cervical spine radiographs following trauma. *Ann Emerg Med* 17:792, 1988.
15. McNamara RM, Heine E, Esposito B: Cervical spine injury and radiography in alert, high-risk patients. *J Emerg Med* 8:177, 1989.

16. Saddison D, Vanek VW, Racanelli JL: Clinical indications for cervical spine radiographs in alert trauma patients. *Am Surg* 57:366, 1991.

17. Hoffman JR, Schriger DL, Mower W, et al: Low-risk criteria for cervical–spine radiography in blunt trauma: A prospective study. *Ann Emerg Med* 21:1454, 1992.

18. Hoffman JR: Personal communication. January 20, 1998.

19. Gatrell CB: "Asymptomatic" cervical injuries: myth (letter)? *Am J Emerg Med* 3:263, 1985.

20. Rhee KJ: The unstable occult cervical spine fracture (letter). *Am J Emerg Med* 10:612, 1992.

21. Thambyrajah K: Fractures of the cervical spine with minimal or no symptoms. *Med J Malaysia* 26:244, 1972.

22. Mace SE: The unstable occult cervical spine fracture: A review. *Am J Emerg Med* 10:136, 1992.

23. Mace SE: Unstable occult cervical-spine fracture. *Ann Emerg Med* 20:1373, 1991.

24. McKee TR, Tinkoff G, Rhodes M: Asymptomatic occult cervical spine fracture: Case report and review of the literature. *J Trauma* 30:623, 1990.

25. O'Malley KF, Ross SE: The incidence of injury to the cervical spine in patients with craniocerebral injury. *J Trauma* 28:1476, 1988.

26. Ross SE, O'Malley KF, DeLong WG, et al: Clinical predictors of unstable cervical spinal injury in multiply injured patients. *Injury* 23:317, 1992.

27. Jacobs LM, Schwartz R: Prospective analysis of acute cervical spine injury: a methodology to predict injury. *Ann Emerg Med* 15:44, 1986.

28. Williams J, Jehle D, Cottington E, Shufflebarger C: Head, facial, and clavicular trauma as a predictor of cervical spine injury. *Ann Emerg Med* 21:719, 1992.

29. Fricker R, Gachter A: Lateral flexion/extension radiographs: Still recommended following cervical spinal injury. *Arch Orthop Trauma Surg* 113:115, 1994.

30. Bracken MB, Shepard MJ, Collins WF, et al: A Randomized controlled trial of methylprednisolone or naloxone in the treatment of acute spinal cord injury. *New Engl J Med* 322:1405, 1990.

31. Shaffer MA, Doris PE: Limitation of the cross table lateral view in detecting cervical spine injuries: A retrospective analysis. *Ann Emerg Med* 10:503, 1981.

32. Ross SE, Schwab W, David ET, et al: Clearing the cervical spine: Initial radiologic evaluation. *J Trauma* 27:1055, 1987.

33. Blahd WH Jr, Iserson KV, Bjelland JC: Efficacy of the posttraumatic cross table lateral view of the cervical spine. *J Emerg Med* 2:243, 1985.

34. Mace SE: Emergency evaluation of cervical spine injuries: CT versus plain radiographs. *Ann Emerg Med* 14:973, 1985.

35. Kim KS, Rogers LF, Regenbogen V: Pitfalls in plain film diagnosis of cervical spine injuries: False-positive interpretation. *Surg Neurol* 25:381, 1986.

36. Acheson MB, Livingston RR, Richardson ML, Stimac GK: High-resolution CT scanning in the evaluation of cervical spine fractures: Comparison with plain film examinations. *AJR* 148:1179, 1987.

37. Clark CR, Igram CM, El-Khoury GY, Ehara S: Radiographic evaluation of cervical spine injuries. *Spine* 13:742, 1988.

38. Shapiro R, Youngberg AS, Rothman SLG: The differential diagnosis of traumatic lesions of the occipito-atlanto-axial segment. *Radiol Clin North Am* 11:505, 1973.

39. Holdsworth FW: Fractures, dislocations and fracture-dislocations of the spine. *J Bone Joint Surg* 52A:1534, 1970.

40. Denis F: The three column spine and its significance in the classification of acute thoracolumbar spinal injuries. *Spine* 8:817, 1983.

41. White AA, Johnson RM, Panjabi MM, Southwick WO: Biomechanical analysis of clinical stability in the cervical spine. *Clin Orthop* 109:85, 1975.

42. Lewis LM, Docherty M, Ruoff BE, et al: Flexion-extension views in the evaluation of cervical-spine injuries. *Ann Emerg Med* 20:117, 1991.

43. Herkowitz HN, Rothman RH: Subacute instability of the cervical spine. *Spine* 9:348, 1984.

44. Wales LR, Knopp RK, Morishima MS: Recommendations for evaluation of the acutely injured cervical spine: A clnical radiologic algorithm. *Ann Emerg Med* 9:422, 1980.

45. Poirier VC, Greenlaw AR, Beaty CS, et al: Computed tomographic evaluation of C1-C2 in pediatric cervical spine trauma. *Emerg Radiol* 1:195, 1994.

46. Davis JW: Cervical injuries—Perils of the swimmer's view: Case report. *J Trauma* 29:891, 1989.

47. McCall IW, Park WM, McSweeny T: The radiologic demonstration of acute lower cervical injury. *Clin Radiol* 24:234, 1973.

48. Webb JK, Broughton RBK, McSweeney T, Park WM: Hidden flexion injury of the cervical spine. *J Bone Joint Surg (Br)* 58:322, 1976.

49. Harris JH Jr, Carson GC, Wagner LK: Radiologic diagnosis of traumatic occipitovertebral dissociation: 1. Normal occipitovertebral relationships on lateral radiographs of supine subjects. *AJR* 162:881, 1994.

50. Harris JH Jr, Burke JT, Ray RD, et al: Low (type III) odontoid fracture: A new radiographic sign. *Radiology* 153:353, 1984.

51. Penning L: Prevertebral hematoma in c-spine injuries. *Am J Radiol* 136:553, 1981.

52. Miles KA, Finlay D: Is prevertebral soft tissue swelling a useful sign in injuries of the cervical spine? *Injury* 17:177, 1988.

53. Templeton PA, Young JWR, Mirvis SE, et al: The value of retropharyngeal soft tissue measurements in trauma of the cervical spine. *Skel Radiol* 16:98, 1987.

54. DeBehnke DJ, Havel CJ: Utility of prevertebral soft tissue measurements in identifying patients with cervical spine fractures. *Ann Emerg Med* 24:1119, 1994.

55. Harris JH: Abnormal cervicocranial retropharyngeal soft-tissue contour in the detection of subtle acute cervicocranial injuries. *Emerg Radiol* 1:15, 1994.

56. Williams CF, Bernstein TW, Jelenko C: Essentiality of lateral c-spine radiographs. *Ann Emerg Med* 10:198, 1981.

57. Woodring JH, Lee C: Limitations of cervical radiography in the evaluation of acute cervical trauma. *J Trauma* 34:32, 1993.

58. Templeton PA, Young JWR, Mirvis SE, Buddemeyer EU: The value of retropharyngeal soft tissue measurements in trauma of adult. *Skel Radiol* 16:98, 1987.

59. Edeiken-Monroe BS, Edeiken J: Imaging of the normal spine, developmental anomalies, and trauma of the spine and extremities. *Curr Opin Radiol* 4:95, 1992.

60. Harris JH: Radiographic evaluation of spinal trauma. *Orthop Clin North Am* 17:75, 1986.

61. Swischuk LE: Anterior displacement of C2 in children: Physiologic or pathologic? *Radiology* 122:759, 1977.

62. Ryan MD, Henderson JJ: The epidemiology of fractures and fracture-dislocations of the cervical spine. *Injury* 23:38, 1992.

63. Fesmire FM, Luten RC: The pediatric cervical spine: Developmental anatomy and clinical aspects. *J Emerg Med* 7:133, 1989.

64. Ferguson J, Beattie TF: Occult spinal cord injury in traumatized children. *Injury* 24:83, 1993.

65. Apple JS, Kirks DR, Merten DF, Martinez S: Cervical spine fractures and dislocations in children. *Pediatr Radiol* 17:45, 1987.

66. Levine AM, Edwards CC: Fractures of the atlas. *J Bone Joint Surg* 73:680, 1991.

67. Levine AM, Edwards CC: Treatment of injuries in the C1-C2 complex. *Orthop Clin North Am* 17:31, 1986.

68. Spence KF Jr, Decker S, Sell KW: Bursting atlantal fracture associated with rupture of the transverse ligament. *J Bone Joint Surg* 52:543, 1970.

69. Smoker WRK, Dolan KD: The "fat" C2: A sign of fracture. *Am J Neurol Res* 8:33, 1987.

70. Pathria MN, Petersilge CA: Spinal trauma. *Radiol Clin North Am* 29:847, 1991.

71. Mirvis SE, Young JWR, Lim C, et al: Hangman's fracture: Radiologic assessment in 27 cases. *Radiology* 163:713, 1987.

72. Daffner RH: Evaluation of cervical vertebral injuries. *Semin Roentgenol* 27:239, 1992.

73. Woodring JH, Goldstein SJ: Fractures of the articular processes of the cervical spine. *AJR* 139:341, 1982.

74. Young JW, Resnik CS, DeCandido P, Mirvis SE: The laminar space in the diagnosis of rotational flexion injuries of the cervical spine. *AJR* 152:103, 1989.

75. Forsyth FH: Extension injuries of the cervical spine. *J Bone Joint Surg* 46A:1792, 1964.

76. Taylor AR: The mechanism of injury to the spinal cord in the neck without damage to the vertebral column. *J Bone Joint Surg* 33B:543, 1951.

77. Davis SJ, Teresi LM, Bradley WG, et al: Cervical spine hyperextension injuries: MR findings. *Radiology* 180:245, 1991.

78. Davis JW, Phreaner DL, Hoyt DB, Mackersie RC: The etiology of missed cervical spine injuries. *J Trauma* 34:342, 1993.

79. Binet EF, Moro JJ, Marangala JP, et al: Cervical spine tomography in trauma. *Spine* 2:163, 1977.

80. Woodring JH, Lee C: The role and limitations of computed tomographic scanning in the evaluation of cervical trauma. *J Trauma* 33:698, 1992.

81. Currarino G, Rollins N, Diehl JT: Congenital defects of the posterior arch of the atlas: A report of seven cases including an affected mother and son. *Am J Neuroradiol* 15:249, 1994.

82. Borock EC, Gabram SGA, Jacobs LM, Murphy MA: A prospective analysis of a two-year experience using computed tomography as an adjunct for cervical spine clearance. *J Trauma* 31:1001, 1991.

83. Roberge RJ, Wears RC: Evaluation of neck discomfort, neck tenderness, and neurologic deficits as indicators for radiography in blunt trauma victims. *J Emerg Med* 10:439, 1992.

84. Alker GJ, Young SO, Leslie EV: High cervical spine and craniocervical junction injuries in fatal traffic accidents. A radiologic study. *Orthop Clin North Am* 9:1003, 1978.

85. Link TM: Substantial head trauma: Value of routine CT examination of the cervicocranium. *Radiology* 196:741, 1995.

86. Orrison WW Jr, Benzel EC, Willis BK, et al: Magnetic resonance imaging evaluation of acute spine trauma. *Emerg Radiol* 2:120, 1995.

87. Schleehauf K, Ross SE, Civil ID, et al: Computed tomography in the initial evaluation of the cervical spine. *Ann Emerg Med* 18:815, 1989.

88. Kirshenbaum KJ, Nadimpalli SR, et al: Unsuspected upper cervical spine fractures associated with significant head trauma: Role of CT. *J Emerg Med* 8:183, 1990.

89. MacDonald RL, Schwartz ML, Mirich D, et al: Diagnosis of cervical spine injury in motor vehicle crash victims: How many x-rays are enough? *J Trauma* 30:392, 1990.

90. Ross SE, Schwab CW, David ET, et al: Clearing the cervical spine: Initial radiologic evaluation. *J Trauma* 27:1055, 1987.

91. Doris PE, Wilson RA: The next logical step in the emergency radiographic evaluation of cervical spine trauma: The five-view trauma series. *J Emerg Med* 3:371, 1985.

92. Kreipke DL, Gillespie KR, McCarthy MC, et al: Reliability of indications for cervical spine films in trauma patients. *J Trauma* 29:1438, 1989.

93. Freemyer B, Knopp R, Piche J, et al: Comparison of five-view and three-view cervical spine series in the evaluation of patients with cervical spine trauma. *Ann Emerg Med* 18:818, 1989.

94. Keats TE, Dalinka MK: *Appropriateness Criteria for Imaging and Treatment Decisions.* Reston, VA: American College of Radiology, 1995.

95. Penning L: Prevertebral hematoma in cervical spine injury: Incidence and etiologic significance. *AJR* 136:553, 1981.

96. Clark WM, Gehweiler JA, Laib R: Twelve significant signs of cervical spine trauma. *Skel Radiol* 3:201, 1979.

97. Paakkala T: Prevertebral soft tissue changes in cervical spine injury. *Crit Rev Diagn Imaging* 24:201, 1985.

98. Gopalakrishnan KC, Elmasri W: Prevertebral soft tissue shadow widening—An important sign of cervical spine injury. *Injury* 17:125, 1986.

99. Waeckerle JF: Occult C-spine injuries (editorial). *Ann Emerg Med* 24:1168, 1994.

SELECTED READINGS

Harris JH, Mirvis SE: *The Radiology of Acute Cervical Spine Trauma,* 3rd ed. Baltimore, Williams & Wilkins, 1996.

Rogers, LF: *Radiology of Skeletal Trauma,* 2nd ed. New York, Churchill Livingstone, 1992, pp. 439–592.

Errico TJ, Bauer RD, Waugh T: *Spinal Trauma.* Philadelphia, Lippincott, 1991.

Sherk HH (The Cervical Spine Research Society Editorial Committee): *The Cervical Spine,* 3rd ed. Philadelphia, Lippincott, 1998.

Gerlock AJ, Kirchner SG, Heller RM, Kaye JJ: *The Cervical Spine in Trauma, Advanced Exercises in Diagnostic Radiology,* vol. 7. Philadelphia, WB Saunders, 1978.

CHAPTER 14

THE THORACOLUMBAR SPINE

RICHARD LEVITAN

Thoracic and lumbar radiographic studies are commonly obtained in the emergency department (ED) either in the investigation of back pain or as part of the evaluation of trauma. Low back pain is the most common musculoskeletal complaint seen in the ambulatory care setting.[1] The lifetime prevalence of sciatica is 40%, while the lifetime prevalence of low back pain is 90%.[2] Back pain is the most common and most costly cause of workers' compensation in the United States. An estimated 9 million lumbosacral radiographic examinations are performed each year.[3,4] For some patients, nontraumatic back pain is due to a serious or potentially life-threatening disorder.

In major trauma, the thoracolumbar spine is visualized incidentally in chest, abdominal, and pelvic radiographs and is deliberately imaged as part of a full spine series. Thoracolumbar fractures occur in 2 to 5% of blunt trauma patients.[4,5] Most of these patients have other major injuries. Although other life threatening injuries often take priority in the initial management of these patients, thoracolumbar fractures can result in neurologic impairment and skeletal instability.

Different segments of the spine vary significantly in their skeletal structure, curvature, and range of motion. These differences influence the location and frequency of fractures as well as disk herniation and nerve root compression. The upper thoracic and lower sacral spine have limited mobility because of the surrounding rib cage and pelvis. The upper thoracic and lower sacral spine also have a kyphotic curvature. In these two regions, the combination of bony protection, limited mobility, and kyphosis minimizes fractures and disk-related pathology. In contrast, the lower thoracic and lumbar sections have significant mobility, both in rotation and flexion-extension. The lordotic curvature in these areas permits symmetrical axial loading, a contributing factor in disk herniation and vertebral burst fractures. Most fractures occur at the junction between the relatively immobile thoracic spine and the relatively mobile lumbar spine. Of all thoracolumbar fractures, two-thirds occur in the area of T12-L2 and more than 90% between T12-L4.

The neurologic sequelae from fractures and other pathology depend on the level of injury. Fractures of the upper and midthoracic spine, even with minimal displacement, almost invariably result in complete cord lesions because the spinal canal is very narrow at this level. The spinal cord itself ends at the L1 or L2 vertebra. The terminal end of the spinal cord is the *conus medullaris*. Below that level, the spinal canal is occupied by the lumbar roots that make up the *cauda equina*. Although the nerve roots of the thoracic spine have limited clinical significance, the lumbosacral roots are critical to the lower extremities as well as anal and bladder sphincter function. The nerve root levels do not exactly correspond with the vertebral levels because the spinal cord is much shorter than the spinal column. Above T10, neurologic injury presents with spinal cord signs and symptoms. Below L2, there are only nerve root findings. At the thoracolumbar junction, neurologic injuries are mixed conus medullaris and nerve root injuries. Of patients with fractures at the thoracolumbar junction, 40% have neurologic deficits because the spinal canal is narrow in this area.[6]

The initial imaging study for almost all patients with thoracic or lumbar spinal injuries are plain radiographs. Computed tomography (CT) is superior for the comprehensive evaluation of spinal fractures.[7] Magnetic resonance imaging (MRI) provides the best direct visualization of the spinal cord, nerve roots, intervertebral disks, and ligaments.[8,9] Myelography has been used to outline the intrathecal space and indirectly provide information about the spinal canal and nerve roots. It involves a C1-2 puncture or lumbar puncture for dye injection. Although myelography is still used in combination with CT, especially in settings where MRI is unavailable, newer high-resolution CT provides evaluation of herniated disks and spinal stenosis without myelographic injection of dye.

CLINICAL DECISION MAKING

ED patients who require thoracic or lumbar radiography can be divided into three groups: those who have sustained major, life-threatening traumatic injuries; those with minor or moderate trauma who are complaining of back pain; and patients with nontraumatic back pain or back pain following minimal trauma such as that due to bending or lifting. Victims of major trauma all require serious consideration of thoracolumbar spinal injury even if there is no complaint of back pain. Patients who have sustained lesser degrees of trauma and have back pain are more frequently seen in the ED. Thoracolumbar radiography is used selectively in these patients because the risk of a fracture is low and the gonadal radiation dose is very high, particularly with radiography of the lumbar spine. Thus, the approach to back

TABLE 14-1

Indications for Radiographs of the Thoracolumbar Spine in Blunt Trauma

Back pain or tenderness
Myelopathy
Cervical spine injury
Glasgow Coma Scale score <15
Alcohol use
Altered sensorium
Major nonthoracolumbar injury
Falls from higher than 10 ft
Ejection from a vehicle
Motorcycle accident >50 mph

pain in patients with mild or moderate trauma differs from that in those with neck pain because the cervical spine is more vulnerable to injury and radiography of the cervical spine should be used liberally. Finally, patients with nontraumatic back pain (or back pain following minimal trauma) are commonly seen in the ED. Most of these patients do not require spinal radiography. However, certain patients are at high risk for significant pathology and should have radiographs. These include patients with known malignancy, preexisting arthropathy, the elderly, intravenous drug users, and patients with HIV infection.

Neurologic impairment and axial skeletal stability are the main concerns that prompt the ordering of thoracolumbar radiographic studies in the ED. Patients with neurologic signs referable to the spinal cord or thoracolumbar roots need emergency radiographic studies. Although plain films are not always definitive, they should be obtained before more advanced studies are ordered. If skeletal pathology is evident, plain films help localize those areas requiring selective study with CT.[10] CT with myelography provides information about impingement on the spinal cord or roots. MRI is the "gold standard" for evaluation of the spinal cord and other nonosseous structures of the spine. MRI is particularly valuable in patients with spinal cord or nerve root compression without bone pathology.[9] Spinal cord and nerve root disease without skeletal abnormalities can be caused by transverse myelitis, spinal cord hemorrhage or infarction, epidural abscess without osteomyelitis, and nerve root compression from disk herniation.

Trauma Patients

Stable trauma patients who have complaints localized to the thoracolumbar spine require anteroposterior (AP) and lateral films as part of their ED evaluation. Falls and motor vehicle accidents, particularly involving vehicle ejection or collisions with motorcyclists, are the most common causes of thoracolumbar fractures.[4,5,11-13] Patients with thoracolumbar fractures usually have other serious injuries. These associated injuries are often more obvious than the vertebral fracture and can distract the clinician from considering a spinal injury. Therefore, in treating the victim of major multisystem trauma,

one must always consider spinal injuries. Vertebral fractures are more common among trauma victims with higher injury severity scores, especially in those with injuries of the cervical spine, major thoracic trauma, pelvic fractures, and fractures of a lower extremity.[5,11,13-15]

Multiple noncontiguous vertebral injuries occur in 4.5 to 17% of spinal injury patients.[15,16] The most common pattern involves a lower cervical fracture associated with a secondary fracture at T12-L5. One-third of patients with upper thoracic spine fractures have a hemopneumothorax, major vessel injury, or ruptured diaphragm. Pelvic fractures occur in 13% of patients with thoracolumbar fractures.[5] Lower extremity and specifically calcaneal fractures often accompany thoracolumbar fractures from vertical plunges.[17] Of patients with thoracolumbar fractures following a vertical plunge, 70.8% had either pelvic or lower extremity fractures, including 31.6% with calcaneal fractures.[18] Of patients with femoral fractures following high-velocity trauma, 3.5% had an associated thoracolumbar fracture.[19]

Radiographs of the thoracolumbar spine are obtained only when the patient does not require immediate interventions or other, more urgent diagnostic studies. In the critical patient who needs emergent surgery, plain films of the chest, abdomen, or pelvis provide preliminary radiographic evaluation of the thoracolumbar spine. CT scans of the thorax and abdomen indicated for other reasons provide another means of examining the spine without delaying the evaluation of more life-threatening injuries. Nevertheless, CT is not an adequate screening study of the spine because AP and lateral spine films are more reliable at localizing injuries, assessing alignment, and detecting vertebral body compression.[20]

Early CT evaluation of the spine is needed for patients with burst fractures, missile injuries, and any fracture associated with neurologic findings. Some authors suggest CT evaluation for all acute vertebral fractures including apparently simple wedge compression fractures.[21,22]

Trauma patients who have unreliable clinical examinations due to head injury, altered mental status, or a distracting major injury should be considered for a complete spine series during their evaluation. Several studies have looked at the reliability of back pain or tenderness on examination as a predictor of thoracolumbar fracture among trauma patients. Back tenderness is absent in 19 to 40% of patients with thoracolumbar fractures.[5,12,13] The lack of back pain or tenderness on examination in the presence of a thoracolumbar fracture occurs in patients with altered mental status, neurologic deficit, and major nonthoracolumbar injury. Patients with Glasgow Coma Scale (GCS) scores of 13 and 14 are three times more likely than patients with a GCS of 15 to have unreliable examinations for back pain or tenderness. Among patients with a GCS of 15, those with major injury were seven times more likely to have an unreliable examination. Therefore the indications for obtaining thoracolumbar films in victims of blunt trauma must be liberal (Table 14-1). Conversely, routine thoracolumbar studies are not indicated in patients who are neurologically intact, with a normal sensorium, no tenderness on examination, and no major nonspinous injury.[13,14]

TABLE 14-2

Indications for Radiographs of the Lumbar Spine in Patients with Low Back Pain

Age older than 55 years
Metastatic disease (especially breast, lung, or prostate cancer)
Osteoporosis
Multiple myeloma
Chronic steroid use
Anklosing spondylitis
Alcoholism
Suspected pyogenic infection (including intravenous drug abuse, diabetes mellitus, fever)

Nontraumatic Back Pain

The largest subset of patients who undergo spinal radiography, most commonly lumbosacral films, are those with nontraumatic back pain or minimal trauma such as bending or lifting. These patients are neurologically intact or have sciatic complaints. In this group, there is a low yield for a relatively high cost and gonadal radiation exposure.[1,2,23,24] Moreover, there is a poor correlation between radiographic abnormalities (e.g., degenerative changes) and clinical complaints. Because low back pain is such a common complaint, one should be selective in deciding which patients require radiographs. In addition, one should be mindful of numerous nonmusculoskeletal causes of back pain, such as aortic aneurysm and urolithiasis. The purpose of obtaining spinal radiographs with patients with nontraumatic back pain is to identify malignancy, infection, or inflammatory spondyloarthropathy. In the primary care setting, fewer than 0.2% of all patients with back pain have one of these conditions.

Patients with back pain or bone tenderness who are at high risk for osseous pathology require radiographs in the ED. This includes the elderly and patients with a history of metastatic disease, osteoporosis, multiple myeloma, intravenous drug abuse, chronic steroid use, tuberculosis, or ankylosing spondylitis (Table 14-2). In these patients, fractures can occur spontaneously or after minor trauma. In Scandinavia, about one in four persons above 75 years of age had a wedge compression fracture.[25,26] Even without trauma, burst fractures with neurologic compromise can occur in osteoporotic patients.[27] Patients with weight loss or other signs suggesting a malignancy should have radiographic studies. Breast, lung, and prostate cancers account for 50% of metastatic lesions in the spine. Plain-film radiographic abnormalities are a late finding, seen only after destruction of 50% of the bony matrix. Alcoholics are also at high risk because their history is unreliable for trauma and chronic alcohol abuse is associated with osteoporosis.

Patients who are prone to develop pyogenic spinal infections, such as intravenous drug users, diabetics, and any patient with localized midline back pain or tenderness associated with fever should have radiography. Plain-film radiographic abnormalities from osteomyelitis take 2 to 4 weeks to develop. Radionuclide bone scanning along with an elevated erythrocyte sedimentation rate (ESR) suggest the diagnosis within 3 days of onset. However, bone scan abnormalities are nonspecific. In addition, fewer than half of the patients with osteomyelitis have elevated leukocyte counts. MRI is the procedure of choice for detecting paravertebral and intraspinal infections.[28]

Spondyloarthropathies such as ankylosing spondylitis should be suspected in patients with back discomfort beginning before the age of 40 years, an insidious onset of symptoms, symptoms lasting at least 3 months, morning stiffness, and improvement with exercise.[23] Finally, patients with chronic back pain lasting longer than 4 to 8 weeks require plain-film studies.

Patients who do not warrant lumbar spine films in the ED for back pain are those who are between 18 and 50 years of age, neurologically intact, afebrile, without history of deceleration or direct trauma, and without risk factors or history of osseous pathology (e.g., metastatic disease, steroids, weight loss).

ANATOMY AND PHYSIOLOGY

The thoracic and lumbar spine is made up of twelve thoracic and five lumbar vertebrae. The bodies and intervertebral disks of the thoracic and lumbar vertebrae increase in size progressively from T1 to L5. The anatomy of the vertebrae must be understood if one is to recognize radiographic landmarks (Fig. 14-1). Posterior to the vertebral body, the paired pedicles meet the paired laminae. The laminae join together medially and form the neural arch enclosing the vertebral canal. The spinous process projects posteriorly from the junction of the laminae. In the thoracic vertebrae, the transverse processes jut out where the laminae and pedicles meet. The superior and inferior articulating facets project above and below the pedicles. In the lumbar vertebrae, the transverse processes project from the junction of the vertebral body and the pedicles.

Intervertebral ligamentous support is provided by the anterior and posterior longitudinal ligaments, capsular ligaments, ligamentum flava, supraspinous ligaments, and interspinous ligaments (Fig. 14-2). The ligamentum flava connects the laminae of the dorsal vertebral arches. The capsular ligaments connect the articular facets at the apophyseal joints. The supraspinous and interspinous ligaments connect the spinous processes. Between the vertebral bodies are the intervertebral disks, made up of the central gelatinous *nucleus pulposus* and surrounded by the *annulus fibrosus*.

The articulations between vertebrae and between the vertebrae and the ribs are numerous and complex. Collectively, there are more than 100 intervertebral and costovertebral articulations. The intervertebral articulations occur at the two superior and two inferior facets of each vertebra. The inferior facet of one vertebra and the superior articulating facet of the vertebra below form the apophyseal joint, which is a true synovial joint. The facets help stabilize one vertebra on top of another.

The "typical" thoracic vertebrae are T2-T9, and the "atypical" ones are T1 and T10-T12. In the typical thoracic vertebra, each rib articulates with the vertebral body and the transverse

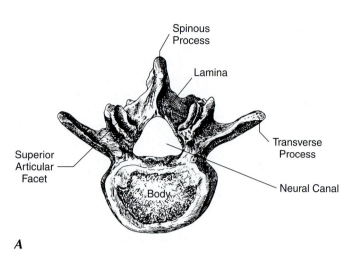

A

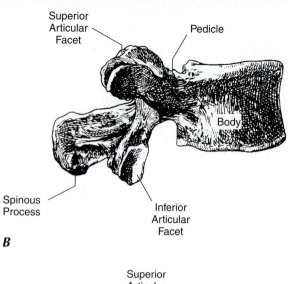

B

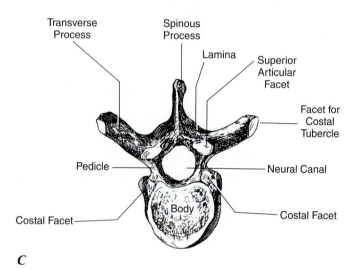

C

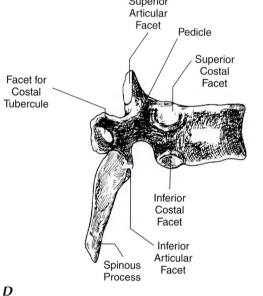

D

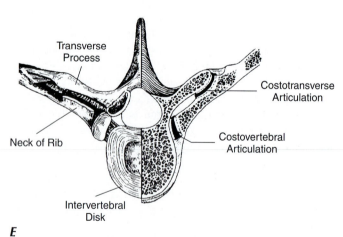

E

FIGURE 14-1. A characteristic lumbar and thoracic vertebra seen from above and from the side. *A* and *B*. Lumbar vertebra. *C* and *D*. Thoracic vertebra. *E*. Costovertebral articulation. (From Pansky B: *Review of Gross Anatomy,* 6th ed. New York: McGraw-Hill, 1996. With permission.)

process. The second through ninth ribs articulate with two vertebrae across the corresponding intervertebral disk. The head of the first rib articulates only on T1 and not on the vertebra above. T10-T12 differ from the other thoracic vertebrae because the ribs here articulate with only one vertebra and have no articulation with the transverse processes. The lumbar vertebrae have larger bodies than the thoracic vertebrae. The lumbar transverse processes are bulkier and longer and they project more perpendicularly from the vertebral body.

Collectively, the neural arches of the vertebrae form the spinal canal, through which the spinal cord and cauda equina run. The spinal cord is enveloped by the closely adherent and well-vascularized pia mater, which is itself enclosed by the arachnoid membrane. The dura mater has an inner meningeal layer overlying the arachnoid and an outer periosteal layer that is adherent to the bone of the vertebral foramen. Located between the two layers of the dura mater is the epidural space and the venous plexus. The nerve roots exit through the intervertebral notches. The spinal cord tapers and ends at the conus medullaris at the level of the L1 vertebra in the adult. The lumbar, sacral, and coccygeal nerve roots travel a significant distance before exiting the spinal canal. These intravertebral spinal roots make up the cauda equina.

Biomechanics. Biomechanically, the spine can be viewed as a three-column structure (Fig. 14-2).[6] The anterior column is made up of the anterior longitudinal ligament, the anterior an-

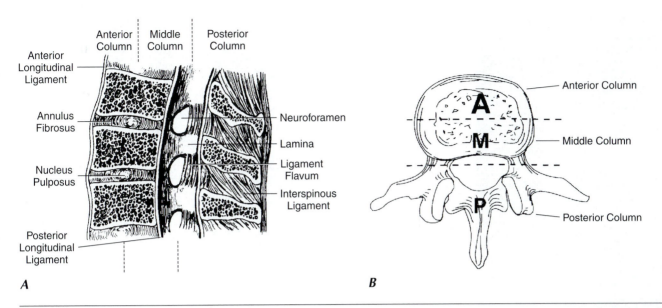

FIGURE 14-2. The three biomechanical columns of the spine. The anterior, middle, and posterior columns include both skeletal and ligamentous structures. *A.* Sagittal section. (From Pansky B: *Review of Gross Anatomy,* 6th ed. New York: McGraw-Hill, 1996. With permission.) *B.* Top view. (From Dee R, Hurst LC, Gruber MA, Kottmeier SA: *Principles of Orthopaedic Practice,* 2d ed. New York: McGraw-Hill, 1997. With permission.)

nulus fibrosus, and the anterior part of the vertebral body. The middle column includes the posterior annulus fibrosus, the posterior vertebral body, and the posterior longitudinal ligament. The posterior column comprises the posterior neural arch (pedicles, laminae, facets, transverse processes, and spinous processes) alternating with the posterior ligamentous complex (supraspinous ligament, interspinous ligament, apophyseal capsule, and ligamentum flava). This biomechanical model is used to understand the classification, mechanisms of injury, and stability of thoracolumbar fractures.

RADIOGRAPHIC TECHNIQUE

The standard views of the thoracic and lumbar spine are the AP and lateral radiographs. (Table 14-3; Figs. 14-3 and 14-4). Additional lumbar views include the oblique radiographs, a coned-down projection of the lumbosacral space, and projections of the thoracolumbar junction. Oblique views provide additional visualization of the apophyseal joints and the intervertebral foramina. The coned-down projections improve visualization of the lumbosacral and thoracolumbar junctions by centering the beam at these locations.

The standard lateral view of the thoracic spine demonstrates the upper thoracic vertebrae poorly because of the superimposed shoulders. The upper thoracic vertebrae are better seen with a Fletcher view, where the patient is slightly rotated from a true lateral position. This brings one shoulder anterior and the other posterior to the spine. Alternatively, a swimmer's projection, with one arm elevated, also improves visualization of the upper vertebrae.

Overlying ribs and pulmonary vasculature partly obscure the thoracic vertebrae on the lateral view. Better delineation of the

thoracic vertebrae on the lateral view is further accomplished by having the patient inhale or exhale slowly during a long radiographic exposure. This "blurs out" superimposed structures.

Although the thoracic and lumbar spine is partially seen on standard films of the AP chest and pelvis, there are important reasons to specifically obtain spinal films. The chest film does not provide good visualization of the lower thoracic vertebrae, and the pelvic film does not usually include the upper lumbar vertebrae. Therefore, the most common area of traumatic pathology (T12-L2) is not usually seen on the chest and pelvic films. Although the AP view of the thoracic spine is similar in orientation to the AP view of the chest, the spine film is exposed to display osseous structures. Subtle but significant widening of the interpedicular distance and differences in vertebral body height or disk spaces can be difficult to see on a chest radiograph. Finally, the lateral spine views provide critical information about the vertebral bodies and their alignment that is not seen on an AP projection. Most missed thoracolumbar fractures occur in victims of major trauma because inadequate spine studies were obtained.[12,14,15]

CT and MRI have several distinct advantages over plain spine films. CT provides the best visualization of posterior neural arch structures.[7] Although CT demonstrates the intervertebral disks and soft tissues, there is limited contrast between the disks and neural structures on an unenhanced CT. This limitation is overcome by combining CT with metrizamide myelography. However, MRI is now the procedure of choice for imaging nonosseous structures and for detecting herniation of the nucleus pulposus and other causes of spinal cord compression. MRI can provide axial, sagittal, and coronal images and permits evaluation of the entire thoracolumbar spine without patient manipulation. MRI using gadolinium-DPTA enhancement improves imaging of the intrathecal space.[9]

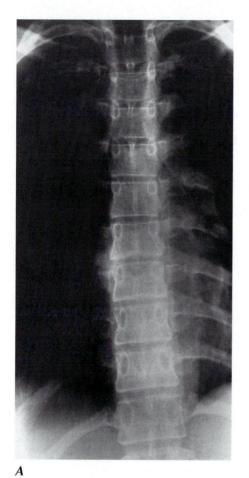

A

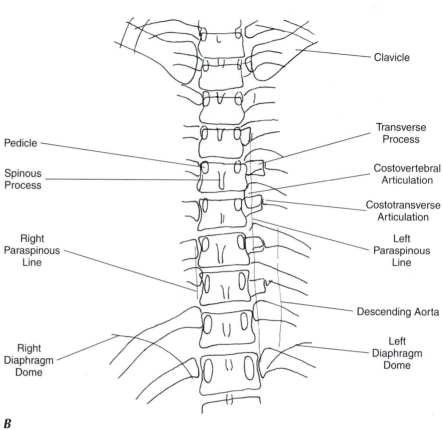

B

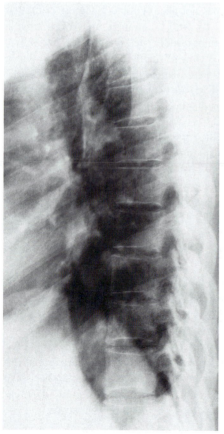

C

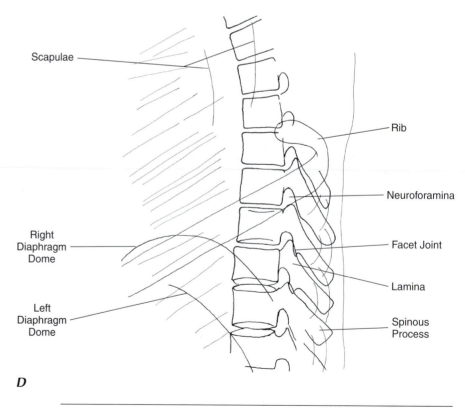

D

FIGURE 14-3.   Thoracic spine. *A* and *B.* AP view. *C* and *D.* Lateral view.

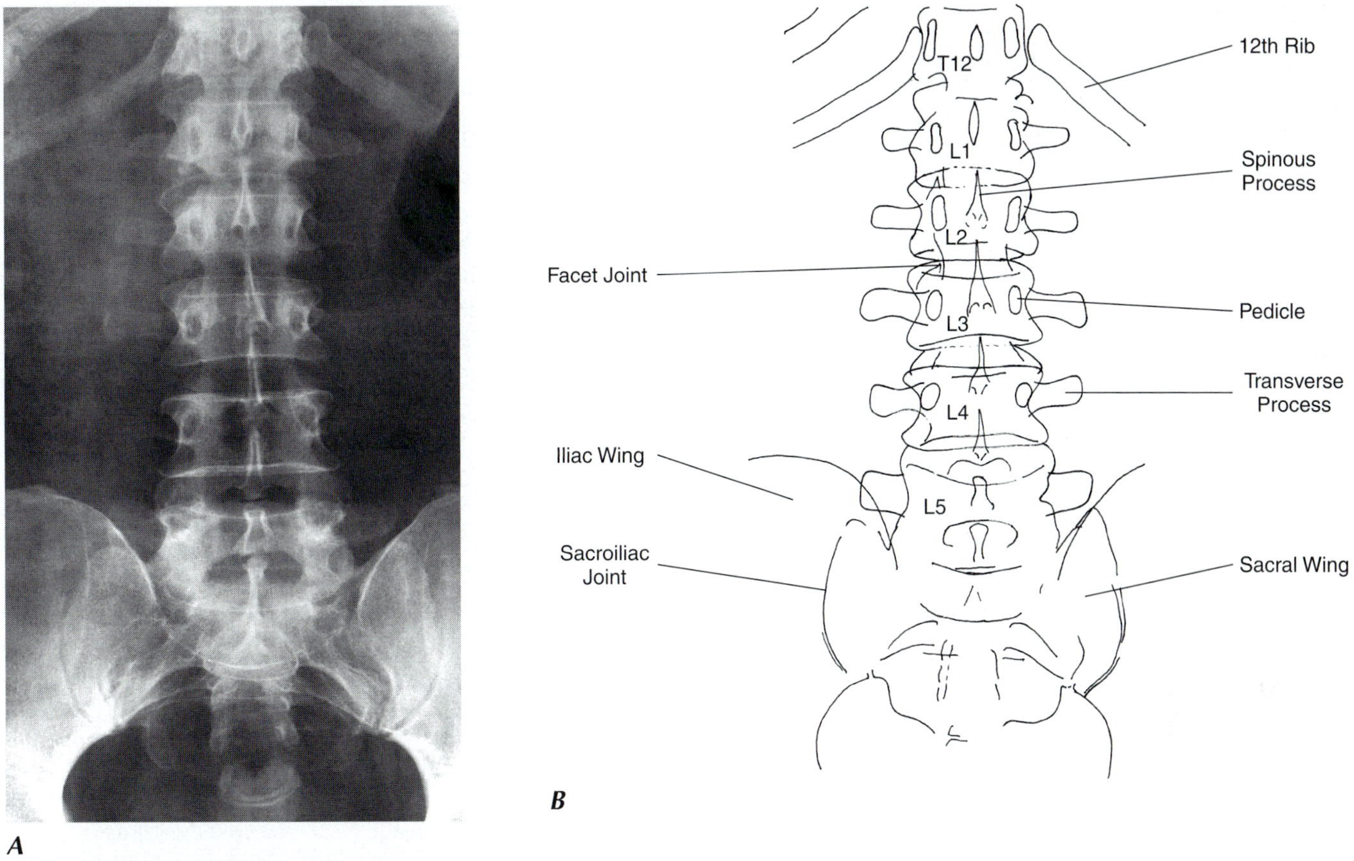
12th Rib
T12
L1
Spinous Process
L2
Facet Joint
L3
Pedicle
Transverse Process
L4
Iliac Wing
L5
Sacroiliac Joint
Sacral Wing
A
B

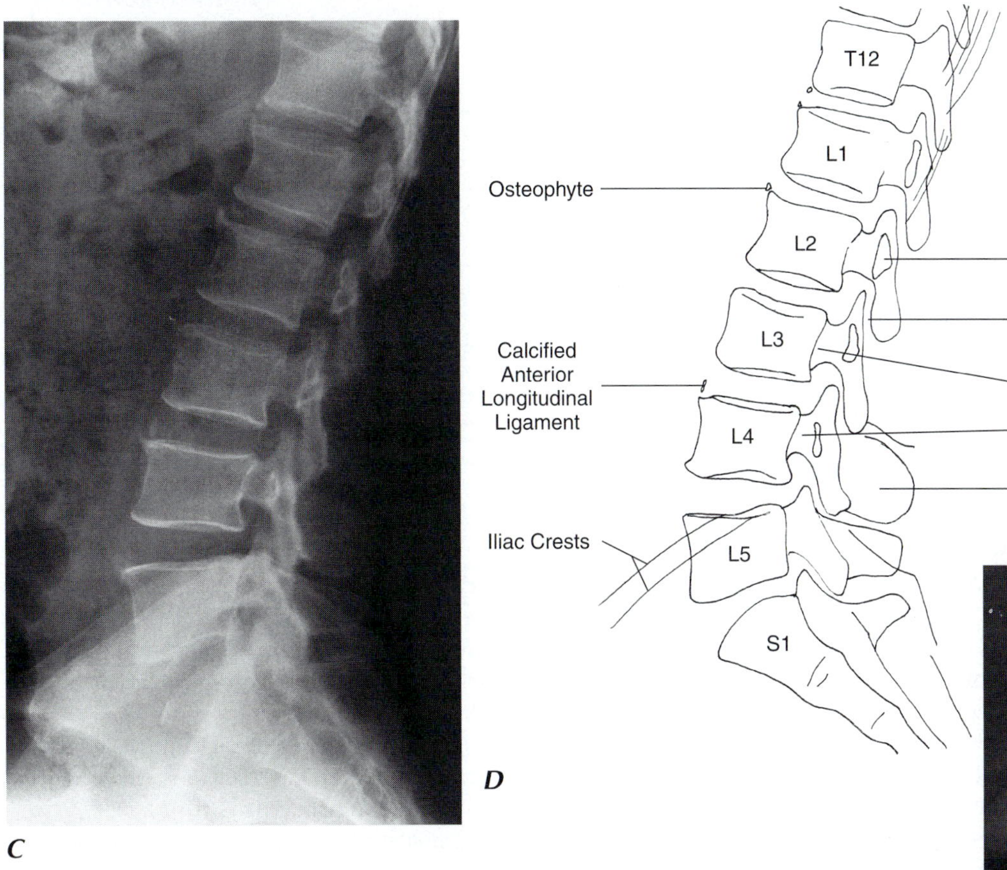
T12
L1
Osteophyte
L2
Transverse Process
L3
Facet Joint
Calcified Anterior Longitudinal Ligament
Posterior Vertebral Body Line
L4
Pedicle
Spinous Process
Iliac Crests
L5
S1
C
D

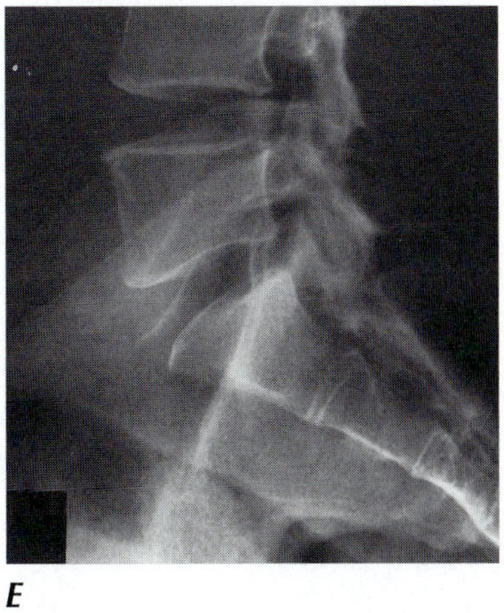
E

FIGURE 14-4. Lumbar spine—normal radiographs. *A* and *B.* AP view. *C* and *D.* Lateral view. *E.* Lumbosacral spot view.

TABLE 14-3

Radiographic Views of the Thoracic and Lumbar Spine

VIEW	TECHNIQUE	ADEQUACY	LIKELY FINDINGS
		THORACIC SPINE	
AP	Patient supine. X-ray beam centered 8 cm inferior to sternal notch	Entire thoracic spine seen Spinous processes centered on vertebral bodies Penetration is adequate to show retrocardiac vertebral bodies	Loss of vertebral body height Interpedicular distance Loss of pedicles (metastatic disease)
Lateral	The patient lies left side down with arms extended forward X-ray beam centered at T7 Slow respiration during long exposure blurs overlying ribs	No rotation; intervertebral disk spaces are open Upper thoracic vertebrae hidden by shoulders	Loss of vertebral body height Vertebral body malalignment
Swimmer's view (recumbent)	The patient lies on one side The lower arm extended superoanteriorly The upper arm is posteriorly or caudally. X-ray beam directed at T2-T3	No rotation; shoulders should not overlap C5 to T5 visible	Upper thoracic, vertebral body fractures, and malalignment
		LUMBAR SPINE	
AP	Patient supine with the hips and knees flexed to increase contact with the table X-ray beam at level of iliac crest	Entire lumbar spine seen No rotation Spinous processes centered on vertebral bodies	Loss of vertebral body height Interpedicular distance Transverse process fractures
Lateral	Patient lies left side down without rotation Hips and knees gently flexed X-ray beam centered at iliac crest	Entire lumbar spine seen No rotation Intervertebral disk spaces open	Loss of vertebral body height Vertebral malalignment Lamina, pedicles, and spinous processes
Oblique	45° oblique position	"Scotty dog" seen at each level	Spondylolysis of the pars interarticularis
Lumbosacral lateral	X-ray beam centered 4 cm inferior to anterior superior iliac crest	Lumbosacral joint is seen No rotation L5-S1 disk space open	Lumbosacral pathology including spondylolisthesis
Thoracolumbar AP and lateral	X-ray beam centered at thoracolumbar junction	T11 to L2 clearly seen without rotation	Injuries at the thoracolumbar junction

RADIOGRAPHIC ANALYSIS

Before thoracolumbar films are systematically examined for pathology, the *technical adequacy* of the films is assessed. Patient position and radiographic penetration must be correct. On the AP view, no rotation is present when the spinous processes are in the midline between the pedicles and the lateral edges of the vertebral bodies. On the lateral film, the intervertebral disk spaces and foramina should be clearly distinguishable and the vertebral bodies should jut forward on the pedicles. On the AP view, penetration is correct if the posterior bony structures

are well delineated behind the vertebral bodies and important soft tissue structures are visible. In the AP thoracic spine, these soft tissue structures include the left and right paraspinous lines. In the AP lumbar spine, the psoas margins should be seen.

The radiographic assessment concentrates on the AP and lateral views (Figs. 14-3 and 14-4). The goal of plain-film examination of the thoracolumbar spine is to identify fractures, neoplasms, infections, and arthropathies (Fig. 14-5).

A systematic approach to radiographic interpretation minimizes missed abnormalities. The ABC'S, an acronym for *a*lignment, *b*ones, *c*artilage and joints, and *s*oft tissues, does not

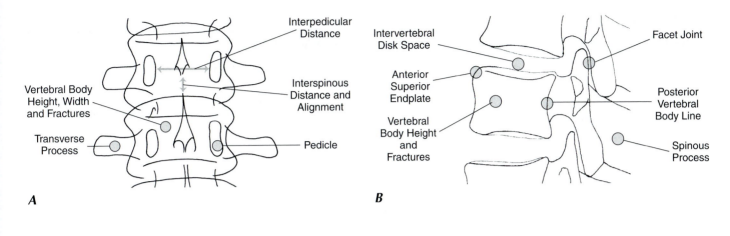

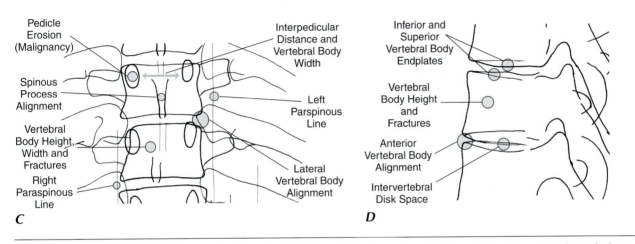

FIGURE 14-5. Sites prone to injury and easily missed injuries. *A.* Lumbar spine—AP view. *B.* Lumbar spine—Lateral view. *C.* Thoracic spine—AP view. *D.* Thoracic spine—Lateral view.

specifically identify the critical components of thoracolumbar radiographic assessment.[32] The acronym BACKPAINS encompasses the ABC'S while adding items critical in the assessment of thoracolumbar pathology (Table 14-4). It stands for *b*ones, *a*lignment, *c*artilage, *k*yphosis, *p*araspinal and *p*soas lines, *a*pophyseal joints, *i*nterpedicular and *i*nterspinous distances, *n*euroforaminae, and *s*coliosis.

The term *cartilage* refers to the intervertebral disks as indirectly evaluated by the disk spaces. The paraspinous and psoas stripes are soft tissue lines seen on the AP views in the thoracic and lumbar spine, respectively. The *paraspinous line* between the paraspinal soft tissues and the lung extends from the diaphragm to the apex on the right side and from the diaphragm to the aortic arch on the left.[33,34] The *psoas stripe* is formed by the psoas major muscle, arising from T12-L4 vertebrae, passing through the pelvis, and inserting on the lesser trochanter of the femur. The *interpedicular distance* (IPD) is the distance between the medial cortical surface of the pedicles on the AP view. The *interspinous distance* (ISD) is the distance between the cortical edges of adjacent spinous processes on the AP and lateral views. The term *neuroforamina* refers to the interverte-

bral foramina and surrounding structures, seen on the lateral view, through which the nerve roots exit. The structures are, in clockwise order, the intervertebral disk, the superior portion of the posterior vertebral body line (of the lower vertebra), the pedicle of the lower vertebra, the superior articular facet of the lower vertebra, the inferior articulating facet of the upper vertebra, the pedicle of the upper vertebra, and the inferoposterior vertebral body line (of the upper vertebra). The cortex of the posterior vertebral body is normally poorly delineated at the insertion of the pedicle.[35]

Anteroposterior View (Thoracic and Lumbar)

Bones that need to be carefully inspected include the vertebral bodies, pedicles, and spinous processes as well as the transverse processes in the lumbar spine (Fig. 14-5). The vertebral bodies are square in the upper thorax and become larger and more rectangular toward the lumbar region. They steadily increase in height and width caudally; they should have sharp, well-defined superior and inferior end plates and a slight, gen-

TABLE 14-4

Systematic Analysis of Thoracic and Lumbar Spine Radiographs—"BACKPAINS"

	AP VIEW	LATERAL VIEW
Bones	Vertebral body height and width Vertebral body cortex, superior and inferior end plates Pedicles and spinous processes Transverse processes (lumbar)	Vertebral height and width Vertebral body cortex, superior and inferior end plates Posterior cortex of each vertebral body (posterior vertebral body line) Pedicles and spinous processes
Alignment	Alignment of lateral margins of vertebral bodies, pedicles, and spinous processes	Alignment of posterior vertebral body line, anterior vertebral bodies and apophyseal joints
Cartilage	Disk space narrowing, widening, or sclerosis	Disk space narrowing, widening, or sclerosis
Kyphosis		Gentle kyphosis is normal in thoracic spine Note any areas of acute kyphosis (thoracic or lumbar spine)
Paraspinal line, psoas stripe	Note focal widening of the paraspinal line (thoracic) Note contour and definition of the psoas stripe (lumbar)	
Apophyseal joints		Inspect articulations of the apophyseal joints
Interpedicular distance, interspinous distances	Compare interpedicular distance at each segment to adjacent vertebra Look for abnormal widening of interspinous distance	
Neuroforamina		Inspect outline of the neuroforamina including the posterior vertebral body line, pedicles, and apophyseal joints
Scoliosis	In areas of scoliosis, check vertebral body end plates, vertebral body and spinous processes alignment, and transverse process (lumbar)	

tle concavity of their lateral edges. The posterior elements are positioned behind the vertebrae. The pedicles and spinous processes have a vertically oriented oval and teardrop shape, respectively, and their cortical margins are smooth and distinct. The oval outline of the pedicles is the waist of the pedicle projecting behind the vertebral body.[36]

The *alignment* of the vertebral bodies, pedicles, and spinous processes is evident on the AP view. Subtle lateral displacement of the bodies, pedicles, or spinous processes at any level indicates instability.[34] The *cartilage* disk spaces increase in height caudally. The disk spaces should be clear and well defined between the vertebral body end plates. At the extremes of the thoracic and lumbar films, the disk spaces are poorly seen because of divergence of the x-ray beam. *Kyphosis* is seen on the lateral view, not the AP view.

The *paraspinous line* is discernible on the left side at T10 in 97% of patients. It varies greatly in width from 5 to 15 mm, depending on the amount of adipose tissue.[33] The paraspinous line is absent on the left above the aortic arch, which is at the T4-T5 level. The left paraspinal shadow is wider in older patients because of tortuosity of the aorta. Regardless of the mea-

surement, which can range up to 22 mm at T6, focal areas of widening are abnormal and warrant further investigation.[37] The paraspinal line is poorly seen on the right side because the pleural reflection has an oblique orientation. On the lumbar AP film, the *psoas margins* diverge laterally and inferiorly from L1 to the pelvis. Disappearance of the psoas margin is a sensitive sign of spinal fracture from T12-L5, although it is nonspecific, since any cause of retroperitoneal hematoma produces the same result.

The IPD and ISD are carefully checked at each level (Fig. 14-6). The IPD normally decreases from T1 to T6 and then increases progressively in the lumbar spine.[38] The ISD increases gradually, moving down the thoracolumbar spine as the vertebrae increase in height. The IPD is abnormal when its width is not intermediate between the IPD of the vertebrae above and below.[39] *Scoliosis* is always abnormal; however, it is usually unrelated to trauma or any other acute process. Scoliosis and angulation localized at only one vertebral level could be due to a lateral vertebral body fracture and requires careful examination of the vertebral end plates and lateral margins at that location.

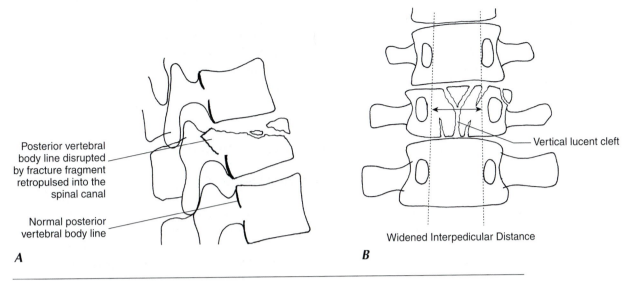

Posterior vertebral body line disrupted by fracture fragment retropulsed into the spinal canal

Normal posterior vertebral body line

A

Vertical lucent cleft

Widened Interpedicular Distance

B

FIGURE 14-6. Radiographic features that distinguish a burst fracture from a wedge compression fracture.

Lateral View

The examination of the *bones* in the lateral projection begins with inspection of the height and width of the vertebrae (Fig. 14-5). The upper thoracic vertebrae are difficult to see without a Fletcher projection or swimmer's view. There is a slight concavity of the anterior and, to a lesser extent, posterior margins of the vertebral body. Although the superior and inferior end plates of the vertebrae are normally parallel, there may be slight loss of height anteriorly in the upper thoracic spine due to the normal kyphosis. The posterior vertebral body line is often poorly defined at the junction of the pedicle and vertebral body; however, the pedicles themselves and the posterior vertebral body line above and below the pedicles should be clearly defined. Above T11, the ribs make the posterior vertebral line difficult to see.[40] The laminae, costovertebral joints, and spinous processes are poorly seen on the lateral view of the thoracic spine because of the rib cage.

Alignment on the lateral view varies from a kyphosis in the thoracic spine to a gradual lordosis in the lumbar spine. This transition should be smooth and without abrupt angulation. Subtle anterolisthesis (anterior slippage) or retrolisthesis (posterior slippage) of one body upon another is significant in a patient with trauma.[34] The intervertebral disk spaces *(cartilage)* are clearly defined by sharp, well-defined end plates. The intervertebral disk height gradually increases in a caudal direction. At the extremes of the film, the intervertebral disk spaces are not clearly seen because they are no longer perpendicular to the x-ray beam.

Although gentle *kyphosis* is normal in the upper thoracic spine, abrupt angulation anywhere in the vertebral column indicates significant pathology. The *apophyseal articulations* are difficult to see in the thorax because of the overlying ribs. The *neuroforamina* should be smooth and similar in appearance from one level to the next. Nonetheless, distortion at the extremes of the thoracic or lumbar film makes it difficult to ac-

curately assess the upper thoracic and lower lumbar neuroforamina. It is especially important to scrutinize the *posterior vertebral body line* in the region of the thoracolumbar junction because this is the most common site for burst fractures.[41] The pedicles and intervertebral disk space are common sites of involvement by malignancy and infection.

Diagnosis of Fractures

The BACKPAINS acronym directs the evaluation of traumatic lesions, specifically identification of burst fractures and subtle nontraumatic pathology (Table 14-4). The eight specific signs of thoracolumbar trauma are incorporated into this acronym: widened paraspinal line, loss of psoas stripe, displacement of vertebrae, scoliosis-kyphosis, widened interspinous space, abnormal intervertebral disk space, widened apophyseal joints, and a widened IPD.[34] Widening of the IDP is characteristic of a vertebral body burst fracture and implies that there are two fractures through the ring of bone forming the vertebral canal. One is a vertical fracture through the vertebral body and the other is through the neural arch.[38]

In a review of thoracolumbar fractures, all fractures from T4-T11 showed displacement of the paraspinal line, and all fractures from L1-L5 showed loss of the psoas shadow.[34] With fractures at T12, approximately 80% had loss of the psoas shadow while the remainder had widening of the paraspinal line. About 70% of all vertebral fractures had accompanying kyphosis or scoliosis with an abnormal adjacent disk space. All fractures with disruption of the posterior ligaments or posterior skeletal structures (i.e., pedicles, laminae, apophyseal joints, or spinous processes) showed one or more of the following four signs: vertebral body displacement, a widened interspinous space, a widened vertebral canal (i.e., IPD), or abnormal apophyseal joints.[34]

Severe *burst fractures* have obvious radiographic abnormalities, including loss of anterior and posterior vertebral body height and vertical lucencies through the body. Widening of the IPD is an indication of a burst fracture that has an associated fracture through the neural arch. Less severe burst fractures may lack these radiographic findings. Distortion, displacement, or lack of definition of the posterior vertebral body line may be the only plain film evidence of a more subtle burst fracture (Fig. 14-6).

Nontraumatic Pathology

When visible on plain films, nontraumatic pathology such as neoplasia, infection, and spondyloarthropathy results in a variety of bone and intervertebral disk changes. Widening of the paraspinal line is frequently seen in nontraumatic pathology.[37] Metastatic lesions usually involve the anterior elements, specif-ically the vertebral bodies and pedicles. Pyogenic infections usually cause destruction of the disk space and erosion of the adjacent vertebral body end plates. Spondyloarthropathy causes bone erosion and new bone formation (sclerosis and osteo-phytes). Any of these processes can result in pathologic frac-tures or abrupt angulation of the spine.

COMMON ABNORMALITIES

Fracture Classification

A simplified three-part classification system of thoracic and lumbar fractures is based on the predominant force applied to the middle vertebral column (Table 14-5).[6,42,43] There are three principal forces that can be applied to the middle vertebral column: compression, distraction, and axial torque. Axial torque is often combined with ei-ther compression or distraction. Each force creates injuries with distinct radiographic fea-tures. Compression injuries primarily involve the vertebral body. Distraction injuries are marked by transverse disruption of posterior ligaments and bony structures. Injuries re-sulting from axial torque are characterized by translation within the transverse plane. The major injuries related to these three types of injury forces are wedge compression and burst fractures resulting from axial compres-sion; seat belt–type injuries, such as Chance fractures, caused by distractive forces; and fracture/dislocations, manifest by translation within the transverse plane due to axial torque.

This three-part classification scheme relates the mechanism of injury and pathomorpho-logic appearance in an easy-to-understand manner, directing a focused radiographic analysis. For example, the presence of a com-pression fracture should always raise the sus-picion of a burst fracture. Compression frac-tures and burst fractures are created by the same axial loading force. Likewise, any trans-verse bone abnormality should lead to a fo-cused search for other signs of distraction in-jury.

There is disagreement as to what constitutes *stability* of the axial skeleton.[42] Many de-scriptions refer only to mechanical stability as it relates to the integrity of the middle and or posterior column. This concept does not ad-dress the potential for a neurologic injury. For example, a "stable" burst fracture could have a fragment retropulsed into the spinal canal with significant neurologic consequences. An "unstable" burst fracture may produce no neu-rologic deficits. A broader and more practical

---

TABLE 14-5

Classification of Fractures of the Thoracic and Lumbar Spine

COMPRESSION FRACTURES (50% TO 70%)

Simple wedge compression fracture	Anterior superior end-plate compression. Usually about 10% loss of vertebral body height.
Severe wedge compression fracture	Usually about 50% loss of vertebral body height. Kyphotic angulation. May compromise spinal canal. Posterior cortex of vertebral body remains intact.
Stable burst fracture	Axial force drives nucleus pulposus into vertebral body. Entire vertebral body involved, including its posterior aspect. Posterior vertebral body line disrupted on the lateral radiograph. Vertebral body fragment often retropulsed into vertebral canal. Posterior column (neural arch) not involved.
Unstable burst fracture	Posterior column fractured. Interpedicular distance is widened on AP radiograph. Most mechanically unstable compression fracture. 55% to 85% of burst fractures are unstable.

DISTRACTION INJURIES (5% TO 15%)

Posterior element fracture or ligament tears—Chance fracture	Horizontal fracture through posterior arch, spinous process, and vertebral body. Ligament injuries cause widening of interspinous distance.

AXIAL TORQUE INJURIES (11% TO 20%)

Fracture/dislocations	Usually combined with compression or distraction forces.

OTHER FRACTURES (15%)

	Isolated fractures of the transverse process (15%). Isolated fractures of posterior elements (<3%)— spinous process, lamina, pars interarticularis, and articular process fractures.

definition considers clinical (not mechanical) stability. Clinical instability is defined as "the inability of the spine under physiologic loads, to maintain relationships between vertebrae so that there is neither initial or subsequent neurologic deficit, no major deformity, and no severe pain."[42] Using this concept of clinical stability, a descriptive division of burst fractures is based on the presence or absence of posterior column disruption and eliminates the confusion about mechanical versus neurologic stability.

The three-part fracture classification system (compression, distraction, axial torque) does not include extension injuries. However, in the thoracic and lumbar spine, unlike the cervical region, extension injuries are extremely rare. Minor injuries—such as transverse process fractures, spinous process fractures, pars interarticularis fractures, and articular process fractures—are also not encompassed by this classification system. Of these latter injuries, only transverse process fractures are reviewed, because the other three collectively account for less than 3% of thoracolumbar fractures.[6]

Compression Injuries

Fractures resulting from axial compression form a continuum from minor wedge compression fractures to severe burst fractures with three-column involvement. Approximately two-thirds of all major thoracolumbar fractures are due to compressive forces.[43] Wedge compression fractures are common in the thoracic spine because the normal kyphosis in this area directs the compressive force into flexion affecting the anterior portion of the vertebral body. Burst fractures are due to symmetrical axial loading with transmission of force from the intervertebral disk to the centrum of the vertebral body.[44] Burst injuries are accordingly seen in areas of the spine where symmetrical axial loading is possible. This includes C1, the lower cervical vertebrae, the thoracolumbar junction, and the lumbar spine.

WEDGE COMPRESSION FRACTURES. Although compression fractures are, by definition, confined to the anterior column, they are clinically unstable when there is involvement of multiple adjacent vertebrae. In addition, there can be delayed neurologic impairment from progressive deformity of the posterior longitudinal ligaments.[42] Wedge compression fractures are characterized as "simple" or "severe" based on the extent of loss of anterior vertebral height, the degree of acute kyphosis, or the presence of a complete fracture through the entire anterior vertebral body. Simple compression fractures involve only the superior portion of the anterior vertebral body, often resulting in less than 10% loss of anterior height (Fig. 14-7). Severe compression fractures cause loss of anterior height greater than 50%, hyperkyphotic angulation, and, rarely, compromise of the AP diameter of the spinal canal (Fig. 14-8).

A wedge compression fracture is best seen on the lateral view. The radiographic findings include loss of anterior vertebral body height, normal posterior vertebral body height, and an intact posterior vertebral body line. The resultant kyphosis

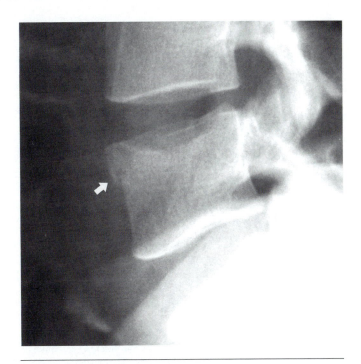

FIGURE 14-7. Minimal wedge compression fracture. The lateral view of L4 shows the fracture involving only the anterosuperior portion of the vertebral body. The fracture has a beak-like deformity. The posterior vertebral body line is intact. (Copyright David T. Schwartz, M.D.)

causes an increase in the ISD. Abnormalities of the vertebral end plate, usually the superior end plate, are best appreciated on the lateral view. There is a characteristic beak-like deformity of the anterosuperior margin of the vertebral body (Fig. 14-7). Uncommonly, end plate disruption is seen on the AP view if there is a significant lateral component to the fracture.[6] Impaction of the trabeculae results in a focal area of increased bone density beneath the affected end plate. This focal area of sclerosis is useful for distinguishing acute fractures from the compression of osteoporotic vertebral bodies that is common in the elderly, particularly involving the middle thoracic vertebrae. Approximately one in four persons above 75 years of age develops osteoporotic compression fractures (Fig. 14-9).[25] Other radiographic signs of an acute fracture include irregularities of the bony cortex and widening of the paraspinal line. Signs of old, healed fractures include focal osteophytosis, bony bridging between deformed vertebrae, and associated calcification of the anterior longitudinal ligament.[30] CT evaluation of acute compression fractures shows an arc-like comminution of the anterior vertebral end plate with an intact posterior vertebral body. If there is a moderate to severe wedge deformity, a CT scan is obtained on a compression fracture to exclude a posterior column fracture or a retropulsed vertebral body fragment. Some authors suggest that CT should be routinely considered in the evaluation of all acute wedge compression fractures.[21,22]

BURST FRACTURES. Burst fractures also result from axial compression. However, burst fractures are distinct from wedge compression fractures in the manner in which the force is applied and in the resultant injury. In a compression fracture, the axial

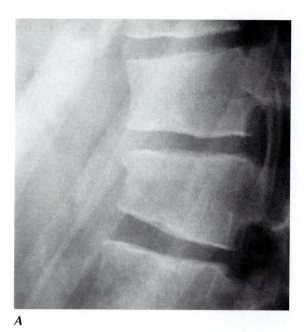

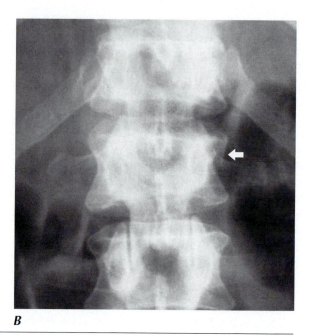

A   *B*

FIGURE 14-8.   Moderate wedge compression fracture. *A.* This patient has a more severe wedge compression fracture of L1, with greater loss of anterior vertebral body height. The posterior vertebral body line is intact. CT confirmed that the posterior portion of the vertebral body was intact. *B.* An AP view of a moderate compression fracture at L1. The fracture involves the left lateral side of the superior end plate (*arrow*). Loss of vertebral body height is minimal, and the interpedicular distance is normal. The mechanism of injury includes both anterior compression and lateral bending.

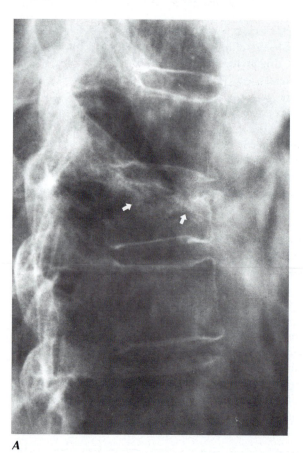

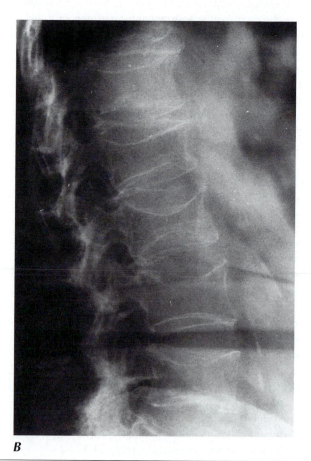

A   *B*

FIGURE 14-9.   Osteoporotic compression fractures. *A.* An acute fracture of a thoracic vertebral body is seen in this osteoporotic woman. The acute nature of the fracture is indicated by the impaction of the superior end plate, causing increased bone density. *B.* Multiple old fractures are seen in the lumbar spine. The superior end plates are depressed, but there is no increase in bone density. Ligamentous calcification is another sign of an old fracture.

TABLE 14-6

Radiographic Distinction Between a Wedge Compression Fracture and a Vertebral Body Burst Fracture

WEDGE COMPRESSION FRACTURE	BURST FRACTURE
Compression of the vertebral body <50%	Compression of the vertebral body >50%
No evidence of posterior cortex fracture	Posterior cortex fracture seen
No interpedicular widening	Widening of the interpedicular space (>1 mm compared to vertebrae above or below)
No loss of posterior vertebral height	Loss of vertebral height (>1 mm) compared to vertebra above
Compression angle <20°	Compression angle >20°
Posterior body vertebral angle <100°	Posterior body vertebral angle >100°

load is directed on the anterior vertebral body, whereas in a burst fracture, the axial load is symmetrically applied to the intervertebral disk. Most burst fractures occur at the thoracolumbar junction and adjacent lumbar vertebrae. The nucleus pulposus is incompressible, distributing any axial force to the adjacent vertebral end plate. With enough force, the end plate bulges and then ruptures, driving the nucleus pulposus into the centrum of the vertebral body.[42] The vertebral body then bursts apart, creating characteristic vertical and horizontal fractures (Fig. 14-10). Fragmentation of the posterior vertebral body results in retropulsion of fracture fragments into the spinal canal. Neurologic impairment occurs in 65% of burst fractures.[41] Burst fractures vary in the degree of vertebral body comminution, retropulsion of fragments, and the presence or absence of posterior column disruption. Burst fractures are divided into those with posterior column disruption and those without posterior column disruption. The latter type involve only the vertebral body; the posterior neural arch is spared.

Radiographically, burst fractures are distinguished from wedge compression fractures by scrutiny of the posterior aspect of the vertebral body (Table 14-6; Fig. 14-6). On the lateral radiograph, the height of the posterior aspect of the vertebral body is easily recognized.[21] On CT, 88% of burst fractures have a sagittally oriented fracture line involving the inferior half of the vertebral body.[41] Wedge compression fractures do not have vertical fracture lines. Depending on the degree of displacement, this vertically oriented fracture can be seen on the AP view as a vertical cleft.[44]

On the lateral view, a burst fracture causes disruption of the normally well-defined cortical line of the posterior aspect of the vertebral body by a displaced fragment of a fractured vertebral body (Fig. 14-10A). The fragmentation of the posterior vertebral body usually occurs between the pedicles and most often involves the superoposterior portion of the vertebral body. On the lateral view, this appears as displacement, disruption, or poor definition of the posterior cortex of the vertebral body. Abnormalities of the posterior vertebral body line were found

by Daffner et al. to be present in all 114 pure burst fractures and in 78% of lateral flexion burst fractures.[35] Posterior displacement of the posterior vertebral body line, usually of its superior portion, was the most common abnormality (68%), followed by rotation of the posterior vertebral line (23%) and obliteration of the line (10%). In another series of burst fractures, 90% were correctly identified from either a distorted or absent posterior vertebral line.[40] The *posterior vertebral body angle* (PVBA) is also useful in detecting subtle burst fractures.[45] The PVBA is the angle between the posterior vertebral body line and the superior or inferior vertebral end plate seen on the lateral view. This angle was greater than 100° in 75% of subtle burst fractures otherwise undetected on plain films. Failure to visualize the posterior vertebral body line (the vanishing-line sign) also raises the suspicion of a burst injury.[37,39] However, failure to visualize the posterior vertebral body line due to overlying ribs is quite common above T11.[40] When one is examining abnormalities of the posterior vertebral body line, it is helpful to compare the area of concern with adjacent vertebrae.

Loss of anterior height greater than 50% and/or kyphosis greater than 20° is characteristic of burst fractures (Fig. 14-10B). These findings are due to severe axial load and anterior column injury and can also be seen in severe wedge compression fractures; they suggest potential instability. Nearly four out of five burst fractures, however, have less than 50% loss of height, and approximately 5% have no measurable loss of height at all.[41] Plain-film discrimination of burst fractures without posterior column disruption from wedge compression fractures may not be possible in 14 to 17% of cases.[21,22]

Some 55 to 85% of burst fractures have an associated fracture of the neural arch causing disruption of the posterior column.[7,21,41] Widening of the IPD is a sensitive and specific sign of posterior column disruption. The IPD at each level should be between the IPDs of the vertebrae above and below. Widening of the IPD on the AP film has a 100% positive predictive value and a 99% negative predictive value for fractures through the body and the lamina or pedicle.[38] The widened IPD coupled with the other signs of burst injury already mentioned usually allow for easy recognition of burst fractures with posterior column displacement.

In summary, the classic unstable burst fracture is a three-column injury: (1) centripetally oriented disruption of the vertebral body, (2) unilateral or bilateral laminar fractures that abut the spinous process, (3) marked anterior wedging, (4) vertically oriented vertebral body fracture, (5) increased interpedicular distance, and (6) significant narrowing of the spinal canal by retropulsed fragments of the vertebral body.[41]

The axial images provided by CT are superior to plain films in the evaluation of burst fractures. On plain films, overlying bony structures obscure the area of greatest interest—the posterior vertebral body and spinal canal. Although posterior column disruption is usually evident on plain films, the specific

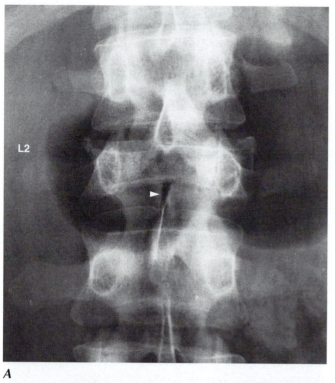

A

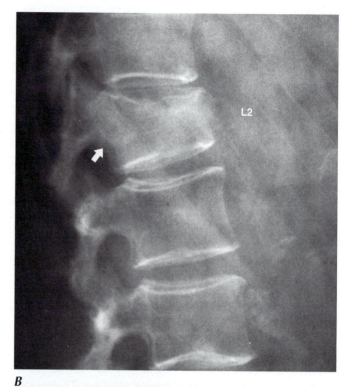

B

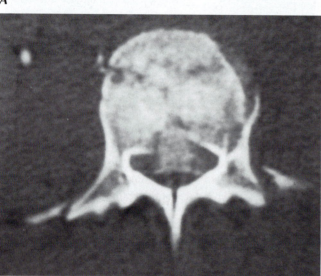

C

FIGURE 14-10. Unstable burst fracture. This young man fell four stories and landed feet first. He presented with bilateral calcaneal fractures, back pain, and weakness in both lower extremities. *A.* On the AP radiograph, there is marked loss of L2 vertebral body height and widening of the interpedicular distance. There is a distinct midline vertical lucency *(arrowhead).* In addition, there are transverse process fractures at L1 and L2. *B.* On the lateral image, there is loss of vertebral body height and angulation. The posterior vertebral body line is disrupted *(arrow).* *C.* The CT slice through L2 shows a comminuted fracture of the entire vertebral body with retropulsion of a fracture fragment into the spinal canal. The interpedicular distance is widened, and consequently there is a fracture through the posterior neural arch (a cleft through the spinous process). *D.* Postoperative radiograph showing the fixation device that supports the vertebral column. (Copyright David T. Schwartz, M.D.)

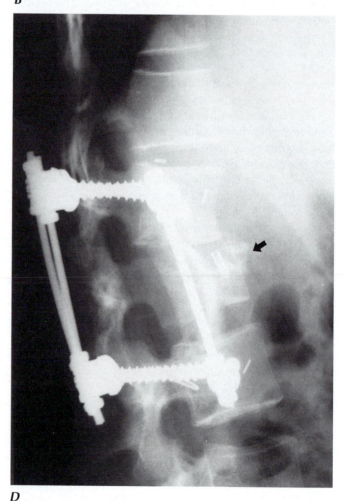

D

fracture of the neural arch usually cannot be determined. On CT, the full extent of injury to the vertebral body is apparent. Retropulsion of fragments into the spinal canal is obvious, and specific fractures of the neural arch are identified (Fig. 14-10C). However, the radiographic appearance of a retropulsed fragment in the spinal canal does not always correlate with clinical neurologic status; minimal retropulsion may be found in a neurologically devastated patient, and significant compromise of the canal may be associated with minor deficits. The degree of canal narrowing on CT defines only the final position of posteriorly displaced fragments and may not indicate the extent of displacement at the time of injury.[11,41] More severe narrowing of the canal and greater neurologic injury are found in burst fractures associated with disruption of the posterior column.

Distraction Injuries

Injuries resulting from distraction of the middle column are much less common than those resulting from axial loads. Distraction injuries account for 5 to 15% of injuries.[6,43] The first report of this type of injury, associated with a lap-type seat belt came from Chance in 1948.[46] A variety of related injuries, consisting of various fractures and ligamentous disruptions, have since been described (Figs. 14-11 and 14-12).

All distraction injuries share a common etiology—namely, tensile distraction of the posterior and middle columns with or without anterior column compression. Most of these injuries were originally reported with isolated lap seat belts.[47] The incidence of this injury has declined with combined shoulder–lap belt use. However, solitary lap seat belts are still present in the rear seats of many vehicles. In addition, many three-point restraints are worn incorrectly, particularly by children.[48] Another mechanism that produces this injury is a fall onto a rigid object, such as a brick wall or a fence.

Distraction injuries cause horizontal fractures through the vertebral body and posterior elements. The fracture is easily seen on the lateral view. The AP view may show a horizontal fracture through the pedicles, transverse processes, or spinous processes. Disruption of the posterior elements, through either bone or ligaments, causes widening of the interspinous distance in both AP and lateral views.[43] On the lateral view, there may be widening of the neuroforamina, posterior disk space, and apophyseal joints. Extreme cases result in marked kyphosis. Spontaneous reduction of these injuries can occur in which the only radiographic finding is a subtle widening of the interspinous distance, apophyseal joints, or neuroforamina. Most patients with distraction injuries have no neurologic deficits unless there is a significant associated dislocation. Recognition of distraction injuries is important, not only because of potential mechanical instability and rare neurologic injury but also because of their common association with intraabdominal injury.[48] In one study, 63% of children with lap seat belt ecchymosis to the anterior abdomen had abdominal, pelvic, or lumbar injuries.

Axial Torque Injuries

Axial torque injuries, also known as *fracture/dislocations,* result from axial torque on the spine, frequently in conjunction with a compression or distraction force (Figs. 14-13 and 14-14). Accordingly, these injuries share radiographic features with the compression or distraction injuries already described. Fracture/dislocations are seen following high-speed auto accidents and falls from great heights. Another mechanism is a direct blow to the spine with massive force, such as direct impact by a falling tree or a high-speed auto-pedestrian collision.[6]

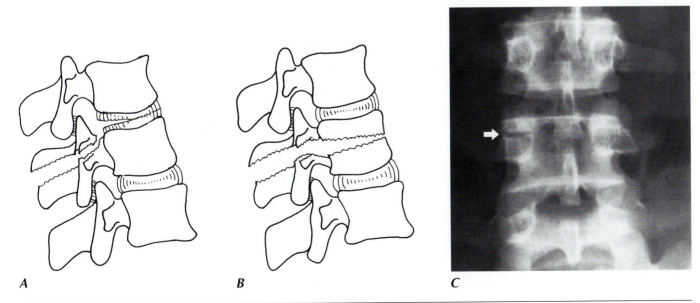

A   *B*   *C*

FIGURE 14-11.   Distraction injury. *A.* The fracture line extends through the intervertebral disk and the posterior vertebral elements (pedicles, laminae, transverse processes, and spinous process). This is a classic "Chance fracture." *B.* The fracture splits the entire vertebra including the vertebral body. *C.* This patient was a rear-seat passenger who was using a lap-type seat belt when she was involved in a motor vehicle accident. There is a horizontal fracture through the right pedicle of L4. (Courtesy of Murray K. Dalinka, M.D., University of Pennsylvania.)

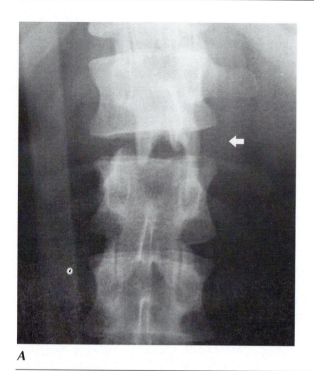

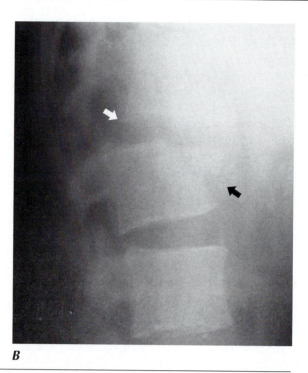

A   *B*

FIGURE 14-12.   Distraction injury. *A.* On the AP view, L1 and L2 have been pulled apart and the posterior ligaments are torn. The inferior articular facets of L1 are visible. There is a horizontal fracture through the transverse processes of L2. The pedicles and vertebral body of L2 are intact.   *B.* On the lateral view, there is an anterior compression fracture of L2 and anterior displacement of L1

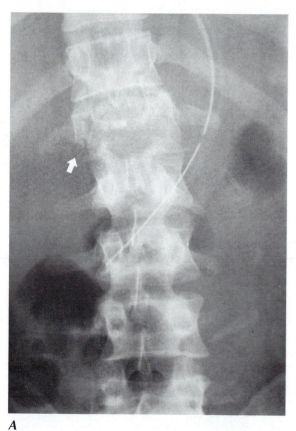

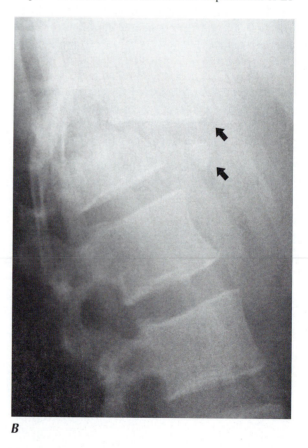

A   *B*

FIGURE 14-13.   Axial torque injury—fracture/dislocation. *A.* The AP radiograph of a pedestrian who was struck by a car. There is an L1 burst fracture with loss of vertebral body height, a vertical lucency through the vertebral body, and disrupted pedicles. Rotation causes a change in alignment of the spinous processes above and below L1. There are multiple transverse process fractures at L1 through L5. *B.* On the lateral view, there is marked anterior dislocation of T12 on L1. (Courtesy of Murray K. Dalinka, M.D., University of Pennsylvania.)

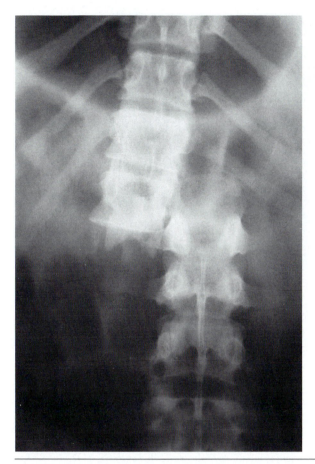

FIGURE 14-14. Complete dislocation. This patient was crushed between two moving subway cars. There is complete dislocation of L1 on L2.

Fracture/dislocations make up 11 to 20% of thoracolumbar fractures.[6,7,43] The predominant radiographic findings—malalignment or discontinuity of contiguous structures—are usually obvious on plain films. After the vertebral bodies are inspected for alignment, the spinous processes are checked for malalignment on the AP film so as not to overlook rotational dislocation. This is of particular importance when there is multicolumn disruption from compressive or distractive forces, because dislocation is likely to be present. Since the spinal canal is defined by the successive neural arches, dislocation of vertebrae causes encroachment of the spinal canal and almost invariably results in significant neurologic injury.

Minor Fractures

The *transverse process fracture* is the most common minor fracture in the lumbar spine, representing nearly 15% of all thoracolumbar fractures.[6] By themselves, these injuries have no significant mechanical or neurologic consequences; however, they are often associated with other injuries. Of patients with transverse process fractures, up to 21% have abdominal visceral injury, 16% have other spinal injuries, and 11% have fatal injuries.[49] Hematuria is present in many of these patients, due to

the proximity of the urinary tract structures to the spine. There is also a high incidence of pelvic fractures (29%), especially with fracture of the L5 transverse process. Fracture of the L2 transverse process is associated with renal artery thrombosis because of its location adjacent to the renal pedicle.[50]

Radiographically, transverse process fractures are usually vertically oriented or oblique, although horizontal fractures do occur with distraction injuries (Fig. 14-15). Overlying intestinal gas and feces often make recognition of fracture lines difficult, but indistinct psoas margins and scoliosis convex to the side of the fracture are indirect signs of the fracture.[50] Scoliosis results from unopposed contraction of the ipsilateral quadratus lumborum muscle, which inserts on the transverse processes.

Fractures of the Thoracic Spine

Fractures of the thoracic spine are considerably less common than fractures of the thoracolumbar junction. They are usually seen in severe trauma. The initial chest radiograph should be scrutinized for signs of injury to the thoracic spine, although this is difficult in an underpenetrated chest film obtained by portable radiography. The radiographic findings are similar to those on the AP view of the thoracolumbar junction: malalignment, loss of vertebral body height, vertebral body and interpedicular widening, and spinous process displacement (Figs. 14-16 and 14-17). An important soft tissue clue to a fracture is focal widening of the paraspinal stripe. The hemorrhage can be so extensive as to mimic the hemomediastinum suggestive of a traumatic aortic injury.

Nontraumatic Disorders

MALIGNANCY AND INFECTION. Plain films are insensitive for diagnosing early signs of neoplasm or infection. Only after de-

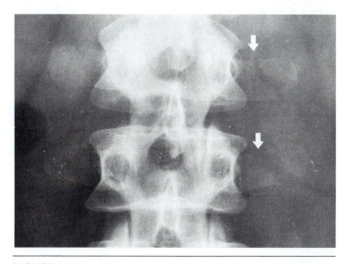

FIGURE 14-15. Transverse process fractures of L2 and L3 on the left.

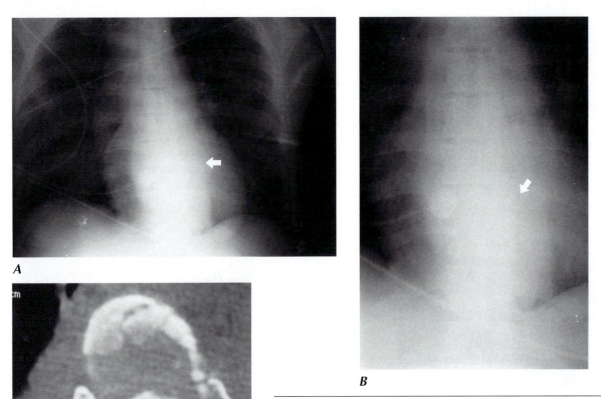

A

B

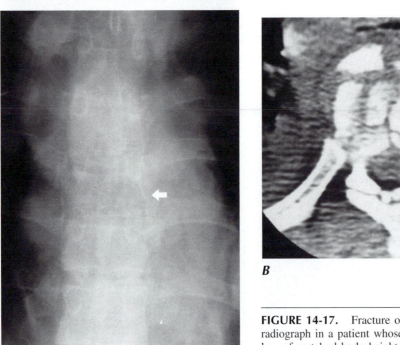

C

FIGURE 14-16.   Thoracic spine injury. This patient was paraplegic after a fall from a great height. *A.* The initial chest radiograph shows widening of the left paraspinal line (*arrow*) and a focal bulge of the right paraspinal line. *B.* On closer inspection of the chest film, there is malalignment of the thoracic vertebral column (*arrow*). *C.* CT reveals complete dislocation of the thoracic spine. (Copyright David T. Schwartz, M.D.)

A

B

FIGURE 14-17.   Fracture of the thoracic spine. *A.* Detailed view of the initial chest radiograph in a patient whose car rolled over. He had a right pneumothorax. There is loss of vertebral body height and poor definition of the T8 vertebra. *B.* CT revealed a burst fracture of T8. (Copyright David T. Schwartz, M.D.)

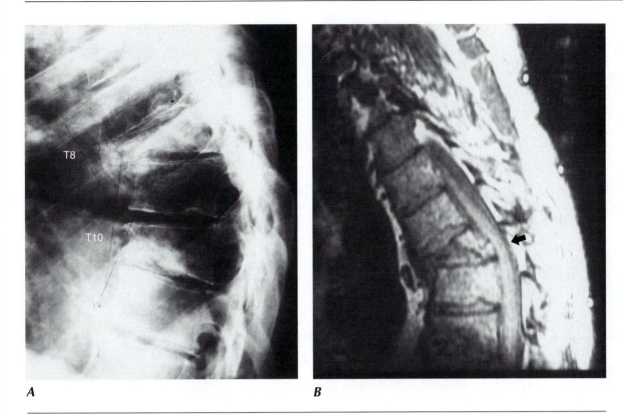

FIGURE 14-18.   Neoplasia. *A.* A patient with collapsed thoracic vertebral bodies typical of malignancy. Two noncontiguous vertebrae are involved (T8 and T10). The adjacent intervertebral disk spaces are preserved. *B.* MRI reveals narrowing of the spinal canal due to the abrupt angulation at T8. (Courtesy of Murray K. Dalinka, M.D., University of Pennsylvania.)

struction of 50% of the bone is neoplasm evident. Osteomyelitis is not visible on plain radiographs for several weeks, and epidural abscess can occur without skeletal involvement. A detailed history, physical examination, and selective use of advanced imaging studies such as CT, bone scan, or MRI are necessary to recognize these diseases before plain-film abnormalities are seen. Soft tissue signs, such as displacement of the paraspinal line or loss of the psoas shadow, are clues to the diagnosis. Ultimately, these diseases cause abnormalities of bone density. Both infection and malignancy create poorly marginated areas of bone destruction. Neoplasm typically affects the vertebral body and pedicles (Figs. 14-18 through 14-23). Although malignancy may involve multiple vertebral levels, it does not bridge the disk space. These radiographic features help to distinguish cancer from osteomyelitis. Infection originates in the disk space and spreads to adjacent vertebral bodies (Fig. 14-24). This results in disk-space narrowing and destruction of the adjacent vertebral bodies. CT is much more sensitive than plain films for detecting irregularities in bone density. MRI is best for imaging the spinal cord and nerve roots (Fig. 14-25).

SPONDYLOARTHROPATHY.   Radiographic recognition of ankylosing spondylitis, as well as an appreciation of its complications, is important. Radiographic evidence of end-stage disease is the pathognomic "bamboo spine" (Fig. 14-26). Early signs include narrowing of the sacroiliac and facet joints, osteoporosis, squaring of the lumbar vertebral bodies, and the for-

mation of syndesmophytes. Because of the rigidity of the ankylosed spine, any fracture is potentially unstable and there is a high incidence of neurologic injury. Even in the absence of trauma, complaints of pain or neurologic symptoms should be investigated aggressively.

SPONDYLOLISTHESIS AND SPONDYLOLYSIS.   Nontraumatic spondylolisthesis typically occurs in the lower lumbar spine. Spondylolisthesis is usually associated with spondylolysis, which is a defect in the pars interarticularis (Fig. 14-27). Spondylolysis is possibly the result of repetitive stresses to the lower back, although congenital defects in that area may be contributory. Spondylolisthesis results in forward slippage of the affected vertebra. The degree of spondylolisthesis is expressed as the percentage of the vertebral body that has advanced anteriorly (e.g., 25%). It most commonly involves L5-S1. Spondylolisthesis is frequently discovered as an incidental finding on roentgenograms. The relationship between back pain and these radiographic abnormalities is unclear, because at least 50% of patients with spondylolisthesis are asymptomatic.

COMMON VARIANTS

Common variants can simulate fractures and complicate radiographic interpretation in the thoracic and lumbar spine. Degenerative changes are ubiquitous in older patients. The com-

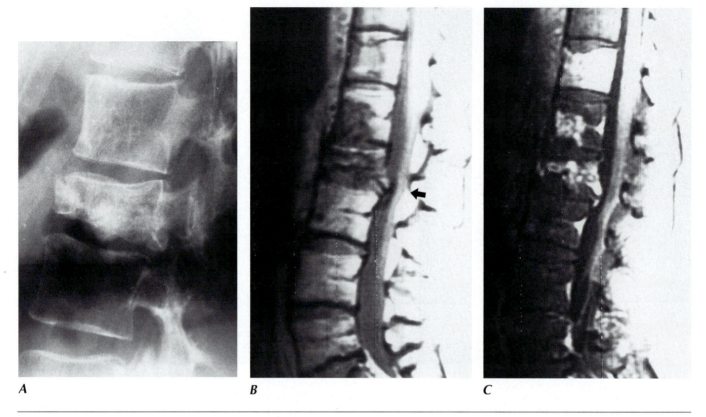

A   *B*   *C*

FIGURE 14-19. Metastatic cancer causing a pathologic fracture. *A.* The lateral radiograph shows collapse of L2. The adjacent disk spaces are preserved, as is typical of malignancy. *B.* A T1-weighted MRI reveals decreased signal intensity at L1 and impingement of the spinal canal. There is also disease in L1 that was not evident on the plain films. *C.* A T2-weighted MRI shows increased signal at L1 and L2.

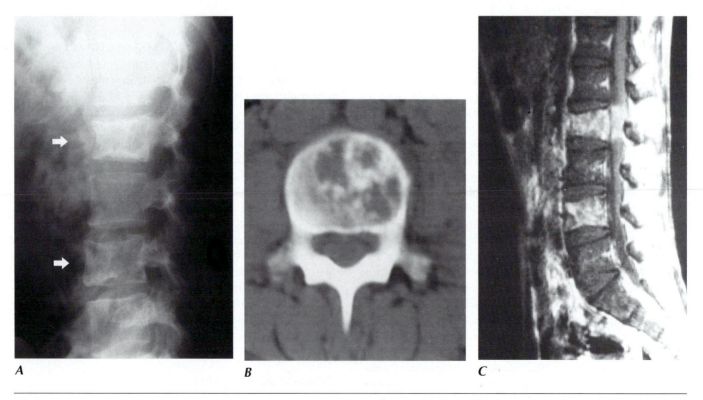

A   *B*   *C*

FIGURE 14-20. Lymphoma. *A.* A 19-year-old man with nontraumatic low back pain returned to the ED for the third time. Radiographs of the lumbar spine showed irregularity in the bone density at L2 and L4 with mild loss of vertebral body height. Diagnostic evaluation revealed lymphoma. *B.* CT reveals mottled lucencies of the vertebral body. *C.* MRI demonstrates increased signal intensity at L2 and L4. (Copyright David T. Schwartz, M.D.)

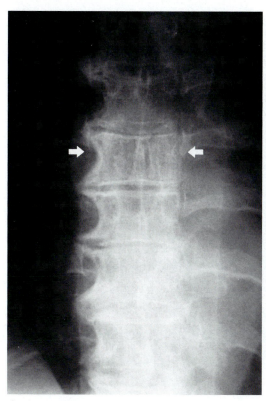

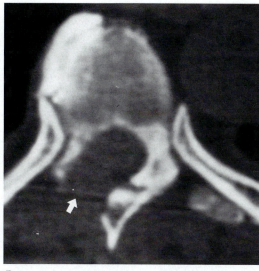

A

B

FIGURE 14-21.   Metastatic cancer. A 55-year-old woman presented with midthoracic back pain and mild weakness and paresthesia in both lower extremities. *A.* The only radiographic sign of this patient's malignancy is the disappearance of the pedicles at T8. *B.* CT reveals erosion of the left pedicle and lamina due to metastatic lung cancer. The primary tumor was not visible on the chest radiograph. (Copyright David T. Schwartz, M.D.)

bination of joint-space narrowing, lipping of the anterior margins of the vertebral body end plates, osteophyte formation, and ligamentous calcification all suggest chronic degenerative changes. Kyphosis and/or scoliosis can be congenital, due to chronic compression fractures or other healed fractures, or a manifestation of acute injury. Congenital and chronic conditions are distinguished from acute injuries by the absence of acute bone and soft tissue radiographic signs as well as the history and physical examination.

Spina Bifida Occulta

Spina bifida occulta is the incomplete fusion of the neural arch. It is most commonly seen in the lower lumbar spine or lumbosacral junction. On the AP film, a vertical lucency is seen that is sometimes misinterpreted as a vertical fracture through the vertebral body. Numerous clues suggest the correct diagnosis. Fractures occur almost exclusively at the thoracolumbar junction and not at L5 and S1. The defect is in the posterior elements, not the body, and can often be seen projecting beyond the borders of the body. The margins of the defect are smooth and well corticated and do not have the appearance of an acute fracture. The IPD is normal and the lateral film lacks signs consistent with a burst fracture.

Vertebral Body Variants

Limbus vertebrae and Schmorl's nodes are congenital vertebral body defects found only in the lumbar spine. The *limbus ver-*

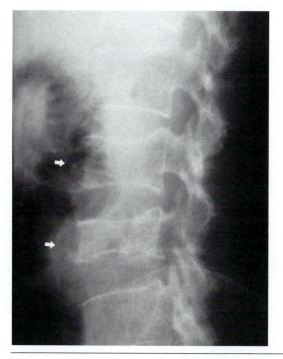

FIGURE 14-22.   Multiple myeloma. An elderly man with osteopenia and lumbar compression fractures at L2 and L3. The radiographic appearance is similar to that of osteoporosis. In this patient, medical evaluation revealed multiple myeloma.

tebrae is a small triangular fragment, most commonly at the anterosuperior edge of the vertebral body. The sclerosed parallel margins of the defect, along with its typical location, size

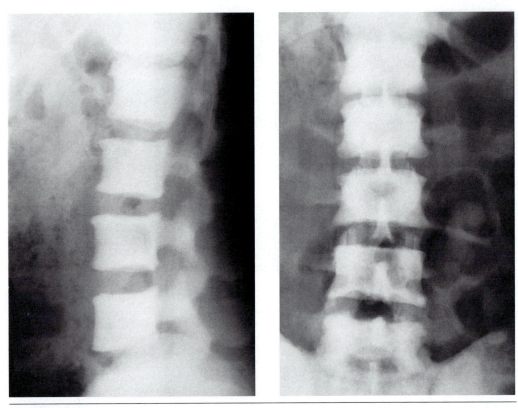

FIGURE 14-23.   Diffuse osteoblastic metastasis in a 45-year-old man with prostate cancer. Because of the radiographic appearance, this is referred to as "ivory vertebrae." (Copyright David T. Schwartz, M.D.)

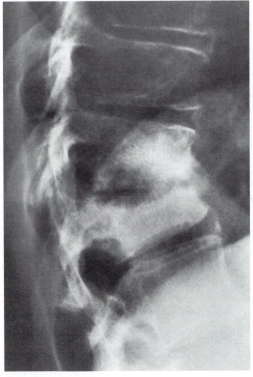

A

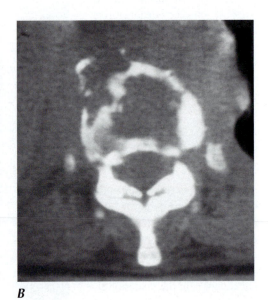

B

FIGURE 14-24.   Vertebral osteomyelitis in an intravenous drug user who presented with back pain. *A.* Lateral film of the thoracic spine shows characteristic findings of vertebral osteomyelitis. The hematogenous infection first localizes in the intervertebral disk and then spreads to the contiguous vertebral bodies. This results in erosion of adjacent vertebral bodies and narrowing of the disk space. *B.* CT reveals fragmentation of the vertebral body.

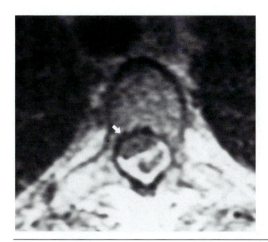

FIGURE 14-25. MRI of epidural abscess with spinal cord compression. An intravenous drug user complained of back pain and paresthesias of the lower extremities. She had a low-grade fever and back tenderness. Her plain radiographs were normal. Within several hours of presentation, her legs became weak. On MRI, an epidural abscess was seen displacing the cord and surrounding cerebrospinal fluid (high signal intensity). The patient made a nearly complete recovery following emergency surgical drainage.

FIGURE 14-26. Ankylosing spondylosis. Continuous ossification of the outer portion of the annulus fibrosus creates the characteristic "bamboo spine" appearance. *C.* Osteoarthritis causes marginal bridging osteophytes.

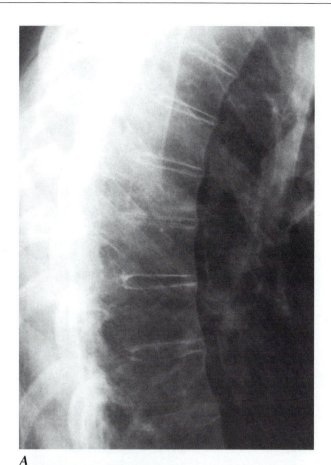

A

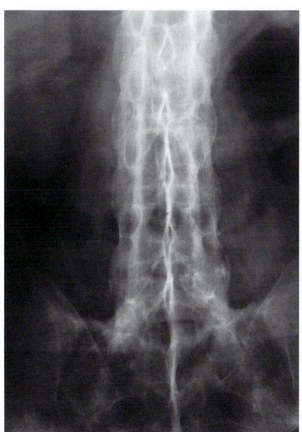

B

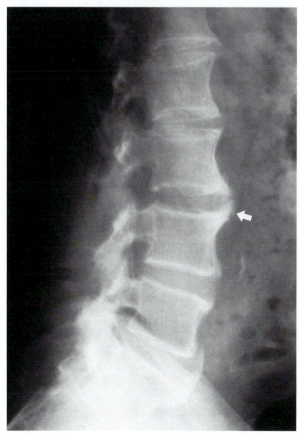

C

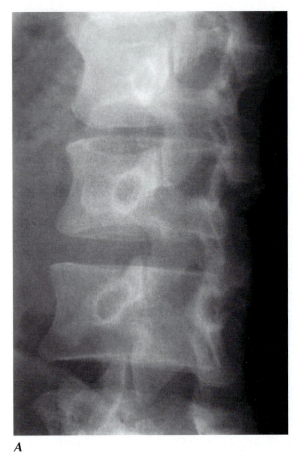

A

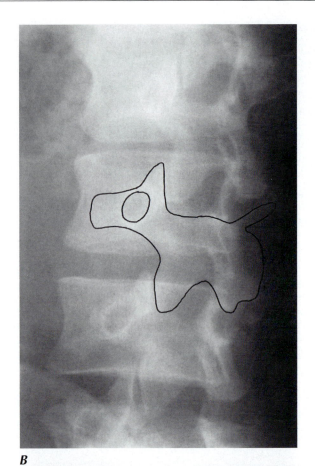

B

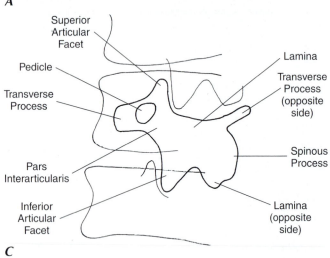

Superior
Articular
Facet

Pedicle

Transverse
Process

Pars
Interarticularis

Inferior
Articular
Facet

Lamina

Transverse
Process
(opposite
side)

Spinous
Process

Lamina
(opposite
side)

C

FIGURE 14-27.   Spondylolysis of the lumbar spine. On a normal oblique lumbar radiograph, the posterior spinal elements of one side form a "Scotty dog." *D.* Spondylolysis is erosion of the pars interarticularis, the neck of the Scotty dog (*arrow*). This is not an acute injury. (Copyright David T. Schwartz, M.D.)

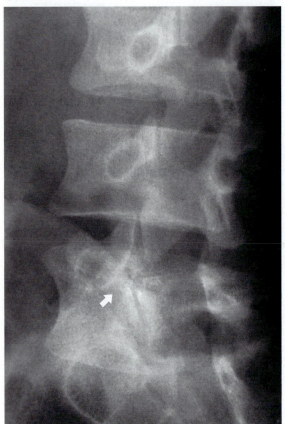

D

and shape, help to distinguish it from a fracture. *Schmorl's nodes* are irregular lucencies in the central portion of the vertebral end plate seen on the lateral view. Usually, multiple vertebrae are affected. In rare instances, Schmorl's nodes result from inflammatory or metastatic disease.

In addition to these specific variants, there are a wide variety of anomalies involving the costovertebral articulations and transverse processes of the lower thoracic and lumbar spine. Examples include rudimentary ribs, anomalous pseudarthoses, and asymmetrical or unilaterally absent transverse processes. Their smooth cortical margins and typical appearance distinguish these entities from acute fractures.

ERRORS IN INTERPRETATION

Trauma

The overall incidence of missed thoracolumbar injuries is estimated to be between 5 and 11%. In many of these instances, no thoracolumbar spine films were obtained. Many of these patients had other significant major injuries, including fractures of the cervical spine, or had depressed consciousness due to intoxication or head injury.

Errors in radiographic interpretation commonly involve a failure to appreciate the severity of injury, specifically the failure to distinguish burst from wedge compression fractures. In a large study of 1019 patients with thoracolumbar fractures, 35 (3%) had neurologic deterioration in the hospital.[51] Of this group, 81% had burst fractures. In a smaller study of 73 patients, 4 out of 28 (12%) patients with burst fractures who were neurologically intact initially went on to develop motor deficits within 48 h.[11] The ability of plain films to discriminate between wedge compression and burst fractures has been questioned. Some 14% of burst injuries have no definitive signs on plain films.[21] Campbell et al. found that plain films had an 83% sensitivity in detecting potentially unstable lumbar fractures.[22] Other traumatic lesions often overlooked are transverse process fractures of the lumbar spine and horizontally oriented fractures due to distraction of the posterior column.

Two traumatic lesions that are easy to overlook include transverse process fractures of the lumbar spine and distraction injuries in which the fracture plane is oriented horizontally. *Transverse process fractures* can be difficult to identify because of overlying bowel gas and feces. On the AP view, clues to this injury when a clear fracture line is not evident are loss of the psoas stripe and scoliosis convex to the side of the fracture.

In *distraction injuries* the fracture plane disrupts the posterior ligamentous complex, with or without a fracture of the posterior bony structures. Two clues to this injury on the AP view are a widened interspinous distance and a horizontal fracture line through the spinous process, pedicles, or transverse processes. On the lateral view, horizontally oriented fractures through the body, pedicles, or spinous process can be seen. Disruption of the posterior ligamentous complex without fracture causes disruption of the normal appearance of the apophyseal joints. An increase in height of the neuroforamina is seen when

the fracture plane is not entirely within the vertebral body and pedicles.

Nontraumatic Lesions

Missed nontraumatic lesions are due to the failure to appreciate subtle changes in the vertebral cortex, disk space, and soft tissues. In the presence of neurologic signs of cord compression, advanced studies should be obtained even if plain films are normal. When plain films show an abnormality, such as a nontraumatic compression fracture, it can be difficult to decide whether the lesion is malignant or benign on the basis of the radiographs alone. Paraspinal and intraspinal infections are inadequately studied with plain radiographs. MRI, and to a lesser extent CT, adds substantially to the diagnostic evaluation of these patients.[28,52]

Mistaking normal variants for pathologic conditions is another pitfall in thoracolumbar radiographic interpretation. Degenerative or chronic osteoporotic changes can be misinterpreted as an acute compression injury if the vertebral margins are not carefully inspected. Anatomic variants—such as spondylolysis, limbus vertebrae, anomalous pseudarthrosis, spina bifida occulta, and Schmorl's nodules—can simulate fractures. Knowledge of these entities, familiarity with the appearance of acute fractures, and close inspection of the margins of the area of concern are necessary for proper interpretation.

CONTROVERSIES

Fracture classifications, biomechanical injury models, and the concept of stability have been debated for decades. The routine use of CT to define fractures and the growing use of MRI to determine ligamentous and neurologic injury are helping to resolve many issues. The debate regarding surgical versus conservative management of various fractures has little relevance to the emergency physician, since all patients with plain-film or CT evidence of a burst fracture require specialist consultation at the time of injury.[11,51]

Overuse of Radiographs

The appropriate number of lumbosacral radiographs to obtain in screening patients with low back pain is debated. After reviewing 68,000 radiographic examinations over a 10-year period, Nachemson showed that clinically unsuspected positive findings in patients 20 to 50 years of age were obtained in approximately 1 out of 2500 radiographic examinations.[53] From the perspective of gonadal radiation exposure, a five-view lumbosacral series (with oblique films and a lumbosacral coned-down spot projection) is equivalent to *daily* chest radiographs for 6 or more years depending on the technique and equipment.[12,54] Even among the elderly or those at risk for osseous pathology, in whom the additional radiation exposure is irrelevant, additional plain films add little to the evaluation of back pain. Scavone found that in using a two-view series, there were 19 missed diagnoses out of 972 cases (2.4%) in a comparison with to the five-view series.[29] Of these 19 missed diagnoses, 13 involved unilateral spondylolysis, 5 were bilateral spondylolysis, and 1 was a congenital abnormality. These are of little importance to acute medical care. In this era of widespread availability of CT and MRI, the routine use of oblique views has little justification. If patients have clinical indications for operative intervention, advanced studies need to be obtained.

Burst Fracture Detection

The plain-film detection of burst fractures is critical for the emergency physician. This is because management of mild wedge compression fractures is analgesia and outpatient referral to a specialist, whereas burst fractures require hospital admission and often transfer to a spinal injury center. The plain-film radiographic sign of a widened IPD is 100% sensitive for detecting a burst fracture with posterior column involvement.[38] This injury is usually accompanied by the other signs of burst injury on plain film and is not likely to be overlooked.

The challenge is to identify burst fractures that involve the posterior vertebral body without a fracture of the neural arch. These fractures can be difficult to distinguish from wedge compression fractures. From 15 to 38% of burst fractures have no posterior column involvement.[7,41] The IPD is normal (Table 14-6). In many cases, the posterior vertebral body line is abnormal.[45] The sensitivity of disruption of the posterior vertebral body line for detecting these fractures is uncertain.

The question is whether plain radiographs are sufficient to exclude or to diagnose an unstable vertebral body fracture. Two recent articles involving large numbers of patients have reexamined the sensitivity of plain films compared with CT scans in the diagnosis of burst fractures.[21,22] Ballock et al. looked at 29 burst fractures documented by CT and reviewed the plain films on these patients, comparing them with 38 wedge compression fractures. Examiners were radiologists and orthopedic surgeons. Measurements were taken of anterior vertebral body height, posterior vertebral body height, and IPD.[21] Anterior wedging was measured as the ratio of the anterior height to the posterior height, expressed as a percentage. There was no statistically significant difference in the amount of anterior wedging between the two groups: 28% ($\pm$17%) and 21% ($\pm$9) for burst and compression fractures, respectively. The IPD was not widened in 13/29 (45%) burst fractures, and no loss of posterior height was present in 4/29 (14%) burst fractures. Fourteen percent of burst fractures had neither sign and would have been misclassified using only plain-film analysis. Among the 16 mild burst fractures with less than 30% anterior wedging (the subgroup of fractures most likely not to be evaluated with CT scan), the sensitivity of plain-film diagnosis of burst fracture was only 63%. Disruption of the posterior vertebral body line was not specifically evaluated in this study because it could not be measured; therefore it is difficult to estimate how many of the unrecognized burst fractures would have been identified. How-

ever, the posterior vertebral body line was "frequently obscured by overlying ribs, scapula, or bowel gas."

Campbell et al. compared plain-film findings with CT scans in 53 patients with lumbar spine fractures, 39 of which were labeled as unstable.[22] Specific criteria used to evaluate plain films included vertebral displacement, widening of the interlaminar or interspinous space, widening of the facet joints, widening of the IPD, disruption of the posterior vertebral body line, and loss of anterior height greater than 50%. Examiners included two skeletal radiologists, one neuroradiologist, one general radiologist, and two neuroradiology fellows. Only 30 of the 53 fractures were correctly identified as unstable on plain films by all six readers. The sensitivity for detection of unstable fractures was 83%.

Clearly, recent studies challenge the 100% sensitivity of plain films for detecting unstable fractures. In addition, from 15 to 45% of burst fractures do not involve a posterior element fracture and their diagnosis on plain film is less reliable.[6,7,21,22,38] Some of these "subtle burst fractures" are not discernible on plain films, even with close scrutiny of the posterior vertebral body line. Therefore, CT should be used liberally in most patients with apparent wedge compression fractures and burst fractures. However, the routine use of CT scans in apparently simple wedge compression fractures has been criticized as cost-prohibitive, given the rarity of subtle burst injuries and the greater frequency of compression fractures. In the setting of trauma or in the osteoporotic elderly patient with acute localized pain, CT examination may be appropriate following plain-film identification of fracture, including all but the most minor wedge compression, to detect posterior vertebral body involvement, which signifies a potentially unstable fracture.

REFERENCES

1. Liang M, Komaroff AL: Roentgenograms in primary care patients with acute low back pain: A cost-effectiveness analysis. *Arch Intern Med* 142:1108, 1982.
2. Frymoyer JW: Back pain and sciatica. *N Engl J Med* 318:291, 1988.
3. Kelen GD, Noji EK, Doris P: Guidelines for use of lumbar spine radiography. *Ann Emerg Med* 15:245, 1986.
4. Samuels LE, Kerstein MD: "Routine" radiographic evaluation of the thoracolumbar spine in blunt trauma patients: A reappraisal. *J Trauma* 34:85, 1993.
5. Cooper C, Dunham M, Rodriguez A: Falls and major injuries are risk factors for thoracolumbar fractures: Cognitive impairment and multiple injuries impede the detection of back pain and tenderness. *J Trauma* 38:692, 1995.
6. Denis F: The three column spine and its significance in the classification of acute thoracolumbar spinal injuries. *Spine* 8:817, 1983.
7. McAffee PC, Yuan HA, Frederickson BE, Lubicky JP: The value of computed tomography in thoracolumbar fractures. *J Bone Joint Surg Am* 65:461, 1983.
8. Petersilge CA, Pathria MN, Emery SE, Masaryk TJ: Thoracolumbar burst fractures: Evaluation with MR imaging. *Radiology* 194:49, 1995.

9. Weisz GM, Lamond TS, Kitchener PN: Spinal imaging: Will MRI replace myelography? *Spine* 13:65, 1988.

10. Keene JS, Goletz TH, Lilleas F, et al: Diagnosis of vertebral fractures. A comparison of conventional radiography, conventional tomography, and computed axial tomography. *J Bone Joint Surg Am* 64:586, 1982.

11. Trafton PG, Boyd CA: Computer tomography of thoracic and lumbar spine injuries. *J Trauma* 24:506, 1984.

12. Frankel HL, Rozycki GS, Ochsner MG, et al: Indications for obtaining surveillance thoracic and lumbar spine radiographs. *J Trauma* 37:673, 1994.

13. Meldon SW, Moettus LN: Thoracolumbar spine fractures: Clinical presentation and the effect of altered sensorium and major injury. *J Trauma* 39:1110, 1995.

14. Terregino CA, Ross SE, Lipinski MF, et al: Selective indications for thoracic and lumbar radiography in blunt trauma. *Ann Emerg Med* 26:126, 1995.

15. Vaccaro AR, An HS, Lin S, et al: Noncontiguous injuries of the spine. *J Spinal Disord* 5:320, 1992.

16. Calenoff L, Chessare JW, Rogers LF, et al: Multiple level spinal injuries: Importance of early recognition. *AJR* 130:665, 1978.

17. Kilcoyne RF, Mack LA, King HA, et al: Thoracolumbar spine injuries associated with vertical plunges: Reappraisal with computer tomography. *Radiography* 146:137, 1983.

18. Smith GR, Northrup CH, Loop JW: Jumpers' fractures: Patterns of thoracolumbar spine injuries associated with vertical plunges. *Radiology* 122:657, 1977.

19. Rupp RE, Ebraheim NA, Chrissos MG, Jackson WT: Thoracic and lumbar fractures associated with femoral shaft fractures in the multiple trauma patient. *Spine* 5:556, 1994.

20. Glass RB, Sivit CJ, Sturm PF, et al: Lumbar spine injury in a pediatric population. *J Trauma* 37:815, 1994.

21. Ballock RT, Mackersie R, Abitbol JJ, et al: Can burst fractures be predicted from plain radiographs? *J Bone Joint Surg Br* 74:147, 1992.

22. Campbell SE, Phillips CD, Dubovsky E, et al: The value of CT in determining potential instability of simple wedge-compression fractures of the lumbar spine. *Am J Neuroradiol* 16:1385, 1995.

23. Deyo RA, Diehl AK: Lumbar spine films in primary care: Current use and effects of selective ordering criteria. *J Gen Intern Med* 1:20, 1986.

24. Scavone JG, Latshaw RF, Rohrer V: Use of lumbar spine films. Statistical evaluation at a university teaching hospital. *JAMA* 246:1105, 1981.

25. Santavirta S, Konttinen YT, Heliovaara M, et al: Determinants of osteoporotic thoracic vertebral fractures. Screening of 57,000 Finnish women and men. *Acta Orthop Scand* 63:198, 1992.

26. Johansson C, Mellstrom D, Rosengren K, Rundgren A: Prevalence of vertebral fractures in 85-year-olds. *Acta Orthop Scand* 64:25, 1993.

27. Kaplan PA, Orton DF, Aselon RJ: Osteoporosis with vertebral compression fractures, retropulsed fragments, and neurologic compromise. *Radiology* 165:533, 1987.

28. Sadato N, Numaguchi Y, Rigamonti D, et al: Spinal epidural abscess with gadolinium-enhanced MRI Serial follow-up studies and clinical correlations. *Neuroradiology* 36:44, 1994.

29. Scavone JG, Latshaw RF, Weidner WA: Anteroposterior and lateral radiographs: An adequate lumbar spine examination. *AJR* 136:715, 1981.

30. Hall FM: Back pain and the radiologist. *Radiology* 137:861, 1980.

31. Wiesel SW, Tsourmas N, Feffer HL, et al: A study of computer assisted tomography: The incidence of positive CAT scans in an asymptomatic group of patients. *Spine* 9:549, 1984.

32. Driscoll PA, Nicholson DA, Ross R: ABC of emergency radiology: Thoracic and lumbar spine. *BMJ* 307:1552, 1993.

33. Lien HH, Kolbenstvedt A: The thoracic paraspinal shadow: Normal appearances. *Clin Radiol* 33:31, 1982.

34. Gehweiler JA, Daffner RH, Osborne RL: Relevant signs of stable and unstable thoracolumbar vertebral column trauma. *Skeletal Radiol* 7:179, 1981.

35. Daffner RH, Deeb ZL, Rothus WE: The posterior vertebral body line: Importance of detection of burst fractures. *Am J Radiol* 148:93, 1987.

36. Phillips JH, Kling TF, Cohen MD: The radiographic anatomy of the thoracic pedicle. *Spine* 19:446, 1994.

37. Lien HH, Kolbvenstvedt A, Lund G: The thoracic paraspinal shadow: A review of the appearances in pathological conditions. *Clin Radiol* 35:215, 1984.

38. Martijn A, Valdhuis EF: The diagnostic value of interpediculate distance assessment on plain films in thoracic and lumbar spine injuries. *J Trauma* 31:1393, 1991.

39. Jelsma RK, Kirsch PT, Rice JR, Jelsma LF: The radiographic description of thoracolumbar fractures. *Surg Neurol* 18:230, 1982.

40. Wang SC, Grattan-Smith A: Thoracolumbar burst fractures: Two "new" plain film signs and C.T. correlation. *Australas Radiol* 31:404, 1987.

41. Atlas SW, Regenbogen V, Rogers LF, Kim KS: The radiographic characterization of burst fractures of the spine. *AJR* 147:575, 1986.

42. Panjabi MM, Oxland TR, Kifune M, et al: Validity of the three-column theory of thoracolumbar fractures: A biomechanical investigation. *Spine* 20:1122, 1995.

43. Magerl F, Aebi M, Gertzbein SD, et al: A comprehensive classification of thoracic and lumbar injuries. *Eur Spine J* 3:184, 1994.

44. Roaf R: A study of the mechanics of spinal injuries. *J Bone Joint Surg Br* 42:810, 1960.

45. McGrory BJ, VanderWilde RS, Currier BL, Eismont FJ: Diagnosis of subtle thoracolumbar burst fractures: A new radiographic sign. *Spine* 18:2282, 1993.

46. Chance CQ: Note on a type of flexion fracture of the spine. *Br J Radiol* 21:452, 1948.

47. Smith WS, Kaufer H: Patterns and mechanisms of lumbar injuries associated with lap seat belts. *J Bone Joint Surg Am* 51:239, 1969.

48. Sivit CJ, Taylor GA, Newman KD, et al: Safety-belt injuries in children with lap-belt ecchymosis: CT findings in 61 patients. *AJR* 157:111, 1991.

49. Sturm JT, Perry JF: Injuries associated with fractures of the transverse processes of the thoracic and lumbar vertebrae. *J Trauma* 24:597, 1984.

50. Gilsanz V, Miranda J, Cleveland R, et al: Scoliosis secondary to fractures of the transverse processes of lumbar vertebrae. *Radiology* 134:627, 1980.

51. Gertzbein SD: Neurologic deterioration in patients with thoracic and lumbar fractures after admission to the hospital. *Spine* 15:1723, 1994.

52. Yuh WT, Zachar CK, Barloon TJ, et al: Vertebral compression fractures: Distinctions between benign and malignant causes with MR imaging. *Radiology* 172:215, 1989.

53. Nachemson AL: The lumbar spine: An orthopedic challenge. *Spine* 1:59, 1976.

54. Antoku S, Russell WJ: Dose to the active bone marrow, gonads, and skin from roentgenography and fluoroscopy. *Radiology* 101:669, 1971.

CHAPTER 15

FACIAL RADIOLOGY

CARLOS FLORES / DAVID T. SCHWARTZ

Injuries to the facial soft tissues and skeleton are common, occurring in 51% of patients admitted to the hospital as a result of motor vehicle collisions and accounting for 2% of all operative procedures.[1,2] Injuries range from simple soft tissue injuries requiring limited intervention to massive facial trauma with significant functional and cosmetic consequences. Trauma to the airway, major craniofacial blood vessels, and the central nervous system make facial injuries life-threatening.

Facial fractures occur in two main clinical settings: motor vehicle collisions and interpersonal violence. The proportion in each category varies according to the population studied. Motor vehicle collisions account for 15 to 80% of facial trauma. Motorcycle accidents are more frequently associated with complex facial trauma. Blows sustained during interpersonal violence account for 5 to 59% of facial injuries.[2-12] Facial injuries are also sustained during falls (8 to 28%), sporting and recreational events (7 to 11%), and occupational accidents (1%).[2-4,13-16] Facial injuries occur in up to 80% of victims of multiple trauma.[17]

Assault and interpersonal violence are frequent causes of facial fractures in adults under 50 years of age.[1,4-6,8-10,12] Persons 20 to 30 years old are the most frequently injured.[5-12] Among men, most assaults occur outside the home (fights); among women, they occur most frequently inside the home and are perpetrated by a known assailant (domestic violence).[3,9] Falls are a frequent cause of facial fractures in adults over 50 years of age.[1,3,5-12]

Children suffer most craniofacial injuries from falls (59%) and impacts with surrounding objects (20%).[3] Fractures of the facial skeleton are less common in children than in adults. In children, mandibular fractures are the most commonly reported, and fractures to the nasal skeleton are also common. Fractures of the midface are infrequent.[18-20]

Of all facial fractures, *nasal fractures* account for 28 to 44%, *midface fractures* account for 27%, and *mandibular fractures* account for 15 to 76%.[2-4,6] Isolated fractures of the orbital rim and zygoma are less frequent, accounting for approximately 5 to 10% of facial fractures.[2,14]

Conventional radiology remains the initial means of evaluating facial injuries. Computed tomography (CT) has improved the ability to diagnose facial fractures and concomitant soft tissue injuries. Three-dimensional CT provides great spatial detail and is used by the surgeon in operative planning.

CLINICAL DECISION MAKING

The evaluation of facial trauma begins by assessing the airway, breathing, and circulation. Although major facial fractures are dramatic, they are frequently associated with other injuries requiring more immediate intervention. The one immediate life threat associated with facial fractures is airway compromise. Emergency management of unstable neurologic or hemodynamic conditions necessitates delayed treatment of facial injuries.[21] Nevertheless, there should not be undue delay in the care of facial injuries in order to avoid a poor cosmetic and functional outcome.[22]

The physical examination helps to identify fracture patterns and guides the decision to obtain facial radiographs. The examiner begins with careful observation of facial symmetry, contour, and external appearance in addition to palpation of the facial skeleton.[17,23,24] Certain clinical findings are characteristic of particular facial fractures (Table 15-1). Palpable bony depression, a visible deformity or asymmetry, orbital emphysema, abnormalities of extraocular muscle movements, and dental malocclusion require further evaluation. Ecchymosis, swelling, and tenderness are suggestive but not diagnostic of facial fractures.[25,26]

Some facial injuries are associated with characteristic motor and sensory abnormalities. Supraorbital ridge fractures cause injury to the supraorbital nerve, which results in frontal (forehead) hypesthesia. Injuries to the infraorbital nerve due to fractures of the zygomaticomaxillary complex (ZMC) or isolated fractures of the orbital floor cause infraorbital facial and gingival hypesthesia. The eye and extraocular muscle function must be examined in detail.

When a facial fracture is suspected, plain-film radiography is the initial screening tool. There are few well-studied guidelines for ordering facial films. One exception is the evaluation of nasal trauma. A careful history and physical examination are sufficient to diagnose and treat nasal fractures. Radiographic findings do not influence treatment. Some authors recommend abandoning nasal films for the evaluation of isolated nasal trauma.[27-30]

CT should be considered if plain-film radiography reveals a facial fracture or if there is a high index of suspicion despite negative films. Two-dimensional CT in the axial and coronal plains is excellent for demonstrating facial fractures.[31-33]

TABLE 15-1

Clinical Findings of Facial Fractures

FRACTURE TYPE	CLINICAL FINDINGS
Supraorbital rim fracture	Edema, ecchymosis, hypesthesia.
Frontal sinus fracture	Loss of consciousness, other facial fractures common, edema, orbital emphysema, intracranial air, CSF leak.
Orbital "blowout" fracture	Enophthalmos, hypesthesia, limitation of ocular motion, diplopia, chemosis, subconjunctival hemorrhage, periorbital edema, orbital emphysema, traumatic telecanthus, globe rupture, visual disturbance, retrobulbar hematoma, hyphema, retinal detachment, optic nerve injury.
Zygomaticomaxillary complex fracture (tripod fracture)	Asymmetrical facial flattening, edema, ecchymosis, malocclusion, epistaxis, diplopia, hypesthesia, facial mobility, dish-face deformity, facial nerve injury.
Zygomatic arch fracture	Edema, facial asymmetry, trismus.
Nasal fracture	Epistaxis, edema, septal hematoma.
Mandibular fracture	Malocclusion, inability to open the mouth, intraoral ecchymosis, crepitus, deviation of the chin (toward fractured side), laceration of the external auditory meatus, gingival laceration, dental trauma, oral hematoma.

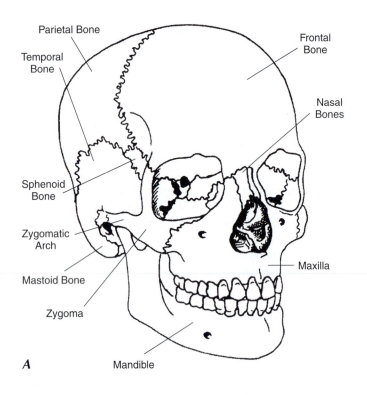

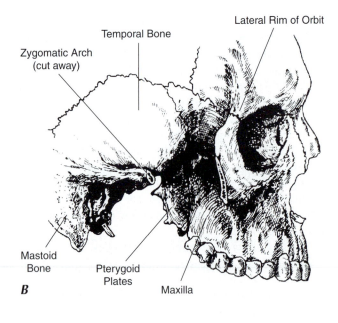

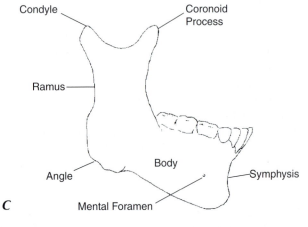

FIGURE 15-1.   *A.* The craniofacial skeleton. *B.* Lateral view of the facial skeleton. The zygomatic arch is cut away, revealing the posterior portion of the maxilla and the pterygoid plates of the sphenoid bone. (*A* and *B.* From Pansky B: *Review of Gross Anatomy,* 6th ed. New York: McGraw-Hill, 1996. With permission.) *C.* Mandible. (From Scaletta TA, Schaider JJ: *Emergent Management of Trauma.* New York: McGraw-Hill, 1996. With permission.)

Conventional radiography is sufficient to identify simple fractures of the zygoma, maxilla, frontal bone, and nose. CT is superior in defining complex facial fractures involving the posterior wall of the frontal sinus, the nasoethmoid-orbital (NEO) complex, the orbits, the ZMC, and complex midface fractures (e.g., LeFort fractures).[34]

Injuries to the eye occur in about 25% of patients with fractures to the orbit.[35,36] CT demonstrates soft tissue injuries with excellent clarity, especially in the orbital and periorbital areas. CT can detect orbital hemorrhage, lens dislocation, a ruptured globe, extraocular muscle entrapment, and intraorbital foreign bodies.[37]

ANATOMY

The skull is composed of 22 bones, which are subdivided into cranial and facial bones. The bones of the cranium are the occipital, sphenoid, frontal, ethmoid, parietals, and temporals. The bones of the face are the maxilla, palatines, zygomas, and mandible.[38,39] The vomer, nasal bones, inferior nasal conchae, and lacrimals are also considered facial bones (Fig. 15-1).

Structurally, the facial skeleton can be viewed as consisting of three vertical and three horizontal supportive struts (Fig. 15-2).[40,41,42] Midfacial fractures follow predictable patterns, with fractures that run perpendicular to these supportive struts. These struts are zones of relative strength that protect the face and cranium against traumatic forces. They also serve to transmit the forces of mastication from the maxilla to the frontal bone.

The anterior vertical strut extends up from the maxilla, along the medial wall of the maxillary sinus and the medial wall of the orbit, to the frontal bone. The middle vertical strut extends up from the premolar teeth, along the lateral wall of the maxillary sinus and lateral wall of the orbit, to the frontal bone. The posterior vertical strut extends up from the posterior maxilla along the posterior walls of the maxillary sinuses and the pterygoid plates to the base of the skull (Fig. 15-1*B*).

The upper horizontal strut is formed by the superior orbital rims and base of the frontal bone. The middle horizontal strut runs along the zygomatic arches and inferior orbital rims. The inferior horizontal strut consists of the hard palate.

RADIOGRAPHIC TECHNIQUE

Each standard radiographic projection provides only a partial view of the facial skeleton, and the evaluation of the facial skeleton requires several radiographs (Table 15-2).[43,44] These radiographs are grouped into several series: the facial series, orbital series, nasal series, and mandibular series.

The *facial series* includes the occipitomental view (Waters), the occipitofrontal view (Caldwell), lateral view, and the submental vertical (SMV or "bucket-handle") view (Figs. 15-3 to 15-7). The *orbital series* includes the occipitomental view (Waters), occipitofrontal view (Caldwell), and two oblique orbital views (Fig. 15-8).

The *nasal series* includes two coned-down lateral radiographs of the nasal bones and the anterior maxillary view (Waters view) (Table 15-3) (Fig. 15-9). The *mandibular series* includes posteroanterior (PA), Towne, and bilateral oblique views. If available, panoramic tomography (Panorex) is helpful in evaluating mandibular fractures (Table 15-4) (Figs. 15-10 and 15-11).

Obtaining good-quality films depends on proper patient positioning (Fig. 15-3). Unfortunately, the patient's medical condition may preclude optimal positioning and adversely affect the quality of the films. The anatomic landmark used to position the patient for the frontal views of the face is the *orbitomeatal line*—which connects the lateral canthus of the eye and the external acoustic meatus and roughly parallels the zygomatic arch.

Occipitomental (Waters) View

The patient is positioned either prone or upright for this view. The upright position is preferred because it demonstrates air-fluid levels in the maxillary sinuses.

The upright occipitomental view is a PA view with the patient's neck extended and the chin resting on the film cassette. The orbitomeatal line is at a 37 to 40° angle with the plane of the film (Fig. 15-3*A*).[45] This positioning places the dense petrous portion of the temporal bone below the maxillary sinus. In patients who cannot sit or stand, the anteroposterior (AP) reverse occipitomental view is used, in which the patient is supine. This AP view magnifies the facial skeleton.[46]

The occipitomental view (Waters) provides the best examination of the midface. This view shows the orbits in their entirety, the maxillary sinuses, nasal skeleton, malar bodies, and frontal sinuses (Fig. 15-4).[25,32,35,40,47]

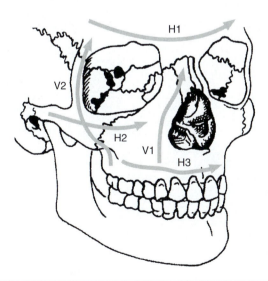

FIGURE 15-2. Supportive struts of the facial skeleton. The three horizontal struts are the base of the frontal bone (H1), the zygomatic arch and inferior orbital rim (H2), and the hard palate (H3). The three vertical struts are the medial walls of the orbit and maxillary sinus (V1), the lateral walls of the orbit and maxillary sinus (V2), and the pterygoid plates (posterior wall of the maxillary sinus) (not visible).

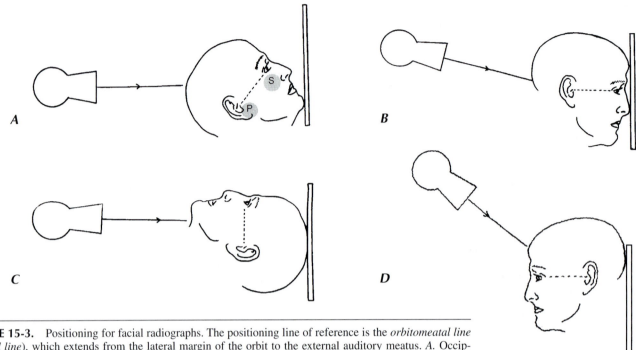

FIGURE 15-3. Positioning for facial radiographs. The positioning line of reference is the *orbitomeatal line* (*dashed line*), which extends from the lateral margin of the orbit to the external auditory meatus. *A.* Occipitomental view (Waters view). The orbitomeatal line makes an angle of about 40° to the x-ray beam. The petrous bone (p) projects below the maxillary sinus (s). The preferred positioning is with the patient upright, as shown here. *B.* Occipitofrontal view (Caldwell view). The x-ray beam is directed at an angle of 15° to the orbitomeatal line. *C.* Submental vertical (SMV) view. The x-ray beam is directed perpendicular to the orbitomeatal line. *D.* AP axial Towne view of the mandibular condyles. The x-ray beam is directed at an angle of 35° to the orbitomeatal line and is centered midway between the temporomandibular joints. (From Fischer HW: *Radiographic Anatomy: A Working Atlas.* New York: McGraw-Hill. With permission.)

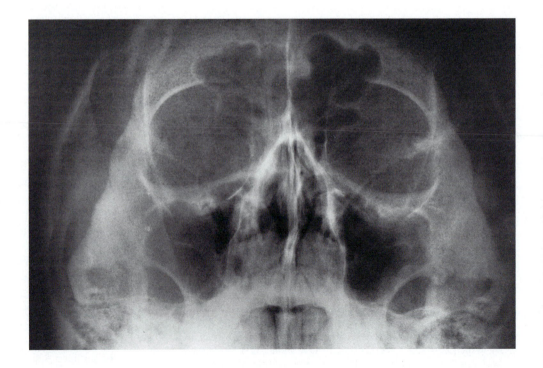

TABLE 15-2

Radiographic Views of the Face—Midface and Orbits

VIEW	POSITION	ADEQUACY	ANATOMIC AREAS SEEN
Occipitomental (Waters)	Sitting or standing (upright). Orbitomeatal line at a 40° angle with the film. X-ray beam is perpendicular to the film. Supine (alternative positioning).	Petrous bones below maxillary sinus. No rotational malalignment.	Maxillary sinus, nasal septum, zygomatic arch, orbital floor, inferior orbital rim, lateral orbital rim. Detects most midface fractures.
Occipitofrontal (Caldwell)	Prone, sitting, or standing. Orbitomeatal line is perpendicular to the film, forehead is against the film cassette. X-ray beam is angled at 15° caudad.	Petrous bones obscure inferior orbits and maxillary sinus. No rotational malalignment.	Frontal sinus, superior orbital rim, ethmoid air cells, lamina papyracea (medial orbital wall), frontal calvarium. Lateral wall of maxillary sinus (below petrous bone).
Lateral	Seated or standing (upright). Midsagittal line is parallel to the film. Interpupillary line is perpendicular to the film.	Includes frontal sinus to mandible. Includes nasal bones to sella turcica. No rotational malalignment (left and right sides of the face superimposed).	Anterior wall of frontal sinus, lateral rims of orbits, sphenoid sinus, maxillary sinus, frontal sinus, pterygoid plate.
Oblique orbital	Seated or semiprone. Midsagittal line forms an angle of about 50° with the film.		Lateral orbital rim (ipsilateral and contralateral).
Submental vertical (SMV) "bucket handle"	Sitting or supine. Hyperextended neck. X-ray beam directed to chin and film cassette above vertex of skull.	Both zygomatic arches visible. Overpenetrated film shows maxillary, sphenoid, and ethmoid sinus; lateral walls of orbit.	Zygomatic arches (lateral orbital wall), maxillary sinus (anterior and lateral wall), sphenoid sinus.

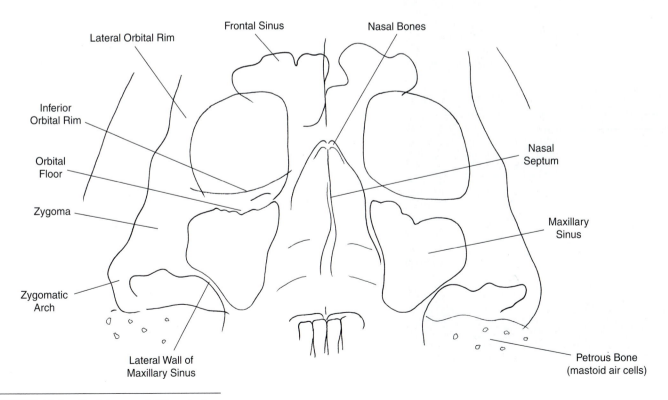

FIGURE 15-4. Occipitomental (Waters) view.

Occipitofrontal (Caldwell) View

For the occipitofrontal (Caldwell) view, the patient can sit, stand, or be prone. The patient's forehead is placed against the film cassette and the orbitomeatal line is perpendicular to the film. The x-ray beam is directed 15° caudad to the film cassette (Fig. 15-3*B*).

In this view, the petrous pyramids obscure the maxillary sinus and inferior orbital rim. The occipitofrontal view delineates the frontal region of the face, including the orbits, lamina papyracea, frontal sinuses, and ethmoid sinuses (Fig. 15-5).

Lateral View

To obtain a lateral view, the side of the patient's face is placed against the film cassette and the interpupillary line is perpendicular to the film. The lateral view includes the areas between the frontal sinuses and the mandible and from the nasal bones to the base of the skull. It demonstrates the frontal sinuses, orbits, maxillary sinus, and pterygoid plates (Fig. 15-6).

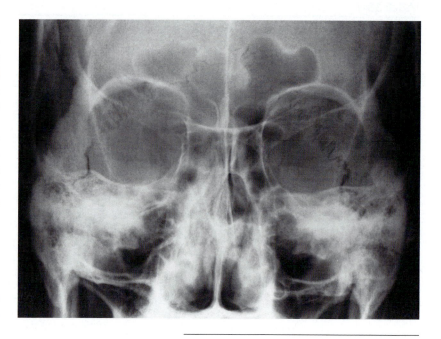

FIGURE 15-5.   Occipitofrontal (Caldwell) view.

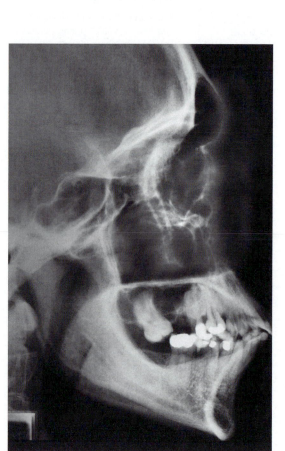

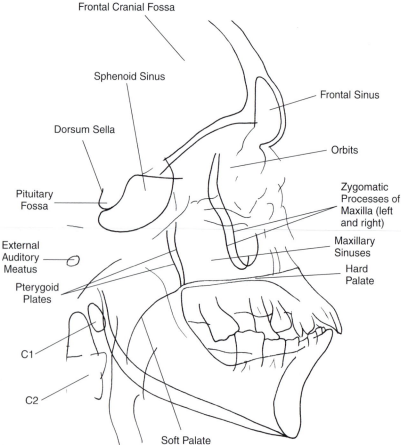

FIGURE 15-6.   Lateral facial view.

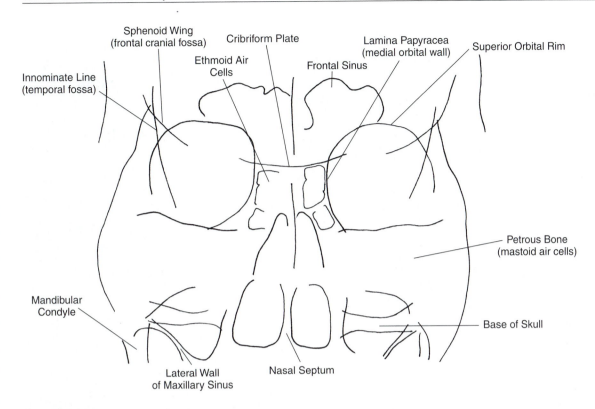

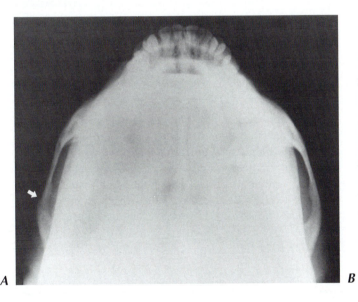

A

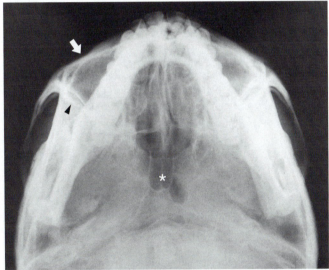

B

Submental vertical ("Bucket-Handle") View

For the submental vertical (SMV), basal, or "bucket-handle" view, the patient can be sitting or supine. The neck is hyperextended, and the film cassette is placed flat against the vertex of the skull. The x-ray beam is directed under the patient's chin to the vertex of the skull. The orbitomeatal line is parallel to the plane of the film (Fig. 15-3*C*). This view is used to examine the zygomatic arches (Fig. 15-7). Using more penetrated radiographic technique, the SMV view visualizes the maxillary, sphenoid, and ethmoid sinuses as well as the lateral walls of the orbits.

FIGURE 15-7. Submental vertical (SMV) view (basal view). *A.* "Bucket handle" view. Standard underpenetrated technique shows the zygomatic arches. In this patient, there is slight depression of the right zygomatic arch due to blunt trauma (*arrow*). *B.* Greater penetration shows a basal view of the facial skeleton, including the sphenoid sinus (*asterisk*), the anterior walls of the maxillary sinuses (*arrow*), and the lateral walls of the orbits (*arrowhead*).

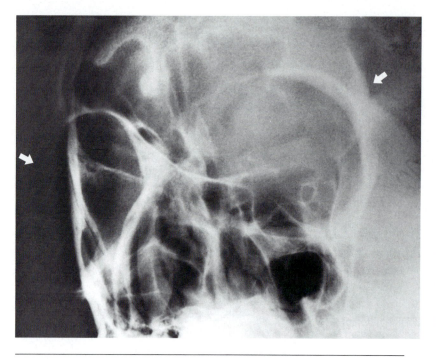

FIGURE 15-8. Oblique orbital view. Lateral orbital rims (*arrows*).

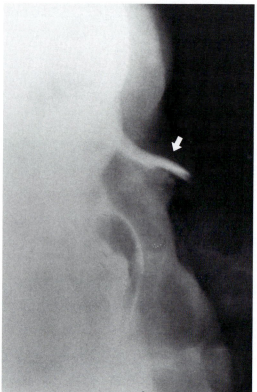

FIGURE 15-9. Lateral nasal view. Nasal bone (*arrow*).

Oblique Orbital View

The oblique orbital views are supplementary for evaluating the orbits. They delineate fractures of the lateral orbital rim (Fig. 15-8). With regard to facial trauma, the oblique orbital view does not add significant information to that obtained from other facial views.

Nasal Series

The nasal series consists of an occipitomental (Waters) view and two coned-down lateral views of the nasal bones (Table 15-3). The *lateral nasal view* uses a narrow field of view and provides greater detail of the side of the nose closest to the film (Fig. 15-9). Both left and right lateral nasal views are obtained. The *occipitomental view* (Waters) provides a frontal image of the nasal septum and the left and right nasal bones. The Waters view demonstrates medial or lateral displacement of a fracture. An additional *axial view* uses either an occlusal or extraoral film.

TABLE 15-3

Radiographic Views of the Face: Nasal Series

VIEW	POSITION	ADEQUACY	ANATOMIC AREAS SEEN
Coned-down lateral views	Semiprone with head in the lateral position. Midsagittal line is parallel to the film. Central ray is aimed at the bridge of the nose.	Centered on nasal bones. Rotational alignment.	Nasal bones. Nasal maxillary suture.
Occipitomental (Waters) view	Sitting or standing. Orbitomeatal line at a 40° angle with the film. Central ray is perpendicular to the film.	No rotational malalignment. Petrous bones below maxillary antrum.	Nasal septum. Nasion (bridge of nose). Lateral walls of nasal cavity.

Mandibular Series

The mandibular series includes two oblique views, a PA view, and an AP axial (Towne) view (Table 15-4).

ANTEROPOSTERIOR OBLIQUE VIEWS.   The patient is supine with the affected side down. The cassette is in contact with the mandible, affected side down. The chin is extended 30°, and the angle of the x-ray beam is approximately 35° cephalad. The side of the mandible closest to the film is visualized (Figure 15-10*A* and *B*). Oblique views of both sides of the mandible are obtained.

POSTEROANTERIOR VIEW.   The patient is prone or sitting with the forehead and nose against the film cassette. The x-ray beam is directed perpendicular to the film. This view demonstrates the mandibular rami and body (Figure 15-10*C*).

AP AXIAL (TOWNE) VIEW.   The patient is supine. The orbito-meatal line is perpendicular to the film and the x-ray beam is directed at 30° caudad (Fig. 15-3*D*). This view shows the mandibular condyles, rami, and the temperomandibular fossa (Fig. 15-10*D*).

PANORAMIC TOMOGRAPHY (PANOREX).   Panoramic tomography (Panorex) produces tomograms of curved objects. The film visualizes the entire mandible, using two techniques. In one, the patient and the film rotate in opposite directions while the x-ray tube remains stationary. In the other, the x-ray tube and film rotate in the same direction around a stationary patient (Fig. 15-11).

This view offers better visualization of the entire mandible than a conventional mandibular series. The Panorex view eliminates the overlapping of bony structures and soft tissues seen in the conventional series.[48,49]

Computed Tomography

CT examination of the face consists of thin (1.5- or 3.0-mm) sections in both axial and coronal planes (Fig. 15-12). The axial images of a facial CT are oriented in a true axial plane. The orientation of a cranial CT is slightly oblique, such that the slices are in a plane parallel to the base of the skull. For coronal slices, the patient is either prone or supine and the patient's neck is hyperextended. Neck extension must be avoided if there is a concomitant injury to the cervical spine. Coronal images can be reformatted from axial sections, although this results in significant loss of resolution. It is preferable to obtain coronal sections with the patient prone rather than supine. This is because when the patient is prone, fluid in the maxillary sinus collects at the inferior portion of the sinus. In the supine position, fluid collects in the superior portion of the maxillary sinus, which can obscure an orbital floor fractures.

Coronal sections are used to evaluate fractures in the axial (horizontal) and sagittal planes, such as an orbital floor fracture. Axial sections are used to evaluate injuries in the coronal and sagittal planes, such as fractures of the anterior or lateral walls of the maxillary sinus.[50] A complete facial CT study includes both bone windows and soft tissue windows.

TABLE 15-4

Radiographic Views of the Face: Mandible

VIEW	POSITION	ADEQUACY	ANATOMIC AREAS AND FRACTURES SEEN
Posteroanterior (PA)	Prone or sitting. Nose on the film. Midsagittal line is perpendicular to the film.	No rotational malalignment.	Entire mandible, tempromandibular joint, condyles, rami, and body. Symphysis and angle fractures.
Oblique views	Supine with affected side down. Extended chin at 30° for a view of the body of the mandible. Extended chin at 15° for a general survey of the mandible.	Opposite mandible is not superimposed; cervical spine is not superimposed.	One half of the mandible. Body and angle fractures.
AP axial view (Towne)	Supine. Orbitomeatal line is perpendicular to the film. Central ray is at 30°.	Centered; no rotational malalignment.	Mandibular condyles, tempromandibular fossa. Condylar fractures.
Panoramic tomography (Panorex)	Sitting upright.	No rotational malalignment.	Entire mandible.

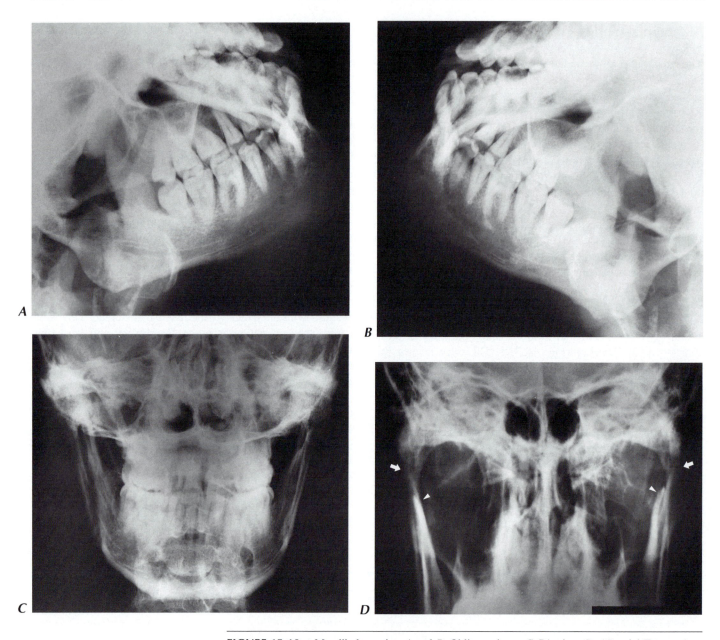

FIGURE 15-10.   Mandibular series. *A* and *B*. Oblique views. *C*. PA view. *D*. AP axial Towne view. Mandibular condyles (*arrows*). Coronoid processes (*arrowheads*)

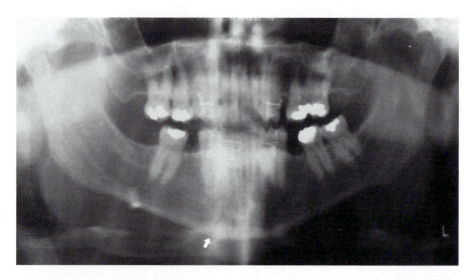

FIGURE 15-11.   Panoramic tomography of mandible (Panorex). There is a nondisplaced fracture of the mandibular symphysis (*arrow*).

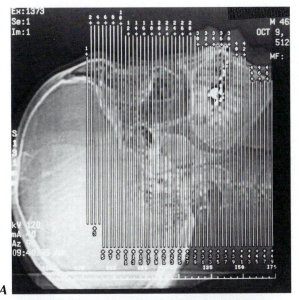

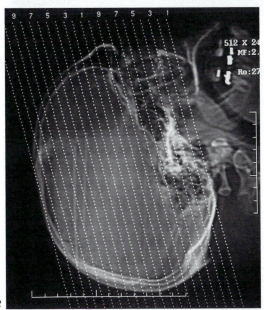

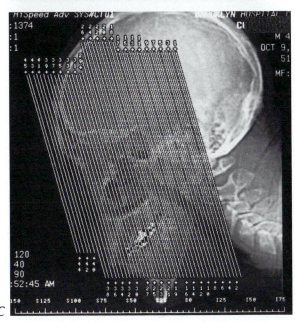

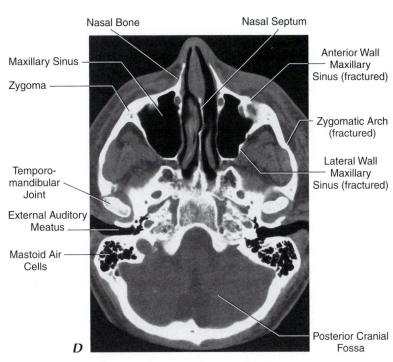

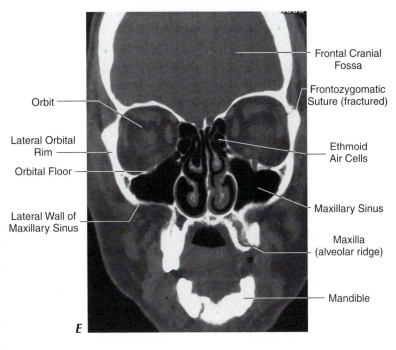

FIGURE 15-12. Facial CT. *A.* Axial facial slices are oriented in the true axial plane of the patient. Slice thickness is 3 mm. *B.* Axial head CT slices are oriented in a slightly oblique angle that follows the base of the skull. *C.* Coronal facial slices are perpendicular to the axial cuts. The patient is either prone, as shown here, or supine. *D.* CT axial slice. *E.* CT coronal slice.

RADIOGRAPHIC ANALYSIS

The radiographic anatomy of the facial skeleton is complex. The numerous overlapping skeletal and soft tissue shadows make analyzing these films challenging. It is not feasible to trace every radiographic contour in the hope of detecting a fracture. An approach based on the identification of commonly occurring fracture patterns is better suited to the evaluation of facial radiographs (Table 15-5 and Fig. 15-13).

Adequacy

The physician must first assess whether the radiographs are of adequate technical quality. In the frontal views (occipitomental and occipitofrontal), the nasal septum, the midpoint of the mandible, and the odontoid process are aligned in the center of the film. The orbital rims are of equal size and shape. In a correctly positioned occipitomental (Waters) view, the petrous portions of the temporal bone are below the maxillary sinus. The left-right orientation of all of the films must be correct. If the radiographs are not labeled consistently, the dental fillings can be used as radiographic landmarks to determine the correct orientation of each view.

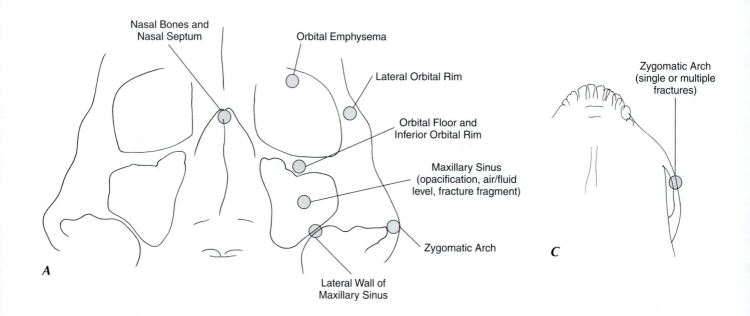

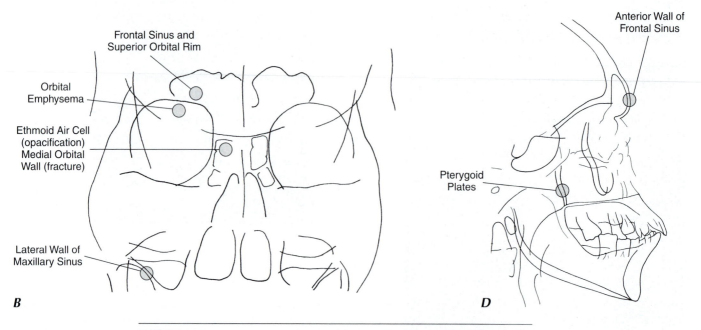

FIGURE 15-13. Sites prone to injury and easily missed injuries. *A.* Waters view. *B.* Caldwell view. *C.* Submental vertical view. *D.* Lateral view.

TABLE 15-5

Systematic Evaluation of Facial Radiographs

Waters view Adequacy	Left-right correctly labeled in all views (check dental work). Petrous bones projected inferior to the maxillary sinuses. No rotation.
Soft tissues	Maxillary sinus air-fluid level or opacification. Orbital emphysema. Infraorbital soft tissue swelling.

Bones	Elephant's head in profile—Dolan lines.
	    Orbital floor and inferior orbital rim (elephant's ear).
	    Lateral orbital rim (elephant's forehead).
	    Zygomatic arch (elephant's trunk).
	    Lateral wall of the maxillary sinus (elephant's chin).
	Nasal septum.

Caldwell view (Review top to bottom)	Frontal sinuses and superior orbital rim. Orbital emphysema. Ethmoid air cells (opacification) and medial orbital wall. Lateral orbital rim and frontozygomatic suture. Inferior orbital rim and orbital floor. Lateral wall of the maxillary sinus (inferior portion).

SMV view	Zygomatic arch fracture.
	    If only a single break is seen, there must be another
	    midface fracture, such as a tripod (ZMC) fracture.

Lateral view	Pterygoid plates (LeFort fractures). Anterior wall of the frontal sinus.

The order in which the radiographic views are reviewed is as follows: occipitomental (Waters), occipitofrontal (Caldwell), SMV (if a zygomatic arch fracture is suspected), and lateral.

Occipitomental (Waters) View

The occipitomental (Waters) view demonstrates most midface fractures. It is optimal for visualizing the maxillary sinuses, the orbits, and the nasal septum. It also provides a view of the zygomatic arches.

BONES. Three lines described by Dolan assist in evaluating the Waters view. They focus attention on the regions of the midface that are most often fractured (Fig. 15-14A). The first line, *the orbital line,* begins at the frontozygomatic suture, then follows the lateral, inferior, and medial margins of the orbit to the arch of the nasion (bridge of the nose), and continues to the other side of the face. This line resembles a rounded W. On the Waters view, the inferior orbital rim appears as an indistinct gray line that is located superior to the thin white line of the orbital floor (Fig. 15-15). The second Dolan line, the *zygomatic line,* follows the lateral margin of the lateral orbital rim, and continues along the superior border of the zygomatic arch. The third Dolan line, the *maxillary line,* begins medially at the lateral wall of the maxillary sinus and continues laterally along the inferior margin of the zygomatic arch. These three lines can be imagined to form the face, ear, and trunk of an elephant's head in profile (Fig. 15-14B).

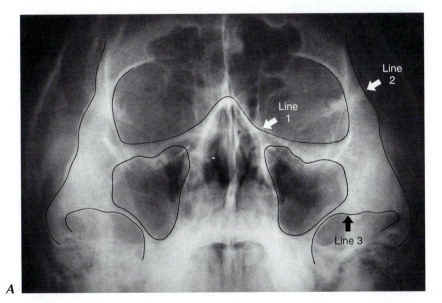

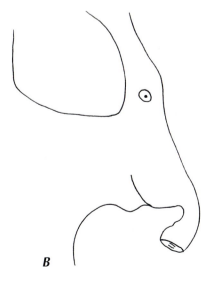

FIGURE 15-14. Visual aids to the interpretation of the Waters view. *A.* Dolan and Jacoby's three lines of reference direct attention on the contours disrupted in most midface fractures. Line 1 follows the inferior and lateral orbital rims and the superior surface of the nasal bones; it has a curved-W appearance. Line 2 follows the lateral orbital rim and the superior surface of the zygomatic arch. Line 3 follows the lateral wall of the maxillary sinus and the inferior surface of the zygomatic arch. *B.* On each side of the face, these three lines together form the image of an elephant's head in profile. (Adapted from Batnitzky S, McMillan JH: Facial trauma, in McCort JJ: *Trauma Radiology.* New York: Churchill Livingstone, 1990, p. 304. With permission.) (Dolan DD, Jacoby CG: Facial fractures. *Semin Roentgenol* 13:37; 1978.)

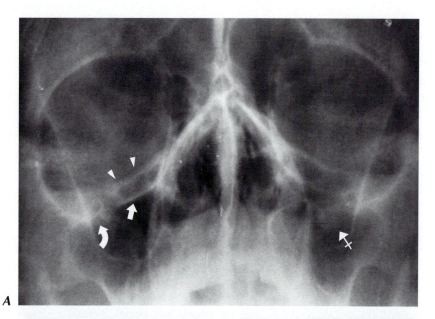

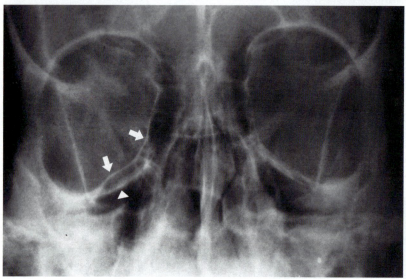

FIGURE 15-15. Appearance of the orbital floor on optimal Waters and Caldwell views. *A.* Waters view. The right orbital floor appears as a well-defined fine white line *(arrow)* that is inferior to the more indistinct grayish shadow of the inferior orbital rim *(arrowheads)*. The circular foramen for the infraorbital nerve is seen laterally *(curved arrow)*. On the left, the orbital floor is indistinct and displaced inferiorly owing to an orbital floor fracture *(crossed arrows)*. *B.* Caldwell view. The posteromedial portion of the orbital floor and the medial orbital wall appear as fine, bright white lines *(arrows)*. The inferior orbital rim is less well defined and located inferior to the orbital floor *(arrowhead)*. On many normal facial radiographs, the orbital floor is not as well seen as in these examples. Therefore, it is often difficult to base the diagnosis of an orbital floor fracture solely on finding an indistinct line on the plain radiographs.

Common midface fracture sites are identified using these three radiographic lines. The *orbital line* helps evaluate the frontozygomatic suture, the lateral orbital rim, and the infraorbital rim and orbital floor. Fractures of the nasal bone and frontal process of the maxilla are detected where the orbital line traverses the nasal skeleton. The *zygomatic line* evaluates the frontozygomatic suture, lateral orbital wall, and the body and arch of the zygoma. The *maxillary line* identifies fractures of the lateral wall of the maxillary sinus and zygomatic arch.[51]

MAXILLARY SINUSES.   Opacification of the maxillary sinus is an important radiographic sign of a fracture. Sinus opacification is due to the accumulation of blood or fluid within the antrum of the sinus. On a supine view, this appears as diffuse opacification of the sinus. On an upright view, fluid in the sinus is more readily detected because it produces a distinctive air-fluid level. In addition, on an upright radiograph, a small amount of fluid is still detectable as an air-fluid level, whereas on a supine radiograph, a small amount of fluid produces only minimal increase in opacity of the sinus. Opacification of a sinus is also present in inflammatory sinus disease. However, in the setting of facial trauma, fluid in the sinus is presumed to be hemorrhage due to a facial fracture (Fig. 15-16).

Asymmetry or discontinuity of the walls of the maxillary sinuses suggests a fracture. The presence of an abnormal bright white linear density within the maxillary sinus represents a bone fragment displaced into the sinus (Fig. 15-17).

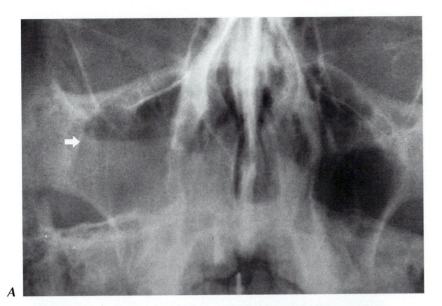

A

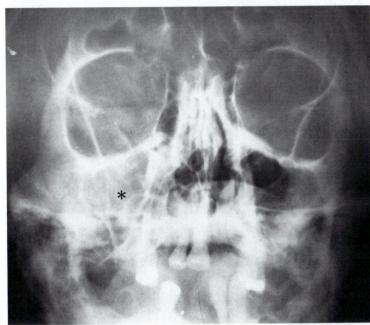

B

FIGURE 15-16. Maxillary sinus opacification and air-fluid level. *A.* On an upright Waters view, a maxillary sinus air-fluid level is the most distinctive radiographic sign of a right-sided orbital floor fracture *(arrow).* *B.* On a supine Waters view, there is diffuse opacification of the maxillary sinus *(asterisk).* When there is only a moderate amount of fluid in the sinus or when there is overlying soft tissue swelling, maxillary sinus opacification can be difficult to diagnose with certainty on a supine Waters view. An upright Waters view showing an air/fluid level is more reliable.

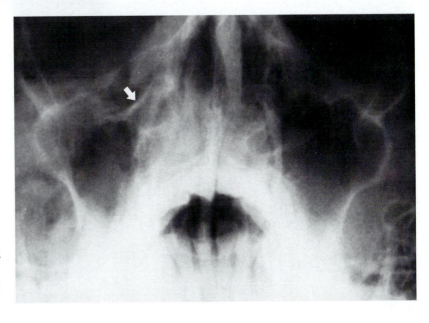

FIGURE 15-17. The bright white line. A fragment of the orbital floor is displaced into the maxillary sinus. When a fracture fragment is seen end-on, it appears as a bright white line.

OTHER SOFT TISSUE SIGNS. *Soft tissue swelling* of the malar area (cheek) causes a diffuse opacification of the involved side of the face, including the region of the maxillary sinus. A well-defined line representing the upper margin of the swollen facial tissues is often seen just above the inferior orbital rim (Fig. 15-18). Facial swelling can be difficult to distinguish from diffuse sinus opacification on a supine radiograph. On an upright radiograph, a distinctive air-fluid level is readily distinguished from overlying soft tissue swelling.

Orbital emphysema (intraorbital air) in the setting of facial trauma is diagnostic of a fracture through one of the adjacent sinuses—the maxillary sinus, the ethmoid air cells, or, rarely, the frontal sinuses. Orbital emphysema appears as a radiolucent (dark) crescent lying adjacent to the superior orbital rim (Fig. 15-19).

Occipitofrontal (Caldwell) View

The occipitofrontal (Caldwell) view shows the frontal portion of the cranium, frontal sinuses, orbital rim, frontozygomatic suture, lamina papyracea, nasal septum, and greater and lesser wings of the sphenoid (Fig. 15-5). Two parallel lines are often seen at the medial border of the orbit; these represent the medial orbital wall (lamina papyracea) and the posterior lacrimal crest. The more lateral line is the lamina papyracea.[52] The orbital floor, when visible, is a white line projected above the inferior orbital rim (Fig. 15-15B). The upper part of the maxillary sinus is obscured by the petrous bone. The inferior portion of the lateral wall of the maxillary sinus is visible below the petrous bone.

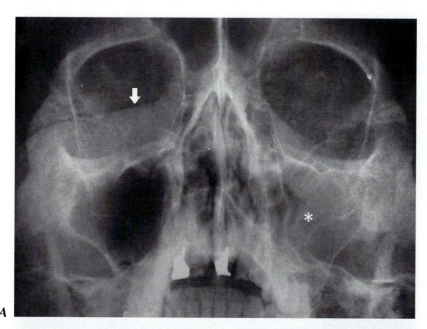

A

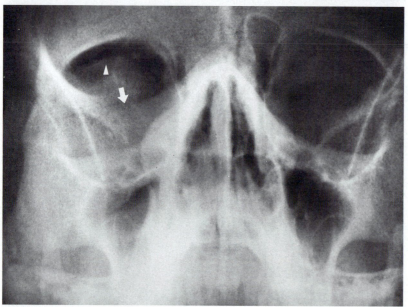

B

FIGURE 15-18. Facial soft tissue swelling. *A.* Soft tissue swelling causes diffuse opacification over the right midface and lower portion of the orbit *(arrow).* This is a nonspecific sign and is not always associated with a fracture. There is also diffuse opacification of the left maxillary sinus *(asterisk).* Since this patient did not have facial trauma on the left, this maxillary sinus opacification is not due to a fracture but is instead the result of an inflammatory condition such as sinusitis. *B.* In another patient, soft tissue swelling is seen over the right maxillary sinus *(arrow).* Orbital emphysema is also seen *(arrowhead).*

Two additional lines are prominent on the radiograph, although they have little significance with regard to facial fractures (Fig. 15-5). The *innominate lines* are formed by the greater wings of the sphenoid bone and the walls of the temporal portion of the skull. A horizontal line that traverses the upper part of the orbits is the floor of the frontal cranial fossa. It is formed by the lesser wings of the sphenoid bone and the cribriform plate.

Important soft tissue signs of a fracture visible on the Caldwell view include orbital emphysema and opacification of the ethmoid air cells. In the setting of trauma, ethmoid air-cell opacification indicates a medial orbital wall fracture (Fig. 15-20).

The Caldwell view is examined from top to bottom (Table 15-5). First, the frontal sinuses and superior orbital rims are examined. Then the superior orbits are examined for orbital emphysema. The ethmoid air cells are examined for opacification due to fluid or blood. Next, the lateral orbital rims and frontozygomatic sutures are assessed, followed by the inferior orbital rims and orbital floors. Finally, the lateral walls of the maxillary sinuses, located below the petrous bones, are examined for evidence of a fracture.

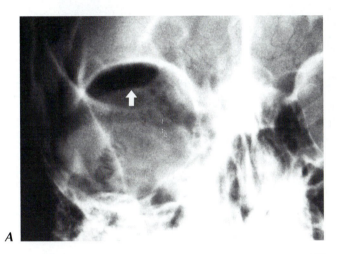

A

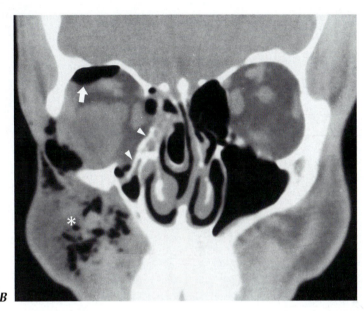

B

FIGURE 15-19. Orbital emphysema. *A.* An air collection in the upper portion of the orbit can be seen on either the Caldwell or Waters view. This is a sign of a fracture into an adjacent sinus, usually the maxillary sinus, through the orbital floor or the ethmoid air cells through the medial orbital wall. *B.* A coronal CT demonstrates the orbital air collection. There are fractures through the orbital floor and medial orbital walls (*arrowheads*). Air in the facial soft tissues is also seen (*asterisk*).

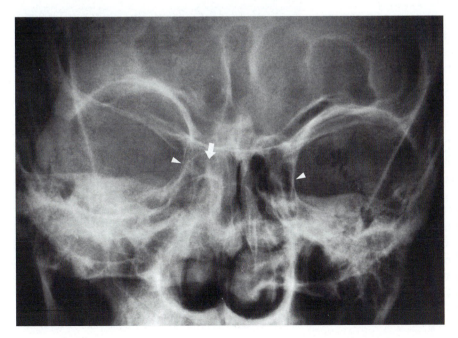

FIGURE 15-20. Ethmoid air cell opacification. Fluid (blood) has filled the right ethmoid air cells as seen on the Caldwell view *(arrow)*. The medial orbital wall (lamina papyracea) is normally a fine white line on the Caldwell view *(arrowheads)*. Loss of this well-defined line is also a sign of a medial orbital wall fracture. The medial orbital wall fracture was confirmed on the coronal CT (see Fig. 15-19*B*).

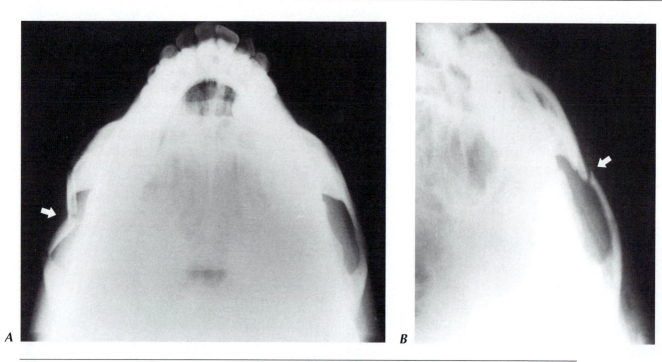

A
B

FIGURE 15-21.   SMV view demonstrating zygomatic arch fractures. *A.* With an isolated zygomatic arch fracture, two or, more commonly, three breaks in the zygomatic arch are present. *B.* A single break in the zygomatic arch occurs only as part of a more extensive midface fracture such as a tripod fracture or LeFort III fracture.

Submental Vertical View

The SMV or "bucket-handle" view is used to evaluate fractures of the zygomatic arch (Fig. 15-7). The zygomatic arch forms a rigid ring with the adjacent temporal portion of the skull. Therefore, it is impossible to have a single fracture in this ring of bone. With an isolated fracture of the zygomatic arch, at least two breaks must be seen. Usually, there are three breaks, creating a V-shaped depressed fragment. If a single break is seen in the zygomatic arch, then a second break must be present elsewhere in the midface. This second fracture is usually in the maxilla or body of the zygoma bone, such as that occurring in a tripod (ZMC) fracture (Fig. 15-21).

With an overpenetrated exposure (the "basal view"), the anterior and lateral walls of the maxillary sinuses, the lateral walls of the orbits, and the sphenoid sinus can be evaluated (Fig. 15-7*B*).

Lateral View

The lateral view identifies fractures of the anterior and posterior walls of the frontal sinus (Fig. 15-6). The anterior maxillary wall, anterior nasal spine, and alveolar ridge are also seen. It is important to evaluate the posterior facial buttresses, which are formed by the posterior walls of the maxillary sinuses and the pterygoid plates. These appear as one or two parallel lines. Fractures through the pterygoid plates are seen in LeFort fractures (Fig. 15-22). The angle and body of the mandible and the subcondylar process are also seen. If a supine cross-table lateral view is obtained, an air-fluid level in the sphenoid sinus suggests a basilar skull fracture.

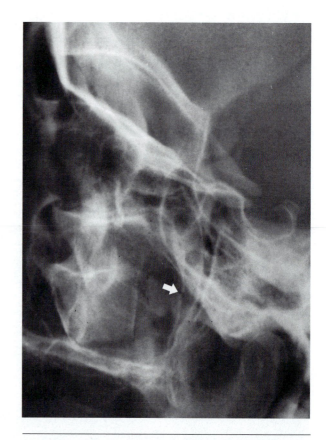

FIGURE 15-22.   Pterygoid plate fracture on lateral view in LeFort fracture. A fracture through the posterior walls of the maxillary sinuses (pterygoid plates) is characteristic of all LeFort fractures and is seen on the lateral facial view *(arrow)*.

COMMON ABNORMALITIES

With regard to facial fractures, it is useful to divide the facial skeleton into three regions. The upper third of the face includes the frontal bone, the frontal sinus, and the supraorbital rim. The middle third includes the nasal bones, zygoma, maxilla, and orbits. The lower third is the mandible.

Fractures of the Upper Third of the Face

SUPRAORBITAL RIM FRACTURES.   Fractures of the supraorbital rim are detected on the occipitomental (Waters) and occipitofrontal (Caldwell) views. These fractures usually involve the frontal sinus. Radiographically, there is a break in the dense cortical line representing the supraorbital rim. Other findings include clouding of the frontal sinus and pneumocephalus (Fig. 15-23).

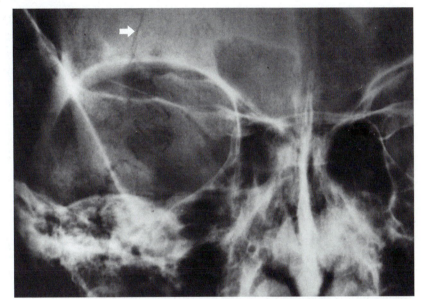

FRONTAL SINUS FRACTURES.   The frontal sinus is fully developed by the age of 19 years. Unilateral agenesis is common, and approximately 4% of individuals have bilateral agenesis. The anterior wall of the frontal sinus is thick and the posterior wall is thin.[53,54] Frontal sinus fractures frequently accompany fractures of the frontal portion of the skull. Loss of consciousness occurs in approximately 70% of patients, and 28% have two or more additional facial fractures, such as maxillary fractures (33%), zygomatic fractures (16%), and orbital NEO fractures (12%). Orbital emphysema and intracranial air are commonly seen. Frontal sinus fractures can be difficult to palpate because of overlying soft tissue swelling.

Isolated fractures of the anterior wall of the frontal sinus occur in 18% of frontal sinus fractures. They are detected on the occipitofrontal (Caldwell) and lateral views. On the occipitofrontal view, the fracture appears as a radiolucent cleft. Opacification of the frontal sinus suggests a fracture, as does an air-fluid level.

Fractures of the posterior wall of the frontal sinus are common albeit difficult to detect on standard radiographic views. Approximately 75% of patients with frontal sinus fractures have involvement of both walls. Patients with fractures of the anterior wall of the frontal sinus require CT evaluation to detect a fracture of the posterior wall because such fractures often violate the cranial cavity.

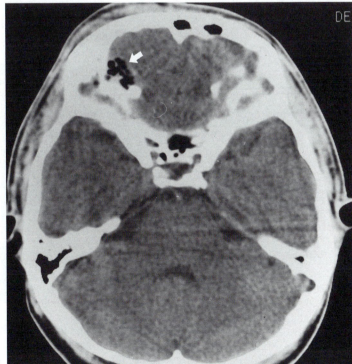

FIGURE 15-23.   Superior orbital rim fracture. *A.* A direct blow to the forehead caused this linear fracture through the superior orbital rim lateral. *B.* A head CT revealed air within the frontal cranial fossa, indicating that this was an open fracture.

Fractures of the Middle Third of the Face

Fractures of the middle third of the face are the most common facial fractures. Midface fractures include orbital fractures, malar and zygomatic arch fractures, nasal fractures, and LeFort fractures (bilateral).

ORBITAL FRACTURES.   Orbital fractures can be classified into those that involve the orbital rim and those that involve the orbital walls. The most common orbital fracture is a "blow-out" fracture involving the orbital floor. Orbital fractures also occur as a component of other midface fractures, such as a tripod fracture (ZMC fracture) or LeFort fracture. Orbital fractures are best evaluated with the occipitomental (Waters) and occipitofrontal (Caldwell) views.

"Blowout" Fractures of the Orbital Floor.   Blowout fractures involve the orbital floor and medial wall of the orbit. The orbital rim is spared. Two theories exist about the mechanism of injury responsible for these fractures. The *hydraulic theory* postulates that the force of a blow to the orbit is transferred through the globe to the walls of the orbit. The orbital floor is fractured because it is the weakest portion of the orbit, weaker than the globe itself (Fig. 15-24). The *buckling theory* proposes that there is a direct blow to the inferior rim of the orbit, causing the orbital floor to buckle and fracture.

There are several clinical signs indicative of a blowout fracture (Table 15-6). With a large orbital floor fracture, the orbital contents herniate into the maxillary sinus, which causes enophthalmos. Infraorbital hypesthesia occurs with injury to the infraorbital nerve. Limitation of ocular motion on upward or occasionally downward gaze results from entrapment of either the inferior rectus muscle or adjacent fat pad. The resultant diplopia often corrects over time as orbital swelling subsides. Ocular injury is frequently associated with blowout fractures. Ocular injuries include hyphema, subconjunctival hemorrhage, retrobulbar hemorrhage, retinal detachment, and vitreous hemorrhage.

The occipitomental (Waters) view is the most useful radiograph in the diagnosis of an orbital floor fracture (Figs. 15-25 to 15-28 and Table 15-6). There may be orbital floor fragmentation with depression of the fragment. The depressed fragment

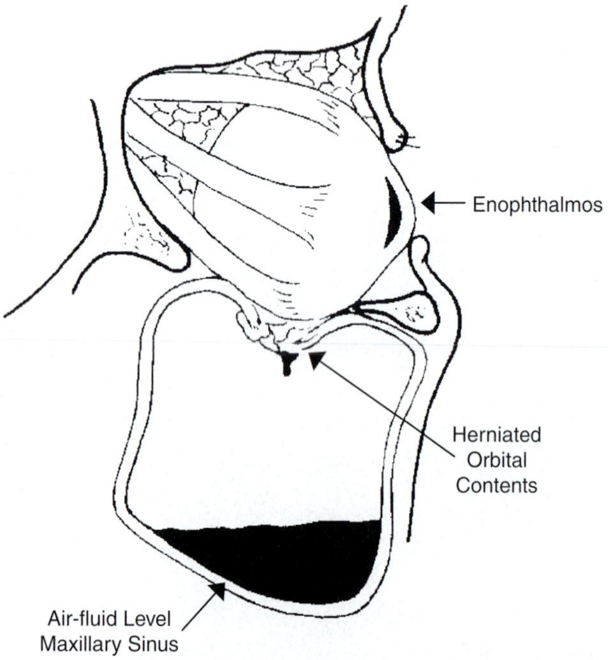

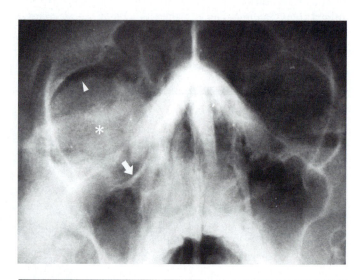

FIGURE 15-25.   Orbital floor fracture. On the Waters view, there is soft tissue swelling *(asterisk)* and orbital emphysema *(arrowhead)*. The orbital floor fracture fragment appears as an oblique bright white line displaced like a "trap door" into the maxillary sinus *(arrow)*. The maxillary sinus is minimally opacified. The Caldwell view and coronal CT are shown in Fig. 15-19.

Enophthalmos

Herniated Orbital Contents

Air-fluid Level Maxillary Sinus

FIGURE 15-24.   Mechanism of injury causing a blowout fracture of the orbital floor. A frontal impact to the orbit increases intraorbital pressure. The orbit fractures at its weakest part—the orbital walls— rather than the globe. Alternatively, a blow to the inferior orbital rim causes the orbital floor to buckle and fracture. (From Scaletta TA, Schaider JJ: *Emergent Management of Trauma.* New York: McGraw-Hill, 1996. With permission.)

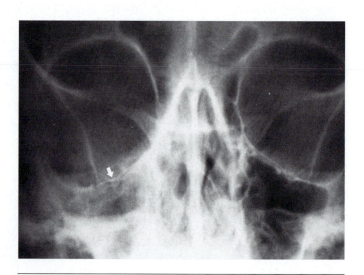

FIGURE 15-26.   Orbital floor fracture. Irregularity and widening of the orbital floor is seen on this Caldwell view. Increased opacity of the maxillary sinus is due to either blood in the sinus or, more likely, overlying soft tissue swelling.

is depressed laterally near the infraorbital groove, and appears as an oblique line or "trap-door" at the "roof" of the maxillary sinus. Soft tissue prolapse through the floor of the orbit into the maxillary sinus may be seen (the *teardrop* sign).[55] Polyps or retention cysts in the sinus cavity can have a similar radiographic appearance. An increase in the distance between the orbital rim and orbital floor greater than 2 mm as compared with the uninjured side is another radiographic finding. Maxillary sinus opacification or an air-fluid level is frequently seen. Orbital emphysema is also common and may be the only radiographic evidence of this fracture (Figs. 15-15 to 15-19).

The accuracy of conventional radiology in diagnosing orbital floor fractures varies. In one series of 30 patients with blowout fractures, the occipitofrontal (Caldwell) view was positive in 87% of the cases and the occipitomental (Waters) view was positive in 83%. The combined rate was 97%.[56] If the diagnosis is unclear, CT in the axial and especially coronal planes accurately detects the fracture and reveals its extent (Figs. 15-27B and 15-28B). CT can also identify concomitant globe and soft tissue injuries.

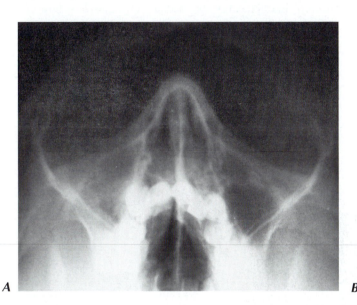
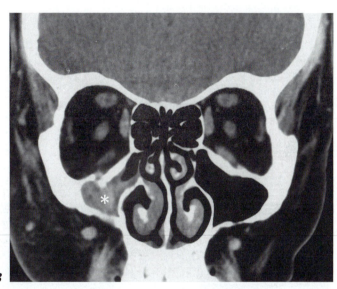

A   *B*

FIGURE 15-27. Orbital floor fracture. *A.* The fracture is not visible on this Waters view. The right maxillary sinus is opacified. *B.* On coronal CT, the depressed fracture fragment appears as a "trap door." The maxillary sinus is filled with blood (*asterisk*).

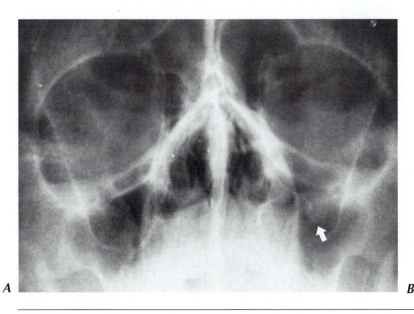
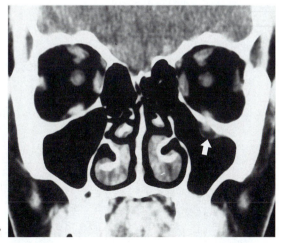

A   *B*

FIGURE 15-28. Orbital floor fracture. *A.* A depressed fragment of the left orbital floor is faintly visible on this Waters view. Herniation of orbital soft tissues produces a "teardrop" sign at the roof of the maxillary sinus (*arrow*). *B.* On coronal CT, a break in the orbital floor is seen and there is a soft tissue collection at the roof of the maxillary sinus. The inferior rectus muscle is entrapped.

TABLE 15-6

Radiographic Signs of a Blowout Fracture

Waters view—orbital floor fracture
1. Orbital floor (fine white line) is obliterated, widened, or displaced downward ("trap-door" sign).
2. Bright white line seen within the maxillary sinus represents the orbital floor fragment.
3. Maxillary sinus air-fluid level or diffuse opacification.
4. Overlying soft tissue swelling (nonspecific).
5. Herniation of orbital contents into the roof of the maxillary sinus ("teardrop" sign).
6. Orbital emphysema (especially medial wall fracture; also orbital floor and frontal sinus).
7. Inferior orbital rim and lateral wall of the maxillary sinus are intact.

Caldwell view—medial orbital wall fracture
1. Opacification of ethmoid air cells (medial orbital wall fracture).
2. Fracture or obliteration of the medial orbital wall (lamina papyracea).

(Copyright David T. Schwartz, M.D.)

Medial Orbital Wall Fractures.   Medial orbital wall fractures are common. Most are associated with other midface fractures. They are present in 20 to 40% of patients with orbital floor blowout fractures. In one study of 273 patients with fractures of the medial orbital wall, only 10% of cases had an isolated fracture of the medial wall, 36% had a fracture of the orbital floor, 28% had a ZMC (tripod) fracture, and 26% had other complex facial fractures.[57]

Patients with fractures of the medial orbital wall present with diplopia, enophthalmos, visual disturbance, and epistaxis. Approximately 2% of these patients have some visual loss. Associated findings include subconjunctival hemorrhage and hyphema.[58] Entrapment of the medial rectus muscle is rare.

Radiographically, fractures of the medial orbital wall cause opacification of the adjacent ethmoid sinus, orbital emphysema, and displacement of the lamina papyracea (Fig. 15-20). The occipitofrontal (Caldwell) view best demonstrates these findings. Conventional radiography diagnoses these fractures accurately in 6 to 16% of cases and is suggestive in 27% of cases. CT is definitive for detecting these injuries (Fig. 15-29).

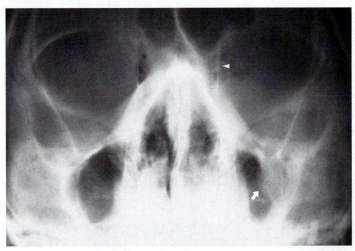

A

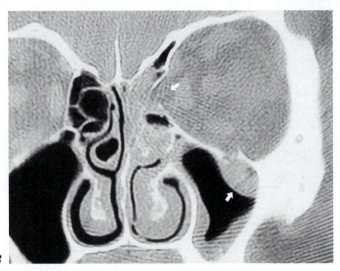
B

FIGURE 15-29.   Fracture of the medial orbital wall. *A.* Opacification of the left ethmoid air cells indicates a fracture of the medial orbital wall *(arrowhead)*. A break in the medial orbital wall is not directly seen. There is disruption of the orbital floor and soft tissue collection in the adjacent maxillary sinus *(arrow)*. *B.* On coronal CT, fractures of the medial orbital wall and orbital floor are seen with hemorrhage into the adjacent paranasal sinuses. *C.* In another patient, coronal CT demonstrates a fracture of the medial orbital wall with hemorrhage into the ethmoid air cells. The orbital floor is intact in this patient.

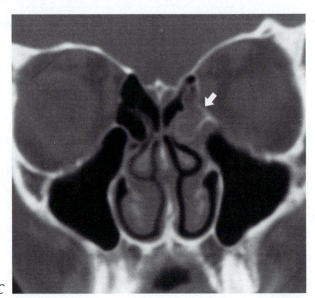
C

Orbital Rim Fractures. Fractures of the orbital rim occasionally occur as isolated injuries but are more often part of complex facial fractures, (e.g., ZMC or LeFort fractures). An isolated orbital rim fracture usually involves the inferolateral orbital rim and is the result of direct trauma to the area. Inferior orbital rim fractures usually involve the orbital floor.

Zygomaticomaxillary Complex Fractures (Tripod Fractures)

The zygoma is a dense bone that articulates with the frontal, maxillary, temporal, and sphenoid bones. These articulations form the zygomatic arch, the lateral wall of the orbit, the inferior rim of the orbit, and the orbital floor. Trauma to the zygoma will cause fractures of these weaker articulations and the walls of the maxillary sinus rather than a fracture to the body of the zygoma itself. For this reason, the term *zygomaticomaxillary complex* (ZMC) best describes fractures to this area. These fractures are also called *tripod fractures* because they extend through the three supportive struts of the zygoma: the zygomatic arch, the lateral orbital rim, the inferior orbital rim, and the anterior and lateral walls of the maxillary sinus (Figs. 15-2 and 15-30). ZMC fractures are the most common fractures involving the maxilla.

ZMC fractures present clinically with asymmetrical facial flattening, edema, and ecchymosis (Table 15-1). The temporalis muscle or the coronoid process of the mandible can become entrapped, causing trismus. Other symptoms include malocclusion, unilateral epistaxis, diplopia, and hypesthesia of the infraorbital nerve.

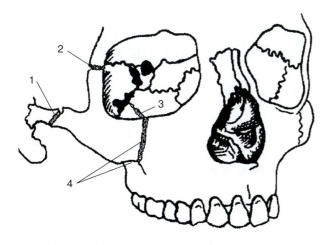

FIGURE 15-30. Fracture of the zygomaticomaxillary complex (tripod fracture). There are fractures through the supporting struts of the malar bone: (1) the zygomatic arch, (2) lateral orbital rim (frontozygomatic suture), (3) inferior orbital rim and orbital floor, and (4) the anterior and lateral walls of the maxillary sinus. (Adapted from Pansky B: *Review of Gross Anatomy,* 6th ed. New York: McGraw-Hill, 1996. With permission.) (Adapted from Rogers LF: *Radiology of Skeletal Trauma,* 2d ed. New York: Churchill Livingstone, 1992. With permission.)

TABLE 15-7

Radiographic Signs of a ZMC (Tripod) Fracture— Waters View

Check Dolan's lines (elephant face in profile):
1. Inferior orbital rim and orbital floor fracture.
2. Frontozygomatic suture diastasis or lateral orbital rim fracture.
3. Zygomatic arch fracture (single break, confirm on the SMV view).
4. Lateral wall of maxillary sinus fracture.
   May see bright white line of displaced fragment within the maxillary sinus.

Soft tissue signs:
1. Maxillary sinus air-fluid level or diffuse opacification.
2. Orbital emphysema.

Key: ZMC, zygomaticomaxillary complex; SMV, submental vertical. (Copyright David T. Schwartz, M.D.)

ZMC fractures are best demonstrated with the occipitomental (Waters) view (Table 15-7 and Figs. 15-31, 15-32, and 15-33). The occipitofrontal (Caldwell) and SMV views provide supplementary information. Soft tissue signs of a fracture are often present including opacification or an air-fluid level within the maxillary sinus, and orbital emphysema.

Careful examination of the three *Dolan's lines* on the Waters view (the elephant's head in profile) is key to the identification of a ZMC fracture (Fig. 15-14). Tracing the *orbital line* (elephant's ear) will reveal a fracture through the lateral orbital rim or diastasis of the frontozygomatic suture. By continuing along the inferior portion of the orbital line, a fracture through the inferior orbital rim and orbital floor is seen. There may be a displaced fracture fragment into its maxillary sinus, appearing as a fine white line. The *zygomatic line* (elephant's forehead and trunk) follows the lateral orbital rim to the superior margin of the zygomatic arch. Fractures are commonly present in both of these regions. The *maxillary line* (elephant's chin and trunk) follows the lateral wall of the maxillary sinus to the inferior margin of the zygomatic arch. Fractures are expected in both of these regions. A bone fragment may be displaced into the maxillary sinus, which appears as a fine white line.

The amount of displacement of the zygoma should be assessed. Inferior displacement causes an apparent increase in vertical length of the orbit. The *railroad sign* is a double line on the lateral aspect of the orbit resulting from displacement of the frontal process of the zygoma.

On the SMV view, a single break in the zygomatic arch is seen (Fig. 15-33*B*). Because the zygomatic arch forms part of a rigid ring of bone with the adjacent skull and temporal fossa, a single break in this ring implies that a second break must be present outside of the zygomatic arch (i.e., in the walls of the maxillary sinus). The Caldwell view is helpful in detecting a fracture through the lateral wall of the maxillary sinus below the petrous bone.

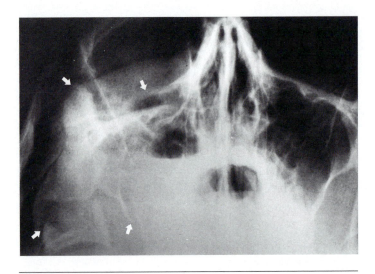

FIGURE 15-31. Displaced tripod fracture. On the Waters view, there is soft tissue swelling and a maxillary sinus air-fluid level. Fractures are seen through the inferior orbital rim, lateral orbital rim, zygomatic arch, and lateral wall of maxillary sinus *(arrows)*.

ISOLATED MAXILLARY FRACTURES. Isolated maxillary fractures are uncommon. Patients have swelling and malocclusion. These fractures often involve the anterolateral wall of the maxillary sinus. Radiographically, there is a fracture line through the anterolateral wall of the maxillary sinus with opacification or an air-fluid level in the antrum of the maxillary sinus. The fracture itself can be difficult to see on standard radiographs; CT is the best imaging study for detection.

ISOLATED FRACTURES OF THE ZYGOMATIC ARCH. Isolated fractures of the zygomatic arch are common. The occipitomental (Waters) and SMV views are used to identify such fractures, which usually appear as a slight buckling or a comminuted fracture (Fig. 15-34). Isolated fractures of the zygomatic arch are typically broken in three places, with a depressed V-shaped fracture. Impingement on the temporalis muscle can cause trismus.

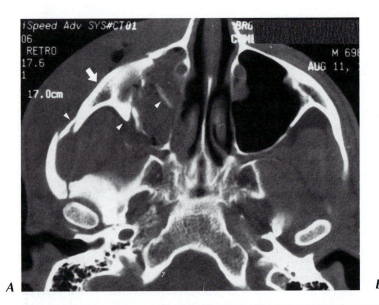

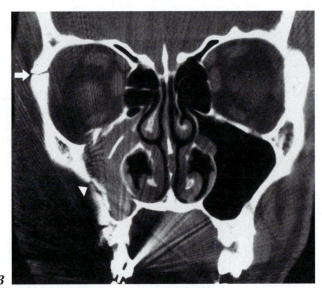

A   *B*

FIGURE 15-32. Displaced tripod fracture. CT images. *A.* An axial CT shows the "floating" body of the zygoma bone *(arrow)*, separated from the facial skeleton by fractures through the anterior and lateral walls of the maxillary sinus and the zygomatic arch. The zygomatic arch is fractured in several places. The maxillary sinus is completely opacified and a bone fragment is seen within the sinus *(arrowhead)*. *B.* The coronal CT shows the separated body of the zygoma with fractures through the lateral orbital rim (frontozygomatic suture) *(arrow)*, orbital floor, and lateral wall of the maxillary sinus *(arrowhead)*. The maxillary sinus is opacified and the bright white line of a bone fragment is seen within the sinus.

FIGURE 15-33. Tripod fracture, nondisplaced. *A.* The Waters view reveals a single fracture through the anterior portion of the zygomatic arch *(arrow)*. The lateral wall of the maxillary sinus appears buckled in comparison with the right side *(arrowhead)*. This area is obscured by overlying teeth. *B.* The "bucket handle" view reveals a single fracture in the zygomatic arch. The presence of a single break in the zygomatic arch implies that there must be another fracture in the contiguous facial skeleton, such as a tripod fracture. *C.* On the oblique orbital view, there is a fracture through the lateral orbital rim at the frontozygomatic suture *(arrow)*. This fracture was also seen on the Caldwell view. *D.* On axial CT, the nondisplaced fracture appears as a buckling of the zygomatic arch and anterior and lateral walls of the maxillary sinus. There is no hemorrhage in the maxillary sinus. *E.* The coronal CT shows the fracture of the lateral orbital rim. Fractures of the orbital floor and lateral wall of the maxillary sinus are not well demonstrated. *F.* A three-dimensional surface-rendered CT reconstruction graphically displays the anatomy of the tripod fracture. A fracture of the mandibular condyle is also visible *(arrow)*.

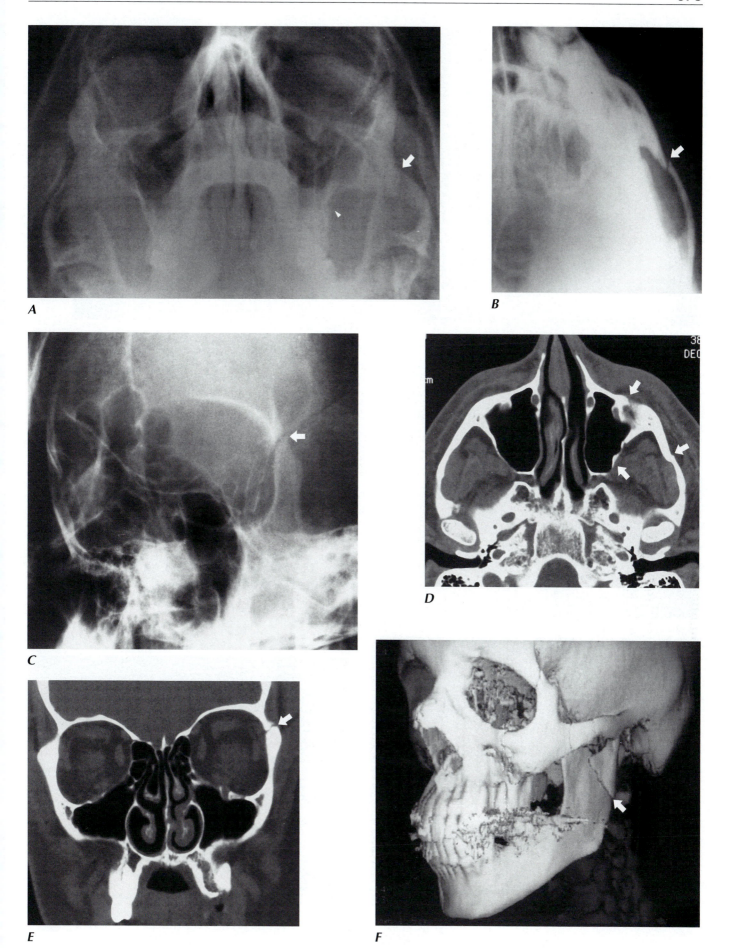

A

B

C

D

E

F

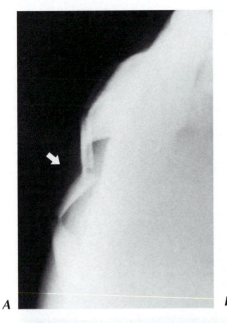

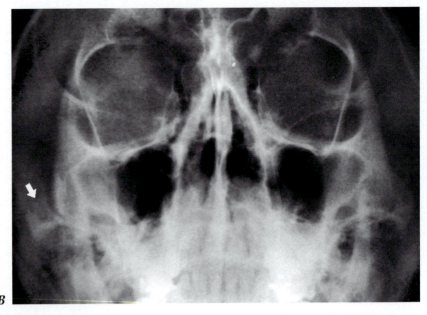

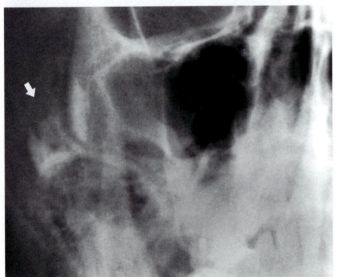

FIGURE 15-34. Isolated zygomatic arch fracture. *A.* This injury is best seen on the SMV view. A V-shaped depressed fracture is typical. *B.* On the Waters view, there is distortion of the zygomatic arch (the "elephant's trunk") (*arrow*). *C.* Closeup of the zygomatic arch fracture on the Waters view (*arrow*). *D.* Comparison with the opposite normal side helps to confirm the injury. *E.* Axial CT at the level of the zygomatic arch.

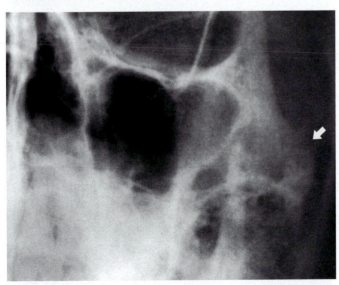

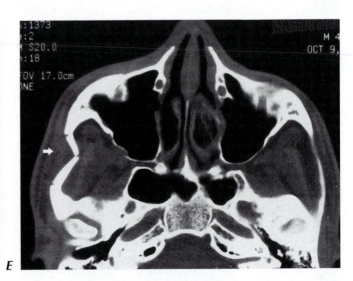

Nasal Bone Fractures

Most nasal fractures are diagnosed clinically—radiography at the time of injury is generally unnecessary. Transverse fractures of the nasal bones are common and best identified in the coned-down lateral view (Fig. 15-35). The nasomaxillary suture and nasociliary grooves mimic fracture lines. On the occipitomental (Waters) view, there is disruption of the nasal arch and deviation or fragmentation of the nasal septum.

Nasoethmoid-Orbital Fractures

NEO fractures involve the nasal bones, the frontal aspect of the maxilla, the lacrimal bone, and the lamina papyracea. These are comminuted fractures that are frequently associated with other facial fractures (94%) and intracranial injury (70%). These fractures can also involve the globe and the medial canthus.

Clinical diagnosis is established by physical examination, including palpation of the medial orbital rim. Motion and bony crepitus of this area is characteristic of a NEO fracture. An intercanthal distance of wider than 35 mm is indicative of this fracture, and distances wider than 40 mm are diagnostic of a displaced NEO fracture.[59,60]

With plain radiography, the only findings may be orbital emphysema and ethmoid air cell clouding. CT is the technique of choice for the diagnosis of NEO fractures.

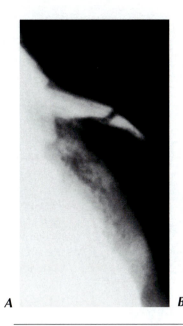
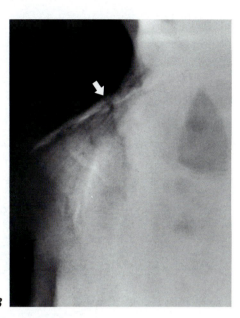

A *B*

FIGURE 15-35. Nasal fracture. *A.* A mildly displaced nasal bone fracture. *B.* A comminuted but nondisplaced nasal bone fracture.

LeFort Fractures

LeFort fractures are bilateral midface injuries (Table 15-8). The LeFort fracture classification is based on cadaver experiments. It does not explain all patterns of bilateral midface fractures, and many injuries are not defined by the LeFort classification. Some authorities believe that the LeFort I fracture is the only type that occurs in pure form as originally described by René LeFort. The other fractures usually occur in combination, such that there is one fracture type on one side of the face and a different fracture type on the other side. With mixed patterns of injury, the fracture is classified based on the most severe fracture. In all LeFort fractures, the fracture line extends through the pterygoid plate (posterior facial strut) (Fig. 15-36).

Patients with LeFort fractures have facial swelling, malocclusion, and hypesthesias. With more severe LeFort fractures, the face appears flattened ("pancake face" or "dish face"). With a nondisplaced LeFort fracture, the patient's face can appear more normal. The characteristic finding on physical examination is midface mobility. To determine the presence of facial mobility, the examiner places one hand on the forehead for stabilization and then moves the maxilla by firmly grasping the

TABLE 15-8

Radiographic Signs of LeFort Fractures

Waters view
Bilateral midface fractures are characteristic of all LeFort fractures.
Bilateral maxillary sinus air-fluid levels or opacification are usually present.
LeFort I
    Bilateral lateral wall of the maxillary sinus fractures.
    Bilateral medial wall of the maxillary sinus fractures (can be difficult to see).
    Nasal septum fracture (inferior).
LeFort II (pyramidal fracture)
    Nasion fracture.
    Bilateral inferior orbital rim and orbital floor fractures.
    Bilateral fractures of the lateral walls maxillary sinuses.
LeFort III (craniofacial separation)
    Nasion fracture.
    Bilateral lateral orbital wall fractures (frontozygomatic suture diastasis).
    Bilateral zygomatic arch fractures.

Lateral view
    Pterygoid plate fractures occur in all LeFort fractures.
    LeFort I may show a horizontal vomer (nasal septum) fracture extending through the anterior nasal spine and anterior wall of the maxillary sinus.

(Copyright David T. Schwartz, M.D.)

alveolar ridge with the other gloved hand. The size of the mobile portion of the midface indicates the type of LeFort fracture.

LeFort I Fractures.   The LeFort I fracture is a horizontal fracture just above the level of the hard palate; it extends from the base of the vomer across the lateral walls of both maxillary sinuses and posteriorly through the pterygoid plate. There is separation of the hard palate from the rest of the facial skeleton—a "floating palate." The fragment is usually displaced posteriorly, causing dental malocclusion. The occipitomental (Waters) view demonstrates bilateral maxillary sinus air-fluid levels, fractures through the lateral walls of both maxillary sinuses, and fractures through the base of the nasal septum and medial walls of the maxillary sinuses. On the lateral view, the fracture through the lower portion of the nasal septum extends posteriorly to the pterygoid plate (Fig. 15-37).

LeFort II Fractures.   The LeFort II fracture is also known as a "pyramidal" fracture. The LeFort II fracture begins at the bridge of the nose (the nasion) and runs on both sides of the face through the medial walls of the orbits to the orbital floors; it crosses inferiorly and laterally down the anterior and lateral walls of the maxillary sinuses. Posteriorly, it extends to the pterygoid plate. The pyramidal fragment is usually displaced posteriorly, resulting in a dish-face deformity. This displacement is best demonstrated on the lateral view. CT provides additional detail on the extent of the fracture and soft tissue injuries (Fig. 15-38).

LeFort III Fractures.   The LeFort III fracture extends from the nasion across the superior portions of the orbits. The fracture continues laterally through the lateral walls of the orbits (frontozygomatic sutures) and then inferiorly to cross the zygomatic arches. Posteriorly, the fracture extends through the orbital portion of the ethmoid air cells to the inferior orbital fissures and continues posteriorly through the pterygoid plates. The entire midfacial skeleton is detached as a unit; the fracture is also known as *craniofacial separation.* LeFort II and III fractures often occur in combination (Fig. 15-38).

Facial Smash.   In cases of severe facial injury, the facial skeleton is markedly fragmented without a defined pattern. This injury has been termed a "facial smash." It is sometimes also referred to as a "LeFort IV fracture", although it is not included in the original classification of LeFort (Fig. 15-39).

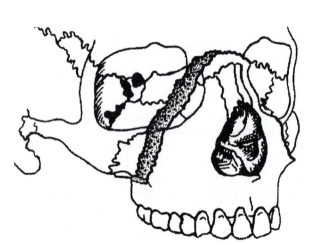

A. LeFort I

B. LeFort II (Pyramidal Fracture)

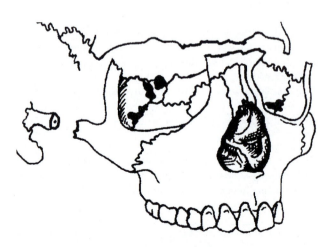

C. LeFort III (Craniofacial Separation)

FIGURE 15-36.   LeFort fractures. *A.* A LeFort I fracture separates the lower maxilla. The fracture extends through the lateral, medial, and posterior walls of both maxillary sinuses. *B.* The LeFort II fracture separates the nasal skeleton and most of the maxilla. Because of its shape, it is also called a pyramidal fracture. *C.* The LeFort III fracture extends through the nasion and superior portions of both orbits. It is also called a craniofacial separation.

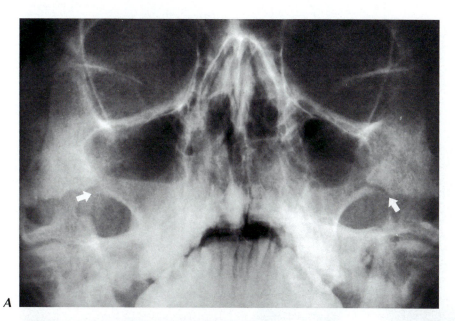

A

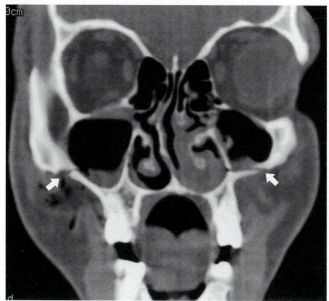

B

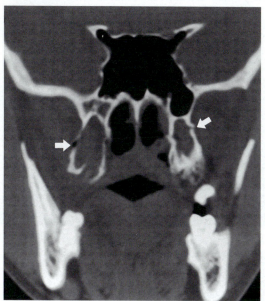

C

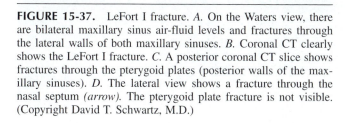

FIGURE 15-37. LeFort I fracture. *A.* On the Waters view, there are bilateral maxillary sinus air-fluid levels and fractures through the lateral walls of both maxillary sinuses. *B.* Coronal CT clearly shows the LeFort I fracture. *C.* A posterior coronal CT slice shows fractures through the pterygoid plates (posterior walls of the maxillary sinuses). *D.* The lateral view shows a fracture through the nasal septum *(arrow).* The pterygoid plate fracture is not visible. (Copyright David T. Schwartz, M.D.)

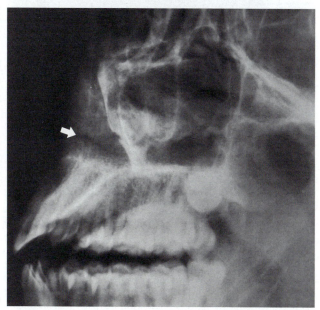

D

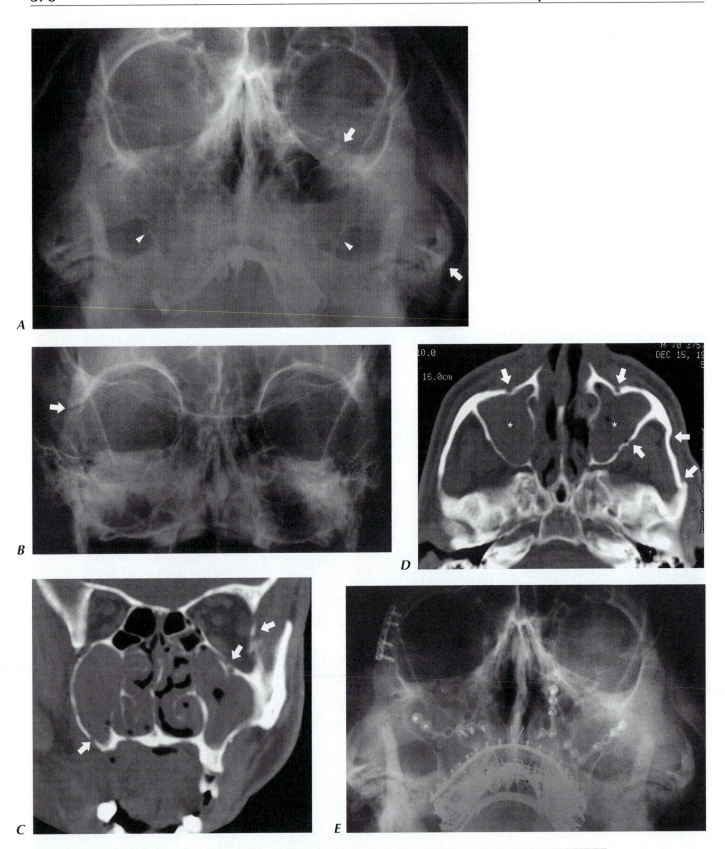

FIGURE 15-38. LeFort II–III fracture. *A.* On the Waters view, there is bilateral maxillary sinus hemorrhage with an air-fluid level on the left and diffuse opacification on the right. An inferior orbital rim fracture and a distal zygomatic arch fracture are on the left *(arrows)*. There are fractures of both sides of the lateral walls of the maxillary sinuses *(arrowheads)*. *B.* The Caldwell view reveals a fracture of the right lateral orbital rim. *C.* A coronal CT image shows bilateral maxillary sinus opacification, fracture of the lateral wall of the right maxillary sinus, a left orbital floor fracture, and lateral orbital rim fracture. *D.* The axial CT shows bilateral maxillary sinus fractures, and left zygomatic arch fractures *(asterisks)*. *E.* Post-operative radiographs show fixation with multiple miniplates and screws. (Copyright David T. Schwartz, M.D.)

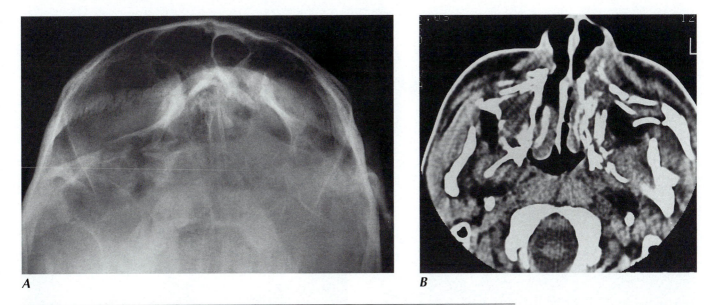

FIGURE 15-39. Facial smash. *A.* A suboptimal Waters view shows multiple comminuted midface fractures. *B.* An axial CT image depicts the severe fracture comminution and displacement.

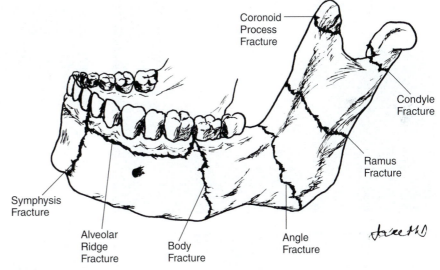

FIGURE 15-40. Sites of mandibular fractures

COMMON		UNCOMMON	
Body	21%	Ramus	3%
Angle	20%	Coronoid process	3%
Condyle	36%	Alveolar ridge	3%
Symphysis	14%		

In about 50% of cases, there are multiple fractures.

Mandibular Fractures

Mandibular fractures are common. Fractures of the body of the mandible are the most frequent, accounting for 27 to 41% of mandibular fractures. Fractures of the angle of the mandible are the second most common and account for 23 to 30% of mandibular fractures, followed by fractures of the condyles (20 to 29%), symphysis (8 to 14%), ramus (2 to 5%), coronoid process (2%), and alveolus (1 to 2%) (Fig. 15-40).[5,8,10] The ringlike structure of the mandible transmits the traumatic force away from the point of impact. The result is that 50 to 60% of patients sustain multiple fractures from a single blow.[5,8,11] Combinations of mandibular fractures that occur frequently include bilateral condylar fractures, bilateral fractures of the angles of the mandible, bilateral fractures of the mandibular body, and fractures of the body and contralateral angle.

Malocclusion, jaw pain, and inability to open the mouth fully are clinical signs of a mandibular fracture. Other findings include crepitus on jaw motion, deviation of the chin (toward the fractured side), laceration of the external auditory meatus, gingival lacerations, fractures or displacement of the teeth, and intraoral ecchymosis or hematoma in the lingual sulcus.[61]

Some 15 to 21% of patients develop complications from their fractures. These range from infectious complications such as abscess and osteomyelitis to permanent malocclusion.

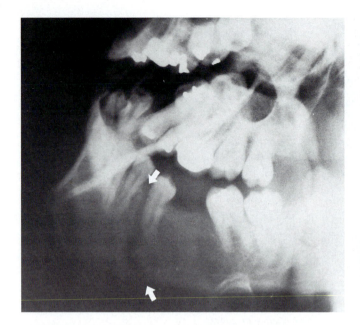

FIGURE 15-41. Mandibular body fractures are best seen on the oblique view *(arrow)*.

Plain-film mandibular radiographs provide the initial evaluation of mandibular fractures (Figs. 15-41 to 15-45). Panoramic tomography is an alternative or supplementary technique (Fig. 15-11). Panoramic tomography requires the patient to be fully cooperative and hemodynamically stable. It is often unavailable in the emergency department. Although CT does not provide additional information for fractures of the angle or body, it is useful for fractures of the mandibular condyles and subcondylar areas (Fig. 15-33*F*).[62]

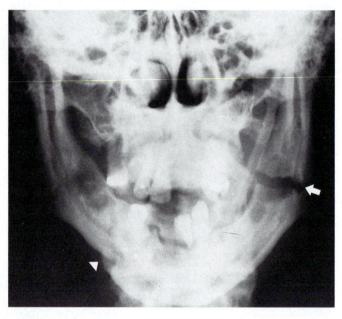

FIGURE 15-43. Fractures through the angle of the mandible are best seen on the PA view *(arrow)*. In this patient, there is also a contralateral mandibular body fracture that is not clearly seen *(arrowhead)*.

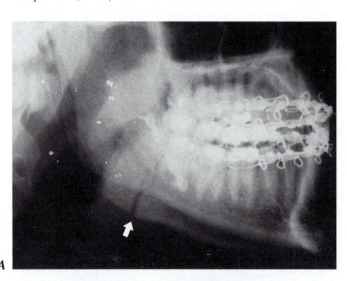

A

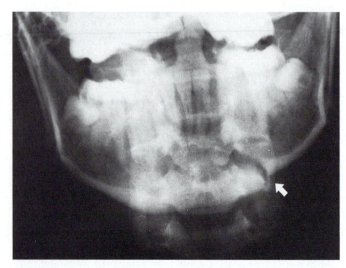

FIGURE 15-42. A fracture through the posterior portion of the mandibular body is seen on the oblique view (*A*) and on Panorex (*B*). This oblique view was obtained after the patient's jaw was wired.

B

FIGURE 15-44. Fractures of the mandibular symphysis are seen on the PA view.

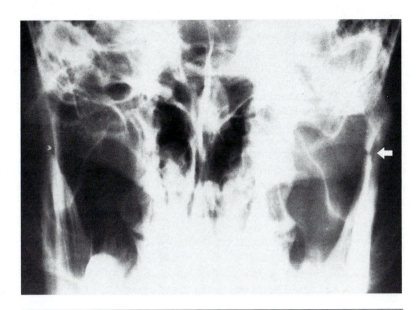

FIGURE 15-45. A fracture of the mandibular condyle is seen on the AP axial (Towne) view. This patient also had a fracture of the mandibular body (Fig. 15-41).

ERRORS IN INTERPRETATION

The complex facial anatomy and many radiographic shadows make plain-film interpretation challenging. Detailed clinical evaluation and a knowledge of fracture patterns is necessary to diagnose facial injuries correctly.

There are several common radiographic findings that can be misinterpreted as representing an injury. A groove on the lateral wall of the maxillary sinus that carries the posterosuperior alveolar nerve and maxillary artery should not be mistaken for a fracture. It has a characteristic appearance and is present bilaterally (Fig. 15-46). A groove for the antero-superior alveolar nerve runs diagonally from the nasal fossa toward the infraorbital foramen and should not be mistaken for a fracture. Underdeveloped sinuses appear opacified and can be confused with either inflammatory disease or blood in the sinus indicative of a facial fracture. Finally, the nasomaxillary suture and nasociliary lines can mimic a fracture line on the lateral nasal views. Contiguous areas of the skull, cervical spine, and mandible should be examined for concomitant injuries (Fig. 15-47).

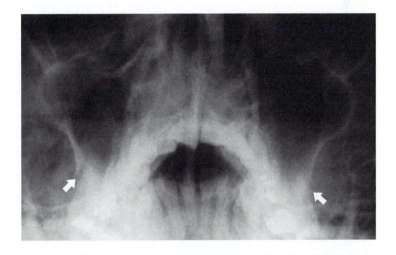

FIGURE 15-46. Pseudofracture of the lateral wall of maxillary sinus. An apparent break in the lateral wall of the maxillary sinus can be caused by a normal neurovascular groove or overlying soft tissues (*arrows*).

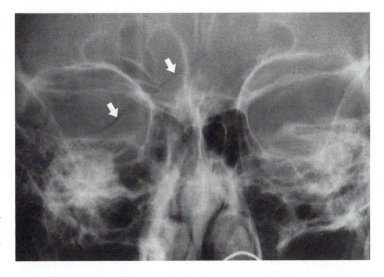

FIGURE 15-47. Missed skull fracture on a facial radiograph. A linear occipital skull fracture is seen projected through the facial skeleton.

ADVANCED STUDIES

Three-dimensional CT uses multiple slices to reconstruct a three-dimensional image (Fig. 15-33*F*). This image can be rotated to provide different views of the injury. The technique gives the surgeon a three-dimensional view, previously impossible with plain films or conventional CT, that is used in operative planning. Three-dimensional CT is time-consuming and expensive, and the radiation exposure is increased. Moreover, this technique does not demonstrate all fractures. Injuries to the orbit are better delineated by conventional CT, as are injuries to the posterior maxillary wall and posterior wall of the frontal sinus.

REFERENCES

1. Nakhgevany KB, LiBassi M, Esposito B: Facial trauma in motor vehicle accidents: Etiological factors. *Am J Emerg Med* 12:160, 1994.
2. Nakamura T, Gross C: Facial fractures: Analysis of five years experience. *Arch Otolaryngol* 97:288, 1973.
3. Hussain K, Wijetunge DB, Grubnic S, Jackson IT: A Comprehensive analysis of craniofacial trauma. *J Trauma* 36:34, 1994.
4. Tanaka N, Tomitsuka K, Shionoya K, et al: Aetiology of maxillofacial fracture. *Br J Oral Maxillofac Trauma* 32:19, 1994.
5. James RB, Fredrickson C, Kent JN: Prospective study of mandibular fracture. *J Oral Surg* 39:275, 1981.
6. Haug RH, Prather J, Indresano AT: An epidemiologic survey of facial fractures and concomitant injuries. *J Oral Maxillofac Surg* 48:926, 1990.
7. Turvey TA: Midfacial fractures: A retrospective analysis of 593 cases. *J Oral Surg* 35:887, 1977.
8. Ellis E, Moos KF, el-Attar A: Ten years of mandibular fractures: An analysis of 2137 cases. *Oral Surg Oval Med Oval Pathol* 59:120, 1985.
9. Ellis E, el-Attar A, Moos KF: An analysis of 2067 cases of zygomatico-orbital fractures. *J Oral Maxillofac Surg* 43:417, 1985.
10. Bochlogyros P: A retrospective study of 1521 mandibular fractures. *J Oral Maxillofac Surg* 43:597, 1985.
11. Chuong R, Donoff RB, Guralnick WC: A retrospective analysis of 327 mandibular fractures. *J Oral Maxillofac Surg* 41:305, 1983.
12. Lund K: Fractures of the zygoma: A follow-up study of 62 patients. *J Oral Surg* 29:557, 1971.
13. Wiesenbaugh JM: Diagnostic evaluation of zygomatic complex fractures. *J Oral Surg* 28:204, 1970.
14. Covington DS, Wainwright DJ, Teichgraeber JF, Parks DH: Changing patterns in the epidemiology and treatment of zygoma fractures: 10-year review. *J Trauma* 37:243, 1994.
15. Hubbard TJ, Dado DV, Izquierdo R: Massive craniofacial injuries from recreational fireworks: A report of three cases. *J Trauma* 33:767, 1992.
16. Schultz RC, de Camera DL: Athletic facial injuries. *JAMA* 252:3395, 1984.
17. Humphreys BF: Otolaryngologic emergencies. *Emerg Med Clin North Am* 4:605, 1986.
18. Kaban LB: Diagnosis and treatment of fractures of the facial bones in children 1943–1993. *J Oral Maxillofac Surg* 51:722, 1993.
19. Anderson PJ: Fractures of the facial skeleton in children. *Injury* 26:47, 1995.
20. Hunter JG: Pediatric maxillofacial trauma. *Pediatr Clin North Am* 39:1127, 1992.
21. Press BH, Boies LR, Shons AR: Facial fractures in trauma victims: The influence of treatment delay on ultimate outcome. *Ann Plast Surg* 11:121, 1983.
22. Thaller SR, Kawamoto HK: Care of maxillofacial injuries: Survey of plastic surgeons. *Plast Reconstr Surg* 90:562, 1992.
23. Sheperd SM, Lippe M: Maxillofacial trauma: Evaluation and management by the emergency physician. *Emerg Med Clin North Am* 5:371, 1987.
24. Altreuter RW: Facial form and function: Film versus physical examination. *Ann Emerg Med* 15:240, 1986.
25. Finkle DR, Ringler SL, Lutteneton CR, et al: Comparison of the diagnostic methods used in maxillofacial trauma. *Plast Reconstr Surg* 75:32, 1985.
26. Kassel EE, Noyek AM, Cooper PW: CT in facial trauma. *J Otolaryngol* 12:2, 1983.
27. Logan M, O'Driscoll K, Masterson J: The utility of nasal bone radiographs in nasal trauma. *Clin Radiol* 49:192, 1994.
28. Clayton MI, Lesser THJ: The role of radiography in the management of nasal fractures. *J Laryngol Otol* 100:797, 1986.
29. Nigam A, Goni A, Benjamin A, et al: The value of radiographs in the management of the fractured nose. *Arch Emerg Med* 10:293, 1993.
30. Coluciello SA: The treacherous and complex spectrum of maxillofacial trauma: Etiologies, evaluation, and emergency stabilization. *Emerg Med Rep* 16:59, 1995.
31. Mayer JS, Wainwright DJ, Yeakley JW, et al: The role of three-dimensional computed tomography in the management of maxillofacial trauma. *J Trauma* 28:1043, 1988.
32. Pathria MN, Blaser SI: Diagnostic imaging of craniofacial fractures. *Radiol Clin North Am* 27:839, 1989.
33. Gentry LR, Manor WF, Turski PA, Strother CM: High-resolution CT analysis of facial struts in trauma: 2. Osseous and soft tissue complications. *AJR* 140:533, 1983.
34. Russell JL, Davidson MJ, Daly BD, Corrigan AM: Computed tomography in the diagnosis of maxillofacial trauma. *Br J Oral Maxillofac Trauma* 28:287, 1990.
35. Berardo N, Leban SG, Williams FA: A comparison of radiographic treatment methods for evaluation of the orbit. *J Oral Maxillofac Surg* 46:844, 1988.
36. Ioannides C, Treffers W, Rutten M, Noverraz P: Ocular injuries associated with fractures involving the orbit. *J Craniomaxillofac Surg* 16:157, 1988.
37. Lustrin ES, Brown JH, Novelline R, Weber AL: Radiologic assessment of trauma and foreign bodies of the eye and orbit. *Neuroimaging Clin North Am* 6:219, 1996.
38. Hollinshead WH: *Textbook of Anatomy,* 3d ed. New York: Harper & Row, 1974.
39. Eisenberg R, Dennis CA, May CR: *Radiographic Positioning.* Boston: Little Brown, 1989.
40. Harris JH, Harris WH, Novelline RA: *The Radiology of Emergency Medicine,* 3d ed. Baltimore: Williams & Wilkins, 1993.
41. Harris JH, Ray RD, Rauschkolb EN, Rappaport NH: An approach to midfacial fractures. *Crit Rev Diag Imaging* 21:105, 1984.
42. Gentry LR, Manor WF, Turski PA, Strother CM: High–resolution CT analysis of facial struts in trauma: 1. Normal anatomy. *AJR* 140:523, 1983.
43. Hodgkinson DW, Lloyd RE, Driscoll PA, Nicholson DA: ABC of emergency radiology. Maxillofacial radiographs. *BMJ* 308:46, 1994.
44. Ballinger PW (ed): *Merrill's Atlas of Radiographic Positions and Radiologic Procedures,* 7th ed. St. Louis: Mosby–Year Book,

45. Rogers LF: *The Radiology of Skeletal Trauma,* 2d ed. New York: Churchill Livingstone, 1992.

46. Dolan KD, Jacoby CG: Facial fractures. *Semin Roentgenol* 13:37, 1978.

47. Chayra GA, Meador LR, Laskin DM: Comparison of panoramic and standard radiographs for the diagnosis of mandibular fractures. *Oral Maxillofac Surg* 44:677, 1986.

48. Ching M, Hase MP: Comparison of panoramic and standard radiographic radiation exposures in the diagnosis of mandibular fractures. *Med J Aust* 147:226, 1987.

49. Johnson DH: CT of maxillofacial trauma. *Radiol Clin North Am* 22:131, 1984.

50. Debalso AM, Hall RE, Margarone JE: Radiographic evaluation of maxillofacial trauma, in Debalso AM (ed): *Maxillofacial Imaging.* Philadelphia: Saunders, 1990.

51. Mathog RH: Management of orbital blow-out fractures. *Otolaryngol Clin North Am* 24:79, 1991.

52. Helmy ES, Koh ML, Bays RA: Management of frontal sinus fractures. *Oral Surg Oral Med Oral Pathol* 69:137, 1990.

53. Wallis A, Donald PJ: Frontal sinus fractures: A review of 72 cases. *Laryngoscope* 98:593, 1988.

54. Keene J, Doris PE: A simple radiographic diagnosis of occult blow-out fractures. *Ann Emerg Med* 14:335, 1985.

55. Hammershlag SB, Hughes S, O'Reilly GV, Weber AL: Another look at blow-out fractures of the orbit. *AJR* 139:331, 1982.

56. Nolasco FP, Mathog RH: Medial orbital wall fractures: Classification and clinical profie. *Otolaryngol Head Neck Surg* 112:549, 1995.

57. Sanderov B, Viccellio P: Fractures of the medial orbital wall. *Ann Emerg Med* 17:973, 1988.

58. Paskert JP, Manson PN, Iliff NT: Nasoethmoidal and orbital fractures. *Clin Plast Surg* 15:209, 1988.

59. Daly BD, Russell JL, Davidson MJ, Lamb JT: Thin section computed tomography in the evaluation of naso-ethmoidal trauma. *Clin Radiol* 41:272, 1990.

60. Bringhurst C, Herr RD, Aldous JA: Oral trauma in the emergency department. *Am J Emerg Med* 11:486, 1993.

61. Creasman CN, Markowitz BL, Kawamoto HK, et al: Computed tomography versus standard radiography in the assessment of fractures of the mandible. *Ann Plast Surg* 29:109, 1992.

62. Laine FJ, Conway WF, Laskin DM: Radiology of maxillofacial trauma. *Curr Probl Diagn Radiol* 22:145, 1993.

63. Gillespie JE, Isherwood I, Barker GR, Quayle AA: Three-dimensional reformations of computed tomography in the assessment of facial trauma. *Clin Radiol* 38:523, 1987.

CHAPTER 16

EMERGENCY IMAGING OF THE BRAIN

DANIEL C. HUDDLE / MARK GLAZER / DIANE B. CHANEY

Imaging has revolutionized neurodiagnosis in virtually all areas of central nervous system (CNS) disease. Computed tomography (CT) was the first major advance in neuroimaging over two decades ago. In most areas of emergency radiology, CT is considered an "advanced" study for which the emergency physician does not need to interpret the radiographic images. However, with regard to imaging of the brain, it is important for emergency physicians to recognize the basic structures and pathologic findings shown on a head CT.

Magnetic resonance imaging (MRI) has further advanced the imaging evaluation of CNS pathology. However, MRI has limited application in the emergency setting. For two of the leading neurologic emergencies, acute head trauma and nontraumatic subarachnoid hemorrhage, CT rather than MRI is the diagnostic test of choice.

CLINICAL DECISION MAKING

CT examinations are requested from the ED for various traumatic and nontraumatic disorders. A noncontrast CT scan is the best study to diagnose a surgically correctable intracranial hemorrhage. Patients selectively undergo CT imaging for focal neurologic deficits, new-onset seizures, suspected subarachnoid hemorrhage, and acute mental status changes unexplained by metabolic or toxicologic disorders. Patients with meningitis do not always require CT imaging unless there is the possibility of a focal intracranial lesion. Important information for the emergency physician is the presence of intracranial blood or significant mass effect, both of which are detected by a noncontrast CT study. If additional information is required, a contrast CT or MRI should be obtained in a timely fashion.

Physicians are generally able to predict CT abnormalities based on the clinical examination. Nonetheless, this ability to predict abnormalities clinically is not entirely reliable. Of patients predicted to have a remote or low likelihood of a lesion demonstrable on CT, 6.7% will still have intracranial abnormalities.[1]

CT versus MRI

The majority of urgent or emergent neuroimaging is performed by CT. CT is the preferred modality for detecting such acute injuries as intracranial hemorrhage or aneurysmal subarachnoid hemorrhage. With the exception of acute blood collections, MRI is generally more sensitive than CT in detecting central nervous system (CNS) pathology. For the patient with a suspected tumor, infection, or subacute or chronic bleed as well as for those with unexplained symptoms and a normal CT, MRI may be needed. However, MRI of the brain is rarely necessary on an emergent basis.

Head Trauma

Plain-film examination of the skull was formerly used for the evaluation of head trauma. CT has virtually eliminated the need for skull films in the ED.[2] Skull fractures are detected in approximately 66% of patients with severe head trauma. However, between 25 and 35% of patients with severe head trauma have no evidence of a skull fracture.[3] CT is the preferred study for skull fractures because it identifies both the fracture and the underlying brain injury. The use of plain skull films to diagnosis or exclude a skull fracture has limited application.[4]

In the ED, head trauma patients are stratified into groups at low, medium, or high risk for intracranial injury (Table 16-1).[2] The low-risk group needs no radiographic evaluation. High-risk patients are candidates for emergency CT scanning and neurosurgical consultation. Moderate-risk patients include a diverse group with loss of consciousness or amnesia surrounding the event, severe headache, nausea, vomiting, alcohol or drug intoxication, seizures, or possible depressed skull fracture. The management of the moderate-risk group is less straightforward. These patients may be clinically observed or have CT scanning. While much of the literature supports scanning all but trivial head injuries, no consensus has been reached.[5-8]

The low-risk group includes patients with trivial head trauma who have essentially no likelihood of intracranial injury. Low-risk patients are essentially asymptomatic, although they can have a mild headache, dizziness, or scalp injury. These patients can be sent home with head injury instructions as long as there is a responsible person who is capable of observing the patient for 24 h.

It is important to recognize that the above-mentioned "low-risk" group is not the same as the "mild head injury" patients described by some investigators. "Mild head injury" includes all patients with a Glasgow Coma Scale (GCS) score of 13 to

TABLE 16-1

Management Strategy for Radiographic Imaging in Patients with Head Trauma[*]

LOW-RISK GROUP	MODERATE-RISK GROUP	HIGH-RISK GROUP
Possible findings:	Possible findings:	Possible findings:
Asymptomatic	History of change of consciousness at the	Depressed level of consciousness (not
Headache	time of injury or subsequently	clearly due to alcohol, drugs, or other
Dizziness	History of progressive headache	cause [e.g., metabolic and seizure])
Scalp hematoma	Alcohol or drug intoxication	Focal neurologic signs
Scalp laceration	Unreliable or inadequate history of injury	Decreasing level of consciousness
Scalp contusion or abrasion	Age younger than 2 years (unless injury is very	Penetrating skull injury or palpably
Absence of moderate-risk	trivial)	depressed fracture
or high-risk criteria	Posttraumatic seizure	
	Vomiting	
	Posttraumatic amnesia	
	Multiple trauma	
	Serious facial injury	
	Signs of basilar fracture[†]	
	Possible skull penetration or depressed	
	fracture[‡]	
	Suspected physical child abuse	
Recommendations:	Recommendations:	Recommendations:
Observation alone:	Extended close observation (watch for	Patient is a candidate for neurosurgical
Discharge patients	signs of high-risk group)	consultation, emergency CT
with head injury	Consider CT examination and	examination, or both
information sheet	neurosurgical consultation	
(listing head trauma	Skull series may (rarely) be helpful if	
precautions) and a	positive, but do not exclude	
second person to	injury if normal	
observe them		

[*]Physician assessment of the severity of injury may warrant reassignment to a high-risk group. Any single criterion from a higher-risk group warrants reassignment of the patient to the highest risk group applicable.
[†]Signs of basilar fracture include drainage from ear, drainage of CSF from nose, hemotympanum, Battle sign, and raccoon eyes.
[‡]Factors associated with open and depressed fracture include gunshot, missile, or shrapnel wounds; scalp injury from firm pointed objects (including animal teeth); penetrating injury of eyelid or globe; object stuck in the head; assault (definite or suspected) with any object; leakage of CSF; and sign of basilar fracture.
SOURCE: From Masters SJ, McClean PM, Arcarese JS, et al: Skull x-ray examinations after head trauma. N Engl J Med 316: 84, 1987, with permission. Copyright 1987 Massachusetts Medical Society. All rights reserved.

15. Placing patients with a GCS score of 13 in the same risk group as patients with a score of 15 does not provide the discrimination required for precise clinical decision making. Patients with a GCS score of 15 have a far less likelihood of intracranial pathology than those with a score of 13. In one study, 40% of patients with a score of 13 had an abnormal CT and 10% required surgical intervention.[6] Although regarded as "mild head trauma" in some schemes, the ED patient with a GCS score of 13 or 14 is not at "low risk" for intracranial injury. Trauma patients in the ED with GCS scores of 13 or 14 should all undergo emergency CT scanning. If there is an obvious metabolic or toxicologic cause for the altered level of consciousness, and the likelihood of a traumatic intracranial injury appears remote, it is appropriate to delay obtaining a CT while the patient is closely observed for neurologic improvement.

In some studies, even patients with a GCS score of 15 have significant intracranial injury requiring surgical intervention. One study showed that 7.1% of patients presenting with minor head trauma and a score of 15 had an abnormal CT. Risk fac-

tors for intracranial injury in patients with a score of 15 include age over 40 years and a complaint of severe headache.[9] A similar study showed that in patients with a score of 15, up to 5.9% can have an abnormal CT scan. Pathology included epidural hematoma, subdural hematoma, subarachnoid hemorrhage, contusion, intraventricular hemorrhage, linear fracture, depressed skull fracture, basilar skull fracture, and pneumocephalus.[10]

Stein recommends routine CT scanning for all head-injured patients with loss of consciousness or posttraumatic amnesia, citing an incidence of intracranial lesions of 11.7% in patients with a GCS score of 15.[6] The incidence of intracranial lesions was 18.3 and 40.3% in patients with GCS scores of 14 and 13, respectively. Miller prospectively studied patients with a score of 15 who had loss of consciousness or amnesia of the event.[5] Of the 1382 patients evaluated, abnormalities were found in 84 (6.1%). Three patients required surgery (0.2%)—two for depressed skull fractures. Miller's work suggests that patients do not need a CT scan if they present only with a history of loss of consciousness or amnesia and do not have physical evidence of trauma or neurologic symptoms. Mendelow et al. found intracranial hematomas in 1.3% of alert and oriented patients admitted to the hospital after a transient loss of consciousness.[11]

If loss of consciousness is to be a discriminating factor in the decision to obtain a CT, the episode must be clearly defined. With *true* loss of consciousness the patient has an amnestic component to his or her episode. This event probably requires CT evaluation. If the patient is "stunned" or has visual changes but can remember all events, including the moment of impact, this probably does not represent a true loss of consciousness and thus by itself does not mandate CT evaluation.

The use of the GCS as a sole criterion for determining who needs a CT can be problematic because patients can have an intracranial injury and still have a GCS score of 15. In addition to loss of consciousness, other factors that should prompt the consideration of CT evaluation include age over 40 years, coagulopathy or anticoagulant medications, and alcohol intoxication. Chronic alcoholics and the elderly have fragile bridging veins due to cerebral atrophy and thus have an increased risk of subdural hematoma from seemingly trivial trauma. Other factors include progressive headache, intoxication, an unreliable history of injury, age younger than 2 years, seizure, vomiting, amnesia, multiple trauma, serious facial injuries, skull fracture (including basilar fractures), skull penetration, child abuse, and focal neurologic signs. Patients who have focal neurologic abnormalities or an opening or penetrating injury should receive a CT even if the GCS score is 15.[12]

A GCS score of 15 must be defined narrowly and applied only to patients with a completely normal mental status. The patient's verbal and motor responses must not be slowed. It is possible that in some studies showing intracranial injury in patients with a GCS score of 15, the score was not rigorously defined.

There is essentially no indication for a contrast-enhanced head CT in the initial evaluation of trauma patients. The goal in the ED is to promptly identify abnormalities such as skull fractures and hemorrhage that do not require enhancement for identification. MRI has a low sensitivity for acute blood collections and skull fractures and therefore has no role in the acute trauma setting. Subacute and chronic blood collections can be demonstrated with MRI; in the stable patient, MRI may be considered in the setting of remote trauma.

CHILDREN. Guidelines for imaging children must be more liberal. Pietrzak recommends a low threshold for radiographic imaging in blunt head injuries in children younger than 2 years of age.[13] The incidence of intracranial pathology is high in the pediatric victim of intentional trauma. In children with stairway-related trauma, 22% sustain significant injuries including concussion (16%), skull fracture (7%), cerebral contusion (3%), and subdural hematoma (1%).[14]

Epidural hematomas can occur after relatively minor head trauma in alert children with no focal neurologic abnormalities. Schutzman reported that of the 53 children who developed traumatic epidural hematomas, 26 were alert. Twenty (38%) were alert with normal vital signs and a normal neurologic examination on diagnosis. The incidence of intracranial pathology in-

creases if there are neurologic abnormalities or if there is an altered mental status at the time of diagnosis.[15]

Not all children with minor head trauma require CT evaluation. In children older than 2 years with a GCS score of 15, a history of minor head trauma, no loss of consciousness, no skull fracture, and no neurologic abnormalities, CT is not required and the child can be sent home.[16]

THE INTOXICATED PATIENT. The intoxicated patient with minor head trauma presents a dilemma. The incidence of intracranial injury on CT among intoxicated patients with minor head trauma is 8.4%.[17] In the absence of an intracranial injury, a GCS score of 13 or 14 could certainly be due to inebriation. The intoxicated patient is often difficult to assess and commonly used clinical parameters and neurologic scores are unable to predict which intoxicated patients have intracranial injuries.

DELAYED DIAGNOSES. Patients who return to the ED after an initial evaluation of a head injury remain at risk for having intracranial pathology. Of returning patients, up to 14% have CT abnormalities.[18] A subdural hematoma can occur on a delayed basis following an initially normal CT scan. Development of focal neurologic signs typically leads to reevaluation, but the correct diagnosis can be significantly delayed (average, 47 days).[19] Therefore, a repeat CT scan may be indicated in the patient suffering minor head trauma with persistent or evolving symptoms.

DISPOSITION. For the emergency physician, the low-risk patient is one who has sustained minimal trauma, has had no amnesia and no loss of consciousness, no persistent nausea, and a GCS score of 15. This patient does not require a head CT and can be sent home with head injury instructions as long as a responsible adult can observe him or her for 24 h. Both the patient and the caregiver should receive the head injury instructions. A normal CT scan in a patient with a normal neurologic examination and normal sensorium has an excellent negative predictive value for delayed neurologic complications.[20]

Some cost-saving strategies use CT in the patient with a mild head injury to avoid the expense of hospital admission for clinical observation.[21] CT scanning in selected cases of minor head trauma essentially excludes intracranial pathology, thus allowing patients to be safely sent home.[22]

Nontraumatic Disorders

HEADACHE. Foremost in the emergency physician's mind is determining whether the headache patient with a normal neurologic examination has a subarachnoid hemorrhage (SAH). Nonvascular causes of cephalalgia need not always be diagnosed in the ED. Frequently the cause of the headache can be safely determined on a delayed basis once SAH is excluded. Therefore, the physician *must* determine if the headache warrants a head CT and lumbar puncture to exclude a hemorrhage.

The importance of using CT in the detection of subarachnoid hemorrhage is emphasized in formal guidelines for the evaluation of the headache patients.[23]

The patients with a sudden-onset "thunderclap" headache require a CT to exclude SAH. Unfortunately, many patients do not have textbook presentations. Although the patient may complain of the "worst headache of my life," this alone is an unreliable predictor. Nonetheless, a severe headache that clearly departs from a typical headache raises the concern of SAH. Up to 39% of patients with a subarachnoid hemorrhage have a prodromal minor leak, termed a *sentinel bleed*. A sentinel bleed precedes a major vascular leak or rupture by a few hours to weeks.[24] A SAH tends to be associated with headache, nausea, vomiting, photophobia, and a stiff neck. In addition, patients taking anticoagulants, those with uncontrolled hypertension, and those using illicit drugs have an increased risk for intracranial hemorrhage and should be scanned more liberally. Immunocompromised patients with headache should be studied for mass lesions or CNS infections (e.g., toxoplasmosis).

The CT is sensitive for subarachnoid hemorrhage and newer CT scans have improved sensitivity. Newer-generation CT scans are 93.1% sensitive for SAH if performed within 24 h of the onset of symptoms. Sensitivity is reduced to 83.8% if the CT scan is performed more than 24 h later.[25] In another study, CT performed within 12 h of onset had a sensitivity of 100%; when done more than 12 h after symptom onset, the sensitivity was 81.7%.[26] In a prospective study, 2 of 119 (1.7%) of patients scanned within 12 h of the onset of minor symptoms of a SAH had a negative CT.[27]

Therefore, almost all SAHs are detected within 12 h of symptoms by new-generation CT alone. This calls into question whether the patient with a low clinical suspicion for SAH who has a negative CT obtained within 12 h of the onset of headache still requires a cerebrospinal fluid (CSF) examination to exclude SAH.[28] This issue remains controversial and needs further investigation. The judicious practice of lumbar puncture to exclude SAH in the patient with normal CT scans should be considered in many cases.

FOCAL NEUROLOGIC FINDINGS.   Patients with focal neurologic findings undergo CT to look for hemorrhage, ischemic infarction, or neoplasm. Although a CT scan may not detect a cerebral infarction early after the onset of a focal neurologic deficit, a scan is indicated to exclude other etiologies such as a hemorrhagic stroke, tumor, abscess or extraaxial hemorrhage.

SEIZURES.   Adults presenting with new-onset seizures require CT as part of their initial evaluation to detect masses, mass effect, or hemorrhage. For purposes of the initial ED evaluation, a noncontrast study is usually sufficient. A contrast-enhanced CT or MRI may ultimately be required. CT should also be considered in the patient with a known seizure disorder having an alteration in seizure activity pattern or who experienced head trauma during a seizure. This is especially true if the patient has a known malignancy, abnormal neurologic examination, or seizure activity lasting longer than 15 min.[29,30]

VERTIGO.   Vertigo is caused by central lesions of the CNS or more commonly peripheral conditions of the vestibular (acoustic) nerve or labyrinth. Central and peripheral causes are distinguished by history and physical examination. Patients with peripheral causes of vertigo are more likely to have dizziness associated with a change in head position, hearing loss, or tinnitus. Patients with a central cause of vertigo complain of weakness, difficulty with speech, and diplopia. On examination, there may be cranial nerve palsies, motor weakness, reflex changes, ataxia, dysmetria, decreased sensation, abnormalities of gait and station, and vertical or multidirectional nystagmus.

Patients with suspected central causes of vertigo require neuroimaging.[31] CT can detect cerebellar or brainstem hemorrhage and larger cerebellar infarctions. MRI is better than CT at detecting lesions in the brainstem and posterior fossa because CT images are degraded by artifacts caused by the thick adjacent skull.

CNS INFECTION.   Symptoms suggestive of CNS infection include fever, headache, neck stiffness, and altered mentation. In the absence of focal neurologic findings, mental obtundation, and papilledema, patients can undergo lumbar puncture (LP) without CT. Certain patient groups are at higher risk of infectious mass lesions and deserve additional caution. These patients include those with antecedent sinus or middle ear infection, those at risk for septic embolization due to bacterial endocarditis, and patients with HIV infection.[32] If the LP is deferred until after a CT is completed, the patient should receive empiric antibiotic treatment against common bacterial pathogens causing meningitis. A noncontrast CT is sufficient to detect intracerebral lesions causing mass effect prior to LP, although small intracerebral abscesses and posterior fossa lesions are more readily detected with intravenous contrast.

Skull Radiography

The use of skull radiographs in the evaluation of head trauma is largely discouraged. Nonetheless, there may be limited indications for skull films in children younger than 24 months. Although a linear skull fracture in the alert patient increases the risk of an intracranial hematoma, the information from skull radiographs changes the medical management in fewer than 1% of cases.

Of patients with minor head trauma (GCS score 13 to 15) who receive skull radiographs, up to 11% have a skull fracture.[33] Of patients with a skull fracture, 5% have an intracranial injury requiring surgery. Despite this, patient management is still rarely altered by the results of plain radiographs, for when intracranial injury occurs, there are usually other findings to suggest pathology.

Bell and Loop analyzed the yield of the skull radiographs in detecting skull fractures in adults and children.[34] They defined clinical criteria associated with skull fracture. The majority of fractures were noted in patients with loss of consciousness or amnesia for longer than 5 min, vomiting, focal neurologic findings, physical findings of a basilar skull fracture, and serious head injuries. Applying the Bell and Loop criteria, up to one-third of skull films could have been avoided without missing any fractures. This study did not suggest the elimination of skull radiographs so much as avoiding the overuse of radiographs. In this study, only 10% of the patients were younger than 12 years, making generalizations to younger children difficult. In summary, the routine use of skull films in adults is unwarranted.

Children. The indications for skull films in children are controversial. For the child older than 24 months, CT is the primary imaging modality. In the infant, the skull is easily fractured. Skull radiography is used by some physicians to evaluate young children with mild head trauma who do not have indications for CT. If a skull fracture is detected, CT evaluation should follow. A recent series found that although skull fractures were detected by such routine screening of infants with mild head trauma, their prognosis was uniformly excellent.[35]

Risk factors for skull fracture in children are cephalohematoma, suspected child abuse, drowsiness, and infancy.[36] In a landmark study of 1187 fractures in 4465 children, Harwood-Nash concluded that a skull fracture alone without mental status or neurologic abnormalities was of limited significance and does not require hospital admission.[37]

Infants are at increased risk for skull fracture. In one study, 35 asymptomatic infants were evaluated in the ED following head trauma. Falls accounted for 88% of the cases. Skull radiographs were normal in 30 patients, equivocal in 2, and positive for a parietal fracture in 3. Although cranial CT revealed no intracranial pathology, the authors concluded that infants who present following minor head trauma should undergo plain-film evaluation for skull fracture.[38] Since a skull fracture increases the risk of intracranial hemorrhage, even relatively asymptomatic infants with a skull fracture warrant CT evaluation or in-hospital observation.[39,40]

The identification of a skull fracture in the infant may provide additional information. For example, skull fracture may suggest child abuse. The detection of a skull fracture also identifies those children at risk for developing a leptomeningeal cyst. For these reasons, plain skull radiographs after minor trauma in children younger than 2 years can be considered unless the injury is extremely trivial or if CT is indicated. CT should be ordered in children when significant trauma is reported or if neurologic deficits are apparent.

ANATOMY OF THE BRAIN

A basic knowledge of gross cerebral anatomy is essential for understanding cross-sectional anatomy as depicted on CT. The brain is divided into supratentorial and infratentorial structures. The supratentorial structures include the cerebral hemispheres, basal ganglia, and the third and lateral ventricles. Structures below the tentorium include the midbrain, cerebellum, fourth ventricle, and brainstem.

CEREBRUM. The cerebrum consists of the frontal, temporal, parietal, and occipital lobes (Fig. 16-1). The *interhemispheric fissure* and *falx* separate the right and left hemispheres. The *Sylvian fissures* separate the frontal and parietal lobes, which lie anterior and superior, and the temporal lobes. The *anterior cranial fossa* is occupied by the frontal lobes; the *middle cranial fossa* is occupied by the temporal lobes. The cerebral cortex is a distinct superficial layer of gray matter, separate from the underlying white matter of the cerebral hemispheres.

There are several deep gray matter structures known as the *basal ganglia*. The *caudate nuclei* are located lateral to the frontal horns of the lateral ventricles and continue posteriorly as an arch along the margins of the lateral ventricles. The thalami have a medial location and lie adjacent to the midline third ventricle. The *globus pallidus* and *putamen* (collectively called the *lentiform nucleus*) are lateral to the deep white matter tracts, the *internal capsule*. More peripherally, the white matter lateral to the lentiform nucleus is termed the *external capsule*. This structure is difficult to visualize on CT.

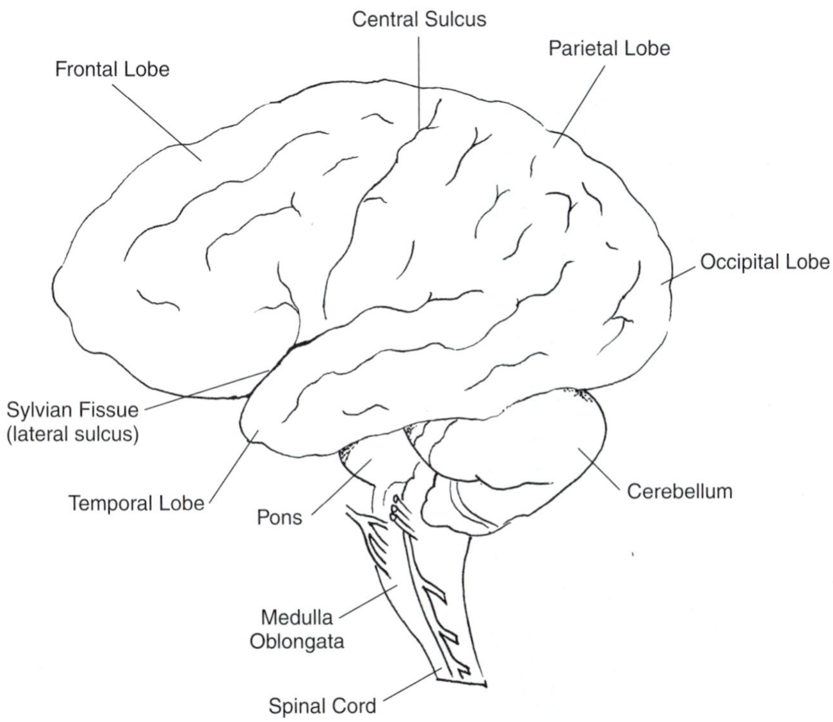

CEREBELLUM. The *posterior cranial fossa* contains the cerebellar hemispheres, the lower brainstem (*pons* and *medulla*), and the fourth ventricle. Superficial gray matter and deep white matter are seen in the cerebellar cortex. The *cerebellar tonsils* are the most inferior and medial aspect of the cerebellum. They extend into the foramen magnum.

FIGURE 16-1. Brain anatomy; external view.

BRAINSTEM.　　The *midbrain* (mesencephalon) lies between the diencephalon (*thalamus, hypothalamus*) and the pons (Fig. 16-2). It is demarcated anteriorly by the *cerebral peduncles* and the interpeduncular fossa. The posterior tectal plate has four distinct rounded protuberances (the superior and inferior colliculi) and is also know as the *quadrigeminal plate*. The *pons* (metencephalon) is caudal to the midbrain and is surrounded anteriorly and laterally by the prepontine and lateral pontine cisterns. The *fourth ventricle* is immediately posterior to the pons in the midline. Projecting posteriorly and laterally from the pons are the middle cerebellar peduncles, which extend into the cerebellar hemispheres. The *medulla* is the most caudal component of the brainstem. The medulla is poorly shown on CT due to artifact from the surrounding bone of the calvarium and foramen magnum. The brainstem is better visualized by MRI.

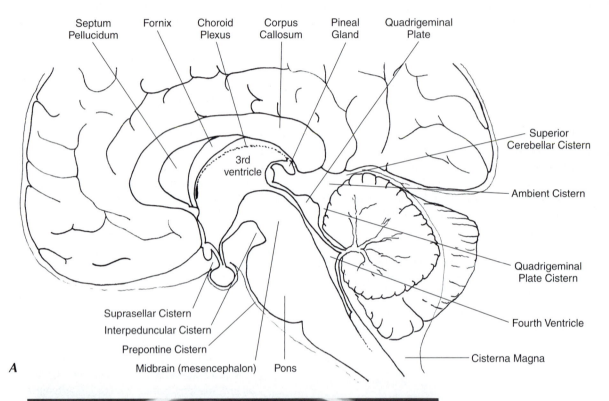

Septum Pellucidum　Fornix　Choroid Plexus　Corpus Callosum　Pineal Gland　Quadrigeminal Plate

3rd ventricle

Superior Cerebellar Cistern

Ambient Cistern

Quadrigeminal Plate Cistern

Fourth Ventricle

Cisterna Magna

Suprasellar Cistern
Interpeduncular Cistern
Prepontine Cistern
Midbrain (mesencephalon)　Pons

A

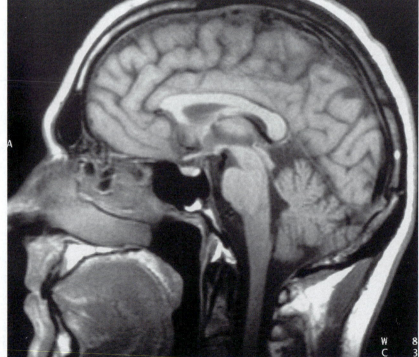

B

FIGURE 16-2.　*A.* Midsagittal section of brain showing brainstem, cisterns, and ventricles. The ambient cistern includes the superior cerebellar cistern, the quadrigeminal plate cistern, and the lateral pontine cisterns. The septum pellucidum is a thin membrane between the anterior horns of the lateral ventricles. (Copyright David T. Schwartz, MD) *B.* Midsagittal MRI.

VENTRICLES AND CISTERNS. The spaces containing CSF are the ventricles and the subarachnoid space. These CSF spaces are readily visualized by CT. The *ventricular system* consists of four interconnected compartments within the brain containing CSF (Fig. 16-3). Each of the paired *lateral ventricles* has a frontal (anterior) horn, a body, a temporal (inferior) horn, and an occipital (posterior) horn. The bodies of the lateral ventricles have a crescent configuration and lie beneath the *corpus callosum*. The medial and inferior aspects of the frontal horns are connected to the third ventricle by the paired *foramina of Monro*. The *third ventricle* is midline and is an ovoid, slit-like space located between the two thalami. Anteriorly and inferiorly, the third ventricle has a funnel-shaped extension to the hypothalamus and pituitary stalk known as the *infundibulum*. Posteriorly and inferiorly, the third ventricle extends into the *aqueduct of Sylvius*, which connects to the *fourth ventricle*. The fourth ventricle is in the midline between the two middle cerebellar peduncles and is located posterior to the pons and anterior to the cerebellum. CSF fluid exits the ventricular system at the caudal extent of the fourth ventricle through the midline *foramen of Magendie* and the two lateral *foramina of Luschka*.

Surrounding the midbrain, brainstem, and cerebellum, the subarachnoid space widens into several interconnecting spaces called *cisterns* (Fig. 16-2). The nomenclature of these cisterns is variable depending on whether gross or cross-sectional anatomy is being used. The cisterns surrounding the midbrain, pons, and superior aspect of the cerebellum are referred to as the *perimesencephalic cisterns*. The *suprasellar cistern* is located in the midline just above the sella turcica. On CT, the suprasellar cistern looks like a five-pointed star and is sometimes referred to as the "pentagonal cistern." This cistern extends slightly posteriorly and superiorly to the space between the cerebral peduncles of the midbrain and is called the *interpeduncular cistern*. Just posterior to the midbrain tectum (the quadrigeminal plate) is the *quadrigeminal cistern*, which has a crescent shape on CT. It extends superiorly above the cerebellum into the *superior cerebellar cistern*. This extends laterally around the pons. This entire superior and posterior cisternal space is also know as the *ambient cistern*. Anterior to the pons is the *prepontine cistern*. The most inferior of the cisternal spaces, below the cerebellum and posterior to the medulla, is the *cisterna magna* or *cerebellomedullary cistern*. The CSF enters the cisterna magna through fenestrations in the inferior extent of the fourth ventricle. From here, CSF flows to all the subarachnoid spaces bathing the brain and spinal cord.

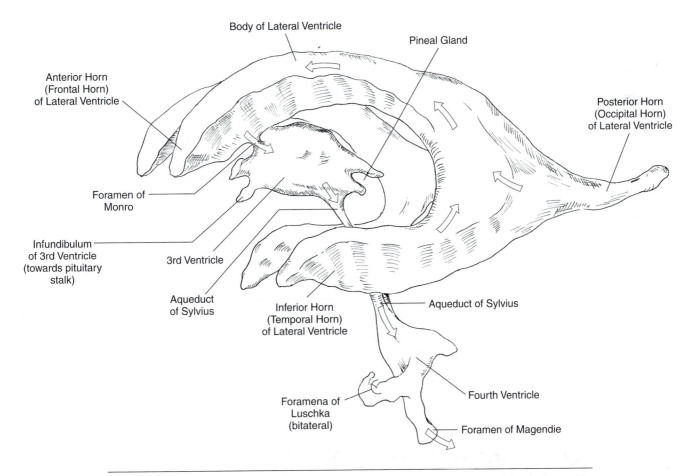

FIGURE 16-3. Anatomy of the ventricular system of the brain. A cast of the ventricles is shown. The substance of the brain has been removed. The flow of CSF (cerebral spinal fluid) is shown by arrows.

VASCULAR ANATOMY.   The cerebrum and cerebellum are supplied by branches of the anterior cerebral artery (ACA), middle cerebral artery (MCA), and posterior cerebral artery (PCA). The ACA supplies the medial frontal lobes and anterior aspect of the parietal lobes. The MCA supplies the posterior parietal lobes, the cortex underlying the Sylvian fissures (the *insula*), and portions of the temporal lobes. The PCA provides flow to the parietal, occipital, and temporal lobes as well as portions of the thalamus and midbrain. These six major cerebral arteries are connected by anastomotic branches (the anterior and posterior communicating arteries) that form the *circle of Willis* at the base of the cerebrum, anterior to the midbrain. The deep structures of the brain (e.g., basal ganglia, deep white matter) are supplied by small perforating branches that arise from the circle of Willis and the larger trunks of the ACA, MCA, and PCA.

CT CROSS-SECTIONAL ANATOMY

The orientation of CT slices is not in a true axial plane. CT slices are in an oblique (tilted) plane that follows that base of the skull. The level and anatomy of the various CT slices is relatively constant. Each slice can be located on a midsagittal section of the brain (Fig. 16-4). Eight typical levels show the primary anatomic landmarks (Fig. 16-6). Each slice is named for a distinctive structure seen in the image. The features of some slices are likened to commonplace objects—the quadrigeminal cistern to a smiling face, the midbrain to a heart, and the suprasellar cistern to a five-pointed star. The levels shown use thin sections through the base of the brain (5 mm rather than 10 mm) because the structures are smaller in that region. There may be minor variations depending on the particular patient, the amount of age-related atrophy, and variations in the tilt of the CT slices. The anatomy of each slice should be correlated with the gross anatomy described above.

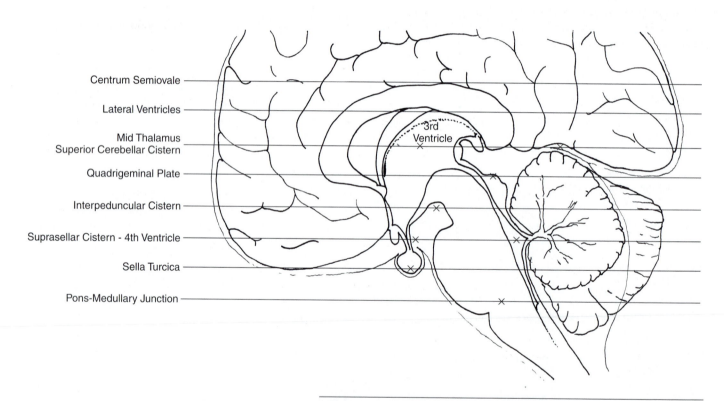

FIGURE 16-4.   Cross-sectional anatomy; × sagittal section locator. Typical slices through the middle and lower brain. In this region, slices are often 5 mm thick. (Copyright David T. Schwartz, MD)

RADIOGRAPHIC TECHNIQUE

Plain Skull Films

A skull series includes a minimum of two radiographs: a frontal [posteroanterior (PA)] view and a lateral view. A third projection, Towne view, is frequently added (Fig. 16-5).

The *frontal view* is obtained with the patient's forehead closest to the film. It provides the best view of the orbits, the frontal bones, and portions of the parietal and occipital bones.

The *lateral view* is obtained 90° perpendicular to the frontal projection. This view shows the parietal bones, the squamous portion of the temporal bones, and part of the occipital bone. It detects skull fractures in these regions.

The *Towne view* is useful for evaluating the occipital bone, the petrous bones, and the mastoid air cells. This view detects fractures of the base of the skull. Towne view is obtained with the x-ray beam angled approximately 25° to 35° caudad with respect to the orbitomeatal line.[41]

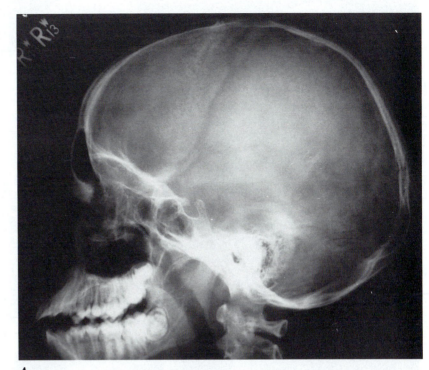

A

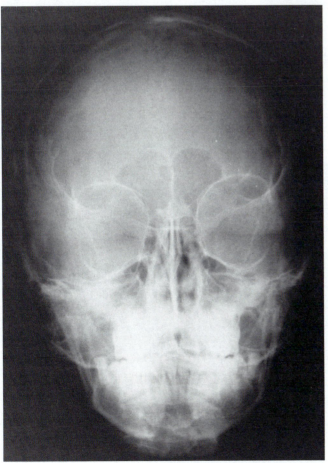

B

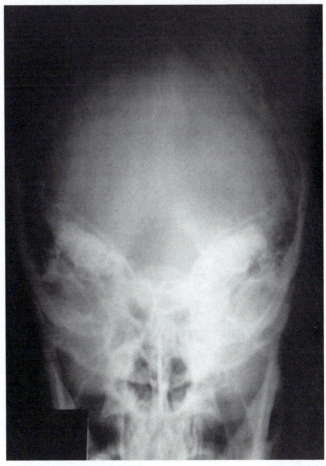

C

FIGURE 16-5. Skull series. *A*. Lateral view. *B*. AP view. *C*. Towne view.

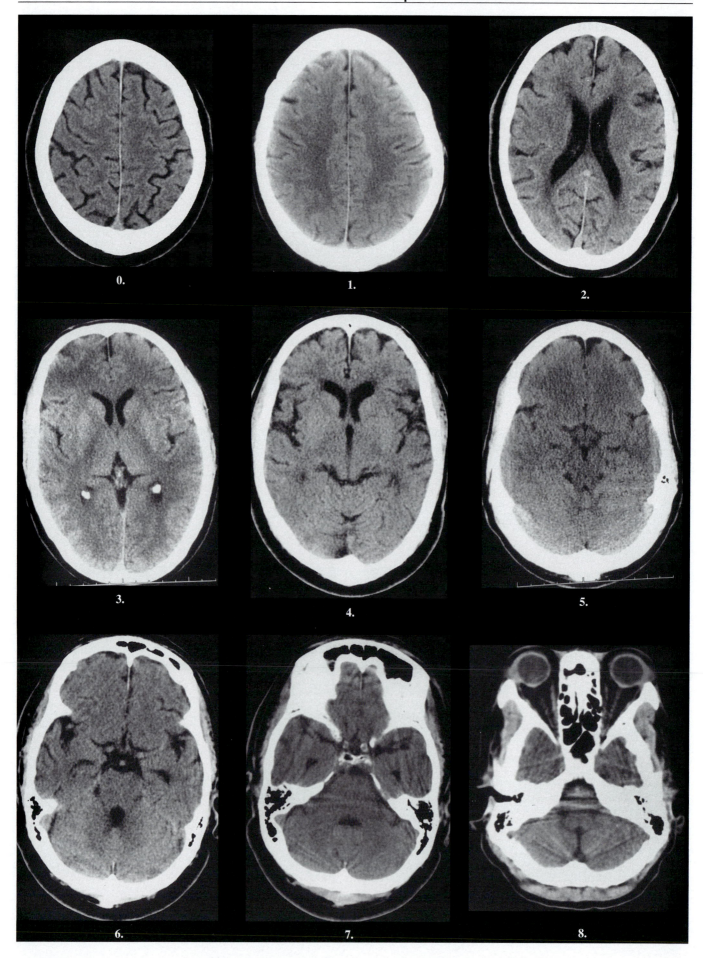

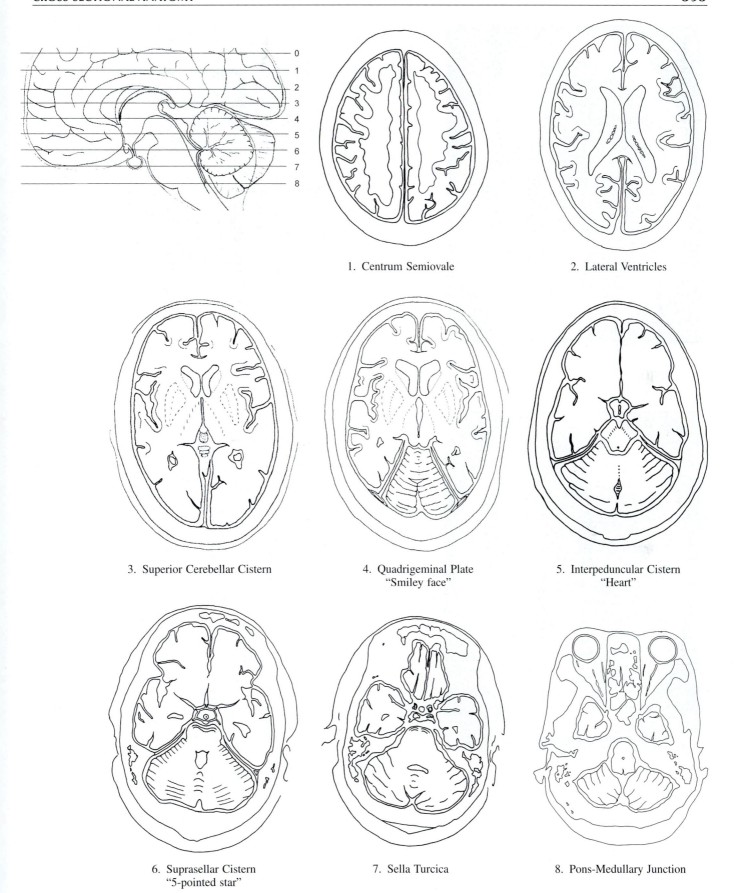

1. Centrum Semiovale

2. Lateral Ventricles

3. Superior Cerebellar Cistern

4. Quadrigeminal Plate
"Smiley face"

5. Interpeduncular Cistern
"Heart"

6. Suprasellar Cistern
"5-pointed star"

7. Sella Turcica

8. Pons-Medullary Junction

FIGURE 16-6.   Cross-sectional CT Anatomy. Characteristic slices through the middle and lower brain.

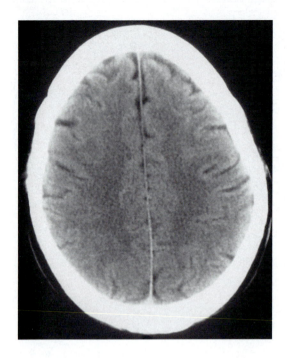

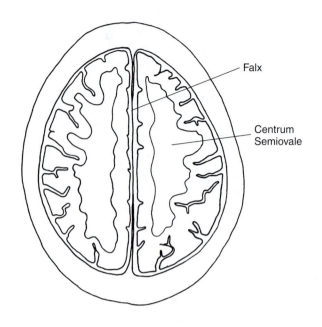

1. Centrum Semiovale

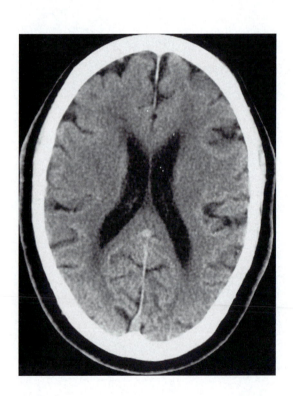

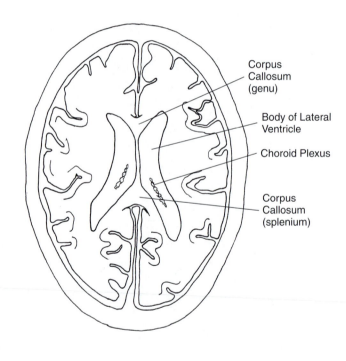

2. Lateral Ventricles

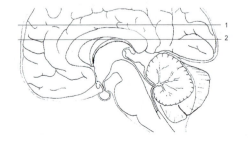

FIGURE 16-6. (*continued*)   Normal CT anatomy. Standard axial images.

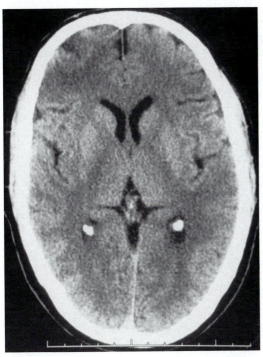

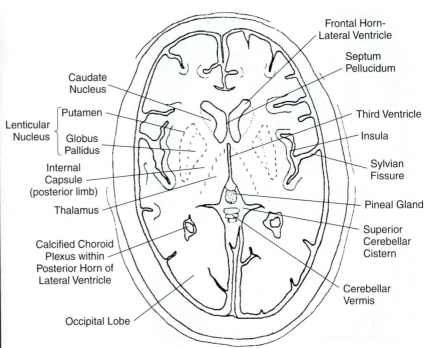

Frontal Horn-
Lateral Ventricle

Septum
Pellucidum

Caudate
Nucleus

Putamen

Lenticular
Nucleus

Globus
Pallidus

Third Ventricle

Insula

Sylvian
Fissure

Internal
Capsule
(posterior limb)

Thalamus

Pineal Gland

Superior
Cerebellar
Cistern

Calcified Choroid
Plexus within
Posterior Horn of
Lateral Ventricle

Cerebellar
Vermis

Occipital Lobe

3. Superior Cerebellar Cistern

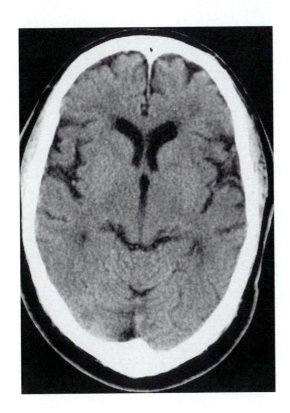

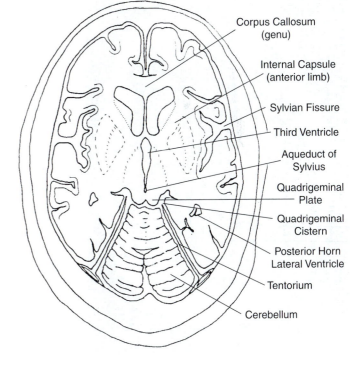

Corpus Callosum
(genu)

Internal Capsule
(anterior limb)

Sylvian Fissure

Third Ventricle

Aqueduct of
Sylvius

Quadrigeminal
Plate

Quadrigeminal
Cistern

Posterior Horn
Lateral Ventricle

Tentorium

Cerebellum

4. Quadrigeminal Plate

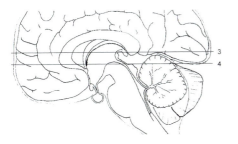

3

4

FIGURE 16-6. (*continued*)

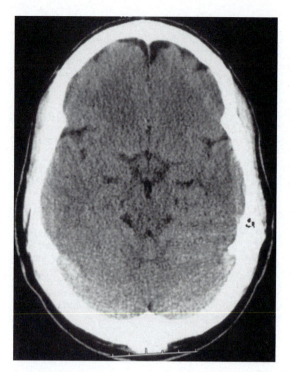

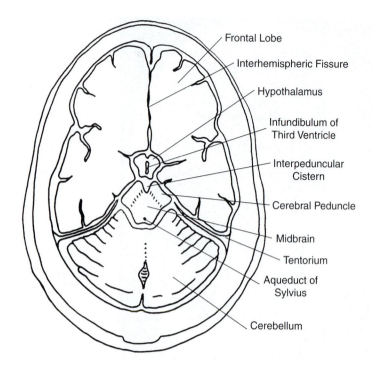

5. Interpeduncular Cistern

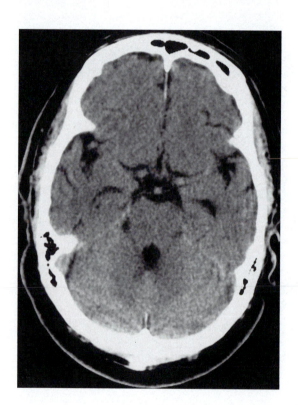

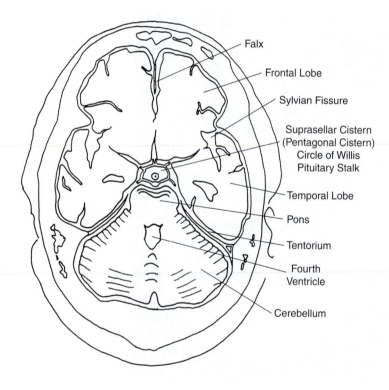

6. Suprasellar Cistern

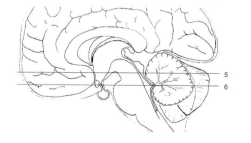

FIGURE 16-6. (*continued*)

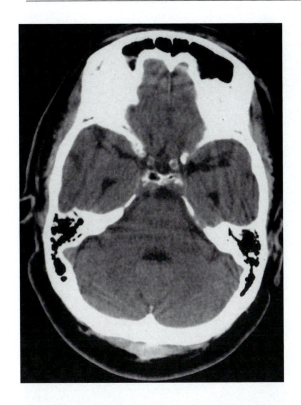

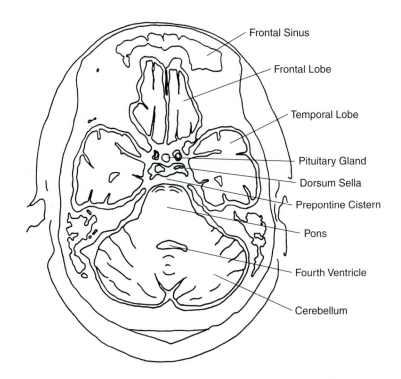

Frontal Sinus

Frontal Lobe

Temporal Lobe

Pituitary Gland

Dorsum Sella

Prepontine Cistern

Pons

Fourth Ventricle

Cerebellum

7. Sella Turcica

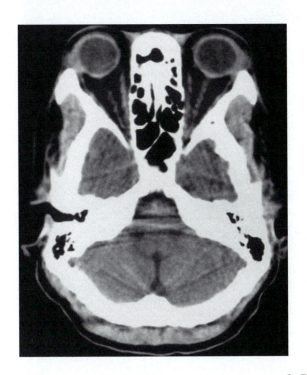

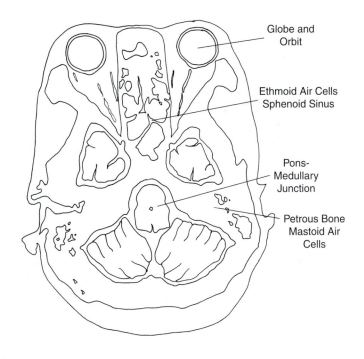

Globe and
Orbit

Ethmoid Air Cells
Sphenoid Sinus

Pons-
Medullary
Junction

Petrous Bone
Mastoid Air
Cells

8. Pons-Medullary Junction

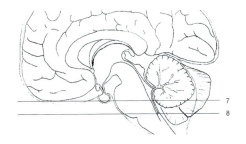

7
8

FIGURE 16-6. (*continued*)

Computed Tomography

A standard CT of the head is obtained using 5-mm to 10-mm sequential slices from the skull base to the vertex of the skull. The upper portion of the orbits is included on the inferior slices. The scanning plane is oriented along a line from the lateral canthus of the eye to the external acoustic meatus, called the *canthomeatal* or *orbitomeatal line.* This is tilted approximately 15 to 20° relative to the patient's true axial plane (Fig. 16-7). This imaging plane parallels the base of the skull, which minimizes artifacts created by the dense bones of the skull base. Standard MRI images are obtained in the patient's true axial plane without this angulation (Fig. 16-8).

The production of CT images depends on inherent differences in the radiographic density of sampled tissues. Air, fat, water, and bone are the standard density references measured in CT imaging. Densities are expressed in Hounsfield units (HU), in which water has a value of 0 HU, air is −1000 HU, and dense cortical bone is +1000 HU (Table 16-2).

CT has greater ability than conventional radiography to distinguish slight differences in the density of various body tissues. It is impossible to display such a wide range of radiographic densities on a single image. Therefore, each CT slice must be displayed in several images, known as *windows,* which vary according to the particular tissues (brain tissue or bone) being evaluated. There are two parameters that determine the CT image display: *window width* and *window level.* The window level is the tissue density shown as a middle gray. Window width is the range of tissue densities displayed over the film's entire gray scale from black to white. A narrow window width permits discrimination of slight differences in tissue

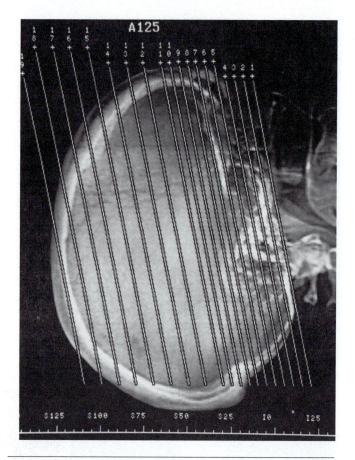

FIGURE 16-7. Scout image (topogram) of standard head CT. The reference or "scout" view is obtained for localizing each axial image. Note angulation of the image slices along the skull base and the orbitomeatal line. Compare this with the true axial plane used for MR images. Slice thickness is 10 mm for the upper half of the brain and 5 mm for the lower half.

TABLE 16-2

Standard CT Reference Attenuation Values

TISSUE	CT DENSITY (HU)*
Air	−1000
Fat	−100
Water (CSF)	0
Brain	+20–30
Acute blood collections	+50–90
Bone	+1000

*Densities are given in Hounsfield units (HU).

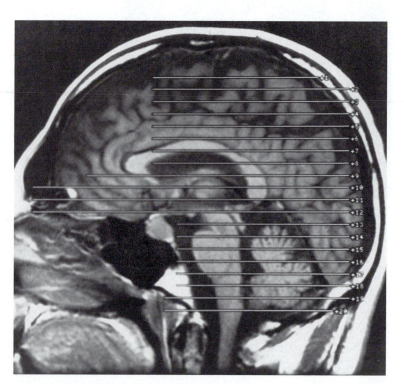

FIGURE 16-8. Scout image of head MRI. The images are obtained in a true axial plane.

radiodensity; however, tissue densities outside this narrow range will be either pure black or pure white. If the window width encompasses a wide range of tissue densities, subtle differences in radiodensity are not visible. However, it is possible to discriminate tissues with greater differences in radiodensity.

Two or three window settings should be routinely obtained in cases of head trauma. *Brain windows* have a narrow window width and are able to display subtle differences in brain tissue. *Bone windows* have a very wide window width set at the level of bone density; they visualize fractures and other bone pathology. A third trauma window is called a *subdural* or *blood window*. It is used routinely for trauma in some institutions. In other hospitals, it is provided when specifically requested. A subdural window is slightly wider than the brain widow. This makes the brain look more uniformly gray but improves the discrimination between blood and bone and can improve the detection of a small subdural hematoma lying next to the skull (Fig. 16-9).

If there is suspicion of cerebellar or brainstem pathology (e.g., intractable vomiting, vertigo, or cranial nerve abnormalities), thin (3 or 5-mm) CT slices through the posterior fossa should be obtained. In some institutions, this is standard for all CT studies. CT is less effective at imaging the posterior fossa because of the bone artifacts at this level. MRI is better for evaluating posterior fossa structures.

Patients with otorrhea or suspected fractures of the skull base should undergo thin-section (3-mm to 1.5-mm) CT images of the temporal bones and skull base in order to detect subtle fractures that can be missed on routine images. Facial trauma also warrants thin-section images to better evaluate fractures. These thin-section bone studies are not required in the emergency setting.

Intravenous Contrast Agents

Radiographic contrast agents do not cross the blood-brain barrier. Therefore, normal brain and spinal cord do not exhibit contrast enhancement. Intravascular contrast agents accumulate within blood vessels, within structures that do not have a blood-brain barrier (e.g., the meninges), and within regions of the brain where the blood-brain barrier is disrupted. Contrast enhancement is normally seen in large blood vessels such as the main cerebral arteries at the circle of Willis, and the pial blood vessels on the surface of the brain. Dural structures such as the falx and tentorium also show contrast enhancement. Abnormal structures that exhibit contrast enhancement include vascular lesions (arteriovenous malformations and aneurysms); dural and cranial nerve neoplasms (meningiomas and acoustic neuromas), which do not have a blood-brain barrier; and cerebral lesions associated with neovascularization and breakdown of the blood-brain barrier (tumors and abscesses).

Most cranial pathology is detected using noncontrast CT either by demonstrating the lesion itself (tumor mass, hematoma) or by recognizing anatomic changes caused by the lesion (surrounding edema, midline shift, effacement of the ventricles or sulci). Many lesions become more evident with intravenous contrast infusion and, in some instances, a lesion may be detected

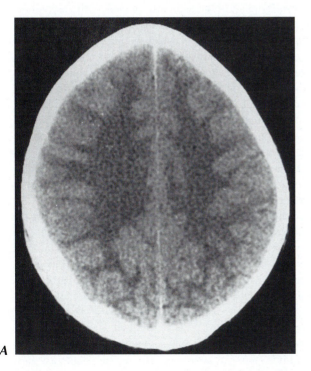
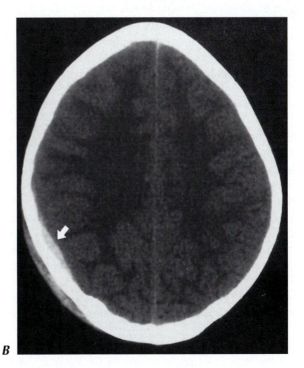

A *B*

FIGURE 16-9. CT "windows." *A.* Standard "brain" windows may be inadequate to demonstrate a small subdural hematoma. *B.* Same slice as in *(A)*, filmed with "subdural" settings—wider window width. Subdural windows augment the difference in density between the acute blood and the adjacent skull. The subdural hematoma *(arrow)* in the right parietal area is now evident.

TABLE 16-3

Indications for Craniocerebral CT and Intravenous Contrast

Traumatic
  Noncontrast CT
    Intraaxial blood (shear, contusion, hematoma)
    Extraaxial blood (subdural, epidural, subarachnoid)
    Parenchymal edema (nonhemorrhagic contusion)
Nontraumatic
  Noncontrast CT
    Stroke (exclude hemorrhage)
    Aneurysmal subarachnoid hemorrhage
    Meningitis to exclude a mass lesion (prior to LP)
  Pre- and postinfusion CT
    Tumor (known CNS tumor, metastatic evaluation)
    Infection (abscess, empyema)
    Vascular lesion (aneurysm, AVM)

KEY: CT, computed tomography; LP, lumbar puncture; CNS, central nervous system; AVM, arteriovenous malformation.

only after contrast is given. If there is a possibility of intracranial hemorrhage, noncontrast images are obtained first because on a contrast scan, enhancing structures (e.g., vessels, tentorium, choroid plexus, dura, venous sinuses) cannot be distinguished from acute blood collections.

The decision to use intravenous contrast is based on the clinical situation (Table 16-3). The detection of primary brain tumors, metastases, or abscesses is aided by the use of contrast material. Noncontrast images should be obtained initially, followed by a contrast-enhanced scan. If the diagnosis is not established by the noncontrast study, a contrast-enhanced study should be obtained. If acute hemorrhage is suspected, contrast should not be administered without first obtaining noncontrast images.

Magnetic Resonance Imaging

In the nonemergency setting, MRI has surpassed CT for imaging most neurologic disorders. MRI offers greater tissue density discrimination than CT. Images can be obtained in axial, coronal, sagittal, and oblique planes. The lack of ionizing radiation is also desirable. However, the long scanning times, the incompatibility with pacemakers or aneurysm clips, and the high cost of imaging has limited the use of MRI in the acute setting. Patients on ventilators or other life-support devices must have MRI-compatible equipment. Finally, CT offers better visualization of acute blood collections and craniofacial fractures.

Magnetic resonance angiography (MRA) is a noninvasive means of imaging the larger vascular structures of the brain. MRA detects flow within the vessels selected for imaging. It is a noninvasive means of screening patients for vascular lesions such as aneurysms and arteriovenous malformations.

TABLE 16-4A

Targeted Analysis of a Cranial CT Scan

Trauma—Look for extraaxial blood collections adjacent to the skull, scalp swelling, coup and contrecoup injuries
Stroke—Scrutinize region where neurologic deficit is localized
  Look for cytotoxic edema, vasogenic edema, hemorrhage
Headache (SAH)—Look for blood in perimesencephalic cisterns

RADIOGRAPHIC ANALYSIS

Neuroimaging studies must be evaluated in a systematic manner. This systematic approach is modified by a search for expected abnormalities. The clinical presentation determines the areas to be examined most closely (e.g., head trauma, headache, or stroke) (Table 16-4A). With head trauma, the examiner looks for extraaxial bleeding adjacent to the skull at the site of impact. Localized soft tissue swelling of the scalp directs examination of the subjacent skull, subdural space, and brain. The brain opposite the point of impact is examined for a contrecoup injury. With a sudden headache, the examiner looks for SAH in the perimesencephalic (basilar) cisterns. In a patient with focal neurologic findings, the examiner looks closely at the involved region of the brain for mass effect or changes in the density of brain tissue, i.e. abnormal lucency (decreased attenuation) or hemorrhage.

There are two complementary strategies to interpreting CT images. One is to review each individual CT slice in its entirety, identifying all of the anatomic elements. The second approach is to concentrate on one anatomic structure and follow it through all of the slices in which it appears. The first approach is important in assuring a complete review of each image, whereas the latter technique provides full evaluation of a particular lesion or anatomic structure. Both methods are used in evaluating a CT study.

The interpretation of a head CT begins with an *initial review* of the images to identify obvious abnormalities or abnormalities expected based on the clinical presentation. This is followed by a *systematic analysis* of the entire study (Table 16-4B). Each image is fully examined and pathologic findings are correlated with the adjacent images. The first images to be reviewed are the *brain windows,* because these show best the anatomic detail of the brain. In a trauma study, this is then followed by an examination of the *subdural windows* to look for small extraaxial blood collections adjacent to the calvarium. Then the *bone windows* are reviewed. Last, the contrast images when obtained are examined and correlated to the noncontrast study.

Adequacy.   The systematic analysis begins with an assessment of the study's *technical adequacy.* The region of interest must be fully included. If the base of the brain or the posterior fossa is important, thin (3 or 5-mm) cuts are obtained through this region. The orientation of the slices parallels the base of the

TABLE 16-4B

Systematic Analysis of a Cranial CT Scan

Review each individual slice in its entirety
Examine lesions and anatomic structures in all adjacent slices

Technical adequacy	Correct slices, correct windows
	Correct positioning (no head tilt, no patient movement)
Scout lateral topogram	Check slice orientation
	Look for fractures and other bone lesions
Anatomic landmarks	Identify anatomic landmarks of each slice:
	Brain structures, CSF spaces, calcifications (pineal, choroid plexus)
Symmetry	Assess overall symmetry of slice:
	Identify midline structures
	Falx, third and fourth ventricles, septum pellucidum, pineal
	Look for shift of midline structures
Brain tissue	Density should be uniform
	Gray matter (cortex and basal ganglia)
	White matter (subcortical)
	Gray-white interface
	Reduced with cytotoxic edema (ischemia)
	Accentuated in vasogenic edema (tumors, abscesses)
	Lesions (intraaxial and extraaxial)
	Decreased density—edema (cytotoxic, vasogenic)
	Increased density—blood, calcification (basal ganglia)
	Distortion of brain tissue (mass effect or volume loss)
CSF spaces	Ventricles, cisterns, cortical sulci, and fissures
	Ventricular enlargement—atrophy, hydrocephalus
	Basilar cistern effacement—herniation
	Increased density—blood, calcification (choroid plexus)
	Decreased density—air (open skull fracture)
Skull and soft tissues	Scalp swelling, sinuses, orbits, fractures
Subdural windows	Small extraaxial blood collections adjacent to the skull
Bone windows	Skull fractures, orbits, sinuses, mastoid air cells
	Intracranial air
Contrast study	Enhancing lesions—tumors (intraaxial and extraaxial),
	abscesses, abnormal vascular structures
	Normal enhancing structures (blood vessels, dura)

skull. If the patient's head is tilted to the left or right, the CT slices are asymmetrical. Motion of the patient during the study greatly degrades the CT images. In a critically ill patient, technically optimal images may be impossible to obtain.

Topogram. The scout *lateral skull image* is reviewed. Although this is mainly used to orient the CT slices, some skull fractures, craniotomy defects, and other bone lesions can be seen on this view. Occasionally, a fracture is more easily seen on the scout view.

Anatomy. Each CT slice is examined completely, beginning with the brain window images. First, the level of the slice is identified by looking for *anatomic landmarks*—brain structures surrounded by CSF (Fig. 16-5). CSF is readily distinguished from brain tissue. Some normal structures, such as the pineal gland and choroid plexus in the posterior horns of the lateral ventricles, are often calcified and easily identified.

Symmetry and Midline. First, the overall *symmetry* of the slice is noted. A quick way to identify abnormalities is to compare one side of the brain with the other. The examiner should identify *midline structures,* such as the falx, the third and fourth ventricles, the septum pellucidum, and the pineal gland. These midline structures can reveal slight degrees of midline shift, which is of great clinical significance.

Brain Tissue. Each of the cranial tissues is sequentially examined beginning with brain tissue, followed by the CSF spaces, and finally the skull and surrounding soft tissues. First, the *brain parenchyma* is examined in detail. CT can discriminate somewhat between white and gray matter as well as detect hemorrhage, edema, and other pathologic lesions. The overall *symmetry* of the brain tissue within the CT slice is evaluated. Asymmetry can be due to either a mass lesion or focal loss of brain tissue (prior infarction, trauma, or surgical procedures).

Next, the *density* of the various portions of the brain is assessed—the gray matter of the cerebral cortex and basal ganglia, and the subcortical white matter. Similar anatomic structures should have similar density. For example, gray matter in the frontal lobe should have an appearance similar to that of gray matter in the parietal lobe. The *gray-white interface* should be distinct. Loss of the interface between gray and white matter is a subtle early sign of cytotoxic edema due to infarction or trauma.

Intracranial lesions cause distortion of anatomic structures and alterations in radiographic density. Edema, hemorrhage, and calcification produce abnormal brain density. *Cerebral edema* causes decreased attenuation of brain tissue. *Cytotoxic edema* is due to ischemia and involves both the gray and white matter. It tends to be localized to a particular vascular distribution and has only a mild amount of mass effect. *Vasogenic edema* (peritumoral edema) spreads along the white matter and spares the gray matter. This can produce an abnormal accentuation of the gray-white interface with finger-like projections of low-density white matter extending outward between the gray matter on the surface of the cortical gyri. When this pattern is seen, a

TABLE 16-5

Differential Diagnosis of a High-Density Mass on CT

Hemorrhage
Calcified tumor (primary or metastatic)
Calcified vascular malformation (aneurysm, AVM)
Hypercellular tumor (lymphoma, germ cell tumor, PNET)
Postinfectious calcification (toxoplasmosis, cytomegalovirus)

KEY: AVM, arteriovenous malformation; PNET, primitive neuroectodermal tumor.

contrast study should be performed to detect an underlying mass lesion such as a neoplasm or abscess.

Increased density is caused by hemorrhage, calcification, and some tumor masses (Table 16-5). Hemorrhage has a density of approximately 40 to 60 HU on CT, whereas calcium typically has a Hounsfield number in the hundreds. High-density material outside of the brain parenchyma is due to an extraaxial blood collection (subdural or epidural hematoma or subarachnoid blood) or calcified tumors (e.g., meningioma). Bone windows and subdural windows help distinguish blood from calcification or bone since both blood and calcium have a similar density (white) on brain-window images and different densities on subdural or bone windows.

CSF Spaces.   Next, the *CSF spaces* are examined for asymmetry, distortion, and change in density. On the supratentorial slices, the two lateral ventricles and the third ventricle are identified and the cortical sulci and sylvian fissures are examined. The lower cuts show the fourth ventricle and the cisterns surrounding the brainstem. Increased density (whiteness) is due to hemorrhage or calcification (choroid plexus or pineal gland). If only a small amount of blood is mixed with CSF, the admixture becomes isodense to brain tissue and is evident only by the "absence" of CSF in an area where CSF should be found. Abnormal lucency (blackness) in the CSF space is caused by air (pneumocephalus), a sign of an open skull fracture. Mass lesions cause distortion or effacement of these CSF spaces. The CSF spaces can be enlarged focally or diffusely. Enlargement is due either to loss of brain tissue or an increased amount of CSF (hydrocephalus). Compression of the CSF compartments is an indication of mass effect or herniation.

Skull and Soft Tissues.   Finally, the *skull* and surrounding *soft tissues* are examined. Scalp or facial swelling serves as a clue to a nearby intracranial traumatic lesion. The paranasal sinuses, mastoid air cells, and orbits are seen on the lower CT slices. Fractures and fluid collections are more easily seen on bone windows. Intracranial air collections are also better seen on bone windows.

Other Images.   Any abnormality noted on one brain-window slice is correlated with the adjacent images. Depending on the nature of the suspected lesion, the corresponding slices in the

other window settings (blood or bone windows) and the contrast-enhanced scan (if performed) are also examined.

After the brain windows are fully evaluated, the remaining images are reviewed. In the trauma patient, the *subdural windows* are scrutinized for blood collections adjacent to the skull, since these can be missed on the brain windows. The *bone windows* are examined for fractures, pockets of air, and abnormal fluid collections within the paranasal sinuses, mastoid air cells, or orbits. In the nontrauma setting, the *contrast study* is examined for areas of abnormal enhancement.

COMMON CNS ABNORMALITIES

Emergency CNS disorders include both traumatic injuries and nontraumatic conditions. Most traumatic injuries result from blunt rather than penetrating injury. Nontraumatic disorders encompass a broad range of diseases including vascular events, neoplasia, and infectious disorders. Congenital and degenerative disorders are not discussed in this chapter.

The radiographic and clinical manifestations of brain injuries are divided into manifestations of the primary traumatic or nontraumatic lesion and those due to secondary changes that evolve after the primary insult.[42,43] *Primary traumatic injury* is the damage sustained immediately at the time of injury (e.g., skull fractures, direct neuronal damage, and intracranial hemorrhage). *Secondary injuries* are the delayed manifestations of brain injury, such as cerebral edema, ischemia, delayed hemorrhage, and herniation. Secondary injuries are seen with both traumatic and nontraumatic conditions. Vascular spasm can cause or worsen cerebral infarction. Pressure differences between intracranial compartments due to mass lesions cause shifting of the brain, resulting in herniation. Cerebral herniation further compromises vascular supply, resulting in additional ischemia and edema and creating an irreversible vicious cycle.

The two major manifestations of brain injury that are amenable to diagnosis by CT are hemorrhage and edema.

Imaging Blood

Detection of intracranial hemorrhage by CT is usually straightforward, although smaller hemorrhages can be difficult for the inexperienced observer to detect. Numerous conditions are considered when intracranial blood is detected (Table 16-6). The collection may be focal (hematoma) or diffuse (subarachnoid hemorrhage).

Clotted blood appears with differing radiographic density depending on its "age" (Table 16-7). Acute clotted blood is seen as an area of high density relative to the brain parenchyma irrespective of its location (subdural, subarachnoid, or intraparenchymal) or cause. This hyperdense stage persists for usually 1 to 2 weeks, but can last up to 4 to 6 weeks.

During the subacute phase (from 1 to 6 weeks), as the blood elements are broken down, the blood collection becomes isodense (having a density similar to that of brain parenchyma).

TABLE 16-6

Types of Intracranial Hemorrhage

TRAUMATIC	NONTRAUMATIC
Shear injury	Hypertensive hemorrhage
Subdural	Hemorrhagic infarct
Epidural	Subarachnoid (aneurysmal)
Contusion, hematoma	Tumor (primary or metastatic)
Subarachnoid	Miscellaneous
	Coagulopathy
	Drug-induced
	Amyloid angiopathy

TABLE 16-7

Characteristics of Intracranial Blood on CT

STAGE	APPROXIMATE AGE*	CT APPEARANCE
Hyperacute	Onset to hours	Variable (mixed, hypodense, or hyperdense)
Acute	Hours to 7–10 days	Hyperdense
Subacute	1 to 4 weeks	Isodense
Chronic	>4 to 6 weeks	Hypodense

*Times vary depending on such factors as clotting times, hematocrit, etc.

The blood collection may be inapparent on the CT scan or visible only because it distorts normal anatomic structures. In the chronic stage (greater than 4 to 6 weeks), blood manifests as an area of decreased density (hypodensity) relative to brain.

MRI is able to detect intracranial hemorrhage; however, during the acute phase (up to 24 h), when blood is composed primarily of oxyhemoglobin, MRI is relatively insensitive to its detection.[44] Therefore, CT is the preferred test during the acute stages of intracranial hemorrhage.

Imaging Cerebral Edema

Tissue injury results in the accumulation of fluid in or around injured cells. On CT, brain edema appears as a region of decreased density relative to normal parenchyma. There are two main classes of cerebral edema. *Cytotoxic edema* is seen with direct neuronal injury caused by ischemia due to vascular occlusion. This type of edema is intracellular and involves both gray and white matter. Its location is a reliable indicator of the vascular territory involved. *Vasogenic edema* occurs in association with neoplastic tumors, focal infections, or in later stages of cerebral infarction. This type of edema is due to disruption of the blood-brain barrier; it accumulates in white matter and spares the cortical gray matter.

Edema is seen on both CT and MRI. On CT, tissue edema is seen as an ill-defined region of hypodensity. There is no enhancement of the edema itself, although a tumor or infection within the region of vasogenic edema may enhance. MRI is more sensitive and even small areas of edema are readily detected.

TRAUMATIC HEAD INJURY

Skull Fractures

Although skull fractures can be diagnosed by plain-film examination, the clinical value of finding an isolated fracture is limited.[34] CT detects most skull fractures, supplanting plain films in nearly all clinical settings. Skull fractures are described as linear, depressed, comminuted, or diastatic. They can involve the calvarium and the skull base. A combination of fracture types can coexist.

Linear fractures are the most common type. They are also the type of fracture most often associated with epidural hematomas.[4] A linear skull fracture appears on both plain films and CT as a well-defined, linear lucency (Fig. 16-10). Fracture lines lack the corticated borders characteristic of sutures and vascular grooves. Linear fractures may be missed on CT if the fracture lies in the same plane as the CT slices. The scout topogram may reveal the fracture.

Diastatic fractures cause widening of the cranial sutures. Normally, sutures are no wider than about 2 mm. Diastatic fractures are usually seen adjacent to a linear skull fracture.

A *depressed* fracture is identified by the overlapping margins of the involved bones (Fig. 16-11A to C). CT can determine the depth of depression and identify underlying brain injury.

Basilar skull fractures involve the petrous portion of the temporal bone, the sphenoid bone, or the frontal or occipital bone (Fig. 16-11D). These fractures are often difficult to see on CT. Indirect signs of a basilar skull fractures are air-fluid levels in the sphenoid sinus or mastoid air cells and pneumocephalus. If clinical findings suggest a skull-base fracture (e.g., hemotympanum, "raccoon's eyes"), a noncontrast CT is obtained to detect underlying brain injury or hemorrhage. Thin CT cuts (1.5 to 3 mm) are usually needed to demonstrate the fracture, although this is not necessary in the ED.

In children, a *leptomeningeal cyst* is an uncommon complication of a skull fracture, occurring in about 1% of all skull fractures.[47] CSF pressure results in gradual protrusion of the leptomeninges through the skull defect. The "cyst" is composed of CSF beneath the arachnoid membrane. Mass effect prevents normal apposition and healing of the fracture margins.

Primary Intraaxial Injury

CONTUSIONS AND HEMATOMAS. Intracerebral contusion or hematoma is an accumulation of blood within the brain parenchyma. *Contusions* are usually ill-defined areas of pe-

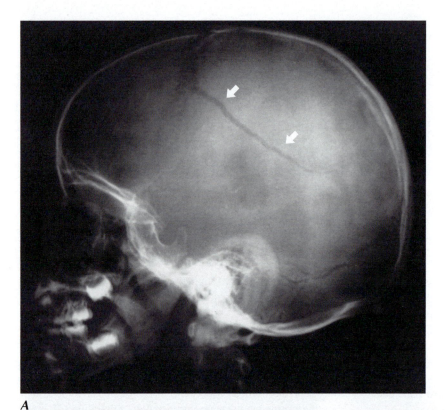

A

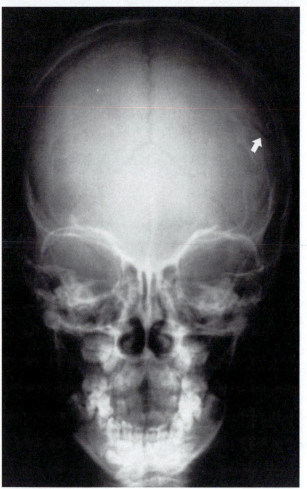

B

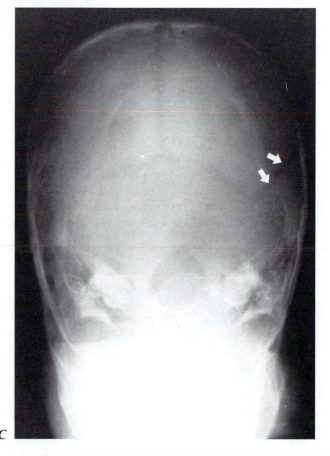

C

FIGURE 16-10.   Linear skull fracture. AP *(A)*, lateral *(B)*, and Towne *(C)* views obtained following blunt head trauma reveal a linear fracture of the left parietal bone *(arrows)*. Note the sharp margins of the fracture and lack of sclerotic margins, which help distinguish a fracture from a vascular groove.

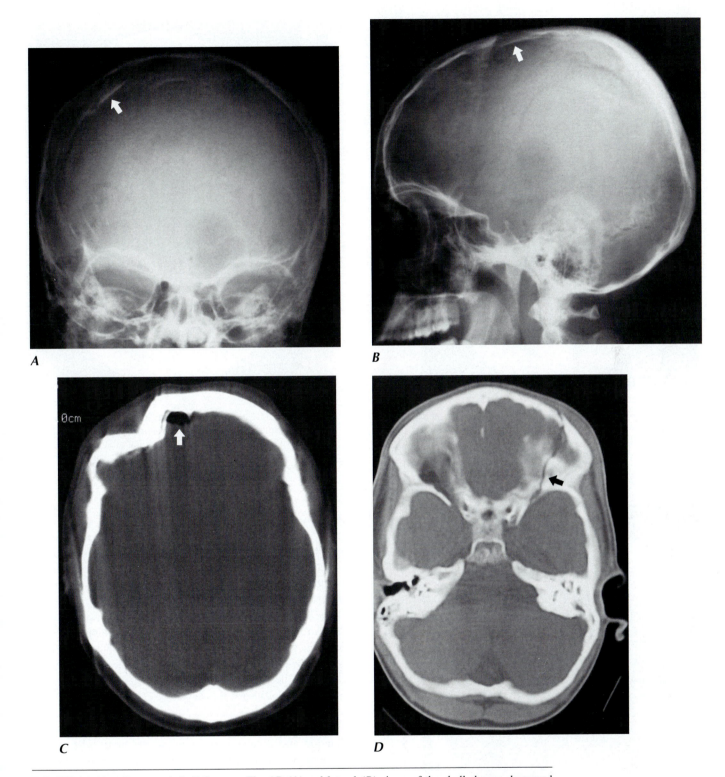

A

B

C

D

FIGURE 16-11.   Depressed skull fracture. The AP *(A)* and lateral *(B)* views of the skull show a depressed fracture of the right parietal bone *(arrows)*. The fracture is more evident on the frontal projection. Overlapping of the fracture fragments results in increased radiographic density. *C*. CT of a depressed skull fracture in another patient. Bone windows show air within the cranium *(arrow)*. *D*. In a third patient, a *basilar skull fracture* involving the frontal cranial fossa was only visible on CT *(arrow)*.

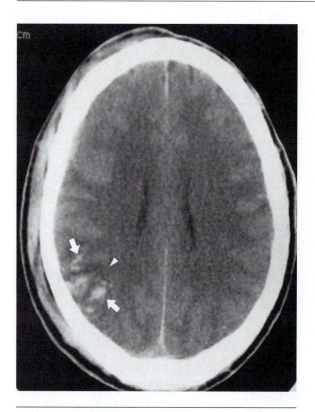

FIGURE 16-12. Cerebral contusion in a 36-year-old male following a motor vehicle accident. A noncontrast head CT demonstrates ill-defined hyperdensities *(arrows)* in the right parietal lobe consistent with hemorrhagic contusions. Low-density edema surrounds the hemorrhage *(arrowhead)*.

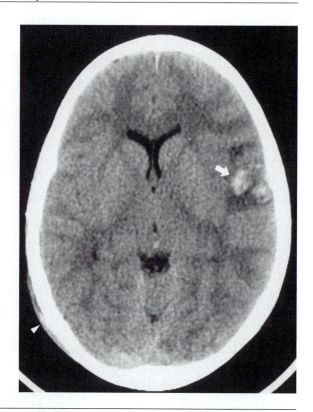

FIGURE 16-13. Coup-contrecoup injury in a 6-year-old boy following blunt head trauma. A noncontrast CT demonstrates soft tissue swelling in the right parietooccipital area representing the "coup" injury *(arrowhead)*, with acute hemorrhage in the left temporoparietal lobe—the "contrecoup" injury *(arrow)*.

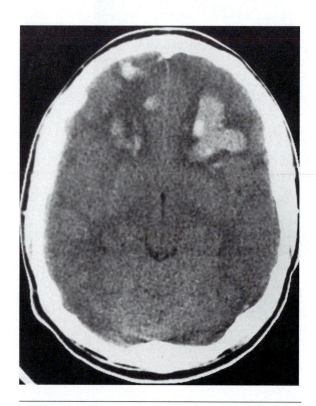

FIGURE 16-14. Cerebral hematoma in a 22-year-old man after a motor vehicle accident. The noncontrast CT demonstrates multiple acute, hyperdense hematomas. The cortical sulci are poorly visualized, suggesting diffuse cerebral edema.

techial hemorrhage involving the superficial cortex (Fig. 16-12). The underlying white matter is usually spared. A contusion is often a contrecoup injury occurring opposite the site of direct injury (the coup injury). The parenchyma immediately beneath the site of impact (coup injury) typically shows a non-hemorrhagic injury (Fig. 16-13).

Cerebral hematomas are well-circumscribed collections of blood in the parenchyma (Fig. 16-14). Development of a hematoma may be delayed. Most intracerebral hemorrhages require neurosurgical consultation to determine if operative intervention is needed. The location of the bleed and the patient's clinical status influence this decision.

SHEAR INJURY. Shear injuries result from severe rotational acceleration and deceleration forces on the brain. The "shear" commonly occurs at the junction of the gray and white matter (the subcortical area) in the frontal and temporal lobes, but it may also affect the deep gray matter (basal ganglia) or brainstem (Fig. 16-15).

Shear injuries appear on CT as small collections of "acute" blood, ranging in size from a few millimeters to several centimeters. Only 20 to 25% of shear injuries are initially hemorrhagic and therefore are difficult to see on CT.[48] If the mechanism of injury is sufficient to produce shearing injuries and the initial CT is negative, follow-up studies or MRI should be obtained. Shear injuries are a sign of severe diffuse axonal injury.

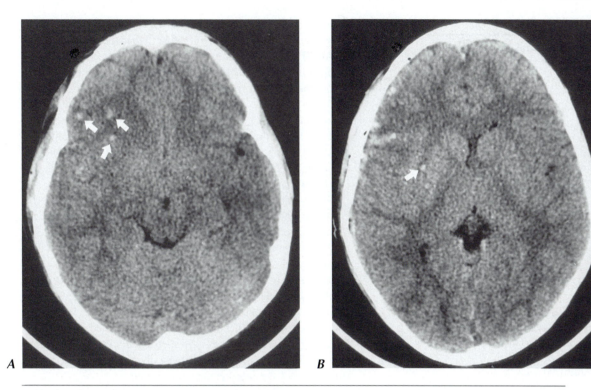

FIGURE 16-15.   Shear injury in a 5-year-old girl after a motor vehicle accident. The noncontrast CT *(A)* shows numerous punctate subcortical hyperdensities in the right frontal lobe typical of shear injuries *(arrows)*. The image at the level of the basal ganglia *(B)* shows additional shear injuries within the external capsule *(arrow)*.

Primary Extraaxial Injury

An accumulation of blood outside of the brain parenchyma is termed an *extraaxial* collection. It can be subdural, epidural, and subarachnoid (Table 16-8). The meninges covering of the brain consists of the pia mater, arachnoid membrane, and dura mater (Fig. 16-16). The pia mater is closely adherent to the brain and conforms to the convolutional markings. The *subarachnoid space* is located beneath the arachnoid membrane and above the pia mater. The *subdural space* is external to the arachnoid membrane and does not conform to the gyri or sulci. The *epidural space* lies between the inner table of the skull and the outer (periosteal) layer of dura.

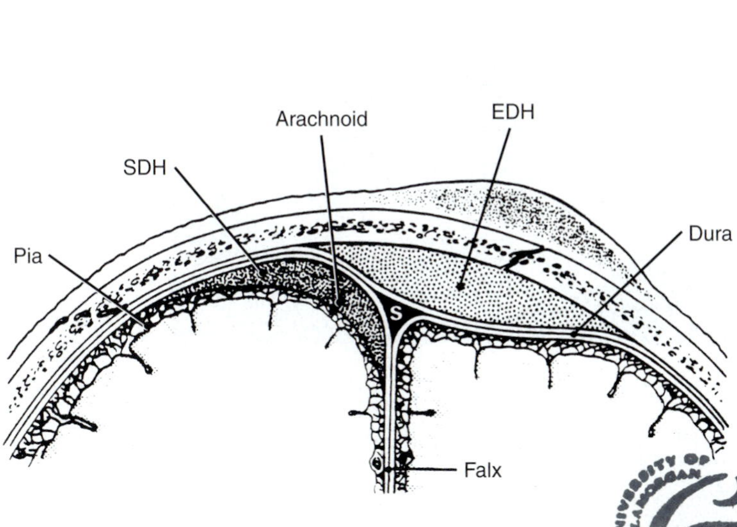

SUBDURAL HEMATOMAS.   Subdural hematomas (SDH) have a wide spectrum of clinical manifestations, ranging from subtle personality changes to coma. SDHs tend to be associated with a higher morbidity and mortality than epidural hematomas owing to the frequent underlying brain injury. Occasionally, the patient is initially asymptomatic and delays seeking medical attention.

SDHs are located between the inner dural layer and the arachnoid membrane and usually result from tearing of the bridging veins between the dura and brain parenchyma. Associated skull

FIGURE 16-16.   Subdural hematoma *(SDH)* versus epidural hematoma *(EDH)*. Coronal schematic through the level of the superior sagittal sinus *(S)* illustrates the relationship of a SDH and an EDH to normal meningeal anatomy. Note how the dura is a bilayered structure composed of an inner (i.e., meningeal) layer and an outer (i.e., periosteal) layer. These two layers split to form the dural sinuses, falx, and tentorium. The outer dural layer serves as the periosteum of the inner table of the skull. The EDH is located between the outer dural layer and the skull. The outer dural layer also forms the superficial wall of the major dural venous sinuses, whereas the side walls are formed by the inner dural layer. Therefore, an EDH rarely crosses cranial sutures because the periosteum is firmly bound at the sutural margin. A SDH is located between the inner dural layer and the arachoid. It can cause compression of subarachnoid space and displaces the cortical veins against the brain surface. Although an EDH tends to cross the midline, a SDH is impeded by the falx. Similarly, an EDH can extend from the supratentorial to the infratentorial space, whereas a SDH is limited by the tentorium. As illustrated in this case, an EDH is frequently associated with an overlying skull fracture and scalp soft-tissue swelling. (From Gean AD: Imaging of Head Trauma. New York, Raven Press, 1994, with permission.)

TABLE 16-8

Features of Traumatic Extraaxial Hematomas

Epidural hematoma
   Biconvex (lens) shape
   Usually arterial origin (middle meningeal artery)
   Usually does not cross suture lines
   May cross midline
   Frequently associated with a skull fracture
   Supratentorial location most common
   Neurosurgical emergency
Subdural hematoma
   Crescentic shape
   Venous origin (bridging veins)
   May be spontaneous (dural AVM, minor trauma in high-risk
      patients)
   May cross suture lines
   Does not cross midline (unless in posterior fossa)
   Usually not associated skull fracture
   May mimic or coexist with EDH
   Surgical management depends on clinical status
   Often associated with brain parenchymal edema
Traumatic subarachnoid hemorrhage
   Interdigitates into cortical sulci and fissures
   Usually supratentorial
   Usually does not cross midline
   Frequently seen in conjunction with traumatic SDH, EDH
   Resolves spontaneously

KEY: AVM, arteriovenous malformation; EDH, epidural hematoma; SDH, subdural hematoma.

fractures are infrequent. SDHs are most commonly located in the supratentorial compartment rather than in the posterior fossa.

An SDH appears as a crescent-shaped collection of blood conforming to the convexity of the cerebral hemispheres. Blood within the subdural space has smooth margins and does not extend into the sulci. The blood collection may extend along the entire hemisphere. The falx prevents blood from crossing the midline. In the posterior fossa, an SDH may cross the midline. An SDH can sometimes mimic or coexist with an epidural hematoma (EDH); the radiographic distinction between the two can be difficult to discern.

SDHs can be acute, subacute, or chronic. The *acute* stage is easily detected as a crescent-shaped hyperdense blood collection. Mass effect or midline shift depends both on the size of the collection and the amount of underlying brain edema. The cortical sulci should be seen at the inner margin of the blood collection (Fig. 16-17). Brain-window settings can make a small acute SDH appear as a region of thickening of the body calvarium. If an extraaxial hematoma is suspected, both brain and blood (subdural) windows must be obtained (Fig. 16-9). Parafalcine SDHs appear as asymmetrical thickening of the falx (Fig. 16-18). In adults, these are usually confined to the posterior aspect of the interhemispheric fissure.

Subacute SDHs can be difficult to see on CT scans because the blood collection has a radiographic density similar to that of normal brain parenchyma. The presence of mass effect along the cerebral convexity and the inability to visualize the cortical sulci next to the inner table of the skull are key findings (Fig. 16-19). MRI is more sensitive than CT in detecting small subacute and chronic subdural collections.

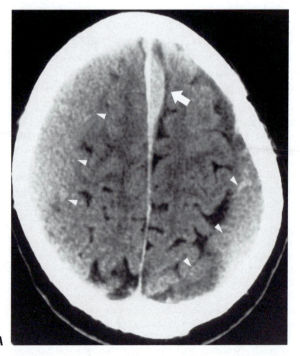
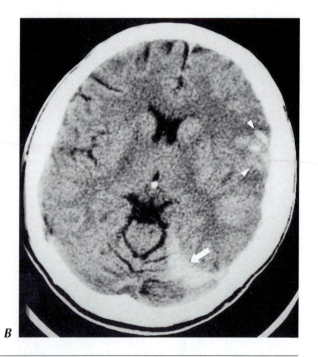

A   *B*

FIGURE 16-17.   Parafalcine and tentorial subdural hematomas. Noncontrast CT *(A)* obtained for dizziness and ataxia. Acute blood is seen adjacent to the anterior falx *(arrow)*; compare the thickness of the normal falx posteriorly. Isodense subdural collections border both cerebral hemispheres *(arrowheads)*. In a different patient *(B)*, blood lies on the tentorium *(arrow)* and subtle contusion *(arrowheads)* due to a motor vehicle accident is seen.

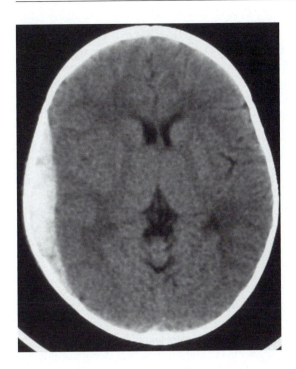

FIGURE 16-18. Acute subdural hematoma in a 1-year-old female following a fall. The noncontrast CT shows a large, hyperdense, extraaxial blood collection. The crescentic configuration is characteristic of a subdural hematoma. The underlying brain parenchyma is flattened from mass effect.

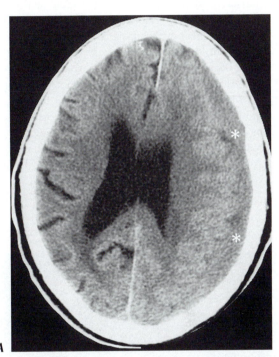

FIGURE 16-19. *A.* Subacute subdural hematoma in an 80-year-old man presenting with mental status changes. The noncontrast CT demonstrates indistinct cortical sulci over the left hemisphere with mild distortion of the lateral ventricle. The density of the hematoma *(asterisks)* is similar to that of brain parenchyma. *B.* In an 84-year-old woman with headaches, bilateral subdural collections *(asterisks)* are seen. The density of the collections is isodense to slightly hypodense, suggesting a late subacute stage. Midline shift may be absent when bilateral collections are present. *C.* Large right frontal isodense subdural hematoma *(asterisks)* following a fall injury. There is mass effect on the frontal lobe with flattening of the cortical sulci.

A

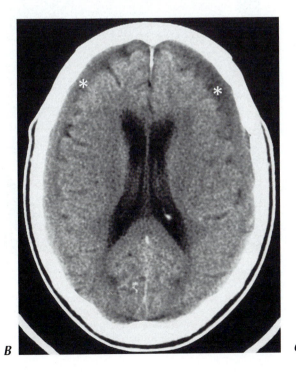

B

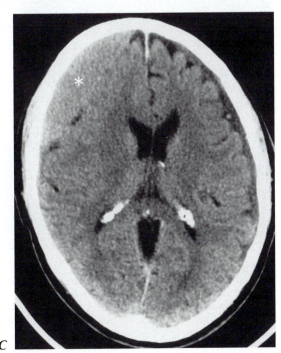

C

The *chronic* stage is recognized by a hypodense extraaxial collection. The density is similar to that of CSF in the ventricles (Fig. 16-20). Differentiating between a *hygroma* (a subdural CSF collection resulting from a tear in the arachnoid) and chronic subdural *hematoma* can be difficult. MRI is useful for making this distinction.

EPIDURAL HEMATOMA. An epidural hematoma (EDH) is a neurosurgical emergency. An EDH is usually arterial in origin and accumulates rapidly. Immediate diagnosis and treatment are essential for survival and optimal patient outcome. Initially, the severity of injury can be underestimated because of the characteristic lucid interval that precedes rapid neurologic deterioration. The mortality rate with an EDH is higher than with an SDH if treatment or diagnosis is delayed.

Blood in the epidural space appears as a biconvex or lens-shaped density (Fig. 16-21). A skull fracture is associated with the EDH in 85 to 95% of cases.[4] The fracture lacerates the middle meningeal artery, resulting in arterial bleeding. The most common location is the temporoparietal area, although an EDH can also occur in the frontal or occipital regions. EDHs that occur in the posterior fossa are usually venous.

TRAUMATIC SUBARACHNOID HEMORRHAGE. SAH is a common sequela of head trauma. Damage to the leptomeningeal vessels results in extravasation of blood into the space beneath the arachnoid membrane. In contrast to SDHs, subarachnoid blood collects within the cortical sulci, conforming to the contour of the subarachnoid space. Traumatic hemorrhage is typically located along the cerebral convexities near the site of trauma, whereas aneurysmal SAH is usually located in the basilar cisterns.

On CT, traumatic SAH has a linear or curvilinear appearance corresponding to the configuration of the cortical sulci or fissures (Fig. 16-22). Small amounts of blood in the subarachnoid space result in only a slight increase in density, making these CSF-containing structures appear isodense relative to the adjacent brain parenchyma.

INTERHEMISPHERIC BLOOD COLLECTIONS. The falx is a thin membrane of dura within the interhemispheric fissure. Posteriorly, the falx converges with the tentorium. The posterior aspect of the falx is usually thicker and more readily seen.[46]

Hyperdensity within the interhemispheric fissure is as an indicator of subarachnoid or subdural hemorrhage, the so-called

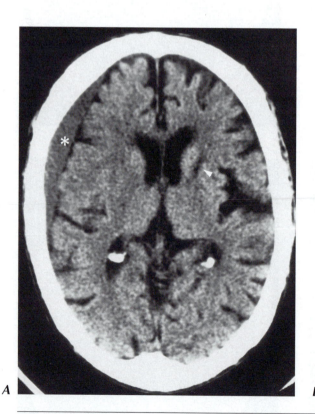
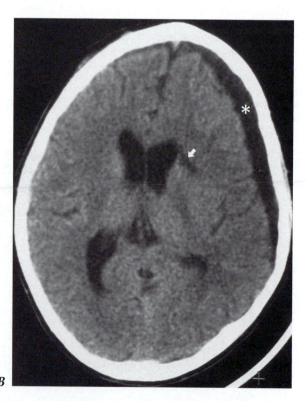

A   *B*

FIGURE 16-20. Chronic subdural hematoma. *A.* A noncontrast CT demonstrates the slightly hypodense extraaxial hematoma *(asterisk)* consistent with a late subacute to chronic subdural hematoma. There is mild mass effect on the brain with effacement of sulci. Note lack of midline shift. Incidentally noted is a small lacunar infarct in the anterior limb of the left internal capsule *(arrow)*. *B.* Chronic left-sided subdural hematoma *(asterisk)* producing mass effect and midline shift. The density of the collection is similar to the density of CSF in the ventricles. Note the small infarct of the caudate nucleus *(arrow)*.

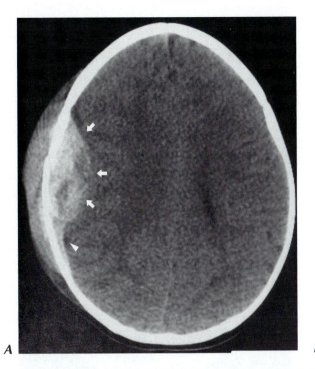
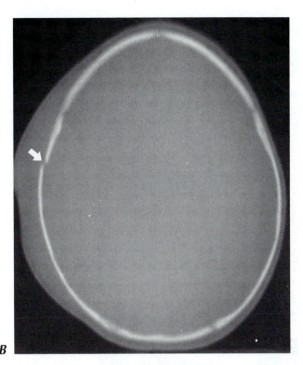

A   *B*

FIGURE 16-21. Epidural hematoma. This noncontrast head CT *(A)* shows a hyperdense extraaxial collection along the right frontoparietal region. The "lens" or "biconvex" configuration is characteristic of blood in the epidural space *(arrows)*. Note the coexisting subdural collection posteriorly *(arrowhead)*. The mixed density of the epidural collection in this patient suggests probable active bleeding at the time of scanning. The bone-window image *(B)* shows a minimally depressed fracture *(arrow)*.

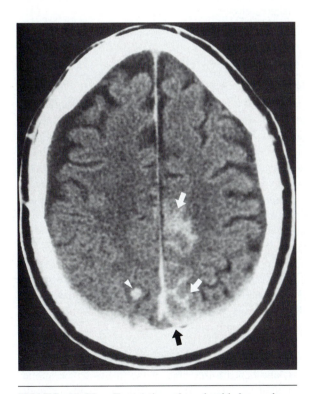

FIGURE 16-22. Traumatic subarachnoid hemorrhage. This noncontrast CT following head trauma demonstrates hyperdense blood conforming to the sulci of the medial left parietal lobe *(arrows)*. A linear or curvilinear configuration is characteristic of blood in the subarachnoid space. Note the small shear injury *(arrowhead)*. Subdural blood is seen posteriorly and adjacent to the falx *(black arrow)*.

TABLE 16-9

Differential Diagnosis of Interhemispheric Hyperdensity

Calcification of falx
Calcified parafalcine mass (meningioma)
Subdural hemorrhage
Subarachnoid hemorrhage
Diffuse cerebral edema (relative hyperdensity of falx)

"falx sign" (Table 16-9).[47] However, since the falx is seen in many normal patients,[46,48] the identification of hyperdensity alone within the interhemispheric fissure does not necessarily indicate hemorrhage. Distinguishing a normal falx from SAH can be difficult. In adults, SAH occurs more frequently along the anterior aspect of the falx, and it causes an asymmetrical density within the fissure.[48] Hyperdense blood interdigitating into the adjacent cortical sulci further supports the presence of subarachnoid blood.

In children, a posteriorly located interhemispheric subdural hematoma appears as hyperdensity of the falx (Fig. 16-23). This occurs in shaken-infant syndrome.[47,49,50] Diffuse cerebral edema is also a manifestation of child abuse. This also results in a relative hyperdensity of the falx, and which has a similar appearance to a subdural blood collection adjacent to the falx.

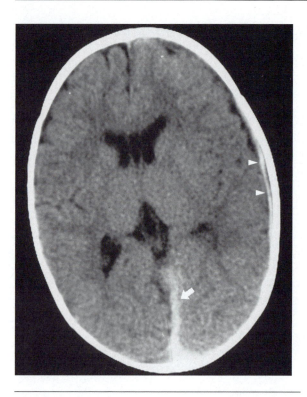

FIGURE 16-23. Interhemispheric subdural hematoma. A noncontrast CT of this infant shows acute subdural blood within the interhemispheric fissure *(arrow)*. Blood in this location raises the possibility of child abuse. A thin subdural hematoma borders the left parietal lobe *(arrowheads)*.

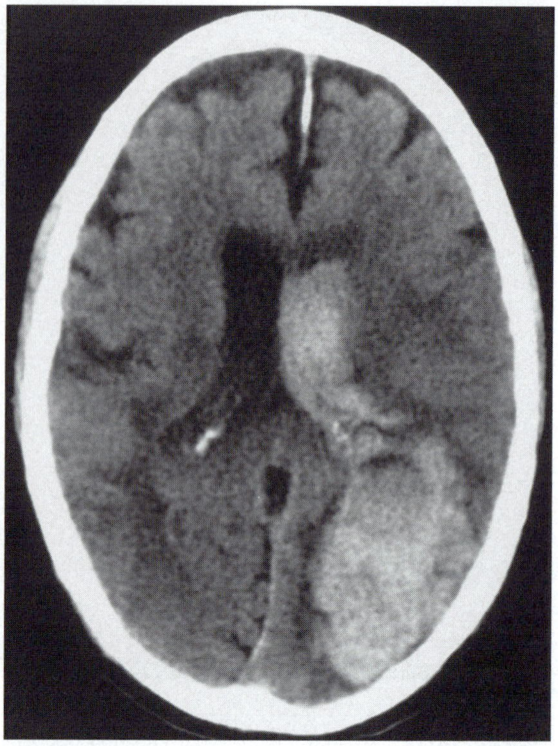

FIGURE 16-24. Intraventricular hemorrhage. This noncontrast CT demonstrates acute blood in the body of the left lateral ventricle with a large parenchymal hemorrhage in the left parietooccipital region. This patient had lymphoma and coagulopathy.

INTRAVENTRICULAR HEMORRHAGE. Hemorrhage into the ventricular compartment results from disruption of the subependymal veins (most common), reflux of subarachnoid blood, or extension of parenchymal hemorrhage. Acute intraventricular blood is a hyperdense collection within the ventricles that produces either a fluid-fluid level or a cast of the ventricle (Fig. 16-24). As time passes, the blood density more closely approximates the density of CSF, making the hemorrhage difficult to identify. During the subacute and chronic stages, detection of hemorrhage is improved by MRI.

Intraventricular hemorrhage can cause hydrocephalus. Clot formation impedes the flow of CSF through the ventricles or inhibits resorption of CSF in the arachnoid villi.

Secondary (Delayed) CNS Injury

The delayed effects of a traumatic injury can be more devastating than the primary injury itself. Delayed injuries include edema, ischemia, infarction, delayed hemorrhage, and brain herniation. These secondary insults result in further brain injury. For example, mass effect can cause herniation, which creates a vicious cycle of additional vascular compromise, ischemic injury and swelling. Secondary injury occurs in both traumatic and nontraumatic disorders.

BRAIN HERNIATION. The diagnosis of herniation is based on clinical findings. If it is suspected, treatment should begin prior to obtaining an imaging study. Moreover, CT findings of herniation are initially subtle or absent. Some types of herniation are difficult to detect by CT. This is largely due to the limited imaging planes (axial) of CT as compared to the multiplanar capability of MRI. It is important that CSF be seen within all of the cisternal spaces and ventricles. Obliteration of these compartments is an indication of mass effect, herniation, or other pathology such as SAH.

Six types of brain herniation are described (Fig. 16-25).[44,54] Herniation may be difficult to see on CT, showing only subtle changes such as mild asymmetry of the cisterns. The subfalcine and uncal patterns are often detectable. Tonsillar herniation is difficult to see on CT due to bone artifacts at the level of the foramen magnum.

Subfalcine Herniation. Herniation of the cingulate gyrus of the frontal lobe beneath the edge of the falx is called subfalcine, or cingulate herniation (Fig. 16-26). The displaced gyrus can exert pressure on branches of the anterior cerebral arteries, resulting in further ischemia or infarction of the brain.

Uncal Herniation. Uncal herniation results from the displacement of the medial aspect of the temporal lobe (the un-

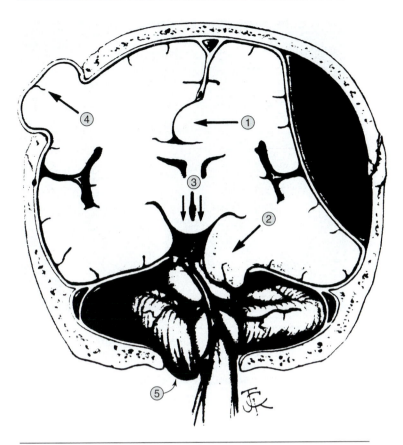

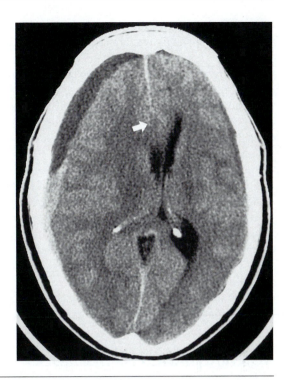

FIGURE 16-25. Classification of brain herniation (coronal schematic). In this diagram, subfalcial, uncal, and downward herniation are caused by a large left epidural hematoma, tonsillar herniation is caused by a right posterior fossa subdural hematoma, and external herniation is caused by a parenchymal contusion. *1.* Subfalcial herniation (note the left cingulate gyrus being displaced to the right beneath the falx); *2.* uncal herniation (note the mass effect on the left oculomotor nerve as it exits between the posterior cerebral artery and superior cerebellar artery); *3.* downward herniation; *4.* external herniation (note the right frontal lobe mushrooming through the skull defect); *5.* tonsillar herniation. Upward herniation is not illustrated. (From Gean AD: Imaging of Head Trauma. New York, Raven Press, 1994, with permission.)

FIGURE 16-26. Subfalcine herniation. 75-year-old man presenting with mental status changes. This noncontrast CT demonstrates a mixed-density subdural hematoma bordering the right hemisphere. Hyperdense blood layers dependently within the low-density collection. This appearance suggests rebleeding within a chronic hematoma, which has resulted in mass effect with subfalcine herniation *(arrow)* and effacement of the ventricles.

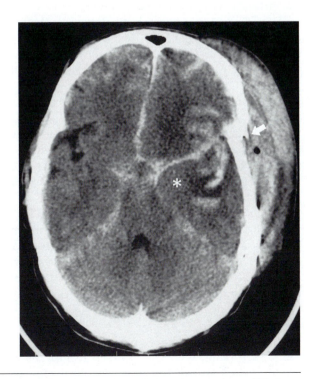

cus) across the tentorial margin. On CT, there is effacement or asymmetry of the lateral border of the suprasellar cistern (Fig. 16-27). The posterior cerebral artery (PCA) courses along the medial temporal lobe and can be compressed, resulting in further ischemia or infarction. Adjacent to the posteroinferior cerebellar artery is the third cranial nerve. A unilateral third-nerve palsy ("blown pupil") is an important early clinical sign of uncal herniation.

Central Herniation. Central herniation is also termed *downward herniation.* Diffuse mass effect in the supratentorial compartment causes downward pressure on the cerebral hemispheres and brainstem. The suprasellar cistern is effaced, as are the cisternal spaces surrounding the midbrain and brainstem. Clinically, patients present with slightly constricted, sluggishly

FIGURE 16-27. Uncal herniation. A noncontrast CT shows massive extracranial soft tissue swelling following head trauma with a depressed skull fracture *(arrow).* Note deviation of the left medial temporal lobe toward midline *(asterisk).* The cisterns are filled by extensive traumatic subarachnoid hemorrhage (white).

reactive pupils. Progression causes impingement on the brainstem's vascular supply and brainstem infarction.

Upward Herniation.   Upward displacement of structures results from a mass in the posterior fossa. The superior cerebellar, quadrigeminal, and ambient cisterns are effaced. The superior cerebellar artery courses over the superior aspect of the cerebellum and can be compressed. This pattern is difficult to see on axial views.

Tonsillar Herniation.   Tonsillar herniation results from pathology of the posterior fossa. The cerebellar tonsils are displaced downward through the foramen magnum. The posteroinferior cerebellar artery lies next to the tonsils and can be compressed causing further cerebellar ischemia.

External Herniation.   Severe edema or swelling of the brain parenchyma with an associated skull fracture can result in external protrusion of brain (Fig. 16-28).

NONTRAUMATIC CNS DISORDERS

Ischemic Cerebrovascular Disease (Nonhemorrhagic Stroke)

Thromboembolic disease accounts for over 90% of ischemic strokes.[52–54] Half of these are due to vascular thrombosis related to atherosclerosis and half are due to embolization from a cardiac or endovascular source. Secondary intraparenchymal hemorrhage develops in a small percentage of cases.

A recent concept is to consider a stroke as a "brain attack" analogous to a "heart attack." This stems from efforts to treat stroke in its earliest stages when thrombolytic therapy is potentially effective. Evaluation of these patients consists of emergency head CT to exclude hemorrhage or other lesions such as a tumor or infarction. Thrombolytic therapy is administered if symptoms began within 3 h. Thrombolytic therapy may be complicated by hemorrhage within the ischemic tissue, and this approach remains controversial. Ideally, there should be no CT signs of cerebral infarction since this indicates that more than 3 h has elapsed since the stroke began. These patients have an increased risk of hemorrhagic transformation.

Brain ischemia causes accumulation of fluid within the injured cells, which is known as *cytotoxic edema,* which involves both gray and white matter. Acute ischemic brain tissue appears as a region of decreased density relative to normal parenchyma with loss of the normal gray-white interface. The location of edema corresponds to the involved vascular territory (Fig. 16-29). Cytotoxic edema produces only a slight amount of mass effect.

After several days, strokes are easily recognized on both CT and MRI. However soon after its onset, a stroke can be difficult to demonstrate radiographically. During the first 6 h after the onset of the stroke, CT is usually negative.[55] The major role of CT is to exclude hemorrhage as well as to look for other causes for the acute neurologic deficit. Acute hemorrhage is

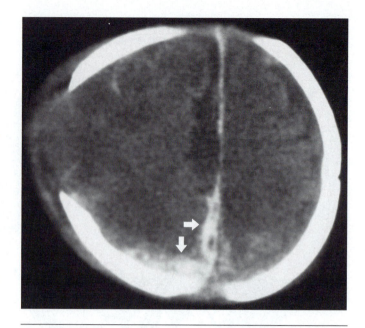

FIGURE 16-28.   External brain herniation. Massive cerebral edema following child abuse has resulted in herniation of the cerebral cortex through the skull fracture. There is acute subdural blood layering along the interhemispheric fissure and adjacent hemisphere *(arrows)*.

TABLE 16-10

Characteristics of Stroke on Computed Tomography

Hyperacute (onset to 24 h)
    Normal CT if under 6 h
    Normal CT in 20–50% of cases at 24 h
    Cytotoxic edema—begins at 6–12 h
        Loss of gray–white matter differentiation
        Subtle low-attenuation areas
        Slight mass effect—effacement of sulci
    May be hemorrhagic

Acute (24 h–7 days)
    Wedge-shaped area of low attenuation involving both gray and
        white matter
    Increasing edema with mass effect—maximal at 3–5 days
    May become hemorrhagic

Subacute (1–8 weeks)
    Contrast enhancement due to neovascularization without intact
        blood-brain barrier
        Gyral pattern of enhancement is characteristic
        Homogeneous and ring-enhancing patterns also occur
    Less mass effect (begins to resolve after approximately 1 week)
    May become hemorrhagic

Chronic (months to years)
    Volume loss—encephalomalacia
        Ex vacuo dilatation of the ventricle
    No longer contrast-enhancing
        Intact blood-brain barrier in areas of neovascularization
    Calcification (uncommon)

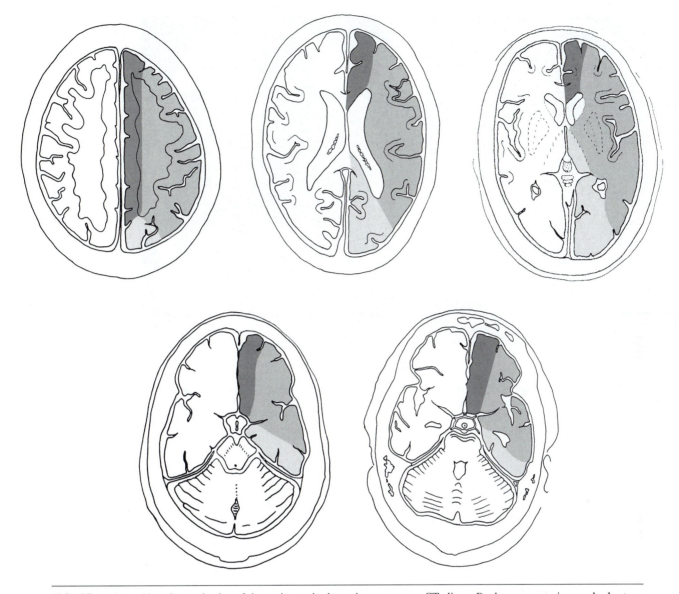

FIGURE 16-29. Vascular territories of the main cerebral arteries as seen on CT slices. *Dark gray*—anterior cerebral artery. *Medium gray*—middle cerebral artery. *Light gray*—posterior cerebral artery.

readily detected by CT. MRI is more sensitive than CT in detecting a stroke in the earliest stage. Abnormalities are detected by MRI as soon as 2 h after the onset of symptoms.[56,57] However, MRI may be unable to detect acute hemorrhage (less than 12 h old), and this is generally the most significant issue in the ED.[44]

The imaging characteristics of strokes are dependent on the time interval since the onset of symptoms. Four phases are distinguished (Table 16-10).[58] Strokes in the hyperacute phase (less than 24 h since onset) are the most important in the ED. The acute phase extends up to 1 week, the subacute phase up to 2 months, and the chronic phase follows.

HYPERACUTE STROKE. Within the first 24 h, the stroke is inapparent on CT in 20 to 30% of cases. Changes are more consistently visualized during the following 24 to 48 h. Early visibility of the abnormality depends on the amount of ischemic tissue. The earliest changes are seen after 6 to 12 h. These consist of decreased density within the ischemic area, loss of the gray-white interface, and minimal brain tissue swelling causing effacement of the cortical sulci (Fig. 16-30).[55] These early findings are due to cytotoxic edema, in which fluid accumulates intracellularly owing to failure of the ischemic cell membrane to maintain sodium and water homeo-stasis. Both gray and white matter are affected, accounting for the diminished difference in radiographic density and loss of the gray-white interface. The amount of edema accumulation is small, and therefore mass effect is minor.

It is important to scrutinize the CT scans of patients with acute stroke for these CT signs of ischemia-infarction. They are associated with an increased risk of hemorrhagic transformation in patients treated with thrombolytic agents. These CT signs are considered a contraindication to the use of thrombolytics.[59,60]

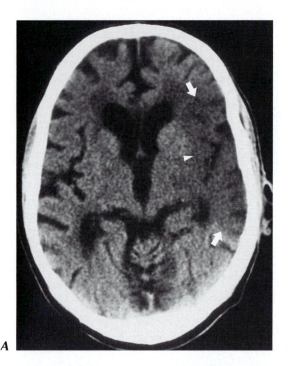 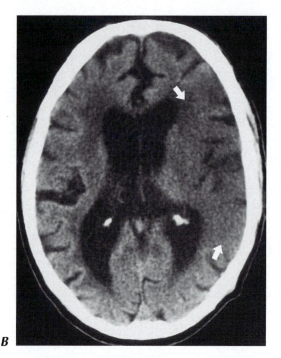

A   B

FIGURE 16-30.   Hyperacute cortical infarct. Noncontrast CT in a 70-year-old male *(A)*. There is large region of low density in the left posterior frontal and superior temporal lobes and insula, corresponding to the distribution of the middle cerebral artery *(arrows)*. There is only minimal effacement of the cortical sulci and sylvian fissure. Note loss of the insular ribbon on the left *(arrowhead)*. Image at next higher level *(B)* shows edema extending superiorly into the left parietal lobe. Note the wedge-shaped pattern characteristic of a stroke.

The *insula* is a region of cerebral cortex at the base of the sylvian fissure. It is supplied predominantly by small perforating branches of the middle cerebral artery. This region is particularly prone to ischemic injury. The result of early ischemic injury in the area supplied by the middle cerebral artery can be loss of the gray-white matter interface beneath the insula (termed *insular ribbon*) or adjacent lentiform nucleus (Fig. 16-31).[61,62]

A hyperdense clot is occasionally seen within the involved cerebral artery. This finding supports the diagnosis of acute stroke (Fig. 16-32).[63,64] However, this should be interpreted with caution because chronic atherosclerotic changes can have a similar appearance (Fig. 16-33).

The detection rate of hyperacute stroke with MRI is substantially greater than with CT. This is due to the greater sensitivity of MRI in detecting tissue signal abnormalities. Signal changes are detected as early as 2 h, especially with the use of gadolinium contrast enhancement.[65,66] Contrast infusion with CT does not assist in detecting early strokes.

ACUTE STROKE.   As the stroke enters the acute phase (24 h to 7 days), there is increasing cerebral edema due to loss of vascular integrity and the blood-brain barrier. CT demonstrates a well-defined, wedge-shaped region of decreased density localized to the particular vascular territory involved (Fig. 16-34). Substantial mass effect can occur, which is maximal at 3 to 5 days. With large infarctions, mass effect can cause fatal herniation.

The hemorrhage may be present on the initial CT scan or detected on follow-up scans (Fig. 16-35). Embolic strokes are especially prone to hemorrhagic transformation after the embolus breaks apart and blood flow to injured brain tissue is reestablished.

SUBACUTE STROKE.   Between 1 and 8 weeks after the stroke, the degree of mass effect diminishes. Contrast-infused CT scans show a characteristic pattern of enhancement that conforms to the contour of the cortical gyri. This is due to reestablished blood flow through either damaged blood vessels or neurovascularization with an undeveloped blood-brain barrier. The presence of contrast enhancement distinguishes a subacute stroke from an acute or chronic stroke. Occasionally, enhancement has a homogeneous or ring pattern similar to that of a tumor. If the distinction between tumor and infarction cannot be made clinically, serial CT studies or MRI can help resolve the issue.

CHRONIC STROKE.   Chronic infarcts are characterized by loss of brain tissue, known as *encephalomalacia* (Fig. 16-36). On CT, encephalomalacia appears as a distinct region of hypodensity similar in density to CSF. If the injury is sufficiently large, the adjacent ventricle becomes dilated (*ex vacuo dilatation*) and the cortical sulci overlying the infarct become enlarged. Contrast enhancement is absent during the chronic stages of infarction because the blood-brain barrier is reestablished as the infarction heals.

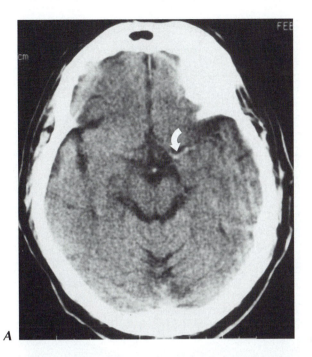

A

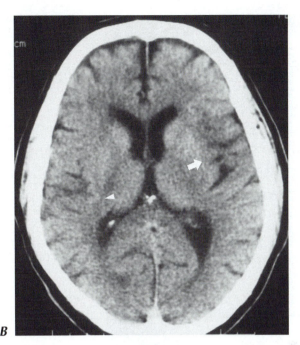

B

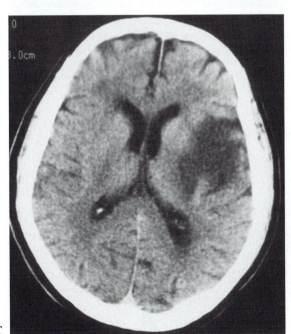

C

FIGURE 16-31. Insular ribbon sign in 71-year-old man with slurred speech (*A* and *B*). There is a region of subtle hypodensity in the left posterior frontal and anterior temporal lobes and loss of the normal insular ribbon (*arrows*). This illustrates the "insular ribbon sign" consistent with a hyperacute infarct of the middle cerebral artery (MCA). There is a normal insular ribbon on the right (arrowhead). The left middle cerebral artery is denser than that on the contralateral side, probably representing clot or thrombus in the vessel (*curved arrow*). This finding is inconsistently seen in early infarcts. A CT scan obtained 3 days later (*C*) confirms an acute left MCA infarct.

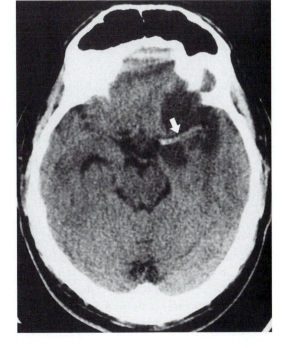

FIGURE 16-32. Hyperdense artery. This noncontrast CT shows an acute infarct in the inferior left frontal, and anterior temporal lobes (middle cerebral artery distribution). The left MCA is abnormally dense, suggesting clot or thrombus (*arrow*). This finding is seen infrequently with acute stroke but helps support the diagnosis.

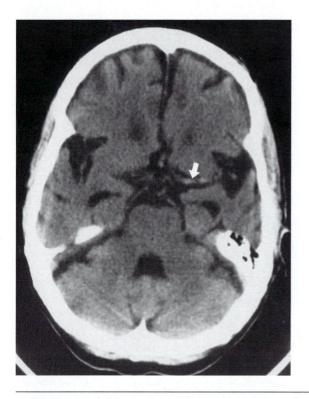

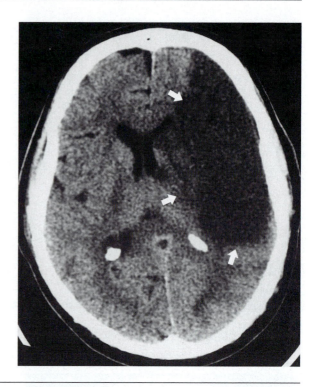

FIGURE 16-33.   Atherosclerotic middle cerebral artery (MCA). The left MCA *(arrow)* appears abnormally dense relative to the opposite side. This finding could be mistaken for a hyperdense vessel seen in association with stroke.

FIGURE 16-34.   Acute infarct. This noncontrast CT shows a large, wedge-shaped region of edema in the left hemisphere. During the subacute phase of stroke, the margins of the infarct become better defined. There is mild midline shift, ventricular compression, and sulcal effacement.

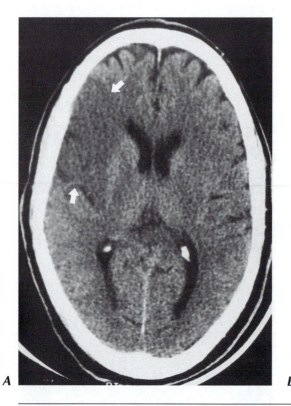

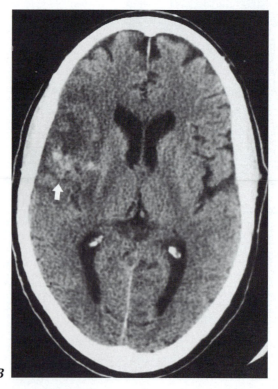

A   *B*

FIGURE 16-35.   Hemorrhagic transformation. This noncontrast CT **(A)** shows edema and effacement of sulci in the right frontoparietal area *(arrows)* consistent with a hyperacute infarct. No hemorrhage is visible on this scan. The follow-up study obtained 4 days later *(B)* demonstrates areas of acute hemorrhage within the region of infarction *(arrow)*.

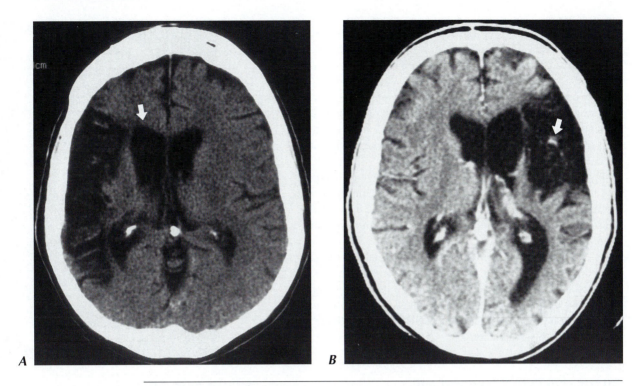

FIGURE 16-36. Chronic infarct. *A.* Prominence of cortical sulci, lack of mass effect and ex vacuo dilation of the ventricle *(arrow)* are findings consistent with a chronic infarct (right middle cerebral artery distribution). *B.* Calcification in the tissue may be seen in chronic strokes *(arrow)*. This should not be mistaken for hemorrhage.

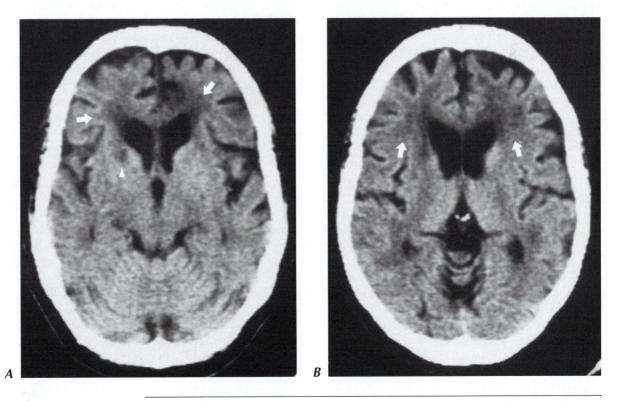

FIGURE 16-37. Small vessel ischemic disease in a 75-year-old with dementia and hypertension. There are ill-defined areas of low density in the subcortical and periventricular white matter of both hemispheres *(arrows)*. A focal hypodensity in the basal ganglia *(arrowhead)* is typical of a lacunar infarct.

WHITE MATTER ISCHEMIC DISEASE AND LACUNAR INFARCTS.
White matter ischemic changes occur frequently in diabetic and
hypertensive patients. This is termed *small vessel ischemic disease* and is presumably due to progressive atherosclerosis of
smaller perforating vessels. The region of white matter infarction may be focal or diffuse (Fig. 16-37). Diffuse white matter
ischemic disease is ill defined on CT. These lesions occur in
the periventricular white matter or in the subcortical white matter at the gray-white junction.

Focal lesions due to ischemic disease involving the small
perforating vessels at the base of the cerebral hemispheres are
termed *lacunar infarcts* or *lacunes*. These may be up to 15 mm
in size. They are located in the basal ganglia or the white matter of the internal capsule.

In contrast to cortical infarcts, the age of small-vessel ischemic disease is difficult to determine by CT. Cavitation with
well-defined CSF density suggests that the infarct was a remote
event. The extent of white matter changes related to chronic
ischemia is best demonstrated with MRI, but determining its
age is difficult in many cases.

Intraparenchymal Hemorrhage

Clinically, intraparenchymal hemorrhage can present in a similar fashion to cerebral infarction. CT imaging is needed to
make the diagnosis. Causes of intraparenchymal hemorrhage
include systemic hypertension, drug-induced hemorrhage, coagulopathy, and amyloid angiopathy. Intracranial bleeding can
also be due to rupture of a vascular malformation or aneurysm.
Although vascular rupture usually presents with headache, an
acute focal neurologic deficit can also occur.

HYPERTENSIVE HEMORRHAGE.   The most common cause of
acute nontraumatic intracerebral hemorrhage is hypertension.[67]
The mechanism by which arteries spontaneously rupture in hypertension is unclear. The deep perforating vessels (thalamo-
perforating and lenticulostriate arteries) are those most often
involved. The putamen and thalamus are the most common sites
of hemorrhage, followed by the cerebellum and the pons.[68] The
hemorrhage can extend into the ventricles or subarachnoid
space.

CT demonstrates a region of hyperdensity corresponding to
the acute blood collection. A location near the basal ganglia
strongly suggests a hypertensive bleed (Fig. 16-38). The configuration is often linear or elongated. Large bleeds can produce significant mass effect and midline shift. An old hypertensive hemorrhage appears as a linear or elongated CSF cavity
near the basal ganglia.

DRUG-RELATED HEMORRHAGE.   An acute intracranial hemorrhage can be precipitated by various drugs of abuse, especially
cocaine. Hemorrhage may be due to a precipitous rise in blood
pressure or rupture of a preexisting aneurysm or vascular malformation.[69,70] Ischemia or infarction can occur as a result of
vasospasm, as well as an arterial or venous thrombosis.[71,72]

There is no distinct radiographic appearance of drug-induced

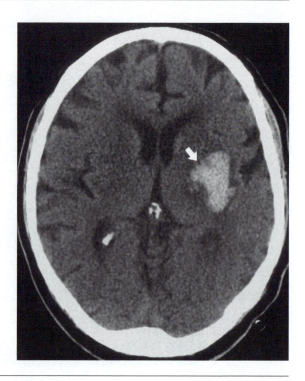

FIGURE 16-38.   Hypertensive hemorrhage. There is a large
hyperdensity (acute blood) with surrounding edema in the left
basal ganglia, the characteristic location of a hypertensive hemorrhage.

hemorrhage. Both parenchymal and subarachnoid blood can be
seen. A centrally located parenchymal hemorrhage can appear
similar to a hypertensive bleed. Drug-related SAH is indistinguishable from that due to non–drug-related aneurysm rupture.
Peripherally located hemorrhages can be due to mycotic
aneurysms resulting from intravenous drug use. This can mimic
amyloid angiopathy of the older patient. Solitary, multiple, or
bilateral hemispheric hemorrhages can occur from cocaine
use.[73,74]

Aneurysms and Nontraumatic Subarachnoid Hemorrhage

Ruptured aneurysms account for the majority of nontraumatic
SAHs. Arteriovenous malformations or venous angiomas are
less common causes. Most aneurysms are located near arterial
bifurcations within the circle of Willis. The most common locations are at the anterior communicating artery and the junction of the posterior communicating and the internal carotid arteries. Other sites are at the middle cerebral artery bifurcations
and the vertebrobasilar arteries. Multiple aneurysms occur in
approximately 20% of cases;[77,78] therefore a second lesion
should be sought after the initial aneurysm is detected.
Aneurysms are most commonly detected in young and middle-
aged adults.

Patients with other vascular abnormalities such as fibro-
muscular dysplasia, polycystic kidney disease, connective tissue
disorders, and coarctation of the aorta have a higher incidence

of intracranial aneurysms. Infection of a vessel wall can produce a mycotic aneurysm.

IMAGING TECHNIQUES. The most common manifestation of aneurysmal rupture is a SAH. A noncontrast CT scan is the initial study for detecting acute hemorrhage. A wide range of detection rates (60 to 90%) for aneurysmal hemorrhage is reported.[77,79] A negative CT more often occurs in patients with a small warning leak or "sentinel bleed." Patients with sentinel bleeds are the ones in whom the clinical diagnosis is most difficult but who stand to benefit most from prompt diagnosis. The prognosis is considerably worse if diagnosis and treatment are delayed until a subsequent major hemorrhage. CT is less sensitive at detecting small SAH if 12 to 24 h have passed since the time of the bleed. Extravasated blood eventually becomes isodense and difficult to detect. A normal head CT therefore does not exclude an acute SAH. In patients in whom the clinician suspects a ruptured aneurysm, an LP should be performed if the CT study is negative.

Acute aneurysmal hemorrhage appears as high-density material in the subarachnoid spaces or basilar cisterns. Occasionally, blood is seen in the brain parenchyma, the ventricles, or the subdural space. The location of the subarachnoid blood correlates with the site of the aneurysm.[77,78] Aneurysms of the anterior communicating artery cause bleeding in the anterior interhemispheric fissure (Fig. 16-39). Blood in one of the sylvian fissures suggest a middle cerebral artery aneurysm (Fig. 16-40). An aneurysm of the posterior circulation is suspected when there is blood in the fourth ventricle and posterior fossa (Fig. 16-41). Subarachnoid blood in conjunction with blood in the subdural space suggests a dural aneurysm or vascular malformation.[78] Extensive hemorrhage precludes localization of the aneurysm.

Conventional cerebral angiography is the "gold standard" for aneurysm detection. A complete evaluation entails injection of both carotid arteries and both vertebral arteries. If the patient's condition does not permit a complete four-vessel study, the vessel suspected of rupturing (based on CT findings) is selectively imaged.

Magnetic resonance imaging has poor sensitivity for acute SAH. Blood in the CSF is in an oxygenated state and has a similar MR signal to the surrounding CSF. However, after 1 to 2 days, MRI has increased sensitivity and offers an advantage over CT.

If an aneurysm is strongly suspected on the basis of focal neurologic signs such as palsy of the third cranial nerve or, a family history of aneurysms or polycystic kidney disease and the CT and CSF examinations are negative, additional studies are indicated. If the aneurysm is sufficiently large, it can be seen on a contrast-enhanced CT. An aneurysm appears as a focal hyperdense structure adjacent to the vessel of origin (Fig. 16-42). Conventional angiography is accurate but invasive and must be used selectively in screening patients for nonbleeding aneurysms. Alternatively, MRI with MR angiography is noninvasive and is able to detect small aneurysms (≥3 mm).[80] An aneurysm smaller than 5 mm has a low risk for rupture.[78]

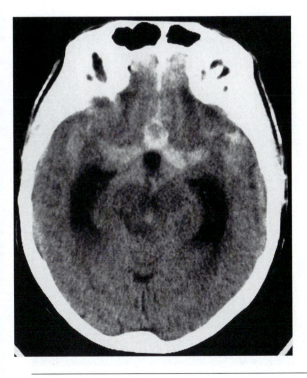 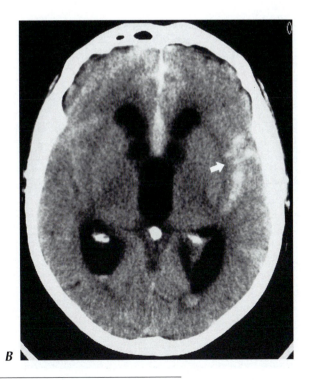

B

FIGURE 16-39. Anterior communicating artery aneurysm. Noncontrast image *(A)* demonstrates extensive subarachnoid hemorrhage in the basilar cisterns *(arrow)* and within the interhemispheric fissure *(arrowhead)*. The image at a higher level *(B)* also shows blood in the sylvian fissure *(arrow)*. Angiography confirmed an anterior communicating artery aneurysm.

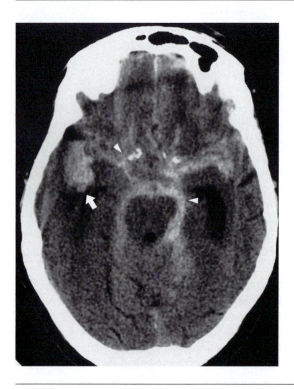

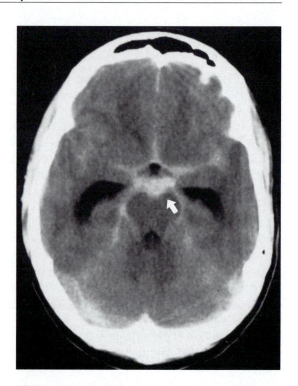

FIGURE 16-40. Middle cerebral artery aneurysm. Image at the level of the basilar cisterns demonstrates diffuse subarachnoid hemorrhage *(arrowheads)* with a larger, focal collection of blood in the right sylvian fissure *(arrow)*. These findings imply a right MCA aneurysm, which was confirmed by angiography.

FIGURE 16-41. Vertebrobasilar artery aneurysm in a 38-year-old man evaluated for seizure activity. This noncontrast image demonstrates diffuse subarachnoid hemorrhage within the basilar cisterns. Blood is most prominent in the prepontine cistern *(arrow)*. Angiography confirmed an aneurysm of the distal left vertebral artery.

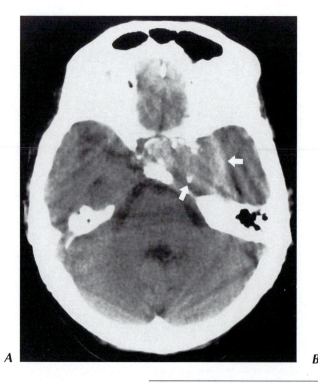

A

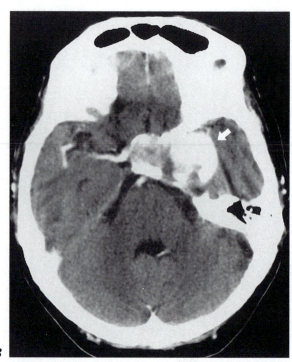

B

FIGURE 16-42. Cavernous carotid artery aneurysm. The noncontrast CT *(A)* demonstrates a heterogenous mass lesion contiguous with the cavernous sinus on the left *(arrows)*. Postcontrast image *(B)* shows dense, irregular enhancement. Angiography confirmed a left cavernous carotid artery aneurysm.

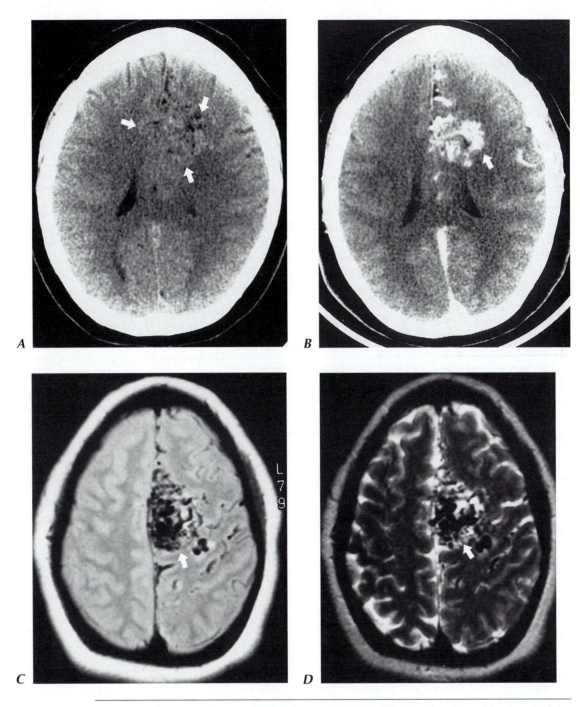

FIGURE 16-43. Arteriovenous malformation (AVM) in a 26-year-old woman with seizure activity. This noncontrast image *(A)* demonstrates an isodense "mass" in the frontal lobes at midline *(arrows)*. Several punctate hypodensities (vessels) are seen within the lesion. The postcontrast image *(B)* shows dense enhancement of vessels *(arrow)*. MRI *(C and D)* demonstrates flow "voids" corresponding to vascular flow within the AVM *(arrow)*. Lack of edema and mass effect are typical of an AVM.

Vascular Malformations

The incidence of intracerebral hemorrhage from vascular abnormalities such as an arteriovenous malformation (AVM) or cavernous hemangioma is lower than that of aneurysm. There are four types of vascular malformations: AVM (most common), venous angioma, cavernous malformation, and capillary telangiectasia. AVMs are the most likely to be symptomatic, and they present clinically as a result of intraparenchymal hemorrhage. Bleeding may extend into the subarachnoid space and ventricles. Most AVMs are located in the cerebral hemispheres.[77,78]

CT AND MRI. Most vascular abnormalities are diagnosed with CT and MRI. With a large AVM, contrast-enhanced CT demonstrates an abnormal collection of disorganized, dilated vessels (Fig. 16-43). Small malformations may be masked by surrounding hemorrhage.

ANGIOGRAPHY. MRA is sufficient for documenting the location and general vascular distribution of an AVM. The determination of precise flow dynamics within the AVM, which is necessary to plan embolization or surgical intervention, requires conventional angiography.

Intracranial Tumors

Neoplastic disease of the CNS may originate in the brain or metastasize from non-CNS sites. Symptoms related to brain tumors include headaches, gait disturbances, confusion, visual disturbances, nausea, vomiting, and seizures. A stroke-like presentation with acute onset of a focal neurologic deficit can also occur. In addition to identifying the tumor itself, it is important to look for secondary findings such as hemorrhage, mass effect, or herniation. Distinguishing an intraaxial from an extraaxial tumor helps in determining the type of neoplasm (Table 16-11).

The incidence of both primary and metastatic tumors increases with age. Approximately 80 to 85% of all intracranial tumors are found in adults.[81] In older patients, the incidence of metastatic disease is roughly equal to that of primary brain tumors. Supratentorial tumors are predominant in adults. Infratentorial tumors occur more frequently in children. Metastatic disease is uncommon in children.

A distinguishing radiographic feature of tumors is *vasogenic edema*. The primary lesion causes a defect in the blood-brain barrier, resulting in the accumulation of fluid in the extracellular space. Vasogenic edema principally affects the white matter and spares the cortical gray matter. If there is a large amount of vasogenic edema, the overlying cortical sulci are effaced. This can obscure the cortical gray-white interface, so that the lesion can be mistaken for cytotoxic edema due to a stroke.

The urgency with which a patient is scanned for a suspected tumor depends on the clinical presentation. If the patient has signs of herniation or a focal neurologic deficit, CT is usually sufficient to make an immediate diagnosis. In most cases, a noncontrast CT demonstrates the tumor and any signs of a mass effect, midline shift, hemorrhage, or hydrocephalus.

In a stable patient or the patient with vague symptoms or clinical findings, MRI can reveal lesions undetected by CT, such as mild edema, small tumors, and unsuspected metastases. Posterior fossa lesions are better seen with MRI.

On CT, most tumors appear as ill-defined, low-density regions representing both the tumor mass and surrounding vasogenic edema. Unlike metastases, which are usually located at the gray-white junction, primary tumors typically occur in the white matter. Contrast enhancement is needed to distinguish the margins of the tumor from the surrounding edema (Fig. 16-44). Certain tumors present on CT as high-density masses (Table 16-9). These include highly cellular tumors such as lymphoma, germ cell tumors, and hemorrhagic tumors. Melanoma, glioblastoma multiforme, thyroid carcinoma, and renal cell carcinoma can be hemorrhagic. Oligodendroglioma and choroid plexus tumors commonly contain calcification, which can be mistaken for hemorrhage. Differentiation between a tumor and other lesions such as stroke or infection may be impossible with a single study. Follow-up scans may be required.

PRIMARY NEOPLASM. In adults, the primary tumors most frequently found are gliomas, ranging from the low-grade astrocytoma to the highly malignant glioblastoma multiforme (Fig. 16-45). Gliomas account for roughly half of adult primary CNS tumors. Other common nonglial tumors include meningiomas

TABLE 16-11

Characteristics of Intra- and Extraaxial Mass Lesions

Extraaxial (e.g., meningioma, dural metastasis, hematoma)
    Appears contiguous with adjacent skull
    Bone changes (hyperostosis, destruction) are often seen
    Extraaxial space is widened around mass
    May indent cerebral cortex
Intraaxial (e.g., glioma, abscess, parenchymal hematoma)
    Separate from skull
    Usually lacks skeletal changes
    Extraaxial space may be narrowed around mass
      (brain is expanded outward)

(Fig. 16-45), acoustic schwannomas (neuromas), and pituitary adenomas.

Primary CNS lymphoma is seen in immunocompromised patients such as transplant recipients and patients with AIDS. These usually present as parenchymal masses in the basal ganglia and periventricular white matter (Fig. 16-46). The hypercellular nature of these tumors results in an isodense or hyperdense appearance on CT. The multiplicity of lesions is often mistaken for metastatic disease. Basal ganglion involvement suggests CNS lymphoma, especially in the immunocompromised patient.

In children, there are several histologic types of brain tumors. Both gliomas (astrocytomas, ependymomas, choroid plexus tumors) and nonglial tumors occur. Medulloblastoma is the most common nonglial tumor. It is derived from undifferentiated primitive stem cells and is termed a *primitive neuroectodermal tumor*. Medulloblastomas, which are highly malignant, are found in the posterior fossa (Fig. 16-47). Other nonglial tumors seen in children are craniopharyngiomas, teratomas, dermoids, and hamartomas.

METASTATIC DISEASE.   Metastases present as either small homogeneously enhancing nodules or ring-enhancing lesions (Table 16-12). Breast, lung, and colon carcinoma and melanoma commonly metastasize to the brain (Fig. 16-48). The presence of multiple lesions strongly supports the diagnosis of metastases, although solitary metastases do occur. CNS metastases from systemic lymphoma appear similar to metastases from other tumors (Fig. 16-49). Dural or leptomeningeal invasion is common and can be seen in combination with discrete parenchymal lesions. Intracranial metastases are uncommon in children except those with neuroblastomas, Ewing's sarcomas, and Wilms' tumors.

TABLE 16-12

Differential Diagnosis of Ring-Enhancing Lesions

Common
    Cerebral abscess (bacterial, fungal, toxoplasmosis)
    Tumor (primary or metastatic)
Uncommon
    Resolving infarct
    Resolving hematoma
    Multiple sclerosis

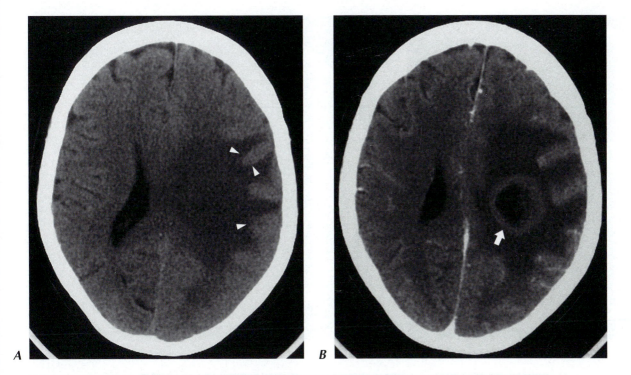

FIGURE 16-44. Vasogenic edema in a 71-year-old woman with mental status changes. This noncontrast CT *(A)* demonstrates extensive edema throughout the white matter of the left hemisphere and extending between the cortical gray matter *(arrowheads)*. Sparing of gray matter is characteristic of vasogenic edema. The postcontrast image *(B)* shows mild enhancement of the tumor margins *(arrow)* of this glioblastoma multiforme.

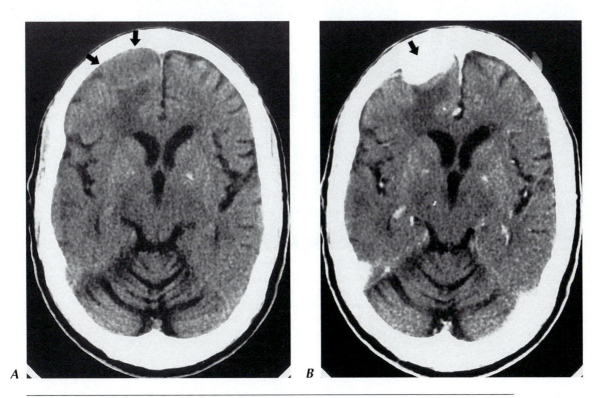

FIGURE 16-45. Meningioma. The noncontrast image *(A)* shows loss of cortical sulci in the right frontal lobe *(arrows)*. Subtle hypodensity (edema) is seen in the frontal white matter. The postinfusion image *(B)* shows dense enhancement of the meningioma *(arrow)*. The tapered margins of the mass are typical of an extraaxial lesion.

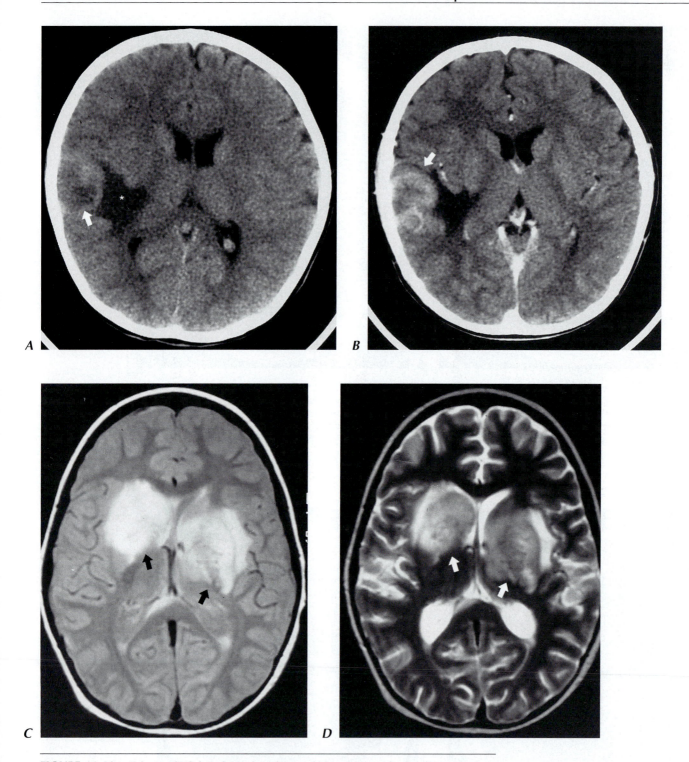

FIGURE 16-46.   Primary CNS lymphoma in a 6-year-old boy who received a liver transplant. Noncontrast CT *(A)* demonstrates a minimally hyperdense mass *(arrows)* with surrounding edema in the superficial aspect of the right parietal lobe *(asterisk)*. The postcontrast image *(B)* demonstrates subtle enhancement of the mass. MRI *(C and D)* of a different patient shows lymphomatous involvement of the basal ganglia, which is a characteristic location.

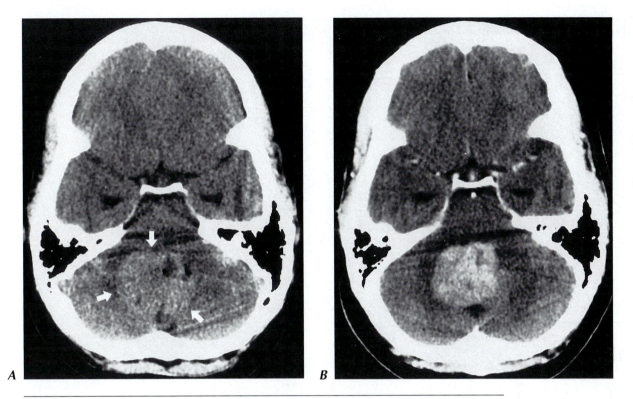

FIGURE 16-47.   Medulloblastoma. The noncontrast image *(A)* demonstrates an ill-defined, slightly hyperdense lesion in the posterior fossa *(arrows)*. The fourth ventricle is compressed and indistinct. The postcontrast image *(B)* shows dense enhancement of the tumor.

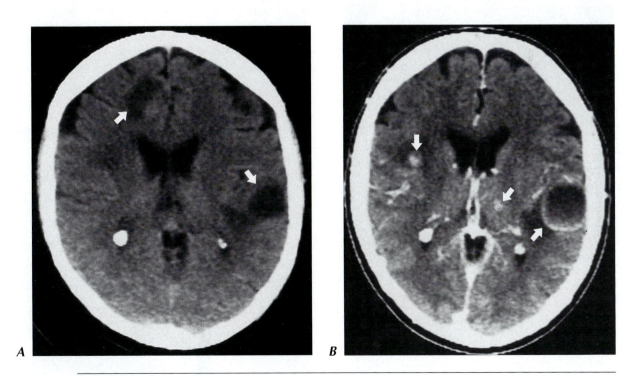

FIGURE 16-48.   Intracranial metastases in a 56-year-old woman with known lung carcinoma and mental status changes. The precontrast image *(A)* shows patchy areas of low attenuation in the subcortical white matter of the right frontal lobe and presumed cortical involvement of the left parietal lobe. The postcontrast image *(B)* demonstrates multiple small enhancing nodules and a large ring-enhancing lesion. Multiplicity of lesions is typical of metastases.

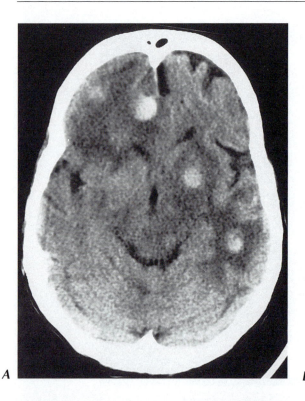

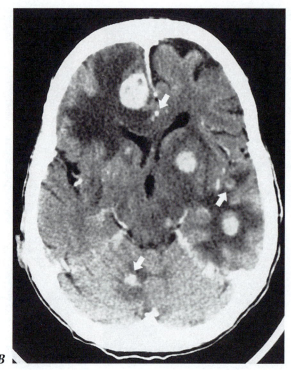

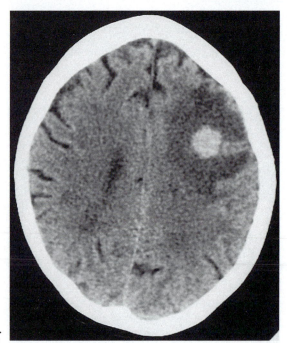

FIGURE 16-49.   Metastatic lymphoma in a patient with systemic lymphoma. The noncontrast CT *(A)* demonstrates several high-density lesions (hemorrhagic) with surrounding edema in both hemispheres. The postcontrast study *(B)* demonstrates several small enhancing lesions *(arrows)* from lymphomas that were not evident on the noncontrast study. Metastases from nonlymphomatous sources can produce similar findings. In a patient with known colon carcinoma *(C)*, the solitary hyperdense lesion in the left frontal lobe is a hemorrhagic metastasis (noncontrast CT).

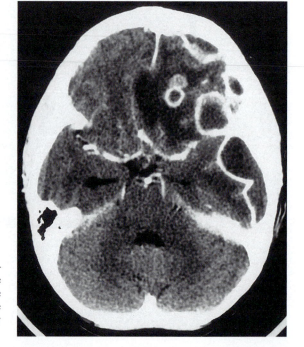

FIGURE 16-50.   Brain abscess. A postcontrast CT image shows multiple ring-enhancing lesions with surrounding edema in the left frontal lobe. Large extraaxial collections with enhancing margins represent empyemas. Note the subfalcine herniation and deviation of the left uncus toward midline secondary to mass effect.

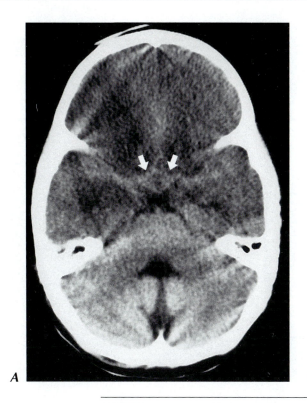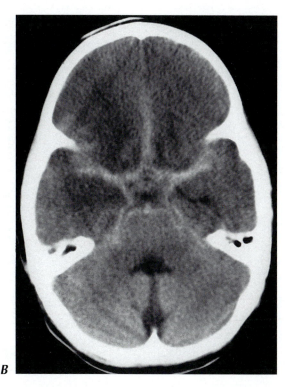

A   *B*

FIGURE 16-51.   Meningitis. A noncontrast CT *(A)* of an infant with suspected meningitis shows patchy areas of low density in the frontal and temporal lobes. The basilar cisterns are poorly visualized and are outlined anteriorly by subtle hyperdensity *(arrows)*. The corresponding postcontrast image *(B)* shows extensive enhancement within the cisterns corresponding to diffuse leptomeningeal enhancement.

Central Nervous System Infection

BRAIN ABSCESS.   MRI is more sensitive at detecting CNS infection than CT. Intracranial abscess forms by spread from contiguous sites of infection (e.g., mastoiditis, sinusitis), hematogenous spread (e.g., infective endocarditis, septic emboli from intravenous drug abuse), penetrating head trauma, and AIDS. On CT, it can be difficult to determine if a lesion is an abscess or tumor, even after contrast administration. On noncontrast CT scan, an abscess appears as a focal area of low density within the subcortical white matter. With contrast CT, the walls of the abscess enhance and there is a central necrotic area of lower density (Fig. 16-50). MRI can demonstrate intraventricular or subarachnoid spread of infection and accurately reveal the extent of disease.[82]

MENINGITIS.   During the acute stage of meningitis, the CT scan is usually normal. As the infection progresses, impaired resorption of CSF can cause communicating hydrocephalus.[83] In severe cases, meningeal inflammation causes arterial spasm resulting in cerebral ischemia or infarction. Meningitis is associated with parenchymal involvement (meningoencephalitis).

On CT, inflammation causes the meninges to be densely enhancing and appear thickened. Meningeal enhancement occurs during the early stages of infection, prior to the development of encephalitis.[84] Obliteration of the basilar cisterns by enhancing debris is typical of tuberculous meningitis (Fig. 16-51). MRI is more sensitive than CT in detecting early or subtle parenchymal changes.

ENCEPHALITIS.   Many viral and some bacterial organisms can cause encephalitis. In adults, herpes simplex virus type 1 (HSV-1) is responsible for about 12% of cases of encephalitis. The CT shows nonfocal, low-attenuation lesions, usually within the frontal and temporal lobes. Involvement of the insular cortex is a distinctive feature. Parenchymal hemorrhage is occasionally seen.[83]

Herpes simplex virus type 2 predominates in neonates. This is acquired from maternal genital infection. There is a diffuse parenchymal edema affecting both hemispheres (Fig. 16-52). Edema obscures the gray-white interface and effaces the cortical sulci.

OPPORTUNISTIC INFECTIONS.   In the immunocompromised host, mucormycosis and aspergillosis produce areas of parenchymal hemorrhage and calcification.[84] These infections can be complicated by intracerebral arterial occlusion.

HIV INFECTION.   *Toxoplasma gondii, Cryptococcus neoformans, Candida albicans, Coccidiomycosis, Mycobacterium avium intracellulare, Mycobacterium tuberculosis,* and syphilis are seen with increased frequency in HIV-infected patients. CT findings include nonspecific, ill-defined areas of hypodensity (Fig. 16-53). Multiple ring-enhancing lesions are seen with toxoplasmosis often involving the basal ganglia.

Progressive multifocal leukoencephalopathy results from papovavirus infection and is seen in the subcortical and periventricular areas bilaterally, sparing the cortex. Although a

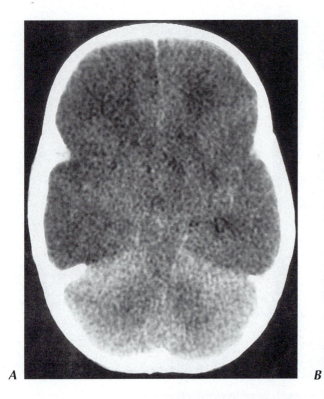

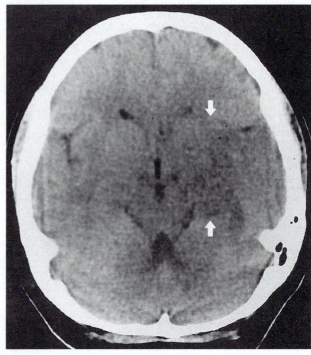

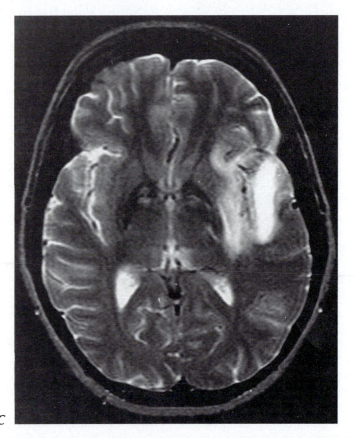

FIGURE 16-52.   Herpes encephalitis. *A.* Noncontrast image in a neonate with herpes. The ventricles, cortical sulci, and cisterns are indistinct, consistent with global cerebral edema. *B.* Noncontrast CT in an adult patient shows subtle low density in the left temporal lobe and insula *(arrows)*. *C.* MRI better illustrates the parenchymal edema.

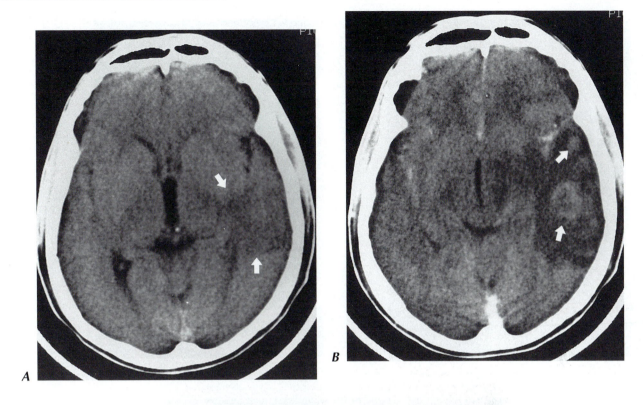

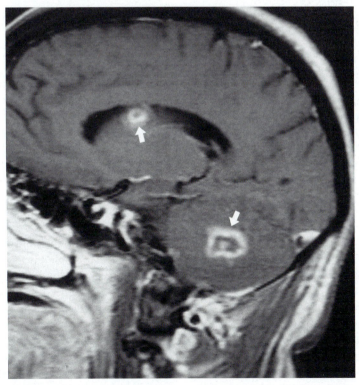

FIGURE 16-53. Toxoplasmosis. A noncontrast CT *(A)* shows an ill-defined area of edema in the left temporal lobe. The postcontrast image *(B)* shows a subtle ring-enhancing lesion *(arrows)* with surrounding edema. Contrast-enhanced MRI in a different patient *(C)* shows multiple ring-enhancing lesions *(arrows).* (MRI courtesy of Ruth G. Ramsey, M.D. University of Chicago)

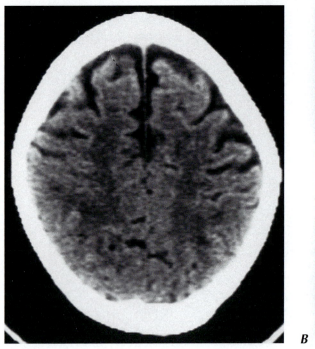 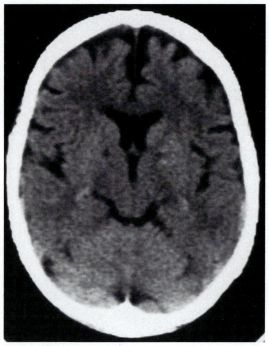

A   *B*

FIGURE 16-54.   HIV encephalopathy in a 41-year-old AIDS patient with mental status changes. Noncontrast images *(A* and *B)* demonstrate diffuse hypodensity of the white matter and multiple subcortical lucencies. Given the clinical history, this is presumed to be HIV encephalopathy.

multifocal pattern is typical, a more confluent and asymmetrical pattern can be seen.

HIV encephalopathy causes nonenhancing low-density lesions within the deep white matter of the frontal lobes (Fig. 16-54). The nonspecific appearance is similar to other white matter disorders such as small vessel ischemic disease. CT scans may show only diffuse atrophy without focal lesions.

Hydrocephalus

Hydrocephalus results from either overproduction of CSF, obstruction to CSF flow, or decreased CSF absorption. The term *hydrocephalus* is sometimes used erroneously to describe any dilation of the ventricular system. More accurately, there is dilation of the ventricles secondary to an increased volume of CSF. Enlargement of the ventricles due to cerebral atrophy should not be called hydrocephalus. This is better termed *ex vacuo dilatation of the ventricles* or *hydrocephalus ex vacuo.* When the nature of the ventricular enlargement is uncertain, the term *ventricular prominence* is appropriate.

Various measurements of ventricular size and shape have been devised to help distinguish hydrocephalus from atrophy. Overall measurements of ventricular dimensions are frequently misleading because ventricular size varies with age. For the experienced observer, determination of hydrocephalus is subjective and based on the overall appearance of the ventricles. The frontal horns of the lateral ventricles are normally tapered as

they project anteriorly. This tapered conformation is also seen in cerebral atrophy. In hydrocephalus, the frontal horns are rounded. Two measurements are used in quantifying the changes due to hydrocephalus: the frontal horn ratio (FHR) and the ventricular angle (Fig. 16-55).[85,86] The *frontal horn ratio* measures the greatest frontal horn diameter perpendicular to its long axis. This is increased with hydrocephalus. The *ventricular angle* is the angle of the frontal horn relative to the midline and is abnormally decreased with hydrocephalus. These parameters remain relatively normal in ventricular enlargement due to atrophy. The prominence of the cortical sulci suggests that ventricular dilation is due to cerebral atrophy rather than true hydrocephalus. Last, the temporal horns of the lateral ventricles tend to be dilated and prominent with hydrocephalus and have a narrower and more normal appearance with cerebral atrophy.

Hydrocephalus is classified as either communicating or noncommunicating.[86] *Noncommunicating hydrocephalus* is also termed *intraventricular obstructive hydrocephalus. Communicating hydrocephalus* is due to obstruction to CSF flow outside of the ventricular system, usually at the basilar cisterns but also in the subarachnoid space over the cerebral convexities and at the arachnoid villi. Communicating hydrocephalus is therefore also termed *extraventricular obstructive hydrocephalus* and is sometimes incorrectly called "nonobstructive hydrocephalus."

With noncommunicating hydrocephalus, the obstruction can be at any point within the ventricular system but is most common in the third ventricle or the aqueduct of Sylvius.

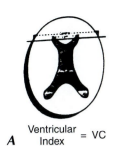

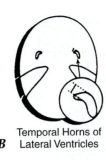

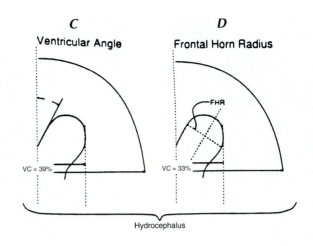

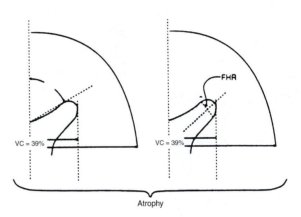

FIGURE 16-55. Methods to distinguish hydrocephalus from atrophy on CT. *A.* The *ventricular index* is the ratio of the ventricular diameter at the frontal horns to the diameter of the brain. This is not very sensitive or specific. *B.* Disproportionate enlargement of the *temporal horns* is a reliable sign. In hydrocephalus, there is greater dilatation of the temporal horns. *C.* The *ventricular angle* measures the divergence of the frontal horn. The ventricular angle is reduced in hydrocephalus *(top).* *D.* The *frontal horn radius* measures the widest diameter of the frontal horn. This measurement is increased with hydrocephalus *(top)* and reduced with atrophy *(bottom).* No single measurement is completely accurate in the diagnosis of hydrocephalus. The size of the temporal horns, the ventricular angle, the frontal horn radius, and the size of the ventricles relative to the cortical sulci should all be assessed. (From Barkovich AJ, ed: Pediatric Neuroimaging, 2nd ed. New York, Raven Press, 1995, with permission.)

Dilatation of the lateral ventricles and third ventricle with a normal-sized fourth ventricle indicates noncommunicating hydrocephalus due to obstruction to flow of CSF between the third and fourth ventricles. Posterior fossa tumors can cause noncommunicating hydrocephalus due to extrinsic compression of the ventricular system. In young children, stenosis of the aqueduct of Sylvius is a common cause.

Communicating hydrocephalus is characterized by uniform dilation of all of the ventricles. Communicating hydrocephalus is distinguished from ventricular enlargement secondary to cerebral atrophy by noting that with atrophy the cortical sulci are dilated, whereas in communicating hydrocephalus, the sulci are effaced. Causes of communicating hydrocephalus include SAH, inflammation or infection of the meninges, or any other process that impedes flow of CSF in the subarachnoid space or absorption of CSF through the arachnoid villi.

Hydrocephalus that results from overproduction of CSF is uncommon. It is usually due to an intraventricular choroid plexus papilloma.

An increase in intraventricular pressure causes leakage of CSF from the ventricles into the surrounding white matter. This transependymal extravasation is termed *interstitial edema.* On CT, it appears as a decreased density of the white matter surrounding the ventricles. On MRI, it causes a region of increased signal intensity (Fig. 16-56). In older patients, periventricular lucency secondary to white matter ischemic disease produces a similar radiographic appearance. This can create diagnostic difficulty in elderly patients, who frequently have both white matter abnormalities and ventricular enlargement.

SHUNT MALFUNCTION. Ventriculoperitoneal shunt function should be evaluated with serial CT examinations. Shunt function cannot be determined accurately by a single study. The integrity of the shunt tubing and reservoir are checked by testing the shunt manually and by plain-film examination that encompasses the entire course of the shunt tubing. This can show detachment of parts of the shunt or breaks in its continuity.

NORMAL-PRESSURE HYDROCEPHALUS. Normal-pressure hydrocephalus (NPH) is a clinical triad of urinary incontinence, ataxia, and dementia. These patients have enlarged ventricles without increased ventricular pressure. Some patients may improve clinically after shunting. NPH is often difficult to distinguish from dilation of the ventricles due to diffuse cortical atrophy or from true hydrocephalus.

PSEUDOTUMOR CEREBRI. Pseudotumor cerebri typically occurs in young females. The patient presents with headache or visual changes and has papilledema. On LP, there is an abnormally elevated opening pressure. Imaging studies may be normal or show "slit ventricles." Pseudotumor cerebri is not a radiographic diagnosis because it is difficult to discriminate normal from abnormally small ventricles in a young person.

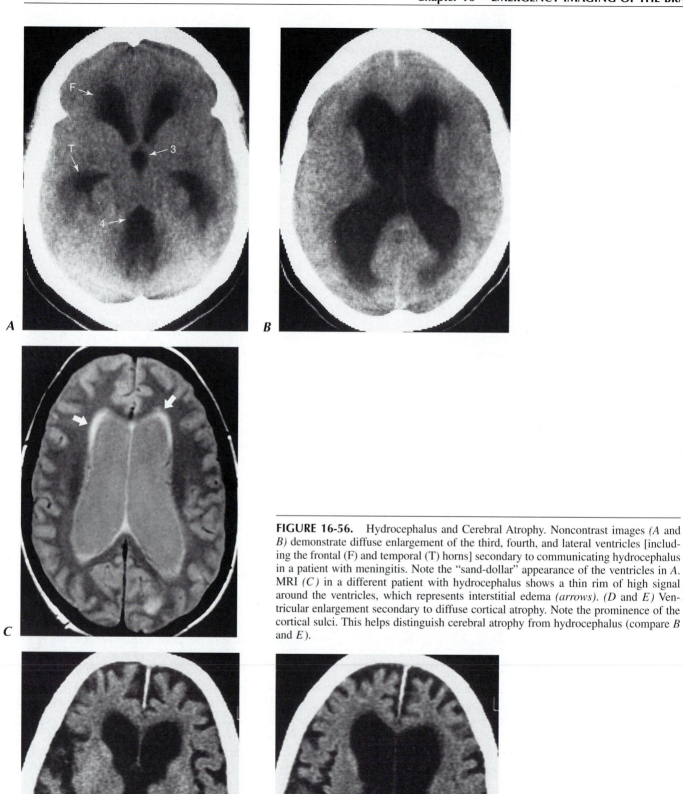

FIGURE 16-56. Hydrocephalus and Cerebral Atrophy. Noncontrast images *(A* and *B)* demonstrate diffuse enlargement of the third, fourth, and lateral ventricles [including the frontal (F) and temporal (T) horns] secondary to communicating hydrocephalus in a patient with meningitis. Note the "sand-dollar" appearance of the ventricles in *A.* MRI *(C)* in a different patient with hydrocephalus shows a thin rim of high signal around the ventricles, which represents interstitial edema *(arrows). (D* and *E)* Ventricular enlargement secondary to diffuse cortical atrophy. Note the prominence of the cortical sulci. This helps distinguish cerebral atrophy from hydrocephalus (compare *B* and *E).*

ERRORS IN INTERPRETATION

CT Artifacts

Artifacts inherent in CT scanning are a common source of CT misinterpretation. *Partial-volume averaging* occurs when a CT slice partly includes both a high-density structure, such as bone, and a low-density structure such as brain. The computer averages these two densities numerically so that the density seen on the CT slice had an intermediate value. This can produce a visible "lesion" on the images.

Beam-hardening artifacts occur when the various wavelengths of the x-ray beam are unequally absorbed as they pass through different cranial tissues. Dense cortical bone absorbs a disproportionate amount of longer-wavelength (softer) x-rays. This produces the darkening and loss of anatomic detail usually seen between the petrous bones in the posterior fossa (Fig. 16-57). Beam hardening also causes *streak artifacts* (alternating dark and white lines) that radiate from thickened points of the skull. Most scanners automatically correct for beam hardening caused by the uniformly dense bone of the calvarium. When this is overcorrected, a *cupping artifact* results. This causes the surface of the brain that lies just beneath the skull to appear abnormally bright, mimicking the appearance of an acute blood collection on the surface of the brain. *Patient motion* during the scan seriously degrades the image quality and also causes streak artifacts, which are due to inconsistency in the x-ray path through the patient.[87]

Calcification

Calcific densities can be mistaken for acute hemorrhage (Table 16-5). Most blood collections are not as well defined as calcifications. Follow-up studies show that the blood resolves over a period of several days, whereas calcifications do not change. On a contrast scan, bone and calcium can look similar to enhancing blood vessels or other enhancing lesions.

Fractures and Vascular Grooves

Skull fractures lack sclerotic borders, whereas vascular grooves have well-marginated sclerotic borders. A linear skull fracture that is parallel to the plane of CT scanning can be missed on routine CT images of the head. For this reason, the lateral scout topogram is carefully reviewed.

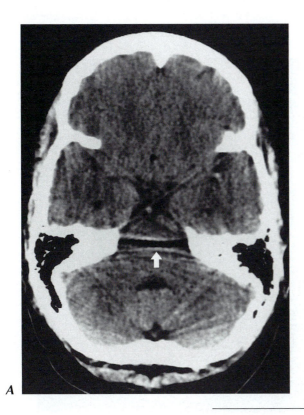
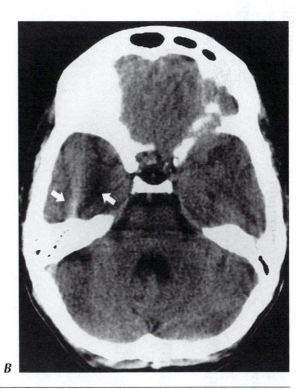

A   *B*

FIGURE 16-57. Beam-hardening artifact. Noncontrast CT image *(A)* shows a black line between the petrous bones *(arrow)*. This represents beam hardening of x-rays as they are absorbed by the dense bone, obscuring the details of the pons. Artifact *(B)* produces abnormal high and low density in the right temporal lobe *(arrow)*.

COMMON VARIANTS

There are several common anatomic variants that should be recognized. Benign calcification or thickening of the tentorium or falx is frequently seen and should not be mistaken for subdural blood (Fig. 16-58). This is more frequently seen in adults. Focal calcification of the falx can mimic a parafalcine meningioma.

Physiologic calcification of the basal ganglia is seen in older adults and should not be misinterpreted as hemorrhage (Fig. 16-59). Basal ganglion calcifications occur in patients with hypoparathyroidism, Wilson disease, Fahr disease (idiopathic basal ganglion calcification), and lead toxicity.

Vascular grooves and venous lakes appear as irregular, nonlinear defects in the skull (Fig. 16-60). These can be mistaken for fractures or metastases. In general, vascular markings follow an irregular course and lack the sharp margins characteristic of fractures.

Cavum septum pellucidum is an anatomic variant that results when the normal embryologic fusion of the two leaves of the septum pellucidum fails to occur. There is persistence of this potential space (Fig. 16-61).

The cisterna magna is a retrocerebellar fluid collection that, if prominent, can be mistaken for other pathologic entities such as a Dandy-Walker cyst, an arachnoid cyst, or a cystic tumor. This is a normal midline CSF collection posterior to the medulla and posteroinferior to the cerebellum. It should not be contiguous with the fourth ventricle (Fig. 16-62).

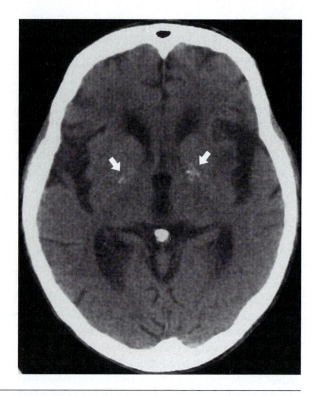

FIGURE 16-59.   Calcification of the basal ganglia. Punctate densities are present in the basal ganglia bilaterally *(arrows)*. Note the symmetrical distribution. Benign physiologic calcifications occur with increased frequency in older adults.

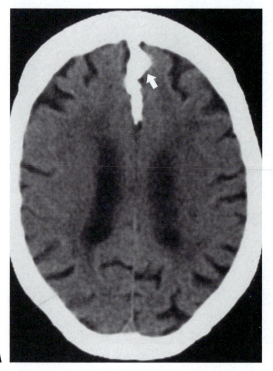

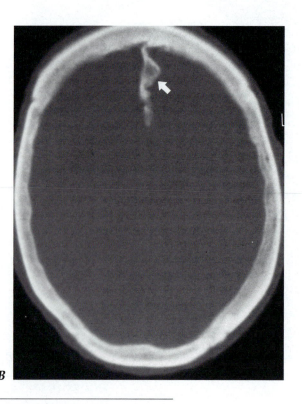

A   *B*

FIGURE 16-58.   Falx calcification. A densely calcified falx *(arrow)* could be misinterpreted as an interhemispheric subdural hemorrhage. The high density of calcium is visible on both the standard soft tissue window image *(A)* and the bone window image *(B)*. Acute hemorrhage has a lower density than calcium and should not be visible on bone images.

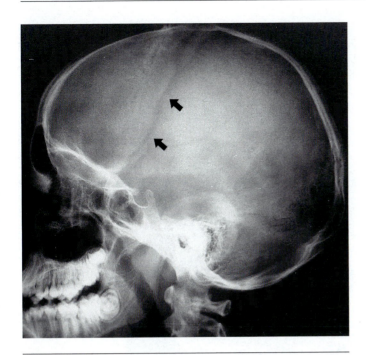

FIGURE 16-60. Vascular grooves. Cranial sutures and vascular grooves *(arrows)* have an irregular course over the calvarium, with ill-defined margins. Linear skull fractures are usually straight, with sharply defined borders (see Fig. 16-10).

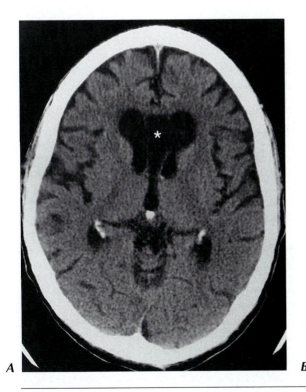
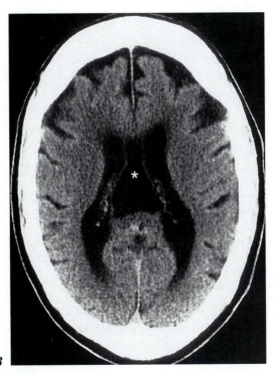

A *B*

FIGURE 16-61. Cavum septum pellucidum. Incomplete midline fusion of the septum pellucidum *(A)* is a common variant. The cavum lies between the frontal horns *(asterisk)*. An image at a slightly higher level *(B)* shows the posterior extension of the cavum between the lateral ventricles, termed *cavum vergae (asterisk)*.

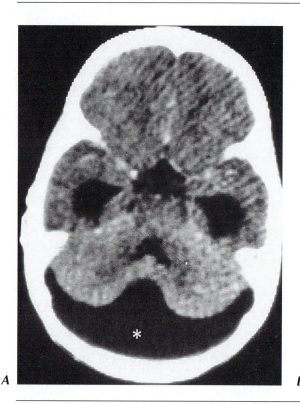
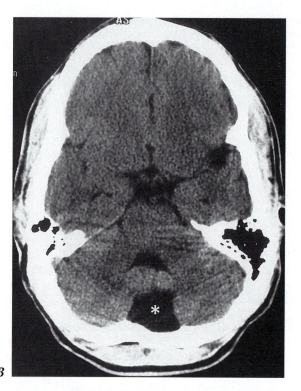

FIGURE 16-62. Cisterna magna. Noncontrast CT *(A)* of an infant brain shows a retrocerebellar CSF collection *(asterisk).* There is no communication with the fourth ventricle. CT of a different patient shows a smaller midline retrocerebellar CSF collection *(B).* This entity is difficult to distinguish from retrocerebellar arachnoid cysts on CT. Lack of mass effect would be atypical of a cystic tumor in this location.

REFERENCES

1. Reinus WR, Zwemer FL Jr: Clinical prediction of emergency cranial computed tomography results. *Ann Emerg Med* 23:1271, 1994.

2. Masters SJ, McClean PM, Arcarese JS, et al: Skull x-ray examinations after head trauma. *N Engl J Med* 316:84, 1987.

3. Macpherson BC, Macpherson P, Jennett B: CT evidence of intracranial contusion and haematoma in relation to the presence, site and type of skull fracture. *Clin Radiol* 42:321, 1990.

4. Osborn AG: Craniocerebral trauma, in Osborn AG: *Diagnostic Neuroradiology.* St. Louis: Mosby–Year Book, 1994, pp. 199–247.

5. Miller EC, Derlet RW, Kinser D: Minor head trauma: Is computed tomography always necessary? *Ann Emerg Med* 27:290, 1996.

6. Stein SC, Ross SE: The value of computed tomographic scans in patients with low risk head injuries. *Neurosurgery* 26:638, 1990.

7. Stein SC, O'Malley KF, Ross SE: Is routine computed tomography too expensive in mild head injury? *Ann Emerg Med* 20:1286, 1991.

8. Yealy DM, Hogan DE: Imaging after head trauma: Who needs what? *Emerg Med Clin North Am* 9:707, 1991.

9. Mikhail MG, Levitt MA, Christopher TA, Sutton MC: Intracranial injury following minor head trauma. *Am J Emerg Med* 10:24, 1992.

10. Borczuk P: Predictors of intracranial injury in patients with mild head trauma. *Ann Emerg Med* 25:731, 1995.

11. Mendelow AD, Teasdale G, Jennett B, et al: Risks of intracranial haematoma in head injured adults. *Br Med J Clin Res Ed* 287:1173, 1983.

12. Vollmer DG, Dacey RG Jr: The management of mild and moderate head injuries. *Neurosurg Clin North Am* 2:437, 1991.

13. Pietrzak M, Jagoda A, Brown L: Evaluation of minor head trauma in children younger than two years. *Am J Emerg Med* 9:153, 1991.

14. Chiaviello CT, Christoph RA, Bond GR: Stairway-related injuries in children. *Pediatrics* 94:679, 1994.

15. Schutzman SA, Barnes PD, Mantello M, Scott RM: Epidural hematomas in children. *Ann Emerg Med* 22:535, 1993.

16. Mitchell KA, Fallat ME, Raque GH, et al: Evaluation of minor head injury in children. *J Pediatr Surg* 29:851, 1994.

17. Cook LS, Levitt MA, Simon B, Williams VL: Identification of ethanol-intoxicated patients with minor head trauma requiring computed tomography scans. *Acad Emerg Med* 1:227–34, 1994.

18. Voss M, Knottenbelt JD, Peden MM: Patients who reattend after head injury: A high risk group. *BMJ* 311:1395, 1995.

19. Snoey ER, Levitt MA: Delayed diagnosis of subdural hematoma following normal computed tomography scan. *Ann Emerg Med* 23:1127, 1994.

20. McMicken DB: Emergency CT head scans in traumatic and atraumatic conditions. *Ann Emerg Med* 15:274, 1986.

21. Shackford SR, Wald SL, Ross SE, et al: The clinical utility of computed tomographic scanning and neurologic examination in the management of patients with minor head injuries. *J Trauma* 33:385, 1992.

22. Cummins RO, LoGerfo JP, Inui TS, Weiss NS: High-yield referral criteria for posttraumatic skull roentgenography. Response of physicians and accuracy of criteria. *JAMA* 244:673, 1980.

23. American College of Emergency Physicians: Clinical policy for the initial approach to adolescents and adults presenting to the emergency department with a chief complaint of headache. *Ann Emerg Med* 26:821, 1996.

24. LeBlanc R: The minor leak preceding subarachnoid hemorrhage. *J Neurosurg* 66:35, 1987.

25. Sames TA, Storrow AB, Finkelstein JA, Magoon MR: Sensitivity of new-generation computed tomography in subarachnoid hemorrhage. *Acad Emerg Med* 3:16, 1996.

26. Sidman R, Connolly E, Lemke T: Subarachnoid hemorrhage diagnosis: Lumbar puncture is still needed when computed tomography scan is normal. *Acad Emerg Med* 3:827, 1996.

27. van der Wee N, Rinkel GJ, Hason D, van Gijn J: Detection of subarachnoid hemorrhage on early CT: Is lumbar puncture still needed after a negative scan? *J Neurol Neurosurg Psychiatry* 58:357, 1995.

28. Singal BM: A tap in time? *Acad Emerg Med* 3:823, 1996.

29. Warden CR, Brownstein DR, Del Beccaro MA: Predictors of abnormal findings on computed tomography of the head in pediatric patients presenting with seizures. *Ann Emerg Med* 29:518, 1997.

30. Reinus WR, Wippold FJ, Erickson KK: Seizure patient selection for emergency computed tomography. *Ann Emerg Med* 22:1298, 1993.

31. Froehling DA, Silverstein MD, Mohr DN, Beatty CW: Does this dizzy patient have a serious form of vertigo? *JAMA* 217:385, 1994.

32. Tso EL, Todd WC, Groleau GA, Hooper FJ: Cranial computed tomography in the emergency department evaluation of HIV-infected patients with neurologic complaints. *Ann Emerg Med* 22:1169, 1993.

33. Murshid WR: Role of skull radiography in the initial evaluation of minor head injury: A retrospective study. *Acta Neurochir (Wien)* 129:11, 1994.

34. Bell RS, Loop AW: The utility and futility of radiographic skull examination for trauma. *N Engl J Med* 284:236, 1971.

35. Greenes DS, Schutzman SA: Infants with isolated skull fractures: What are their clinical characteristics and do they require hospitalization? *Ann Emerg Med* 30:253, 1997.

36. Leonidas JC, Ting W, Binkiewicz A, et al: Mild head trauma in children: When is roentgenogram necessary? *Pediatrics* 69:139, 1982.

37. Harwood-Nash CE, Hendrick EB, Hudson AR: The significance of skull fracture in children. A study of 1,187 patients. *Radiology* 101:151, 1971.

38. Ros SP, Cetta F: Are skull radiographs useful in the evaluation of asymptomatic infants following minor head injury? *Pediatr Emerg Care* 8:328, 1992.

39. Steiger HJ: Assessment and treatment of minor cranio-cerebral injuries. *Schweiz Rundsch Med Prax* 81:879, 1992.

40. Yealy DM, Hogan DE: Imaging after head trauma: Who needs what? *Emerg Med Clin North Am* 9:707, 1991.

41. Ramsey RG: The plain skull film. In Ramsey RG, ed: *Neuroradiology,* 3d ed. Philadelphia: Saunders, 1993, pp. 6–102.

42. Gean AD: *Imaging of Head Trauma.* New York: Raven Press, 1994, pp. 1–25.

43. Gentry LR, Godersky JC, Thompson B: MR imaging of head trauma: Review of the distribution and radiopathologic features of traumatic lesions. *AJR* 150:663, 1988.

44. Bradley WG: MR appearance of hemorrhage in the brain. *Radiology* 189:15, 1993.

45. Gean AD: Neuroradiologic evaluation of head injury, in Gean AD, ed: *ASNR Core Curriculum Course in Neuroradiology.* 1994, pp. 109–117.

46. Zimmerman RD, Yurberg E, Russell EJ, Leeds NE: Falx and interhemispheric fissure on axial CT: 1. Normal anatomy. *AJNR* 3:175, 1982.

47. Dolinskas CA, Zimmerman RA, Bilaniuk LT: A sign of subarachnoid bleeding on cranial computed tomograms of pediatric head trauma patients. *Radiology* 126:409, 1978.

48. Zimmerman RD, Russel EJ, Yurberg E, Leeds NE: Falx and interhemispheric fissure on axial CT: II. Recognition and differentiation of interhemispheric subarachnoid and subdural hemorrhage. *AJNR* 3:635, 1982.

49. Caffey J: The whiplash shaken infant syndrome: Manual shaking by the extremities with whiplash-induced intracranial and intraocular bleedings, linked with residual permanent brain damage and mental retardation. *Pediatrics* 54:396, 1974.

50. Zimmerman RA, Bilaniuk LT, Bruce D, et al: Interhemispheric acute subdural hematoma: A computed tomographic manifestation of child abuse by shaking. *Neuroradiology* 16:39, 1987.

51. Gean AD: Brain herniation, in Gean AD, ed: *Imaging of Head Trauma.* New York: Raven Press; 1994, pp. 249–297.

52. Harrison CL, Dijkers M: Traumatic brain injury registries in the United States: An overview. *Brain Injury* 6:203, 1992.

53. Osborn AG. Stroke, in Osborn AG, ed: *Diagnostic Neuroradiology.* St. Louis: Mosby–Year Book, 1994, p. 331.

54. Grossman RI: Clinical concepts in cerebrovascular disease: Clinical approach and management for diagnostic imaging. *RSNA Syllabus: Special Course in Neuroradiology.* 1994, pp. 9–29.

55. Elster AD: CT and MR imaging of stroke. *ASNR Core Curriculum Course in Neuroradiology.* 1994, pp. 43–48.

56. Yuh WT, Crain MR, Loes DJ, et al: MR imaging of cerebral ischemia: Findings in the first 24 hours. *AJNR* 12:621, 1991.

57. Yuh WT, Crain MR: Magnetic resonance imaging of acute cerebral ischemia. *Neuroimag Clin North Am* 2:421, 1992.

58. Weingarten K: Computed tomography of cerebral infarction. *Neuroimaging Clin North Am* 2:409, 1992.

59. Tissue plasminogen activator for acute ischemic stroke. The NINDS rt-PA Stroke Study Group. *N Engl J Med* 333:1581, 1995.

60. del Zoppo GJ: Acute stroke—On the threshold of a therapy. *N Engl J Med* 333:1632, 1995.

61. Tomura N, Uemura K, Inugami A, et al: Early CT finding in cerebral infarction: Obscuration of the lentiform nucleus. *Radiology* 168:463, 1988.

62. Truwit CL, Barkovich AJ, Gean-Marton A, et al: Loss of the insular ribbon: Another early CT sign of acute middle cerebral artery infarction. *Radiology* 176:801, 1990.

63. Bastianello S, Pierallini A, Colonnese C, et al: Hyperdense middle cerebral artery CT sign. *Neuroradiology* 33:207, 1991.

64. Leys D, Pruvo JP, Godefroy O, et al: Prevalence and significance of hyperdense middle cerebral artery in acute stroke. *Stroke* 23:317, 1992.

65. Crain MR, Yuh WT, Greene GM, et al: Cerebral ischemia: Evaluation with contrast-enhanced MR imaging. *AJNR* 12:631, 1991.

66. Elster AD, Moody DM: Early cerebral infarction: Gadopentetate dimeglumine enhancement. *Radiology* 177:627, 1990.

67. Bozzola FG, Gorelick PB, Jensen JM: Epidemiology of intracranial hemorrhage. *Neuroimag Clin North Am* 2:1, 1992.

68. Gokaslan ZL, Narayan RK: Intracranial hemorrhage in the hypertensive patient. *Neuroimag Clin North Am* 2:171, 1992.

69. Jacobs IG, Roszler MH, Kelly JK, et al: Cocaine abuse: Neurovascular complications. *Radiology* 170:223, 1989.

70. Landi JL, Spickler EM: Imaging of intracranial hemorrhage associated with drug abuse. *Neuroimag Clin North Am* 2:187, 1992.

71. Osborn AG: Intracranial hemorrhage, in Osborn AG, ed: *Diagnostic Neuroradiology*. St. Louis: Mosby–Year Book, 1994, pp. 154–198.

72. Brown E, Prager J, Lee HY, Ramsey RG: CNS complications of cocaine abuse: Prevalence, pathophysiology and neuroradiology. *AJR* 159:137, 1992.

73. Green RM, Kelly KM, Gabrielsen T, et al: Multiple intracerebral hemorrhages after smoking "crack" cocaine. *Stroke* 21:957, 1990.

74. Ramsey RG: Stroke and atherosclerosis, in Ramsey RG, ed: *Neuroradiology*, 3d ed. Philadelphia: Saunders, 1993, pp. 431–494.

75. LeBlanc R, Preul M, Robitaille Y, et al: Surgical considerations in cerebral amyloid angiopathy. *Neurosurgery* 29:712, 1991.

76. Awasthi D, Voorhies RM, Eick J, Mitchell WT: Cerebral amyloid angiopathy presenting as multiple intracranial lesions on magnetic resonance imaging: Case report. *J Neurosurg* 75:458, 1991.

77. Osborn AG: Intracranial aneurysms, in Osborn AG, ed: *Handbook of Neuroradiology*. St. Louis: Mosby–Year Book, 1991, pp. 79–84.

78. Lowie SP: Intracranial hemorrhage in aneurysms and vascular malformations. *Neuroimag Clin North Am* 2:195, 1992.

79. Watanabe AT, Mackey JK, Lufkin RB: Imaging diagnosis and temporal appearance of subarachnoid hemorrhage. *Neuroimag Clin North Am* 2:53, 1992.

80. Atlas SW, Listerud J, Chung W, Flamm ES: Intracranial aneurysms: Depiction on MR angiograms with a multifeature–extraction, ray-tracing post-processing algorithm. *Radiology* 192:129, 1994.

81. Osborn AG: Brain tumors and tumor-like masses, in Osborn AG, ed: *Diagnostic Neuroradiology*. St. Louis: Mosby–Year Book, 1994, pp. 401–408.

82. Haines AB, Zimmerman RD, Morgello S, et al: MR imaging of brain abscesses. *AJNR* 10:279, 1989.

83. Enzmann DR: Viral Meningoencephalitis, in *ASNR Core Curriculum in Neuroradiology: Part II. Neuroplasms and Infectious Disease.* 1996, pp. 179–185.

84. Cox J, Murtagh FR, Wolfong A, Brenner J: Cerebral aspergillosis: MR imaging and histopathologic correlation. *AJNR* 13:1489, 1992.

85. Heinz ER, Ward A, Drayer BP, Dubois PJ: Distinction between obstructive and atrophic dilatation of ventricles in children. *J Comput Assist Tomogr* 4:320, 1980.

86. Barkovich AJ: Hydrocephalus, in Barkovich AJ, ed: *Pediatric Neuroimaging,* 2d ed. New York: Raven Press, 1995, pp. 439–476.

87. Lee SH, Rao KCVG, Zimmerman RA: *Cranial MRI and CT,* 3d ed. New York: McGraw-Hill, 1992, pp. 17–19.

SELECTED READINGS

Gean AD: *Imaging of Head Trauma.* New York: Raven Press, 1994.

Cwinn AA, Grahovac SZ: *Emergency CT Scans of the Head: A Practical Atlas.* St. Louis: Mosby, 1998.

Greenberg JO: *Neuroimaging: A Comparison to Adams and Victor's Principles of Neurology.* New York: McGraw-Hill, 1995.

Kretschmann HJ, Weinrich W: *Cranial Neuroimaging and Clinical Neuroanatomy,* 2d ed. New York: Thieme Medical Publishers, 1992.

Lee SH, Rao KCVG, Zimmerman RA: *Cranial MRI and CT,* 4th ed. New York: McGraw-Hill, 1999.

Osborn AG: *Diagnostic Neuroradiology.* St. Louis: Mosby, 1994.

Ramsey RG: *Neuroradiology,* 3d ed. Philadelphia: WB Saunders, 1993.

Schnitzlein HN, Murtagh FR: *Imaging Anatomy of the Head and Spine,* 2d ed. Baltimore-Munich: Urban and Schwarzenberg, 1990.

Woodruff WW: *Fundamentals of Neuroimaging.* Philadelphia: WB Saunders, 1993.

CHAPTER 17

PULMONARY CHEST RADIOGRAPHY

Mary Jo Wagner / Robert Wolford / Brian Hartfelder / David T. Schwartz

Chest radiographs are the most frequently ordered radiographic studies in the emergency department (ED). Of all ED patients, 16% receive a chest radiograph.[1] Chest radiography is helpful in selected patients with dyspnea, cough and fever, chest pain, and thoracic trauma. Pulmonary disorders with distinctive radiographic findings include pneumonia, tuberculosis, pulmonary edema, pneumothorax, and lung tumors.

Many pulmonary diseases result in the accumulation of fluid within the lung. The difference in radiographic density between normal aerated lung and diseased, fluid-filled lung allows pulmonary disorders to be detected on plain radiographs. Identifying the pattern of pulmonary opacification is a large part of chest radiograph interpretation. However, the pattern of fluid accumulation is usually not diagnostic of one particular disease, and a given radiographic pattern generally suggests a number of diagnostic possibilities. Other chest radiographic patterns include those that cause decreased lung density and those that cause abnormalities of the mediastinum, hilum, pleura, or chest wall.

Chest radiograph interpretation also depends on knowing the radiographic findings associated with particular pulmonary diseases. For example, in a patient with cough and fever, looking specifically for signs of pulmonary infection makes radiograph interpretation accurate and efficient.

CLINICAL DECISION MAKING

Asthma or Chronic Obstructive Pulmonary Disease

The exacerbation of acute asthma or chronic obstructive pulmonary disease (COPD) is a common cause of ED visits. Chest radiography rarely contributes to the management of these patients. Chest radiographs are used to exclude pulmonary infections and such complications as pneumothorax and pneumomediastinum.

NEW-ONSET WHEEZING. Patients presenting to the ED for the first time with bronchospasm should receive a chest radiograph as part of their ED evaluation to exclude alternative causes of wheezing such as congestive heart failure, aspirated foreign body, and pneumonia. Among children with a first episode of wheezing, 94% of chest films are normal or consistent with reactive airway disease.[2,3] Only 6% of these chest films show pathologic findings. Most commonly, radiographic pathology (e.g., pneumonia) is associated with abnormal vital signs or abnormal auscultatory findings such as rales or localized decreased breath sounds.

EXACERBATION OF ASTHMA AND COPD From 50% to more than 90% of chest radiographs of adults and children with acute exacerbation of asthma or COPD are normal or show only hyperinflation and do not affect patient management.[4–7] Aronson classified adult ED asthmatics or COPD patients as either complicated or uncomplicated.[5] Criteria for complicated asthmatics included recent fever or chills, immunosuppression, cancer, intravenous drug abuse, prior cardiothoracic surgery, cardiac disease, or other pulmonary disease (including COPD). No chest film in the uncomplicated asthma admissions resulted in changes in patient management. In the complicated asthmatics, 30% of admission radiographs prompted changes in management. These criteria were validated in a prospective study at the same institution.[8]

Sherman et al. proposed the following indications for admission chest radiographs in patients with asthma or COPD: white blood cell count $>15 \times 10^9$; polymorphonuclear leukocyte count $>8 \times 10^9$; a history of congestive heart failure; coronary artery disease; chest pain; or edema.[9] When Sherman's criteria were retrospectively applied to the ED visits of adult COPD patients, 16% had significant abnormalities on their chest radiographs.[10] The white blood cell count, presence of chest pain, and history of coronary artery disease were not statistically associated with radiographic abnormalities. A history of congestive heart failure, fever, presence of rales, pedal edema, and jugular venous distention were associated with significant chest film findings.

Despite the absence of clear indications for chest radiographs in this setting, reasonable indications for radiography include abnormal findings on physical examination of the chest, abnormal vital signs, immunosuppression, and clinical findings suggestive of congestive heart failure (Table 17-1).

Respiratory Infections

Chest radiographs are often ordered to diagnose serious causes of cough such as pneumonia, tuberculosis, and lung cancer. The

TABLE 17-1

Indications for Chest Radiography in Patients with Asthma or COPD Exacerbations

1. Presence of "high-risk" historical, clinical, or laboratory findings
   Fever
   Abnormal vital signs
   WBCs >15,000 c/mm^3 and PMNs >8000 c/mm^3
   History of congestive heart failure
   History of coronary artery disease
   Chest pain
   Peripheral edema
   Immunosuppressed or HIV infection
   History of intravenous drug abuse
   Prior thoracic surgery
   Localizing physical examination findings suggestive of
      pulmonary infection
2. First episode of wheezing in a child
3. Poor response to intensive bronchodilator treatment
4. Admission

clinical diagnosis of pneumonia is sometimes unsupported by radiographic findings. Melbye et al. studied adult ED patients diagnosed as having a lower respiratory infection, asthma, or COPD exacerbation with convalescent serology and chest radiographs.[11] Only one of eight patients with *Streptococcus pneumoniae* and two of seven patients with *Mycoplasma pneumoniae* infections had radiographic findings. Normal chest films also occur in children with viral or bacterial lower respiratory infections.[12]

Chest radiographs are sometimes used to differentiate bacterial from viral infections. It is assumed that the two etiologic classes of organisms produce identifiable radiographic patterns. Viral or atypical organisms (*Mycoplasma, Chlamydia*) are associated with diffuse airspace filling and interstitial patterns, whereas most bacterial organisms (*S. pneumoniae*) are associated with localized airspace filling. However, the radiographic pattern of the pneumonia does not reliably differentiate viral from bacterial pathogens.[13,14]

Several scoring systems and clinical decision rules have been developed to identify patients who are likely to have chest films demonstrating pneumonia[15] (Table 17-2). Gennis et al. developed criteria to guide the ordering of chest films in adult ED patients with acute respiratory illnesses.[16] The presence of an abnormal vital sign [temperature >37.8°C (100.0°F), pulse >100 beats per minute, respirations >20 breaths per minute] was 97% sensitive for detecting radiographic infiltrates.

Another clinical decision rule for adult ED patients was developed by Heckerling et al.[17] Five predictors for radiographic infiltrate were identified: temperature >37.8°C, pulse >100 beats per minute, presence of rales, decreased breath sounds, and the absence of asthma. The number of variables present predicted the probability of an infiltrate (Table 17-3).

Despite the development of such decision rules, physician judgment is more sensitive than any of the rules but also is less specific.[18] Physician judgment and all decision rules possessed high negative predictive values.

TABLE 17-2

Indications for Chest Radiography in Patients with Possible Community-Acquired Pneumonia

Children
Fever or abnormal chest auscultation
   or
Physician judgment

Adults
Gennis rule
   Any abnormal vital sign:
      Temperature >37.8°C
      Pulse >100/min
      Respirations >20/min
or
Diehr score ≥0
   Add points for each variable present:
      Rhinorrhea (−2)
      Sore throat (−1)
      Night sweats (1)
      Myalgias (1)
      Sputum (1)
      Respirations >25/min (2)
      Temperature >37.7°C (2)
or
Heckerling score ≥2
   Add 1 point for each variable present:
      Temperature >37.8°C
      Pulse >100/min
      Rales
      Decreased breath sounds
      Absence of asthma
or
Physician judgment

TABLE 17-3

Heckerling Score: Predicted Probability of Radiographic Infiltrate in Patients Suspected of Having Pneumonia

NUMBER OF ABNORMAL VARIABLES	PREDICTED PROBABILITY (%) (PREVALENCE 12.4–30%)
0	1–3
1	3.1–9.1
2	9.2–24.2
3	24.5–50.6
4	51.0–76.6
5	76.9–91.3

SOURCE: From Heckerling et al.,[17] with permission.

Reasonable indications for radiography in patients with symptoms of respiratory infections include abnormal chest findings on physical examination, abnormal vital signs, immunosuppression (e.g., AIDS, malignancy, alcoholism). However, physician judgment remains critical in determining the role of chest radiography in these patients. Furthermore, the absence of an infiltrate does not exclude a pneumonia requiring antibiotics.

Chest Pain or Shortness of Breath

In patients with dyspnea and chest pain, chest films have a high incidence of abnormalities. Buenger reviewed 5000 ED chest radiographs, 25% of which were ordered for the complaints of chest pain, dyspnea, or congestive heart failure.[19] Significant radiographic findings were found in 79% of patients suspected of having congestive heart failure. The incidence of abnormal findings varied for dyspnea (55%), chest pain and dyspnea (34%), and chest pain alone (25%).

Two other studies showed that patients with chest pain have a high incidence of radiographic abnormalities. Russell analyzed ED patients with anterior chest pain and found that 17% of them had radiographic abnormalities that either contributed to the diagnosis or influenced management (e.g., pulmonary edema).[20] In another study of adult ED patients with chest pain, 44% of all chest films had an abnormality. Of these abnormalities, 52% were significant (e.g., pulmonary vascular congestion, cardiomegaly).[21]

Thoracic Trauma

Because chest injuries are a common cause of trauma-related deaths, a chest radiograph must be obtained on all patients who have suffered significant blunt or penetrating trauma to the torso. In addition, patients who are unconscious, going to the operating room or in respiratory distress also require a chest film.[22]

Thompson et al. evaluated patients with penetrating chest wounds to compare the physical examination with radiology in detecting hemothoraces and pneumothoraces.[23] Chest radiography was necessary to reliably exclude large hemopneumothoraces, small hemothoraces, and small pneumothoraces.

The initial chest film obtained during the resuscitation of the trauma patient is usually a supine portable radiograph. It is often assumed that most significant abnormalities are detected by this radiographic technique. However, Hehir et al. found that 25% of survivors and 47% of patients who died in the hospital had significant chest injuries that were missed by the initial study.[24] McLellan similarly found that 30% of significant chest injuries found on autopsy were missed on a single anteroposterior (AP) chest film.[25]

Routine Admission and Preoperative Chest Radiographs

ED patients are frequently admitted to the hospital. Often, if a chest film has not been obtained during the patient's ED evaluation, it is frequently obtained upon his or her admission.[26,27] However, patients without chest symptomatology or abnormal chest physical findings and who are younger than 40 years of age are unlikely to have an abnormal chest radiograph on hospital admission.

One prospective study grouped adult patients admitted to the hospital from the ED as being at "high risk" (age ≥65 years, history of cigarette use, altered mental status or HIV infection)

TABLE 17-4

Indications for "Routine" Admission Chest Radiographs

1. Planned thoracic surgery or procedure
2. Age <40 years with chest symptoms, or history of hemoptysis and/or abnormal chest physical examination or persistent chest symptoms
3. Age ≥40 years and chest symptoms or abnormal chest examination

and as "low risk" (absence of high-risk criteria).[28] Some 75% of all patients (82% of high-risk versus 61% of low-risk patients) had abnormalities found on their "routine admission" chest films. However, many of these abnormalities were chronic and of limited clinical consequence. Only 4% of patients (all high-risk) had their hospital management altered by the radiographic findings.

Patient age, hemoptysis, and abnormal physical examination findings are also important predictors of acute findings on the chest film.[29] In one study, 2.9% of patients below 40 years of age who did not have abnormalities on physical examination, hemoptysis, or other indications for chest radiography had acute findings on their chest film (mediastinal mass, pneumonia). Patients 40 years of age or older more frequently (37%) had acute radiographic findings and normal chest physical examinations (Table 17-4).

RADIOGRAPHIC TECHNIQUE

The preferred radiographic studies of the chest are the posteroanterior (PA) and lateral views (Table 17-5). Ideally, the patient is standing. The standard distance between the x-ray source and film is 6 ft. Equipment in the radiology suite produces high-energy x-rays that provide proper penetration with a short exposure time. This decreases motion artifact and reduces the radiographic opacity of skeletal structures so that they do not obscure overlying lung and soft tissues. Portable equipment cannot produce high-energy x-rays and therefore does not have these advantages.

The PA Radiograph

The PA projection is obtained with the x-ray beam passing through the thorax from posterior to anterior. The anterior chest is positioned flat against the film cassette. The upper arms are abducted and the dorsa of the hands are placed on the hips. In this position, the scapulae are rotated laterally to reduce their overlap on the lungs. The patient inspires maximally and maintains this position throughout the exposure.

The Lateral Radiograph

For the standard lateral view, the patient is positioned with the left chest wall against the film cassette (a left lateral radio-

TABLE 17-5

Radiographic Views of the Chest

VIEW	POSITION	ADEQUACY	LIKELY FINDINGS
Posteroanterior (PA)	Patient standing. Anterior chest against film cassette. Scapulae rotated laterally. Horizontal x-ray beam.	Entire thorax seen. Correct penetration. Full inspiration. No rotation.	In combination with lateral, will identify most pathology. Confirm and localize infiltrates and other lung lesions.
Left lateral	Left lateral chest wall placed against film cassette. Arms elevated.	Entire thorax seen. Correct penetration. Full inspiration. No rotation.	Hilar adenopathy. Small pleural effusions. Interlobar fissures thickened in pulmonary edema. Heart size.
Anteroposterior (AP) (portable)	Patient supine or upright with back against film cassette.	Entire thorax seen. Correct penetration. Full inspiration. No rotation.	Most gross pathology. Limited in comparison to PA view.
Apical lordotic	Patient inclined 60° with posterior surface of shoulders against cassette.	Clavicles projected above lung apices.	Apical pathology— tuberculosis, tumors.
Lateral decubitus	An AP view with patient lying in lateral decubitus position. Arms extended above head.	Thoracic cavity well visualized. Arms do not overlap thorax.	Pleural effusion. Pneumothorax. Air trapping (bronchial obstruction).

graph). However, if the pathology is known to be in the right lung, the exposure can be obtained with the patient in the right lateral position. The film is marked by the radiology technician as to which lateral projection was obtained. With a lateral radiograph, the patient is standing or sitting upright with the arms extended forward and upward to minimize overlap with the lungs. If the pathology is in the anterior mediastinum, the arms can be extended posteriorly.

Portable Chest Technique

In unstable patients, an AP portable chest radiograph is performed with the patient lying either flat or upright on a stretcher. Upright positioning is preferred whenever possible. With the portable radiograph, patients are less able to inspire completely, rotation is more frequent, and a longer exposure time is required, thus increasing motion artifact. The focus-to-film distance is shortened to 40 in., causing magnification of the anterior structures. The cardiac diameter is about 15 to 20% larger than on the posteroanterior (PA) view.

Many trauma victims and critically ill patients cannot be placed in a sitting position; therefore a supine AP radiograph must be obtained. This further compromises the radiographic technique. The patient's ability to inhale maximally is additionally restricted. The heart and upper mediastinum appear

wider than on an upright film. The recognition of a pneumothorax is hindered because free air moves to the nondependent anterior thorax, which is perpendicular to the x-ray beam. The detection of hemothoraces and pleural effusions is limited for similar reasons.

Supplementary Chest Radiographic Views

Other radiographic views aid in specific situations (Table 17-5). These include the lateral decubitus, expiratory, lordotic, rib, and sternal projections.

Lateral Decubitus Radiograph.   The lateral decubitus radiograph is not actually a lateral view but an AP projection obtained with the patient in either the left or right lateral decubitus position. When one is evaluating for pleural effusions or bronchial obstruction with air trapping, the side of the thorax with pathology is placed in the dependent position. In the evaluation of a pneumothorax or to show the lung that is obscured by pleural fluid, the affected side of the thorax is placed in the nondependent position.

Expiratory View.   An expiratory view is sometimes obtained in addition to the standard inspiratory view in patients suspected of having a small pneumothorax or a bronchial foreign body.

The expiratory view is obtained at maximal end-expiration. The radiographic density of the lung increases during expiration, resulting in greater contrast between the lung and pneumothorax. Additionally, the lung is displaced further from the chest wall, enhancing visualization of the visceral pleural edge. When a radiolucent bronchial foreign body is suspected, an expiratory view can detect air trapping. There is less of a decrease in lung volume during expiration on the obstructed side.

Apical Lordotic View. The lordotic view provides better visualization of the lung apices. The lordotic view is obtained with the patient inclined at 60° with the x-ray beam passing from anterior to posterior. This moves the clavicles and the costochondral junction above the apices of the lungs.

Rib and Sternum Views. A standard rib series includes an AP and oblique thoracic views and a lower rib AP view. Sternum views include a lateral radiograph and a slightly oblique PA view in which the sternum is not superimposed on the vertebrae.

RADIOGRAPHIC ANATOMY—THE NORMAL CHEST RADIOGRAPH

The pulmonary structures seen on a plain chest radiograph include the lungs, hila, pulmonary vasculature, and proximal tracheobronchial tree (Fig. 17-1). Cardiovascular structures within the mediastinum include the heart, thoracic aorta, superior and inferior vena cava, and main pulmonary arteries and veins. Peripheral thoracic structures include the chest wall, diaphragm, and thoracic spine. Although a comparison of the left and right sides of the thorax is often helpful in assessing a questionable radiographic abnormality, many anatomic structures are not symmetrical.

Anatomy of the Lungs

The right lung is divided into upper, middle, and lower lobes. The left lung has only upper and lower lobes. The lingula, a portion of the left upper lobe, corresponds to the middle lobe of the right lung. Interlobar fissures separating these lobes appear as fine white lines on the chest radiograph (Fig. 17-2). The entire length of the fissure is not usually seen. Both lungs have a *diagonal fissure* (also called an *oblique* or *major fissure*) between the upper and lower lobes. The right lung is also divided by a *horizontal fissure* (or *minor fissure*), which separates the upper and middle lobes. The diagonal fissures are seen on the lateral film and the horizontal fissure is seen on both the PA and lateral film.

The lung is further divided into segments (Fig. 17-3). The segmental divisions are based on the branching of the bronchial tree, and no intrapulmonary septa separate these segments. Therefore, although a pneumonia may remain predominantly in an individual segment, such as the anterior segment of the left lower lobe, because there are no connective tissue boundaries between segments, the pneumonia readily spreads beyond a single segment.

Normal Lung Markings

Normal lung markings are comprised of pulmonary blood vessels and therefore have the features of vascular structures. Lung markings have a branching appearance and get progressively

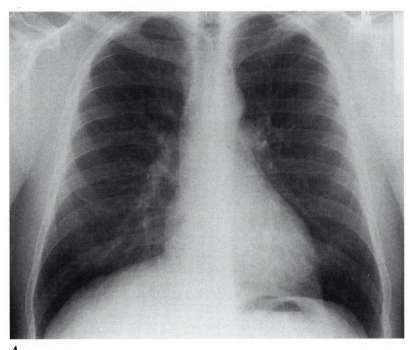

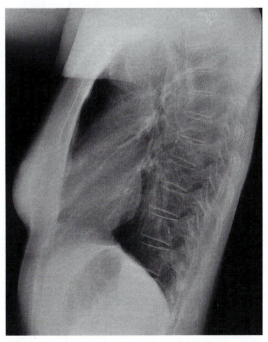

A   *B*

FIGURE 17-1. PA and lateral chest radiographs.

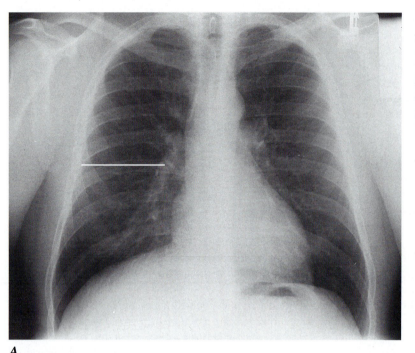
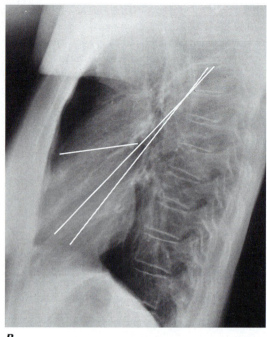

A   *B*

FIGURE 17-2.   Interlobar fissures. On the PA radiograph, only the horizontal (minor) fissure is seen. On the lateral radiograph, both oblique (major) fissures and the horizontal fissure are seen. The approximate locations of the fissures are depicted. The entire length of the fissures are not usually seen.

smaller from the central regions of the lung to the periphery (Fig. 17-4). They become faint and disappear within about 1 cm of the pleural surface. Lung markings that extend to the pleural surface are abnormal. Because the lung is a three-dimensional structure, overlap of pulmonary blood vessels creates a reticular (netlike) appearance. Confluence of vascular shadows can sometimes have a cystic appearance, which should not be misinterpreted as abnormal. The margins of vascular markings are normally well defined.

When pulmonary blood vessels are seen on end, they appear as white dots (Fig. 17-4). These white dots can be differentiated from small calcified granulomas by noting that blood vessels seen on end have the same cross-sectional diameter as nearby blood vessels, while granulomas are larger. This distinction is easier to make in the peripheral zones of the lung.

The proximal segments of the bronchial tree are visible on chest radiographs when they are seen directly on end. They appear as small circles of about the same diameter as nearby blood vessels and normally have "pencil-line thin" walls (Fig. 17-4).

The overall lung density is greater in the medial (central) portions of each lung because the lung is thicker in these regions. In addition, the radiographic density of the

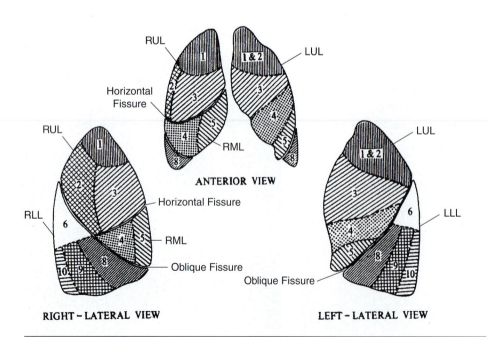

FIGURE 17-3.   Pulmonary lobes and segments. Right upper lobe (RUL): apical (1), anterior (2), posterior (3). Right middle lobe (RML): lateral, (4) medial (5). Right lower lobe (RLL): superior (6), medial basal (7), anterobasal (8), lateral basal (9), posterobasal (10). Left upper lobe (LUL): apical posterior (1 and 2), anterior (3), superior lingular (4), inferior lingular (5). Left lower lobe (LLL): superior (6), medial basal (7), anterobasal (8), lateral basal (9), posterobasal (10). (From Pansky B: *Review of Gross Anatomy,* 6th ed. McGraw-Hill, 1996,with permission.)

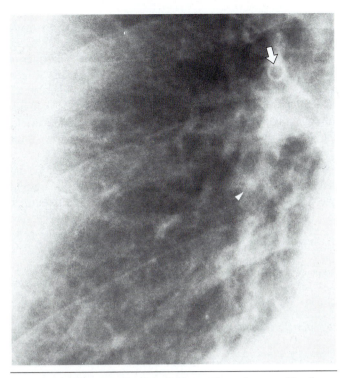

FIGURE 17-4. Normal lung markings. The pulmonary blood vessels successively branch and become finer toward the lung periphery. The overlapping lung markings create a reticular pattern. The confluence of shadows can have a cystlike appearance. The small round white dot is a blood vessel seen on end *(arrowhead)*. Near the hilum, a bronchus is seen end-on *(arrow)*. The wall of the bronchus is normally "pencil-line thin."

two lungs should be symmetrical, such that each portion of one lung should appear the same as the equivalent portion of the opposite lung. This left-to-right comparison is made using the lung seen between two ribs—for example, the interspace between the fourth and fifth ribs. Because the heart is not located symmetrically within the chest, equivalent portions of each lung should be determined with reference to the midline of the thorax, not the distance from the mediastinum.

Normal lung markings vary greatly from person to person, and the physician must avoid overreading prominent but normal lung markings as abnormal. An understanding of the changes expected with airspace-filling and interstitial lung disorders helps differentiate normal but prominent lung markings from abnormal lung markings. Nonetheless, this differentiation can be difficult to make in subtle cases. Abnormal lung markings often have blurred, indistinct margins. They do not branch or become successively smaller from the central to the peripheral regions of the lung and may extend all the way to the pleural surfaces. Abnormal lung markings often have a fine reticular pattern. However, overlapping normal vascular marking can also create a fine reticular pattern. Identification of other radiographic findings associated with but easier to distinguish from increased lung marking can also be helpful. These findings include thickening of the wall of a bronchus seen on end, air bronchograms, thickening of the interlobar fissures, and a pleural effusion. In the elderly and in patients who smoke cigarettes or who have prior pulmonary disease, thin fibrotic lines and thin-walled bullae are common.

Centrally, the main pulmonary arteries and veins radiate outward from the hilum. However, in the middle and lower portions of the lungs, the pulmonary veins run in a horizontal direction (Fig. 17-5). In both lungs, the pulmonary arteries of the lower lobe run for 2 to 4 cm before dividing. On the lateral radiograph, both lower lobe pulmonary arteries overlap as they extend posteriorly and inferiorly from the hilum (Fig. 17-1*B*). The increased vascular density in these regions should not be misinterpreted as abnormal. In addition, subtle abnormalities can be difficult to discern in this area.

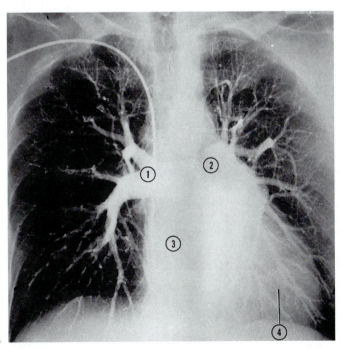

A

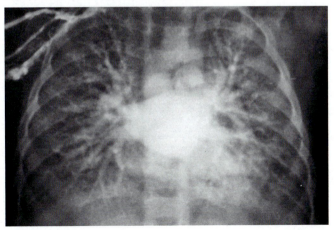

B

FIGURE 17-5. Normal pulmonary angiogram showing the anatomy of the central pulmonary vasculature. *A.* The arterial phase shows the major upper and lower lobe pulmonary artery branches and the subsequent segmental divisions. The left side is partly obscured by the mediastium. (1) Right pulmonary artery; (2) left pulmonary artery; (3) right ventricle; (4) left ventricle. (From Pansky B: *Review of Gross Anatomy,* 6th ed. New York: McGraw-Hill, 1996. With permission.) *B.* The venous phase shows the left and right superior and inferior pulmonary veins emptying into the left atrium (LA). (From Fischer HW: *Radiographic Anatomy: A Working Atlas.* New York: McGraw-Hill, 1988. With permission.)

The Heart, Mediastinum, and Hilum

The mediastinum is divided into superior, anterior, middle, and posterior regions. The superior region includes the trachea, aortic arch, and nearby lymphatics. The hilum makes up the middle region and consists mostly of pulmonary vascular structures. The anterior mediastinum is the heart. The posterior mediastinum contains the descending aorta and the esophagus.

On the PA radiograph, the left and right mediastinal contours represent the heart and great vessels (Fig. 17-6). The lateral radiograph provides a different view of the mediastinal structures (Fig. 17-7).

THE HEART.   The contours of the cardiac silhouette are made up by specific heart chambers (Fig. 17-6). On the PA film, the right heart border is formed by the right atrium. The inferior vena cava forms the inferior corner of the right heart border, where it intersects the right hemidiaphragm. The right ventricle is not seen because it is an anterior structure. The left side of the cardiac silhouette is formed largely by the left ventricle. The left atrial appendage is located in a slight concavity at the superior part of the left heart border.

On the lateral radiograph, the right ventricle forms the anterior aspect of the heart (Fig. 17-7). The posterior margin of the heart is the left atrium (superiorly) and the left ventricle (inferiorly). The inferior vena cava is sometimes seen where the heart intersects the diaphragm.

The *cardiothoracic ratio* provides an estimate of heart size. It is determined by measuring the cardiac width at its widest point and comparing this to the greatest thoracic diameter as measured from the inner margins of the ribs. The normal heart is less than half the width of the thoracic diameter, (i.e., a cardiothoracic ratio ≤50%) (Fig. 17-8).

THE SUPERIOR MEDIASTINUM AND MEDIASTINAL PLEURAL REFLECTION LINES. Several distinct radiographic lines are seen within the mediastinum (Fig. 17-9). Absence or distortion of these lines can indicate pathology. The superior mediastinum should be less than 7.5 cm in width on a normal PA chest film. However, in determining mediastinal pathology, the "visual impression" of an abnormally wide mediastinum is more accurate than its actual measurement.[30]

The tracheal air shadow should be in the midline. It can be displaced slightly toward the right at the level of the aortic arch. The right tracheal wall extends from the thoracic inlet to the right tracheobronchial angle. The right tracheal wall is outlined by the *right paratracheal stripe*, which is a thin layer of connective tissue between the right tracheal wall and the right lung. Normally, it is less than 5 mm wide. Inferiorly, the right paratracheal stripe ends in a slight bulge, the arch of the azygos vein, which crosses over the right mainstem bronchus. The right

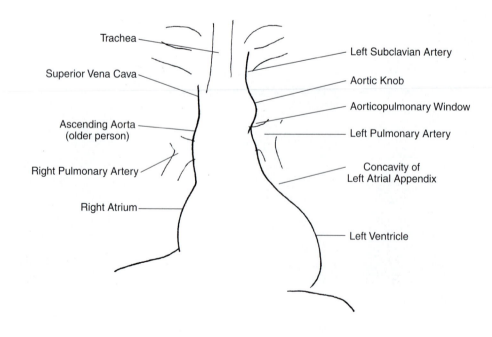

FIGURE 17-6.   Heart and mediastinal borders on the PA radiograph.

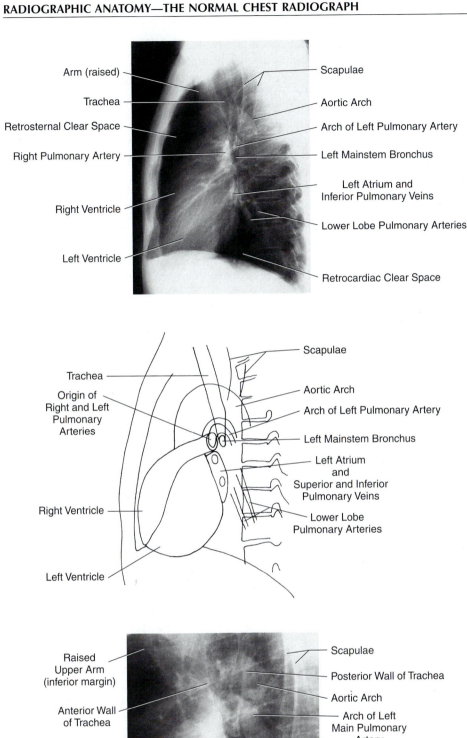

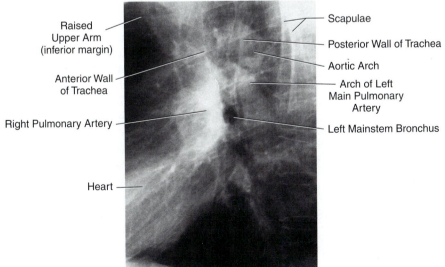

FIGURE 17-7. Heart and mediastinum on the lateral radiograph.

paratracheal stripe is widened or obliterated by fluid or blood in the mediastinum or by lymphadenopathy. There is no distinct left paratracheal stripe because the left tracheal wall is adjacent to mediastinal soft tissues.

The faint shadow of the *superior vena cava* is sometimes seen at the right border of the superior mediastinum. The left margin of the superior mediastinum is the *left subclavian artery,* which makes a gentle concave curve and disappears at the superior cortex of the clavicle.

The *ascending aorta* occupies the lower right side of the superior mediastinum. In an older individual with a tortuous aorta, the ascending aorta makes a convex curve on the right mediastinal contour. The aortic arch curves to the left and posteriorly and then downward, forming a prominent rounded shadow on the PA chest radiograph—the *aortic knob.* Inferior to the aortic arch and superior to the left pulmonary artery is a concavity called the *aorticopulmonary window.* This space can be filled in by lymphadenopathy or fluid (blood) in the mediastinum (Fig. 17-10).

The left (lateral) margin of the *descending aorta* makes a distinct shadow below the aortic knob and extending down to the diaphragm. The medial (right) margin of the descending aorta lies within the mediastinal soft tissues and does not cast a radiographic shadow. The *left paraspinal line* parallels the left side of the vertebral bodies and extends from the diaphragm to the aortic arch. It lies medial to the left margin of the descending aorta. A right paraspinal line is seen less frequently.

In the midline below the carina, the medial surface of the right lung lies posterior to the heart, adjacent to the esophagus. This prominent pleural reflection line is called the *azygo-esophageal recess.* Although the azygo-esophageal recess often parallels the descending aorta, it should not be misinterpreted as the medial border of the descending aorta.

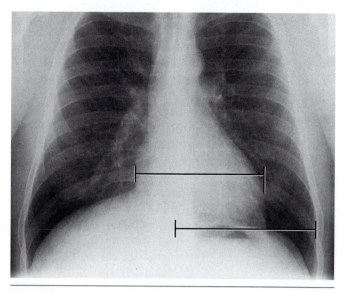

FIGURE 17-8. Cardiothoracic ratio. The widest diameter of the heart is compared with the width of half the thorax at its widest point measured to the inner margin of the ribs. Normally, the cardiac diameter is less than the diameter of the hemithorax.

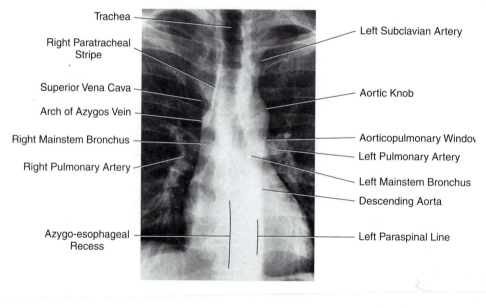

Trachea		Left Subclavian Artery
Right Paratracheal Stripe		
Superior Vena Cava		Aortic Knob
Arch of Azygos Vein		
Right Mainstem Bronchus		Aorticopulmonary Window
Right Pulmonary Artery		Left Pulmonary Artery
		Left Mainstem Bronchus
		Descending Aorta
Azygo-esophageal Recess		Left Paraspinal Line

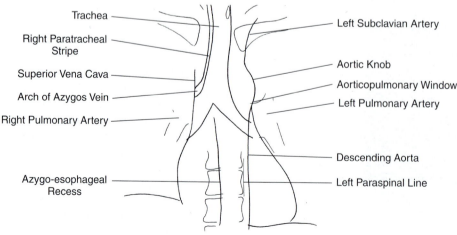

FIGURE 17-9. Mediastinal pleural reflection lines on PA radiograph.

The Lateral Radiograph. On the lateral view, the tracheal air column extends from the thoracic inlet to the carina (Fig. 17-7). The thin anterior and posterior walls of the trachea are visible. Thickening of the posterior tracheal wall is a sign of lymphadenopathy. The left mainstem bronchus is frequently seen end-on at the termination of the tracheal air column. Two thin lines representing the scapular bodies seen end-on should not be misinterpreted as the posterior tracheal wall. The superior portion of the arch of the aorta is visible on the lateral view. In an older individual with an elongated tortuous aorta, the descending aorta is seen overlying the thoracic vertebral bodies.

THE HILUM. The hilum is composed of the left and right main pulmonary arteries and the superior pulmonary veins. The inferior pulmonary veins enter the left atrium below the hilum. The main pulmonary artery bifurcates within the pericardium and its divisions follow the course of the mainstem bronchi. The inferior branch of the right main pulmonary artery provides most of the lateral border of the lower right hilum. The superior branch of the right pulmonary artery lies medial to the vein, so that the right superior pulmonary vein produces the lateral border of the upper right hilum. On the left, the pulmonary artery and its branches form the margins of the left hilum (Fig. 17-11). The left and right hila should be roughly symmetrical although the left hilum is superior to the right hilum by about 2 cm.

At the division of the trachea, the mainstem bronchi are asymmetrical. The left mainstem bronchus is more horizontal and the left upper lobe bronchus arises more distally as compared with the right side.

The Lateral Radiograph. On the lateral radiograph, the right and left hila are superimposed (Fig. 17-7). The left upper lobe bronchus is seen on end and its superior margin is outlined by the arch of the left pulmonary artery. The right upper lobe bronchus is usually less distinct. Anterior to the lower portion of the trachea, the opacity of the overlapping right pulmonary artery and vein is seen. The posterior tracheal wall is visible on the lateral chest film and normally has a width of 2 to 4 mm. The inferior pulmonary veins are seen end-on entering the left atrium below the hila and form an opacity that should not be mistaken for a parenchymal mass.

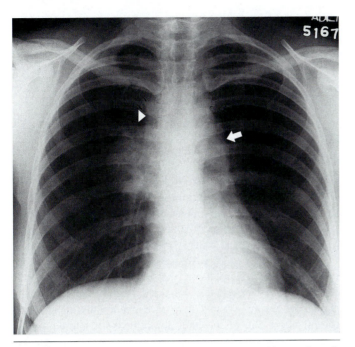

FIGURE 17-10. Abnormal mediastinal contours. The aorticopulmonary window is obliterated by lymphadenopathy *(arrows)*. There is a large rounded right hilar mass. The right paratracheal stripe is widened *(arrowhead)*.

The Diaphragm

The diaphragm attaches to ribs 7 to 12. The apex ("dome") of the right side of the diaphragm is usually 1.5 to 2.5 cm higher than the left. The left and right domes of the diaphragm make smooth, convex curves from the lateral rib margins to the mid-

line. Both the cardiophrenic (medial) sulci and the costophrenic (lateral) sulci are normally clear and sharp (Fig. 17-1A).

The Lateral Radiograph. On the lateral radiograph, the left and right diaphragmatic domes can be distinguished by four criteria (Figs. 17-1B and 17-7). In any given radiograph, one, two or all of these criteria may be present. First, the right diaphragm is usually 1 to 3 cm higher than the left. Second, the gastric air bubble is located under the left hemidiaphragm. Third, the heart lies against the anterior portion of the left hemidiaphragm, so that the left dome of the diaphragm disappears (is "silhouetted out") anteriorly, whereas the right dome of the diaphragm is normally visible all the way to the anterior chest wall.

Fourth, because on the standard lateral radiograph the patient is positioned with the left side of the chest against the film cassette (a "left lateral" radiograph), the right side of the chest is further from the film and is magnified (appears larger). The right ribs are therefore larger and usually more posteriorly located than the left ribs. Both of the diaphragmatic domes can be followed posteriorly to its respective costophrenic sulcus. The right costophrenic sulcus intersects with the right ribs, which are larger and more posterior than the left ribs.

RADIOGRAPHIC ANALYSIS

There are two complementary approaches to the interpretation of chest radiographs: (1) a systematic examination of the film; and (2) a targeted analysis looking for radiographic patterns of pulmonary diseases (Table 17-6). In a *systematic analysis,* each tissue density is examined in all regions of the film—bones, soft tissues, and airspaces. Although theoretically, no finding

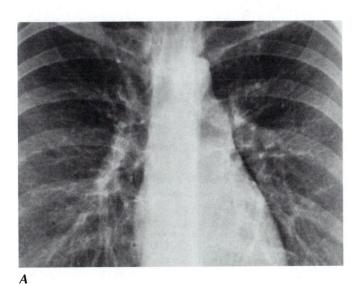

A

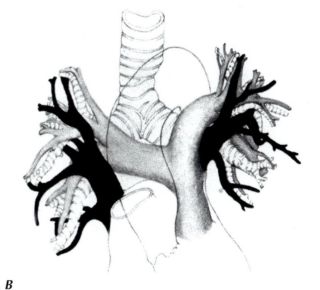

B

FIGURE 17-11. Normal hilar anatomy. *A.* The normal hilum has a branching vascular appearance in which the vascular divisions are successively thinner and less radiodense. The pulmonary arteries of the lower lobes extend 2 to 4 cm before branching. Two-thirds of the vascular density of the hilum is in its lower half. The hila are roughly symmetrical, although the left side is slightly higher than the right, and the left hilum is partly hidden by the mediastinum. *B.* The pulmonary arteries are shown in gray. The superior pulmonary veins are shown in black. The aorta is outlined and transparent. The superior vena cava is cut away. On the right, the pulmonary artery and vein are anterior to the right mainstem bronchus. On the left, the pulmonary artery arches over the left mainstem bronchus. (*B.* From Novelline RA: *Squire's Fundamentals of Radiology,* 5th ed. Cambridge, MA: Harvard University Press, 1997, with permission.)

TABLE 17-6

How to Read a Chest Radiograph

Systematic analysis	Adequacy Bones Soft tissues Lungs	Adequacy Central—mediastinum Middle—lungs Periphery—chest wall
Targeted analysis	Pattern recognition	Airspace filling Interstitial patterns Lymphadenopathy
	Diagnosis-based approach	Pneumonia Congestive heart failure Pneumothorax

should be missed using this technique, the systematic review is laborious and time-consuming for less experienced interpreters. Normal structures can be misinterpreted as pathologic and subtle abnormalities are often missed. Nonetheless, the systematic approach compels the examiner, after an initial inspection of the radiograph, to carefully reexamine the bones, soft tissues, and all airspaces.

An accurate and efficient technique of chest radiograph interpretation involves a *targeted analysis*. The targeted analysis

TABLE 17-7

Systematic Analysis of the Frontal Chest Radiograph

Adequacy	Assess penetration, rotation, inspiration
Bones and chest wall	Ribs, clavicles, shoulders, thoracic vertebrae Chest wall masses, subcutaneous air, breasts
Soft tissues	
Heart	Heart size (cardiothoracic ratio) Cardiac contours (heart chambers)
Mediastinum	Mediastinal widening Trachea midline Mediastinal contours—aortic knob, descending aorta, 　aorticopulmonary window, left subclavian artery, superior 　vena cava Pleural reflection lines—right paratracheal stripe, left 　paraspinous line
Hila	Lymphadenopathy, masses, increased vascularity, calcification
Diaphragm	Assess contour, effusion (costophrenic sulci) Intraabdominal abnormalities (free air)
Lungs	Inspect each region of both lungs using symmetry 　Lung markings (normal branching vascular structures) 　Airspace filling: 　　Opacification, silhouette signs, indistinct lung markings, 　　　air bronchograms 　Interstitial processes: 　　Reticular or nodular patterns, septal lines (Kerley A or B 　　　lines) 　Pleural regions—thickening, effusion, or pneumothorax

is based on (1) knowledge of the pathologic radiographic patterns seen in the thorax and (2) an understanding of the radiographic findings expected with the suspected pulmonary disease. Using *pattern-recognition,* a differential diagnosis is based on the particular radiographic pattern identified. This approach is especially important for the radiologist whose only information about the patient is derived from the radiograph. Most often, pulmonary abnormalities are associated with increased lung opacity (airspace filling and interstitial lung disorders). In other cases, there is decreased pulmonary opacity or abnormalities of the mediastinum, pleura, or chest wall.

A *diagnosis-based approach* to the interpretation of chest radiographs depends on knowledge of the radiographic findings associated with the diagnoses under consideration. For example, suspicion of a pneumothorax leads to careful inspection of the lung adjacent to the chest wall for signs of collapsed lung. Suspicion of pneumonia prompts examination for focal areas of opacity, blurring of the margins of the heart or diaphragm, indistinct lung markings, and "air-bronchograms." In addition, regions of the film where focal infiltrates are difficult to detect are closely reviewed. A diagnosis-based approach should not be used exclusively, because this can lead one to miss unexpected but significant findings such as a small asymptomatic neoplasm in the lung apex hidden by the overlapping clavicle.

A *systematic approach* to reading the chest radiograph is presented in this section. *Radiographic patterns* of chest diseases are presented in the following section. *Specific thoracic diseases* are discussed in the Common Abnormalities section and in Chap. 18, "Cardiovascular Imaging."

Systematic Analysis of the PA Radiograph

In a systematic approach, each tissue density is examined in every region of the film (Table 17-7). First the bones, then the soft tissues, and then the lungs are examined. Next, extraneous structures—such as electrocardiographic leads, nasogastric tubes, and endotracheal tubes—are identified and their proper positioning verified. An alternative *geographic approach* looks first at the central areas of the film (the heart and mediastinum), then outward to the lungs, and finally to the peripheral regions of the chest wall.

In interpreting a chest radiograph, it is important to consider that the radiographic image is a two-dimensional representation of a three-dimensional object. Overlap of thoracic structures can create confusing radiographic shadows, and the interpreter should attempt to distinguish the individual components of any questionable findings.

ADEQUACY.   Three factors determine the technical adequacy of a PA chest film: penetration, positioning of the patient without rotation, and complete filling of the lungs with air (Table 17-8). The radiographic exposure (penetration) is correct if the outlines of the lower thoracic vertebral bodies are faintly visible behind the heart. If the film is overpenetrated (too dark), an infiltrate may be obscured. If the film is underpenetrated (too light), the lung marking will appear too prominent and mimic pulmonary opacities.

To determine whether the patient was properly positioned without rotation, the alignment between an anterior midline landmark (the midpoint between the clavicular heads) and a posterior midline landmark (the tips of the spinous processes of the thoracic vertebrae) is assessed. If the patient was rotated at the time of exposure, the heart and mediastinum will appear wide and distorted. In addition, it is more difficult to detect mediastinal shift accurately. The trachea should not be used to assess rotation because it is a soft tissue structure that can be shifted by pathologic processes.

With a complete inspiration that fills the lungs with air, the right cardiophrenic sulcus is located below the posterior costovertebral junction of the tenth or eleventh rib. The ribs are counted beginning with the first rib. Because the posterior portions of the upper two or three ribs overlap, an accurate rib count is made by first finding the anterior ends of the first, second, and third ribs. These upper ribs are then traced back, one by one, to their posterior junctions with the vertebrae. The posterior aspects of the third, fourth, and lower ribs is then correctly identified. When the level of inspiration is not adequate, the vessels in the lower portions of both lungs are crowded and can mimic an infiltrate. Assessment of cardiac enlargement is difficult because the heart appears enlarged and horizontal.

In some patients, inspiration to the level of the tenth rib is not sufficient for the radiograph. Therefore, it is more accurate to assess the overall appearance of the film (i.e., whether the vascular markings at both lung bases are crowded and the heart appears horizontal) rather than to rely solely on rib counting to determine level of inspiration.

BONES.   The scapula, humerus, shoulder joint, and clavicle are examined for fractures, lesions, and asymmetry. Evaluation of these structures is limited because the radiographic technique is designed to minimize skeletal opacity. The ribs are studied individually from posterior to anterior, following the cortex of each rib carefully. The sternum and thoracic spine are superimposed and overlie the heart, which limits their evaluation. Specific studies for the ribs, shoulders, or thoracic spine are obtained if further evaluation is necessary.

SOFT TISSUES.   The soft tissues of the *chest wall* are examined for subcutaneous emphysema and asymmetry. The presence and symmetry of the breast shadows are noted because they alter the apparent density in the lower portions of the lungs. The diaphragm and abdomen are examined for subdiaphragmatic free intraperitoneal air and other abdominal abnormalities.

The *mediastinum* and *heart* are then assessed. The mediastinum is examined for widening, masses, and emphysema. The aorta, its proximal branches, and the superior vena cava are examined. The caliber and position of the trachea and carina are assessed. Pleural reflection lines, such as the right paratracheal stripe, are identified. The cardiothoracic ratio and cardiac contours are examined, looking for signs of heart chamber enlargement.

The *hila* are assessed for enlargement and masses. The pulmonary arteries and veins are evaluated for engorgement. Enlarged lymph nodes have a rounded contour and indicate infection or malignancy. Tumor masses are commonly unilateral and asymmetrical.

THE LUNGS.   The lungs are examined for areas of increased or decreased opacity. The lung markings should be well-

TABLE 17-8

Evaluation of Technical Adequacy of the Frontal and Lateral Chest Radiograph

	PA OR AP VIEW	LATERAL VIEW
Entire thorax seen	Lung apices, lateral chest walls, and entire diaphragm including both lateral costophrenic sulci.	Lung apex, anterior and posterior chest wall, and entire diaphragm including both posterior costophrenic sulci.
Penetration correct	Lower thoracic vertebral bodies faintly visible behind heart.	Lower thoracic vertebral bodies faintly visible.
Inspiration full	Posterior end of right tenth or eleventh rib is just above right cardiophrenic sulcus.	No crowding of lower lung markings (retrocardiac).
No rotation	Tips of the spinous processes aligned with midpoint between the clavicular heads. Do not use trachea to assess rotation.	Posterior right ribs are 1 to 3 cm posterior to the left ribs. Sternum seen edge-on.

TABLE 17-9

Useful Findings on the Lateral Chest Radiograph

Confirm and localize intrapulmonary opacities—pneumonia and other lesions (especially retrocardiac and retrosternal)
Hilar abnormalities—especially lymphadenopathy
Small pleural effusions—posterior costophrenic sulcus
Thickened interlobar fissures—pulmonary edema
Heart chamber enlargement (right ventricle, left ventricle, left atrium)
Aortic abnormalities (tortuosity, aneurysm)

Copyright David T. Schwartz, M.D.

TABLE 17-10

Systematic Analysis of the Lateral Chest Radiograph

Adequacy	Penetration, inspiration, rotation
Bones	Vertebral bodies, ribs, sternum, scapulae
Soft tissues	Heart, aorta, hila, trachea, diaphragm
Lungs	Review airspaces from front to back: Retrosternal Lung overlying the heart Retrocardiac Lung overlying the vertebrae* Interlobar fissures

*The lower vertebral bodies should normally appear more radiolucent (darker) because there is less overlying soft tissue and more overlying air (lung).

defined. Subtle focal abnormalities are detected by comparing each intercostal space with the corresponding region of the opposite lung. Areas of increased opacity are inspected for evidence of an alveolar or interstitial process. The air–soft tissue interfaces of the lung with the heart, diaphragm and aorta are evaluated. Loss of a sharp interface suggests opacification of lung tissue or a pleural effusion.

The thorax is examined for signs of volume loss, such as mediastinal or tracheal shift, diaphragm elevation, and shift of an interlobar fissure. Hyperinflation, of one lung (e.g., bronchial obstruction) can also cause a shift of intrathoracic structures. Finally, the pleural surfaces, including the interlobar fissures, are inspected for thickening, effusion, and pneumothorax.

Systematic Analysis of the Lateral Radiograph

Abnormalities that are seen on the PA view should be identified on the lateral view to confirm their presence and determine their anatomic location (Table 17-9). The bones, soft tissues, and lungs are examined in a systematic fashion (Table 17-10). First, the technical adequacy of the film is assessed, although the criteria used are not as well defined as with the PA radiograph (Table 17-8). Next, the sternum, vertebral column, and ribs are evaluated.

Examination of the soft tissues includes the heart, aorta, mediastinum and hila, trachea, and diaphragm. Cardiac enlargement is assessed, especially the right ventricle, left ventricle, and left atrium. Abnormalities of the aortic contour can be seen on the lateral film. Hilar abnormalities, especially lymphadenopathy, is often more readily identified on the lateral film. The left and right domes of the diaphragm are distinguished and should be clearly defined. A small pleural effusion that is not visible on the PA radiograph will blunt the posterior costophrenic sulcus on the lateral film.

Finally, the lungs are examined, going from anterior to posterior. Special attention is given to areas of the lungs that are not well seen on the PA view—the retrocardiac and retrosternal regions. The radiodensity of the vertebral bodies normally decreases from superior to inferior. If the inferior vertebral bodies appear more dense, there is often an overlying intrapulmonary opacity. The interlobar fissures are identified, including the left and right major fissures and the right minor fissure. Thickening of the fissures is readily identified on the lateral radiograph and is a sign of pulmonary edema.

Systematic Analysis of the AP Portable Radiograph

The approach to interpretation of the AP portable radiograph is similar to that of the standard PA radiograph, although several significant differences must be recalled. The technical adequacy of the film is often suboptimal. The radiograph is frequently underpenetrated. The patient may be rotated and often has not taken a full inspiration, (see Chap. 20, Fig. 20-1).

Several distortions are commonly seen on the AP portable film (Table 17-11). An upright rather than supine film should be obtained whenever possible. There is less cardiac and mediastinal enlargement, the level of inspiration is better, and lung lesions are better seen. In addition, pleural effusions and pneumothoraces are easier to detect on an upright film.

Finally, overlying extrathoracic objects are common, such as clothing, spine immobilization boards, tubes, monitoring wires and clips. These produce artifacts that obscure or mimic pathologic findings.

TABLE 17-11

Distortions Seen on the AP Portable Radiograph

Cardiac enlargement
Mediastinal widening
Rotation of the patient (apparent shift of trachea and mediastinum)
Poor inspiration (crowded lung markings at the bases, enlarged heart)
Suboptimal exposure (over- or underpenetrated)
Longer exposure time causes blurring due to patient movement
Lower-energy x-rays increase opacity of overlying bones
Overlying extrathoracic objects are common
Pneumothorax and pleural effusions difficult to see (supine film)

Copyright David T. Schwartz, M.D.

RADIOGRAPHIC PATTERNS OF CHEST PATHOLOGY

Identification of specific radiographic patterns suggests certain diagnoses. Most pulmonary disorders detected by conventional radiography cause opacity of the lung. Other lung diseases cause increased radiolucency (decreased opacity) on the chest radiograph. Other radiographic manifestations of cardiopulmonary diseases include hilar enlargement and pleural changes (e.g., effusions, thickening).

Disorders causing increased opacity of lung tissue are divided into those that cause airspace filling and those that increase the density of interstitial tissues. Atelectasis (collapse) can also increase the opacity of the lung due to loss of aeration. Increased opacity is also caused by a pleural effusion (ex-trapulmonary and intrathoracic) and chest wall masses (extrathoracic). Disorders causing decreased pulmonary opacity include emphysema, bullae, and diminished vascularity (e.g., pulmonary embolism). Decreased opacity is also caused by a pneumothorax and loss of chest wall tissue (e.g., mastectomy).

Radiographic Terminology

The terminology used to describe pulmonary findings on a chest radiograph has been standardized (Table 17-12).[31] *Airspace filling* results from accumulation of fluid or cellular material within the alveoli without causing destruction of lung parenchyma.[32] The term *infiltrate* denotes areas of the lung that are filled with inflammatory or neoplastic cells. Radiographic-

TABLE 17-12

Commonly Used Terms in Pulmonary Radiography

Acinar pattern   A collection of round, poorly defined, discrete or partly confluent opacities in the lung, each 4 to 8 mm in diameter, which, when together, produce an extended, inhomogeneous shadow.

Air bronchogram   The radiographic shadow of an air-filled bronchus surrounded by airless lung—a finding indicative of an airspace-filling pathologic process in which there is patency of the more proximal airway.

Atelectasis   Radiologic evidence of diminished volume affecting all or part of a lung, which may or may not include loss of normal lucency in the affected part of lung.

Bulla   Any sharply demarcated lucency 1 cm or more in diameter within the lung, the wall of which is less than 1 mm thick.

Coalescent   Joined together—said of multiple opacities joined to form a single opacity but still individually identifiable.

Consolidation   An essentially homogeneous opacity in the lung characterized by little or no loss of volume, effacement of blood vessel shadows, and sometimes by the presence of an *air bronchogram*.

Density   The opacity of a radiographic shadow to visible light; film blackening.

Honeycomb pattern   A number of closely approximated ring shadows representing airspaces, 5 to 10 mm in diameter with walls 2 to 3 mm thick, that resemble a true honeycomb—a finding whose occurrence implies "end-stage" lung.

Infiltrate   A poorly defined opacity in the lung that neither destroys nor displaces the gross morphology of the lung and is presumed to represent an infiltrate in the pathologic sense (infiltration of lung parenchyma by cellular material).

Interstitium   A continuum of loose connective tissue throughout the lung comprising three subdivisions: (1) the bronchovascular (axial), surrounding the bronchioles and arteries from the lung root to the level of the respiratory bronchiole; (2) the parenchymal (acinar), situated between alveolar and capillary basement membranes; and (3) the subpleural, interlobular septa, and deep intraparenchymal septal bands. Parts 1 and 3 can become radiographically visible with a pathologic process. Part 2 is microscopic and is not distinguishable radiographically.

Lobule   (formerly, secondary pulmonary lobule)   The smallest division of lung tissue completely surrounded by connective tissue septa; approximately 1 to 2 cm in diameter. Comprises the airspaces and airways of several terminal bronchioles. The primary pulmonary lobule (lung distal to the terminal bronchiole) is no longer believed to be a distinct anatomic unit.

Lucency   Any circumscribed area that appears more black than its surroundings. Usually applied to the shadows of air or fat when surrounded by more effective absorbers such as muscle or exudate.

Mass   Any pulmonary or pleural lesion represented by a discrete opacity greater than 30 mm in diameter.

Nodule   Any pulmonary or pleural lesion represented by a sharply defined, discrete, nearly circular opacity 2 to 30 mm in diameter.

Opacity   Any circumscribed area that appears more nearly white than its surroundings. Usually applied to the shadows of pulmonary collections of fluid, tissue, and so on whose attenuation exceeds that of the surrounding aerated lung.

Pneumonia   Consolidation or any of various other forms of pulmonary opacification presumed to represent pneumonia in the pathologic sense.

Pulmonary edema   Opacification (often bilaterally symmetrical and perihilar in distribution) representing alveolar filling and/or interstitial fluid accumulation.

Reticular pattern   A collection of innumerable small, linear opacities that together produce a netlike appearance.

Segment   One of the principal anatomic subdivisions of the lobes of the lung (usually 10 on the right and 9 on the left).

Shadow   Any perceptible discontinuity in film blackening ascribable to the attenuation of the x-ray beam by a specific anatomic absorber or lesion on or within the body of the patient. An opacity or lucency.

Silhouette sign   The effacement of an anatomic soft tissue border by consolidation of the adjacent lung or accumulation of fluid in the contiguous pleural space.

ally, an infiltrate causes opacification of the lung with ill-defined margins. However, the term *infiltrate* is actually a histologic term rather than a radiographic term. For example, filling of a portion of the lung with edema fluid rather than cellular material results in an ill-defined opacity even though it is not an "infiltrate" in the pathologic sense. To call a focal lung opacification an *infiltrate* has a connotation that might not be pathologically correct. The descriptor "ill-defined opacity" is therefore preferred over the term *infiltrate* in describing radiographic findings.[33] *Consolidation* refers to a relatively uniform opacification of the airspaces of the lung.

Some disease processes cause opacification of the lung by infiltration or edema of the lung interstitium. Normally, the interstitial connective tissue of the lung is not radiographically visible. An *interstitial* radiographic pattern is produced when the connective tissue is pathologically infiltrated by inflammatory or neoplastic cells or is filled with edema fluid. The pat-

TABLE 17-13

Disorders that Cause Airspace Filling

Focal (segment or lobe)
  Pneumonia
    Bacterial pneumonia
    Aspiration pneumonia
    Tuberculosis
    Viral or mycoplasmal pneumonia
  Pulmonary embolism with hemorrhage or infarction
  Neoplasm
    Bronchoalveolar cell carcinoma
    Postobstructive pneumonia (bronchial carcinoma)
  Atelectasis
  Blunt trauma (pulmonary contusion)

Diffuse or multifocal
  Pulmonary edema
    Congestive heart failure
    Renal failure (fluid overload)
    Noncardiogenic pulmonary edema (ARDS) (shock lung)*
      Sepsis
      Near-drowning
      Opiate overdose
      Head trauma
  Pneumonia
    Bacterial, viral, mycoplasmal, fungal, aspiration, rickettsial
    Pneumocystis carinii (AIDS)
    Tuberculosis
  Hemorrhage
    Goodpasture syndrome, bleeding diatheses, DIC
  Neoplastic
    Bronchoalveolar cell carcinoma
    Lymphoma
  Other
    Toxic inhalations (nitrogen dioxide, sulfur dioxide)
    Alveolar proteinosis
    Neonatal respiratory distress syndrome
    Desquamative interstitial pneumonitis

*Partial listing.
Key: ARDS, adult respiratory distress syndrome; AIDS, acquired immunodeficiency syndrome; DIC, disseminated intravascular coagulation.

tern may be linear or reticular, nodular or cystic. It is more accurate simply to describe the radiographic pattern rather than use the term *interstitial infiltrate*. Many interstitial pulmonary disorders, such as viral pneumonitis, result in both interstitial and airspace inflammation.

Airspace-Filling Disorders

Airspace filling can be focal, diffuse, or patchy (multifocal) (Table 17-13). Because many diseases that cause filling of the alveoli spread through interalveolar connecting channels, the margins are typically ill-defined. Focal airspace filling is often referred to as being localized to a specific segment of the lung, even though there are no physical boundaries between lung segments and the opacity does not usually conform to an exact anatomic segment (Figs. 17-12 and 17-13). When the pathologic process is stopped at an anatomic boundary, primarily an interlobar fissure, the opacity has a sharp border. When airspace filling is caused by a pulmonary edema, it often develops centrally adjacent to the hilum, having a "bat wing" or a "butterfly" pattern (Fig. 17-14).

There are two characteristic radiographic findings associated with airspace filling. The *air bronchogram* is seen when an air-filled bronchus is surrounded by fluid-filled lung. The thin-walled pulmonary bronchi and bronchioles are not normally visible (Fig. 17-12). Pathologic processes that cause air bronchograms include diseases, including pneumonia and pulmonary edema, that cause fluid to accumulate in the alveoli but not the bronchi. An air bronchogram is not seen when fluid also accumulates within the bronchus.

The *silhouette sign* is caused by the obliteration of a normal air–soft tissue interface by the accumulation of fluid in the adjacent lung or in a contiguous pleural space. More accurately, the silhouette sign is actually the *loss* of a normal silhouette between a soft tissue organ (heart, aorta, or diaphragm) and the lung. Since fluid in the alveoli has the same radiodensity as the contiguous solid organ, the normal distinct border is lost. For example, a pneumonia in the right middle lobe obliterates or "silhouettes out" the right heart border and a lingular pneumonia silhouettes out the left heart border (Fig. 17-13).

Interstitial Patterns

Some pulmonary disorders result in the accumulation of fluid or cells in the interstitial tissues of the lung. There are several classification schemes for interstitial lung diseases. In one scheme, interstitial processes are divided into four categories—the nodular, fine reticular (linear), honeycomb (coarse reticular), and cystic (ring) (Table 17-14).

There is often a difference between an interstitial lung disorder as demonstrated on a radiograph and interstitial disorders in the pathologic sense. For the pathologist, interstitial disorders cause infiltration of the lung interstitium by cellular material. This is often accompanied by infiltration of the airspaces, as in viral pneumonia. Therefore, interstitial lung diseases often result in a radiographic pattern of airspace filling. It is more precise to describe the appearance of the radiographic pattern

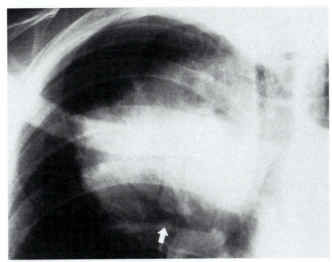

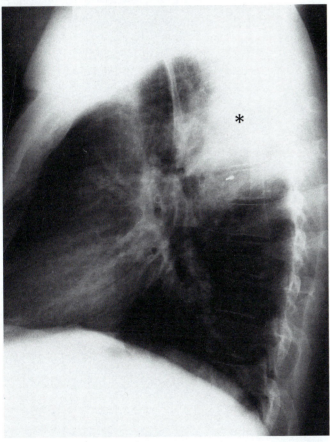

FIGURE 17-12. Air bronchogram. *A.* A branching air bronchogram is seen in this patient with a right-upper-lobe pneumonia *(arrow).* The air-filled bronchus is visible because it is surrounded by fluid-filled alveoli. *B.* The lateral view reveals that the infiltrate is in the posterior segment of the right upper lobe *(asterisk).* (Copyright David T. Schwartz, M.D.)

(e.g., a fine linear pattern or a nodular pattern) rather than to presume to identify a pathologic process (e.g., an "interstitial infiltrate").

NODULAR PATTERN. The *nodular pattern* consists of multiple discrete, small pulmonary opacities (<1 cm diameter) through-

TABLE 17-14

Diseases that Cause Interstitial Patterns

Fine nodular pattern (Miliary)
 Miliary tuberculosis
 Histoplasmosis
 Pneumoconiosis (silicosis, asbestosis)
 Sarcoidosis
 Other disorders causing a fine reticular pattern

Reticular or linear pattern
 Acute
  Pulmonary edema (congestive heart failure, uremia)
  Pneumonia (viral, mycoplasmal)
 Chronic*
  Idiopathic pulmonary fibrosis
  Sarcoidosis
  Collagen vascular diseases (rheumatoid, scleroderma)
  Lymphangitic carcinomatosis
  Pneumoconiosis (silicosis, asbestosis)
  Drug reactions
  Hypersensitivity pneumonitis
  Eosinophilic granuloma

Honeycomb or coarse reticular pattern*
 Scleroderma
 Idiopathic pulmonary fibrosis
 Other disorders causing a chronic fine reticular pattern
Cystic or ring interstitial pattern
 Cystic bronchiectasis

*Partial listing.

out the lungs. The nodules result from the infiltration of a foreign substance or pathogen into the interstitium. The nodular interstitial pattern is seen with miliary tuberculosis, histoplasmosis, pneumoconiosis, and sarcoidosis (Fig. 17-15).

FINE RETICULAR PATTERN. A *reticular* or *linear pattern* describes a pattern of thin linear markings. The fine reticular pattern usually results from enlargement of interstitial connective tissue septa. Three types of septal lines were described by the radiologist Peter Kerley. *Kerley A lines* represent thickening of deep septal bands that radiate from the hilum and are more prominent in the upper lungs. *Kerley B lines* are thickened interlobular septa that appear as short parallel lines perpendicular to the pleura. The most common cause of thickened interlobular septa is pulmonary edema, although they are also seen with lymphangitic carcinomatosis and interstitial fibrosis. *Kerley C lines* form a fine netlike pattern of lines most prominently at the lung base. Kerley C lines are actually Kerley B lines (thickened interlobular septa) seen on end (Fig. 17-16).

Although a large number of lung diseases cause a reticular pattern, the acute onset of a reticular pattern is due either to interstitial pulmonary edema or atypical (e.g., viral) pneumonitis (Table 17-14).

COARSE RETICULAR PATTERN—HONEYCOMB LUNG. The *honeycomb pattern* or *coarse reticular pattern* is caused by marked thickening or fibrosis of the lung interstitium. The thick lines

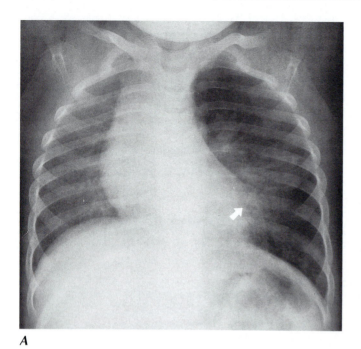

A

FIGURE 17-13. The silhouette sign. Pneumonia in the lingula of the left lung. The left border of the heart is not seen because it is "silhouetted out" by the fluid-filled lingula *(arrow)*. On the lateral view, the pulmonary opacity is seen overlying the heart. This confirms that the pneumonia does not involve the lower lobe, in which case the infiltrate would be behind the heart.

surround airspaces. The size of the airspaces range from minuscule to 1 cm, but is generally consistent in any particular patient. This pattern is seen in patients with pulmonary fibrosis that is idiopathic or due to any of a number of interstitial lung diseases (Fig. 17-17). A coarse reticular pattern also occurs when an airspace-filling disorder such as pulmonary edema or pneumonia occurs in a patient with underlying emphysema.

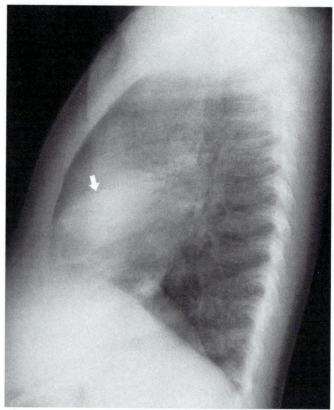

B

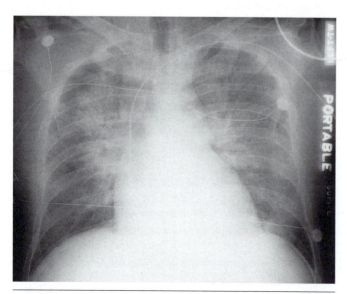

FIGURE 17-14. Diffuse airspace filling. There is a centralized "bat wing" distribution that is characteristic of pulmonary edema. Opacification of the lung is inhomogeneous owing to interspersed aerated alveoli and bronchi.

FIGURE 17-15. Nodular interstitial pattern. Innumerable calcified granulomas in a patient with histoplasmosis.

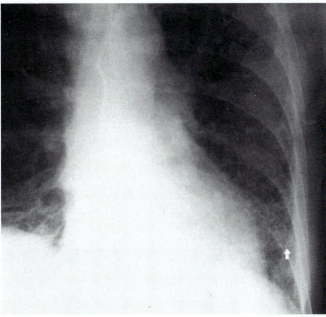

A

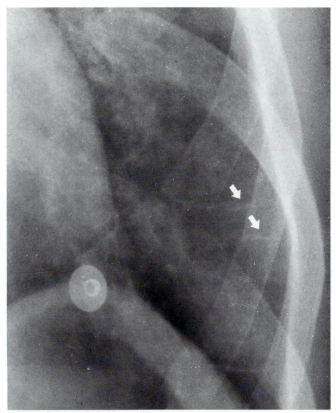

B

FIGURE 17-16. Fine reticular pattern. *A.* A fine reticular pattern is seen at the lung bases in this patient with mild congestive heart failure. Kerley B lines (thickened interlobular septa) are present adjacent to the pleural margin *(arrow)*. *B.* Detail showing Kerley B lines in another patient with mild congestive heart failure (Copyright David T. Schwartz, M.D.)

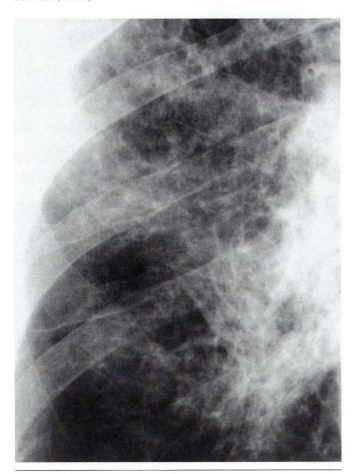

FIGURE 17-17. Coarse reticular pattern. Thick, fibrotic bands are seen in this patient with idiopathic pulmonary fibrosis.

CYSTIC (RING) PATTERN. A *cystic* or *ring interstitial pattern* is usually seen with cystic bronchiectasis. If the rings are larger than 1 cm (compared with the honeycomb pattern above), the radiograph is diagnostic for bronchiectasis. The radiographic findings are caused by dilatation of the bronchi from recurrent infections (Fig. 17-18).

Pulmonary Masses

A *pulmonary mass* is any well-defined opacity greater than 3 cm in diameter, and a *nodule* is 2 mm to 3 cm in diameter. A solitary pulmonary nodule is usually due to one of three disorders—malignant neoplasm, benign tumor, or infectious granuloma. Calcification that is uniformly distributed in the mass is uncommon in malignancy. A nodule smaller than 1 cm is rarely lung cancer, because nodules this small must be highly calcified in order to be visible. A lesion with an irregular edge and particularly a *corona radiata* (a stellate lesion appearing with strands spreading into the adjacent lung) is indicative of bronchial carcinoma (Fig. 17-19).

Multiple pulmonary nodules are caused by malignancy, infection, or inflammatory conditions (Table 17-15). The margins of the lesions are generally well defined (Fig. 17-20). Multifocal airspace disease can also have the appearance of multiple pulmonary nodules, although the margins of the lesions are ill defined.

A *cavity* is any gas-filled space surrounded by a wall at least 1 mm thick. Malignant and infectious cavities tend to have thicker, irregular walls than benign diseases.

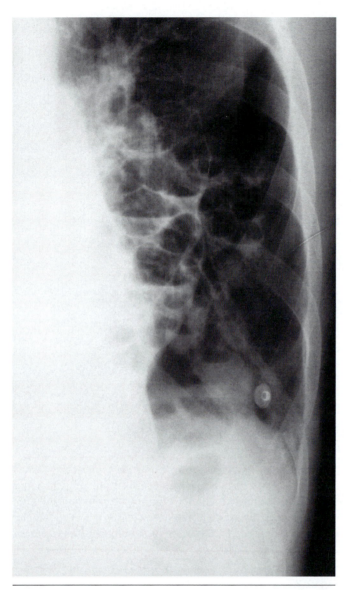

FIGURE 17-18. Cystic interstitial pattern. Curvilinear bands (ring-like shadows) represent thickened bronchial walls of dilated bronchi in this patient with cystic bronchiectasis.

TABLE 17-15

Diseases that Cause a Multinodular Pattern

Neoplasm
    Metastatic—renal, gastrointestinal, ovarian, uterine,
        testicular, melanoma, etc.
    Lymphoma
    Kaposi sarcoma (AIDS), etc.
Benign tumors
Fungal or parasitic infection
Septic emboli
Rheumatoid nodules
Wegener granulomatosis

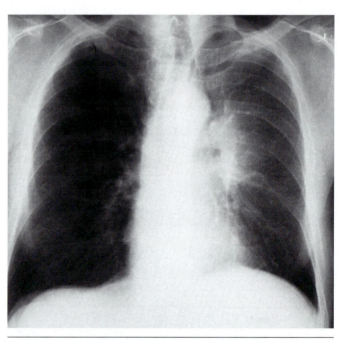

FIGURE 17-19. Corona radiata. A patient with bronchial carcinoma. The perihilar mass has radiating bands that extend outward to the lung periphery. This appearance is highly suggestive of malignancy.

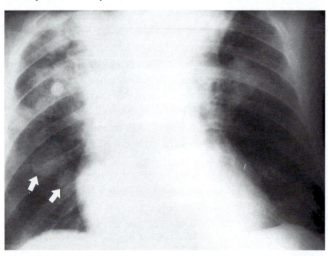

A

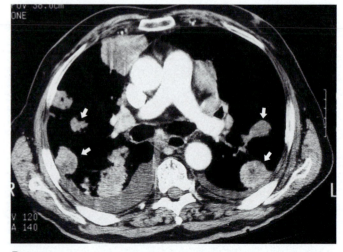

B

FIGURE 17-20. Multinodular pattern. Multiple pulmonary nodules are seen in this patient with lymphoma. The margins of the nodules are generally well defined *(arrows)*. *B.* CT clearly demonstrates the nodules, which are 1.5 to 3 cm in diameter.

Atelectasis

Atelectasis, also called *collapse,* has many causes (Table 17-16). The most clinically significant form of atelectasis is obstruction of a major airway. Bronchial obstruction is caused by an endobronchial tumor, an aspirated foreign body, or a mucous plug. Because of the extensive collateral airflow between alveoli, only when there is obstruction of a major bronchus, such as a bronchus to entire lobe, will collapse of lung ensue. When the bronchus is obstructed, air that is trapped in the distal lung is gradually reabsorbed into the pulmonary circulation. For this reason, bronchial obstructions result in *resorptive atelectasis.* Radiographically, there are signs of volume loss affecting the involved portion of lung. Signs of atelectasis include shift of a fissure, mediastinal shift, elevation of the diaphragm, compensatory hyperinflation of adjacent lung tissue, and, frequently, increased opacity of the involved lung (Table 17-17).

Collapse of each of the various lobes of the lung results in a characteristic radiographic picture. There is loss of lung volume and shift of an interlobar fissure. For example, with the "Golden S" sign (named for Dr. R. Golden), the horizontal fissure is pulled superiorly, around the mass, forming a reverse S-shaped curve (Fig. 17-21).[34]

Other causes of atelectasis include a lack of pulmonary surfactant in the newborn, hypoventilation, and extrinsic compression. *Discoid atelectasis* is so named because of the linear opacity seen on chest radiography. It results from hypoventilation in the basal portions of the lungs, typically in patients in whom deep inspiration is decreased (e.g., a bedridden patient, a patient splinting from rib fractures). An effusion or pleural-based mass causes extrinsic compression of lung tissue and is known as *compressive atelectasis.*

Decreased Pulmonary Opacity

Abnormal radiolucency of the lung has various causes. It can be generalized, focal, or unilateral (Table 17-18). Generalized lucency is usually due to small airways diseases, such as asthma or COPD, that cause alveolar hyperinflation. Focal lucency is seen in patients with bullous emphysema. *Bullae* are gas-filled spaces with thin walls (<1 mm) in which parenchymal tissue is destroyed and alveolar size is greatly increased. Diminished blood flow to a portion of lung will also result in focal radio-

TABLE 17-16

Diseases that Cause Atelectasis

Bronchial obstruction
  Neoplasm
  Foreign body
  Mucous plugging
Extrinsic compression (pleural effusion, masses)
Scarring with adhesions
Hypoventilation (discoid atelectasis)
Lack of surfactant in neonates

TABLE 17-17

Radiographic Signs of Lobar Atelectasis

Displaced fissure (the principal direct sign)
Loss of aeration causing increased opacity (not always present)
Indirect signs of volume loss:
  Elevated hemidiaphragm
  Shift of the trachea, heart, or hilum
  Compensatory hyperinflation of adjacent lung
  Rib cage narrowing

TABLE 17-18

Disorders that Cause Decreased Pulmonary Density

Asthma
Emphysema
Bullae
Pneumothorax
Pulmonary embolism—oligemia in involved segment

lucency. This is seen infrequently with a massive pulmonary embolism.

Unilateral lucency is seen when there is overexpansion of a lobe or entire lung. This can be caused by progressive air trapping distal to a bronchial obstruction. It also occurs with compensatory hyperinflation adjacent to a collapsed lobe. Unilateral lucency is also seen where there is air in the pleural space, as occurs with a pneumothorax.

Hilar Abnormalities

The hilum is a difficult area in the interpretation of chest radiographs because there is wide variation in the normal hilar appearance from one individual to another. In addition, there are no strict criteria or discrete measurements to distinguish normal hila from abnormal ones. An understanding of normal hilar anatomy as seen on the PA and lateral radiographs and the various pathologic changes that are seen in the hilum forms the basis of radiographic interpretation of the hila.

The hilum is made up mostly of the major pulmonary vasculature—the main pulmonary arteries and the superior pulmonary veins (Fig. 17-11). The hila therefore have a branching vascular appearance in which the radiographic density gradually diminishes from the center toward the periphery. In addition, because the lower half of each lung has greater volume and receives more blood flow than the upper half, the lower half of each hilum has greater vascular density than the upper half.

The use of symmetry in comparing the left to the right hilum is helpful in identifying hilar abnormalities. However, there are normally some differences between the two hila. Although both hila are roughly the same size, the right side appears larger because the medial portion of the left hilum is partly obscured by the mediastinum, heart, and aorta. In addition, the left hilum is located 1 to 2 cm superior to the right hilum.

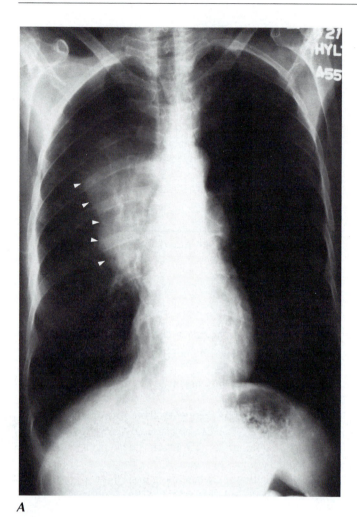

A

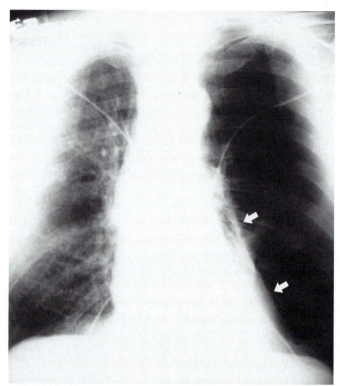

B

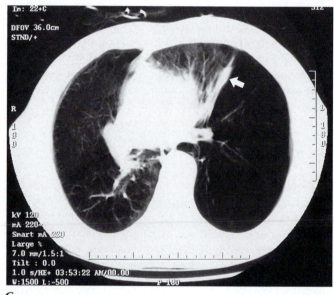

C

FIGURE 17-21.   Lobar atelectasis. *A.* The "Golden S" sign. There is right upper lobe collapse due to lung carcinoma. A mass is present at the right hilum. Just superior to the mass is the density of the collapsed upper lobe. The well-defined lateral margin of the collapsed lobe is formed by the minor fissure that has been pulled up. The combined lateral margins of the mass and the adjacent collapsed lobe have a reversed S shape *(arrowheads)*. Volume loss is also indicated by slight rightward tracheal deviation. *B.* Collapse of the left lower lobe results in an elongated triangular density adjacent to the left side of the mediastinum behind the heart *(arrows)*. The left upper lobe has expanded to fill the entire left hemithorax. Because of its hyperexpansion, the lung is abnormally lucent. The lobar collapse developed gradually and is of long standing, as indicated by the lack of mediastinal shift or elevation of the diaphragm. *C.* CT shows the collapsed lower lobe adjacent to the heart and the hyperexpanded lucent left upper lobe.

Hilar enlargement can be due to increased vascularity (arterial or venous), hilar lymphadenopathy, or hilar masses. Obviously enlarged hila are abnormal, although this is an insensitive criterion by which to judge hilar enlargement. Three criteria that are more sensitive at detecting hilar abnormality are (1) a rounded rather than branching vascular shape, (2) an abrupt fall-off of radiodensity rather than a gradually tapering appearance, and (3) alteration in the proportionate radiodensity of the upper and lower halves of each hilum. The normal proportionality is one-third upper and two-thirds lower (Table 17-19).

The *lateral radiograph* is often helpful in determining whether the hila are abnormal. Normally, an area of increased

radiodensity is seen just anterior to the distal trachea (Fig. 17-7). This is the right main pulmonary artery and the origin of the left main pulmonary artery. The regions immediately posterior and inferior to the distal trachea should be radiolucent. Increased density in these regions is abnormal and is usually due to lymphadenopathy. A discrete area of increased density slightly below the hila is due to the inferior pulmonary veins where they enter the left atrium. This should not be misinterpreted as a pulmonary mass or nodule.

HILAR LYMPHADENOPATHY.   Hilar enlargement that has a rounded or lumpy contour rather than a branching vascular appearance is indicative of hilar lymphadenopathy (Table 17-20).

TABLE 17-19

Criteria to Evaluate the Hilum on the PA Chest Film

1. **Shape:** A branching vascular pattern is normal. Rounded contours that are not part of vessels are mass lesions (tumors or lymph nodes).
2. **Radiodensity:** Radiodensity progressively diminishes toward the periphery.
3. **Proportionate size:** Normally, two-thirds of the radiodensity is in the lower half of the hilum and one-third of the radiodensity is in the upper half.
4. **Absolute size:** Obviously enlarged hila are likely to be abnormal, but there are no definite measurements that serve as a guide. Left and right should be roughly the same size.

From Freedman M: *Clinical Imaging: An Introduction to the Role of Imaging in Clinical Practice.* New York, Churchill Livingstone, 1988, with permission.

The hilar density falls off abruptly rather than gradually. In addition, the upper half of the hilum often has an abnormally greater proportion of the hilar radiodensity. The lateral film is especially helpful in questionable cases of hilar adenopathy. The distal trachea appears encased in and outlined by soft tissue representing subcarinal and retrotracheal adenopathy (Fig. 17-22).

Unilateral hilar lymphadenopathy or asymmetrical adenopathy results from infections (viral, fungal, or primary tuberculosis), lymphoma, or metastasis (Fig. 17-10). Bilateral symmetrical adenopathy is seen in patients with sarcoidosis (Table 17-21).

INCREASED HILAR VASCULARITY. Increased hilar vascularity can be due to engorgement of either the pulmonary arteries or pulmonary veins (Table 17-20) (see Chap. 18, "Cardiovascular Imaging"). Pulmonary venous engorgement is a sign of pulmonary venous hypertension. This is most commonly due to congestive heart failure (left ventricular failure). It is also seen with mitral valve stenosis or insufficiency and in such rare conditions as left atrial myxoma and pulmonary venoocclusive disease. Radiographically, there is hilar enlargement in a branching vascular pattern. There is disproportionate enlargement of the upper half of the hila. This is due to the greater contribution of the superior pulmonary veins to the upper half of the hila.

Pulmonary artery enlargement is due to either increased pressure or increased blood flow. Pulmonary artery hypertension is idiopathic (primary pulmonary hypertension) or secondary (e.g., pulmonary embolism or COPD). The hila are enlarged in a branching vascular pattern and the perihilar blood vessels taper rapidly, creating a "pruned tree" appearance. There is cardiac enlargement primarily involving the right atrium and right ventricle. Increased pulmonary blood flow is difficult to detect on plain chest radiograph unless it is marked. It occurs with left-

to-right cardiac shunts due to an atrial septal defect or ventricular septal defect. There is hilar vascular enlargement with associated cardiac enlargement and increased peripheral vascular lung markings.

Pleural Processes

The visceral pleura is a thin membrane covering the lung surface. The pleura reflect back over the inner surface of the chest wall, forming the parietal pleura. Normally, there is a minute amount of serous fluid separating the parietal and visceral pleura.

A *pleural effusion* is an abnormal collection of fluid between the pleural layers. A moderate-sized effusion is easily identified by its characteristic homogenous opaque appearance at the base of the lungs. On an upright chest radiograph, the superior surface of the pleural effusion curves upward around the lung because surface tension causes a meniscus to form (Fig. 17-23). The diaphragm is silhouetted out by the pleural effusion. A lateral decubitus film confirms that the pleural effusion is free-flowing and amenable to thoracentesis. A small pleural effusion is seen best on the lateral film. Small effusions obliterate the normally sharp costophrenic sulcus.

Pleural thickening occurs in a variety of circumstances, including loculated pleural effusions, asbestos exposure, and after thoracic surgery. Pleural thickening is seen as a linear or curved density just medial to the chest wall (Figs. 1-1*A* and 23-24 in Chaps. 1 and 23). In the apices, the pleura do not fol-

TABLE 17-20

The Abnormal Hilum—Radiographic Diagnosis

Lymphadenopathy and **tumor masses** (i.e., bronchogenic carcinoma) are rounded, nonbranching structures. The radiodensity falls off abruptly at the margin of the tumor or lymph node. The proportionate size of the hilum is usually abnormal, with relatively greater than expected radiodensity where the mass or enlarged lymph node is located.

Increased pulmonary venous pressure (pulmonary venous hypertension) is caused by congestive heart failure, mitral stenosis, and mitral regurgitation. Radiographically, there is relatively increased radiodensity in the upper half of the hilum due to engorgement of the superior pulmonary veins. The inferior pulmonary veins enter the left atrium below the level of the hilum and do not contribute radiodensity to the hilum on the PA film.

Increased pulmonary arterial pressure (pulmonary artery hypertension): The central pulmonary arteries are enlarged and hilar density tapers abruptly. Etiologies include primary pulmonary hypertension, pulmonary embolism, chronic lung diseases.

Increased pulmonary blood flow occurs in left-to-right intracardiac shunts (ventricular or atrial septal defect), high fever, pregnancy. It causes increased central and peripheral pulmonary vascular markings (peripheral lung markings become readily visible in the most peripheral 1 to 2 cm of the lung). Increased pulmonary blood flow must be two to three times greater than normal to be radiographically visible.

Decreased pulmonary blood flow causes small hila and diminished vascular lung markings. This is seen in cyanotic congenital heart diseases, such as tetralogy of Fallot.

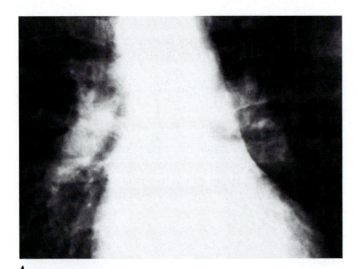

A

B

FIGURE 17-22. Hilar enlargement due to lymphadenopathy. There is bilateral symmetrical hilar adenopathy in a patient with sarcoidosis. *A.* On the PA radiograph, the hila are enlarged and have a rounded, lumpy appearance. *B.* On the lateral radiograph, the enlarged lymph nodes highlight the margins of the distal trachea, particularly the posterior tracheal wall and the subcarinal region. The soft tissue density anterior to the trachea is also increased. (Copyright David T. Schwartz, M.D.)

low the same plane as the ribs. This causes the apical pleura to appear prominent even on a normal film. Apical pleural thickening is caused by scarring, tumor, or tuberculosis.

TABLE 17-21

Hilar Adenopathy—Differential Diagnosis

Bilateral
    Sarcoidosis—the prime diagnosis for bilateral *symmetrical* adenopathy
    Lymphoma—(usually asymmetrical)
    Infection—viral, TB, fungal, etc. (usually asymmetrical)
    Metastatic—oat cell, renal, melanoma, breast (usually asymmetrical)
Unilateral (also bilateral asymmetrical)
    Tuberculosis ("primary" tuberculosis, AIDS patients)
    Fungal, atypical mycobacterium, viral, tularemia
    Metastatic or primary hilar tumor (bronchogenic carcinoma)
    Lymphoma
    Sarcoidosis, silicosis, drug reaction

The Diaphragm

Elevation of part or all of one side of the diaphragm is occasionally seen. A congenital defect in which part of the diaphragm muscle is replaced by a membranous sheet, gives the contour of the diaphragm a smooth bulge (eventration). This is most frequently seen on the medial side of the right hemidiaphragm. Elevation of an entire hemidiaphragm occurs from paralysis of the phrenic nerve, hepatomegaly, a subdiaphragmatic abscess, or significant bowel distention. A subpulmonic pleural effusion can be mistaken for an elevated hemidiaphragm.

The diaphragm is flattened by disorders that cause increased intrathoracic volume, most commonly chronic overexpansion of the lungs in patients with COPD or an acute exacerbation of asthma.

The Ribs

Rib fractures and osseous lesions can be detected on standard chest radiographs. However, a dedicated rib radiographic series is better for defining a lesion fully and detecting subtle abnormalities. The indications for obtaining rib radiographs to detect fractures are controversial. Although painful, rib fractures in themselves are less significant than associated pulmonary and neurovascular injuries. The diagnosis of a rib fracture can be made clinically. Nondisplaced rib fractures may not be radiographically visible.

A grossly displaced rib fracture is easily identified (Fig. 17-24), but close inspection is necessary to identify subtle buckle fractures. Local pleural thickening is caused by a hematoma at the site of the fracture. One technique that aids detection of a nondisplaced rib fracture is to hold the radiograph upside down, which can make a fracture more conspicuous. A significant number of rib fractures are not seen initially on plain film radiographs; these are often visible on later chest radiographs because of callus formation.

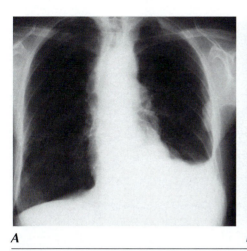
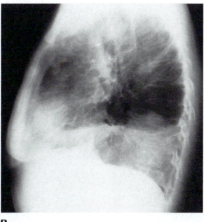
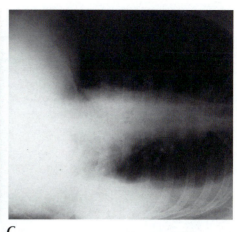

A   *B*   *C*

FIGURE 17-23. Pleural effusion. *A.* Left pleural effusion on a PA radiograph. The diaphragm is "silhouetted out" and the superior margin of the effusion forms an upturned meniscus with the lateral chest wall. Note the left pleural-based mass. *B.* On the lateral radiograph, the effusion obliterates the left side of the diaphragm. The margin of the right side of the diaphragm is clear, including the posterior costophrenic sulcus. *C.* A left lateral decubitus radiograph shows that the free-flowing effusion layers out along the left lateral chest wall.

pathogens is suggestive but by no means pathognomonic (Table 17-22). *S. pneumoniae* incites an inflammatory response that spreads via interconnecting channels throughout the acini, resulting in a focal *airspace-filling pattern* (Fig. 17-25). With severe infection, the disease spreads to involve an entire lobe and is known as a *lobar pneumonia* (Table 17-23).

TABLE 17-22

Pneumonia—Radiographic Patterns*

Lobar (segmental) pneumonia—pneumococcus, *Klebsiella*
    Infection originates in alveolar sacs and spreads via
        interconnecting passages.
Bronchopneumonia (lobular)—*S. aureus,* aspiration, *Pseudomonas*
    Nidus of infection in bronchus spreads distally, producing a
        multifocal, patchy airspace pattern often in a segmental
        distribution. Bronchopneumonia is more accurately
        distinguished from lobar pneumonia histologically than
        radiographically.
Interstitial—viral, mycoplasmal, etc.
    "Atypical" pneumonia can have an interstitial pattern, diffuse or
        patchy airspace filling, or segmental consolidation.

*The radiographic pattern has a poor correlation with etiologic agent.

FIGURE 17-24. Rib fractures. Displaced fractures of the left ribs (3, 4, 5, and 6). There is an adjacent pulmonary contusion.

COMMON ABNORMALITIES

Pneumonia

In community-acquired pneumonia, the most common pathogen is *Streptococcus pneumoniae*. In young, healthy adults (<40 years), atypical pneumonia (most commonly due to *Mycoplasma pneumoniae*) is common. The vast majority of nosocomial pneumonia is caused by aerobic gram-negative bacilli (predominantly *Enterobacteriaceae* and *Pseudomonas* spp.).[35] The radiographic pattern produced by these various

TABLE 17-23

Lobar Pneumonia—Radiographic Signs

Homogeneous opacity except for:
    Air bronchogram
    Air alveologram (0.5- to 1-cm lucent area due to an air-filled
        acinus)
Border is indistinct and distribution is nonsegmental because
    infection spreads via interconnecting pores.
Sharp border where the infiltrate abuts an interlobar fissure.
Silhouette sign—obliterates the normal air/fluid interface when the
    infiltrate lies against the heart, diaphragm, or aorta.
Obliterates normal vascular markings.

Copyright David T. Schwartz, M.D.

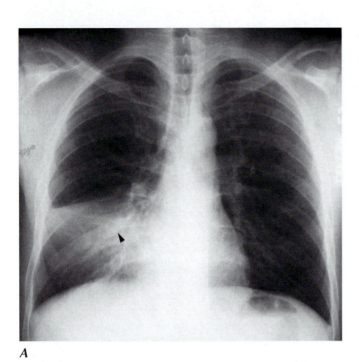

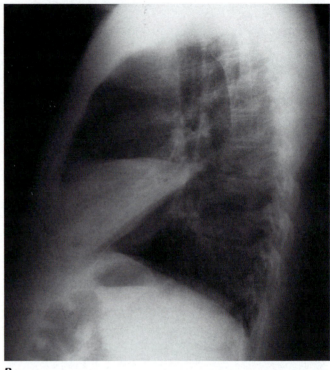

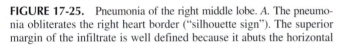

A   *B*

FIGURE 17-25. Pneumonia of the right middle lobe. *A*. The pneumonia obliterates the right heart border ("silhouette sign"). The superior margin of the infiltrate is well defined because it abuts the horizontal fissure. An air bronchogram is present (*arrowhead*). *B*. On the lateral view, the entire right middle lobe is opacified. It has a well-defined triangular shape because it abuts the horizontal and oblique fissures.

S. aureus pneumonia tends to begin in the bronchus and spread distally via the airways, creating the radiographic pattern known as *bronchopneumonia* or *lobular pneumonia.*[36] Lobular pneumonia produces "patchy" opacities (Fig. 17-26). *S. aureus* also causes abscesses, cavitation, and pleural effusion.

Atypical and viral pneumonias are often grouped together owing to their similar radiographic appearance—bilateral diffuse or patchy infiltrates (Fig. 17-27). An atypical pneumonia can also have a lobar radiographic pattern.[37]

Gram-negative organisms provoke a strong inflammatory response, creating large amounts of exudate in the airspaces. *Klebsiella pneumoniae* has a predilection for involving one anatomic lobe, causing expansion of the lobe and bulging of the fissures. Gram-negative organisms can also show a lobular pattern.

The radiographic appearance of pneumonia often lags behind the clinical symptoms and signs. Moreover, radiographic signs of pneumonia persist after clinical resolution of the disease. Therefore, a normal radiograph in the presence of a clinical diagnosis of pneumonia or a persistent infiltrate in a pa-

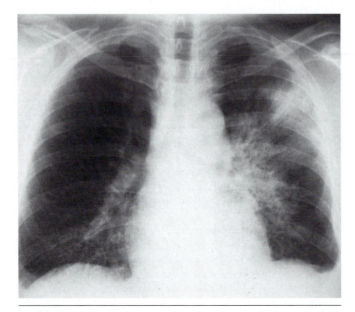

FIGURE 17-26. Lobular pneumonia. A patchy infiltrate extends from the left hilum.

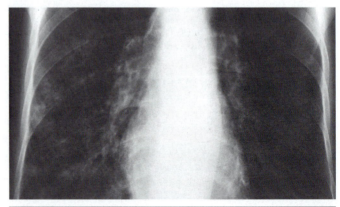

FIGURE 17-27. Bilateral interstitial infiltrates. A fine reticular pattern is seen more prominently on the right lung than the left in this patient with viral pneumonitis.

tient who is clinically improving does not alter medical management.

Tuberculosis

Patients with pulmonary tuberculosis (TB) can have a number of different radiographic patterns. *Primary tuberculosis* is the initial infection caused by *Mycobacterium tuberculosis* and is often only mildly symptomatic. *Postprimary disease* or *reactivation tuberculosis* is characterized by fatigue, night sweats, and hemoptysis. Multiorgan system involvement (e.g., kidney failure) is seen in patients with *disseminated tuberculosis.*[38]

In *primary tuberculosis,* the most common radiographic findings include a localized infiltrate, pleural effusion, and hilar or mediastinal lymphadenopathy. Among patients with culture-documented primary TB, 10 to 15% have negative chest radiographs at the time of presentation.[39,40] Focal consolidation is the most common radiographic manifestation and is similar to the pattern of a typical bacterial pneumonia (Fig. 17-28). Although slow to clear, radiographic changes do not persist after the initial infection in two-thirds of patients.[41] Residual parenchymal changes are generally seen as a small calcified nodule called a *Ghon focus* or *Ghon complex.* Lymphadenopathy is more common in children than in adults, and the diagnosis of primary TB should be considered in children with a slowly resolving infiltrate and hilar adenopathy.

The typical radiographic findings of *reactivation (postprimary) tuberculosis* are an upper lobe parenchymal infiltrate frequently associated with cavitation and scarring (Fig. 17-29). This is caused by reactivation of the dormant pathogen, which tends to reside in the upper lobes. Reactivation TB occurs in up to 15% of infected patients.[41] The cell-mediated inflammatory response due to previous sensitization of the patient results in granuloma formation with caseous necrosis. Cavitation

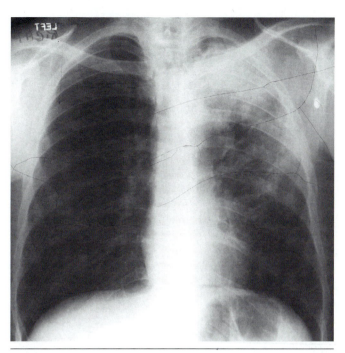

FIGURE 17-29. Postprimary (reactivation) tuberculosis. Active postprimary tuberculosis involves the left upper lobe. There is cavity formation.

occurs when the necrotic tissue of a tubercle opens into a bronchiole. Cavitation indicates active disease. It is difficult to determine conclusively whether the radiograph of a patient with postprimary TB represents active or inactive disease. Clinical symptoms and cultures, not radiologic findings, are used to determine disease activity.[39]

Hematogenous spread of TB throughout the lung causes *miliary tuberculosis.* It is more likely to complicate primary TB. Diffuse small nodules (2 to 3 mm) are seen throughout the lungs (Fig. 17-30). These radiographic findings are often not seen until 6 weeks after the initial dissemination. Without therapy, miliary TB can be fatal. In nearly all survivors, the radiographic changes resolve.[41]

AIDS

Pulmonary symptoms such as cough, dyspnea, and fever often leads to ED visits by HIV-infected patients. The chest radiograph is an important part of the evaluation of these patients. Many of the opportunistic infections seen in immunocompromised patients involve obvious radiographic changes. Nonetheless, diagnosing specific infections on the basis of the chest radiograph is virtually impossible. Further studies, including cultures and tissue histology, are required to make a definitive diagnosis.

Pneumocystis carinii pneumonia (PCP) is seen in 60 to 80% of AIDS patients. Its frequency is decreasing, due largely to antibiotic prophylaxis.[42] PCP is often the initial manifestation of AIDS in the HIV-positive individual. The typical radiographic appearance shows bilateral, diffuse, perihilar, or basilar infiltrates (Fig. 17-31). Lymphadenopathy and pleural effusions are rarely seen. Up to 50% of patients with PCP have

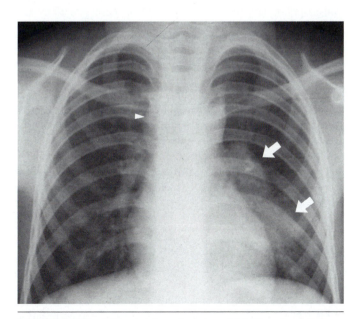

FIGURE 17-28. Primary tuberculosis in a child. There is a left lower lobe infiltrate and left hilar lymphadenopathy *(arrows).* Right paratracheal adenopathy causes a widened right paratracheal stripe *(arrowhead).*

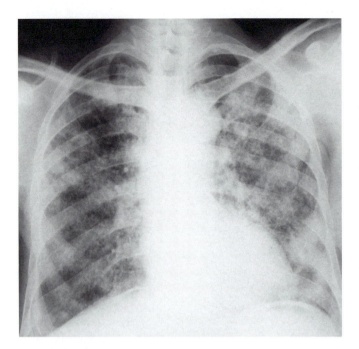

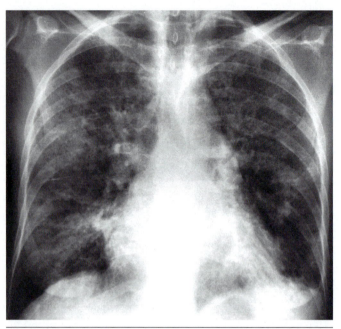

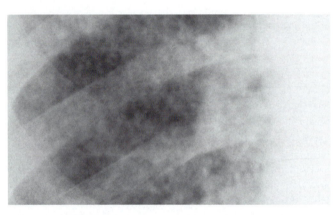

FIGURE 17-31.   *Pneumocystis carinii* pneumonia. There is diffuse airspace filling throughout both lungs.

FIGURE 17-30.   Disseminated (miliary) tuberculosis. There are innumerable tiny nodules throughout both lungs. In some regions, the disease has progressed to ill-defined patchy opacities.

atypical radiographic findings. Usually these are unilateral or focal infiltrates. Cavitation and pneumatoceles are occasionally seen and can cause a pneumothorax. Normal radiographs are seen in up to 39% of patients with PCP at the time of initial presentation.[43]

Mycobacterium infections are common in HIV-infected patients. *Mycobacterium avium intracellulare* is seen in about 20% of AIDS patients. Radiographic findings include diffuse patchy alveolar infiltrates, mediastinal lymphadenopathy, and scattered pulmonary nodules. *M. tuberculosis* is seen in approximately 10% of AIDS patients and is often the presenting illness.[44] AIDS patients often have a radiographic pattern suggestive of primary TB, even though they are experiencing a reactivation of previous disease. This is due to deficient cell-mediated immunity. There is hilar and mediastinal lymphadenopathy. Apical and cavitary lesions may not be seen, because these manifestations require an intact immune system.[45]

Typical bacterial pneumonia is the most common pulmonary infection in HIV-positive patients, occurring at a rate greater

than five times that of the non-HIV population. *S. pneumoniae* is the most common organism. AIDS patients are more likely than immunocompetent hosts to have multilobar involvement.

Fungal infections are seen in about 5% of AIDS patients. The incidence varies with geographic location. *Cryptococcus neoformans* is the most common. Radiographic findings include single or multiple nodules that progress to confluence or cavitation. *Histoplasma capsulatum* appears as diffuse interstitial and airspace infiltrates. *Coccidioides immitis* is usually seen as diffuse nodular or interstitial infiltrates. *Candida albicans,* the most common fungal infection in AIDS patients, rarely causes pulmonary infections. With all of these infections, the initial radiograph can appear normal. Cytomegalovirus (CMV) pneumonia is seen frequently, but CMV is rarely the sole pathogen. Its radiographic appearance is identical to that of *P. carinii.*

Noninfectious diseases also cause chest radiographic abnormalities in AIDS patients. Kaposi's sarcoma presents with hilar and mediastinal adenopathy, poorly defined nodular infiltrates, and large pleural effusions. AIDS-related lymphoma typically appears as hilar and mediastinal adenopathy, parenchymal infiltrates, or pleural effusions. Lymphocytic interstitial pneumonia is radiographically indistinguishable from a diffuse infectious process.

Asthma and Chronic Obstructive Pulmonary Disease

Most chest radiographs of patients with asthma or exacerbations of COPD are either normal, demonstrate hyperinflation (air trapping), or show chronic abnormalities. Chest films should be obtained in patients not responding to bronchodilator therapy, those with "high-risk" factors, or those with their first episode of wheezing (Table 17-1). The primary role of chest radiography is to detect concurrent pulmonary conditions or other diseases that cause wheezing, such as pulmonary edema or pneumonia (Table 17-24).

Hyperinflation due to air trapping is the most common radiographic abnormality. Nonetheless, air trapping is an expected finding and simply reflects the obstructive airways dis-

ease. Radiographic signs of air trapping include increased lung volume with hyperlucency, flattening of the diaphragm, and a vertical cardiac silhouette. On the lateral film, there is an increased retrosternal airspace and widening of the intercostal spaces, with the ribs becoming horizontally oriented (Fig. 17-32). Increased perihilar markings frequently appear in asthmatic patients due to peribronchial edema. Patients with COPD

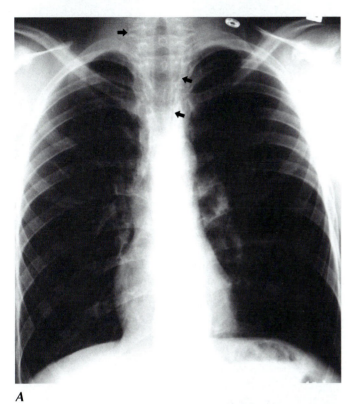

A

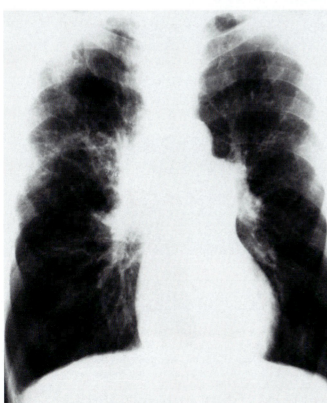

B

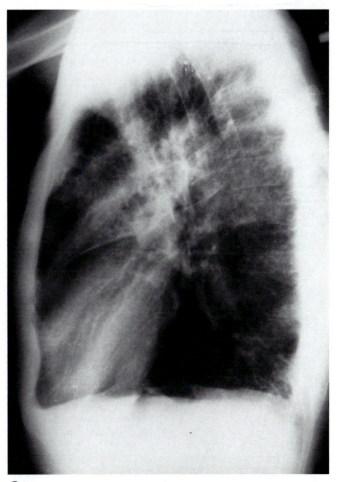

C

FIGURE 17-32. Asthma and COPD. *A.* In this young patient with an acute asthma exacerbation, the lungs are hyperexpanded and abnormally lucent. The diaphragm is flattened and the heart appears relatively small. Air is present within the mediastinum, outlining the left tracheal wall and extending into the neck *(arrows). B.* The radiograph in this middle-aged patient with COPD shows hyperexpanded lucent lungs with coarse fibrotic lines in both lungs, predominantly in the upper lobes. The patient has cor pulmonale. The pulmonary arteries are enlarged, producing hilar enlargement in a branching vascular pattern. The heart is enlarged, even though the cardiothoracic ratio is not increased. This is because of the increased thoracic diameter. *C.* On the lateral view, the diaphragm is flattened and there is an increased AP diameter of the thorax. The hilar vasculature is prominent. (*B* and *C* Copyright David T. Schwartz, M.D.)

TABLE 17-24

Frequency of Radiographic Findings in Patients with Asthma and COPD

FINDING	FREQUENCY
Normal	50–87%
Hyperinflation	7–22%
Pneumonia/infection	3–22%
Pleural thickening	12–14%
New cardiac enlargement	8–10%
Atelectasis	3–4%
Congestive heart failure	0–6%
Elevated hemidiaphragm	1–5%
New mass	≤2%
Pneumothorax	≤2%
Pneumomediastinum	≤1%
Effusion	≤1%

also have an increased anteroposterior diameter, emphysematous bullae, and fibrotic areas in the lung. Atelectasis can result from infection or mucous plugging, especially in children.

Pneumomediastinum

A pneumothorax or pneumomediastinum is occasionally seen in patients with obstructive lung disease. Radiographic signs of pneumomediastinum can be subtle. Lateral displacement of the mediastinal pleura by mediastinal air creates a linear density paralleling the mediastinal contour. This is usually more apparent on the left (Fig. 17-33). On the lateral film, pneumomediastinum can be seen in the retrocardiac airspace. Mediastinal air can dissect into the soft tissues of the neck and chest wall.

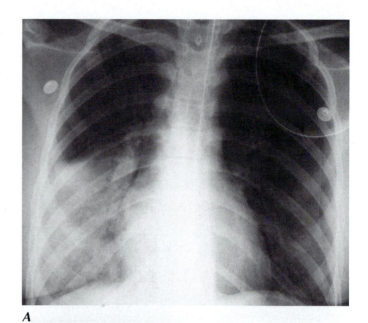

A

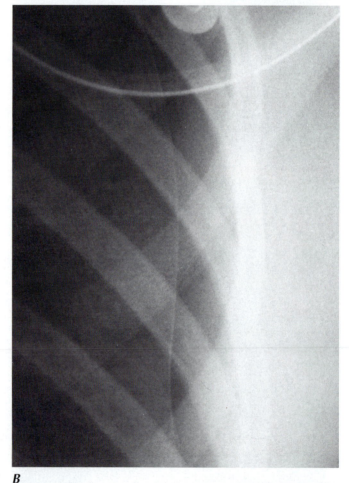

B

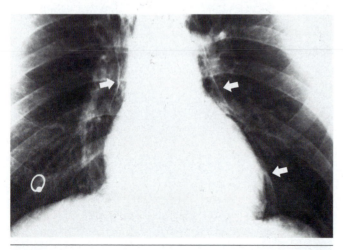

FIGURE 17-33.   Pneumomediastinum. Mediastinal air lifts the parietal pleura off the mediastinum, creating fine white lines adjacent to the left and right heart and mediastinal borders *(arrows)*. Streaks of air extend into the soft tissues of the neck (not shown). A nipple ring is seen.

FIGURE 17-34.   Pneumothorax. *A.* A subtle medium-sized left pneumothorax is difficult to see. Note that the collapsed left lung is not more radiodense than the right lung. *B.* A detailed view of the lower left thorax shows the fine white line of the edge of the collapsed lung that parallels the lateral chest wall. A small hemothorax is present, causing the horizontal shadow over the left costophrenic sulcus. The pleural effusion does not have a curved meniscus because the pneumothorax releases surface tension forces that are normally present between the apposed visceral and parietal pleural surfaces.

Pneumothorax

With a pneumothorax, there is air within the pleural space, causing collapse of the lung. Although various chest radiograph measurements have been devised to quantify the size of a pneumothorax, none are accurate. It is generally sufficient to describe a pneumothorax as either small, medium, or large. A small pneumothorax involves only the apex of the lung; a medium pneumothorax extends completely down the lateral thoracic wall; and a large pneumothorax causes complete or nearly complete collapse of the lung.

A pneumothorax is most reliably diagnosed by identifying the fine visceral pleural edge of the collapsed lung (Fig. 17-34). Lung markings are absent beyond the edge of the pneumothorax and the pneumothorax is slightly more radiolucent than the adjacent lung. Although it might be expected that the collapsed lung would appear denser than the opposite normal lung, this is only the case when there is near total collapse of a lung. This is because the radiographic density of the lung is determined by the amount of the vascular lung markings. With

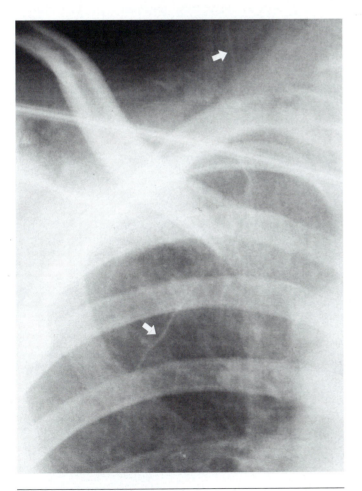

FIGURE 17-35. Pseudopneumothorax. The fine white vertical line overlying the right upper thorax mimics a pneumothorax. However, the line can be followed superiorly, outside of the thorax, indicating that this is not an intrathoracic process. In addition, lung markings are present beyond the line. The line is due to a fold in the clothing lying underneath this immobilized victim of blunt trauma.

a pneumothorax, the blood flow to the collapsed lung diminishes in proportion to the extent of collapse; therefore the radiographic density of the collapsed lung is normal.

It is sometimes difficult to detect a small pneumothorax because the thin pleural margin follows and is obscured by the ribs. Comparison of expiratory and inspiratory films can facilitate detection of a questionable pneumothorax. During expiration, lung tissue becomes denser and the visceral pleural line is easier to see.[46] Expiratory films are needed only if the diagnosis is in question. On the other hand, a skin fold or overlying clothing or bed sheet sometimes mimics the fine white line of a pneumothorax. This is especially a problem with portable chest radiographs. These extraneous lines can be distinguished from a pneumothorax by noting that they extend outside of the thorax and that peripheral lung markings are present (Fig. 17-35).

In the supine patient, pleural gas collects anteriorly. A moderate-sized pneumothorax will cause widening of the costophrenic sulcus (the *deep sulcus sign*) (see Fig. 20-2 in Chap. 20, "Priorities in Trauma").[47] A lateral decubitus film can be used to detect a pneumothorax in a patient who cannot sit upright. In the lateral decubitus position, gas in the pleural space rises along the upper edge of the lateral chest wall. Computed tomography (CT) readily detects a pneumothorax in a supine patient. This is often seen in the superior slices of an abdominal CT performed on a stable victim of blunt trauma. Although such a small pneumothorax itself might not be clinically significant, a chest tube should be inserted if endotracheal intubation is anticipated, because positive-pressure ventilation can rapidly create a tension pneumothorax.

A *tension pneumothorax* occurs when pressure within the pleural space progressively increases, causing decreased systemic venous return and hypotension. Radiographic signs of a tension pneumothorax are depression of the diaphragm and shift of the mediastinum and trachea away from the collapsed lung (Fig. 17-36).[48] However, the diagnosis must be made clinically in a patient with hypotension, unilaterally absent breath sounds, and tracheal deviation. Treatment with emergency thoracostomy should not be delayed while awaiting radiographic confirmation. Conversely, radiographic signs of a tension pneumothorax may be seen in a patient who is clinically stable. Although the patient does not clinically have a tension pneumothorax, a chest tube should be inserted expeditiously to avert sudden deterioration.

Trauma

Many pulmonary complications of blunt and penetrating trauma are readily diagnosed by chest radiography, including pneumothorax, hemothorax, and pulmonary contusion. *Pneumothoraces* result from pulmonary laceration, bronchial tear, bleb rupture, rib fracture, and chest wall penetration.[49] The presence of subcutaneous emphysema in a victim of blunt trauma implies that a pneumothorax is present even if it is not visible on the portable chest radiograph.

A *hemothorax* appears on an upright radiograph as blunting of the costophrenic sulcus or loss of the diaphragmatic margin.

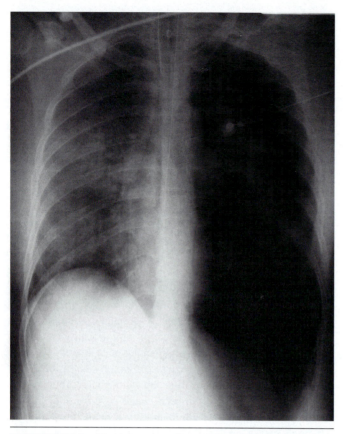

FIGURE 17-36.   Tension pneumothorax. There is marked depression of the left hemidiaphragm and mediastinal shift toward the right. The increased density of the right lung is due to its being compressed. A small simple pneumothorax was converted into a tension pneumothorax by positive-pressure ventilation via the endotracheal tube.

On a supine radiograph, diffuse homogeneous haziness is seen on the involved side of the thorax if a sufficiently large quantity of blood is present. Approximately 25% of traumatic hemothoraces have an associated pneumothorax.

Pulmonary contusions represent accumulations of edema and blood in the airspaces of the lung. Most pulmonary contusions are caused by rapid deceleration injuries such as motor vehicle collisions, falls, and blasts with concussive shock waves. Pulmonary contusions should be suspected in trauma patients with respiratory difficulty or hypoxia as well as rib or sternal fractures. Pulmonary contusions are almost always present in patients with flail chest. They appear as areas of inhomogeneous opacification of the lung (Fig. 17-37), are usually seen within minutes of injury, and can progress over several hours. The extent of injury is difficult to assess from the plain radiograph. Clinical findings, such as hypoxia, are better indicators of the severity of injury.[50,51]

ERRORS IN INTERPRETATION

Errors in interpretations are classified as "false positives" (normal findings simulating disease) and "false negatives" (a pathologic process that is present yet missed). A commonly missed diagnosis is a small pulmonary nodule or lesion. Lesions smaller than 10 mm in diameter are missed on a chest radi-

ograph in up to 50% of cases. Lesions larger than this can be missed if there are overlying shadows, if the lesion is retrocardiac or behind a rib or clavicle, or adjacent to the pleura. Because of the superimposition of the heart and the increased vascularity in the inferior portions of the lungs, lesions are more often missed in the lower lobes than the upper lobes.[52]

Sometimes normal shadows seen on a chest radiograph are misinterpreted as nodules or masses. Calcification of the costal cartilages, vertebral osteophytes, a prominent nipple shadow, or an asymmetrical diaphragm can mimic a pulmonary lesion. A raised skin lesion such as a mole or lipoma may appear as an indistinct region of increased density on the radiograph.[53] Other structures that can simulate an intrapulmonary opacity are asymmetrical breast shadows and a pericardial fat pad.[48]

Vascular markings, such as an end-on view of a pulmonary blood vessel, can simulate a pulmonary mass.[54] Suboptimal radiographic technique causes significant changes in the lung markings. If a patient has a poor inspiratory effort, there is crowding of the vascular markings in the lower portions of both lungs, mimicking pulmonary opacification. If the film is improperly penetrated, the lung markings and lesions can be obscured (if the film is overpenetrated) or normal vascular markings can appear abnormally prominent (if the film is underpenetrated) and be mistakenly interpreted as an infiltrate. This is particularly true in the right lower lobe, where the pulmonary vessels are normally quite prominent. On the lateral film, overlap of the right and left lower pulmonary vessels can also mimic an abnormal opacity. Lung lesions are often "hidden" by overlapping structures in the retrocardiac area, retroclavicular regions, and posterior costophrenic sulcus.

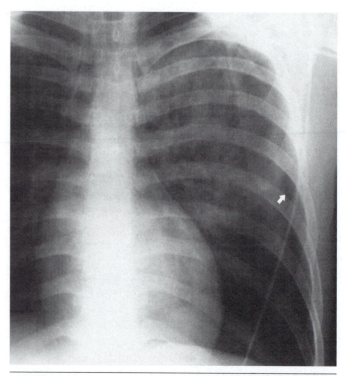

FIGURE 17-37.   Pulmonary contusion. In this victim of blunt trauma, inhomogeneous opacification of the left upper lung is due to a pulmonary contusion. A medium-sized pneumothorax is also present (*arrow*).

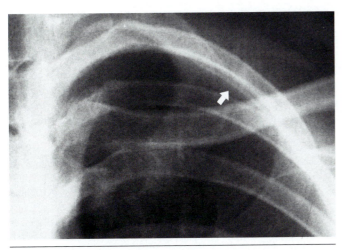

FIGURE 17-38. Rib companion shadows. A fine white line lies just under the second rib, where the pleura is separated from the rib by a thin layer of connective tissue. This should not be misinterpreted as a small pneumothorax. This determination is confirmed by seeing the companion shadow on both sides of the thorax.

Superimposition of electrode patches, clothing, or bed linens can create lines that may be improperly attributed to a pulmonary process. A line caused by a hospital gown at the edge of the lung can mimic a pneumothorax (Fig. 17-35). Tracing the entire length of these lines reveal that they extend outside of the thoracic cavity.

A pneumothorax can be simulated by other shadows. Extrapleural fat between the parietal pleura and the chest wall occasionally mimics a pneumothorax. This is called a *rib companion shadow;* it is usually bilateral and seen at the upper thoracic ribs (Fig. 17-38).[48]

COMMON VARIANTS

Numerous anatomic variants are seen in chest radiography. The azygos lobe fissure is seen in approximately 1% of the population. It is formed during embryogenesis as the azygos vein migrates through the apex of the right lung to the right tra-

TABLE 17-25

Radiographic Appearance of the Thymus in Children

Thymic notch	Distinct indentation at the junction of the thymus and the heart
Sail sign	Triangular density radiating from the mediastinum, especially on the right
Thymic wave	Rippled appearance of the left side of the cardiac silhouette due to indentation of the soft thymus by the costal cartilage, especially on the left

cheobronchial angle. The azygos lobe often appears more radiodense than the surrounding areas (Fig. 17-39). There are several other accessory lobes and fissures that are seen infrequently.

Another common variant seen in young children is a prominent thymus. In a child up to 3 years old, the thymus is superior to the heart and its inferior portion is often continuous with the cardiac shadow. The two lobes of the thymus have a pyramidal shape, but the right lobe is usually larger and more prominent. The prominent right edge of the triangular thymus creates the radiographic *sail sign.* It is seen in 9% of infants (Fig. 17-40).[55] On a lateral radiograph, the thymus has a distinct inferior edge and its density fills the retrosternal space anterior to the heart (Table 17-25). The thymus can be confused with cardiomegaly. Identifying the cardiac shadow on the lateral film will clarify the radiographic findings. The relative position of the thymus changes with the respiratory phase. If a question arises as to the diagnosis, inspiratory and expiratory films can be helpful.[56]

Variants of the diaphragm can be mistaken for a pathologic process. Commonly, the diaphragm is incompletely muscularized, with part of the muscle replaced by a thin membrane. With *eventration,* there is an elevated hump in the anterior medial

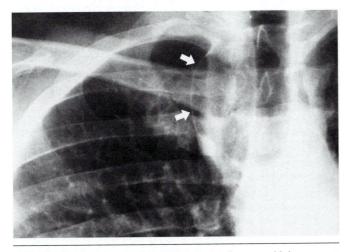

FIGURE 17-39. Azygos fissure. An azygos fissure and lobe are seen in the upper right lung.

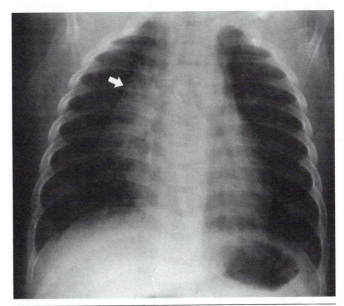

FIGURE 17-40. Normal thymus in a young child. The *sail sign* of a normal thymus is seen on the right in a 2-year-old child.

portion of the diaphragm, usually on the right. Complete even-tration is indistinguishable from an elevated hemidiaphragm.

ADVANCED STUDIES

Techniques—including helical CT, magnetic resonance imaging, nuclear scintigraphy, and ultrasonography (US)—play an important role in evaluating pulmonary pathology. *Computed tomography* is used to better define masses, vascular pathology, and skeletal abnormalities. It is used to clarify questionable findings on a plain radiograph, including a solitary pulmonary nodule or a widened mediastinum in a trauma patient. Helical (spiral) CT allows complete scanning of the chest with one breath-hold (32 s). These volumetric data are used to create axial, coronal, or three-dimensional images. Enhancement of the vascular structures is obtained with contrast. This provides an accurate, noninvasive technique for the evaluation of the aorta and the medium-sized pulmonary vessels.[57]

Magnetic resonance imaging (MRI) of the thorax is useful in the evaluation of hilar masses. It can distinguish between vascular structures and solid masses. It is indicated in patients in whom a CT is not diagnostic. MRI is also used in the evaluation of tracheal obstruction, particularly in children, because it offers images in the coronal and sagittal planes.[58]

Nuclear medicine studies are useful in studying pulmonary radiology. Ventilation/perfusion scanning is used for patients with suspected pulmonary embolism. Gallium scintigraphy is used to identify infectious or inflammatory processes in the lung. Infections caused by *P. carinii* and *M. avium intracellulare* can be identified on a gallium scan when the chest radiograph is normal. Gallium scanning is also used to evaluate sarcoidosis, mediastinal lymphoma, and occasionally adenocarcinoma.[59] Bone scans help to identify occult rib or sternal fractures as well as skeletal metastatic disease.[60]

Ultrasonography is used to evaluate pleural effusions. US is useful for identifying the size and boundaries of a pleural effusion and is sensitive for even minute effusions.[61] Real-time US can be used to guide thoracentesis. In cases of a loculated or small effusion, US is often necessary.

REFERENCES

1. Stussman BJ: *National Hospital Ambulatory Medical Care Survey: 1995 Emergency Department Summary. Advance Data from Vital and Health Statistics of the Centers for Disease Control and Prevention, no. 285.* Hyattsville, MD: National Center for Health Statistics. 1997.
2. Walsh-Kelly CM, Kim MK, Hennes HM: Chest radiography in the initial episode of bronchospasm in children: Can clinical variables predict pathologic findings? *Ann Emerg Med* 28:391, 1996.
3. Gershel JC, Goldman HS, Stein RE, et al: The usefulness of chest radiographs in first asthma attacks. *N Engl J Med* 309:336, 1983.
4. Zieverink SE, Harper AP, Holden RW, et al: Emergency room radiography of asthma: An efficacy study. *Radiology* 145:27, 1982.
5. Aronson A, Gennis P, Kelly D, et al: The value of routine admission chest radiographs in adult asthmatics. *Ann Emerg Med* 18:1206, 1989.
6. Dalton AM: A review of radiological abnormalities in 135 patients presenting with acute asthma. *Arch Emerg Med* 8:36, 1991.
7. Ismail Y, Loo CS, Zahary MK: The value of routine chest radiographs in acute asthma admissions. *Singapore Med J* 35:171, 1994.
8. Tsai TW, Gallagher EJ, Lombardi G, et al: Guidelines for the selective ordering of admission chest radiography in adult obstructive airway disease. *Ann Emerg Med* 22:1854, 1993.
9. Sherman S, Skoney JA, Ravikrishnan KP: Routine chest radiographs in exacerbations of chronic obstructive pulmonary disease. *Arch Intern Med* 149:2493, 1989.
10. Emerman CL, Cydulka RK: Evaluation of high-yield criteria for chest radiography in acute exacerbation of chronic obstructive pulmonary disease. *Ann Emerg Med* 2:680, 1993.
11. Melbye H, Berdal BP, Straume B, et al: Pneumonia—A clinical or radiographic diagnosis? *Scand J Infect Dis* 24:647, 1992.
12. Friis B, Eiken M, Hornsleth, Jensen A: Chest X-ray appearances in pneumonia and bronchiolitis. *Acta Paediatr Scand* 79:219, 1990.
13. Korppi M, Kiekara O, Heiskanen-Kosma T, Soimakallio S: Comparison of radiological findings and microbial aetiology of childhood pneumonia. *Acta Paediatr* 82:360, 1993.
14. Courtoy I, Lande AE, Turner RB: Accuracy of radiographic differentiation of bacterial from nonbacterial pneumonia. *Clin Pediatr (Phila)* 28:261, 1989.
15. Diehr P, Wood RW, Bushyhead J, et al: Prediction of pneumonia in outpatients with acute cough—A statistical approach. *J Chronic Dis* 37:215, 1984.
16. Gennis P, Gallagher J, Falvo C, et al: Clinical criteria for the detection of pneumonia in adults: Guidelines for ordering chest roentgenograms in the emergency department. *J Emerg Med* 7:263, 1989.
17. Heckerling PS, Tape TG, Wigton RS, et al: Clinical prediction rule for pulmonary infiltrates. *Ann Intern Med* 113:664, 1990.
18. Emerman CL, Dawson N, Speroff T, et al: Comparison of physician judgment and decision aids for ordering chest radiographs for pneumonia in outpatients. *Ann Emerg Med* 20:1215, 1991.
19. Buenger RE: Five thousand acute care/emergency department chest radiographs: Comparison of requisitions with radiographic findings. *J Emerg Med* 6:197, 1988.
20. Russell NJ, Pantin CF, Emerson PA, Crichton NJ: The role of chest radiography in patients presenting with anterior chest pain to the Accident & Emergency Department. *J R Soc Med* 81:626, 1988.
21. Templeton PA, McCallion WA, McKinney LA, Wilson HK: Chest pain in the accident and emergency department: Is chest radiography worthwhile? *Arch Emerg Med* 8:97, 1991.
22. Committee on Trauma, American College of Surgeons: Resource document 5: Roentgenographic studies, in *ATLS: Advanced Trauma Life Support, Program for Physicians. 1993 Instructor Manual,* 5th ed. Chicago: American College of Surgeons, 1993.
23. Thomson SR, Huizinga WK, Hirshberg A: Prospective study of the yield of physical examination compared with chest radiography in penetrating thoracic trauma. *Thorax* 45:616, 1990.
24. Hehir MD, Hollands MJ, Deane SA: The accuracy of the first chest x-ray in the trauma patient. *Aust NZ J Surg* 60:529, 1990.
25. McLellan BA, Ali J, Towers MJ, Sharkey PW: Role of the trauma-room chest x-ray film in assessing the patient with severe blunt traumatic injury. *Can J Surg* 39:36, 1996.
26. Sagel SS, Evens RG, Forrest JV, et al: Efficacy of routine screening and lateral chest radiographs in a hospital-based population. *N Engl J Med* 291:1001, 1974.
27. Hubbell FA, Greenfield S, Tyler JL, et al: The impact of routine admission chest x-ray films on patient care. *N Engl J Med* 312:209, 1985.

28. White CS, Austin JH, Lubetsky HW, Cole RP: The impact of routine chest radiography on the management of patients admitted from an emergency service. *Invest Radiol* 25:720, 1990.

29. Benacerraf BR, McLoud TC, Rhea JT, Cope RP: An assessment of the contribution of chest radiography in outpatients with acute chest complaints: A prospective study. *Radiology* 138:293, 1981.

30. Caskey CI, Templeton PA, Zerhouni EA: Current evaluation of the solitary pulmonary nodule. *Radiol Clin North Am* 28:511, 1990.

31. Tuddenham WJ: Glossary of terms for thoracic radiology: Recommendations of the Nomenclature Committee of the Fleischner Society. *AJR* 143;509, 1984.

32. Armstrong P: Basic patterns in lung disease, in Armstrong P et al (eds): *Imaging of Diseases of the Chest,* 2d ed. St. Louis: Mosby, 1995, pp. 58–124.

33. Friedman PJ: Radiologic reporting: The description of alveolar filling, *AJR* 141:617, 1983.

34. Golden R: The effect of bronchostenosis upon the roetgen-ray shadows in carcinoma of the bronchus. *AJR* 13:21, 1925.

35. Donowitz GR, Mandell GL: Acute pneumonia, in Mandell GL, Bennett JE, Dolin R (eds): *Principles and Practice of Infectious Diseases,* 4th ed. New York: Churchill Livingstone, 1995, pp. 619–637.

36. Montgomery JL: Pneumonia: Pearls for interpreting patients' radiographs. *Postgrad Med* 90:58, 1991.

37. Scanlon GT, Unger J: The radiology of bacterial and viral pneumonia. *Radiol Clin North Am* 11:317, 1973.

38. Carden DL, Smith JK: Pneumonias. *Emerg Med Clin North Am* 7:25, 1989.

39. Woodring JH, Vandiviere HM, Fried AM, et al: Update: The radiographic features of pulmonary tuberculosis. *AJR* 146:497, 1986.

40. Schaaf HS, Beyers N, Gie RP, et al: Respiratory tuberculosis in childhood: The diagnostic value of clinical features and special investigations. *Pediatr Infect Dis J* 14:189, 1995.

41. McAdams HP, Erasmus J, Winter JA: Radiologic manifestations of pulmonary tuberculosis. *Radiol Clin North Am* 33:655, 1995.

42. McGuiness G: Changing trends in the pulmonary manifestations of AIDS. *Radiol Clin North Am* 35:1029, 1997.

43. Opravil M, Marincek B, Fuchs WA, et al: Shortcomings of chest radiography in detecting Pneumocystis carinii pneumonia. *J Acquir Immune Defic Syndr* 7:39, 1994.

44. Poulton TB: Chest manifestations of AIDS. *Am Fam Physician* 45:163, 1992.

45. Small PM, Hopewell PC, Schecter GF, et al: Evolution of chest radiographs in treated patients with pulmonary tuberculosis and HIV infection. *J Thorac Imaging* 9:74, 1994.

46. Seow A: Comparison of upright inspiratory and expiratory chest radiographs for detecting pneumothoraces. *AJR* 166:313, 1996.

47. Gordon R: The deep sulcus sign. *Radiology* 136:25, 1980.

48. Freedman M: Pneumothorax, in Freedman M (ed): *Clinical Imaging: An Introduction to the Role of Imaging in Clinical Practice.* New York: Churchill Livingstone, 1988, pp. 136–144.

49. Schmidgall JR, Jui J: Diagnostic techniques in the evaluation of chest injury. *Top Emerg Med* 10:19, 1988.

50. Hoff SJ, Shotts SD, Eddy VA, Morris JA: Outcome of isolated pulmonary contusion in blunt trauma patients. *Am Surg* 60:138, 1994.

51. Johnson JA, Cogbill TH, Winga ER: Determinants of outcome after pulmonary contusion. *J Trauma* 26:695, 1986.

52. Kelsey CA, Moseley RD, Brogdon BG, et al: Effect of size and position on chest lesion detection. *AJR* 129:205, 1977.

53. Gronner AT, Ominsky SH: Plain film radiography of the chest: Findings that simulate pulmonary disease. *AJR* 163:1343, 1994.

54. Cole TJ, Henry DA, Jolles H, Proto AV: Normal and abnormal vascular structures that simulate neoplasms on chest radiographs: Clues to the diagnosis. *Radiographics* 15:867, 1995.

55. Meza MP, Benson M, Slovis TL: Imaging of mediastinal masses in children. *Radiol Clin North Am* 31:583, 1993.

56. Day DL, Gedgaudas E: Symposium on Nonpulmonary Aspects in Chest Radiology. The thymus. *Radiol Clin North Am* 22:519, 1984.

57. Naidich DP: Helical computed tomography of the thorax. Clinical applications. *Radiol Clin North Am* 32:759, 1994.

58. Shepard JO, McLoud TC: Imaging the airways: Computed tomography and magnetic resonance imaging. *Clin Chest Med* 12:151, 1991.

59. Kramer EL, Divgi CR: Pulmonary applications of nuclear medicine. *Clin Chest Med* 12:55, 1991.

60. LaBan MM, Siegel CB, Schultz LK, Taylor RS: Occult radiographic fractures of the chest wall identified by nuclear scan imaging: Report of seven cases. *Arch Phys Med Rehabil* 75:353, 1994.

61. Heller M, Jehle D: Other emergency department applications, in *Ultrasound in Emergency Medicine.* Philadelphia: Saunders, pp. 135–205.

SELECTED READING

Armstrong P, Wilson AG, Dee P, Hansell DM: *Imaging of Diseases of the Chest,* 2d ed. St. Louis: Mosby–Year Book, 1995.

Felson, B: *Chest Roentgenology.* Philadelphia: Saunders, 1973.

Fraser RS, Paré JAP, Fraser RG, Paré PD: *Synopsis of Diseases of the Chest,* 2d ed. Philadelphia: Saunders, 1994.

Reed JC: *Chest Radiology: Plain Film Pattern and Differential Diagnosis,* 3d ed. St Louis: Mosby–Year Book, 1991.

CHAPTER 18

CARDIOVASCULAR IMAGING

WILLIAM J. BRADY, JR. / TOM P. AUFDERHEIDE / PHOEBE A. KAPLAN

The chest radiograph is frequently used in the emergency department (ED) to evaluate patients with traumatic and nontraumatic cardiovascular conditions. Despite numerous advances in radiographic imaging, the chest film remains a fundamental diagnostic tool, and the emergency clinician must understand the radiographic findings associated with various cardiovascular disorders. For some patients, other diagnostic imaging studies such as echocardiography, computed tomography (CT), magnetic resonance imaging (MRI), nuclear scintigraphy, or angiography are indicated.

RADIOGRAPHIC ANATOMY

The Heart

On the posteroanterior (PA) chest radiograph, the position of the heart is variable. On average, one-third of the heart lies to the right of the midline (Fig. 18-1A and B). The right heart border is composed almost entirely of the right atrium (RA) (Fig. 18-2A, B and C). Above the right atrium lies the superior vena cava. The right ventricle (RV) is an anterior structure and is not seen in profile on the frontal radiograph. The left heart border represents the left ventricle (LV). At the upper portion of the left heart border is a slight concavity. Enlargement of the left atrial appendage creates a bulge in this area. The left atrium (LA) is not normally seen in the PA view.[1,2]

On the lateral view, the anterior border of the cardiac silhouette is the right ventricle (Fig. 18-3A and B). The posterior and inferior cardiac borders are formed by the left ventricle. The inferior vena cava is usually superimposed on the posteroinferior border of the left ventricle, but occasionally it extends just posterior to the left ventricular outline at the junction with the diaphragm. The LA forms the superior portion of the posterior border of the heart.

Normally, the cardiac valves are not seen. Only when they are heavily calcified do the cardiac valves become visible (Fig. 18-4A and B).

Heart Size.   On the PA view, heart size is estimated by the *cardiothoracic ratio.* (see Chap. 17, Fig. 17-8) The width of the heart is determined by measuring the distance between two vertical lines drawn tangential to the widest points on the right and left cardiac borders. The width of the thoracic cavity is measured at the widest point between the inner rib margins. A cardiothoracic ratio of greater than 50% indicates cardiac enlargement.[2]

Estimating cardiac size from the chest radiograph has several limitations. Only the PA projection can be used to calculate the cardiac size. The anteroposterior (AP) view often produces an artificially enlarged cardiac silhouette, especially when taken in the supine position or with an incomplete inspiration. If the patient is rotated, the heart size cannot be reliably assessed. Chronic obstructive pulmonary disease (COPD) increases the thoracic width due to hyperinflation of the lungs, making the cardiothoracic ratio unreliable because the heart appears disproportionately small (see Chap. 17, Fig.17-32B).

The lateral chest radiograph is also used to assess cardiomegaly. An increase in the size of the LV causes the inferoposterior border of the heart to encroach upon or overlie the thoracic spine, obliterating the retrocardiac clear space. Right ventricular enlargement is noted when the retrosternal clear space is partially or completely filled. Massive left ventricular enlargement displaces the RV anteriorly, also obliterating the retrosternal clear space.

The Aorta

The thoracic aorta is divided into three segments—the ascending aorta, the aortic arch, and the descending aorta. The ascending aorta extends superiorly from the left ventricular outflow tract. The ascending aorta is not normally seen on the PA radiograph because it is contained within the mediastinal soft tissues. In older individuals, the aorta becomes elongated and tortuous, and the ascending aorta forms a curved contour on the right mediastinal border. The aortic arch extends across the midline into the left side of the mediastinum. The posterior portion of the aortic arch makes a prominent rounded shadow on the left mediastinal border known as the *aortic knob.* With aging, the aortic knob is enlarged and makes a distinct impression on the left side of the distal trachea. The descending aorta parallels the thoracic vertebral bodies. The left lateral margin of the descending aorta appears as a prominent vertical line. The right side of the descending aorta is not radiographically visible.

On the lateral film, only the aortic arch is seen in younger individuals. With aging, the widely curved descending aorta lies adjacent to the vertebral column and is visible.

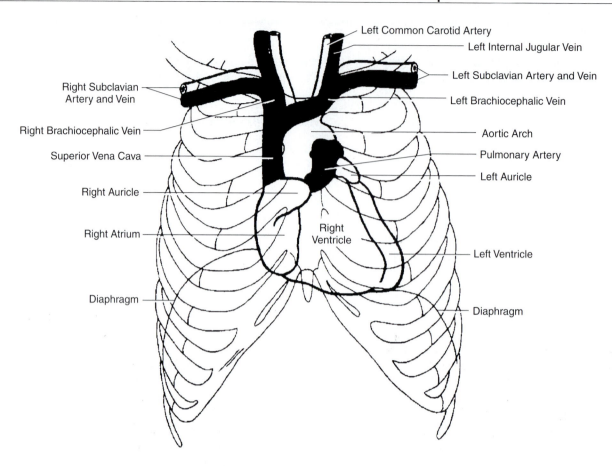

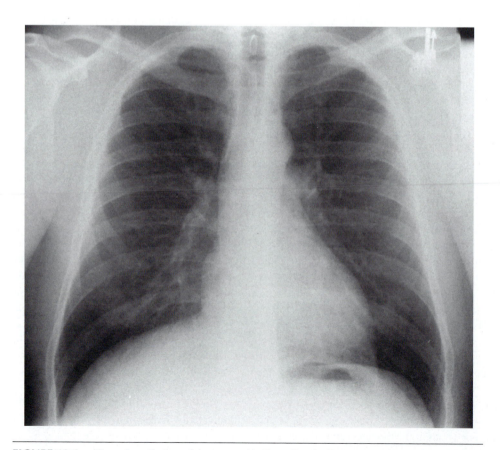

FIGURE 18-1.   Normal cardiothoracic anatomy. (*A.* From Pansky B: *Review of Gross Anatomy,* 6th ed. New York: McGraw-Hill, 1996. With permission.)

The Mediastinum

The mediastinum is bounded anteriorly by the sternum, posteriorly by the vertebral column, superiorly by the thoracic inlet, and inferiorly by diaphragm. The heart is the largest mediastinal structure. The right mediastinal contour includes, from superior to inferior, the right brachiocephalic vessels and superior vena cava (SVC), the ascending aorta (in older individuals), the right main pulmonary arteries, the RA, and the inferior vena cava. The left mediastinal contours include the left subclavian artery, the aortic knob, left main pulmonary arteries, concavity of the left atrial appendage, and the LV (Fig. 18-2).

Pleural Reflection Lines. Mediastinal soft tissue structures create radiographically visible shadows when they are adjacent to aerated lung (Figs. 18-2 and 18-3). They are known collectively as the *mediastinal pleural reflection lines.* The *right paratracheal stripe* is seen in up to 95% of patients and has a normal width of up to 5 mm.[3] Widening of the right paratracheal stripe can result from lymphadenopathy, mediastinal fluid, or excessive paratracheal fat. There is no left paratracheal stripe because the left side of the trachea is within the mediastinal soft tissues and not against the lung.

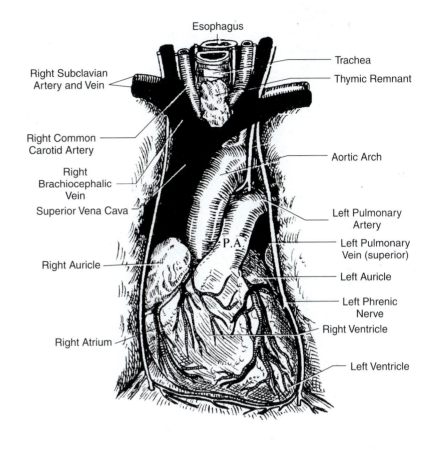

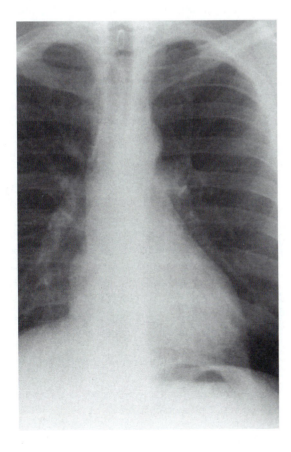

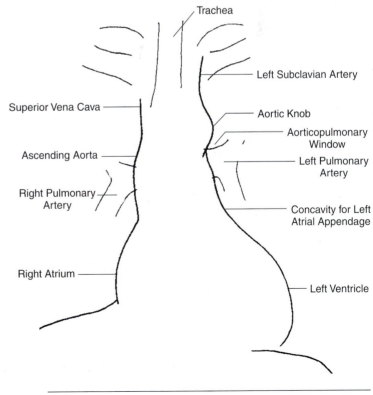

FIGURE 18-2. Anatomy of the heart and great vessels. (From Pansky B: *Review of Gross Anatomy,* 6th ed. New York: McGraw-Hill, 1996. With permission.)

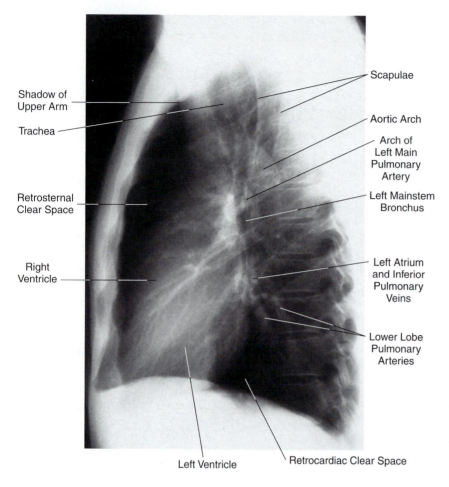

Shadow of
Upper Arm

Trachea

Retrosternal
Clear Space

Right
Ventricle

Scapulae

Aortic Arch

Arch of
Left Main
Pulmonary
Artery

Left Mainstem
Bronchus

Left Atrium
and Inferior
Pulmonary
Veins

Lower Lobe
Pulmonary
Arteries

Left Ventricle   Retrocardiac Clear Space

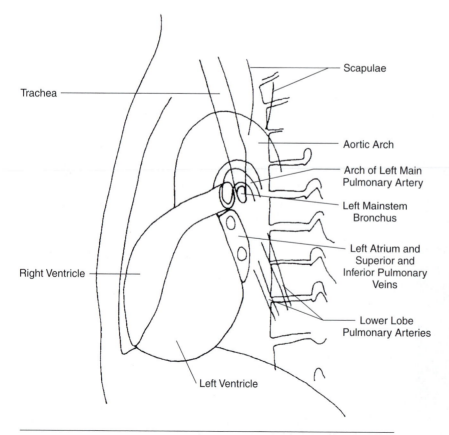

Trachea

Right Ventricle

Left Ventricle

Scapulae

Aortic Arch

Arch of Left Main
Pulmonary Artery

Left Mainstem
Bronchus

Left Atrium and
Superior and
Inferior Pulmonary
Veins

Lower Lobe
Pulmonary Arteries

FIGURE 18-3.   Cardiac and mediastinal structures on the lateral radiograph.

The *left paraspinal line* parallels the lateral margin of the vertebral bodies and lies midway between the vertebrae and the descending aorta. It extends inferiorly from the aortic arch to the level of the diaphragm. The right paraspinal line is less frequently seen.

The *left subclavian artery* arises from the aortic arch, passing upward and lateral to the trachea. On the PA chest film, the left subclavian artery appears as an arcuate opacity extending from the aortic knob to a point at or just above the superior margin of the left clavicle.

The *azygos vein* originates in the upper lumbar region at the level of the renal veins. In the thorax, it ascends anterior and to the right of the thoracic vertebrae. At the level of the carina, the azygos vein arches anteriorly over the right mainstem bronchus and inserts into the SVC. The arch of the azygos vein is visible on the PA radiograph, where it appears as an oval-shaped soft tissue density at the superior border of the right mainstem bronchus and is continuous with the inferior end of the right paratracheal stripe.

The *aorticopulmonary window* is the space below the arch of the aorta and above the left pulmonary artery. This space normally contains fat, the ligament of the ductus arteriosus, the left recurrent laryngeal nerve, and lymph nodes. Obliteration of this normal space suggests mediastinal pathology (e.g., lymphadenopathy, fluid, or blood).

Hilum

The central vascular structures on both sides of the mediastinum form the hila of the lungs. The right hilar vessels appear to extend further into the lung than those on the left because the medial part of the left hilum is obscured by the mediastinum. The left pulmonary artery arches over the left main bronchus, making the left hilum slightly higher than the right. The right main pulmonary artery is contained within the soft tissues of the mediastinum. Its ascending and descending (interlobar) branches are the right hilar arterial vessels. The right hilar complex also includes the right superior pulmonary vein, the right mainstem bronchus and its proximal branches, and surrounding connective tissue. The left hilum is composed of the left upper lobe pulmonary artery, which arches over the left upper lobe bronchus, the interlobar artery, and the left superior pulmonary vein.

Pulmonary Vasculature

The lungs and bronchial tree are air-filled and cast little or no shadow in a normal chest radiograph. Normal "lung markings" are vascular and have a branching and tapering appearance on the radiograph. If a blood vessel is oriented parallel to the x-ray beam, it appears as a dense round spot. The pulmonary vessels closer to the mediastinum are larger than those in the lung periphery. The vessels at the far periphery of the lung, within 1 cm of the pleural surface, are normally too small to be radiographically visible.

RADIOGRAPHIC ANALYSIS

An initial review is performed to identify any striking abnormalities. Because the presence of an obvious abnormality can distract the viewer from more subtle changes, the initial review must be followed by a comprehensive analysis of the radiograph. The technical adequacy of the film is evaluated. The film is assessed for correct penetration, an adequate inspiration, and the absence of rotation. A systematic review of the radiograph follows, looking at the bones, soft tissues, and lungs. In patients with suspected cardiovascular disease, the focus is on the heart, the great vessels and mediastinum, the hila, and the pulmonary vasculature (lung markings) (Table 18-1).

Analysis of the Frontal Radiograph

The Heart. Cardiac size is estimated by the *cardiothoracic ratio*. Evidence of specific heart chamber enlargement is then sought. Bulging of the right heart border represents right atrial enlargement. The left heart border represents the LV, which is

TABLE 18-1

Radiographic Analysis of the Cardiovascular System

Heart and aorta	Heart size and cardiac chambers Aortic knob, ascending and descending aorta
Lungs	Pulmonary vasculature—lung markings Pulmonary parenchyma—examine both the interstitium and air spaces Interlobar fissures—especially on lateral view
Hila	Main pulmonary arteries and veins Abnormal masses or lymph nodes
Mediastinum	Mediastinal contours (major vessels): aorta, inferior vena cava, superior vena cava, left subclavian artery Mediastinal pleural reflection lines Trachea
Diaphragm	Both diaphragms sharply visible to intersection with chest wall (pleural effusion blunts costophrenic sulcus)

enlarged if the left heart border is near the left chest wall. The upper portion of the left heart border normally has a slight concavity. Straightening or a bulge in this region is indicative of left atrial enlargement. Other signs of left atrial enlargement include widening of the angle between the left and right mainstem bronchi at the carina and a double density along the right heart border. The sites of the cardiac valves (normally not seen) are inspected for calcification (Fig. 18-4*A* and *B*).

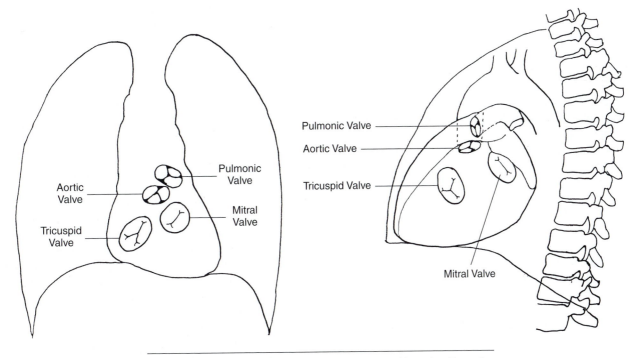

FIGURE 18-4. Heart valve positions on the PA and lateral radiographs.

The Great Vessels.   The great vessels form the margins of the superior mediastinum. On the right side is the SVC. On the left side is left subclavian artery and the aortic knob. The aortic knob should be well defined and have a transverse diameter of 2 to 3 cm. The left margin of the descending aorta is seen paralleling the vertebral column. In an elderly patient with a tortuous aorta, the aortic knob is enlarged, and a curve representing the ascending aorta is seen along the right mediastinal border.

Mediastinal Lines.   The mediastinal borders are normally sharp and clearly defined. Widening of the superior mediastinum suggests lymphadenopathy or a mediastinal fluid collection (blood). The *right paratracheal stripe* should measure 2 to 4 mm in width and the arch of the azygos vein less than 1 cm in width. The *aorticopulmonary window* is located between the inferior margin of the aortic arch and the left pulmonary artery and is normally a clear concave space. It is obliterated or bulging in the presence of lymphadenopathy or mediastinal fluid. The outline of the descending aorta and left paraspinal line should be noted. Finally, the contour and position of the trachea, carina, and mainstem bronchi are observed.

The Hila.   The normal hila are branching vascular structures that become successively smaller and less radiopaque. The left and right hila should be of equal dimensions at the same distance from the midline. The right hilum appears larger than the left because the proximal portion of the left hilum is partly obscured by the left side of the heart. Because the lower portions of the lungs are larger than the upper, the vascularity of the lower hilum is greater than the upper in a ratio of two-thirds to one-third. Vascular prominence of the hilum can be arterial or venous. Pulmonary venous engorgement causes abnormal prominence of the upper zones of the hila, where the superior pulmonary veins are located. This is seen in congestive heart failure and mitral stenosis. Pulmonary arterial engorgement is seen in pulmonary artery hypertension, in which the proximal pulmonary arteries are engorged and then rapidly taper, like a "pruned tree." Hilar prominence due to lymphadenopathy or tumors causes a rounded, lumpy contour rather then the normal branching vascular appearance.

The Lungs.   Symmetry of the lungs is used to assess an area of questionable abnormality by comparing the area in question with the opposite lung.

The lung markings are evaluated for a normal branching vascular pattern and the presence of abnormal interstitial markings. With the patient upright, vascular markings are normally thinner and less prominent in the upper portions of the lungs owing to the effect of gravity. Relatively increased vascular markings in the superior portions of the lungs is called *cephalization* and suggests pulmonary venous hypertension due to congestive heart failure. Some examiners look at the PA radiograph upside-down to help assess cephalization. More prominent lung marking are expected in the lower portions of the lung; therefore, if prominent lung markings are seen in the lower portions of an upside-down radiograph, cephalization is present.

Lung markings normally disappear within about 1 cm of the pleural surface. The interstitial connective tissue of the lung is not normally visible. Lung markings that extend to the pleural surface are abnormal and usually represent thickened interlobular septa (Kerley B lines). Increased interstitial markings are characterized by a fine, reticular pattern throughout the lung.[4,5]

The Diaphragm.   Both domes of the diaphragm should be identified. The surface of the diaphragm should be clearly outlined except where the heart and pericardial fat are in contact with the diaphragm. The costophrenic sulci should be sharp. Pleural effusions are seen with various cardiovascular and pulmonary disorders (e.g., congestive heart failure).

Analysis of the Lateral Radiograph

The lateral radiograph is used to assess heart chamber enlargement, identify small pleural effusions, and better characterize pulmonary opacities.

The Heart.   An increase in size of the RV fills the retrosternal airspace. Enlargement of the LV causes the inferoposterior border of the heart to encroach upon the thoracic spine. Left atrial enlargement causes a bulge from the superior posterior heart border. Calcification of the cardiac valves is also seen on the lateral film.

The Mediastinum.   The aorta, trachea, and hilum are examined on the lateral radiograph. Aortic aneurysms and tortuosity of the aorta can be seen. Increases in the size or density of the hilum due to vascular engorgement or lymphadenopathy can sometimes be more reliably identified on the lateral radiograph than on the PA film. Tracheal displacement and thickening of the posterior tracheal wall can also be seen on the lateral radiograph.

The Lungs.   The lateral radiograph is helpful in identifying and localizing intraparenchymal pulmonary disease, especially in the retrosternal, retrocardiac, and posterior costophrenic regions. Thickening of the interlobar fissures is easily detected on the lateral radiograph and is a sign of pulmonary edema.

The Diaphragm.   Both sides of the diaphragm should be sharply defined and visible to their intersection with the posterior chest wall. Both posterior costophrenic sulci are carefully inspected for pleural effusion or fibrosis.

Synthesis of Radiographic Findings

In patients with cardiovascular disease, the heart, aorta, lungs, hila, mediastinum, and diaphragm are reviewed on both the PA and lateral radiographs (Table 18-1). This information is then synthesized into a diagnosis. For example, if the PA radiograph demonstrates cardiomegaly, prominent upper hilar vascularity, and Kerley B lines and the lateral radiograph confirms cardiomegaly with encroachment of the inferoposterior border of the heart on the thoracic spine, thickened interlobar fissures, and a small pleural effusion, the radiographic findings are consistent with left ventricular hypertrophy and left ventricular failure with pulmonary edema.

COMMON ABNORMALITIES

Congestive Heart Failure

The chest film in the patient with congestive heart failure (CHF) may reveal cardiac enlargement, upper-zone redistribution of pulmonary blood flow, interstitial and alveolar pulmonary edema, and pleural effusions. *Cardiomegaly* and *pulmonary edema* are the most characteristic radiographic findings.

CARDIOMEGALY. Cardiomegaly is either *focal,* where a single heart chamber is enlarged, or *global,* with overall expansion of the heart. Numerous pathophysiologic processes cause cardiac enlargement. Many disease states initially produce single-chamber enlargement and then progress to generalized cardio-megaly. For example, patients with mitral valve stenosis (MVS) initially demonstrate left atrial (LA) enlargement. With disease progression, generalized cardiomegaly results. In other cases, such as patients with a dilated cardiomyopathy due to myo-carditis, the chest radiograph shows generalized cardiac enlargement from the outset.

Specific patterns of chamber enlargement can suggest an underlying cardiac disorder (Table 18-2). With left ventricular (LV) enlargement, the PA view demonstrates extension or bulging of the lower left heart border (Fig. 18-5). The lateral view shows the posteroinferior border of the heart progressing further posteriorly to the point of approaching or overlapping the spine. An LV aneurysm causes similar findings on the lateral chest radiograph (Fig. 18-6). Echocardiography distinguishes a LV aneurysm from ventricular enlargement.

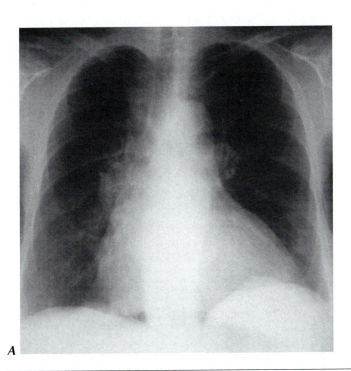
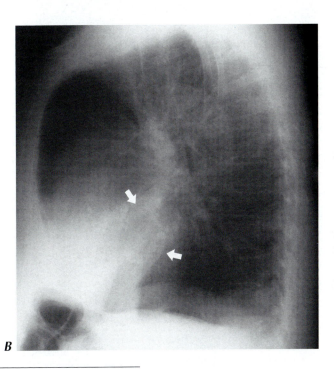

FIGURE 18-5. *A.* Aortic valve stenosis. Cardiomegaly and left ventricular enlargement with elongation of the left heart border and inferior displacement of the apex. *B.* Left ventricular enlargement with displacement of the left ventricle posteriorly toward the spine. Calcification of the aortic and mitral *(arrows)* valves is seen.

TABLE 18-2

Radiographic Features of Specific Chamber and Cardiac Enlargement

Generalized cardiac enlargement	PA: Lateral:	Cardiothoracic ratio > 0.5 (on PA projection) Estimation of left and right ventricular components of cardiomegaly
Left ventricle	PA: Lateral:	Elongation of left heart border, inferior, and leftward displacement of cardiac apex Encroachment of posterior portion of left ventricle onto the spine
Right ventricle	PA: Lateral:	Not helpful Filling of retrosternal airspace
Left atrium	PA: Lateral:	Straightening or bulging of left upper heart border; "double contour" at right heart border Posterior displacement of esophagus; bulging of upper portion of posterior heart border

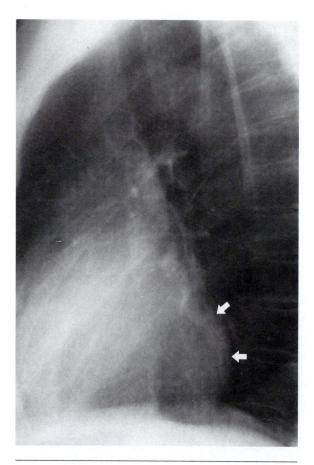

FIGURE 18-6. Left ventricular aneurysm. Lateral chest film demonstrating protrusion of the left ventricle postero-inferiorly with encroachment on the thoracic spine consistent with either LV enlargement or aneurysm *(arrows)*.

In cases of LA enlargement, the upper left heart border (normally concave) flattens or becomes convex (Figs. 18-7, 18-8, and 18-9). With additional enlargement, the LA overlaps the RA, producing a *double-shadow* or *double-contour* appearance. In addition, left atrial enlargement causes splaying of the carina and widening of the subcarinal angle.

With right ventricular (RV) enlargement, the PA chest film is of limited use because the RV lies anteriorly and is not seen on the PA view (Fig. 18-9A). The PA radiograph may show generalized cardiomegaly. On the lateral film, RV enlargement is demonstrated when the retrosternal clear space is either completely or partially filled by the enlarged RV (Fig. 18-9B).

In patients with CHF, the chest film provides information useful in determining the prognosis and chronicity. Approximately one-third of patients with acute myocardial infarction (AMI) have pulmonary vascular congestion or frank pulmonary edema demonstrated on chest film. AMI patients who develop CHF have an increased mortality. The chronicity of the heart disease causing CHF is indicated by the cardiac size. Patients with a first AMI complicated by pulmonary edema have a normal heart size. In fact, AMI is the most frequent cause of pulmonary edema with a normal cardiac size. Patients with AMI with an enlarged cardiac silhouette on the chest radiograph frequently have a preexisting cardiomyopathy, an anterior wall infarct, or multiple-vessel coronary artery disease.[6]

PULMONARY EDEMA. With pulmonary edema, there is accumulation of excess fluid in extravascular pulmonary tissues (Fig. 18-10). Pulmonary edema is most often cardiogenic, resulting from elevated pulmonary venous pressure due LV dysfunction (Table 18-3). Noncardiogenic pulmonary edema

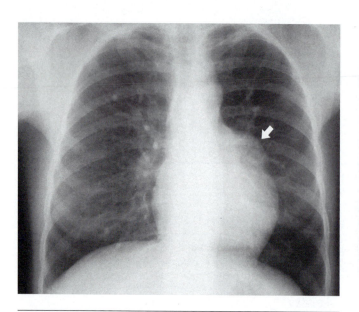

FIGURE 18-7. Mitral valve stenosis. Left atrial enlargement with bulging of the left upper heart border *(arrow)*. Vascular redistribution is noted, indicating stage I pulmonary edema.

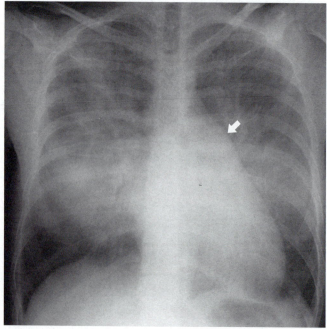

FIGURE 18-8. Mitral valve stenosis with congestive heart failure. "Bat-wing" configuration of acute pulmonary edema. Left atrial enlargement is noted with a bulging of the left upper heart border.

has various causes, including overdoses of heroin or aspirin, sepsis, pulmonary venous or lymphatic obstruction, and uremia with fluid overload. Differentiating cardiogenic from noncardiogenic pulmonary edema solely on the basis of radiographic findings is difficult. A normal-sized heart suggests a noncardiogenic etiology except in the patient with a first AMI.[7]

From a radiographic perspective, cardiogenic pulmonary edema is divided into three phases: stage I, vascular redistribution; stage II, interstitial edema; and stage III, alveolar edema.

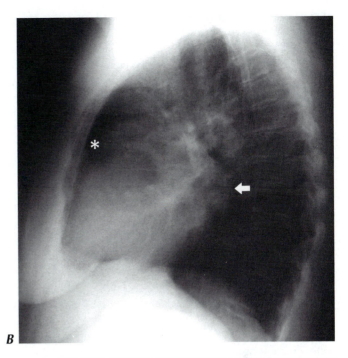

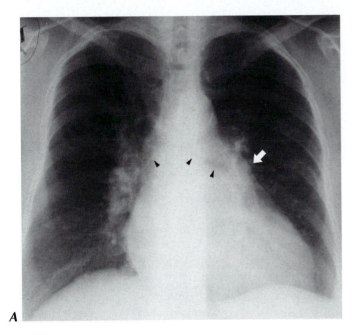

FIGURE 18-9. *A.* Mitral valve stenosis. Cardiomegaly with left atrial enlargement manifest by splaying of the left and right mainstem bronchi *(arrowheads)*, and bulging of the left upper heart border. The hila are prominent due to pulmonary venous hypertension. *B.* Lateral view confirming that the right ventricle is primarily responsible for the cardiac enlargement noted on the PA view. The right ventricular enlargement causes partial loss of the retrosternal clear space *(asterisk).* Left atrial enlargement is present as a bulge in the upper posterior heart border *(arrow).*

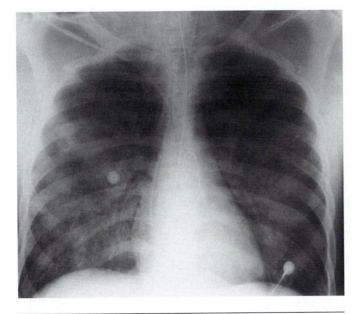

FIGURE 18-10. Congestive heart failure complicating an acute myocardial infarction. Stage III pulmonary edema (alveolar edema) in "butterfly" configuration. The normal cardiac size suggests that this patient had no prior cardiac disease. This large myocardial infarction complicated by pulmonary edema has a poor prognosis.

TABLE 18-3

Radiographic Features of Congestive Heart Failure

Cardiomegaly (global)
Heart chamber enlargement
    Left ventricular enlargement
    Right ventricular enlargement
    Left atrial enlargement

Pulmonary edema
    Stage I
        Apical redistribution of flow: "cephalization"
    Stage II (interstitial edema)
        Blurred pulmonary vascular markings
        Peribronchial cuffing
        Kerley A, B, and C lines
        Subpleural edema—thickened interlobar fissures
        Prominent upper hilar vasculature
            Distended superior pulmonary veins
        Pleural effusion (small; right > left)
    Stage III (alveolar edema)
        Airspace-filling edema, often in "bat-wing" pattern

Stage I (vascular redistribution). In *stage I (vascular redistribution)*, there is an increase in blood flow to the upper regions of the lungs. Normally, vascular markings are thicker and more prominent in the lower lung regions. Upper and lower lung markings are equalized at pulmonary capillary wedge pressures (PCWPs) of 13 to 15 mmHg.[8] Equalization of flow is difficult to identify radiographically. Vascular redistribution to the upper lung zones ("cephalization") develops with PCWPs of 15 to 18 mmHg. Vascular redistribution is apparent when the upper lobe vessels are more dilated than those in the lower lung fields (Fig. 18-8).

Stage II (interstitial edema). In *stage II (interstitial edema)*, edema fluid leaves the vascular space and enters the interstitial lung tissue.[7] This occurs at a PCWP of 18 to 22 mmHg. The lung interstitium is divided into three components. Peribronchovascular tissue consists of sheaths of connective tissue that surround the pulmonary arterioles and bronchioles. Septal tissues consist of connective tissue divisions between the pulmonary lobules at the periphery of the lung and longer bands that run deep within the lung tissue. The third component, the alveolar walls, are microscopic; therefore thickening of the alveolar walls is not perceptible on a radiograph.

Edema in the peribronchovascular connective tissue causes peribronchial "cuffing" and blurring of the margins of the pulmonary blood vessels. Edema in the interlobular and deep septal connective tissues results in Kerley A, B, and C lines. *Kerley A lines* represent enlargement of deep septal bands that are most prominent in the upper lung zones and radiate outward from the hila. *Kerley B lines* are due to thickening of the interlobular septa at the lung periphery. On the chest radiograph, they form short, thin, horizontal lines perpendicular to the pleural surface. (see fig. 17-16*B*) *Kerley C lines* result from the superimposition of Kerley B lines and result in a fine reticular pattern at the lung bases. The accumulation of edema in the subpleural connective tissue causes thickening of the interlobar fissures. This is most prominent on the lateral film (Fig. 18-11). Thickening of the minor (horizontal) fissure is also seen on the PA film. This finding is sometimes incorrectly referred to as "fluid in the fissures." Subpleural edema can accumulate in a focal area and appear as a mass called a *pseudotumor* (Fig. 18-12).

A *pleural effusion* is noted and is usually isolated to the right hemithorax. If the effusion is bilateral, the right-sided fluid collection is usually larger.

Also, in stage II CHF, the *hila become more prominent* due to pulmonary venous hypertension. With progressive elevation of the pulmonary venous pressure, there is engorgement of the superior pulmonary veins, which results in enlargement of the upper zones of the hila.

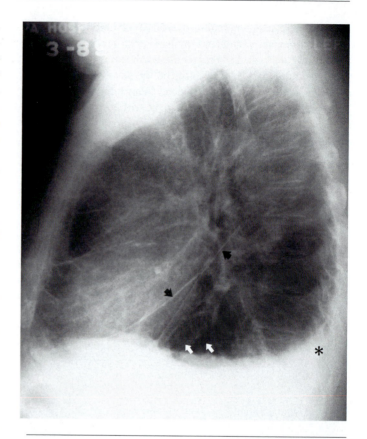

FIGURE 18-11. Lateral view of patient in congestive heart failure (late stage II or interstitial phase) demonstrating the fine reticular pattern of pulmonary edema *(small arrows)*, thickening of the fissures due to subpleural edema *(large arrows)*, and pleural effusion *(asterisk)*.

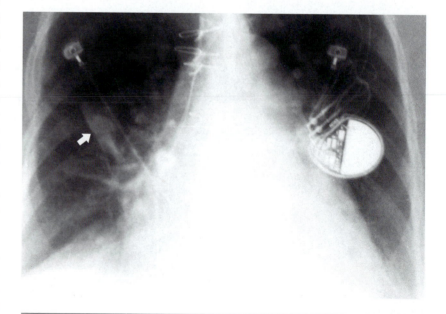

FIGURE 18-12. Pseudotumor sign. A round density is seen in the right upper lung *(arrow)*. This "mass" is actually a fluid collection in the fissure resulting from congestive heart failure.

Stage III (alveolar edema). In *stage III (alveolar edema),* fluid leaves the lung interstitium and enters the airspaces. Alveolar edema develops at a PCWP over 22 to 24 mmHg. Alveolar edema appears as patchy, ill-defined densities throughout both lungs. Alveolar edema is usually most prominent in the perihilar regions, forming a "butterfly" or "bat-wing" appearance (Figs. 18-8*A* and 18-10).

In patients with emphysema, the radiographic manifestations of pulmonary edema are altered due to the destruction of pulmonary parenchyma. Pulmonary edema in the remaining lung tissue appears as a coarse reticular pattern similar to that of pulmonary fibrosis. With diuresis, the coarse reticular pattern disappears. In addition, the cardiothoracic ratio in a COPD patient is falsely small owing to the relative expansion of lung volumes (hyperinflation).

Valvular Heart Disease

The chest radiograph provides indirect information of significant valvular stenosis or insufficiency based on the pattern of heart chamber enlargement and the presence of pulmonary edema. The radiographic findings depend on both the extent and duration of valvular dysfunction. Chronic valvular disease is more likely to result in heart chamber enlargement. Echocardiography provides precise information regarding valve structure and function.

Aortic Valve Stenosis. Aortic stenosis can result from a congenitally bicuspid valve or rheumatic heart disease. LV outflow obstruction caused by aortic stenosis initially results in dilation of the proximal aorta. This is followed by concentric LV hypertrophy. If unchecked, the process culminates in LV enlargement and CHF. On the chest radiograph, poststenotic dilation of the proximal aorta is seen as a lateral bulging of the upper right border of the cardiac silhouette (Fig. 18-13) (Table 18-4).[9] LV hypertrophy appears as a rounding of the cardiac apex (Figs. 18-5*A* and 18-13*A*). The lateral view demonstrates posterior displacement of the LV toward the spine (Figs. 18-5*B* and 18-13*B*). With LV failure, pulmonary edema develops. Radiographic features of LV failure include an overall increase in cardiac size, elongation of the left cardiac border, displacement of the apex leftward and inferiorly, LA enlargement, and pulmonary edema. In cases of prolonged duration, aortic valve calcification can occur. Mitral valve pathology may coexist with aortic stenosis, particularly in patients with rheumatic heart disease.

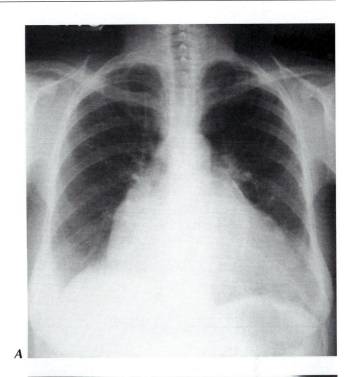

A

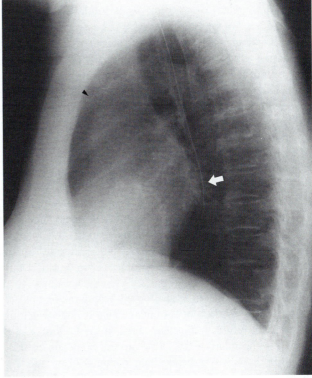

B

FIGURE 18-13. *A.* Multiple valve lesions. PA view demonstrating marked cardiomegaly. Left ventricular enlargement is noted with elongation and a globular configuration of the left heart border as well as inferior and leftward displacement of the cardiac apex. The right heart border is extended laterally due to right atrial enlargement. The left atrial enlargement causes bulging of the upper left heart border, and splaying of the bronchi at the carina. This patient has aortic stenosis, mitral stenosis, and tricuspid insufficiency due to rheumatic heart disease. *B.* Lateral view demonstrating right ventricular hypertrophy (filling of retrosternal air space). There is also bulging of the superior left heart border consistent with left atrial enlargement (*arrow*). Poststenotic dilation of the aorta is present (*arrowhead*).

TABLE 18-4

Radiographic Features of Aortic Valve Dysfunction

Aortic stenosis
    Poststenotic dilation of aorta
    Left ventricular enlargement
        Rounding of cardiac apex and elongation of left heart border
    Cardiomegaly
    Pulmonary edema
    Valvular calcification

Aortic insufficiency
    Widening of thoracic aorta (descending > ascending)
    Left ventricular enlargement
        Rounding of cardiac apex and elongation of left heart border
    Left atrial enlargement
        Straightening or bulging of left upper heart border
    Cardiomegaly
    Pulmonary edema

Aortic Valve Regurgitation.   With aortic regurgitation (aortic insufficiency), backflow of blood causes volume overload in the LV during diastole. This ultimately results in dilation of the LV chamber. On the PA film, the LV enlargement is seen as an inferolateral and leftward displacement of the cardiac apex and elongation of the left heart border (Fig. 18-14). With LV failure, pulmonary edema, LA enlargement, and generalized cardiomegaly occur. The aorta is dilated, especially in the descending segment. Aortic valve dysfunction frequently occurs with other valvular abnormalities, and the chest radiograph may reflect a mixture of pathophysiologic processes.

Mitral Valve Stenosis.   Mitral stenosis causes obstruction to blood flow from the LA to the LV. This results in LA hypertrophy, pulmonary venous congestion, and ultimately CHF. The radiographic hallmark of mitral stenosis is enlargement of the LA. Enlargement of the LA appendage causes straightening or bulging of the left heart border.[10] A "double-density" or overlapping-contour at the right heart border occurs because of overlap of the enlarged LA and the RA. Calcification may be seen in the mitral valve area on the PA and lateral radiographs (Fig. 18-13). Other findings of LA enlargement include widening of the tracheal bifurcation at the carina on the PA film and posterior displacement of the left mainstem bronchus on the lateral film. With significant long-standing obstruction, cardiomegaly and pulmonary edema occur.

Mitral Valve Regurgitation.   Mitral regurgitation results in a backflow of blood into the LA from the LV during ventricular systole, producing overdistention of the LA. LV failure follows because of the increased demand. The PCWP is usually only modestly elevated. Pulmonary edema is infrequently encountered in chronic cases of isolated mitral insufficiency.

Acute mitral regurgitation can result from papillary muscle rupture. It occurs suddenly, several days to weeks after a posterior wall MI.[6] The radiographic findings of acute mitral regurgitation are pulmonary edema without LA enlargement or

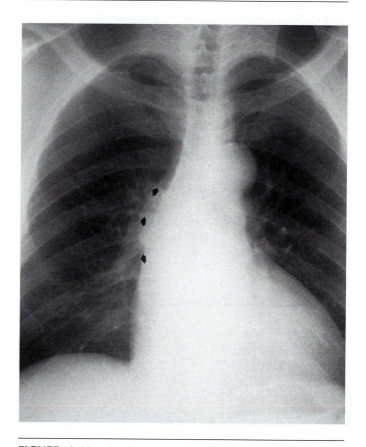

FIGURE 18-14.   Aortic valve regurgitation. Left ventricular enlargement manifest by elongation by the left heart border in a globular configuration and inferior, leftward displacement of the cardiac apex. There is marked dilation of the ascending aorta *(arrows)*.

TABLE 18-5

Radiographic Features of Mitral Valve Dysfunction

Mitral stenosis
    Left atrial enlargement
        Straightening or bulging of left upper heart border
        Overlap with right upper heart border ("double contour")
    Widening of angle between left and right mainstem bronchi at
        the carina
    Posterior displacement of left mainstem bronchus
    Mitral valve calcification
    Cardiomegaly
    Pulmonary edema

Mitral regurgitation
    Acute
        Pulmonary edema
    Nonacute
        Left atrial enlargement
            Straightening or bulging of left upper heart border
            Overlap of right upper heart border with "double contour"
            Massive left atrial enlargement may be seen
        Left ventricular enlargement
            Rounding of cardiac apex and elongation of left heart
               border with globular appearance
        Pulmonary edema (rare)

cardiomegaly. Chronic mitral regurgitation manifests radiographically with LA enlargement similar to that encountered with mitral stenosis. The enlargement of the LA from mitral regurgitation can be pronounced. At times, the LA forms both the upper left and right borders of the cardiac silhouette with the double-contour appearance along the right upper border. The increased size of the LV in mitral regurgitation is seen as both a downward displacement of the cardiac apex and an elongated lower left heart border with a rounded or globular appearance. Because the mitral valve can be both stenotic and insufficient, radiographic features of both abnormalities are sometimes seen (Table 18-5).

Tricuspid Valve Disease. The tricuspid valve can develop stenosis or insufficiency, most often as a result of endocarditis from intravenous drug abuse. Both tricuspid stenosis and insufficiency have similar radiographic appearance, including RV and RA enlargement and SVC dilation. In cases involving right-sided endocarditis, there are scattered lung nodules representing septic pulmonary emboli (Fig. 18-15). RV enlargement is more common in tricuspid regurgitation. RA enlargement is seen as a bulging convexity of the upper right heart border.

Pericardial Disease

The pericardium consists of two tissue layers and a potential space between these two layers. The visceral tissue layer is affixed to the epicardial surface and the parietal layer overlies the visceral pericardium. The pericardial space between these two tissue layers normally contains up to 55 mL of fluid. Acute pericarditis, pericardial effusion, and cardiac tamponade are three clinical entities that increase the amount of pericardial fluid.

Conventional chest radiography is frequently normal in patients with *acute pericarditis*. The chest radiograph can identify the etiology of pericarditis (e.g., a malignancy) or associated complications (e.g., pericardial effusion). In chronic pericarditis, pericardial calcification may be seen on the chest radiograph.

Pericardial effusions are well tolerated if the accumulation of fluid is gradual. However, a rapid buildup of pericardial fluid results in hemodynamic compromise due to cardiac tamponade. On a chest radiograph, cardiomegaly may be caused by either a pericardial effusion or enlargement of the heart itself. The clinical scenario often provides evidence about the cause of cardiac enlargement. For example, an enlarged cardiac silhouette with pulmonary edema suggests a dilated cardiomyopathy rather than a pericardial effusion. A "water bottle" or globular heart configuration is associated with cardiomegaly due to a pericardial effusion, but this is not always reliable (Fig. 18-16A). The "double density" sign indicates the presence of pericardial fluid contrasted against the myocardium of the RV (Fig. 18-16B). Echocardiography is the study of choice in diagnosing pericardial effusion (Fig. 18-16C, D, and E).

Cardiac tamponade results from the accumulation of fluid in the pericardial space that causes a reduction in cardiac out-

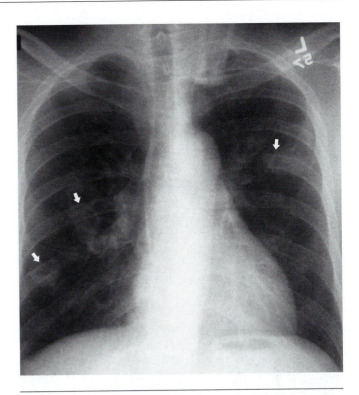

FIGURE 18-15. Septic pulmonary emboli. Multiple nodules scattered about the lungs are consistent with septic pulmonary embolism in an intravenous drug abuser. Cavitation of the lesions is seen (*arrows*).

put. Echocardiographic signs of tamponade include a pericardial effusion with diastolic collapse of the RV or RA. The chest radiograph demonstrates cardiac enlargement with clear lungs. With acute onset, the amount of pericardial fluid is small and the heart size is normal. With gradual onset, the patient has dyspnea, cardiomegaly, and clear lungs.

Pulmonary Hypertension

PA hypertension is either a primary (idiopathic) disorder or occurs secondary to cardiac or pulmonary disease. Chronic cardiopulmonary disorders associated with pulmonary hypertension include long-standing LV failure, mitral stenosis, recurrent pulmonary embolism, interstitial fibrosis, COPD, and adult respiratory distress syndrome.

Radiographic findings of advanced pulmonary hypertension include cardiomegaly, RV enlargement, enlargement of the central pulmonary arteries with rapid tapering or attenuation of the peripheral pulmonary vessels, and oligemic lungs (Fig. 18-17). Fullness of the central pulmonary circulation with "pruning" of the peripheral vessels is classic. Nevertheless, the radiographic appearance varies depending on the extent of disease, the rate of progression, coexisting diseases, and the patient's age. Early in the disease course, the chest film is normal.

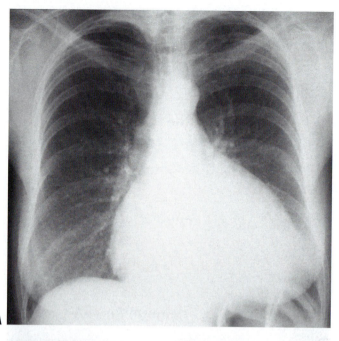

A

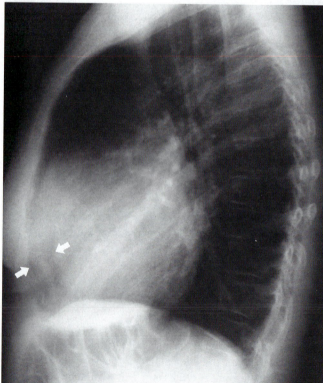

B

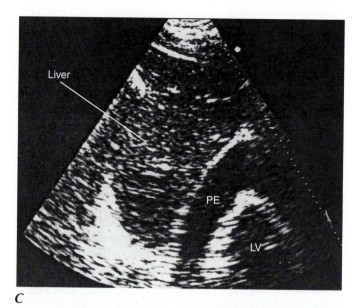

C

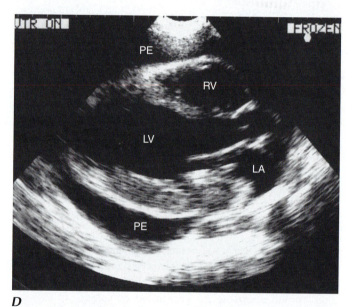

D

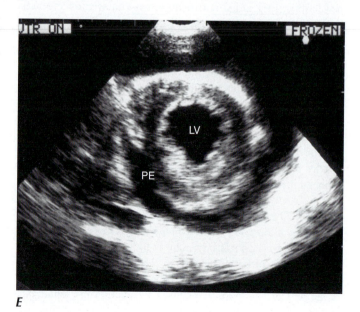

E

FIGURE 18-16.   Pericardial effusion. *A.* PA view shows a "water bottle" configuration of the cardiac silhouette. *B.* Lateral view shows a "double density" sign in the retrosternal area. Pericardial fluid causes expansion of the pericardial space, which is contrasted against the myocardium of the right ventricle. *C.* Transthoracic echocardiogram (subxyphoid view) demonstrating a pericardial effusion surrounding the right ventricle *(PE, pericardial effusion). D.* Transthoracic echocardiogram (parasternal long-axis view) shows a pericardial effusion surrounding the right and left ventricular cavities. *E.* Transthoracic echocardiogram (parasternal short-axis view) shows a pericardial effusion surrounding the left ventricular cavity. *(D* and *E.* Courtesy of James R. Mateer, M.D., Department of Emergency Medicine, Medical College of Wisconsin, Milwaukee, Wisconsin.)

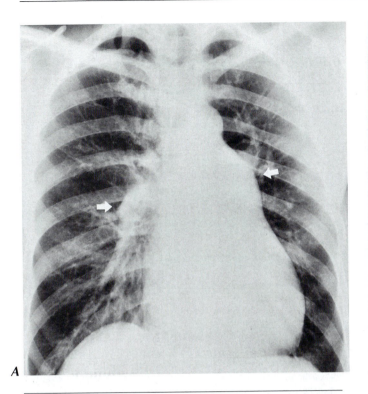

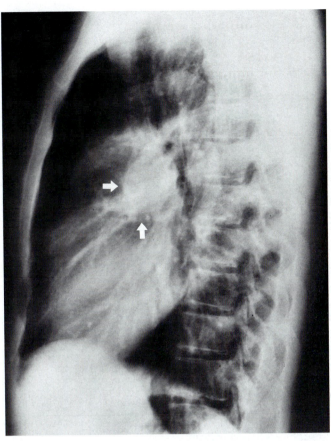

FIGURE 18-17. Pulmonary arterial hypertension. *A.* Radiographic findings include cardiomegaly, prominent right and left pulmonary arteries *(arrows)*, and rapid attenuation of the peripheral pulmonary vessels, known as "pruning." *B.* Note the prominent superimposed right and left pulmonary arteries on this lateral view *(arrow)*.

Pulmonary Embolism

The classic radiographic finding of pulmonary embolism (PE) is a relatively normal chest radiograph in a patient in "dire straits" (Fig. 18-18). However, the chest film frequently does have subtle abnormalities.[11] In fact, although a paucity of chest radiographic abnormalities is the rule during ED evaluation, about 80% of patients demonstrate some radiographic abnormality during hospitalization.[12] Nevertheless, these findings are generally nonspecific and are not diagnostic of PE. Nonspecific findings include discoid atelectasis, elevation of the hemidiaphragm, and a small unilateral pleural effusion (Table 18-6).

A specific although infrequent radiographic finding of PE is the *Westermark sign.* This results from complete occlusion of a central pulmonary artery near the hilum with relative oligemia (a paucity of vascular markings) in the involved area of lung. Relative oligemia can be difficult to identify with certainty. The occluded pulmonary artery is distended by the clot and tapers abruptly (the "knuckle" sign).

If pulmonary infarction has occurred (intraparenchymal hemorrhage), a wedge-shaped, pleural-based opacity called *Hampton's hump* may be seen (Fig. 18-18*B*). This pulmonary opacity can have a similar appearance to pneumonia.

Chest radiography is used to exclude other thoracic causes of dyspnea or chest pain, such as a pneumothorax and pulmonary edema. A chest film is also needed to corroborate the

TABLE 18-6

Radiographic Features of Pulmonary Embolism

Normal chest radiograph
Findings suggestive of pulmonary embolism
    Discoid atelectasis
    Elevation of hemidiaphragm
    Westermark sign
        Localized oligemia
        Ipsilateral dilated and truncated pulmonary artery
Findings suggestive of pulmonary infarction
    Pleural effusion
    Hampton hump (pleural-based, wedge-shaped opacity)

findings on the lung scan. Nonetheless, the chest radiograph is minimally helpful in establishing the diagnosis of PE.

Ventilation perfusion ($\dot{V}/\dot{Q}$) scanning, pulmonary angiography, duplex ultrasonography (US) of the lower extremities, and helical contrast CT are useful in patients with a suspected PE. The $\dot{V}/\dot{Q}$ scan is most effective in patients with a high clinical probability of PE who are stable in terms of their cardiopulmonary function (Fig. 18-18*C*).[13] The $\dot{V}/\dot{Q}$ scan compares perfusion of the lung to ventilation (Fig. 18-19). A difference between areas of perfusion and areas of ventilation is called $\dot{V}/\dot{Q}$

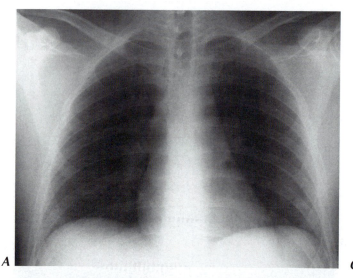

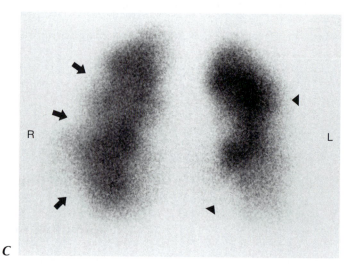

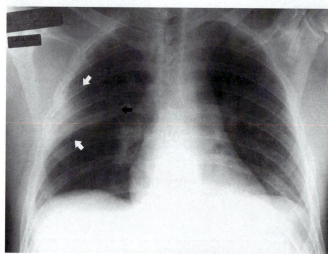

FIGURE 18-18.   Pulmonary embolism. *A.* A middle-aged man with a pulmonary embolism had significant dyspnea and a normal chest radiograph. *B.* A repeat chest radiograph the next day showed a peripheral pleural-based infiltrate with an apex "pointing" to the hilum—Hampton's hump *(arrows). C.* This perfusion scan shows multiple defects at the peripheral right lung and right base *(arrows).* There is also diminished activity at the lateral aspect of the left lung and near the cardiac apex *(arrowheads).* The ventilation scan was normal. The lung scan therefore showed multiple subsegmental and segmental V̇/Q mismatches, and was interpreted as being "high-probability" for pulmonary embolism.

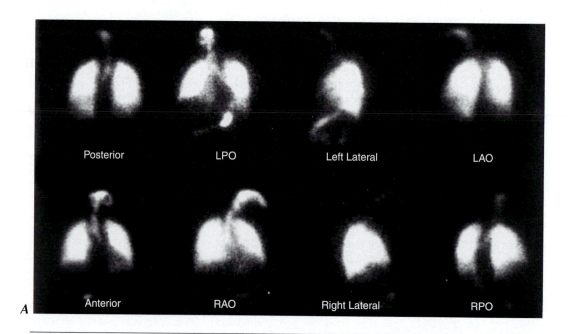

FIGURE 18-19.   Ventilation-perfusion scan Images are taken in light different orientation. *A.* A normal ventilation scan. *B.* An abnormal perfusion scan. There are several areas of decreased activity *(arrows),* especially at the bases of both lungs. These represent multiple "unmatched defects." This patient had multiple pulmonary emboli from malignancy-induced hypercoagulopathy.

mismatch. The major disadvantage of V̇/Q̇ scanning is the low sensitivity and specificity of intermediate- and low-probability scans. Lower extremity duplex US is useful in the patient with equivocal V̇/Q̇ scan results. A lower extremity duplex US that is positive for deep venous thrombosis (DVT) is a diagnostic endpoint. If negative, further diagnostic testing is warranted, often pulmonary angiography. With a positive US, pulmonary angiography is unnecessary.

Spiral CT scan of the chest with a bolus of intravenous contrast is useful in the evaluation of suspected PE (Fig. 18-20).[14,15] It is relatively noninvasive and has greater sensitivity and specificity than the V̇/Q̇ scan. Spiral CT is effective at detecting larger proximal clots, confirming the diagnosis of PE. CT misses smaller peripheral pulmonary emboli and is therefore unable to fully exclude the diagnosis of PE.

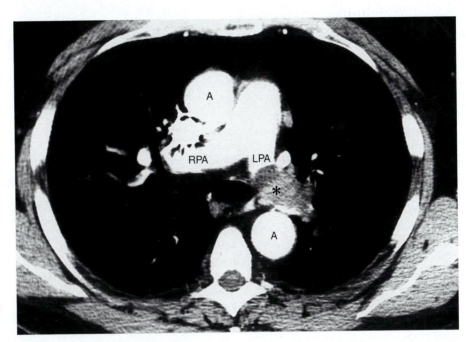

FIGURE 18-20. Pulmonary embolus. This helical CT shows a large embolus in the left pulmonary artery just beyond the bifurcation of the pulmonary trunk. (*RPA*, right pulmonary artery, *LPA*, left pulmonary artery, *A*, aorta. *Asterisk*, pulmonary embolus)

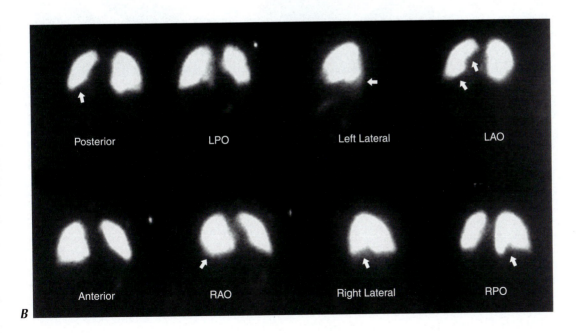

B

Thoracic Aortic Aneurysm

Thoracic aortic aneurysms (TANs) involve either the ascending aorta, aortic arch, or descending aorta. TANs are asymptomatic in approximately 60% of patients and are often discovered incidentally on a chest radiograph obtained for other reasons. TAN can present in a subacute fashion with pulsatile chest discomfort or recurrent laryngeal nerve paralysis. Acute presentations of TAN result from leakage and are manifest as chest pain or catastrophic rupture.

TAN appears as an enlarged distorted aorta, a widened mediastinum, or a mediastinal soft tissue mass (Figs. 18-21 and 18-22). An aortic diameter of 6 cm or more at the level of the arch is consistent with TAN. A normal aortic diameter at the aortic arch is less than 4 cm. However, the chest radiograph is an unreliable means of measuring mediastinal structures, and CT is needed to measure the aortic diameter accurately. The lateral chest film can demonstrate filling of the retrosternal space by an ascending aortic aneurysm. Sometimes, a mass representing a saccular aneurysm is seen arising from the aorta itself (Fig. 18-22*B*). Calcifications within the aortic wall are associated with atherosclerotic aneurysms (Table 18-7). Other findings include displacement of the trachea, depression of the left mainstem bronchus, and leftward displacement of the esophagus (with a nasogastric tube). It is difficult to distinguish an aortic dissection from an aortic aneurysm solely on plain-film findings. Additional imaging studies are necessary to define the exact pathologic process. Patients with TAN should be further evaluated with CT or angiography.

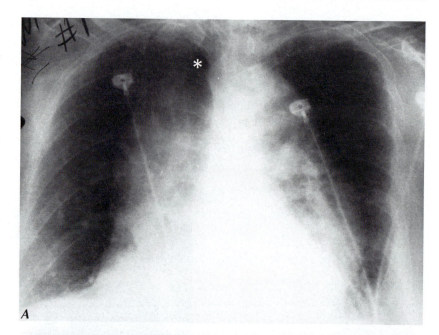

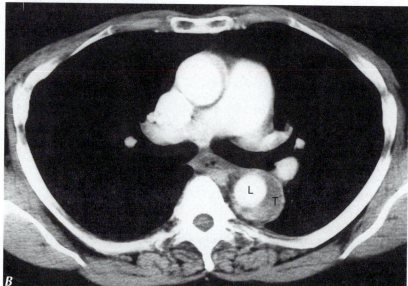

FIGURE 18-21.   Fusiform thoracic aortic aneurysm. *A.* A fusiform thoracic aneurysm is demonstrated by an enormously widened mediastinum and displacement of the trachea to the right (*asterisk*). *B.* CT shows a large mural thrombus (T) within the aneurysm surrounding the aortic lumen (L).

TABLE 18-7

Radiographic Features of Aortic Dissection and Thoracic Aortic Aneurysm

Aortic silhouette
  Widening, blurring, irregularity, or indistinct aortic contour
  Disproportionate enlargement of ascending or descending aorta
  Progressive enlargement when compared with previous radiographs
  Normal aortic appearance in 4 to 20% of aortic dissections
    Aorta is abnormal in all aneurysms (by definition)
Calcium sign (aortic dissection)
  Separation of outer vessel wall and intimal calcifications by 6 mm
Displacement of other thoracic structures
  Trachea or endotracheal tube—rightward and anteriorly
  Left mainstem bronchus—inferiorly
  Esophagus or nasogastric tube—rightward
Evidence of hemorrhage (leaking aneurysm or dissection)
  Widened mediastinum, hemomediastinum
  Pleural effusion (left)

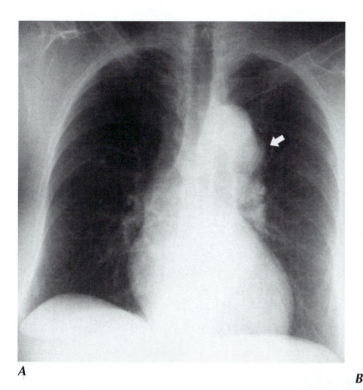

A

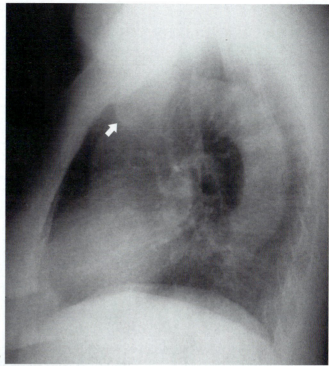

B

FIGURE 18-22. Saccular thoracic aortic aneurysm. *A.* A rounded density distorts the aortic knob and obliterates the aorticopulmonary window *(arrow). B.* The saccular aneurysm is shown as a rounded density *(arrow)* arising from the aortic arch. *C.* The CT shows the aneurysmal dilation of the aortic arch *(arrows).*

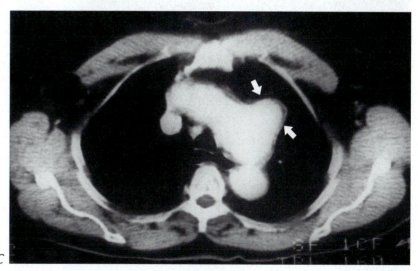

C

Thoracic Aortic Dissection

Thoracic aortic dissection (TAD) is most often seen in patients with long-standing, poorly controlled hypertension. Marfan syndrome is a less frequent cause of aortic dissection. When aortic dissection is acute, the patient presents with sudden chest and back pain. Alternatively, TAD can be chronic, with chest and back pain characterized by a slow progression of the dissection over 2 weeks or more.

Two classification schemes are used for TAD. In the De-Bakey classification, a dissection involving both the ascending and descending aorta is termed type I. Type II dissection is limited to the ascending aorta. A type III dissection starts at or distal to the left subclavian artery and progresses distally.

In the Stanford classification, a type A dissection involves the ascending aorta and may or may not extend to the descending aorta. Type B dissections are limited to the descending aorta. The Stanford classification is simpler and is related to treatment. Type A (ascending) dissections all require surgery. Type B (descending) dissections can be managed medically (control of hypertension) unless continual progression or serious branch vessel involvement (e.g., renal, mesenteric) occurs.

With aortic dissection, the hematoma progresses within the media, forcing the intima inward toward the lumen and away from the outer margin of the aorta. Because TAD is confined to the aortic lumen itself, the chest radiograph does not show direct evidence of the dissection itself. In the 80% of patients, the chest radiograph demonstrates a dilated aorta. This is dif-

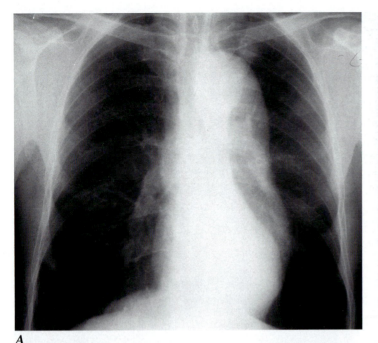

A

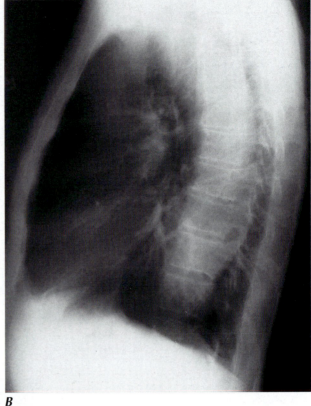

B

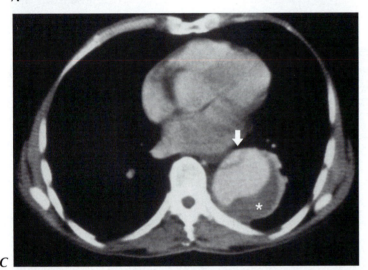

C

FIGURE 18-23. Thoracic aortic dissection. *A.* There is a widened mediastinum, an enlarged aortic knob, and dilation of the descending aorta. *B.* The lateral view shows a dilated aorta. *C.* CT scan shows aortic dissection of the descending thoracic aorta. The intimal flap *(arrow)* separates the true lumen and false lumen. A mural thrombus is present *(asterisk). D.* In a different patient, a thoracic aortic dissection extends inferiorly to involve the abdominal aorta. The true and false lumens are separated by the intimal flap. (*D.* Copyright David T. Schwartz, M.D.)

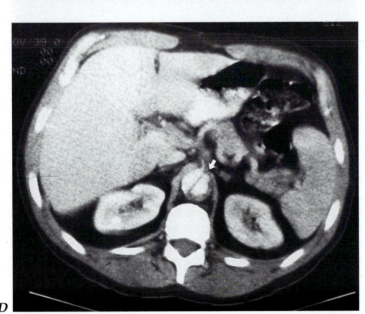

D

ficult to distinguish from a tortuous aorta frequently seen in patients who are elderly or have hypertension. An enlarged aortic silhouette is the most frequently encountered radiographic sign of TAD (Fig. 18-23). There may be blurring or indistinct margins of the aorta, an irregular aortic contour, mediastinal widening, or discrepancy in the diameters of the ascending and descending portions of the aorta. Comparison with prior chest films may reveal an interval increase in the aortic diameter. The chest film is interpreted as "normal" in 4 to 20% of cases, and so a normal chest film does not exclude the diagnosis.[16–18]

Other plain-film radiographic findings of TAD include displacement of adjacent structures and evidence of mediastinal bleeding if the dissection is leaking. The trachea (or endotracheal tube) may be deviated leftward or anteriorly, the left mainstem bronchus depressed inferiorly, and the esophagus (or nasogastric tube) displaced leftward. With leakage, pleural blood appears as mediastinal widening, or a left pleural effusion (Fig. 18-23*A*, Table 18-7).

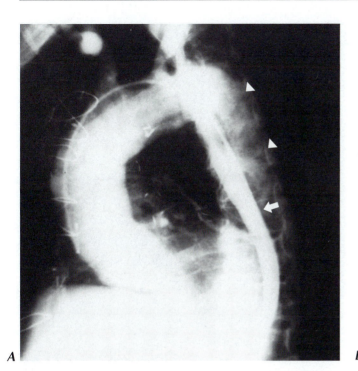

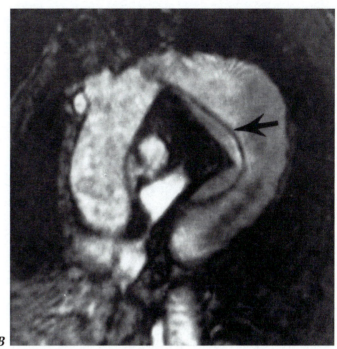

FIGURE 18-24. Thoracic aortic dissection. *A.* This aortogram shows a double lumen in the descending aorta. The true lumen is narrowed and is shown as a dense white stripe *(arrow).* The false lumen is less well opacified *(arrowheads).* (Copyright David T. Schwartz, M.D.) *B.* MRI. An oblique coronal image shows the low signal intimal flap within the distal aortic arch and descending aorta *(arrow).* (From Chen MYM, Pope TL Jr., Ott DJ: Basic Radiology. New York, McGraw-Hill, 1996. With permission.)

Intimal calcifications are often seen in the aortic knob due to age-related atherosclerosis. The position of the calcification relative to the aortic wall can provide evidence of TAD.[16,19] Typically, calcifications are located in the innermost layer of the arterial wall—the intima. With dissection, the intima (and associated calcifications) is displaced away from the outer margin of the aorta. The width of the aortic wall is estimated by measuring the distance from the intimal calcifications to the outer margin of the aortic shadow. A separation wider than 6 mm is suggestive of TAD. However, the oblique orientation of the aortic arch in the thorax may falsely suggest a separation of the calcified intima and the outer layer of the aorta on the chest film. This "calcium sign" is therefore reliable only in the ascending or descending aorta, not the aortic knob.

Patients with suspected TAD need further evaluation with angiography, CT, MRI, or echocardiography.[20] The choice of imaging study depends on the clinical suspicion for the diagnosis, the availability of these studies, patient stability, and preferences of the consultants (radiologist and cardiovascular surgeon). Aortography was formerly considered the test of choice (Fig. 18-24). However, reports of occasional missed diagnosis and false-positive studies reveal that angiography is not 100% accurate.[21–23] Thrombosis of the false lumen can be responsible for false-negative aortograms. Other disadvantages of aor-

tography include the time required for mobilization of an angiography team, the invasive nature of the examination, and the risk of reaction to contrast agents.

The CT scan has a sensitivity of from 83 to 100%, and a specificity approaching 100% (Figs. 18-22C and 18-23C and D).[19,23] Demonstration of the two distinct lumens—a true lumen surrounded by intima and a false lumen (the area within the aortic wall through which the dissection is occurring)—separated by the intimal flap is required to make the diagnosis by CT. CT is noninvasive, widely available, and can identify other mediastinal disorders. CT also reveals thrombosis within the false lumen. The disadvantages of CT include contrast exposure, a lower sensitivity than transesophageal echocardiography or MRI, and the inability to note branch vessel involvement. However, spiral CT scanning offers an accuracy approaching 100% in the diagnosis of TAD.

MRI provides detailed anatomic information of the thoracic aorta in multiple planes without the need for intravenous contrast (Fig. 18-24B). It is able to define the extent of dissection and involvement of major branch vessels. The advantages of MRI include its precise anatomic information and excellent sensitivity and specificity.[19,24] Because of the logistics of obtaining an MRI, its use is limited to stable patients.

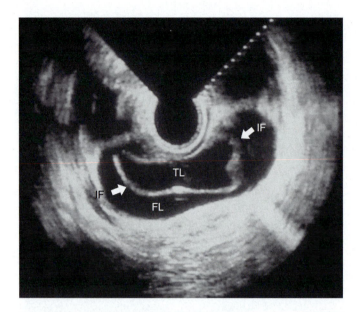

FIGURE 18-25.   Transesophageal echocardiogram. This TEE shows an aortic dissection identifying the intimal flap separating the true and false lumens. The true lumen is distinguished from the false lumen by being completely surrounded by the intimal flap. FL, false lumen; TL, true lumen; IF, intimal flap. (Courtesy of James R. Mateer, M.D., Department of Emergency Medicine, Medical College of Wisconsin, Milwaukee, Wisconsin.)

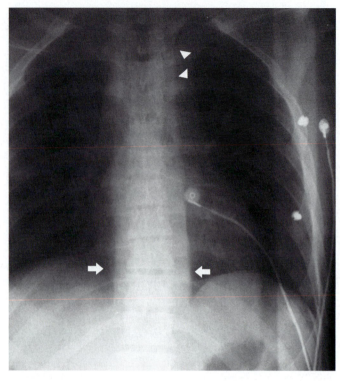

FIGURE 18-26.   Blunt aortic injury. There is an indistinct mediastinum due to mediastinal hemorrhage. There is displacement of the left and right paraspinal lines *(arrows)* due to hemorrhage. The left paraspinal line extends above the aortic knob towards the apex of the lung forming a left apical plaural cap *(arrowheads)*.

Transthoracic echocardiography (TTE) and transesophageal echocardiography (TEE) have been used especially in unstable patients (Fig. 18-25). TTE is generally widely and rapidly available and is noninvasive. It has moderate sensitivity at detecting ascending aortic dissection and can reveal aortic valve involvement and pericardial hemorrhage and tamponade. However, it is poor for detecting descending aortic dissection. TEE is excellent for detecting both descending aorta and aortic arch dissection.

Blunt Traumatic Aortic Injury

Blunt trauma patients who have experienced sudden deceleration such as a high-speed motor vehicle crash or fall from a significant height are at risk for traumatic aortic injury. The sudden deceleration results in a shear force, producing a tear of the aortic wall. In patients who survive to ED arrival, the aortic laceration is incomplete (nontransmural). A complete laceration results in rapid, fatal exsanguination. Only approximately 20% of aortic injury patients survive to ED arrival.

The plain-film chest radiograph is abnormal in nearly all patients with blunt aortic injury (BAI) (Figs. 18-26 and 18-27*A*, Table 18-8).[25,26] The findings include a widened mediastinum, abnormalities of the aortic contour, displacement of adjacent mediastinal structures, and alteration of the mediastinal pleural reflection lines. Most of these signs are due to bleeding into the mediastinum. However, the hemorrhage does not come directly from the torn aorta itself. Bleeding from the aorta would

TABLE 18-8

Radiographic Features of Traumatic Aortic Injury

Hemomediastinum (blood collection within mediastinum)
    Widened mediastinum
        > 8 cm at aortic arch (supine radiograph)
        Mediastinum:chest-width ratio > 0.25
    Blurring of the aortic contour with indistinct margins
    Left apical pleural cap
    Widening of the left paraspinal stripe
    Opacification of the aorticopulmonary window
    Widening of right paratracheal stripe
    Left pleural effusion
Displacement of adjacent structures
    Trachea—rightward and anteriorly
    Left mainstem bronchus—inferiorly
        Angle formed by the left mainstem bronchus and the
            spine > 140°
    Esophagus (nasogastric tube)—rightward and posteriorly
Injury to adjacent thoracic structures
    First or second rib, sternum, scapula, thoracic vertebrae

occur only with a complete aortic tear, which is a rapidly fatal exsanguinating injury. The mediastinal blood comes from torn branch vessels such as intercostal or internal mammary arteries or veins. Therefore, although hemomediastinum is a characteristic finding in traumatic aortic injuries, it is not a direct sign of the injury itself. Only about 25 to 35% of patients with traumatic mediastinal blood have an aortic injury.

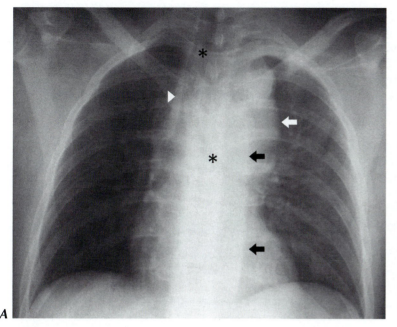

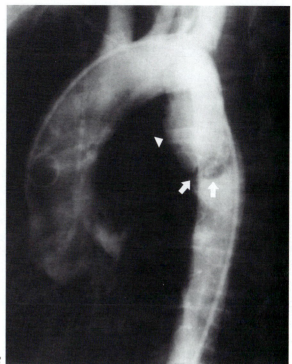

FIGURE 18-27. Blunt aortic injury. *A.* Radiographic signs of mediastional hemorrage include a widened and distorted mediastinum, an aortic knob obscured by surrounding mediastinal blood (*white arrow*), displacement of the left paraspinal line and extension of the line above the aortic arch (*black arrows*), widening of the right paratracheal stripe (*arrowhead*), and deviation of the trachea to the right and depression of the left mainstem bronchus (*asterisks*). *B.* Aortography demonstrates a laceration (*arrows*) of the descending aorta at the ligamentum arteriosum with a hematoma contained by the aortic adventitia—a pseudoaneurysm (*arrowhead*).

The mediastinal hemorrhage is present in the vast majority of cases of BAI, and mediastinal widening is the most common radiographic finding. Widening of the superior mediastinum on a supine portable chest radiograph greater than 8 cm is abnormal.[27] Another criterion for mediastinal widening uses the ratio of the transverse diameter of the mediastinum measured at the level of the aortic arch to the thoracic width measured between the inner rib margins at the same level. A ratio of greater than 0.25 is abnormal.[25] However, the detection of mediastinal widening in the trauma patient is often difficult because of the suboptimal radiographic technique usually seen with an acutely injured patient.[28] Portable AP technique, especially in a supine patient with poor inspiration, produces distortion and magnification of thoracic structures, widening the mediastinum. If the patient is able to sit upright and the mediastinum is normal in width and contour, a repeat AP film can eliminate the need for additional studies. If the upright film is abnormal or the clinical situation makes obtaining an upright film impossible, advanced imaging is required.

With BAI, the aorta may have an abnormal radiographic appearance, including a blurring of the aortic knob with indistinct margins or loss of contour of the aorta. Displacement of adjacent thoracic structures suggests BAI. The trachea may be displaced to the right. The left mainstem bronchus may be displaced inferiorly, such that the angle formed by the left mainstem bronchus and a vertical line parallel to the spine exceeds 140°.[27] Deviation of the esophagus (containing a nasogastric tube) to the right, although an infrequent radiographic finding, is reported to be the most specific abnormality for BAI.[29] Other radiographic evidence of mediastinal hemorrhage includes a left apical pleural cap, displacement of the left paraspinal line (Fig. 18-26), widening of the right paratracheal stripe, and obliteration or filling of the aorticopulmonary window.

Fractures of the thoracic skeleton serve as an indirect marker for BAI, including fractures of the first or second rib, the sternum, scapula, and thoracic vertebrae. Some reports debate the importance of sternal fracture, but continue to emphasize the potential risk of both rib and scapular fractures.[30–33]

Aortography is the test of choice to diagnose BAI (Fig. 18-27B). It demonstrates the aortic pseudoaneurysm and possibly the intimal flap that is most often located at the aortic isthmus (junction of the aortic arch and descending aorta). TEE is being used in some centers for the initial evaluation of patients at risk for BAI. While some authorities recommend aortography or CT in all blunt trauma victims with a major deceleration mechanism, the patient with a normal chest film and little clinical risk can be observed for BAI and monitored with serial chest radiography over several days. With equivocal chest radiographic findings in a patient at risk for aortic injury, additional imaging is often required. In a patient undergoing CT of the abdomen or head, additional slices through the upper chest can be obtained to look for evidence of mediastinal hemorrhage. If this is detected, aortography is needed to confirm an aortic tear, because CT cannot always detect the aortic intimal tear. (See Chap. 20, "Imaging Priorities in Trauma.")

Traumatic Cardiac Injuries

Traumatic cardiac injuries include myocardial contusion, laceration, or rupture. The radiographic methods used to evaluate blunt cardiac trauma include echocardiography and nuclear medicine imaging. Chest radiography has little to offer in such cases other than to exclude other chest injuries, such as pneumothorax or BAI.

The chest radiograph is usually normal or nonspecifically abnormal in patients with cardiac contusion. Cardiac laceration from penetrating injury or rupture from blunt trauma may present in hemorrhagic shock with or without tamponade. The chest radiograph, most often a portable AP view, is an insensitive tool for evaluating such injuries. The chest film is used to exclude a massive pneumothorax or hemothorax as the cause of circulatory failure. Chest radiographic findings occasionally reported in cardiac trauma include enlarged cardiac silhouette in a "water bottle" configuration, widened mediastinum, blurring of the aortic contour, and air-fluid levels in the pericardial area.[34–37]

The best modality for imaging of the heart to look for penetrating chamber injuries or tamponade is a bedside echocardiogram. Unstable patients are best managed empirically with appropriate surgical measures.

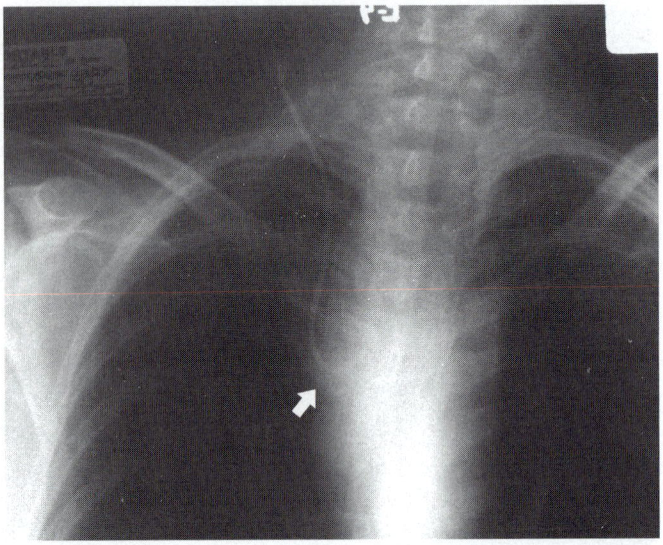

Indwelling Devices

The chest radiograph is used to assess the placement of an indwelling device such as a central venous line (CVL) or cardiac pacemaker. Complications of the placement of these devices are also evaluated with the chest radiograph. The chest radiograph is used to evaluate patients with permanent pacemakers experiencing malfunction. Abnormalities such as lead dislodgment and wire fracture can be identified.

The CVL inserted by the subclavian route should course along the inferior border of the medial portion of the clavicle and turn downward toward the heart at the junction of the medial segment of the clavicle and the right tracheal border. It should follow the right tracheal border, into the subclavian vein and end immediately above the RA. A central venous catheter placed in the internal jugular vein should proceed inferiorly from the neck and follow a similar course as described for the subclavian approach. Incorrect distal tip positioning is seen with the tip curved medially (Fig. 18-28); the tip directed laterally, indicating a perforation of the subclavian vein (Fig. 18-29); the line not following the right paratracheal border (Fig. 18-30); and the tip directed posteriorly (Fig. 18-31). Complications of line placement noted on chest radiography include pneumothorax or hemothorax, mediastinal hemorrhage, and intrathoracic fluid accumulation (Fig. 18-29 and 18-30).

FIGURE 18-28.   Central venous line misplacement. Catheter placed in the right internal jugular vein is misplaced. The distal tip is curved inward, facing medially and directed cranially *(arrow)*.

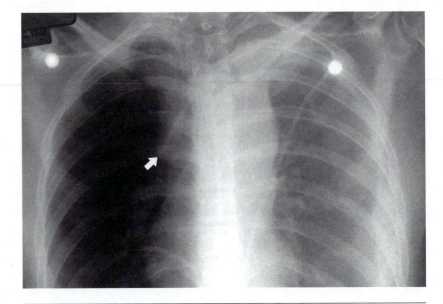

FIGURE 18-29.   Central venous line perforating the superior vena cava. Catheter placement is complicated by a left hemothorax and mediastinal hematoma manifest by mediastinal widening. The distal tip is directed laterally, indicating a perforation of the superior vena cava *(arrow)*.

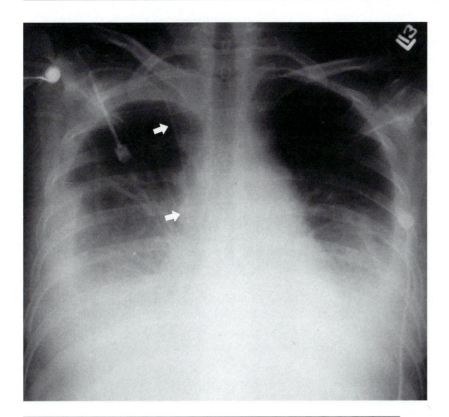

FIGURE 18-30. Central venous line misplaced into the mediastinum *(arrows)*. Catheter misplacement complicated by bilateral pleural effusions and mediastinal widening due to accumulating fluid and/or blood. The catheter does not follow expected course along the inferior portion of the clavicle.

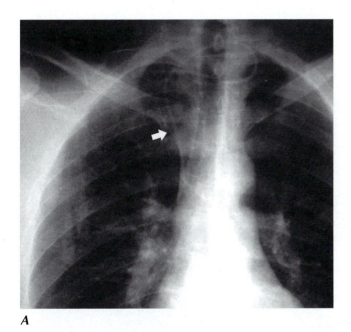

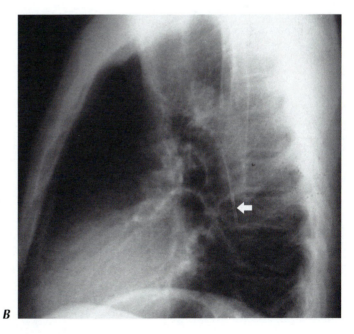

A   *B*

FIGURE 18-31. Central venous line misplaced into the azygos vein. *A.* Misplaced catheter into the azygos vein via the right internal jugular vein. The proper course of the catheter would be to follow the right paratracheal stripe inferiorly in the superior vena cava. Here, the line is laterally displaced below the clavicle, indicating an incorrect position *(arrow). B.* On the lateral view, the line is directed too far posteriorly to be in the superior vena cava, indicating placement in the azygos vein *(arrow).*

The transvenous pacemaker should have the same course as a CVL. On the PA chest film, the pacing wire follows the right tracheal border and enters the RA, arriving in the RV (Fig. 18-32). After entering the RV, the catheter moves toward the patient's left side and crosses the midline with attachment to the endocardium of the RV. The lateral chest film demonstrates the pacing wire's distal tip coursing anteriorly toward the lower portion of the sternum. The pacing wire may be incorrectly placed in the coronary sinus (Fig. 18-33). With a dual-chamber pacemaker, the leads should be properly placed in the RA and RV (Fig. 18-34). In this case, the lateral view demonstrates the distal tip coursing posteriorly, away from the RV. In addition, the chest radiograph may demonstrate an enlarged cardiac silhouette due to myocardial perforation from a pacemaker lead. Abnormalities of the pacemaker leads include dislodgment from the myocardium or the generator unit and lead fracture at any point along the course of the pacemaker lead (Fig. 18-35). "Twiddler's syndrome," in which a patient repeatedly manipulates the generator box, can result in lead fracture and sudden pacemaker failure.

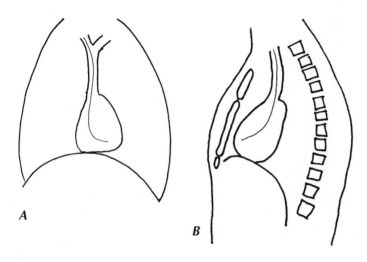

FIGURE 18-32.   Transvenous pacemaker placement. Correct position in the right ventricular cavity. *A*. PA view. *B*. Lateral view).

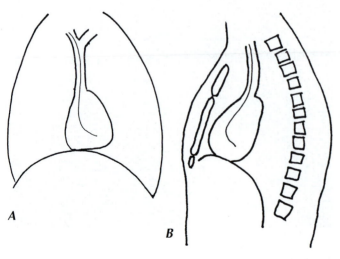

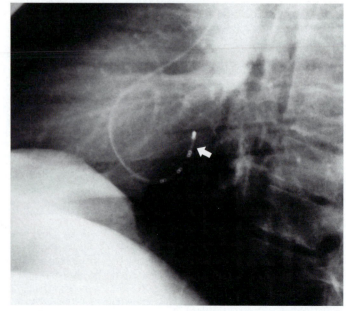

FIGURE 18-33.   Incorrect pacemaker placement. Pacemaker resting in the coronary sinus. *A*. PA view. *B*. Lateral view. Note the posterior orientation of the curl of the pacer wire on the lateral view. *C*. This lateral film shows a pacer wire in the coronary sinus. (Courtesy of R.K. Thakur, M.D., Michigan State University.)

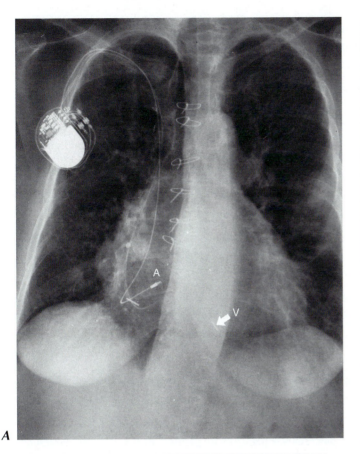

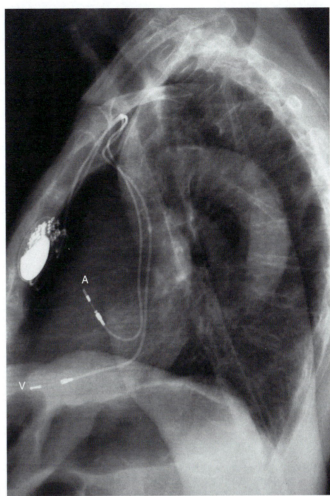

FIGURE 18-34. Dual-chamber pacemaker. *A.* The right atrial pacing wire *(A)* is clearly seen just right of the spine. The right ventricular pacing wire *(V-arrow)* overlies the spine. *B.* On lateral, the atrial pacing wire is above the ventricular pacing wire.

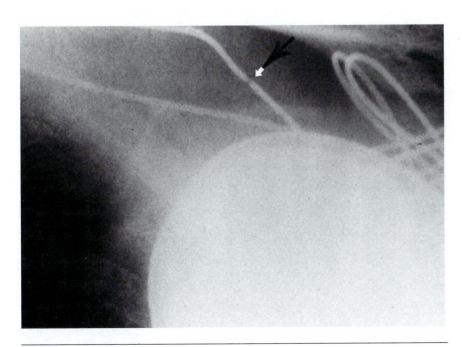

FIGURE 18-35. Fractured pacemaker wire. This magnified image demonstrates a pacing wire fracture *(arrow)* near the generator unit. (Courtesy of Lawrence R. Goodman, M.D., Department of Radiology, Medical College of Wisconsin, Milwaukee, Wisconsin.)

ERRORS IN INTERPRETATION

One of the most frequent errors in interpreting the chest radiograph is the failure to note an abnormality that was unexpected based on the patient's history and physical examination (Table 18-9). The clinician must always examine the entire film and search for incidental findings that are unrelated to the initial chief complaint. For example, in the patient with an exacerbation of CHF, the clinician could miss an osteolytic lesion in the proximal humerus.

Poor radiographic technique and a lack of awareness of its effect on radiograph quality commonly lead to errors in interpretation. Poor inspiratory effort distorts cardiac anatomy, incorrectly suggesting an enlarged heart. Inadequate penetration can simulate interstitial lung disease or CHF.

The portable film can also be a source of interpretive error. The heart size cannot always be assessed with the AP portable film. When taken in the supine position, the portable film may fail to detect a pleural effusion or pneumothorax. In the trauma patient, the aortic silhouette is distorted, simulating or masking an aortic injury.

Subtle findings are easy to miss in the chest radiograph. With CHF, indistinct or blurred upper lung vessels, as well as early redistribution and vascular equalization, can be difficult to identify.

The patient with PE most often has either a normal chest radiograph or a film with a nonspecific abnormality. However, a segmental opacity, which is most often associated with pneumonia, can also occur in pulmonary embolism and so does not exclude the diagnosis of PE.

TABLE 18-9

Common Errors in the Interpretation of Chest Radiographs

SYNDROME	FINDING	COMMENT
Congestive heart failure	Apical redistribution of pulmonary blood flow	Missed
	Left pleural effusion	Incorrectly attributed to CHF
	Cardiomegaly	Incorrectly noted on AP film
Pulmonary embolus	Normal	Incorrectly rules out pulmonary disease
Thoracic aortic dissection or aneurysm	Widened mediastinum	Confused with other mediastinal, nonvascular pathology
	Indistinct aortic knob	Missed
	Separation of calcification and wall	Missed
Blunt aortic injury	Wide and indistinct mediastinum	Missed or attributed to portable radiographic technique
Transvenous pacemaker	Posterior direction of distal tip on lateral view	Missed due to apparent correct placement on PA view

COMMON VARIANTS

Epicardial Fat Pads

Epicardial fat pads are frequently seen on chest radiographs. Fat pad size often depends on the weight of the patient. Although most often seen as ill-defined opacities, epicardial fat pads vary in shape and form and sometimes appear as a small, discrete, round masses. They are most commonly located at the cardiac apex, although they can occur at either the right or left side of the pericardium. These fat collections can be confused with cysts, infiltrates, and neoplasia (Fig. 18-36).

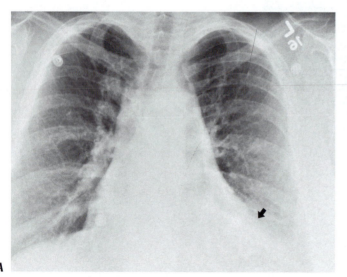

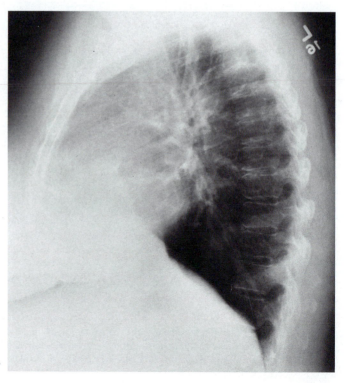

A

B

FIGURE 18-36. Epicardial fat pad. *A.* An epicardial fat pad is located at the cardiac apex. Epicardial fat pads vary in size depending on the weight of the patient and may be located on the right or left side of the pericardium. The cardiac apex is the most common location. These fat collections can be misinterpreted as cysts, infiltrates, effusions, or neoplasms. *B.* Lateral view of the epicardial fat pad.

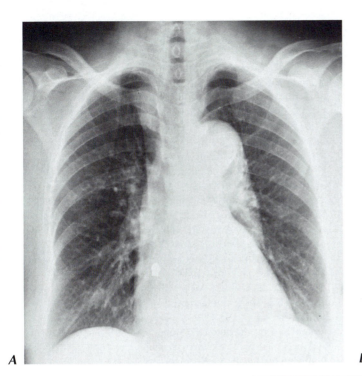

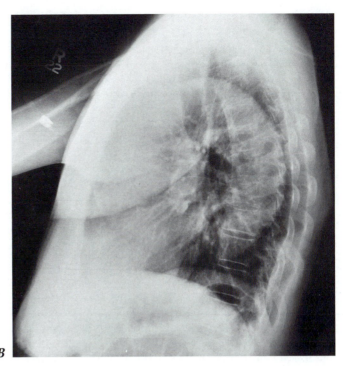

FIGURE 18-37. Tortuous aorta. *A.* A tortuous elongated and ectatic (dilated) aorta is commonly seen in older individuals. The ascending aortic arch is seen on the right side of the mediastinum, and the aortic knob is prominent. *B.* The lateral radiograph shows the elongated aorta overlying vertebral column.

Tortuous Aorta

A tortuous (elongated) and ectatic (dilated) aorta is frequently seen in older individuals. It is usually an incidental finding on chest radiography. The aorta is diffusely dilated in cross-sectional diameter and the aortic knob is prominent. The aorta is also elongated and has a larger arc of curvature in the thorax before it crosses the diaphragm. The ascending aortic segment may appear to the right of the upper right heart border. The descending aorta is prominent, displaced to the left, and visible on both the PA and lateral radiographs. If the aortic diameter is 6 cm or more at the level of the arch, the aorta is considered aneurysmal rather than simply ectatic (Fig. 18-37).

CONTROVERSIES

Few controversies exist regarding the use of the chest radiography in patients with acute cardiovascular complaints or syndromes in the ED.[48] Nevertheless, the use of the chest film in *all* patients presenting in the ED with chest discomfort is certainly questioned. The controversy related to the use of the chest radiograph in patients with cardiovascular disease regarding the proper selection and use of ancillary studies is discussed throughout this chapter (Table 18-10).

TABLE 18-10

Advanced Cardiovascular Imaging Studies

Congestive heart failure	Echocardiography
Valvular lesions	Echocardiography
Pulmonary embolism	Ventilation/perfusion scan
	Pulmonary angiography
	Lower extremity duplex
	ultrasonography
	Helical CT (contrast)
Aortic dissection	CT (contrast, helical)
	Transesophageal echocardiography
	MRI
	Aortography
	Transthoracic echocardiography
	(dissection of ascending aorta)
Traumatic aortic injury	Aortography
	CT (detects blood in mediastinum)
	Transesophageal echocardiography
Central venous line	Ultrasonography to assist line placement
Transvenous pacemaker	Fluoroscopy to assist placement

REFERENCES

1. Cardiac imaging, in Daffner RH (ed): *Clinical Radiology: The Essentials.* Baltimore: Williams & Wilkins, 1993, pp. 119–149.
2. The heart, in Squire LF, Novelline RA (eds). *Fundamentals of Radiology,* 4th ed. Cambridge, MA: Harvard University Press, 1988, pp. 128–155.
3. The normal chest, in Fraser RS, Paré JAP, Fraser RG, Paré PD (eds): *Synopsis of Diseases of the Chest,* 2d ed. Philadelphia: Saunders, 1994, pp. 1–116.
4. Juhl JH: Methods of examination, anatomy, and congenital malformations, in Juhl JH, Crummy AB (eds): *Paul and Juhl's Essentials of Radiologic Imaging,* 5th ed. Philadelphia: Lippincott, 1987, pp. 695–739.
5. Armstrong P: Chest, in Keats TE (ed): *Emergency Radiology,* 2d ed. St. Louis: Mosby–Year Book, 1989, pp. 149–212.
6. Kelley MJ, Newell JD: Chest radiography and cardiac fluoroscopy in coronary artery disease. *Cardiol Clin* 1:575, 1983.
7. Chen JT: The chest roentgenogram and cardiac fluoroscopy, in Schlant R, Alexander RS, Fuster V, et al (eds): *Hurst's The Heart,* 8th ed. New York: McGraw-Hill, 1994.
8. Chen J: The plain radiograph in the diagnosis of cardiovascular disease. *Radiol Clin North Am* 21:609, 1983.
9. Batson GA, Urquhart W, Sideris DA: Radiographic features in aortic stenosis. *Clin Radiol* 23:140, 1972.
10. Simon G: The value of radiology in critical mitral stenosis: An amendment. *Clin Radiol* 23:145, 1972.
11. Figley MM, Gerdes AJ, Ricketts HJ: Radiographic aspects of pulmonary embolism. *Semin Roentgenol* 2:389, 1967.
12. The PIOPED Investigators. The value of ventilation/perfusion scan in acute pulmonary embolism. *JAMA* 263:2753, 1990.
13. Woodard PK, Sostman HD, MacFall JR, et al: Detection of pulmonary embolism: Comparison of contrast-enhanced spiral CT and time-of-flight MR techniques. *J Thorac Imaging* 10:59, 1995.
14. Costello P: Spiral CT of the thorax. *Semin Ultrasound* 15:90, 1994.
15. Spittell PC, Spittell JA, Joyce JW, et al: Clinical features and differential diagnosis of aortic dissection: Experience with 236 cases (1980–1990). *Mayo Clin Proc* 68:642, 1993.
16. Slater EE, DeSanctis RW: The clinical recognition of dissecting aortic aneurysm. *Am J Med* 60:625, 1976.
17. Earnest F, Muhn JR, Sheedy PF: Roentgenographic findings in thoracic aortic dissection. *Mayo Clin Proc* 54:43, 1979.
18. Nienaber C, von Kodolitsch Y, Nicolas V, et al: The diagnosis of thoracic aortic dissection by noninvasive imaging procedures. *N Engl J Med* 328:1, 1993.

19. Cigarroa JE, Isselbacher EM, DeSanctis RW, Eagle KA: Diagnostic imaging in the evaluation of suspected aortic dissection: Old standards and new directions. *N Engl J Med* 328:35, 1993.
20. Wilbers CRH, Carrol CL, Hnilica MA: Optimal diagnostic imaging of aortic dissection. *Tex Heart Inst J* 17:271, 1990.
21. Shuford WH, Sybers RG, Weens HS: Problems in the aortographic diagnosis of dissecting aneurysm of the aorta. *N Engl J Med* 280:225, 1969.
22. Erbel R, Engberding R, Daniel W, et al: Echocardiography in diagnosis of aortic dissection. *Lancet* 1:457, 1989.
23. Nienaber CA, Spielmann RP, von Kodolitsch Y, et al: Diagnosis of thoracic aortic dissection: Magnetic resonance imaging versus transesophageal echocardiography. *Circulation* 85:434, 1992.
24. Mirvis SE, Bidwell JK, Buddemeyer EU, et al: Imaging diagnosis of traumatic aortic rupture: A review and experience at a major trauma center. *Invest Radiol* 22:187, 1987.
25. Mirvis SE: Traumatic disruption of the thoracic aorta: Imaging diagnosis. *Trauma Q* 4:2, 1988.
26. Richardson JD, Wilson ME, Miller FB: The widened mediastinum: Diagnostic and therapeutic priorities. *Ann Surg* 211:731, 1990.
27. Marnocha KE, Maglinte DD, Woods J, et al: Blunt chest trauma and suspected aortic rupture: Reliability of chest radiographic findings. *Ann Emerg Med* 14:644, 1985.
28. Brookes JG, Dunn RJ, Rogers IR: Sternal fractures: A retrospective analysis of 272 cases. *J Trauma* 35:46, 1993.
29. Roy-Shapira A, Levi I, Khoda J: Sternal fractures: A red flag or a red herring? *J Trauma* 37:59, 1994.
30. Hills MW, Delprado AM, Deane SA: Sternal fractures: Associated injuries and management. *J Trauma* 35:55, 1993.
31. Thompson DA, Flynn TC, Miller PW, Fischer RP: The significance of scapular fractures. *J Trauma* 25:974, 1985.
32. McGinnis M, Denton JR: Fractures of the scapula: A retrospective study of 40 fractured scapulae. *J Trauma* 29:1488, 1989.
33. Ziegler DW, Agarwal NN: The morbidity and mortality of rib fractures. *J Trauma* 37:975, 1994.
34. Dee PM: The radiology of chest trauma. *Radiol Clin North Am* 30:291, 1992.
35. DiGugliemo L, Raisaro A, Villa A, et al: Diagnostic imaging of the pericardium. *Rays* 18:164, 1993.
36. Van Gelderen WF: Stab wounds of the heart: Two new signs of pneumopericardium. *Br J Radiol* 66:794, 1993.
37. Thakur RK, Aufderheide TP, Boughner DR: Emergency echocardiographic evaluation of penetrating chest trauma. *Can J Cardiol* 10:374, 1994.

CHAPTER 19

ABDOMINAL IMAGING

MATTHEW SPATES / DAVID T. SCHWARTZ / DANIEL SAVITT

Patients with acute abdominal pain represent approximately 5% of emergency department (ED) visits.[1,2] Between 8 and 13% of ED patients with abdominal pain require surgical intervention. Although most disorders that cause acute abdominal pain have characteristic clinical presentations, the clinical presentation in many patients is atypical. It is often impossible to make a definitive clinical diagnosis based on the history and physical examination alone. The main objective in the ED is to distinguish patients with potentially serious diagnoses that merit further evaluation (inpatient observation, diagnostic imaging, or exploratory laparotomy) from those likely to have less urgent conditions that can be managed on an outpatient basis.[3]

The choice of imaging study (plain film versus CT or ultrasound) depends on the particular diagnoses being considered. Plain abdominal radiography is used selectively for patients likely to have diseases amenable to plain radiographic diagnosis—pneumoperitoneum and bowel obstruction. Because plain radiography is a simple, inexpensive, and noninvasive test, the clinician should maintain a low threshold for ordering plain films in patients who might have these conditions. Although the radiographic findings of free intraperitoneal air and intestinal obstruction are often obvious, the nuances of radiographic technique and interpretation must be fully understood in order to detect more subtle presentations.

For other ED patients—including those with suspected appendicitis, cholecystitis, and renal colic—plain films can generally be omitted and more accurate tests (e.g., CT and ultrasonography [US]) employed. When a disease that requires emergency surgical treatment such as appendicitis, is being considered, the decision to undertake a confirmatory imaging study should be made in concert with the surgeon to minimize delay in definitive treatment.

CLINICAL DECISION MAKING

The emergency physician is first concerned with identifying and excluding life-threatening illness. If the clinical diagnosis indicates a potentially lethal condition—for example, hypotension and back pain due to a leaking abdominal aortic aneurysm (AAA)—radiologic investigation should be omitted in favor of immediate intervention. In many patients, imaging studies are needed to confirm a clinical diagnosis and direct further management. However, imaging studies must be used judiciously to avoid misleading results, unnecessary expense, and delay in patient care.

Plain Abdominal Radiography

The usefulness of plain abdominal radiographs in ED patients with abdominal pain is controversial.[4–13] Several authors have derided abdominal plain films as having limited value, claiming that they provide information that is often as misleading as it is helpful. Only 7 to 15% of abdominal films obtained in adults are abnormal, and few of these abnormalities are clinically significant.[6] Similar results were found in ED patients with abdominal complaints.[5] However, in a prospective study of 96 ED patients with abdominal pain, plain radiographic abnormalities were found in 15% of cases.[8]

Even though a diagnostic yield of about 10% for abdominal radiographs could be considered "low," this yield is similar to that of other ED radiographic studies, such as those of the ankle, knee, and cervical spine (as low as 3%). However, a major shortcoming of plain abdominal radiography is that while skeletal radiographs effectively exclude most fractures, a negative abdominal radiograph does not exclude serious causes of abdominal pain.

Much of the literature on the role of abdominal radiographs is from the 1980s, when plain radiography was the mainstay of diagnostic imaging.[4–11,14–16] Today, with better imaging techniques available, plain radiography should be used only in patients for whom it will offer significant benefit, i.e., those with suspected perforation and obstruction. Radiographs are also indicated in patients who have ingested or inserted into the rectum a radiopaque foreign body (Table 19-1). Occasionally, abdominal plain films have findings suggesting appendicitis, urolithiasis, gallstones, bowel ischemia or infarction, emphysematous cholecystitis, calcified AAA, and abdominal masses. Nonetheless, CT and US are more accurate and should be used instead of plain films in patients suspected of having these illnesses if they require diagnostic imaging.

In older patients, plain abdominal radiographs should be ordered more liberally because of the higher incidence of surgical disease. In addition, the elderly often have atypical signs and symptoms of perforation and obstruction.[17–19] Among 127 patients older than 65 years presenting to an ED, 12% were found to have small bowel obstruction and 7% had pneumoperitoneum. In all but one case, pneumoperitoneum was unsuspected prior to radiologic study.[17]

In children, suggested high-yield criteria for plain abdominal radiographs include prior abdominal surgery, abnormal bowel sounds, abdominal distention, peritoneal signs, and a history of foreign-body ingestion.[20] The presence of any one of

TABLE 19-1

Indications for Abdominal Radiography

Perforation (upright chest radiograph)
Small bowel obstruction
Large bowel obstruction, including volvulus
Radiopaque foreign bodies

Appendicitis (controversial)
Ureterolithiasis (controversial)
Cholelithiasis (controversial)
Pneumobilia (biliary-enteric fistula or
    emphysematous cholecystitis)
Bowel infarction (intramural air)
Soft tissue masses and abscesses (massive)

these clinical variables has 93% sensitivity in uncovering a potential surgical condition. Serious diseases to consider in infants include pyloric stenosis, midgut volvulus, and intussusception. Although these disorders occasionally have suggestive plain radiographic findings, confirmatory imaging is usually needed (e.g., an enteric contrast study or US) (see Chap. 22, "Pediatric Considerations").

Computed Tomography

The diagnostic accuracy of CT makes it a useful test in many ED patients with abdominal pain (Table 19-2).[21] Despite this, CT should not be used indiscriminately. As always, one must determine the best diagnostic testing strategy for the specific diseases under consideration. If a disorder that might require emergency surgery is being considered, the surgeon should be consulted when ordering a CT scan so as to avoid delaying patient care. Finally, the capacity of CT to exclude serious illness is questionable. For example, appendicitis is not excluded unless a normal appendix is visualized. CT cannot reliably exclude bowel ischemia or incomplete small bowel obstruction.

TABLE 19-2

Indications for Abdominopelvic CT

Appendicitis
Diverticulitis
Abdominal aortic aneurysm
Blunt abdominal trauma (solid viscus injury)
Ureterolithiasis (noncontrast helical CT)
Pancreatitis and complications (pseudocyst)
Ischemic bowel (limited sensitivity)
Inflammatory bowel disease
Perforation (negative or equivocal plain radiographs)
Small bowel obstruction (negative or equivocal plain radiographs)
Intraabdominal and retroperitoneal masses, abscesses, fluid (ascites)
Ovarian or uterine masses or abscesses

Patients suspected of having these diagnoses may warrant inpatient observation or laparotomy despite a negative CT scan.

The overall role of CT in ED patients with abdominal pain is not precisely defined. However, the impact of CT on patients with certain specific diagnoses such as appendicitis has been investigated. CT lowers the negative laparotomy rate in patients with suspected appendicitis.[22] Historically, a negative laparotomy rate of about 20% has been accepted. In this study, CT was used in patients with an uncertain diagnosis of appendicitis (about 55% of cases), and the negative laparotomy rate was reduced to 4%. The question of exactly which patients suspected of having appendicitis should undergo CT was not addressed.

In another series, CT was performed on *all* patients with suspected appendicitis, and an overall improvement in patient care and cost savings was achieved.[23] CT was helpful in expediting laparotomy or in discharging patients from the hospital when appendicitis was excluded. However, these were all patients who had been selected by the surgical consultant to require laparotomy or inpatient observation. Therefore, this result cannot be directly applied to a less selected group of ED patients. In addition, this study used a special CT protocol limited to the diagnosis of appendicitis (rectal contrast taking only 15 min to administer, with no intravenous or oral contrast). Nevertheless, both of these studies support the liberal use of CT when appendicitis is suspected but there is some clinical uncertainty.

Ultrasonography

Ultrasonography is an important diagnostic test in ED patients with suspected acute cholecystitis, renal colic, abdominal aortic aneurysm, appendicitis, ectopic pregnancy, or other gynecologic disorders. (Table 19-3).[24] Limited bedside US performed by a trained emergency physician is useful in certain

TABLE 19-3

Indications for Abdominal Ultrasonography

Cholelithiasis
    Acute cholecystitis
    Choledocholithiasis
Gynecologic conditions
    Ovarian cyst
    Ovarian torsion (requires Doppler)
    Tuboovarian abscess
Obstetric conditions
    Ectopic pregnancy
    Intrauterine gestation
    Placenta previa
    Placental abruption
Abdominal aortic aneurysm
Renal colic or hydronephrosis
Acute appendicitis (graded-compression technique)
Ascites
Hepatic lesions (tumor, abscesses)

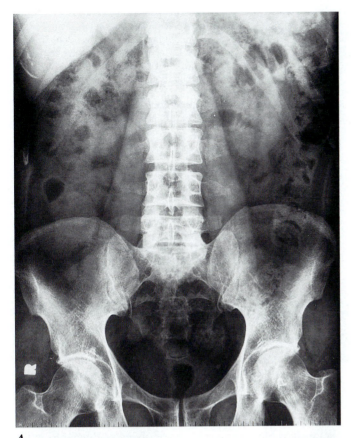

A

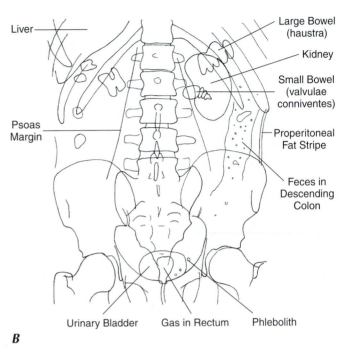

B

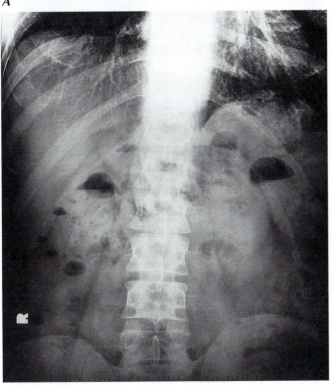

C

FIGURE 19-1. Normal supine and upright abdominal radiographs. *A.* The supine radiograph shows a small amount of air in the small bowel, colon, and rectum. The liver, left kidney, and psoas margins are seen. *C.* The upright radiograph shows a few scattered air-fluid levels and the domes of the diaphragm.

specific applications. These include the identification of gallstones, intrauterine gestation in early pregnancy, AAA, hydronephrosis in suspected renal colic, and ascites. Victims of blunt abdominal trauma are also amenable to sonographic investigation to detect hemoperitoneum or pericardial effusion. Comprehensive US performed in the radiology department can further identify biliary tract disease, appendicitis (special graded-compression technique), ovarian and uterine pathology (including ovarian torsion with the use of Doppler US), pancreatitis, and liver lesions (see Chap. 21, "Ultrasonography").

RADIOGRAPHIC TECHNIQUE

In the evaluation of patients with abdominal pain, three radiographic views are generally obtained: supine and upright abdominal films and an upright chest film (Fig. 19-1). To some extent, the selection of films depends on the suspected diagnoses. The upright abdominal film is used to detect air-fluid levels within the bowel to assist in the diagnosis of mechanical small bowel obstruction. The chest film is indicated to look for pneumoperitoneum and other intrathoracic disorders. If the patient is too ill to obtain an adequate upright chest or ab-

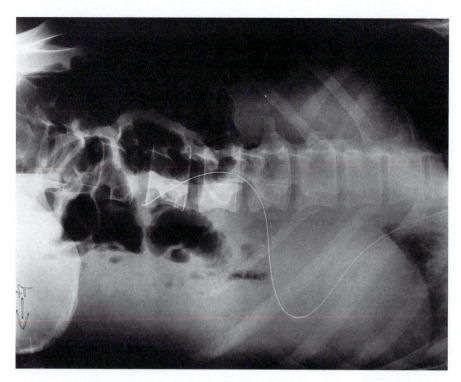

FIGURE 19-2. The left lateral decubitus abdominal radiograph. An AP abdominal radiograph is taken with the patient lying on the left lateral side. The radiograph is exposed with adequate penetration to show the intraabdominal organs. An underpenetrated exposure is needed to demonstrate free intraperitoneal air along the right (upper) side of the abdomen.

allow equilibration of intestinal contents and the development of air-fluid levels.

Chest Radiograph

The chest radiograph should be obtained with the patient in an upright position, using a horizontal x-ray beam. This is necessary to detect free air under the diaphragm. If the patient is seriously ill, a supine or partially upright anteroposterior (AP) chest radiograph is obtained. In this case, a left lateral decubitus radiograph should be added to the series, if pneumoperitoneum is a diagnostic concern. The addition of a lateral chest film increases the yield of plain radiography in the diagnosis of pneumoperitoneum. Finally, the chest radiograph is useful because some patients with acute abdominal pain have intrathoracic disorders such as pneumonia or a pleural effusion.

Left Lateral Decubitus Abdominal Radiograph

The left lateral decubitus abdominal view is helpful in patients unable to stand for an upright abdominal or chest film (Fig. 19-2). It is an AP abdominal radiograph in which the patient is positioned by lying on his or her left side for several minutes. A horizontal x-ray beam is directed at the midabdomen. The side on which the patient lies is the *decubitus* side.

The lateral decubitus radiograph is performed with the left side down, because the liver edge provides excellent contrast for detecting free intraperitoneal air. To see free air, the radiograph should be *underpenetrated* ("chest technique"). Lateral decubitus films performed with standard penetration ("abdominal technique") are used to detect air-fluid levels in patients with suspected small bowel obstruction. The technician should be alerted prior to obtaining the radiograph.

RADIOGRAPHIC ANATOMY

The radiographs in an abdominal series should extend from the diaphragm to the pubic rami and include both lateral abdominal walls (Fig. 19-1). The radiographs show the lower ribs, liver, kidneys, and psoas muscles as well as portions of the gastrointestinal (GI) tract from the esophagogastric junction to the

dominal radiograph, a left lateral decubitus film should be obtained to look for air-fluid levels and signs of pneumoperitoneum.

Depending on the circumstances, not all three films are necessary to evaluate the abdomen. For example, if radiographs are being obtained to detect an ingested radiopaque foreign body or to follow a known ureteral calculus, the supine abdominal radiograph is sufficient. Whether an upright abdominal film is always needed in the diagnosis of a bowel obstruction is debatable.[25,26] In many instances, the findings of bowel obstruction are clear on the supine film. In these cases, an upright film is needed only to clarify questionable findings. However, the difficulty of interpreting radiographic signs of obstruction and the logistics of returning the patient to the radiology suite for additional films make this approach impractical.

Supine Abdominal Radiograph

The supine abdominal radiograph is obtained with a vertical beam directed at the center of a cassette positioned beneath the patient. It should include the entire abdomen between the diaphragm and symphysis pubis as well as the lateral abdominal walls.

Upright Abdominal Radiograph

The upright abdominal film is obtained with a horizontal beam directed at the midabdomen of a standing patient. Upright films are ideally obtained after the patient stands for 5 to 10 min to rectum. Skeletal structures that are seen include the lower ribs, the lumbar and lower thoracic vertebrae, and the pelvis.

Bowel Gas

Stomach and Duodenum. Most bowel gas is from swallowed air, with a small contribution from bacterial fermentation of fecal matter. Normally, there is gas in the stomach and colon and a minimal amount in the small intestine. The stomach lies in the left upper quadrant and is characterized by irregular-appearing rugae along the greater curvature. The mucosal folds of the lesser curvature are more uniform and longitudinally oriented. The stomach has a J-shaped appearance in a tall, thin patient; it has a more horizontal location in an obese patient. The stomach is a mobile structure that is fixed proximally to the esophagus. The distal pyloric region of the stomach has limited mobility because the duodenum is attached to the posterior abdominal wall. On the upright radiograph, there is usually a distinct air-fluid level in the stomach.

Small Bowel. The small bowel occupies a central position in the abdomen. It is characterized by numerous mucosal folds called *valvulae conniventes* (or *plicae circulares*) that circumferentially indent the intestinal wall and cross the entire lumen (Fig. 19-3*A*). The valvulae conniventes are most prominent in the jejunum and taper in the ileum, so that the terminal ileum has a smooth appearance. Small pockets of air in nondistended bowel have a nondescript round appearance. The small bowel is pliable and can fold back on itself, giving it a "bent finger" appearance (Table 19-4).

Large Bowel. The large bowel is mostly located peripherally and has transverse indentations or *haustra* that do not extend completely across the bowel lumen (Fig. 19-3*B*). The ascending and descending portions of the colon are attached to the posterior abdominal wall. The transverse and sigmoid colon are mobile within the peritoneum and often have a more central location. When the patient is supine, gas tends to collect in the transverse colon because of its anterior location. The colon normally contains fecal matter, which has a stippled radiographic appearance.

TABLE 19-4

Radiographic Appearance of the Bowel

Small bowel
   Valvulae conniventes (plicae circularis)
   Central location
   Pliability ("bent finger" appearance)
Large bowel
   Haustra
   Peripheral location (except transverse and sigmoid colon)
   Stippled appearance of fecal material

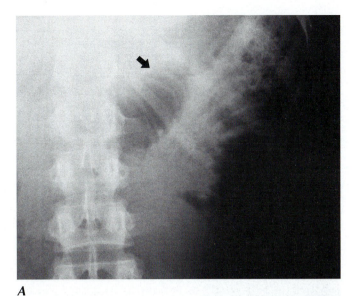

A

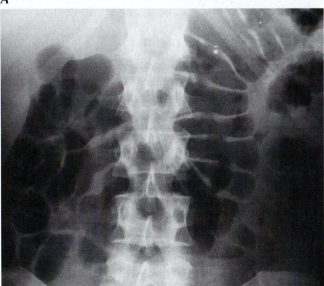

B

FIGURE 19-3. Small bowel and colon. *A.* Mildly dilated small bowel is present left of the midline with several thin valvulae conniventes that traverse the entire diameter of the bowel. *B.* Gas in normal transverse colon showing haustra and sacculations.

Solid Organs and Retroperitoneum

Solid organs are seen on abdominal radiographs because surrounding fat or adjacent gas-filled structures delineate their margins (Fig. 19-1). The inferior hepatic margin is contrasted by bowel gas. The spleen tip is also occasionally visible. The *properitoneal fat stripe,* or flank stripe, is a region of hypodensity located between the lateral abdominal wall and the ascending and descending colon.

   The *retroperitoneum* contains three major compartments—the perirenal spaces and the anterior and posterior pararenal spaces. A retroperitoneal inflammatory process can obscure the properitoneal fat stripe or psoas margin. The kidneys are frequently outlined by the surrounding fat. The kidneys normally span a distance of three to four lumbar vertebrae; the right kid-

TABLE 19-5

Systematic Analysis of Abdominal Radiographs

Adequacy	Three views—supine, upright (or left lateral decubitus), upright chest Entire abdomen seen (pelvis to diaphragm)
Free air	Upright chest film—free air under diaphragm Left lateral decubitus abdominal film Supine abdominal film—massive free air
Bowel gas	Bowel gas pattern—normal, ileus, or obstruction Assess mucosal pattern, location and distention Air-fluid levels on upright film
Other gas collections	Pneumobilia, intramural gas, hepatic portal venous gas Abscesses, retroperitoneal gas
Soft tissues	Solid organs—liver, spleen, kidneys, bladder Psoas margins, properitoneal fat stripe Masses—tumors, abscesses, fluid-filled gut Diaphragm and lungs
Bones and calcifications	Ribs, spine, pelvis, hips Gallstones, urinary stones, pancreas, mesenteric lymph nodes Phleboliths, aorta and major branch arteries (splenic iliac, renal) Tumor calcification, granuloma (hepatic, splenic)
Foreign bodies	Radiopaque (metallic) Radiolucent

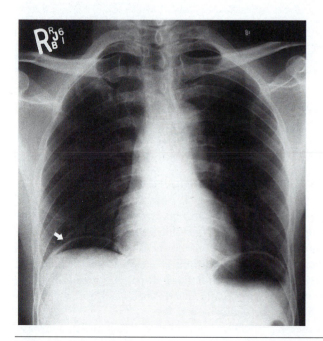

FIGURE 19-4. Pneumoperitoneum. There is obvious free air beneath the right hemidiaphragm and above the superior surface of the liver *(arrow)*. On the left, a large amount of air in the distended stomach mimics the appearance of a pneumoperitoneum.

ney is located a few centimeters inferior to the left kidney. The pancreas is not seen on abdominal radiographs unless it is calcified.

RADIOGRAPHIC ANALYSIS

Interpretation is first directed at identifying a potentially fatal abnormality. A *targeted approach* involves looking for clinically suspected pathologic processes (e.g., free air under the diaphragm, bowel obstruction). A *systematic approach* analyzes the radiograph methodically, sequentially examining gas, soft tissues, and calcified structures (Table 19-5). The evaluation of gas begins with a search for pneumoperitoneum. Next, the bowel gas pattern is evaluated, identifying either a normal, ileus or obstructive pattern. Other pathological sites of gas—such as the biliary system, liver, bowel wall, abscesses, and retroperitoneum—are then sought. Next, soft tissue contours are examined, calcifications identified, and bones inspected. Finally, a search for radiopaque foreign bodies is conducted.

Search for Free Intraperitoneal Air

A systematic evaluation begins with a search for free air under the diaphragm on the upright chest radiograph (Fig. 19-4).[27,28] On the supine abdominal radiograph, massive amounts of free air will outline both sides of the bowel wall. On a left lateral decubitus film, free air is seen between the lateral hepatic margin and right abdominal wall and along the left iliac wing. A "bright light" is needed to examine this area of the film if the radiograph is dark (overpenetrated using "abdominal technique").

Interpretation of Bowel Gas Pattern

The lumen of the bowel normally contains fluid and gas. Intraluminal gas is readily seen on plain abdominal radiographs, whereas intraluminal fluid is not distinguishable from other abdominal soft tissues.

There are six different bowel gas patterns: normal, nonspecific, mild or localized ileus, adynamic ileus, mechanical small bowel obstruction, and mechanical large bowel obstruction.[28] Although a fully developed mechanical small bowel obstruction is usually obvious, in many other cases the interpretation of the radiograph is less certain. The interpretation of bowel gas patterns is subject to considerable interobserver variability.[29,30] In addition, there are often discrepancies between the radiographic findings and clinical diagnosis. For example, a patient with a mechanical small bowel obstruction can have a normal, nonspecific, or mild ileus pattern.

Normal and Nonspecific Bowel Gas Pattern.   In a "normal" abdominal radiograph, gas is seen in the stomach and colon. In the colon, gas is mixed with fecal matter and has a stippled appearance. The small bowel normally contains little or no gas and only a few small, isolated pockets of air.

In the "nonspecific bowel gas pattern," more air has accumulated in the small bowel, although the loops of small bowel are not dilated (<3 cm in diameter) (Fig. 19-1). This gas accumulation is due to mildly disordered intestinal motility. The clinical significance of a nonspecific bowel gas pattern is uncertain and the term has limited usefulness. Some radiologists use the term *nonspecific pattern* when there are a small number of borderline dilated small bowel loops—i.e., a mild ileus. Because this term lacks a clear definition and is of questionable clinical significance, some authors suggest that the term *nonspecific bowel gas pattern* be abandoned.[31,32] Nonetheless, the term is commonly used.

Adynamic Ileus.   In a mild adynamic ileus, intestinal motility is further deranged by an intraabdominal or systemic pathologic process. More fluid and gas accumulates in the small bowel, and one or more loops of small bowel become dilated (>3 cm diameter). In patients with a focal intraabdominal inflammatory process, one loop of bowel may become significantly dilated. This is called a *sentinel loop* or *localized ileus*. The location of the sentinel loop may provide a clue to the nature of the inflammatory process, although this finding is of limited diagnostic accuracy. A sentinel loop in the right lower quadrant *suggests* appendicitis, a sentinel loop in the right upper quadrant *suggests* cholecystitis, and a sentinel loop in the mid-epigastrium *suggests* pancreatitis.

In a fully developed adynamic ileus, intestinal motility is severely deranged and there are multiple loops of dilated bowel containing air and fluid (Fig. 19-5). The upright abdominal film often has several small air-fluid levels. Although clearly pathologic, an adynamic ileus is nonspecific and is seen in such diverse conditions as appendicitis, renal colic, vertebral fractures, pneumonia, and hypokalemia. When the entire small and large bowel is involved, the pattern is sometimes called intestinal *pseudoobstruction* because it is indistinguishable from a distal large bowel obstruction. It is common in debilitated, bed-bound patients.

Mechanical Bowel Obstruction.   In a mechanical bowel obstruction, although there are dilated loops of bowel, the dilatation is present only proximal to the point of obstruction (Fig. 19-6).[28] When obstruction is fully developed, bowel distal to the obstruction collapses and appears gasless. Frequently, the distal bowel is not yet completely devoid of air, although it has a relatively smaller amount of intraluminal gas. When distal bowel gas is present, the radiographic pattern is referred to as an "incomplete small bowel obstruction." This pattern also occurs early after the onset of a complete obstruction. Thus, an incomplete small bowel obstruction can be difficult to distinguish radio-graphically from adynamic ileus.

In a mechanical small bowel obstruction, the upright radiograph shows air-fluid levels that have a different appearance

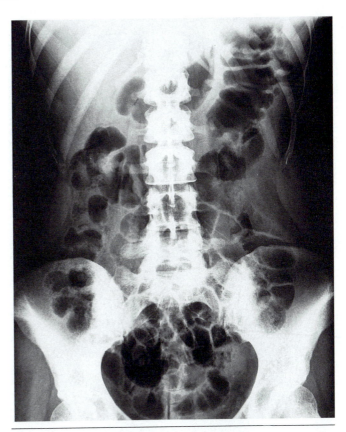

FIGURE 19-5.   Adynamic ileus. A large amount of air is present throughout the stomach, small bowel, colon and rectum. The bowel is mildly distended. Although abnormal, this pattern is seen in a wide variety of pathologic processes.

from those seen in adynamic ileus. The air-fluid levels are usually broader and often have an inverted-U shape. With a *differential air-fluid level,* the air-fluid interface is at two differing levels within an inverted U–shaped loop of bowel. The degree to which these two levels are separated increases the specificity of air-fluid levels for mechanical bowel obstruction.

Other Abnormal Gas Collections

In unusual cases, gas may collect within the hepatobiliary system, bowel wall, or intraabdominal abscesses.[27]

Pneumobilia.   *Pneumobilia* (gas within the biliary tract) is due either to a fistulous connection to the intestines or an infection of the biliary tract with gas-forming organisms (emphysematous cholecystitis). Biliary-enteric fistulas form in patients with chronic gallbladder inflammation. Branching tubular air is seen centrally within the main bile ducts. Occasionally, air is seen in the gallbladder, although the gallbladder is usually collapsed. If a large gallstone has passed through the fistula into the intestines, it can obstruct the intestines, usually at the ileocecal valve. This results in a type of mechanical small bowel obstruction known as *gallstone ileus.* Surgical procedures are the most common cause of pneumobilia, (e.g., choledochojejunostomy or endoscopic papillotomy) (Fig. 19-7).

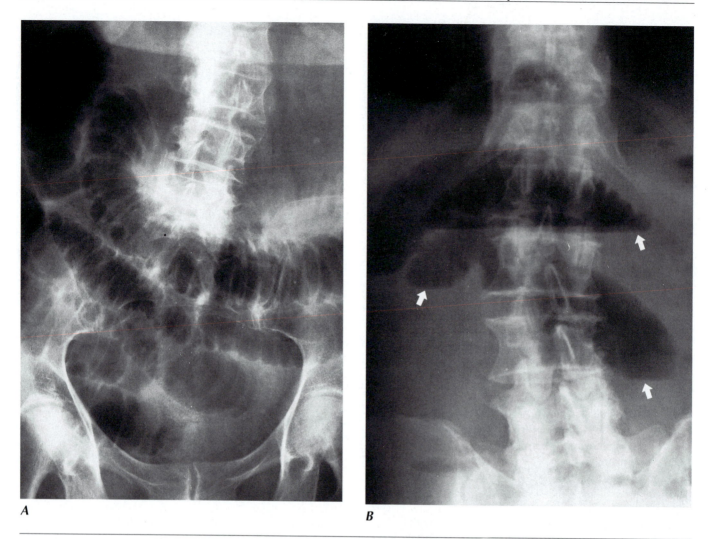

A   *B*

FIGURE 19-6.   Mechanical bowel obstruction involving the distal small bowel. There are moderately distended loops of small bowel and an absence of gas in the large bowel. On the upright radiograph (*B*), distinct air-fluid levels are seen (*arrows*). The absence of gas in the large bowel is evident.

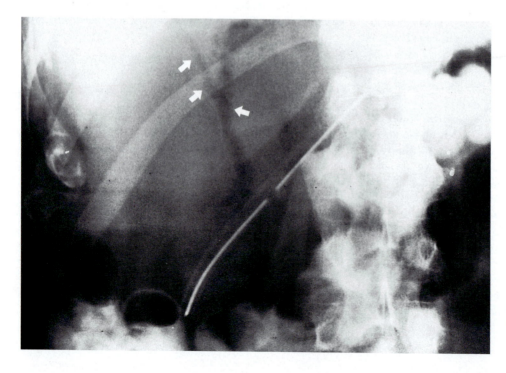

FIGURE 19-7.   Pneumobilia in a patient who had previously had an endoscopic papillotomy. (Copyright David T. Schwartz, M.D.)

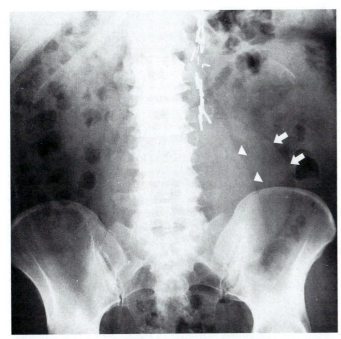

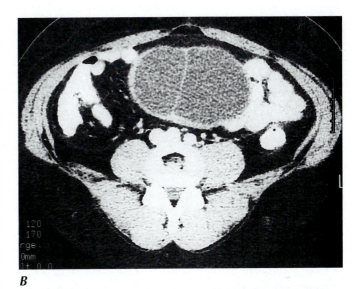

B

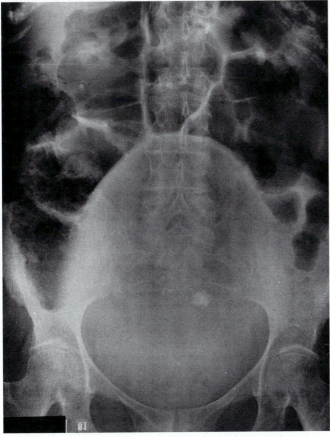

A

C

FIGURE 19-8. A large soft tissue mass is present in the left lower abdomen (*A*) *(arrows)*. Surgical clips are from a prior operation. The mass is intraabdominal rather than retroperitoneal, so the psoas shadow is preserved *(arrowheads)*. On CT, a large cystic ovarian neoplasm is seen (*B*). *C*. A large lower abdominal mass is a distended urinary bladder in a woman taking anticholinergic medication. (Copyright David T. Schwartz, M.D.)

Emphysematous cholecystitis due to infection with gas-forming organisms, complicates 1% of cases of acute cholecystitis, usually in elderly diabetic patients. Gas appears within a distended gallbladder. There is often an air-fluid level on the upright film. Curvilinear streaks of air may be seen within the gallbladder wall.

Intramural Gas. Microperforation and infection can allow gas to enter the wall of severely ischemic or infarcted bowel. *Intramural gas* appears as streaky curvilinear lucencies following the contour of the bowel. This is seen in only 5% of patients with mesenteric ischemia, although it is more frequently apparent on CT. The gas may enter the portal veins and migrate to the liver. *Hepatic portal venous gas* is rarely seen on plain film. It appears as fine, branching linear lucencies within the liver.

A benign form of intramural gas is *pneumatosis cystoides intestinalis.* This often idiopathic condition produces bubbly or occasionally curvilinear streaks within the bowel wall. Some cases are associated with air dissecting from a pneumomediastinum or appearing after colonoscopy.[33]

Abscesses. Gas collections within an intraabdominal abscess are occasionally large enough to see on plain radiographs. Examples include periappendiceal or diverticular abscesses, as well as intrahepatic or subdiaphragmatic abscesses.

Retroperitoneum. Gas may dissect into the retroperitoneum either from a posterior penetrating duodenal ulcer, a traumatic duodenal laceration or from a pneumomediastinum. Retroperitoneal gas appears as streaks that outline the retroperitoneal organs, such as the kidneys. Retroperitoneal gas does not move with changes in patient positioning—i.e., on an upright or lateral decubitus radiograph.

Solid Organ Abnormalities

Solid organ enlargement or a solid mass can displace intraabdominal structures from their normal location (Fig. 19-8). Obscured margins of the *properitoneal fat line* or the *psoas mus-*

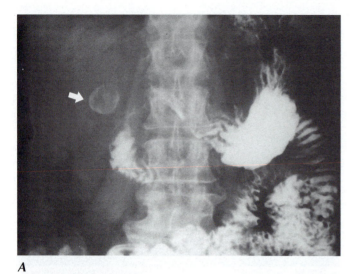

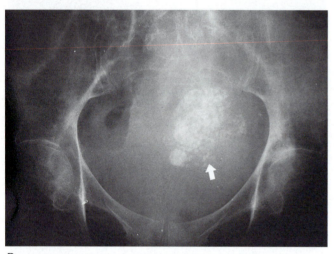

FIGURE 19-9. *A.* A large calcified renal artery aneurysm is seen on the right. Calcification of the wall of the aneurysm gives it a shell-like appearance. This finding was initially misinterpreted as a gallstone. Enteric contrast material is in the stomach and small bowel. *B.* A calcified uterine fibroid (leiomyoma) has a stippled solid pattern of calcification.

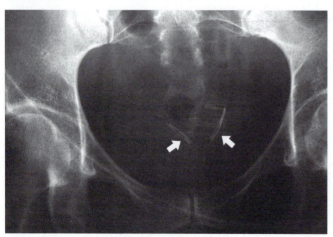

FIGURE 19-10.　Razor blades inserted into the vagina in an attempt to smuggle them into a prison facility.

cles suggest an adjacent intraabdominal inflammatory process or fluid collection.

Calcifications

Calcifications are frequently seen on abdominal radiographs, yet only occasionally are responsible for acute pathology. Calcified structures appear solid, lamellated (layered with a lucent center), cystic, or tubular. Calcifications take a long time to develop, and many are clinically insignificant (Fig. 19-9). Nonetheless, calcifications can be responsible for acute abdominal pain if they suddenly obstruct a hollow viscus such as the ureter, biliary tree, or appendix. Although ureteral stones are calcified in 85% of cases, they are usually small and cannot be reliably identified. Furthermore, the finding of a calcification such as a gallstone does not imply that it is responsible for the patient's symptoms. There must be a compatible clinical presentation or confirmation by a more definitive imaging study.

Chronic pathologic processes such as splenic infarcts, chronic cholecystitis, and chronic pancreatitis can create calcifications. *Phleboliths* are calcium deposits within organized venous thrombi in the pelvis. They are rounded with a central lucency, whereas ureteral stones are typically solid and irregular. Uterine fibroid tumors, mesenteric lymph nodes, and arteries in elderly patients with atherosclerosis are also frequently calcified. Caicified aneurysms have a cystic or fusiform appearance. Hepatic calcifications occur with a primary or metastatic malignancy, a cavernous hemangioma or abscess. Echinococcal cysts, though rare in North America, are the most common cause of hepatic calcifications worldwide.

Metallic Objects

Metallic objects are readily seen on plain radiographs. These may be overlying extraneous objects, surgical clips, and material that has either been ingested or inserted into the rectum or vagina (Fig. 19-10).

COMPUTED TOMOGRAPHY

Radiographic Technique

Standard abdominopelvic CT uses 10-mm thick slices. Thinner slices are obtained in certain circumstances such as suspected appendicitis, for which 5-mm thick slices are taken through the region of appendix. The scan extends from the top of the diaphragm to the lower pelvis and rectum. Helical CT technology improves anatomic resolution and the alignment between CT slices.

Oral and intravenous contrast materials are administered for a standard abdominal CT. Oral contrast is given in small aliquots over a 2 hour period in order to opacify the entire bowel lumen. This is the optimal protocol for the diagnosis of ap-

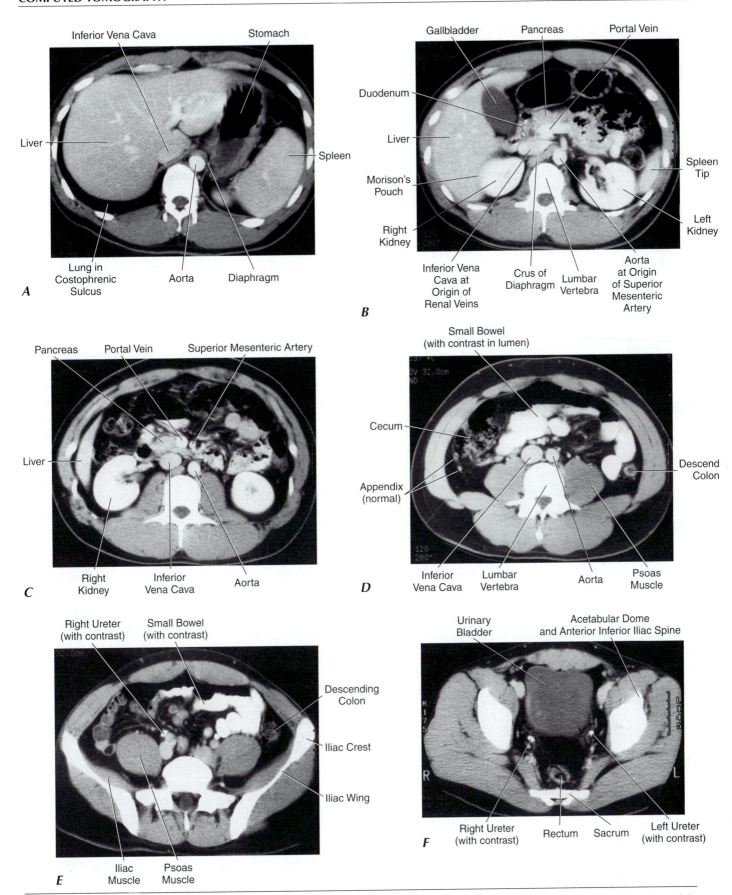

FIGURE 19-11. Normal abdominopelvic CT scan of a 26-year-old man. Both oral and intravenous contrast was administered. *A.* Liver (right and left lobes), tomach, and spleen. *B.* Liver, gallbladder, kidneys, and pancreas. *C.* Kidneys, pancreas, and intestines. *D.* Small bowel, cecum, descending colon, and normal appendix. *E.* Intestines and ureters at level of iliac wings. *F.* Bladder, distal ureters, and rectum at the level of the acetabular domes.

pendicitis or diverticulitis. In patients with blunt abdominal trauma or suspected small bowel obstruction, a shorter period of oral contrast administration can be used (30 to 60 min). Intravenous contrast is delivered rapidly by a power injector, and the scan is performed immediately after the contrast bolus. Rapid scanning augments the enhancement of major arterial structures and is known as *dynamic CT scanning.*

In certain circumstances, a noncontrast CT is performed. For example, a ureteral calculus would be obscured by contrast within the ureter. If the patient has a contraindication to intravenous contrast (allergy, severe asthma; or renal insufficiency) or cannot tolerate oral contrast because of uncontrolled vomiting, a noncontrast CT, even though suboptimal, will often yield adequate information. If the patient is potentially unstable and cannot wait for complete enteric contrast administration or verification of renal function before receiving intravenous contrast, a rapid noncontrast study can be performed as long as the patient can be adequately monitored. This is the case in a stable patient with severe blunt abdominal trauma or a patient with a gradually leaking but "stable" AAA.

Cross-Sectional Anatomy

The upper CT slices show the stomach, liver, spleen, gallbladder, and aorta, while the midabdominal slices show the intestines, kidneys, pancreas, and aorta. The bowel lumen contains air, enteric fluid, and oral contrast material. The lower slices show the pelvis, bladder, rectosigmoid colon, and, in females, the uterus. Many structures are seen in several contiguous slices, so that interpretation of a CT requires comparison of adjacent images (Fig. 19-11).

Enteric contrast opacifies the bowel lumen. This helps to distinguish bowel from other soft tissue structures such as intraperitoneal fluid collections, enlarged lymph nodes, and abscesses.

Intravenous contrast enhances the liver, spleen, kidneys, and urinary tract, the bowel wall, and the lumen of major blood vessels. Intravenous contrast is needed to distinguish solid organ parenchyma from intraparenchymal tumors, hematomas, and infarctions. Bowel wall abnormalities are also best seen on contrast CT.

COMMON ABNORMALITIES

1. Perforation
2. Small bowel obstruction
3. Large bowel obstruction
4. Volvulus
5. Gastric outlet obstruction
6. Appendicitis
7. Diverticulitis
8. Inflammatory bowel disease
9. Bowel ischemia
10. AIDS
11. Cholecystitis
12. Choledocholithiasis
13. Pancreatitis
14. Renal colic
15. Abdominal aortic aneurysm
16. Gynecologic emergencies
17. Abscesses, cysts, and masses
18. Ascites
19. Foreign body ingestion
20. Esophageal abnormalities
21. Gastrointestinal hemorrhage
22. Abdominal trauma

Perforation

The upright chest radiograph is the diagnostic imaging study of choice for pneumoperitoneum (Figs. 19-4 and 19-12).[27,28] Free intraperitoneal air is more reliably identified beneath the right hemidiaphragm. On the left side, free air is often difficult to distinguish from gas in the stomach. The upright chest film can detect as little as 1 to 2 mL of intraperitoneal air provided that the patient is able to remain upright for at least 5 min.[34–36] Occasionally, when the air fails to migrate to the most superior part of the diaphragmatic dome, free air is seen only on the lateral chest radiograph.[37,38] Subdiaphragmatic air is not usually visible on an upright abdominal radiograph because the diaphragm is overpenetrated and the x-ray beam is not horizontal in that region of the film.

In 90% of cases, perforation with pneumoperitoneum is due to peptic ulcer disease. Most of the remaining 10% of cases represent cecal perforation due to large bowel obstruction. These two etiologies can often be distinguished from one another by abdominal radiography. Perforation of a peptic ulcer usually shows a normal (small) amount of bowel gas on the abdominal radiograph, whereas cecal perforation is generally accompanied by considerable air-filled, distended bowel owing to an antecedent intestinal obstruction. However, when an ileus develops after peptic ulcer perforation, distended loops of air-filled bowel are also seen.

Perforation of appendicitis or diverticulitis is usually contained within an inflammatory mass and does not cause free intraperitoneal air. Free intraperitoneal air can also be caused by trauma (hollow viscus injury or peritoneal lavage). Rare benign causes of pneumoperitoneum include rupture of blebs from pneumatosis intestinalis, entry of air through the uterus, and dissection from a pneumothorax or pneumomediastinum.[39] Pneumoperitoneum due to surgical procedures or diagnostic studies can persist for up to 4 weeks.[40]

A left lateral decubitus view of the abdomen should be obtained if the patient is too ill to maintain an upright posture for a chest radiograph. Intraperitoneal air migrates to a position between the right hemidiaphragm and the superior hepatic margin. A lucent air collection is seen between the right lateral hepatic margin and the diaphragm (Fig. 19-13). Free air may also be seen in the right iliac fossa. In addition, the left lateral decubitus view aids detection of pneumoperitoneum from a posterior perforation of a peptic ulcer because free air in the lesser

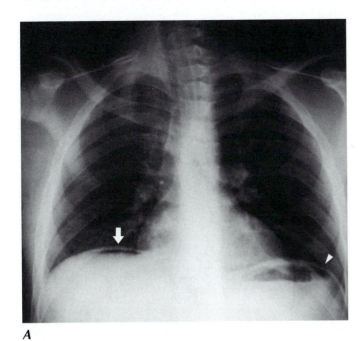

A

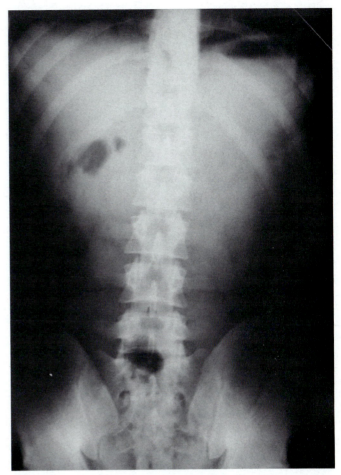

FIGURE 19-12. A small amount of free intraperitoneal air is seen under the right hemidiaphragm *(arrow)*. Free air may also be present on the left, just lateral to the stomach bubble *(arrowhead)*. On the upright abdominal radiograph *(B)*, free air beneath the diaphragm is difficult to see because this area of the film is overpenetrated and the diaphragm lies at the edge of the film, so the x-ray beam is not horizontal.

B

sac can migrate through the foramen of Winslow into the peritoneal cavity.

A technique to improve visualization of a small pneumoperitoneum on a chest radiograph is to have the patient lie in a left lateral decubitus position for about 10 min. Then, the

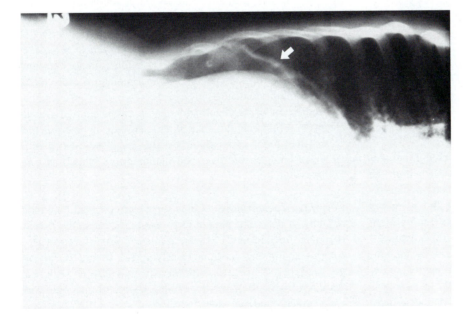

upright chest film is repeated. In this way, the amount of air under the right hemidiaphragm is maximized.[34]

An additional method to improve detection of peptic ulcer perforation is insufflation of about 300 mL of air through a nasogastric tube, followed by repeat chest radiography. This *pneumogastrogram* is helpful when a small quantity of free air is questionably present under the diaphragm on an initial upright chest radiograph.[41,42]

Pneumoperitoneum can be detected on a supine abdominal film if a large amount of free air is present. Air outlining the mucosal and serosal surfaces of the bowel wall is referred to as the *double-wall sign* (Fig. 19-14). Extraluminal air appears as a triangular area of lucency surrounded by the serosal surfaces of three loops of bowel. In the *lucent liver*

FIGURE 19-13. A left lateral decubitus radiograph demonstrating free air between the right hepatic margin, the diaphragm, and the lateral peritoneum. The film is underpenetrated, so the abdominal contents appear white. The patient was too ill to assume an upright position for a chest radiograph. (Copyright David T. Schwartz, MD)

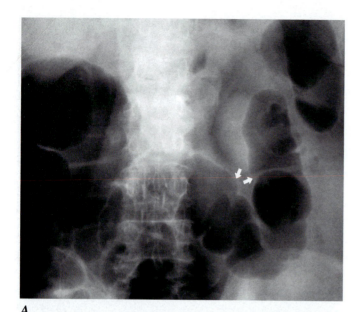

A

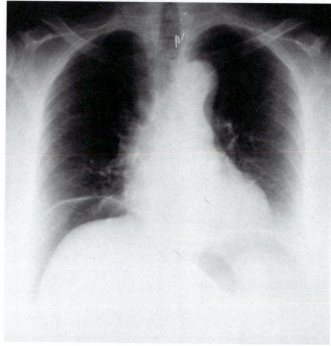

B

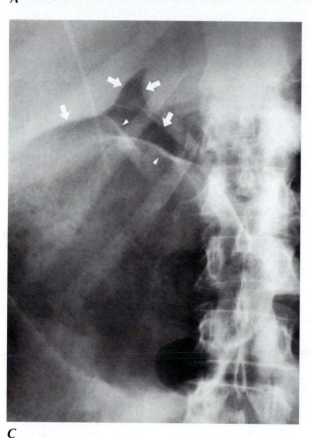

C

FIGURE 19-14. A large pneumoperitoneum in a 68-year-old woman who had been on an extended course of steroids for a rheumatologic condition. On the supine abdominal radiograph, pneumoperitoneum is evident because the air outlines both sides of the bowel wall *(arrows)*. This is known as the *Rigler's sign.* The upright chest radiograph (*B*) demonstrates a large amount of free air beneath the diaphragm. *C.* Another patient with a perforated cecal volvulus showing the *double-bowel-wall sign (arrowheads).* Air outlines the inferior margin of the liver. There is an indentation of the liver margin between the left and right hepatic lobes, producing a triangular appearance—the *doge's cap sign (arrows).* (*C.* Copyright David T. Schwartz, M.D.)

sign, a single, rounded gas density is seen overlying the ventral surface of the liver on supine radiographs. Air within the subhepatic space (Morison's pouch) appears as a triangular hyperlucency above the superior pole of the right kidney known as a *doge's cap.* Free air within the peritoneum can highlight anterior ligamentous structures such as the falciform ligament, lateral umbilical ligaments (forming an inverted V), or the urachus (the fibrous remnant of the fetal allantoic membrane extending from the bladder apex to the umbilicus).[27]

Retroperitoneal air can arise from posterior duodenal ulcer perforation or from dissection originating in the thoracic cavity. This is often difficult to detect on abdominal plain films because the amount of air is small and is obscured by overlying structures. Radiographic signs include rounded, mottled, or linear gas collections outlining the retroperitoneal organs. If plain films are repeated in different positions and the extramural gas fails to migrate, pneumoretroperitoneum is more likely than pneumoperitoneum.

Free air under the diaphragm can be mimicked by basal atelectasis, subphrenic fat, a subphrenic abscess, or interposition of air-filled loops of bowel above the liver. The interposition of bowel between the liver and diaphragm is known as *Chilaiditi syndrome.*

Computed Tomography. CT is superior to conventional radiography in detecting pneumoperitoneum. Because the patient is supine, free air on CT is seen as a gas collection beneath the anterior abdominal wall and overlying the ventral surface of the liver (Fig. 19-15). Extraluminal air may also be seen near the inferior fissure of the liver (porta hepatis) in patients with a perforated duodenal ulcer.[43]

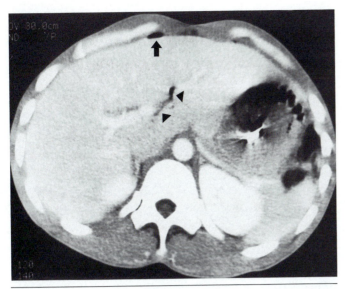

FIGURE 19-15. Free intraperitoneal air seen on CT scan. A small collection of free air is present anterior to the liver *(arrow)*. Another small collection of air is located at the liver hilum *(arrowheads)*, a typical location of air escaping from the duodenum. The patient had a perforated duodenal ulcer. The plain radiographs were negative. (Copyright David T. Schwartz, M.D.)

Small Bowel Obstruction

Mechanical bowel obstruction produces dilatation of bowel proximal to the point of obstruction and collapse of bowel distal to the obstruction (Figs. 19-6 and 19-16).[28,44] Dilated loops of small bowel are greater than 3 cm in diameter. The numerous valvulae conniventes can give the obstructed segment of small bowel the appearance of a *stack of coins*. Gas in the distal bowel is cleared by peristalsis beyond the obstructing lesion. Eventually, the distal bowel is entirely collapsed and devoid of gas. However, early in the clinical course or when the obstruction is incomplete, gas can be present in the distal bowel and rectum (Fig. 19-17). Nevertheless, the quantity of bowel gas distal to the obstruction is less than the amount of gas and distention proximal to the obstruction. An incomplete or early small bowel obstruction can appear similar to a mild ileus or a nonspecific pattern. Gas in the distal bowel or rectum does not exclude a mechanical bowel obstruction. A digital rectal examination does not introduce radiographically significant amounts of air into the rectum.[45]

The presence of distal bowel gas radiographically distinguishes a partial small bowel obstruction from a complete obstruction. This is an important distinction because complete obstructions are more likely to require surgery, whereas incomplete obstructions are more likely to resolve with conservative measures.

The *upright abdominal radiograph* provides additional evi-

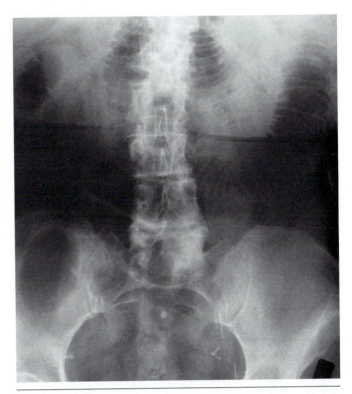

FIGURE 19-16. Small bowel obstruction. Supine abdominal radiograph demonstrating several dilated small bowel loops with a paucity of air in the distal bowel. There are numerous well-defined valvulae conniventes that cross the bowel lumen, giving the segment of bowel the appearance of a "stack of coins." There are surgical clips from prior abdominal surgery.

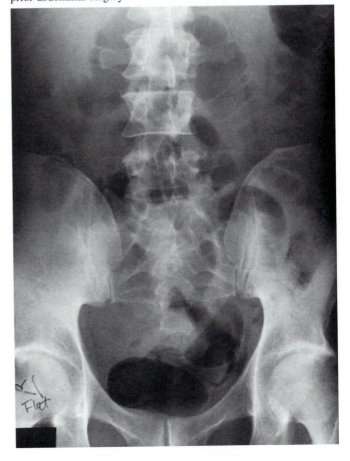

FIGURE 19-17. A partial small bowel obstruction. There is air in both the large and small bowel and the rectum, with a relatively greater amount of gas and distention of small bowel. (Copyright David T. Schwartz, M.D.)

dence of a mechanical bowel obstruction by revealing distinctive air-fluid levels (Fig. 19-18). Air-fluid levels that occur at differing heights within the same bowel loop are known as *differential* or *dynamic* air-fluid levels. Multiple differential air-fluid levels create a radiograph appearance like that of a *step ladder*. Differential air-fluid levels are more characteristic of mechanical obstruction than of adynamic ileus. However, they are only 52% sensitive and 71% specific for mechanical obstruction. The greater the height differential, the more likely it is that mechanical obstruction is present.[46] With a 20 mm height differential, the specificity is increased to 94%, although sensitivity drops to less than 25%. As the obstructed bowel becomes more fluid-filled, only small pockets of air are left, resembling a *string of beads*. On the supine radiograph, these small pockets of air appear as slit-like lucencies perpendicular to the fluid-filled loops of small bowel. This is called the *stretch sign*. A few isolated air-fluid levels can also be seen in patients with adynamic ileus, so air-fluid levels alone are not diagnostic of obstruction.

Although plain radiography is considered an excellent test in the diagnosis of bowel obstruction, only 50% of patients with a mechanical bowel obstruction have diagnostic plain radiographs.[47,48] In 30% of cases, the plain radiographs are "suggestive"; in the remaining 20% of cases, the radiographs are nonspecific or negative. Patients with complete and fully developed bowel obstruction are most likely to have diagnostic radiographs. Causes of negative or nonspecific radiographs include (1) an early or incomplete obstruction, (2) proximal jejunal obstruction, and (3) an obstruction in which the bowel lumen is completely filled with fluid and is therefore not visible on plain radiographs (Fig. 19-19).

Computed Tomography.   CT is highly sensitive in diagnosing small bowel obstruction (SBO). CT can also accurately define the location of the obstruction, the nature of the obstructive lesion, and signs of bowel ischemia. CT detects SBO with a sensitivity of 94% and specificity of 96%.[49–54] CT is less sensitive at detecting low-grade partial obstruction. A specialized small bowel contrast study (*enteroclysis*) is most accurate in diagnosing low-grade obstruction, although this is generally not used in the ED.[48,55]

Bowel obstruction is diagnosed on CT when there are dilated loops of bowel proximal to the point of obstruction and normal or collapsed loops of bowel distal to the obstruction (Fig. 19-19*C*). An abrupt transition point is often seen between the dilated and collapsed small bowel. CT can detect an extraluminal mass, such as an intraperitoneal metastasis, that is causing obstruction. If no obstructing lesion is seen, the cause of obstruction is presumed to be an adhesion. CT is also able to detect internal hernias and closed-loop obstructions that pose a high risk of ischemia (see below).[50,56]

CT can reveal signs of bowel ischemia complicating obstruction with moderate sensitivity (approximately 75%). Thickening of the bowel wall greater than 3 mm indicates ischemia (or an inflammatory or malignant condition of the bowel wall). The *target sign* (two concentric layers of enhancement of the thickened bowel wall), mesenteric edema and

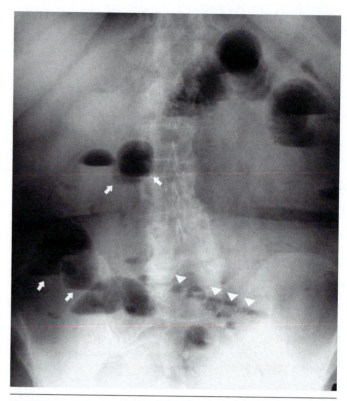

FIGURE 19-18.   The upright abdominal radiograph from the patient shown in Fig. 19-16. There are several collections of air in moderately distended small bowel loops. Differential (dynamic) air-fluid levels are seen *(arrows)* in which the air-fluid levels at each end of a loop of small bowel are at different heights. In addition, there is a series of smaller air collections aligned in a row *(arrowheads)*. This is known as the *string-of-pearls* sign. It represents air trapped under the valvulae conniventes of an obstructed bowel loop. The upright film also helps to confirm the absence of air in large bowel. The supine radiograph (Fig. 19-16) suggests mechanical obstruction, and the findings on the upright film further support this diagnosis.

hemorrhage, intramural gas, ascites and free intraperitoneal air are all signs of intestinal ischemia or infarction.[57–59]

CT is indicated in patients with suspected small bowel obstruction when there is diagnostic uncertainty and equivocal plain radiographs (about 20 to 30% of cases). CT is also indicated when information about the nature of the obstructing lesion is needed to determine treatment. This is the case when the patient has an intraabdominal malignancy and has had prior surgery (risk for adhesions) or radiation therapy (risk for radiation enteritis). In general, when plain films are nondiagnostic, or when expectant (nonsurgical) treatment is planned, CT should be performed to determine the nature of the obstruction (adhesion, tumor, or internal hernia) and to look for signs of ischemia.

Ultrasonography.   Ultrasonography does not have a clear role in the evaluation of patients with suspected bowel obstruction. Signs of SBO on ultrasound include dilated fluid-filled intestinal loops and collapsed distal bowel. There is increased peristalsis in the obstructed bowel, which is seen on US as a rapid whirling motion of lumenal contents. In contrast, peristalsis is absent in adynamic ileus. In evaluating mechanical bowel obstruction, ultrasound has similar or slightly better sensitivity

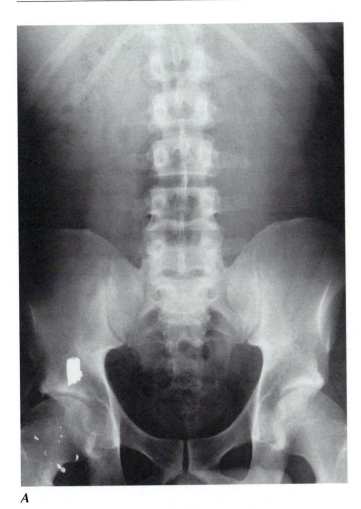

A

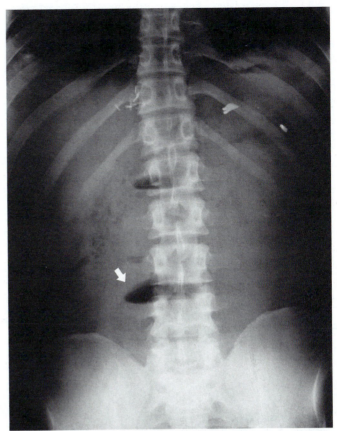

B

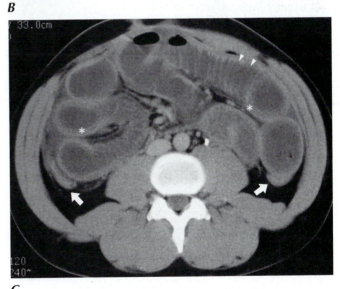

C

FIGURE 19-19. Small bowel obstruction with negative plain films. A 24-year-old man presented with abdominal pain, distention, and vomiting. He had undergone laparotomy 6 months earlier for a gunshot wound. The abdominal radiographs were negative. *A.* There is a small amount of air in both the large and small bowels. Retained bullet fragments and surgical clips are seen. On the upright radiograph (*B*), two small air-fluid levels are seen in the midabdomen *(arrow)*. An abdominal CT scan (*C*) shows multiple dilated fluid-filled loops of small bowel. Note the valvulae conniventes *(arrowheads)*. The large bowel is collapsed *(arrows)*. This CT is diagnostic of a distal small bowel obstruction. Obstruction was not evident on the conventional radiographs because the bowel was almost completely filled with fluid, as shown by CT. Although oral contrast was given, it did not reach the small bowel because of vomiting and slow intestinal transit. The small bowel wall is slightly thickened, suggesting ischemia *(asterisks)*.

compared to plain radiography. In a retrospective study, SBO was detected by ultrasound with 89% sensitivity as compared with 71% for plain films.[60–62]

Strangulation Obstruction

Bowel ischemia is an ominous complication of mechanical obstruction and constitutes a surgical emergency. Suspicion of this diagnosis rests on clinical findings: pain that is constant rather than intermittent, localized tenderness or rebound tenderness, fever, and leukocytosis. Patients with complete obstruction and markedly distended bowel loops are higher risk of bowel wall ischemia. Ischemic loops of bowel are often completely fluid-filled, and a relatively gasless abdomen can signify a strangulation obstruction. This is a difficult diagnosis because the radiographic finding of a gasless abdomen is similar in appearance to a negative abdominal radiograph.

A *closed-loop obstruction* is at especially high risk of ischemia because the mesenteric vascular supply is compressed at

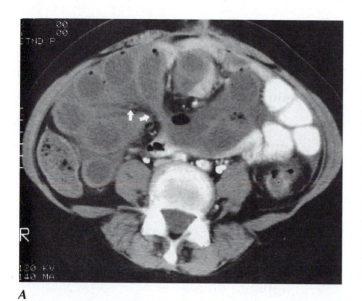

A

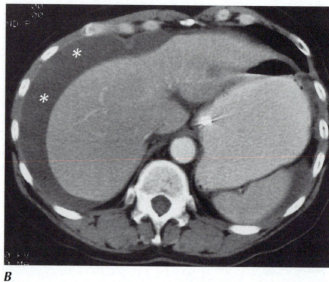

B

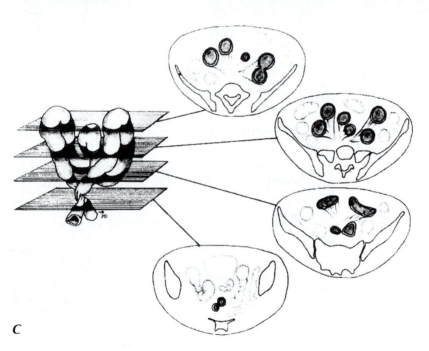

C

FIGURE 19-20. Closed-loop obstruction shown by CT. A 57-year-old woman complained of diffuse abdominal pain. Plain radiographs were negative. *A.* A CT scan shows fluid-filled loops of bowel with bowel wall thickening and mesenteric congestion. Folds of the mesentery converge to the point of volvulus *(arrows)*. At surgery, the patient had an incarcerated internal hernia with ischemic loops of bowel. *B.* A second CT slice shows ascites surrounding the liver *(asterisk)*. This is another sign of ischemic bowel, representing hemorrhagic intraperitoneal fluid. *C.* Schematic diagram of closed-loop obstruction. The superior CT slices show a radial distribution of fluid-filled loops of bowel and engorged mesentery converging toward the site of torsion. At the level of torsion there are two adjacent collapsed loops of bowel. (*A* and *B*. Copyright David T. Schwartz, M.D.) (*C*. From Balthazar EJ: CT of small bowel obstruction. *AJR* 162:258, 1994, with permission.)

the point of obstruction. A closed-loop is caused by torsion of a loop of bowel around a lesion or adhesion. Vascular occlusion also occurs at the neck of an internal or external hernia. Closed-loop obstruction is not reliably detected by plain radiography. However, there are three radiographic signs associated with this condition. These are seen infrequently and are difficult to identify with certainty. One sign is fixation of a single dilated loop of bowel on serial radiographs. Second, an air-filled small bowel volvulus may have a *coffee bean* appearance when the two limbs of the air-distended bowel loop are compressed together side by side. Finally, when completely fluid-filled, the closed loop can mimic a soft tissue mass—the *pseudotumor sign*.[63,64]

The great anatomic resolution of CT permits detection of closed-loop obstruction.[50,57] The involved mesentery radiates

from a central point at the origin of the volvulus. Near the point of the volvulus, two collapsed loops of bowel lie adjacent to one another (Fig. 19-20). The involved bowel is usually fluid-filled and often shows signs of ischemia: a thickened bowel wall and an edematous, congested mesentery.

Gallstone Ileus

Gallstone ileus is a distinct type of mechanical SBO.[65,66] A gallstone erodes into the duodenum, enters the intestinal lumen, and, if the stone is large (>3 cm), can cause an intraluminal blockage, usually at the ileocecal valve. Although this accounts for only 2% of all cases of mechanical bowel obstruction, the incidence is up to 25% in elderly patients who have not had

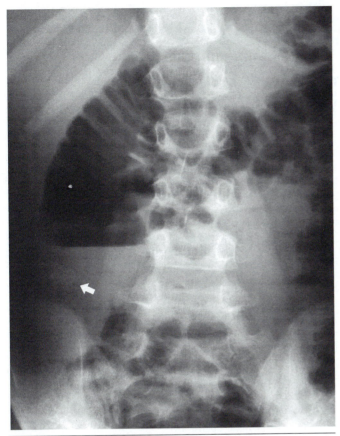

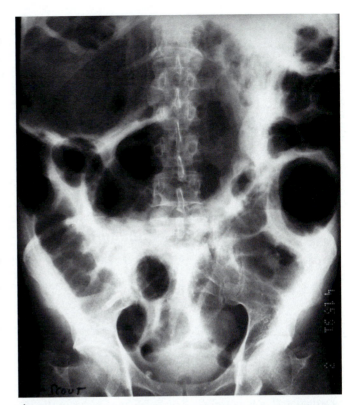

A

FIGURE 19-21. Gallstone ileus in an elderly diabetic patient. The patient presented with symptoms suggestive of a mechanical bowel obstruction. The abdominal plain film revealed dilated loops of small bowel and an ectopic gallstone *(arrow)*. Pneumobilia was not seen. At surgery, the gallstone was found lodged at the ileocecal valve. (See Fig. 19-7, pneumobilia.)

prior abdominal surgery. The radiographic findings are known as *Rigler's triad*—a SBO pattern, ectopic gallstone, and pneumobilia (Fig. 19-21).[67,68] All three signs are seen in only a minority of cases. Air in the biliary tree *(pneumobilia)* is always pathologic. Pneumobilia is a finding of gallstone ileus, emphysematous cholecystitis or prior surgery (endoscopic papillotomy, choledochojejunostomy) (Fig. 19-7).[27]

Large Bowel Obstruction

Small bowel obstruction and colonic obstruction can usually be differentiated on plain radiographs. Dilated loops of small bowel are centrally located and have *valvulae conniventes*. Obstructed large bowel is peripherally located, shows haustral mucosal indentations, and is distended by gas, liquid, and fecal material. In addition, dilated large bowel is of greater diameter than dilated small bowel could attain.

The diagnosis of colonic obstruction depends on seeing distention of large bowel that extends proximally from the site of obstruction to the cecum (Fig. 19-22).[28,69–71] The cecum is characteristically the most distended segment in large bowel

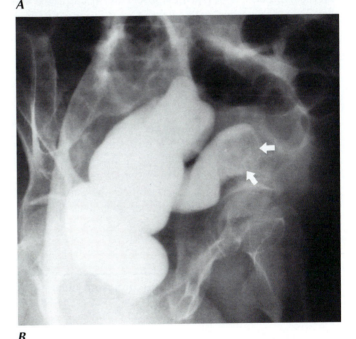

B

FIGURE 19-22. Large bowel obstruction due to sigmoid carcinoma. *A.* There is massively dilated large bowel throughout the abdomen. The patient presented with abdominal distention and constipation without abdominal pain. *B.* Contrast enema demonstrates a mass lesion obstructing the sigmoid colon *(arrows)*. An emergency diverting colostomy was performed. Later evaluation confirmed adenocarcinoma and the patient had a partial colectomy. (Copyright David T. Schwartz, M.D.)

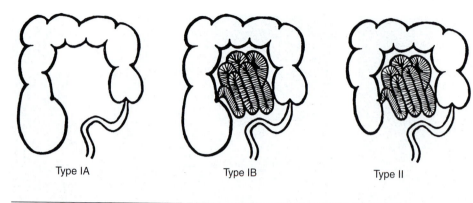

Type IA   Type IB   Type II

FIGURE 19-23.   Three patterns of large bowel obstruction. An obstructing lesion is located at the distal descending colon. In type I, the ileocecal valve is competent and the cecum is markedly distended. In type IA, only the large bowel is distended. In type IB there is concomitant small bowel distention. In type II, the ileocecal valve is incompetent and the cecum is decompressed into the terminal ileum. (From Plewa MC: Emergency abdominal radiography. *Emerg Med Clin North Am* 9:834, 1991, with permission. Adapted from Love L: Large bowel obstruction. *Semin Roentgenol* 8:300, 1973, with permission.)

obstruction. In fact, if the cecum is not the most distended region of large bowel, mechanical obstruction is less likely. Concomitant small bowel distention is often seen with large bowel obstruction. Large bowel air-fluid levels may occur in the absence of gastrointestinal pathology and are therefore of limited significance.

In the presence of a competent ileocecal valve (ICV), a large bowel obstruction can lead to massive colonic dilatation, especially involving the cecum (Fig. 19-23). A transverse cecal diameter of 9 to 13 cm portends imminent perforation.[72,73] A rapidly developing obstruction is more likely to perforate. If the ileocecal valve is incompetent, the cecum will decompress into the small bowel. With an incompetent ICV, there is widespread dilatation of both large and small bowel, resembling an adynamic ileus. A right lateral decubitus or prone radiograph helps distinguish between obstruction and ileus because the descending colon and rectum fills with air in an ileus but not in an obstruction.

Collapse of distal large bowel is often difficult to discern on plain radiographs. When the patient is supine, the descending colon and rectum are dependent and fill with fluid. On a radiograph taken in the prone position, the rectum will fill with air if there is no large bowel obstruction.

The radiographic differentiation of distal large bowel obstruction and diffuse adynamic ileus is difficult. Although several criteria are useful in distinguishing the two, the reliability of these criteria diminishes with rapidly developing colonic obstruction or a long-standing ileus (Table 19-6). If the ileocecal valve is incompetent, the diagnosis is even more difficult because the cecum is decompressed into the small bowel. This fills the small bowel with air, mimicking a diffuse ileus. Large amounts of colonic fecal material are more consistent with a functional alteration in colonic motility than with an obstructive lesion.

Contrast Enema.   Contrast enema is the procedure of choice in evaluating colonic obstruction.[74] It will confirm or refute the diagnosis of obstruction as well as reveal the nature of the obstructing lesion. An intraluminal mass lesion is seen with an obstructing carcinoma, the most common cause of large bowel obstruction (Fig. 19-22*B*). A narrowly tapering "bird's beak" is seen with volvulus. Contrast studies are contraindicated if strangulation, perforation, or peritonitis is suspected. A severe, diffuse adynamic ileus is often difficult to distinguish from a distal large bowel obstruction and is therefore sometimes referred to as a *pseudoobstruction.* Contrast enema readily differentiates an adynamic ileus from a distal colonic obstruction by showing complete filling of the entire colon and often reflux into the terminal ileum.

TABLE 19-6

Distinguishing Large Bowel Obstruction from Ileus

	LARGE BOWEL OBSTRUCTION	ADYNAMIC ILEUS
Distention	Fluid-filled	Gaseous
Fluid in upright position	Mottled	
Haustra	Localized accentuation, diminished overall	Preserved
Septa	Thickened, irregular, increased in local regions	Thin
Colonic wall	Thickened	Thin
Inner colonic contour	Ragged	Smooth

Volvulus

Volvulus is a mechanical obstruction caused by a loop of bowel twisting about its mesentery. It usually involves the sigmoid colon or cecum. A closed-loop obstruction develops, which compromises the vascular supply to the involved segment of bowel. *Sigmoid volvulus* is responsible for 60% of adult forms of volvulus and is characterized by a massively distended sigmoid loop arising out of the pelvis. There is often considerable proximal large bowel and also small bowel distention (Fig. 19-24). *Cecal volvulus* is characterized by a massively dilated cecum that projects into the mid- or upper left abdomen. The distal large bowel is undistended and usually collapsed. Cecal volvu-

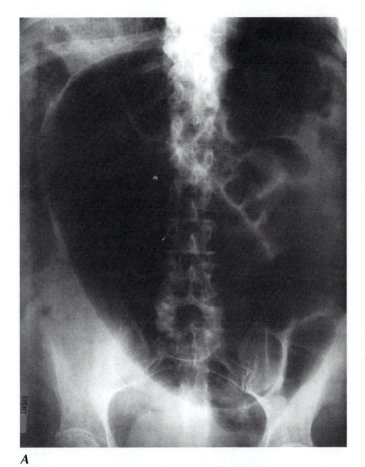

A

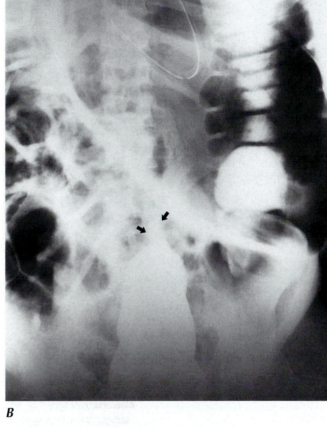

B

Distended Sigmoid Loop

Long Sigmoid
Mesentery that
Predisposes to
Volvulus

Volvulus
Colon and Mesenteric
Vessels Are Occluded at
the Axis of the Volvulus

C

FIGURE 19-24. Sigmoid volvulus. *A.* There is a massively distended coffee bean–shaped loop of bowel that arises from the left lower quadrant and extends to the right upper quadrant. A small amount of air is seen in the proximal colon. *B.* A contrast enema demonstrates the characteristic tapering "bird's beak" in the sigmoid colon *(arrows).* Some contrast has entered the descending colon. *C.* Elongated redundant sigmoid colon can twist around its mesentery. (*C.* From Jones DJ: Large bowel volvulus. *BMJ* 305:358, 1992, with permission.) (*B.* Copyright David T. Schwartz, M.D.)

lus is often accompanied by SBO (Fig. 19-25).[75] Effacement of colonic haustra is common to both forms of volvulus. If plain radiographs are equivocal, a contrast enema is indicated. A volvulus has a "bird's beak" appearance as the contrast column terminates at the point of the mesenteric twist, either at the sigmoid colon or at the cecum.

Additional plain film signs helpful in diagnosing sigmoid volvulus include the location of the apex of the distended loop under the left hemidiaphragm, inferior convergence of the walls of the sigmoid loop to the left of the midline, and a *left flank overlap sign.* This sign occurs when the walls of the volvulus overlap the soft tissues of the descending colon. These three signs have 100% specificity in diagnosing a sigmoid volvulus. A markedly distended ahaustral colonic loop is 94%

sensitive and 20% specific for a volvulus. A *medial summation line* represents the approximated medial walls of the sigmoid volvulus.[76]

Gastric Outlet Obstruction

Gastric outlet obstruction can have varied radiographic manifestations. Depending on the degree of vomiting and the duration of a gastric outlet obstruction, one may see a hugely distended stomach with a large epigastric or left-upper-quadrant air-fluid level (Fig. 19-26). The transverse colon may be displaced inferiorly. A contrast examination confirms a gastric outlet obstruction.

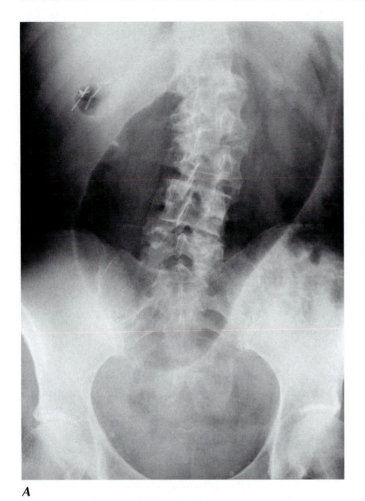

A

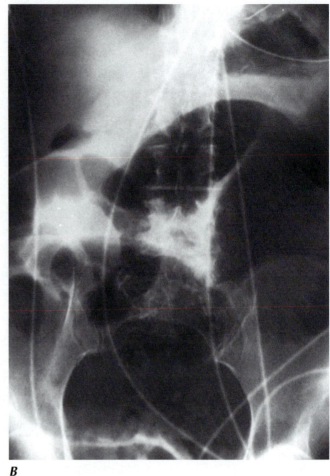

B

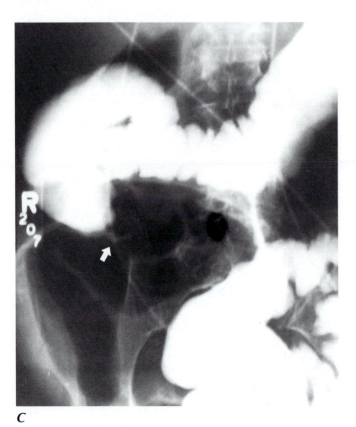

C

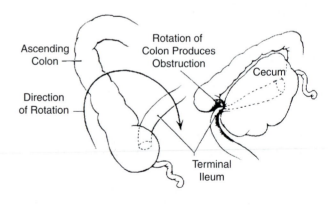

FIGURE 19-25. Cecal volvulus. *A.* An elderly woman presented with a sudden onset of abdominal pain and distention. Supine radiograph showing a large (16-cm) distended cecum arising from the right side of the pelvis. The remainder of the large bowel is collapsed and gasless. *B.* Another patient with cecal volvulus. The massively dilated cecum occupies the left side of the abdomen. There is associated small bowel distention. *C.* A contrast enema reveals filling of the entire colon up to the tapering "bird's beak" at the ascending colon *(arrow). D.* Incomplete fixation of the ascending colon results in a mobile cecum that can twist around the terminal ilium. The volvulus results in a massively distended cecum located in the midabdomen. (D. From O'Mara CS, Wilson TM, Stonesifer GL, Cameron JL: Cecal volvulus. *Ann Surg* 189:724, 1979, with permission.)

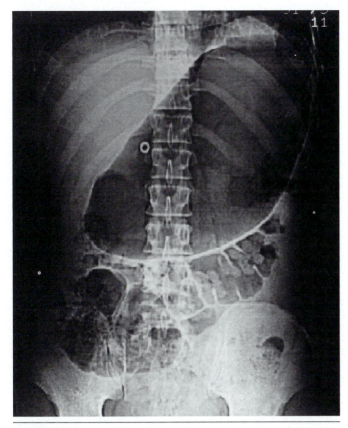

FIGURE 19-26. Gastric outlet obstruction. A supine abdominal radiograph shows a distended air-filled stomach, causing inferior displacement of the transverse colon. The patient was a pedestrian who had been struck by a slow-moving car. Gastric outlet obstruction was due to a duodenal hematoma.

Appendicitis

Appendicitis is diagnosed primarily on clinical grounds.[77] However, in a substantial minority of cases, the diagnosis is uncertain and additional imaging modalities are helpful in deciding management. Some authors recommend the liberal use of diagnostic imaging (CT or US) in all patients with diagnostic uncertainty as a means of reducing both the negative laparotomy rate and the delays inherent in watchful waiting in cases where clinical findings are equivocal.[22,23]

Plain Abdominal Radiography. Plain radiographs play a minor role in the diagnosis of appendicitis. Abdominal radiographs are "abnormal" in as many as 80% of patients with appendicitis, although most of these abnormalities are a pattern of nonspecific ileus.[78] The diagnostic finding of a calcified appendicolith is seen in at most 10% of adults (Fig. 19-27). A right-lower-quadrant soft tissue mass containing gas may represent a periappendiceal abscess. A localized ileus can result in an air-fluid level in the cecum or distal ileum. Diminished motility throughout the small bowel leads to a pattern of diffuse adynamic ileus. An obscured right properitoneal fat line, obliteration of the psoas margin, and rightward scoliosis also suggest acute appendicitis.

Air in the appendix can be either normal or indicative of acute appendicitis. A normal appendix may be air-filled, especially in the presence of an ileus. A noninflamed air-filled appendix has a normal caliber, serpentine appearance, and smooth margins (Fig. 19-28). With acute appendicitis, the margins of the air-filled appendix are irregular, the lumen is dilated, and a fluid meniscus may be present. Nevertheless, acute appendicitis can also occur in the patient whose air-filled appendix appears "unremarkable."

Contrast Enema. In the past, contrast enema had been used to diagnose appendicitis. Complete filling of the appendix with barium is normal. However, failure to fully opacify a normal appendix occurs in 10% of cases. In addition, a barium enema may partially fill the appendix in some patients with acute appendicitis. Because of these limitations, the risk of iatrogenic perforation, and the availability of more accurate tests, contrast enema are no longer indicated in the evaluation of suspected appendicitis.[79]

Computed Tomography. CT is highly accurate in the diagnosis of appendicitis. Sensitivities range from 96 to 98% and specificity from 83 to 89%.[80–83] CT criteria for acute appendicitis include visualization of an abnormally dilated appendix (>6 mm) and appendiceal wall thickening with increased intravenous contrast enhancement (unless the vascular supply has been compromised). An appendicolith is seen in about 30% of cases. Periappendiceal inflammation appears as streaky densities within the perimesenteric fat (Fig. 19-29). Stranding of mesenteric fat is common but nonspecific. A discrete fluid collection suggests a periappendiceal abscess. Such an abscess may warrant surgical exploration even if an abnormal appendix or appendicolith is not seen on CT. Among patients with appendicitis, 75% have an abnormal appendix seen on CT and 28% have either an appendicolith, periappendiceal inflammation, or fluid collection consistent with an abscess. CT excludes appendicitis if a normal appendix without inflammatory

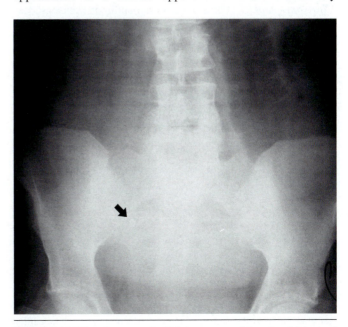

FIGURE 19-27. An appendicolith is seen overlying the right sacral wing *(arrow)* in a patient with appendicitis.

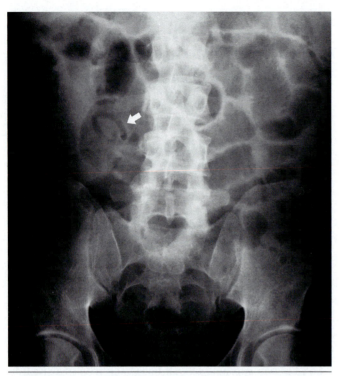

FIGURE 19-28. A supine abdominal radiograph in a patient clinically suspected of having appendicitis. An adynamic ileus is present, with numerous dilated, air-filled loops of small and large bowel. A curved, tubular, air-filled appendix is present in the right midabdomen *(arrow).* An air-filled normal-caliber appendix implies that the lumen of the appendix is not obstructed and that the appendix is not inflamed. Laparotomy for suspected appendicitis was negative.

changes is seen (Fig. 19-11*D*). CT can also diagnose other causes of right lower quadrant pain, including cecal diverticulitis, Crohn's disease, mesenteric adenitis, and ovarian cysts and abscesses.

Ultrasonography. Ultrasound for appendicitis uses a graded-compression technique in which a linear-array transducer is pressed into the right iliac fossa to deflect air-filled bowel over-

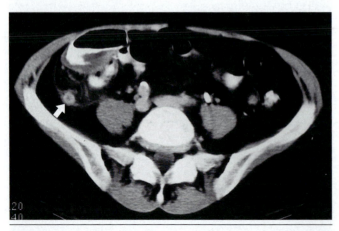

FIGURE 19-29. CT scan showing nonperforated appendicitis. There is an enlarged (1 cm in diameter) appendix with a thickened, enhancing wall *(arrow).* The lumen of the obstructed appendix is not filled with enteric contrast, as is the adjacent cecum. There is mild inflammatory stranding in the periappendiceal mesenteric fat.

lying the appendix.[84–86] Signs of appendicitis include visualization of an enlarged (6 mm or more) noncompressible appendix. In some cases, an appendicolith, periappendiceal inflammation, or abscess is seen (Fig. 19-30). Some radiologists feel that appendicitis cannot be excluded unless a normal appendix is seen, while others feel that demonstration of a normal psoas muscle is adequate to exclude appendicitis. Ultrasound has a sensitivity of 85% and a specificity of 92% for diagnosing appendicitis. In cases of an appendiceal perforation, the sensitivity falls significantly. Ultrasound is highly effective at detecting gynecologic causes of right lower quadrant abdominal pain, including tuboovarian abscess and ruptured ovarian cyst.

Whether CT or ultrasound is more useful in the diagnosis of appendicitis remains unanswered although current practice favors CT in most situations because it is more accurate and less dependent on operator technique. In one study, CT was found to be more accurate.[81] The sensitivity of CT was 96%, versus 76% for ultrasound. Specificity was approximately 90% for both CT and ultrasound. In 20 patients in whom the results from CT and ultrasound were discordant, CT was correct in 17 while ultrasound was correct in only 3. The recent application of helical CT technology has further increased the advantages of CT over US.

Diverticulitis

Diverticulitis most commonly involves the sigmoid colon.[87] Painful attacks of diverticulitis are frequently associated with microperforations of the involved colon that seal off, preventing generalized peritonitis. Plain film findings are rare and none is pathognomonic. If a paracolonic abscess develops, a soft tissue density may be seen in the left lower quadrant. Barium enema is highly sensitive at detecting diverticulae (Fig. 19-31). However, their presence does not make the diagnosis of diverticulitis. Radiographic signs of diverticulitis include extravasation of contrast and segmental narrowing; however, these signs have limited sensitivity and specificity for the diagnosis. Barium enema is used to make the diagnosis only after treatment with bowel rest, intravenous fluids, and antibiotics. During an acute exacerbation, barium enema can result in bowel perforation, and is therefore contraindicated.

CT is the imaging modality of choice in acute diverticulitis (Fig. 19-32). There is localized mural thickening and stranding of nearby mesenteric fat. Diverticulae are visible in 84% of cases and mural thickening greater than 5 mm is present in 70%.[88] CT can differentiate diverticulitis from colon cancer. It can detect abscess formation and perforation with extracolonic gas, which helps to predict failure of medical management.[89]

Inflammatory Bowel Disease

Inflammatory bowel disease usually does not show appreciable changes on conventional radiographs. Intraluminal contrast is required to detect inflammatory changes that can involve any segment of the alimentary canal. A hallmark of Crohn disease on contrast radiography is the *string sign* due to stricture for-

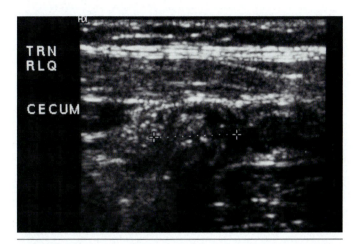

FIGURE 19-30. Right lower quadrant graded-compression sonogram of a 28-year-old man with appendicitis. There is an enlarged (1.3 cm in diameter) noncompressible appendix. To visualize the appendix, the abdominal wall is pressed against the iliac fossa using a linear-array ultrasound transducer.

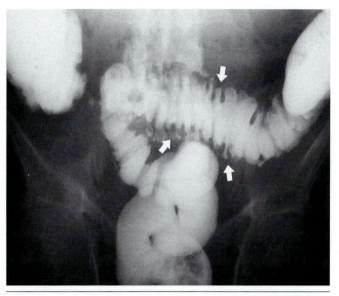

FIGURE 19-31. Barium enema showing diverticulosis. There are many contrast-filled diverticulae of the sigmoid colon *(arrows)*. There is no extravasation of contrast, extrinsic compression, or structure formation, which would be indicative of diverticulitis.

mation, usually in the region of the terminal ileum. Ulcerative colitis is limited to the colon, and a characteristic finding on barium enema is a *lead-pipe* colon—a smooth, cylindrical, ahaustral segment of colon.

CT can visualize inflammatory bowel disease (Fig. 19-33).[90] The normal bowel wall measures 2 to 3 mm in thickness. Bowel wall thickening is seen in various inflammatory bowel conditions (<1 cm in diverticulitis and ulcerative colitis, up to 3 cm in Crohn's disease). A double halo *(target sign)* is seen in both inflammatory bowel disease and infectious or ischemic colitis. Although nonspecific, the target sign helps to exclude colonic neoplasm.[91] CT is useful for identifying complications of Crohn's disease, including strictures, fistulas, and abscesses. Fistulas or sinus tracts allow air to enter the bladder, vagina, or abdominal wall.[92]

In ulcerative colitis, 70% of patients demonstrate a nonhomogeneous pattern of bowel wall thickening due to submucosal deposition of lipid debris. Other common CT findings include a narrowed rectal lumen and stranding of the perirectal fat.

Toxic Megacolon. *Toxic megacolon* is a complication of inflammatory bowel disease. The patient presents with fever, diarrhea, and signs of systemic toxicity.[93,94] The characteristic plain radiographic appearance is dilation of the colon with loss of haustrations and nodular indentations of the mucosa (Fig. 19-34). Toxic megacolon is usually a complication of ulcerative colitis, although it can also occur with infectious enteritis, especially in patients treated with antiperistaltic agents.

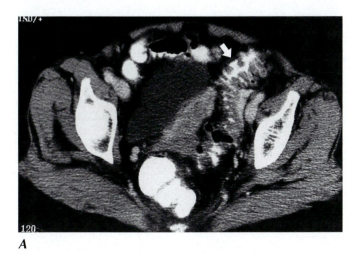

A

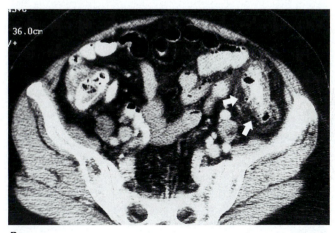

B

FIGURE 19-32. CT of diverticulitis. *A.* There is extensive diverticulosis of the contrast-filled sigmoid colon *(arrow)*. *B.* A slightly superior CT slice shows inflammatory stranding of the mesenteric fat surrounding the distal descending colon *(arrows)*.

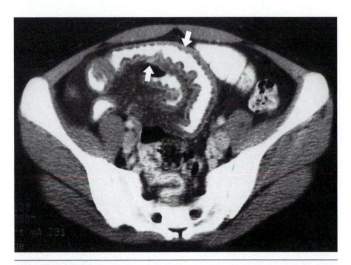

FIGURE 19-33.   Crohn's disease diagnosed on CT in a 26-year-old woman with right-lower-quadrant abdominal pain. The bowel wall of a segment of distal ileum is markedly thickened *(arrows)*. (Copyright David Schwartz, MD)

Bowel Ischemia

Acute bowel ischemia from mesenteric vascular occlusion presents as sudden, severe abdominal pain.[95,96] Acute mesenteric vascular occlusion is caused by embolic disease (e.g., atrial fibrillation), arterial or venous thrombosis (e.g., vascular disease, hypercoagulability), or shock. Bowel ischemia can also com-

plicate mechanical bowel obstruction, especially a closed-loop obstruction. With mesenteric ischemia, the physical examination is relatively unremarkable given the degree of pain. Bowel infarction results in bloody stool, sepsis, and shock.

Plain radiography is usually not helpful. Most often, a nonspecific ileus pattern is seen.[96-98] A gasless abdomen is seen in 10% of cases. *Intramural gas* accumulation appears as mottled or streaky radiolucencies. However, this is seen in only about 5% of cases. The intramural gas can enter the portal veins and migrate to the liver, appearing as fine linear streaks *(hepatic portal venous gas)* (Fig. 19-35). Intramural gas is also seen in a benign condition known as *pneumatosis cystoides intestinalis.* This can be a complication of pneumomediastinum, severe asthma, or colonoscopy, or it may be idiopathic. The patient's symptoms are mild despite the remarkable radiographic picture.[33]

CT and angiography are the imaging modalities of choice in suspected bowel ischemia. *Angiography* is highly accurate for localizing arterial emboli, thrombotic lesions, and vasospasm. The suspected vessel is catheterized under fluoroscopic guidance, and intravenous contrast is injected. Occlusion of a major mesenteric vessel is seen as an abrupt termination or diminution of the contrast flow. Sharp demarcation suggests an embolic etiology, whereas a gradually tapered, irregular cutoff of contrast is seen in cases of *in situ* thrombus formation. Angiography is performed when there is a high clinical likelihood of mesenteric ischemia, because it is both diagnostic and therapeutic. Intraarterial papaverine infu-

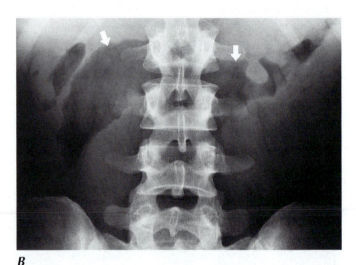

B

FIGURE 19-34.   Toxic megacolon. A 30-year-old man with ulcerative colitis presented with bloody diarrhea, fever, and abdominal distention. *A.* The transverse colon is markedly dilated and does not have normal haustral indentations. The ascending and descending colon was also involved, but this cannot be seen, because when the patient is supine, the ascending and descending colon are filled with fluid. The patient was managed medically. *B.* Five days later, the colon is no longer distended. The transverse colon is ahaustral and has a "lead pipe" appearance. There is a nodular mucosal indentation *(arrow)*. This appearance is characteristic of ulcerative colitis. (Copyright David T. Schwartz, M.D.)

A

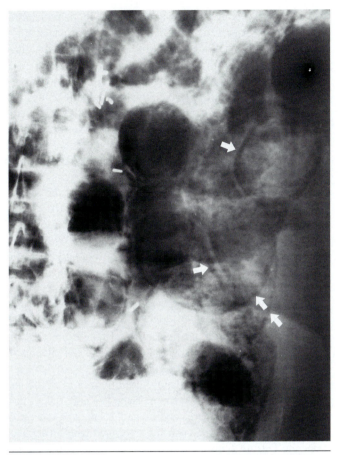

FIGURE 19-35. Pneumatosis intestinalis. Curvilinear streaks of intramural gas surround multiple loops of small bowel. (Copyright David T. Schwartz, M.D.)

to exclude mesenteric ischemia.[99–101] If bowel ischemia is strongly suspected, emergency angiography or laparotomy is indicated. Findings on contrast CT are related to the etiology (e.g., mesenteric vein thrombosis) and complications (e.g., intramural and hepatic portal venous gas). CT findings appear late and indicate severely ischemic or infarcted bowel. Circumferential bowel wall thickening is due to submucosal edema *(target sign)* (Fig. 19-36). The diagnosis of ischemia is strengthened if the involved bowel is in a specific vascular distribution. There is often inflammatory stranding in the surrounding mesenteric fat.

Ischemic colitis encompasses a spectrum of disorders ranging from acute infarction to an indolent chronic pain syndrome due to microvascular disease. Plain radiographs or contrast enema may show characteristic *thumb printing* in the area of vascular compromise. This is due to intramural foci of edema or hemorrhage. Thumb printing appears as rounded indentations perpendicular to the bowel wall.

Acquired Immune Deficiency Syndrome (AIDS)

Patients who are immunocompromised are susceptible to the same illnesses that cause abdominal pain in the immunocompetent person. Persons with HIV-related immunosuppression may also have other infectious or malignant disorders that can cause significant abdominal pain. CT identifies enlarged mesenteric lymph nodes due to lymphoma or tuberculosis as well as many other abdominal disorders. In concert with ultrasound, CT is useful for evaluating acute right upper quadrant pain in patients with AIDS who are at a risk for acalculous cholecystitis, sclerosing hepatic abscesses, and bacillary angiomatosis. Localized extramural air collections are seen in abscesses. Gastrointestinal lymphoma can be complicated by perforation of a hollow viscus. Lymphoma and Kaposi sarcoma can cause bowel obstruction either by a direct mass effect or by

sion can reduce associated vasospasm and restore some blood flow to the ischemic segment.[95,96]

CT has only moderate sensitivity in detecting bowel ischemia (about 75 to 80%) and therefore *cannot* be relied upon

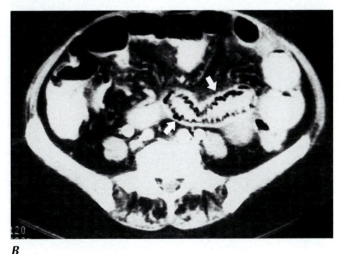

A   *B*

FIGURE 19-36. Ischemic bowel as seen on a CT. *A.* A prominent *target sign (arrows)* is present in several loops of strangulated bowel. The bowel was incarcerated within an internal hernia. The mesentery is edematous and congested as indicated by its uniform fluid density. *B.* In another patient, pockets of intramural gas are seen in a segment of small bowel. (Copyright David T. Schwartz, M.D.)

initiating a lead point in intussusception. CT is helpful in the diagnosis of a pancreatic abscess or hemorrhagic pancreatitis.

Patients with AIDS-related diarrhea rarely require imaging. However, patients with enteritis secondary to *Mycobacterium avium intracellulare* (MAI) are at risk for bowel perforation.[102] In patients with significant abdominal pain and diarrhea, abdominal CT can distinguish infectious enteritis from lymphoma. MAI enteritis causes mesenteric and retroperitoneal adenopathy in addition to marked nodular intestinal mucosal folds. Focal necrotic lesions of the liver and spleen are also seen with MAI. *Mycobacterium tuberculosis* infection is characterized by prominent asymmetrical thickening of the cecum, low-density lymphadenopathy (in comparison to MAI), and a thickened ileocecal valve. Tuberculous peritonitis is seen on CT as hyperdense ascitic fluid with loculations. With *Cryptosporidium* and other protozoal infections, contrast examination or CT characteristically reveals prominent mucosal thickening and narrowing of the bowel lumen.

Cytomegalovirus colitis (CMV) causes small vessel vasculitis and ischemic colitis. Findings of CMV colitis on CT range from circumferential thickening of colon, mucosal ulceration, pericolonic inflammation (stranding), and pneumatosis intestinalis to frank perforation.[77]

Typhlitis refers to inflammatory necrotic lesions of the terminal ileum, appendix, and cecum. There is a high risk of perforation. This formerly rare condition affects both patients with AIDS and those with malignancies associated with severe neutropenia. Diffuse bowel wall thickening, pneumatosis intestinalis, pericolonic fluid, and fascial thickening are all common CT manifestations of typhlitis.[103]

Cholecystitis

Acute cholecystitis is the most common abdominal condition requiring surgical intervention in patients above age 50.[18] The abdominal plain film has limited usefulness because only 15% of gallstones are radiopaque (Fig. 19-37). Clues to the presence of cholecystitis on abdominal plain radiographs include a right upper quadrant *sentinel loop,* scoliosis with concavity to the right, and a right hypochondrial mass. If the gallbladder is significantly enlarged, indentation of the hepatic flexure of the colon may be seen. In 1% of cases of acute cholecystitis, there is gas in the gallbladder wall or lumen of a distended gallbladder (*emphysematous cholecystitis*) (Fig. 19-38).[104,105] Gas in a nondilated gallbladder or in the biliary tree is seen with fistula formation (gallstone ileus) or surgical procedures (Fig. 19-7).

Ultrasonography.   US is the primary imaging study for patients with right upper quadrant pain (Fig. 19-39).[106–109] The sensitivity of ultrasound in detecting cholelithiasis is 97%. The sensitivity falls to 94% in detecting acute cholecystitis.[110] Although ultrasound readily detects gallstones, their mere presence does not prove that they are responsible for the patient's symptoms. The diagnosis of acute cholecystitis is clinical, and imaging confirmation may not be necessary if there is good

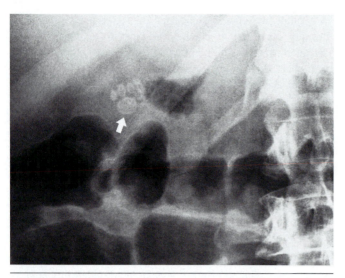

FIGURE 19-37.   Multiple gallstones in the gallbladder are visible because of the rim of calcification. Approximately 15% of gallstones are sufficiently calcified to be seen on plain radiographs.

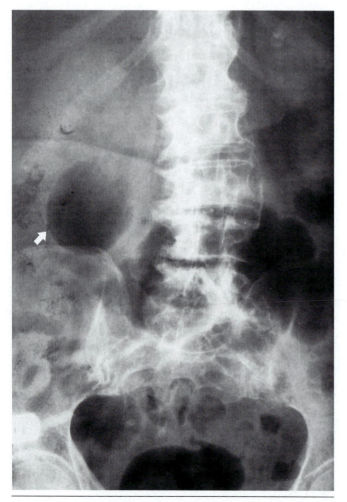

FIGURE 19-38.   Emphysematous cholecystitis. An elderly woman with diabetes presented with fever and right upper quadrant abdominal pain. The abdominal radiograph shows gas within a distended gallbladder, diagnostic of emphysematous cholecystitis. (Copyright David T. Schwartz, M.D.)

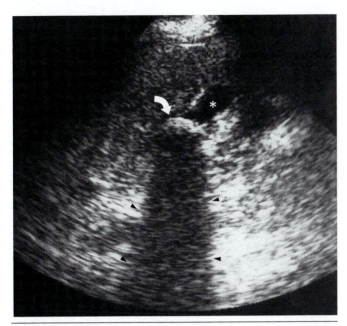

FIGURE 19-39. Right upper quadrant ultrasound demonstrates an echogenic gallstone *(arrow)* in the gallbladder *(asterisk)* that casts a prominent acoustic shadow *(arrowheads)*. There is no gallbladder wall thickening or pericholecystic fluid. This patient showed tenderness when the probe was placed over the inflamed gallbladder (the sonographic Murphy's sign).

clinical evidence for this diagnosis. Sonographic signs of acute cholecystitis are gallbladder wall thickening, pericholecystic fluid, gallbladder distention, and focal tenderness when the sonographer places the probe immediately over the gallbladder (sonographic Murphy's sign). A sonographic Murphy's sign is 75 to 94% sensitive in the detection of acute cholecystitis.[111] Gallbladder wall thickening is often present with cholecystitis

but is nonspecific. It is also seen with chronic cholecystitis, gallbladder cancer, portal hypertension, renal disease, hypoalbuminemia, and right heart failure. Gas within the gallbladder lumen or wall in emphysematous cholecystitis appears as a bright, highly echogenic contour on ultrasound.

Hepatobiliary Scintigraphy. The *hepatoiminodiacetic acid* (HIDA) scan is also used to diagnose acute cholecystitis.[112] A normally functioning gallbladder will take up the radioisotope following intravenous administration. Images obtained 1 h postinjection normally demonstrate contrast in the intrahepatic biliary system, the gallbladder fossa, and the proximal small bowel. This indicates biliary tract patency and reliably excludes cholecystitis. Failure of the of the gallbladder to fill suggests cystic duct obstruction and concomitant cholecystitis (Fig. 19-40).[113] Whether or not HIDA scanning should be performed preferentially over ultrasound in patients with suspected acute cholecystitis is controversial. Those who discourage HIDA scanning cite its poor specificity of 36%, compared with 91% for ultrasound.[114] This same study showed the sensitivity of HIDA scan and ultrasound to be 94 and 89%, respectively. Advocates for HIDA report sensitivity and specificity of 90 and 97% in the diagnosis of acute cholecystitis as compared to 94 and 78% for ultrasound.[110]

Computed Tomography. CT has a limited role in acute cholecystitis. It is not as sensitive as sonography at detecting gallstones. Only 50% of gallstones are sufficiently calcified to be seen on CT. However, in many but not all patients, CT is able to detect the inflammatory changes associated with acute cholecystitis, such as gallbladder wall thickening, pericholecystic fluid, and streaky densities in surrounding tissues (Fig. 19-41).[115]

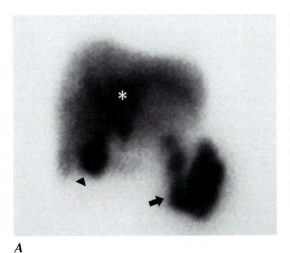
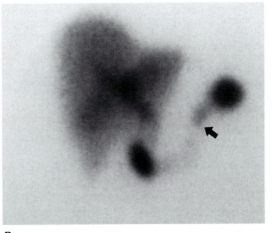

A   *B*

FIGURE 19-40. A hepatobiliary (HIDA) scan is used to diagnose cystic duct obstruction causing acute cholecystitis. *A.* A normal HIDA scan showing tracer taken up by the liver *(asterisk)* and excreted into the biliary system and then into duodenum *(arrow)*. The gallbladder is filled with radioisotope *(arrowhead)*. *B.* A HIDA scan positive for acute cholecystitis. The tracer has been excreted into the duodenum and small bowel *(arrows)* without filling the gallbladder. (Copyright David T. Schwartz, M.D.)

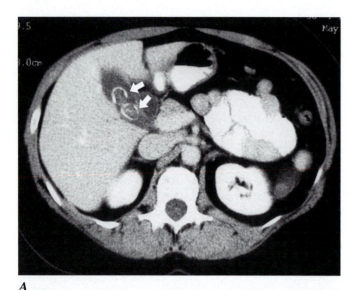

A

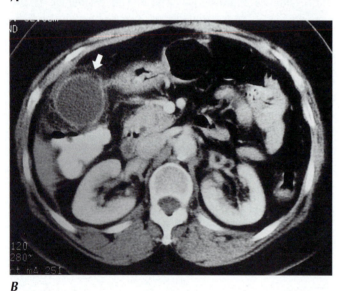

B

FIGURE 19-41. *A.* A CT scan showing two large gallstones that have a rim of calcification. Approximately 50% of gallstones are sufficiently calcified to be seen on CT. *B.* CT of acute cholecystitis in another patient. There is stranding in the pericholecystic tissues (*arrow*) and mild thickening of the gallbladder wall. The gallstones are not visible on CT in this patient but were identified by ultrasound. (*B.* Copyright David T. Schwartz, M.D.)

Choledocholithiasis

Common bile duct stones cause obstruction and bile duct dilatation, with resultant inflammation and infection. Obstruction typically occurs at the ampulla of Vater. CT can reliably detect common bile duct obstruction and dilatation but is less sensitive than ultrasound in detecting a stone.

The ultrasound diagnosis of choledocholithiasis includes common bile duct dilatation greater than 5 mm and intrahepatic bile duct dilation. Definitive diagnosis requires cholangiography to reveal the site and cause of obstruction. This can be done by percutaneous transhepatic cholangiography, by endoscopic retrograde cholangiopancreatography (ERCP) and,

most recently, by magnetic resonance cholangiography. Other causes of common bile duct dilatation include ampullary and pancreatic carcinoma.

Pancreatitis

Pancreatitis is primarily diagnosed by clinical and laboratory information.[116] Plain film signs are rare and nonspecific. These include widening of the proximal duodenum, left lung basilar atelectasis or a left pleural effusion, elevation of the left hemidiaphragm, and obscuration of the left psoas margin. There may be local isolated dilatation of the descending portion of the duodenum or the transverse colon (*sentinel loop*). Mottling due to fat necrosis or gas within the pancreas is rarely seen. Calcifications within the pancreas suggest chronic inflammation.

CT is the preferred study for imaging the pancreas (Fig. 19-42).[117] It is used to grade edema, hemorrhage, or surrounding inflammatory reaction. CT is always positive in moderate to severe cases of pancreatitis. In mild cases, 15 to 30% of CT scans are negative. There is a poor correlation between the CT grade of pancreatitis and the clinical outcome. Importantly, CT demonstrates complications of pancreatitis including cysts, pseudocysts, or abscesses. Cysts are homogeneous structures of low to intermediate density with a clearly defined circumferential margin of epithelial tissue. A pseudocyst is contiguous with the adjacent pancreas and lacks the epithelial boundaries. An abscess is a fluid-filled mass of heterogeneous material of intermediate density that may have an air-fluid level.

Renal Colic

The clinical presentation of renal colic is highly characteristic and an accurate clinical diagnosis can be made in most patients.[118–120] The patient complains of acute onset of severe unilateral flank pain that radiates to the lower abdominal quadrant or groin. The patient appears restless. Nausea and vomiting are common. There is costovertebral angle tenderness but only mild lower abdominal tenderness. Microscopic hematuria is seen in 90 to 95% of patients.[121] With a classic presentation, a clinical diagnosis can be made and treatment—including adequate analgesia and intravenous hydration—initiated without delay. In most cases, pain resolves after several hours in the ED.

The extent to which emergency imaging should be used in patients with suspected renal colic is controversial.[122,123] There is general agreement that imaging should be used to confirm the diagnosis when it is uncertain and to help determine management when the patient has persistent pain or when there is a high probability that a urological procedure will be needed. Diagnostic imaging options include plain abdominal radiograph [kidneys-ureter-bladder (KUB) radiograph], an intravenous urogram (IVU) (also known as intravenous pyelogram), US, and noncontrast helical CT.

There is some controversy, however, about whether a patient with a classic clinical presentation, microscopic hematuria, and

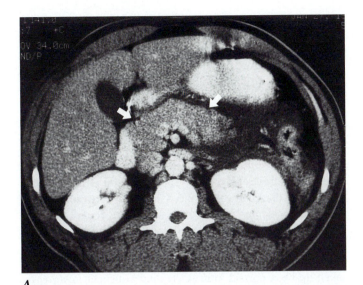

A

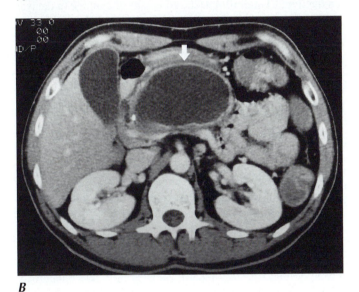

B

FIGURE 19-42. *A.* The pancreas is enlarged and edematous in this patient with pancreatitis. *B.* In another patient with midepigastric pain and fever who had a history of alcoholic pancreatitis, a large pancreatic pseudocyst is seen.

pain resolution after several hours in the ED needs confirmatory imaging. Although some practitioners feel that it is unnecessary, other clinicians prefer to have imaging confirmation even though they are fairly certain of the diagnosis.[122] In a small number of patients, imaging changes the diagnosis or management. In addition, an elective imaging study is generally recommended following a first episode of renal colic in order to exclude other urinary tract disorders such as a tumor or infarction.[124,125] Having this study performed in the ED, especially when clinical follow-up is uncertain, assures that this is accomplished. Other authors suggest that in patients with classic symptoms of renal colic, imaging should be performed only in those who remain symptomatic after 6 h of treatment in the ED.[123]

The main indications for emergency imaging are diagnostic

uncertainty, persistent pain despite adequate treatment, and signs or symptoms of infection. Persistent pain means that the patient may need hospitalization and possibly a procedure to remove the stone (lithotripsy or ureteroscopy). Operative procedures depend on the size and location of the stone. Stones that are 4 mm or smaller, and those located at the ureterovesical junction (UVJ) are likely to pass spontaneously. Stones that are 5 mm or larger in size, especially those of 10 mm or more, and those located at the ureteropelvic junction (UPJ) or midureter, are likely to require a procedure such as lithotripsy or ureteroscopy.

Of the four diagnostic imaging tests for renal colic, the traditional "gold standard" is the IVU. It is highly accurate and clearly displays urinary tract anatomy. In addition, intravenous contrast administration may promote stone passage because it causes a vigorous diuresis (although this effect has not been studied in a controlled manner). The IVU can also detect other urinary tract causes of flank pain such as a renal tumor, cyst, or infarction. Its shortcoming is that it cannot detect non-urinary tract disorders. US and especially CT have the advantage of being able to detect non-urinary tract disorders (appendicitis, ovarian torsion, aortic aneurysm). Finally, an IVU is contraindicated in patients with renal insufficiency, contrast allergy, or pregnancy.

Plain Radiography.   The plain abdominal radiograph is a simple, relatively quick, and inexpensive test used as an initial screening test for patients with possible urolithiasis (Fig. 19-43). However, even though 85% of stones are calcified and potentially detectable by plain radiography, in most patients the stone cannot be identified reliably. Most stones are small (<4mm) and are obscured by overlying bowel gas and bones. The course of the ureter is variable and, without contrast opacification, it is difficult to be certain that a calcification lies within the ureter. Finally, other calcifications, especially phleboliths,

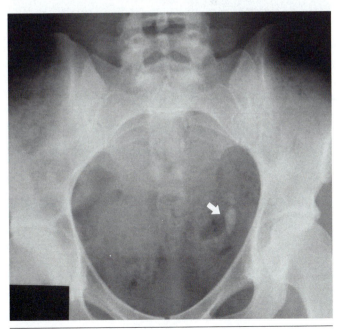

FIGURE 19-43.   Scout film of a patient with suspected ureterolithiasis. Note the large, irregular calcification in the left side of the pelvis *(arrow).*

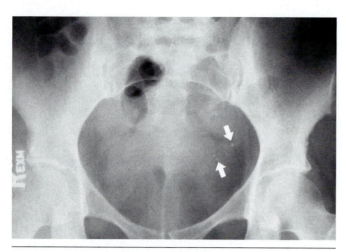

FIGURE 19-44.   The scout abdominal radiograph in another patient shows multiple small pelvic calcifications that are phleboliths. On plain radiography, these are difficult to distinguish from small stones in the distal ureter. The intravenous urogram (IVU) in this patient was negative.

are very common in the pelvis, and are difficult to distinguish from ureteral stones (Fig. 19-44). The true sensitivity and specificity of a KUB is only about 50%.[126–130] The KUB is most useful to follow progressive movement of a stone that has been previously identified by IVU or CT. A KUB may also be useful in patients with prior documented urolithiasis who are ex-

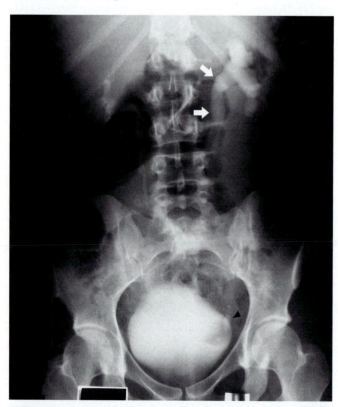

FIGURE 19-45.   This IVU radiograph of the patient shown in Fig. 19-43 was taken 20 min after the contrast injection. There is marked hydronephrosis and hydroureter on the left *(arrows)*. Ureteral obstruction is caused by the large calculus located in the distal ureter. The filling defect of the bladder is due to edema at the ureterovesical junction *(arrowhead)*.

periencing typical symptoms. In such patients, a KUB can identify a stone and show its size and location.

Intravenous Urogram.   The IVU uses time-sequenced contrast-enhanced plain films that highlight the urinary tract (Figs. 19-45 and 19-46).[131] IVU signs confirming renal colic are delayed uptake and excretion of contrast from the involved kidney, hydroureter and hydronephrosis, and identification of the obstructing stone. A normal protocol uses films taken 5, 10, and 20 min postinfusion. A postvoid plain film is obtained to assess the retrovesicular area. The scout film (KUB) is compared with the contrast-enhanced radiographs to identify the obstructing calculus. With high-grade obstruction, excretion of contrast is significantly delayed and the test may take up to 8 hours or longer to complete.

Immediately following the infusion, contrast is promptly taken up by a normal kidney, creating a distinct *nephrogram* on the initial 1-min film. Delayed uptake of contrast (a delayed nephrogram) is a sensitive indicator of ureteral obstruction and renal functional derangement. With acute ureteral obstruction, the delay in uptake is usually only several minutes. With severe, long-standing obstruction, contrast uptake can be delayed 1 h or longer. This is followed by a persistently dense nephrogram. Excretion of contrast into the urinary tract can be delayed up to several hours.

Hydroureter is identified when there is a continuous column of contrast extending from the renal pelvis to the point of obstruction. A normal ureter does not form a continuous contrast column because it tapers and disappears where it is contracted by peristalsis. Although no firm criteria exist, 7 mm is considered the upper limit of normal ureteral diameter in adult males and nulliparous women.

Hydronephrosis causes blunting of the renal calyces and dilation of the renal pelvis and calyces. Comparison with the opposite normal side aids identification of mild hydronephrosis. The degree of hydronephrosis is more dependent on the duration of obstruction than on whether the obstruction is complete or incomplete. In a patient with acute onset of flank pain, moderate or severe hydronephrosis is not expected. With chronic obstruction, hydronephrosis is marked and there may be thinning of the renal parenchyma.

Identification of the ureteral stone defines the cause of obstruction. The dilated ureter is followed to the point of blockage to identify the location of the stone. Ureteral contrast can prevent visualization of a calculus, so the scout film is reviewed to identify the stone. Although about 85% of stones are calcified, only about 65 to 75% of stones are conclusively identified on IVU. Some 10 to 15% of stones are radiolucent (mainly uric acid stones) and are identified on IVU as a filling defect in the contrast-enhanced ureter.

Computed Tomography.   Unenhanced helical CT will likely supplant IVU as the imaging "gold standard in the diagnosis of renal colic."[132–136] The primary CT diagnostic criterion for renal colic as the cause of flank pain is demonstration of a high-attenuation stone within a well-visualized ureter or at the ureterovesical junction. Secondary signs of ureteral obstruction

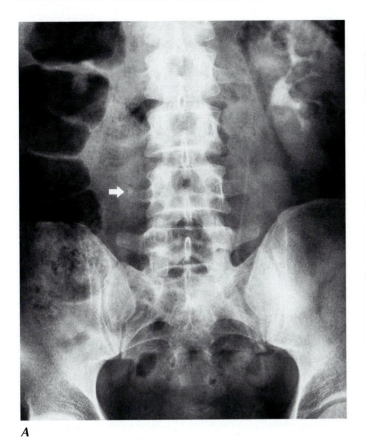
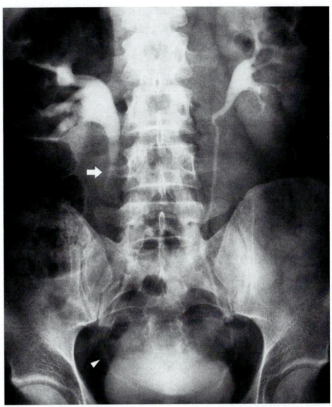

A   *B*

FIGURE 19-46.   Renal colic due to a left midureteral stone. *A.* The 5-min IVU radiograph shows a 5-mm calcification near the right L4 transverse process *(arrow).* The calcification has the typical angular shape and uniform calcification of a kidney stone. On the left, there is a normal nephrogram, which appeared promptly after the contrast infusion. Contrast is seen in the renal pelvis and ureter. A nephrogram is not seen on the right. *B.* The 20-min film shows hydronephrosis and hydroureter on the right extending down to the level of the obstructing calculus *(arrow).* Contrast is seen in the distal ureter, implying that the ureter is not completely obstructed *(arrowhead).* (Copyright David T. Schwartz, M.D.)

are unilateral dilatation of the involved ureter, dilatation of the intrarenal collecting system, and stranding of perinephric fat (Fig. 19-47).[137]

In the evaluation of patients with acute flank pain suggestive of renal colic, CT and IVU are equally efficacious in detecting hydronephrosis and hydroureter, while CT has superior sensitivity in identifying a stone.[132,133] CT can detect 95 to 98% of obstructing stones (including uric acid stones that are not visible on IVU). Secondary signs of ureteral obstruction are seen in 90 to 95% of cases.[137]

Noncontrast CT is ideal in patients allergic to contrast media or in patients with preexisting renal insufficiency. CT offers the further advantage of detecting nonurinary causes of acute flank pain, such as appendicitis, diverticulitis, and an AAA. However, the diagnostic accuracy of a noncontrast CT for these other disorders is reduced in comparison to a contrast CT. For example, the sensitivity of CT for the diagnosis of appendicitis is reduced from 98 to 90% without the use of oral and intravenous contrast.[82,83]

One area of CT interpretation difficulty, particularly in medical centers less experienced in the CT diagnosis of urolithiasis, is distinguishing distal ureteral stones from pelvic phleboliths. A rim of edematous ureteral tissue or localization of the stone at the UVJ often helps make this distinction. Occa-

sionally, administration of intravenous contrast may be necessary to trace the path of the ureter.

Ultrasonography.   Ultrasound is 77 to 94% sensitive in detecting ureteral obstruction.[138–141] Hydronephrosis is the principal ultrasound finding (see Chap. 21, fig. 21-5). Because ultrasonography is dependent on this single finding, it has less diagnostic sensitivity than IVU or CT. Hydronephrosis might not be seen if the ureteral obstruction is acute or if the patient is dehydrated. In addition, the cause and location of the obstruction can usually not be determined by ultrasonography. Renal or proximal ureteral stones may occasionally be seen. A UVJ stone may be seen on a sonogram of the bladder. US is valuable in pregnant patients and in those with renal insufficiency or contrast allergy (although CT is a better alternative in the latter). Ultrasound can also image the abdominal aorta, gallbladder, appendix, and female pelvic organs. Sonography can detect renal lesions such as tumors and cysts.

Bedside sonography in the ED may have a role in screening patients for further diagnostic testing. In a patient with a high clinical likelihood of renal colic and microscopic hematuria, a rapid bedside sonogram showing hydronephrosis might obviate the need for IVU or CT. If hydronephrosis is not seen and the clinical picture is atypical or there is no hematuria, then

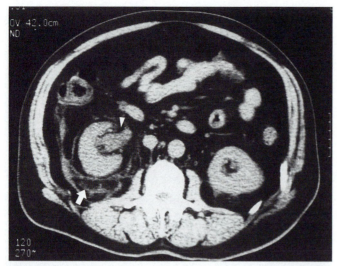

A

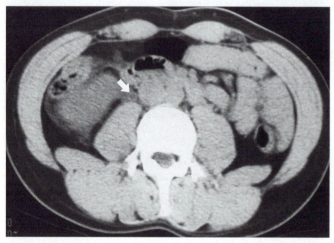

B

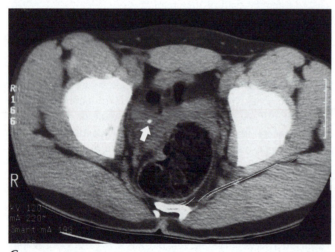

C

FIGURE 19-47. A noncontrast helical CT of a patient with right flank pain. *A.* There is hydronephrosis *(arrowhead)* and stranding of the perinephric fat *(arrow)*. *B.* There is hydroureter on the right *(arrow)*. The left ureter cannot be seen on this noncontrast study. *C.* In the pelvis, there is a 2-mm stone in the distal ureter *(arrow)*. (Copyright David T. Schwartz, M.D.)

a double-contrast CT rather than an IVU or noncontrast CT may be warranted.[142,143]

Abdominal Aortic Aneurysm

Abdominal aortic aneurysms (AAA) may be identified as an asymptomatic incidental finding on physical examination, may cause abdominal or back pain due to gradual leakage or expansion, or present as catastrophic exsanguination when ruptured.[144] The aorta is a high-pressure blood vessel and a tear in its wall would be expected to result in rapid exsanguination. However, gradual leakage from an aortic aneurysm is possible because the aneurysm wall is usually lined with thick, protective mural thrombus. The most common erroneous alternative diagnosis is renal colic, and AAA should always be considered in elderly patients with flank pain.[145,146] AAA leakage can cause microscopic hematuria. Three imaging modalities can be used for AAA—plain radiography, CT, or ultrasound—with the choice of imaging study depending on the clinical scenario.

Hemodynamically unstable patients thought to have a rapidly leaking or ruptured AAA should go directly to the operating room without waiting for imaging studies. For those patients who are stable, the most useful imaging studies for an AAA are CT and US.

On *plain radiographs,* from 55 to 85% of AAAs have enough calcium to be detected. Calcified aneurysms on supine views of the abdomen appear to the left of the vertebrae. A cross-table lateral radiograph can be obtained in patients suspected of having an AAA to look for an eccentric calcified aorta anterior to the vertebral column (Fig. 19-48). When seen, the size of the aneurysm can be estimated. However, this can be misleading if the inner surface of the thrombus rather than the wall of the aneurysm is calcified. Occasionally, leakage from the aneurysm into the retroperitoneum is seen as increased soft tissue density adjacent to the vertebral column, which can obscure the psoas margins.

Computed tomography easily identifies AAAs (Fig. 19-49).[147,148] CT can demonstrate mural thickness, thrombus, contained hemorrhage, and rupture. Intravenous contrast opacifies the aortic lumen, although contrast is not always necessary to detect the aneurysm or leakage. CT signs of a *leaking* AAA include an indistinct aortic wall and extravasation of blood into a retroperitoneal hematoma (Fig. 19-50). The major problem with CT is that a potentially unstable patient is outside the monitored environment of the ED. If a complete double-contrast CT is being performed because of other diagnoses under consideration (e.g., diverticulitis or appendicitis), there can be a significant time delay while the patient is drinking oral contrast over a 2-h period. However, if a leaking AAA is being considered, a rapid noncontrast study can be performed. The appropriate surgical service should be notified that such a patient is in the CT suite so that immediate surgery can be initiated if necessary.

Ultrasonography can detect the presence and size of an aneurysm but gives no information regarding leakage or extension into the renal or iliac vessels. Ultrasound is most often

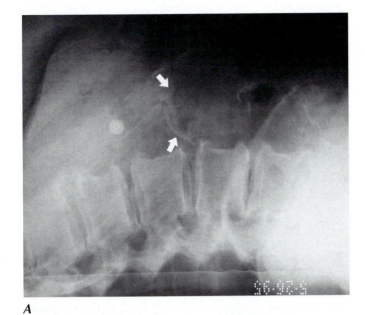

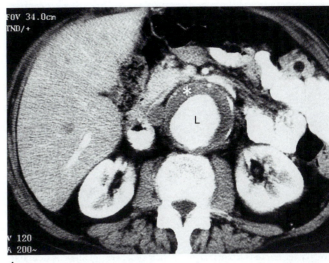

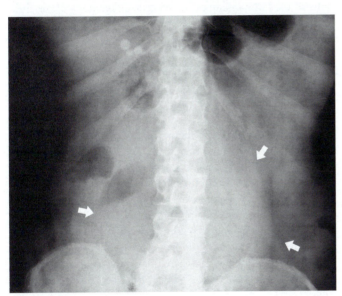

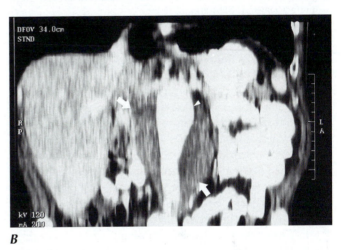

FIGURE 19-48. Abdominal aortic aneurysm. *A.* A cross-table lateral abdominal radiograph shows calcification in the wall of an infrarenal abdominal aortic aneurysm that is 8 cm in diameter *(arrows).* *B.* In another patient, a plain abdominal radiograph demonstrates a leaking abdominal aortic aneurysm detectable by the soft tissue mass seen on both sides of the midabdomen representing retroperitoneal hemorrage *(arrows).*

FIGURE 19-49. *A.* Contrast-enhanced abdominal CT demonstrates a large abdominal aortic aneurysm 7 cm in diameter. The aortic intima is partially calcified and lined with mural thrombus *(asterisk).* The lumen of the aorta is contrast-enhanced (L). There is no evidence of leakage. *B.* Coronal reconstruction of the CT images provides a "CT angiogram" showing contrast in the aortic lumen *(arrowhead)* and surrounding mural thrombus *(arrows).*

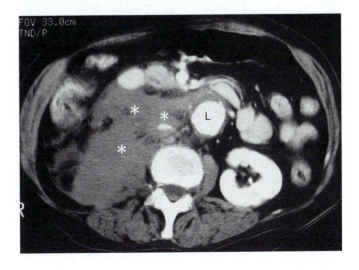

FIGURE 19-50. A leaking abdominal aortic aneurysm. A large amount of blood has collected in the retroperitoneum to the right of the aortic aneurysm *(asterisks).* Contrast material is seen within the aortic lumen (L). Contrast administration is not necessary to show the aortic wall or the retroperitoneal hematoma. The patient was immediately taken to surgery.

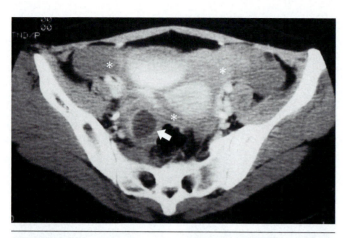

FIGURE 19-51. CT showing a ruptured ovarian cyst in a patient with right lower quadrant abdominal pain who was transiently hypotensive. There is a 3-cm right ovarian cyst (*arrow*) and considerable free fluid in the pelvis surrounding the uterus and bladder (*asterisks*). (Copyright David T. Schwartz, M.D.)

used for confirmation of a suspected AAA, and to electively monitor the size of a known AAA over time. The most consistent indicator of risk of aneurysmal rupture is its diameter. Between 3 and 5 cm, there is less than a 5% chance of rupture; at greater than 6 cm, the risk increases to 16%; and an aneurysm measuring larger than 7 cm has a 76% chance of rupturing.[149]

In the ED, bedside sonography can confirm a suspected AAA. When leaking is suspected, ultrasound does not replace CT in the "stable" patient, nor should it delay laparotomy in the unstable patient. Bedside ultrasound can demonstrate the existence of an aneurysm that may or may not be palpable on physical examination. Bedside ultrasound can be performed rapidly to add support to the diagnosis of AAA in a patient who is too unstable for CT. One caution is that a ruptured AAA may collapse, and its size could be underestimated by US.

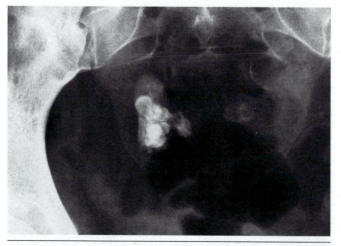

FIGURE 19-52. Abdominal radiograph of a woman with right lower quadrant abdominal pain demonstrating an ovarian teratoma (dermoid cyst) with calcified tooth buds. Doppler ultrasonography demonstrated good blood flow to the ovary, excluding ovarian torsion. (Copyright David T. Schwartz, M.D.)

Gynecologic Emergencies

The possibility of pregnancy and the paucity of clinically useful information about the female pelvic organs on plain radiographs militate against routine roentgenographic imaging in women with a potential obstetric or gynecologic emergency. Transabdominal and especially transvaginal ultrasound of the abdomen and pelvis is frequently helpful in the evaluation of acute abdominal pain in women of childbearing age.[150,151] CT is used to further characterize pelvic pain in nonpregnant females in whom ultrasound studies are equivocal or when nongynecologic disorders such as appendicitis or diverticulitis are suspected.

Gynecologic emergencies include *pelvic inflammatory disease* (PID), ovarian torsion, and ovarian cyst rupture. Although PID is largely a clinical diagnosis, ultrasound is useful in visualizing a *tuboovarian abscess*. Endometritis is suggested on ultrasound by a hypoechoic, poorly defined endometrium. If tubal involvement is present, there is fluid within edematous walls of the fallopian tubes. Increased echogenicity of the fluid suggests purulence rather than a simple hydrosalpinx. Ultrasonographic criteria for tuboovarian abscess include thickening and obscuring of the ovarian margins with pyosalpinx. These findings are best appreciated with transvaginal ultrasound. Although pelvic CT can detect a markedly abnormal ovary or pelvic fluid, it is not as helpful as ultrasound in distinguishing an ovarian cyst, abscess or tumor (Fig. 19-51).

Ovarian torsion is uncommon and generally occurs in an ovary harboring a benign neoplasm. Ovarian torsion threatens reproductive capacity and is a surgical emergency. On ultrasound, it appears as a significantly enlarged solid structure. The normal ovary may appear as a solitary structure, may contain a cyst, or may demonstrate peripheral follicles. It can also contain heterogeneous material with a high signal and shadows suggestive of teratoma (dermoid cyst). Teratomas are also seen on plain radiographs when they contain heavily calcified structures sometimes resembling teeth (Fig. 19-52). Doppler ultrasound *(duplex)* probes are useful to assess ovarian blood flow. The absence of flow strongly suggests torsion (Fig. 19-53).

A hemorrhagic ovarian cyst appears as a hypoechoic cystic structure with a fluid-blood level. The cysts can be uniform or may contain septations. A hyperechoic mass may represent a clot within the cyst. A cystic ovary that undergoes torsion may be indistinguishable from a hemorrhagic cyst. Thickened septa within a hemorrhagic cyst can resemble an ovarian neoplasm. If hemorrhage leads to rupture and hemoperitoneum, the cyst may be undetected or appear as an irregular ovarian mass. Ultrasound reliably detects blood within the pelvis. Initially, blood appears diffusely hypoechoic, gradually becoming more irregular and echogenic during the first day and finally returning to diminished echogenicity as clot resolution occurs.

Intraabdominal Abscesses, Cysts, and Masses

Left untreated, the mortality from an abdominal abscess approaches 100%. The most common plain radiographic finding

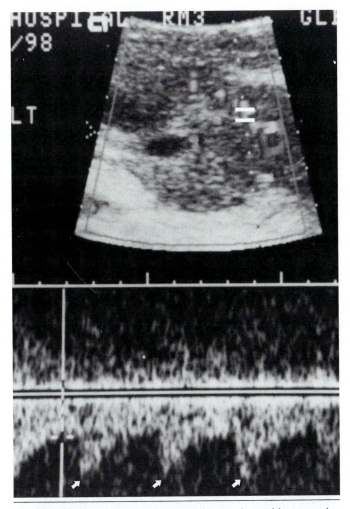

FIGURE 19-53. Doppler ultrasound in a patient with an ovarian cyst, which was causing right lower quadrant abdominal pain. The Doppler probe is placed over the ovarian cyst *(small rectangle)*. The Doppler waveform reveals good pulsatile blood flow, excluding ovarian torsion *(arrows)*. (Copyright David Schwartz, MD)

is a collection of extraluminal air pockets. An air-fluid level increases the specificity of the radiographic diagnosis. Large abdominal masses displace adjacent organs (Fig. 19-8). Subdiaphragmatic abscesses can displace the hemidiaphragm superiorly.

Ultrasound is most useful for evaluating upper abdominal and pelvic fluid collections. Noninfected collections (including cysts) are encapsulated and have few internal echoes. Abscesses appear as ill-defined heterogeneous fluid collections with thickened, irregular borders and prominent internal echoes and debris.[152] Gas is seen within an abscess as a region of increased echogenicity.

CT is more accurate than US in detecting and characterizing abdominal abscesses and fluid collections.[153] On CT, abscesses appear as collections of low-attenuation fluid of intermediate density between water and soft tissue. The intracavitary fluid is more heterogeneous than that within a cyst (Fig. 19-8B). Gas within the collection increases the likelihood of infection (Fig. 19-54 and 19-55). Intravenous contrast enhances the walls of the abscess as well as the surrounding normal parenchyma. CT is superb in its ability to detect retroperitoneal pathology such as a psoas abscess. Both ultrasound and CT can help guide percutaneous drainage procedures.

Ascites

Abdominal plain radiographs are insensitive and nonspecific in visualizing ascites. Ascites is detectable radiographically only when it is massive, by which time the diagnosis is clinically obvious. Ascites has a *ground glass* appearance on plain abdominal radiographs. The ascending or descending colon is displaced from the properitoneal fat stripe as the ascitic fluid collects in the paracolic gutters. Extremely large pelvic fluid collections displace bowel superiorly on upright films.

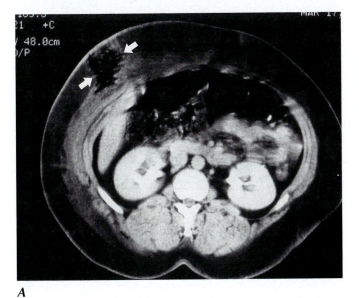
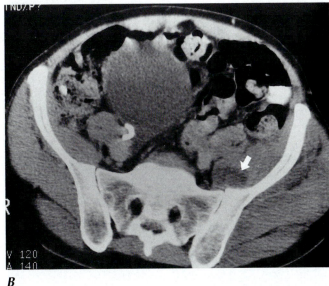

A   *B*

FIGURE 19-54. *A.* CT scan of a patient with abdominal wall cellulitis and a tender fluctuant mass. A collection of gas is seen within the abscess as well as inflammatory changes in the subcutaneus fat *(asterisk)*. The peritoneum is intact. *B.* An ileopsoas abscess is seen in this patient with left lower back pain *(arrow)*.

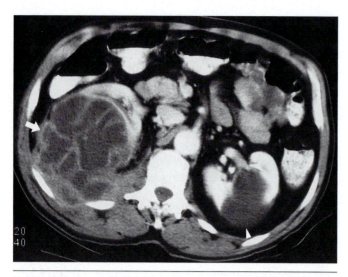

FIGURE 19-55. CT scan of a toxic patient with a tender mass in the right flank. There is a large multilobulated perinephric abscess compressing the right kidney and extending into the surrounding musculature *(arrow)*. A cyst is seen in the left kidney *(arrowhead)*.

On CT, ascites appears as homogeneous free fluid within the abdomen and pelvis (Fig. 19-20*C*). Associated findings include hepatosplenomegaly, a shrunken, cirrhotic liver, diffuse bowel wall thickening, hepatic vein thrombosis, hepatic malignancy, and metastatic disease.

Ultrasound is useful both for detecting ascites and for guiding paracentesis when the fluid collection is not obvious or the patient is coagulopathic. Ascitic fluid appears as a homogeneous echolucent region in dependent intraperitoneal recesses.

Foreign-Body Ingestion

Many ingested or inserted foreign bodies have some degree of radiopacity and can be identified on plain radiographs (Fig. 19-56).[154] Grapes, hot dogs, peanuts, and small pieces of aluminum and wood are not radiopaque. Common childhood ingestions that are easily seen include coins, button batteries, and small toys. Coins lodged in the esophagus are seen *en face* in the frontal plane and on edge in the lateral view.[155] The oppo-

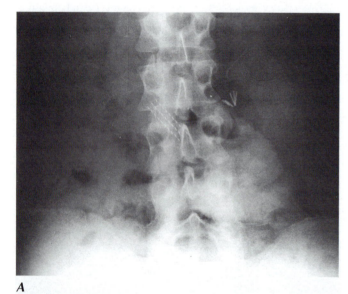

A

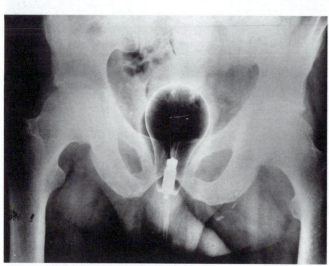

B

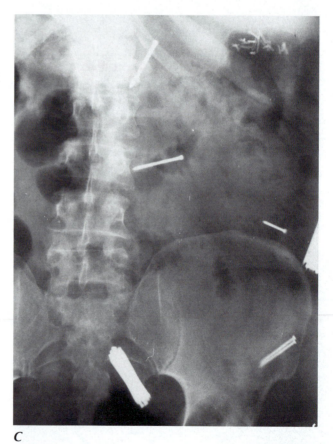

C

FIGURE 19-56. *A.* A patient who had ingested a toothbrush. Only the bristles are visible on the radiograph. This elongated object will not pass out of the stomach and must be removed by endoscopy. *B.* A light bulb inserted into the rectum must be removed carefully (under general anesthesia). *C.* A patient with a psychiatric disorder ingested several nails. Such sharp objects usually become imbedded in fecal material and pass uneventfully through the intestines. (*A.* and *B.* Copyright David T. Schwartz, M.D.)

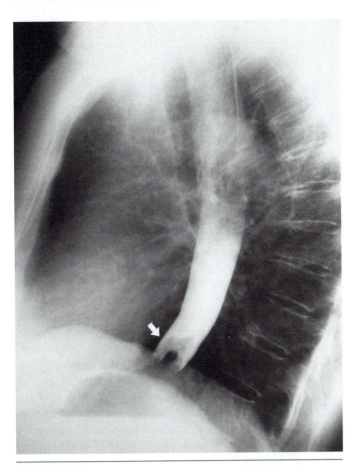

FIGURE 19-57. A food bolus lodged in the distal esophagus was seen on a contrast esophagram. The obstructing material was pushed into the stomach during upper endoscopy. If the patient is completely obstructed and immediate endoscopy is planned, radiographic imaging is not necessary. Barium retained in the esophagus makes endoscopy difficult. Water-soluble contrast causes chemical pneumonitis if aspirated.

site is true of tracheal foreign bodies. On plain frontal radiographs, button batteries demonstrate a "step off" on a lateral view, in contrast to the smooth appearance of coins.[156] Esophageal perforation can occur in children only 6 hours after a button battery is ingested.[157] A food bolus causing esophageal impaction is unlikely to cause immediate perforation but may cause pressure necrosis and delayed perforation (Fig. 19-57). Radiographs of the soft tissues of the neck and chest may show an air-fluid level if there is complete obstruction.

One practice among drug smugglers is "body packing," swallowing securely sealed latex packages filled with illicit drugs. Although cocaine and other drugs of abuse are intrinsically radiolucent, the packets often appear as rounded or oblong intraluminal structures, detectable because of the contrast provided by the packaging.[158] (See Chap. 23, "Toxicologic Emergencies.")

Esophageal Abnormalities

Esophageal disease usually presents with symptoms related to the chest.[159,160] The main radiographic finding of esophageal

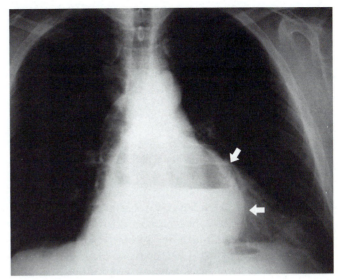

A

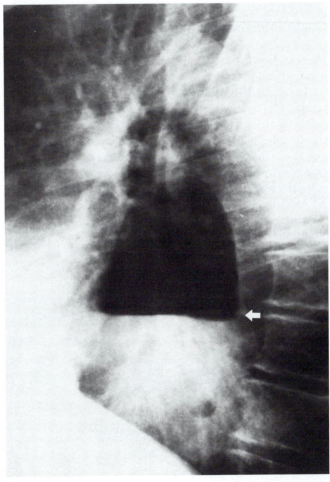

B

FIGURE 19-58. A large hiatal hernia has allowed the stomach to enter the thorax. A stomach air-fluid level is seen in the mediastinum.

perforation on the chest radiograph is pneumomediastinum, although pneumomediastinum most often this results from pulmonary disease. A widened mediastinum suggests mediastinitis, which often complicates esophageal perforation. Other radiographic signs of esophageal perforation include pneumothorax, pleural effusion, and subcutaneous emphysema.[161] *Boerhaave's syndrome* is rupture of the distal esophagus usually following an episode of vomiting. Although the classic clinical triad consists of vomiting, chest pain, and subcutaneous emphysema, 75% of patients have abdominal pain.[162,163]

A *hiatal hernia* may be detected on a plain chest radiograph if it is large enough to cause mass effect. A soft tissue density is typically located at the left posterolateral aspect of the mediastinum (Fig. 19-58). A hiatal hernia is best characterized by an esophagram. *Achalasia* is the most common esophageal motility disorder. Findings of achalasia on plain chest radiography include air-fluid levels within a dilated esophagus. Similar findings are seen in mechanical esophageal obstruction.

Gastrointestinal Hemorrhage

There are no plain radiographic signs of GI hemorrhage. If patients are in hypovolemic shock, they require emergent surgical intervention or perhaps embolization therapy in an interventional radiology suite. Endoscopy and colonoscopy are replacing radiographic imaging for the evaluation of ongoing GI bleeding.[164] GI bleeding that remains undiagnosed after attempts at direct visualization can be further evaluated by angiography or technetium-99m bleeding scans.

Angiography is most useful if the rate of bleeding is between 0.5 and 1.0 mL/min, while the nuclear medicine scans (bleeding scan) detect bleeding between 0.1 and 0.5 mL/min. The angiographic catheter is positioned under fluoroscopic guidance near the site of a suspected bleed. Extravasation of dye con-

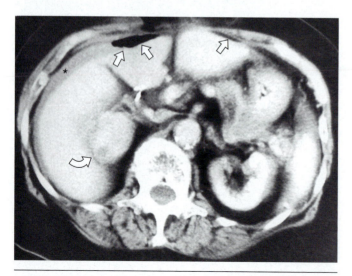

FIGURE 19-59. CT demonstrating a hepatic laceration *(curved arrow)* and intraperitoneal hemorrhage *(asterisk)* in an 85-year-old woman who had fallen at home. Free intraperitoneal air *(arrows)* was due to a laceration of the small bowel.

firms the source. After sufficient collateral flow to the region of hemorrhage has been ensured, the bleeding is stopped by infusion of vasopressin, a potent vasoconstrictor. If this fails, embolization is attempted.[165]

Bleeding scans are performed by infusing a patient's own radioactively labeled erythrocytes or labeled sulfur colloid. A positive scan demonstrates pooling of the radioactive tracer in the involved region of bowel.

Blunt Abdominal Trauma

Although abdominal plain radiographs are of limited help in evaluating victims of blunt trauma, the *chest radiograph* is useful in the trauma patient with intraabdominal injury. It is especially important because physical examination is a poor predictor of the presence of intraabdominal injury. Roughly 20% of patients with a left lower rib fracture after blunt trauma have a splenic injury. Lower right rib fractures warrant concern about hepatic injury. Free air under the diaphragm due to perforation of a hollow viscus is easily seen on an upright chest radiograph. When there is diaphragmatic rupture, herniated abdominal contents are seen within the thoracic cavity.

Computed tomography is the primary imaging modality for stable patients suspected of having an intraabdominal injury from blunt trauma. CT reliably detects hemoperitoneum (96-99% sensitive) as well as injuries to solid organs. CT is 96 to 99% sensitive in its ability to detect hemoperitoneum.[166–170]

Bedside ultrasonography. *Bedside ultrasonography* is used in victims of blunt abdominal trauma to rapidly identify hemoperitoneum. Its principal application is in the hemodynamically unstable patient who would otherwise need a diagnostic peritoneal lavage (DPL) to identify intraperitoneal hemorrhage.[171–173] Ultrasound has the further advantage that serial examinations may be performed to detect ongoing hemorrhage. In some centers, ultrasound has supplanted the use of DPL.[174–176] The accuracy of ultrasound in evaluating blunt trauma is highly operator-dependent.[177] Ultrasound is not as useful as CT in detecting solid organ or retroperitoneal injury. The diagnosis of hemoperitoneum by ultrasound requires routine examination of all dependent regions for free fluid. These include the hepatorenal fossa (Morison pouch), the paracolic gutters, the perisplenic spaces, the perihepatic spaces, and the pelvis.

Computed Tomography. On CT, blood typically has intermediate density (about 45 HU) and may be isodense with adjacent tissue. Streaks of extravasated intravenous contrast material within regions of clot are a sign of active and rapid hemorrhage.

The spleen is the most commonly injured organ in blunt abdominal trauma. Radiographic clues to splenic injury on the chest film include elevation of the left hemidiaphragm, left pleural effusion, or left hemothorax. The ideal imaging modality for detecting splenic injuries is CT.

The liver is the second most commonly injured organ in blunt abdominal trauma. Injury to the left hepatic lobe is rare but should alert one to the possibility of a concomitant pancreatic or duodenal injury. On contrast CT, hepatic lacerations are low in attenuation compared with the normal-appearing liver parenchyma. Lacerations may be linear or irregular (likened to a bear claw) and may be continuous with regions of contusion or hematoma (Fig. 19-59). Hematomas may be intrahepatic or subcapsular.

The kidneys are the third most frequently injured viscera in blunt abdominal trauma. Although hematuria is the hallmark of injury to the genitourinary system, its absence does not exclude damage, especially in the presence of hypotension. Patients going to emergency laparotomy should have a one-shot IVU performed to verify that they have two functioning kidneys or to detect renal parenchymal or ureteral injury. Nonvisualization of a kidney on IVU is strongly suggestive of a renovascular injury.

Hollow viscus injuries are notoriously difficult to see on CT. However, CT may detect bowel wall thickening, fluid, or hematomas around an injured area. Isolated injury to the duodenum or pancreas is relatively rare in blunt abdominal trauma. A pleural effusion on chest film may indicate a duodenal or, more commonly, a pancreatic injury. Free air may be detectable on a cross-table lateral abdominal film as well as on CT. (See Chap. 20, "Radiographic Priorities in Trauma.")

ERRORS IN INTERPRETATION

Plain Abdominal Radiography

Pneumoperitoneum. While free air within the abdomen is abnormal, it does not always indicate a surgical emergency. Benign causes of pneumoperitoneum include recent laparoscopic procedures, peritoneal dialysis, or the introduction of air through the fallopian tubes. Pulmonary conditions such as pneumothorax, recent intubation, and chronic obstructive pulmonary disease can lead to the dissection of air from peribronchial spaces into the mediastinum and then to the retroperitoneum, from which it may follow the course of the mesenteric vessels into the peritoneum. Free peritoneal air can be mimicked by basal atelectasis, subphrenic fat, a subphrenic abscess, or by interposition of air-filled loops of bowel above the liver.

Bowel Obstruction. Air-fluid levels in the diagnosis of bowel obstruction are nonspecific. One or two air-fluid levels on an upright abdominal radiograph in an otherwise fluid-filled abdomen increase the likelihood that an obstructing lesion exists (Fig. 19-19). CT may confirm the diagnosis or uncover alternative pathology.

Calcifications. Calcifications may be the only radiographic clue to significant intraabdominal disease, especially when they outline a large aneurysm or represent an abdominal malignancy. More frequently, calcifications are benign. Bismuth mimicking acute pancreatitis, bubble gum within the stomach, and a rectal foreign body misdiagnosed as colonic cancer are all examples of items that may resemble pathologic calcifications.[178–180]

COMMON VARIANTS

The interposition of radiolucent tissues such as fat or air trapped in skin folds may cause findings that are confused with pathology. A rib shadow, fat beneath the diaphragm, or air within the stomach or intestine can mimic pneumoperitoneum. Colonic interposition, particularly in children, also mimics pneumoperitoneum. These situations are often clarified by insufflating air into the stomach through a nasogastric tube, repositioning the patient, or obtaining a CT. The posterior margins of the lung, lobes of the liver, and stomach contents simulate masses in the abdomen. Gas is occasionally found within the appendix, but this is not necessarily pathologic. Calcifications within the abdomen can mimic gallstones, renal and ureteral stones, or appendicoliths. Calcifications of the costal cartilage that are circular and overlie the gallbladder can be confused with cholelithiasis. Phleboliths and calcified lymph nodes can appear in the right upper or lower quadrants overlying the kidneys and ureters, mimicking gallstones, an appendicolith, or renal stones. Vessels can display segmental calcifications that are confused with pathology.

REFERENCES

1. Brewer RJ, Golden GT, Hitch DC, et al: Abdominal pain—An analysis of 1,000 consecutive cases in a university hospital emergency room. *Am J Surg* 131:219, 1976.
2. Powers RD, Guertler AT: Abdominal pain in the ED: Stability and change over 20 years. *Am J Emerg Med* 13:301, 1995.
3. Lukens TW, Emerman C, Effron D: The natural history and clinical findings in undifferentiated abdominal pain. *Ann Emerg Med* 22:690, 1993.
4. Greene CS: Indications for plain abdominal radiography in the emergency department. *Ann Emerg Med* 15:257, 1986.
5. Eisenberg RL, Heineken P, Hedgcock MW, et al: Evaluation of plain abdominal radiographs in the diagnosis of abdominal pain. *Ann Surg* 197:464, 1983.
6. Rosenbaum HD, Lieber A, Hanson DO, et al: A routine survey roentgenogram of the abdomen on 500 consecutive patients over the age of 40. *AJR* 91:903, 1964.
7. Harris JH Jr: In defense of plain abdominal radiography. *Ann Emerg Med* 11:48, 1982.
8. McCook TA, Ravin CE, Rice RP: Abdominal radiography in the emergency department: A prospective analysis. *Ann Emerg Med* 11:7, 1982.
9. Campbell JPM, Gunn AA: Plain abdominal radiographs and acute abdominal pain. *Br J Surg* 75:554, 1988.
10. Velanovich V: Plain abdominal radiographs and acute abdominal pain. *Br J Surg* 75:1147, 1988.
11. de Lacey GJ, Wignall BK, Bradbrooke S, et al: Rationalising abdominal radiography in the accident and emergency department. *Clin Radiol* 31:453,1980.
12. Mindelzun RE, Jeffrey RB: Unenhaced helical CT for evaluating acute abdominal pain: A little more cost, a lot more information. *Radiology* 205:43, 1997.

13. Baker SR: Unenhanced CT versus plain abdominal radiography: A dissenting opinion. *Radiology* 205:45, 1997.

14. American College of Emergency Physicians: *Cost Effective Diagnostic Testing in Emergency Medicine.* Dallas: American College of Emergency Physicians, 1994.

15. Flak B, Rowley VA: Acute abdomen: Plain film utilization and analysis. *Can Assoc Radiol J* 44:423, 1993.

16. Bohner H, Yang Q, Franke C, et al: Simple data from history and physical examination help to exclude bowel obstruction and to avoid radiographic studies in patients with acute abdominal pain. *Eur J Surg* 164:777, 1998.

17. Bugliosi TF, Meloy TD, Vukov LF: Acute abdominal pain in the elderly. *Ann Emerg Med* 19:1383, 1990.

18. Telfer S, Fenyo G, Holt PR, et al: Acute abdominal pain in patients over 50 years of age. *Scand J Gastroenterol Supp* 144:47, 1988.

19. Cina SJ, Mims WW, Nichols CA, Conradi SE: From emergency room to morgue: Deaths due to undiagnosed perforated peptic ulcers. *Am J Forensic Med Pathol* 15:21, 1994.

20. Rothrock SG, Green SM, Hummel CB: Plain abdominal radiography in the detection of major disease in children: A prospective analysis. *Ann Emerg Med* 21:1423, 1992.

21. Balthazar EJ (ed): Imaging the acute abdomen. *Radiol Clin North Am* 32:829, 1994.

22. Balthazar EJ, Rofsky NM, Zucker R: Appendicitis: The impact of computed tomography imaging on negative laparotomy and perforation rates. *Am J Gastroenterol* 93:768, 1998.

23. Rao PM, Rhea JT, Novelline RA, et al: Effect of computed tomography of the appendix on treatment of patients and use of hospital resources. *N Engl J Med* 338:141, 1998.

24. Nordenholz KE, Rubin M, Kelen GD (eds): The use of ultrasound in the emergency department. *Emerg Med Clin North Am* 15:735, 1997.

25. Mirvis SE, Young JW, Keramati B, et al: Plain film evaluation of patients with abdominal pain: Are three radiographs necessary? *AJR* 147:501, 1986.

26. Simpson A, Sandeman D, Nixon SJ, et al: The value of an erect abdominal radiograph in the diagnosis of intestinal obstruction. *Clin Radiol* 36:41, 1985.

27. Cho KC, Baker SR: Extraluminal air: Diagnosis and significance. *Radiol Clin North Am* 32:829, 1994.

28. Shaffer HA Jr: Perforation and obstruction of the gastrointestinal tract. *Radiol Clin North Am* 30:405, 1992.

29. Markus JB, Somers S, Franic SE, et al: Interobserver variation in the interpretation of abdominal radiographs. *Radiology* 171:69, 1989.

30. Suh RS, Maglinte DDT, Lavonas EJ, et al: Emergency abdominal radiography: Discrepancies of preliminary and final interpretation and management relevance. *Emerg Radiol* 2:315, 1995.

31. Patel NH, Lauber PR: The meaning of a nonspecific abdominal gas pattern. *Acad Radiol* 2:667, 1995.

32. Maglinte DDT: Nonspecific abdominal gas pattern: An interpretation whose time has gone. *Emerg Radiol* 3:93, 1996.

33. Keene JG: Pneumatosis cystoides intestinalis and intramural intestinal gas. *J Emerg Med* 7:645, 1989.

34. Miller RE, Nelson SW: The roentgenological demonstration of tiny amounts of free intraperitoneal gas: Experimental and clinical studies. *AJR* 112:574, 1971.

35. Miller RE: The radiologic evaluation of intraperitoneal gas (pneumoperitoneum). *CRC Crit Rev Radiol Sci* 4:61, 1973.

36. Miller RE, Becker GJ, Slabaugh RD: Detection of pneumoperitoneum: Optimum body position and respiratory phase. *AJR* 135:487, 1980.

37. Woodring JH, Heiser MJ: Detection of pneumoperitoneum on chest radiographs: Comparison of upright lateral and posteroanterior projections. *AJR* 165:45, 1995.

38. Markowitz SK, Ziter FM: The lateral chest film and pneumoperitoneum. *Ann Emerg Med* 15:425, 1986.

39. Miller RE, Becker GJ, Slabaugh RD: Nonsurgical pneumoperitoneum. *Gastrointest Radiol* 6:73, 1981.

40. Nelson RL, Abcarian H, Prasad ML: Iatrogenic perforation of the colon and rectum. *Dis Colon Rectum* 25:305, 1982.

41. Lee CW, Yip AW, Lam KH: Pneumogastrogram in the diagnosis of perforated peptic ulcer. *Aust N Z J Surg* 63:459, 1993.

42. Maull KI, Reath DB: Pneumogastrography in the diagnosis of perforated peptic ulcer. *Am J Surg* 148:340, 1984.

43. Stapakis JC, Thickman D: Diagnosis of pneumoperitoneum: Abdominal CT versus upright chest film. *J Comput Assist Tomogr* 16:713, 1992.

44. Levin B: Mechanical small bowel obstruction. *Semin Roentgenol* 8:281, 1973.

45. Golden DA, Gefter WB, Gohel VK: Digital examination of the rectum as a source of rectal gas. *Radiology* 141:618, 1981.

46. Harlow CL, Stears RL, Zeligman BE, et al: Diagnosis of bowel obstruction on plain abdominal radiographs: Significance of air-fluid levels at different heights in the same loop of bowel. *AJR* 161:291, 1993.

47. Mucha P: Small intestinal obstruction. *Surg Clin North Am* 67:597, 1987.

48. Shrake PD, Rex DK, Lappas JC, et al: Radiographic evaluation of suspected small bowel obstruction. *Am J Gastroenterol* 86:175, 1991.

49. Megibow AJ, Balthazar EJ, Cho KC, et al: Bowel obstruction: Evaluation with CT. *Radiology* 180:313, 1991.

50. Balthazar EJ: CT of small bowel obstruction. *AJR* 162:255, 1994.

51. Maglinte DD, Reyes BL, Harmon BH: Reliability and role of plain film radiography and CT in the diagnosis of small-bowel obstruction. *AJR* 167:1451, 1996.

52. Fukuya T, Hawes DR, Lu CC, et al: CT diagnosis of small bowel obstruction: Efficacy in 60 patients. *AJR* 158:765, 1992.

53. Gazelle GS, Goldberg MA, Wittenberg J: Efficacy of CT in distinguishing small-bowel obstruction from other causes of small-bowel dilatation. *AJR* 162:43, 1994.

54. Frager D, Medwid SW, Baer JW, et al: CT of small-bowel obstruction: Value in establishing the diagnosis and determining the degree and cause. *AJR* 162:37, 1994.

55. Maglinte DDT, Herlinger H, et al: Radiologic management of small bowel obstruction: A practical approach. *Emerg Radiol* 1:138, 1994.

56. Balthazar EJ, et al: Closed-loop and strangulating obstruction: CT signs. *Radiology* 185:769, 1992.

57. Balthazar EJ, Liebeskind ME, Macari M: Intestinal ischemia in patients in whom small bowel obstruction is suspected: Evaluation of accuracy, limitations, and clinical implications of CT in diagnosis. *Radiology* 205:519, 1997.

58. Ha HK, Kim JS, Lee MS: Differentiation of simple and strangulated small-bowel obstructions: Usefulness of known CT criteria. *Radiology* 204:507, 1997.

59. Frager D, Baer JW, Medwid SW, et al: Detection of intestinal ischemia in patients with acute small-bowel obstruction due to adhesions or hernia: Efficacy of CT. *AJR* 166:67, 1996.

60. Young TK, et al: Small bowel obstruction: Sonographic evaluation. *Radiology* 188:649, 1993.

61. Ogata M, Mateer JR, Condon RE: Prospective evaluation of abdominal sonography for the diagnosis of bowel obstruction. *Ann Surg* 223:237, 1996.

62. Czechowski J: Conventional radiography and ultrasonography in the diagnosis of small bowel obstruction and strangulation. *Acta Radiol* 37:186, 1996.

63. Frimann-Dahl J: Strangulating obstruction of the small bowel with special reference to cases with poor roentgen findings. *Acta Radiol* 25:480, 1944.

64. Mellins HZ, Rigler LG: The roentgen findings in strangulation obstruction of the small intestine. *AJR* 71:404, 1954.

65. Reisner RM, Cohen JR: Gallstone ileus: A review of 1001 reported cases. *Am Surg* 60:441, 1994.

66. Day EA, Marks C: Gallstone ileus: Review of the literature and presentations of thirty-four new cases. *Am J Surg* 129:552, 1975.

67. Rigler LG, Borman CN, Noble JF: Gallstone obstruction: Pathogenesis and roentgen manifestations. *JAMA* 117:1753, 1941.

68. Loren I, Lasson A, Nilsson A, et al: Gallstone ileus demonstrated by CT. *J Comput Assist Tomogr* 18:262, 1994.

69. Wittenberg J: The diagnosis of colonic obstruction on plain abdominal radiographs: Start with the cecum, leave the rectum to last. *AJR* 161:443, 1993.

70. Love L: Large bowel obstruction. *Semin Roentgenol* 8:299, 1973.

71. Bryk D: The altered colon and colonic obstruction. *AJR* 115:360, 1972.

72. Lowman RM, Davis L: Evaluation of cecal size in impending perforation of the cecum. *Surg Gynecol Obstet* 103:711, 1956.

73. Novy S, Rogers LF, Kirkpatrick W: Diastatic rupture of the cecum in obstructing carcinoma of the left colon. *AJR* 123:281, 1975.

74. Chapman AH, McNamara M, Porter G: The acute contrast enema in suspected large bowel obstruction: Value and technique. *Clin Radiol* 46:273, 1992.

75. Anderson JR, Mills JO: Caecal volvulus: A frequently missed diagnosis. *Clin Radiol* 35:65, 1984.

76. Burrel HC, Baker DM, Wardrop P, et al: Significant plain film findings in sigmoid volvulus. *Clin Radiol* 49:317, 1994.

77. Lewis FR, Holcroft JW, Boey J, et al: Appendicitis: A critical review of diagnosis and treatment in 1,000 cases. *Arch Surg* 110:677, 1975.

78. Baker SR: Acute appendicitis: Plain radiographic considerations. *Emerg Radiol* 3:63, 1996.

79. Gelfand DW: Questions and answers. *AJR* 164:763, 1995.

80. Balthazar EJ, Megibow AJ, Siegel SE, et al: Appendicitis: Prospective evaluation with high-resolution CT. *Radiology* 180:21, 1991.

81. Balthazar, EJ, Birnbaum BA, Yee J, et al: Acute appendicitis: CT and US correlation in 100 patients. *Radiology* 190:31, 1995.

82. Rao PM, Rhea JT, Novelline RA: Focused appendiceal computed tomography: Technique and interpretation. *Emerg Radiol* 4:268, 1997.

83. Lane MJ, Katz DS, Ross BA, et al: Unenhanced helical CT for suspected acute appendicitis. *AJR* 168:405, 1997.

84. Orr RK, Porter D, Hartman D: Ultrasonography to evaluate adults for appendicitis: Decision making based on meta-analysis and probabilistic reasoning. *Acad Emerg Med* 2:644, 1995.

85. Crady SK, Jones JS, Wyn T, Luttenton CR: Clinical validity of ultrasound in children with suspected appendicitis. *Ann Emerg Med* 22:1125, 1993.

86. Puylaert JB, Rutgers PH, Lalisang RI, et al: A prospective study of ultrasonography in the diagnosis of appendicitis. *N Engl J Med* 317:666, 1987.

87. Ferzoco LB, Raptopoulos V, Silen W: Acute diverticulitis. *N Engl J Med* 338:1521, 1998.

88. Cho KC, Morehouse HT, Alterman DD, Thornhill BA: Sigmoid diverticulitis: Diagnostic role of CT—Comparison with barium enema studies. *Radiology* 176:111, 1990.

89. Ambrosetti P, Grossholtz M, Becker C, et al: Computed tomography in acute left colonic diverticulitis. *Br J Surg* 84:532, 1997.

90. Jacob JE, Birnbaum BA: CT of inflammatory disease of the colon. *Semin Ultrasound CT MRI* 16:91, 1995.

91. Fishman EK, Kavuru M, Jones B, et al: Pseudomembranous colitis: CT evaluation of 26 cases. *Radiology* 180:57, 1991.

92. Goldberg HI, Gore RM, Margulis AR, et al: Computed tomography in the evaluation of Crohn's disease. *AJR* 140:277, 1983.

93. Present DH: Toxic megacolon. *Med Clin North Am* 77:1129, 1993.

94. Beaugerie L, Ngo Y, Goujard F, et al: Etiology and management of toxic megacolon in patients with human immunodeficiency virus infection. *Gastroenterology* 107:858, 1994.

95. McKinsey JF, Gewertz BL: Acute mesenteric ischemia. *Surg Clin North Am* 77:307, 1997.

96. Boley SJ, Brandt LJ (ed): Intestinal ischemia. *Surg Clin North Am* 72:1, 1992.

97. Wolf EL, et al: Radiology in intestinal ischemia: Plain film, contrast, and other imaging studies. *Surg Clin North Am* 72:107, 1992.

98. Klein HM, Lensing R, Klosterhalfen B, et al: Diagnostic imaging of mesenteric infarction. *Radiology* 197:79, 1995.

99. Balthazar EJ, Hulnick D, Megibow AJ, Opulencia JF: Computed tomography of intramural intestinal hemorrhage and bowel ischemia. *J Comput Assist Tomogr* 11:67, 1987.

100. Smerud MJ, Johnson CD, Stephens DH: Diagnosis of bowel infarction: A comparison of plain films and CT scans in 23 cases. *AJR* 154:99, 1990.

101. Yamada K, Saeki M, Yamaguchi T: Acute mesenteric ischemia: CT and plain radiographic analysis of 26 cases. *Clin Imaging* 22:34, 1998.

102. Wyatt SH, Fishman EK: The acute abdomen in individuals with AIDS. *Radiol Clin North Am* 32:1023, 1994.

103. Jones BJ, Fishman EK: CT of the gut in the immunocompromised host. *Radiol Clin North Am* 27:763, 1989.

104. Brandon JC, Glick SN, Teplick SK, et al: Emphysematous cholecystitis: Pitfalls in its plain film diagnosis. *Gastrointest Radiol* 13:33, 1988.

105. Jolly BT, Love JN: Emphysematous cholecystitis in an elderly woman: Case report and review of the literature. *J Emerg Med* 11:593, 1993.

106. Hudson PA, Promes SB: Abdominal ultrasonography. *Emerg Med Clin North Am* 15:825, 1997.

107. Laing FC, Federle MP, Jeffrey RB, Brown TW: Ultrasonic evaluation of patients with acute right upper quadrant pain. *Radiology* 140:449, 1981.

108. Jeffrey RB, Laing FC, Wong W, Callen PW, et al: Gangrenous cholecystitis: Diagnosis by ultrasound. *Radiology* 148:219, 1983.

109. Ralls PW, Colletti PM, Lapin SA, et al: Real time sonography in suspected acute cholecystitis. *Radiology* 155:767, 1985.

110. Shea JA, Berlin JA, Escarce JJ, et al: Revised estimates of diagnostic test sensitivity and specificity in suspected biliary tract disease. *Arch Intern Med* 154:2573, 1994.

111. Bree RL: Further observations on the usefulness of the sonographic Murphy's sign in the evaluation of suspected acute cholecystitis. *J Clin Ultrasound* 23:169, 1995.

112. Grossman SJ, Joyce JM: Hepatobiliary imaging. *Emerg Med Clin North Am* 9:853, 1991.

113. Kim CK, Tse KK, Juweid M, et al: Cholescintigraphy in the diagnosis of acute cholecystitis: Morphine augmentation is superior to delayed imaging. *J Nucl Med* 34:1866, 1993.

114. Johnson H, Cooper B: The value of HIDA scans in the initial evaluation of patients for cholecystitis. *J Natl Med Assoc* 87:27, 1995.

115. Fidler J, Paulson EK, Layfield L: CT evaluation of acute chole-cystitis: Findings and usefulness in diagnosis. *AJR* 166:1085, 1996.

116. Steinberg W, Tenner S: Acute pancreatitis. *N Engl J Med* 330:1198, 1994.

117. Balthazar EJ: CT diagnosis and staging of acute pancreatitis. *Radiol Clin North Am* 27:19, 1989.

118. Abber JC, McAninch JW: Renal colic: Emergency evaluation and management. *Am J Emerg Med* 3:56, 1985.

119. Brown DF, Nadel ES: Acute flank pain. *J Emerg Med* 15:875, 1997.

120. Stewart C: Nephrolithiasis. *Emerg Med Clin North Am* 6:617, 1988.

121. Press SM, Smith AD: Incidence of negative hematuria in patients with acute urinary lithiasis presenting to the emergency room with flank pain. *Urology* 45:753, 1995.

122. Wrenn K: Emergency intravenous pyelography in the setting of possible renal colic: Is it indicated? *Ann Emerg Med* 26:304, 1995.

123. Tasso SR, Shields CP, Rosenberg CR, et al: Effectiveness of selective use of intravenous pyelography in patients presenting to the emergency department with ureteral colic. *Acad Emerg Med* 4:780, 1997.

124. Silber SH, Melendez LH, Shamsian S: Sonographic detection of a renal mass in a young adult: A case for radiologic screening of new onset ureteral colic (letter). *Acad Emerg Med* 4:831, 1997.

125. Hall SK: Acute renal vascular occlusion: An uncommon mimic. *J Emerg Med* 11:691, 1993.

126. Zangerle KF, Iserson KV, Bjelland JC, Criss E: Usefulness of abdominal flat plate radiographs in patients with suspected ureteral calculi. *Ann Emerg Med* 14:316, 1985.

127. Roth CS, Bowyer BA, Berquist TH: Utility of the plain abdominal radiograph for diagnosing ureteral calculi. *Ann Emerg Med* 14:311, 1985.

128. Elton TI, Roth CS, Berquist TH, Silverstein MD: A clinical prediction rule for the diagnosis of ureteral calculi in emergency departments. *J Gen Intern Med* 8:57, 1993.

129. Mutgi A, Williams JW, Nettleman M: Renal colic: Utility of the plain abdominal roentgenogram. *Arch Intern Med* 151:1589, 1991.

130. Boyd R, Gray AI: Role of the plain radiograph and urinalysis in acute ureteric colic. *J Accid Emerg Med* 13:390, 1996.

131. Chen MY, Zagoria RJ, Dyer RB: Radiologic findings in acute urinary tract obstruction. *J Emerg Med* 15:339, 1997.

132. Smith RC, Rosenfield AT, Choe KA, et al: Acute flank pain: Comparison of non-contrast-enhanced CT and intravenous urography. *Radiology* 194:789, 1995.

133. Smith RC, Verga M, McCarthy S, Rosenfield AT: Diagnosis of acute flank pain: Value of unenhanced helical CT. *AJR* 166:97, 1996.

134. Levine JA, Neitlich J, Verga M, et al: Ureteral calculi in patients with flank pain: Correlation of plain radiography with unenhanced helical CT. *Radiology* 204:27, 1997.

135. Dalrymple NC, Verga M, Anderson KR, et al: The value of unenhanced helical CT in the management of acute flank pain. *J Urol* 159:735, 1998.

136. Fielding JR, Steele G, Fox LA, et al: Spiral computerized tomography in the evaluation of acute flank pain: A replacement for excretory urography. *J Urol* 157:2071, 1997.

137. Smith RC, Verga M, Dalrymple N, et al: Acute ureteral obstruction: Value of secondary signs of helical unenhanced CT. *AJR* 167:1109, 1996.

138. Brown DEM, Rosen CL, Wolfe RE: Renal ultrasonography. *Emerg Med Clin North Am* 15:877, 1997.

139. Juul N, Brons J, Torp-Pedersen S, Fredfeldt KE: Ultrasound versus intravenous urography in the initial evaluation of patients with suspected obstructing urinary calculi. *Scand J Urol Nephrol* 137:45, 1991.

140. Sinclair D, Wilson S, Toi A, Greenspan L: The evaluation of suspected renal colic: Ultrasound scan versus excretory urography. *Ann Emerg Med* 18:556, 1989.

141. Haddad MC, Sharif HS, Shahed MS, et al: Renal colic: Diagnosis and outcome. *Radiology* 184:83, 1992.

142. Rosen CL, Brown DEM, Sagarin M, et al: Ultrasonography by emergency physicians in detecting hydronephrosis in patients with suspected ureteral colic (abstr). *Acad Emerg Med* 3:541, 1996.

143. Brown DEM, Rosen CL, Chang YC, et al: Efficacy of a clinical pathway for suspected ureteral colic in reducing IV pyelogram utilization (abstr). *Acad Emerg Med* 3:482, 1996.

144. Ernst CB: Abdominal aortic aneurysm. *N Engl J Med* 328:1167, 1993.

145. Lederle FA, Parenti CM, Chute EP: Ruptured abdominal aortic aneurysm: The internist as diagnostician. *Am J Med* 96:163, 1994.

146. Marston WA, Ahlquist R, Johnson G, Meyer AA: Misdiagnosis of ruptured abdominal aortic aneurysm. *J Vasc Surg* 16:17, 1992.

147. Seigel CL, Cohen RH, Korobkin M, et al: Abdominal aortic aneurysm morphology: CT features in patients with ruptured and non-ruptured aneurysms. *AJR* 163:1123, 1994.

148. Seeger JM, Kieffer RW: Pre-operative CT in symptomatic abdominal aortic aneurysms: Accuracy and efficacy. *Am Surg* 52:87, 1986.

149. Thompson JE, et al: Surgery for abdominal aortic aneurysms, in Bergan J, Yao J (eds.): *Aneurysms: Diagnosis and Treatment.* New York: Grune & Stratton, 1982, pp. 287–299.

150. Phelan MB, Valley VT, Mateer JR: Pelvic ultrasonography. *Emerg Med Clin North Am* 15:789, 1997.

151. Moore L, Wilson SR: Ultrasonography in obstetric and gynecologic emergencies. *Radiol Clin North Am* 32:1005, 1994.

152. Gazelle GS, Mueller PR: Abdominal abscess: Imaging and intervention. *Radiol Clin North Am* 32:913, 1994.

153. Fry, DE: Noninvasive imaging tests in the diagnosis and treatment of intra-abdominal abscesses in postoperative patient. *Surg Clin North Am* 74:693, 1994.

154. Stack LB, Munter DW: Foreign bodies in the gastrointestinal tract. *Emerg Clin North Am* 14:493, 1996.

155. Savitt DL, Wason S: Delayed diagnosis of coin ingestion in children. *Am J Emerg Med* 6:378, 1988.

156. Kuhns DW, Dire DJ: Button battery ingestion. *Ann Emerg Med* 18:293, 1989.

157. Maves MD, Carithers JS, Birck HG: Esophageal burns secondary to disc battery ingestion. *Ann Otol Rhinol Laryngol* 93:364, 1984.

158. Hierholzer J, Cordes M, Tantow H, et al: Drug smuggling by ingested cocaine-filled packages: Conventional x-ray and ultrasound. *Abdom Imaging* 20:333, 1995.

159. Swann LA, Munter DW: Esophageal emergencies. *Emerg Clin North Am* 14:557, 1996.

160. Stark P, Thordarson S, McKinney M: Manifestations of esophageal disease on plain chest radiographs. *AJR* 155:729, 1990.

161. Panzini L, Burrell M, Traube M: Instrumental esophageal perforation: Chest film findings. *Am J Gastroenterol* 89:367, 1994.

162. Henderson JA, Peloquin AJ: Boerhaave revisited: Spontaneous esophageal perforation as a diagnostic masquerader. *Am J Med* 86:559, 1989.

163. Jagminas L, Silverman RA: Boerhaave's syndrome presenting with abdominal pain and right hydropneumothorax. *Am J Emerg Med* 14:53, 1996.

164. Richter JM, Christensen MR, Kaplan LM, et al: Effectiveness of current technology in the diagnosis and management of lower gastrointestinal hemorrhage. *Gastrointest Endosc* 41:93, 1995.

165. Whitaker SC, Gregson RH: The role of angiography in the investigation of acute or chronic gastrointestinal haemorrhage. *Clin Radiol* 47:382, 1993.

166. Colucciello SA: Blunt abdominal trauma. *Emerg Med Clin North Am* 11:107, 1993.

167. Pevec WM, Peitzman AB, Udekwu AO, et al: Computed tomography in the evaluation of blunt abdominal trauma. *Surg Gynecol Obstet* 173:262, 1991.

168. Wing VW, Federle MP, Morris JA, et al: The clinical impact of CT for blunt abdominal trauma. *AJR* 145:1191, 1985.

169. Federle MP: Comparative value of computed tomography in the evaluation of trauma. *Emerg Med Rep* 4:147, 1983.

170. Federle MP, Crass RA, Jeffrey RB, et al: Computed tomography in blunt abdominal trauma. *Arch Surg* 117:645, 1982.

171. Bennett MK, Jehle D: Ultrasonography in blunt abdominal trauma. *Emerg Med Clin North Am* 15:763, 1997.

172. Rozycki GS, Ochner MG, Jaffin JH: Prospective evaluation of the surgeon's use of ultrasound in the evaluation of trauma victims. *J Trauma* 34:516, 1993.

173. Lentz KA, McKenney MG, Nunez DB, et al: Evaluating blunt trauma: Role for ultrasonography. *J Ultrasound Med* 15:447, 1996.

174. McKenney M, Lentz K, Nunez D, et al: Can ultrasound replace diagnostic peritoneal lavage in the assessment of blunt abdominal trauma? *J Trauma* 37:439, 1994.

175. Liu M, Lee C, Fang K: Prospective comparison of diagnostic peritoneal lavage, computed tomographic scanning, and ultrasonography for the diagnosis of blunt abdominal trauma. *J Trauma* 35:267, 1993.

176. Lucciarini P, Ofner D, Weber F, et al: Ultrasonography in the initial evaluation and follow-up of blunt abdominal trauma. *Surgery* 114:506, 1993.

177. Rothlin M, Naf R, Amgwerd M, et al: Ultrasound in blunt abdominal and thoracic trauma. *J Trauma* 34:488, 1993.

178. Bernstein D, Barkin JS: Pepto-Bismol mimicking pancreatic calcification. *Am J Gastroenterol* 87:1677, 1992.

179. Geller E, Smergel EM: Bubble gum simulating abdominal calcifications. *Pediatr Radiol* 22:298, 1992.

180. Khoda J, Lantsberg L, Sebbag G: Foreign body mimicking colon cancer. *Am Fam Physician* 46:1378, 1992.

SUGGESTED READING

Baker SR, Cho KC: *The Abdominal Plain Film,* 2nd ed. Stamford, CT: Appleton & Lange, 1999.

Balthazar EJ (ed): Imaging the acute abdomen. *Radiol Clin North Am* 32:829, 1994.

McCort JJ (ed): *Abdominal Radiology.* Baltimore: Williams & Wilkins, 1981.

Mori PA, Mori KW: Abdomen, in Keats TE (ed): *Emergency Radiology,* 2d ed. Chicago: Year Book, 1989, pp. 243–344.

Novelline RA: Abdomen: non-traumatic emergencies, in Harris JH, Harris WH, Novelline RA (eds): *The Radiology of Emergency Medicine,* 3d ed. Baltimore: Williams & Wilkins, 1993, pp. 819–895.

Plewa MC: Emergency abdominal radiology. *Emerg Med Clin North Am* 9:827, 1991.

Silen W: *Cope's Early Diagnosis of the Acute Abdomen,* 17th ed. Oxford University Press, 1987.

CHAPTER 20

IMAGING PRIORITIES IN TRAUMA

JAMES CISEK / KEITH WILKINSON

Trauma-related injuries are either accidental or intentional (Table 20-1).[1] Trauma is the leading cause of mortality and morbidity among children and young adults. Almost one-fourth of any emergency department (ED) census and one-third of all hospital admissions are directly related to traumatic injuries. The direct and indirect economic losses due to trauma are estimated at nearly $200 billion annually, exceeding the economic toll from heart disease and cancer combined.[2]

GENERAL PRINCIPLES

Although trauma is separated into blunt and penetrating mechanisms of injury, significant overlap exists for any given patient. Knowledge of the circumstances and mechanism of the traumatic event heightens suspicion for certain types of injuries (Table 20-2).[3] Trauma patients often suffer from a combination of vertical, horizontal, and rotational forces.

The biomechanics of blunt injury are complex and most completely studied for motor vehicle collisions.[4] Trauma occurs when an initial external force is applied to the body by a moving object (car, baseball bat) or when the moving human body comes to a rapid halt (automobile collision). The direction of deceleration can be horizontal (car crash) or vertical (fall or jump). In both cases (direct blow or deceleration), a second collision occurs between the supporting structures of the body, such as the skull or chest wall, and movable organs (e.g., brain or heart).

TABLE 20-1

Number of Deaths Caused by Injury in 1992

CAUSE	NUMBER	PERCENT
Motor vehicle	40,982	16
Suicide	30,484	12
Homicide	25,488	10
Falls	12,646	5
Poisonings	7,082	3
Fires, burns	4,803	2
Drowning	4,196	2
Other	19,984	8

SOURCE: U.S. Department of Health and Human Services.[1]

Penetrating injuries are divided between high-energy bullet wounds and lower-energy stab wounds. Many factors are involved in the wounds produced by bullets, including the mass of the bullet and its velocity.[5] The path of the bullet through the patient and the organs injured are highly unpredictable. Although the effects of a stab wound are more predictable than

TABLE 20-2

Traumatic Injury Patterns

MECHANISM OF INJURY	RESULTANT INJURIES
Motor vehicle collision: frontal impact Bent steering wheel Knee imprint in dashboard Bull's-eye fracture of windshield	Cervical spine injury Anterior flail chest Pneumothorax Pulmonary contusion Aortic transection Myocardial contusion Intraabdominal injuries— spleen, liver, etc. Fractures of pelvis, hip, femur, or knee
Motor vehicle collision: side impact	Contralateral neck sprain Cervical spine fracture Lateral flail chest Pneumothorax Traumatic aortic rupture Intraabdominal injuries— spleen, liver, etc. Fractured pelvis or acetabulum
Motor vehicle collision: rear impact	Cervical spine injury
Motor vehicle collision: pedestrian	Head injury Thoracic and abdominal injuries Fractured lower extremities
Fall from height	Calcaneal fractures Axial spine fractures Tibial fractures

SOURCE: Adapted from American College of Surgeons Committee on Trauma,[3] with permission.

TABLE 20-3

Guidelines for Imaging Studies

1. **The more severely injured the patient, the fewer the number of radiographic studies needed in the ED.**
2. **Be systematic in ordering and interpreting films.**
   Avoid the tendency to focus on the dramatic clinical or radiographic findings and potentially miss less evident but potentially lethal injuries.
3. **Captain the radiographic studies as you would the resuscitation.**
   Subspecialists may unduly elevate their particular area of interest and request unnecessary or improperly sequenced studies. Stay focused on the complete picture.
4. **Communicate with the radiologist.**
   The history and clinical concerns provided to the radiologist can focus attention on particular injuries. Be specific when requesting studies and communicating your concerns. The radiologist can help sequence tests to minimize contrast and radiation exposure and reduce the time out of the resuscitation area.
5. **Insist on adequate films.**
   Repeat films or order alternative studies if unable to visualize a needed area. On the other hand, an unyielding determination can be dangerous. The patient may decompensate during prolonged attempts to obtain quality images in the radiology suite.
6. **Avoid studies that do not affect clinical management.**
   Nasal bones, skull, rib, and coccyx films have little use and consume valuable time.
7. **Contrast looks like blood.**
   If a head CT is clinically indicated, it should be obtained before administering intravenous contrast for studies such as abdominal CT scanning or angiography.
8. **You order it. You look at it.**
   The clinician can take advantage of having examined the patient and seen the films. It is an unexplainable embarrassment when a finding was not seen because no one looked at the film. Looking at special studies like CT scans, aortograms, and ultrasounds in concert with the radiologist increases the understanding of both pathology and normal variants.
9. **When in doubt, return to the patient.**
   Serial vital signs and examinations (particularly of the central nervous system and abdomen) can be lifesaving. Return to the ABCs in a patient who deteriorates. If there is a discrepancy between the physical exam and the radiologic findings, reexamine the patient.

those of a gunshot wound, the depth and direction of penetration are often difficult to predict from the surface appearance of the wound.

Host factors must also be considered in the trauma victim. Patients at the extremes of age (infants and the elderly) have increased mortality rates. Concurrent medical problems (cardiac disease, emphysema, obesity, diabetes, malignancy, coagulopathy) increase morbidity and mortality risk. Use of drugs (prescription, nonprescription, illicit) and alcohol can lead to injury, mask an injury, impair the physiologic response to an injury, or cause secondary injury.

Imaging Priorities

The establishment of priorities in radiographic studies for the trauma patient requires sound clinical judgment and a systematic approach (Table 20-3). Diagnostic evaluation should not impede therapeutic intervention; imaging should never delay resuscitation or definitive surgery. A detailed radiographic evaluation is ill advised in the hemodynamically unstable patient. The patient with hypotension and a distended abdomen needs an exploratory laparotomy rather than a computed tomography (CT) scan. Needle decompression and tube thoracostomy should not be delayed in the patient with a suspected tension pneumothorax while waiting for a chest radiograph. If a patient has a pulseless extremity distal to an obvious dislocation, then joint relocation is performed prior to obtaining radiographs. The radiology suite is a poor place for a patient with unstable vital signs or a deteriorating neurologic exam. The one exception is angiographic embolization of pelvic arterial hemorrhage, where the therapeutic benefit to an unstable patient outweighs the risk. The need for studies outside of the resuscitation area must be balanced against the lost opportunity for serial examinations.

Imaging studies focus first on the most serious injuries. In the patient with multisystem trauma, dilemmas arise when there are several suspected concurrent life-threatening injuries, such as a suspected intracranial hematoma, solid viscus injury, aortic injury, and complex pelvic fracture. The priorities for diagnostic imaging for such injuries are determined by the immediacy of life threat.

Missed injuries occur in up to 10% of patients with blunt multisystem trauma.[6] Most of these are musculoskeletal injuries (Table 20-4). Missed injuries tend to occur in more severely injured patients with concomitant head injury or hemodynamic instability. The *tertiary survey* refers to reexamination of the patient to identify less obvious injuries.

Advanced Imaging Modalities

CT has great sensitivity and specificity for injuries of solid abdominal viscera, retroperitoneal structures, the brain, and bones. It is relatively insensitive for hollow viscus injuries of the abdomen (even with oral contrast). CT visualizes the lung parenchyma and can detect pleural effusions and pneumothoraces better than a supine chest radiograph. Conventional CT

TABLE 20-4

Missed Injuries in Major Trauma Patients

Extremity fractures	58%
Abdominal injuries	17%
Spinal fractures	14%
Thoracic injuries	14%
Vascular injuries	6%
Facial fractures	5%

SOURCE: Enderson et al.[6] with permission.

is not sensitive enough to exclude traumatic aortic injury; however, it readily detects mediastinal hemorrhage that is an indirect marker of aortic injury. With further experience, contrast-enhanced helical CT may prove to be sufficiently sensitive to supplant aortography in the diagnosis of traumatic aortic injury.

Angiography has limited, well-defined roles in the imaging of the trauma patient. It is the "gold standard" for the evaluation of a suspected aortic injury in the stable patient. Angiography provides definitive therapy for pelvic arterial bleeding. It is also used to detect arterial injury in patients with penetrating and blunt trauma to an extremity. The disadvantages of angiography are the contrast load, time spent out of the trauma room, invasive nature of the study, and need for a cooperative patient.

Ultrasound (US) is rapidly becoming an integral part of the evaluation of blunt abdominal trauma. It is fast and portable and has excellent sensitivity for detecting free intraabdominal fluid. The disadvantages are the operator-dependent nature of the study, poor retroperitoneal and hollow viscus imaging, and lower specificity for intraabdominal injury compared to CT.

Magnetic resonance imaging (MRI) provides exceptional soft tissue visualization. Its greatest use is in the evaluation of the spine in the stable patient with blunt trauma, particularly if a spinal cord or ligamentous injury is suspected. Lack of access to the patient, getting the patient and equipment to and into the gantry, long study duration, and high cost severely hamper the use of MRI in the acutely injured patient.

THE PATIENT WITH BLUNT TRAUMA

The Trauma Series

Radiographic studies are obtained only after the airway is secured, adequate ventilation is ensured, and the circulation is addressed. This is the primary survey and resuscitation phase of trauma care. Radiographs should never delay resuscitation or operative intervention in the unstable patient. In fact, the number of radiographs obtained in the resuscitation suite should be inversely proportional to the severity of injury.[7] The most unstable patients may require no imaging studies or only a portable abdominal US before exploratory laparotomy.

After the primary survey and resuscitation, all patients sustaining significant blunt force to the torso should rapidly receive supine chest, cross-table lateral cervical spine, and anteroposterior (AP) pelvic radiographs (the *trauma series*). If time permits only a single radiograph, the chest film is the first obtained because it identifies such life-threatening injuries as a massive hemothorax or pneumothorax, which must be quickly treated in the resuscitation suite. The insertion of necessary tubes and lines before obtaining radiographs saves time and avoids the necessity of a second film to check placement. The lateral cervical spine film does not, by itself "clear the neck," and immobilization must be maintained throughout the entire initial management phase.

The trauma series rapidly diagnoses certain treatable, immediately life-threatening injuries. These include a massive hemothorax or pneumothorax, a displaced pelvic fracture at risk for hemorrhage, and gross injury of the cervical spine. Further radiographic studies are delayed until these and other life-threatening processes have been addressed. When a patient must be transferred to another facility for definitive care, radiologic studies beyond the initial trauma series are time-consuming and generally are not warrented.

The Trauma Chest Radiograph

The chest radiograph provides early evidence of such lethal injuries as aortic disruption, diaphragmatic rupture, pulmonary contusion, hemothorax, pneumothorax, esophageal perforation, and tracheal disruption. Although many immediately life-threatening injuries such as a tension pneumothorax, massive hemothorax, flail chest, and sucking chest wound are usually detected on physical examination, a lack of clinical signs does not exclude intrathoracic injury. In fact, certain injuries are notorious for their lack of characteristic physical findings, such as aortic injury and diaphragmatic herniation. Therefore, chest radiography is needed in all victims of major blunt trauma. However, the supine AP chest film identifies only 58% of thoracic injuries in blunt trauma and only 79% of such injuries are seen on an erect AP film.[8] For example, supine portable chest radiography misses up to 30% of significant pneumothoraces.

PORTABLE RADIOGRAPHIC TECHNIQUE.   There are important differences between supine portable chest radiographs and PA films (Fig. 20-1) (see Chap. 17, Table 17-11). The technique is often suboptimal, with exposures frequently under- or over-penetrated. This influences the radiographic appearance of the lung and intrathoracic pathologic processes. The lung markings appear abnormally increased if the film is underpenetrated and intrapulmonary opacifications are obscured if the film is over-penetrated.

Rotation of the patient is frequently present on portable films. This causes distortion of mediastinal structures. Rotation is assessed by observing the alignment of the tips of the spinous processes in relation to the midpoint between the medial clavicular heads. After rotational alignment is determined, tracheal and mediastinal structures are assessed for pathologic shift. It is important not to use the alignment of the trachea with the spinous processes to judge the rotation of the patient, because the trachea is a mobile structure. For example, the trachea would overlie the spinous processes when the patient is rotated in one direction and the mediastinum is shifted in the opposite direction.

Poor inspiration is common in a supine, critically ill patient. Poor inspiration causes the vascular markings of the lung to become crowded, either simulating or obscuring an intrapulmonary pathologic process. The heart and mediastinum appear widened on a supine portable chest film largely because of poor inspiration. Other factors contribute the apparent mediastinal widening on portable radiographs. The AP versus PA technique places the anterior mediastinum further from the x-ray film,

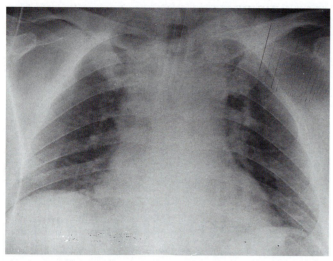

A

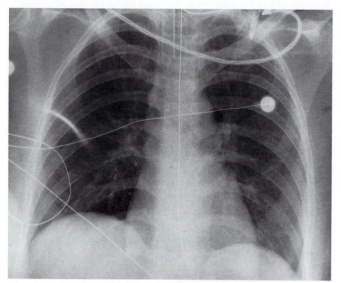

B

FIGURE 20-1. Supine portable chest radiography—the effect of radiographic technique. *A*. With a poor level of inspiration, the lung markings appear crowded, the heart is enlarged, and the mediastinum is indistinct and widened. *B*. With complete inspiration, the heart, lungs and mediastinum have a less distorted appearance.

causing magnification of these anterior structures. With portable equipment, the x-ray source is closer to the patient, 40 in. rather than 72 in. This also causes magnification of anterior structures.

The x-ray energy is lower with portable equipment, which causes overlying bones such as the ribs and scapulae to appear more opaque (white), and this can obscure findings in the lung. In addition, extraneous objects such as immobilization boards, clothing, and monitor leads are frequently present. These objects further compromise radiographic interpretation.

Finally, certain pathologic processes (pneumothorax, hemothorax) are difficult to see because of the supine positioning of the patient. In the supine position, the air from a pneumothorax rises anteriorly. The radiographic findings are subtle and include depression of the diaphragm and more distinct contours

of the mediastinum, diaphragm, and heart on the affected side. The *deep sulcus sign* is a widening and deepening of the costophrenic sulcus on the side of the pneumothorax (Fig. 20-2). Subcutaneous air in the chest wall is an indirect indicator of a pneumothorax in a trauma patient (Fig. 20-3*A*). The supine chest film is insensitive for demonstrating pleural effusions. Up to 1000 mL of blood can accumulate in the supine hemithorax before it is radiographically apparent. Pleural fluid in the supine patient with a hemothorax appears as a diffuse, homogeneous opacification or, if larger, as a layer of increased density along the lateral chest wall (Fig. 20-3). With pulmonary contusion, the opacification is mottled and inhomogeneous due to interposed air-filled alveoli (Fig. 20-4).

SYSTEMATIC ANALYSIS OF THE TRAUMA CHEST FILM. The trauma chest film must be interpreted in a systematic fashion to avoid missing important findings. Review of the film is tailored to the findings expected in the blunt trauma patient. An initial review identifies obvious abnormalities and those that are immediate life threats, such as an aortic injury, massive hemothorax, or pneumothorax. This initial inspection is followed by a complete review of the radiograph.

The first step is to assess the technical quality of the radiograph—the penetration, level of inspiration, and presence of rotation. Suboptimal films that would be unacceptable in other clinical settings are often the best obtainable during a trauma resuscitation.

Each region of the film is examined for trauma-related find-

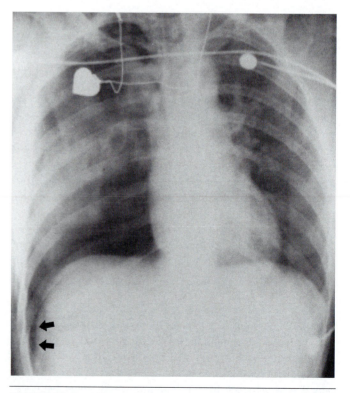

FIGURE 20-2. The deep sulcus sign. In a supine portable chest radiograph, a pneumothorax collects along the anterior thorax, which depresses the lateral margin of the right dome of the diaphragm. The costophrenic sulcus on that side is deep and wide *(arrows)*.

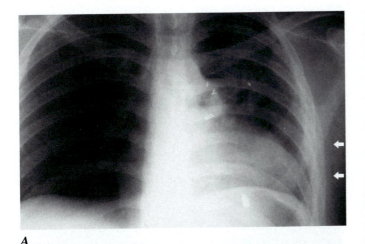

A

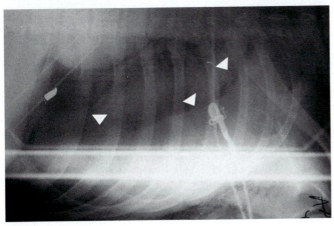

B

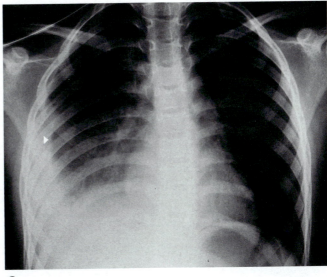

C

FIGURE 20-3. Hemothorax on a supine chest radiograph. *A.* Slightly increased opacity is seen on the left due to the blood that has layered along the posterior thorax. Subcutaneous emphysema is present *(arrows),* which is an indirect indicator of a pneumothorax. *B.* The left lateral decubitus radiograph reveals a moderately large hemothorax *(arrowheads). C.* In another patient with a hemothorax, a semierect portable chest radiograph shows increased opacity over the lower portion of the right side of the thorax. The diaphragm is obliterated by overlying blood, and the lateral margin of the lung is displaced from the chest wall *(arrowhead).*

ings. First, the lungs are inspected, then the mediastinum, and then the peripheral areas that include the chest wall, ribs, spine, and diaphragm.

The Lungs. Increased opacity of the lung regions is due either to a hemothorax or a pulmonary contusion. A pulmonary contusion typically has a mottled, inhomogeneous appearance and is often associated with multiple rib fractures. Homogeneous opacification is characteristic of a hemothorax. In a massive hemothorax, a fluid layer is seen surrounding the lung periphery, obscuring the diaphragm and mediastinal contour.

Radiolucency of the hemithorax is indicative of a massive pneumothorax. The peripheral pleural surface of the thorax is scrutinized for signs of a moderate-sized pneumothorax. There is an absence of lung markings and a fine white line of the visceral pleura paralleling the rib cage. Any vertically oriented line appearing over the thorax is carefully examined because it may represent a pneumothorax. Skin folds and clothing can have a similar appearance, but lung markings are seen lateral to these lines, and clothing folds often extend beyond the chest wall. When the patient is supine, the pneumothorax often collects along the anterior chest wall and is difficult to see. A large anterior pneumothorax depresses the diaphragm and widens the costophrenic sulcus — the "deep sulcus sign" (Fig. 20-2). In all cases of pneumothorax, the position of the trachea is as-

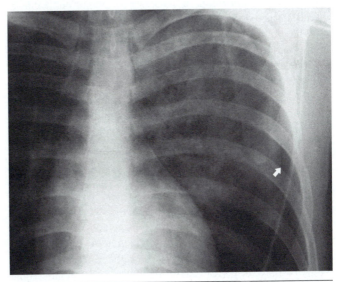

FIGURE 20-4. Pulmonary contusion. In this blunt trauma victim, inhomogeneous opacification of the left upper lung is due to a pulmonary contusion. A medium-sized pneumothorax is also present *(arrow).*

sessed. Shift of the trachea can indicate a tension pneumothorax. When the lung is noncompliant (e.g., emphysema), a tension pneumothorax can be present without complete collapse of the lung (Fig. 20-5).

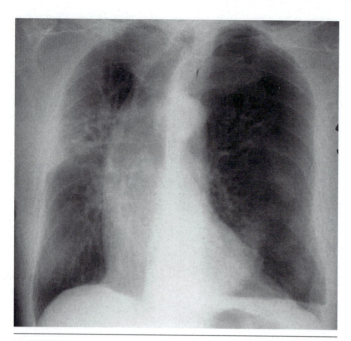

FIGURE 20-5.   Tension pneumothorax. There is marked shift of the mediastinum to the right (note displacement of the trachea, aorta, and heart).

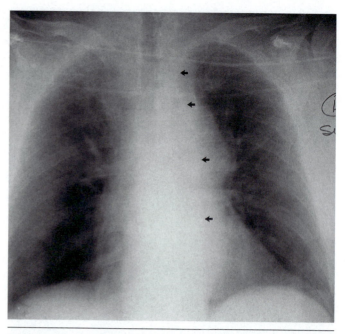

FIGURE 20-6.   Traumatic aortic injury. The superior mediastinum is only slightly widened, but the mediastinal contours, especially the aortic knob, are indistinct. The left paraspinal line is displaced *(arrows)* and extends above the aortic knob toward the apex of the lung. A larger blood collection would form an apical pleural cap. The trachea is displaced to the right, although this is in part due to rotation of the patient. An aortogram must be performed to determine whether there is a tear of the aortic wall.

Heart and Mediastinum.   Technical aspects of the radiograph can significantly alter the mediastinum's radiographic appearance. The primary factors that make interpretation difficult are poor inspiration and rotation. An acute *hemopericardium* causing tamponade is not expected to enlarge the cardiac silhouette, because only a small volume of blood is responsible for this. *Pneumomediastinum* in the setting of blunt trauma can be due to a tracheobroncheal injury or esophageal tear.

Widening of the mediastinum is due to hemorrhage in this region and is an indirect marker of blunt traumatic aortic or brachiocephalic vessel injury (Fig. 20-6). Although the mediastinum may normally be up to 8 cm wide on a supine portable film, the technique of the film must be considered. A poor level of inspiration can cause mediastinal widening in the absence of injury. In addition, a mediastinal hematoma can be present without mediastinal widening. Obscuration of the normal mediastinal contours is another sign of mediastinal blood (see Chap. 17, Fig. 17-9, and Chap. 18, Figs. 18-26 and 18-27). There can be blurring of the aortic knob and descending aorta; opacification of the aorticopulmonary window; widening of the left paraspinal line; extension of the left paraspinal line above the level to the aortic knob up to the lung apex causing an apical pleural "cap"; or widening of the right paratracheal stripe. Signs of mass effect on mediastinal structures include rightward deviation of the trachea and esophagus (with nasogastric tube) and depression of the left mainstem bronchus. If signs of mediastinal hemorrhage are present, the patient must have further radiographic evaluation to look for a great vessel injury, although only a minority of cases (15 to 30%) will have such an injury.

In concluding the examination of the mediastinum, the examiner assesses the trachea to confirm midline positioning. The thoracic vertebral bodies are closely examined for evidence of fracture or dislocation.

Diaphragm and Chest Wall.   The diaphragm, especially on the left side, is examined for signs of rupture including an indistinct contour or displacement of the stomach bubble or tip of the nasogastric tube into the thorax. The chest wall is examined for fractures of the ribs, clavicles, scapulae and proximal humerus. Turning the radiograph 90° so the ribs are vertically oriented helps detect subtle fractures. The soft tissue of the chest wall is examined for subcutaneous emphysema. In the setting of trauma, subcutaneous emphysema is a marker for a pneumothorax. If endotracheal intubation and positive-pressure ventilation is needed, the patient must be carefully observed for the development of a tension pneumothorax or have a chest tube inserted in anticipation of this complication.

Finally, all inserted tubes or catheters—such as an endotracheal tube, nasogastric tube, chest tubes, and central venous catheters—are checked for proper positioning.

The Cervical Spine Radiograph

The lateral cervical spine film is obtained with portable equipment using cross-table technique. The primary role of the initial lateral cervical spine film is to identify obvious abnormalities and to direct early activation of the appropriate surgical specialists. However, a normal cervical spine radiograph does not exclude spine injury in the major trauma patient.[9,10] The lateral radiograph is normal in 10 to 23% of patients with cervical spine injuries.[11] Therefore, the cervical spine must remain

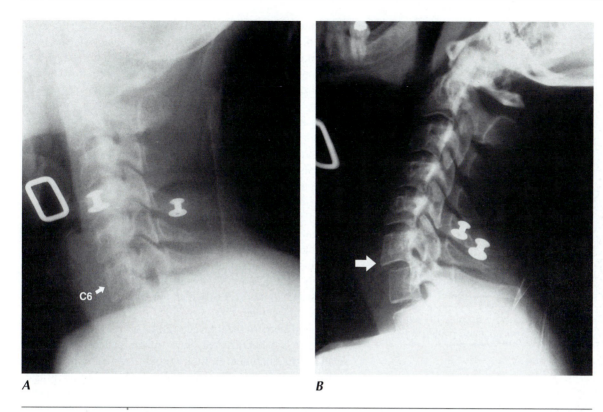

FIGURE 20-7.   Cervical spine radiographs in a major trauma victim using supine cross-table lateral technique. *A.* The initial radiograph is inadequate because C7 is not seen. In addition, C1 is hidden by the base of the skull. *B.* A repeat radiograph with greater traction on the patient's arms reveals anterolisthesis of C6 on C7 *(arrow).*

immobilized despite a normal film. "Clearing" the cervical spine is unnecessary before airway management. Secondary spinal injuries do not occur with careful nasotracheal or orotracheal intubation if in-line spinal immobilization is maintained during intubation.[12–14]

It is often difficult to see all seven cervical vertebrae adequately on the cross-table lateral film in the multiple trauma or combative patient. The application of caudal arm traction helps visualize the C7-T1 area (Fig. 20-7). However, this must be done gently, because forceful traction can distract an unstable spine injury. An obvious injury on the initial lateral view makes repeat radiography to visualize C7 unnecessary and potentially harmful. In a stable patient, the addition of a swimmer's view or right and left supine oblique views can be used when the standard lateral view does not adequately visualize C7 or T1. Moreover, CT can adequately image the cervicothoracic junction. These additional views are appropriate only in a stabilized patient.

A complete three-view cervical spine series in the trauma area is unwarranted in the initial management of severely injured patients. Injuries of the cervical spine are rarely a life threat, and a potentially unstable patient can decompensate during time-consuming diagnostic pursuits.

Cervical radiographs are safely omitted in certain trauma patients. Radiographs are unnecessary in the awake patient with no neck pain, tenderness, altered sensorium, or significant competing source of pain.[15–17] This has limited application in the multisystem trauma patient because of the high likelihood of a distracting injury or altered mentation.

The AP Pelvis Radiograph

An AP radiograph of the pelvis is indicated in all severely injured victims of blunt trauma. A pelvic fracture has significant impact on patient management. Pelvic fractures are a source of major blood loss and require specific interventions for stabilization. These may include the application of an external fixator and pelvic arteriography with embolization of arterial bleeding sites. In men, anterior pelvic fractures are associated with urethral injuries, and insertion of a Foley catheter must be performed with great caution. Finally, the technique of diagnostic peritoneal lavage is altered in the presence of a displaced pelvic fracture. The open supraumbilical technique is used to avoid inserting the catheter into a pelvic hematoma extending up the anterior abdominal wall.

Although the cost-effectiveness of routine pelvic radiography in all victims of blunt trauma has been questioned,[18] the relatively high frequency of fractures and their clinical impact justify pelvic radiography in all severely injured patients. By making pelvic radiography routine, the chance that a pelvic fracture will be missed is reduced. Although unstable pelvic fractures can usually be diagnosed on physical examination by applying bimanual pressure on the anterior iliac crests, this technique is insufficiently reliable to be used to exclude a fracture and to omit radiography in a severely injured patient. Moreover, such manipulation of an unstable pelvis can worsen pelvic hemorrhage and destabilize the patient.

Most displaced pelvic fractures are visible on the AP radiograph (Fig. 20-8). However, because only one radiographic

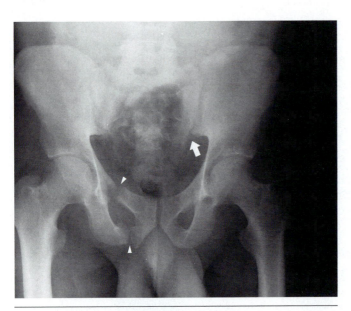

FIGURE 20-8.   Pelvic ring disruption with fractures of the right superior and inferior pubic rami *(arrowheads)* and widening of the contralateral sacroiliac joint *(arrow)*.

view is obtained, displacement can be inapparent on the radiograph. In addition, if the fracture has been reduced after the injury, the extent of instability and initial fracture displacement may not be evident. Only subtle radiographic clues of a severe injury may be present. These include widening of the sacroiliac joint, a vertical fracture through the iliac wing, and an avulsion fracture of the fifth lumbar transverse process.

MANAGEMENT PRIORITIES IN BLUNT TRAUMA

In most patients, the initial trauma series (cross-table lateral cervical spine, supine chest, and pelvic films) are rapidly and safely obtained. However, the patient's condition may prohibit any radiographic studies beyond the trauma series before transport to the operating suite. A rapid bedside abdominal ultrasound may be the only test indicated in the patient with persistent hypotension despite volume resuscitation (Fig. 20-9).

Only if the patient is hemodynamically stable or stabilized after an initial 2-liter volume infusion can imaging studies be performed to determine the full extent of the patient's injuries. Such imaging studies may include an abdominopelvic CT, cranial CT, aortography or chest CT, completion of cervical spine radiographs (or CT), and extremity radiographs.

Airway control and oxygen delivery are the first priorities in management of the blunt trauma patient. Uncontrolled hemorrhage is a leading cause of preventable trauma deaths.[19] The most frequent site of blood loss is the abdomen. Other common sites of hemorrhage include the chest, pelvis, thigh, and external bleeding.

In the hypotensive multiply injured patient, surgically correctable lesions in the abdomen or chest occur more frequently than surgically correctable intracranial lesions.[20,21] Therefore,

the control of hemodynamically destabilizing external and internal bleeding takes precedence over the diagnosis and treatment of intracranial lesions. Fortunately, the number of patients requiring both procedures is small. Furthermore, uncontrolled bleeding and hypotension decrease cerebral perfusion pressure, causing secondary brain injury. If emergent laparotomy is needed in a patient with neurologic injuries, a subarachnoid intracranial pressure (ICP) monitor can be placed concurrently in the operating room. In adults, intracranial injury does not cause hypotension in the neurologically salvageable patient. However, young children and infants can accommodate enough blood in the cranium to become hypotensive.

Bilateral tube thoracostomy can identify and quantify intrathoracic bleeding. Massive hemothorax (>1000 mL) and rapid bleeding (>300 to 500 mL in the first hour) signify that the chest is an important source of bleeding. Despite this, the majority (up to 82%) of patients with a traumatic hemothorax are managed nonoperatively with tube thoracostomy and blood volume replacement.[22]

Diagnostic peritoneal lavage (DPL) or abdominal US is indicated in the hypotensive blunt trauma patient to promptly evaluate the abdomen. Both are rapid tests with a high sensitivity for injury. If the initial aspirate from the DPL is grossly positive (≥10 mL of gross blood), the patient should immediately go for laparotomy.[23,24] If bedside ultrasonography reveals intraperitoneal blood in a hypotensive patient, the patient should immediately go to the operating room.

If a disruption of the pelvic ring is evident on physical examination or the AP pelvic film, the DPL must be done by an open, supraumbilical approach. This minimizes the chance of a false-positive DPL due to placing the catheter into an expanding extraperitoneal hematoma.

If there is a displaced disruption of the pelvic ring and time permits, an external fixator, such as a percutaneous pelvic C clamp, can be applied before laparotomy. If a large or expanding pelvic hematoma is found at laparotomy, the patient is taken to pelvic angiography. Angiography can be done as a portable study in the surgical suite, followed by direct surgical control of arterial bleeding if the patient cannot be sufficiently stabilized to tolerate transportation to an angiography suite. If needed, pelvic angiography should precede aortography.

If the DPL is "positive" by laboratory analysis (red blood cell count >100,000/mm^3) rather than being grossly bloody, an intraabdominal injury requiring surgery may be present but is unlikely to be the cause of hemodynamic instability. In this situation, the treatment of pelvic bleeding is addressed first. The choice of initial external pelvic fixation versus immediate pelvic angiography is controversial and institution-dependent. Most pelvic hemorrhage is venous or osseous. Arterial bleeding amenable to angiography occurs in only 3 to 20% of patients with high-risk pelvic fractures (posterior, open-book, or markedly displaced fractures). Angiography with embolization controls arterial bleeding in 80 to 90% of cases but requires an average of 2.5 hours and does not stop venous or osseous bleeding. External fixation usually slows venous or osseous bleeding and allows closer observation of the patient and evaluation of other injuries. Continued bleeding and hemodynamic insta-

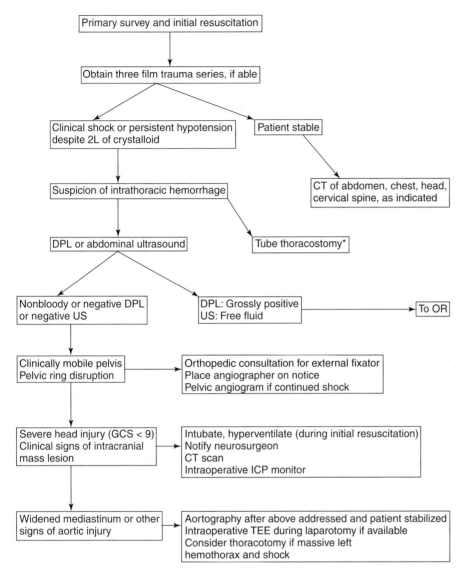

*Chest tube insertion can precede chest radiograph

FIGURE 20-9. Management of the major blunt trauma victim.

bility necessitate pelvic angiography before laparotomy. The mortality rate of a negative exploratory laparotomy is high in the setting of persistent hypotension with a pelvic fracture.[25]

After the immediate circulatory threats are controlled, neurologic injury is addressed. Coma, pupillary asymmetry, lateralizing weakness, or a palpable depressed skull fracture increase the risk of an intracranial lesion requiring surgery. Nearly 40% of brain-injured patients unable to follow commands [Glasgow Coma Scale (GCS) score <9] need surgery for a subdural or epidural hematoma mass lesion. The mortality of an acute subdural hematoma increases from 30% if drained before 4 hours to 90% if drained after 4 hours.[26] A noncontrast head CT should be performed prior to any contrast studies so that the contrast does not obscure a small intracranial hemorrhage.

Traumatic disruption of the aorta is always a concern in the severely injured patient. The patient with an aortic rupture sur-

viving to the ED usually has a contained aortic rupture with an intact adventitia. This patient usually survives the injury for the next 6 to 18 hours. The treatment of extrathoracic hemorrhage and intracranial mass lesions takes priority over aortography. Recently, intraoperative transesophageal echocardiography has been proposed as a rapid technique to detect aortic injury while other destabilizing injuries are being addressed in the operating room.

BLUNT TRAUMA: SYSTEM-SPECIFIC CONSIDERATIONS

Head Trauma

Head injury accounts for 50% of all trauma deaths and 60% of vehicle-related deaths.[27] Indications for head CT scanning are traumatic loss of consciousness, retrograde or antegrade amnesia, progressive headache, vomiting, altered sensorium, evidence of a depressed or basilar skull fracture, and a worsening or focal neurologic exam. Head injuries resulting from falls and assaults are more likely to cause focal mass lesions. Vehicular injuries tend to produce diffuse brain injuries that are not correctable with surgery.

The goal of cranial CT is the rapid identification of surgically correctable lesions. The patient must be hemodynamically stable. Subarachnoid hemorrhage is the most common hemorrhagic injury following head trauma, and subdural hematoma is the most common surgical lesion (Fig. 20-10).[28,29]

Plain films of the skull are generally not indicated in the management of blunt cranial trauma and should not delay CT scanning. Among children, skull films can help in the diagnosis of child abuse (multiple fractures, bilateral fractures, fractures crossing suture lines). Although the issue is controversial, skull films may have a role in children younger than 2 years of age, to screen for a linear skull fracture due to a low-energy impact such as a fall from a low height and with no resulting signs of intracranial injury (i.e., neurologic deficits, irritability, vomiting). A small number of such children will have linear skull fractures. Although these children have an excellent prognosis, relatively asymptomatic children with a linear skull fracture merit close observation either as inpatients or outpatients. They are also at risk for later development of a "growing" skull fracture (leptomeningeal cyst).

Practical factors limit the use of MRI in evaluating intracranial trauma. It is slower, less readily available, and allows

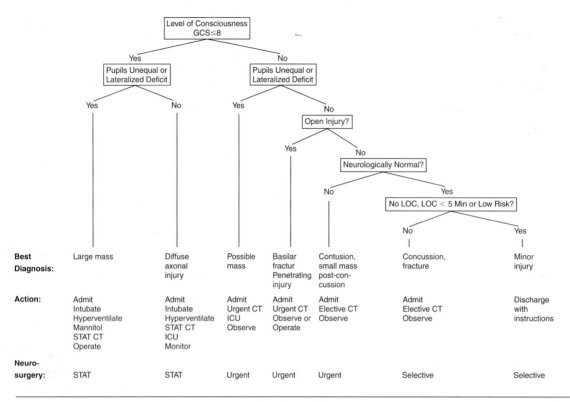

FIGURE 20-10.   Head injury triage. (From American College of Surgeons Committee on Trauma: Head trauma, in *Advanced Trauma Life Support Instructor Manual*. Chicago: American College of Surgeons, 1993, with permission.)

only limited access to the patient. Edema and shear injuries are better seen on MRI, but CT is superior for subarachnoid hemorrhage, pneumocephalus, and skull fractures. Subdural and epidural hematoma are seen well on both.

Cervical Spine and Spinal Cord Injury

The initial cross-table lateral spine radiograph identifies obvious injuries; however, it cannot be relied upon to exclude cervical injury. Once the patient is stabilized, further imaging of the cervical spine should be obtained (Fig. 20-11).

The lateral cervical spine film must be repeated if it is technically suboptimal due to rotation or overlying objects. If there is inadequate visualization of the entire cervical spine, the film is repeated with greater traction on the arms (Fig. 20-7). Alternatively, a swimmer's view or supine oblique view provides partial visualization of this region. However, if the patient is severely injured and especially if CT of the head or abdomen is being performed, a CT through the poorly visualized segments of the cervical spine can be performed with little additional delay.

The open-mouth view is the next most important radiograph, because it identifies such cervical injuries as fractures through the base of the dens and burst fractures of the ring of C1. These are often not evident on the lateral view. Finally, the AP view provides confirmatory evidence of a lower cervical spine injury incompletely identified on the lateral film.

The three-view series, in conjunction with the clinical examination, can clear the cervical spine in victims of limited trauma. However, about 5% of cervical spine injuries have a normal three-view series; therefore, in severely injured multitrauma patients, those with neurologic deficits, or patients with disproportionate neck pain or tenderness, cervical immobilization should be maintained despite normal radiographs.[30]

Missed cervical spine injuries are usually the result of technically suboptimal radiographs rather than misinterpretation of adequately performed studies.[31] Most missed injuries occur at the cervicocranium and cervicothoracic junction. The cervicothoracic junction is often difficult to visualize on the lateral film due to superimposed soft tissues and shoulders. The cervicocranium is a region of complex radiographic anatomy. In severely injured patients, liberal use of CT is warranted in areas poorly seen on conventional radiographs or in areas with questionable abnormalities. Occult cervicocranial fractures can be diagnosed by CT in patients with severe head injury, especially those with intracranial hemorrhage or depressed mentation.[32–34]

CT can miss transversely oriented fractures and has poor sensitivity for ligamentous injuries. CT reconstructions in the sagittal or coronal planes detect transverse fractures. MRI or flexion-extension views are used to detect ligamentous injury.

Special plain-film views like pillar views, tomograms, and flexion-extension views have a limited role in evaluating the multiple trauma victim. The routine use of oblique views in addition to a complete lateral, AP, and open-mouth view does not

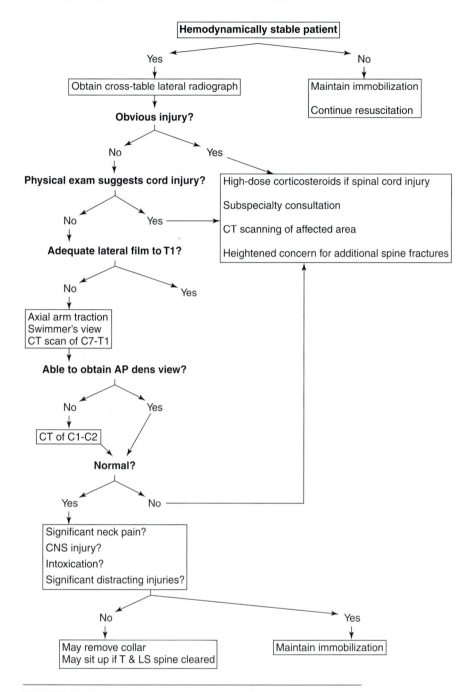

FIGURE 20-11. Evaluation of the cervical spine in blunt trauma.

significantly improve detection of cervical injuries.[35] Oblique views are useful in certain injuries such as unilateral interfacetal dislocation and laminar fractures, although CT better reveals the full extent of the injury.

Flexion-extension views are done when the patient has normal plain films of the cervical spine but has neck pain out of proportion to a muscular strain. Flexion-extension views are also used in the arthritic spine with minor subluxation on the initial lateral view to help distinguish degenerative changes from injury. Flexion-extension views are often done in the presence of a physician, and the patient's neck is never forced into a painful position. Flexion-extension views are not performed with the unstable, incompetent, or intoxicated patient. They are contraindicated in the patient with a potentially unstable fracture on plain films or in the patient with a new neurologic deficit.

MRI is best for assessing the spinal cord, ligament disruption, and disk protrusions. However, MRI is time-consuming and does not allow access to the patient. These factors severely limit its role in initial trauma care.

Blunt Trauma to the Soft Tissues of the Neck

Laryngeal injuries usually occur at the junction of the trachea and cricoid cartilage. These are uncommon and are usually caused by a direct blow or "clothesline" injury. Stridor, hemoptysis, hoarseness, subcutaneous emphysema, and palpable crepitus suggest a major laryngeal injury. The patient must have immediate airway management prior to radiographic studies. Subcutaneous and mediastinal emphysema can be seen on the cross-table view of the cervical spine or AP chest radiographs. Elevation of the hyoid bone above the level of C3 on the cross-table lateral view of the cervical spine view suggests a laryngeal injury.[36] CT of the larynx in the patient with a stable airway is sensitive for identifying the injury.[37] Fiberoptic bronchoscopy is also diagnostic.

Vascular lesions of the neck are due to either direct impact or indirect "whiplash." Most occur at or above the bifurcation of the carotid arteries. They can be difficult to diagnose because 25 to 50% have no external signs of trauma and delayed neurologic deficits are common.[38] Carotid artery injury is suspected in a patient who develops focal neurologic deficits and has a normal CT scan of the brain. Four-vessel angiography or magnetic resonance angiography (MRA) is performed in the patient with a strong suspicion of blunt carotid injury. Multiple vessels are injured in up to 40% of cases.

Facial Trauma

Radiographs are used to confirm suspected facial injuries. Victims of blunt trauma with severe midface fractures need airway protection prior to radiographs. Eagerness to investigate obvious facial deformity can cause unnecessary delay in addressing more life-threatening injuries. Complete facial radiographs are obtained only when the patient's overall condition permits. CT is the procedure of choice for complex facial trauma.

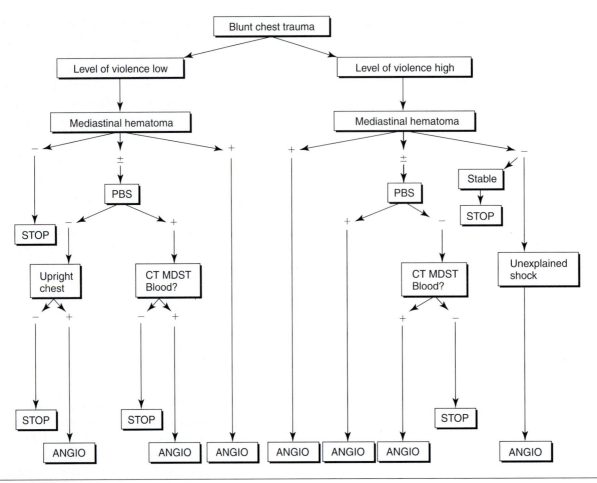

FIGURE 20-12. Assessment of aortic injury in blunt chest trauma. Some traumatologists believe that the chest film is inadequate to exclude an aortic injury with a high-energy mechanism. Stable patients with violent mechanisms, equivocal findings for mediastinal hematoma on chest film, and injuries to the brain, abdomen, or pelvis could be evaluated with mediastinal CT rather than angiography because many such patients require CT imaging of the brain and abdomen. (From Ben-Menachem Y, Fisher RG: Radiology, in Feliciano DV, Moore EE, Mattox KL (eds): *Trauma*, 3rd ed. Stamford, CT: Appleton and Lange, 1996, with permission.) *PBS*, pelvis-brain-spine injury; *CT MDST*, mediastinal CT.

Thoracic Trauma

Many thoracic injuries are detected by physical examination, including rib fractures, flail chest, massive hemothorax or pneumothorax, and tension pneumothorax. The absence of external thoracic trauma on the physical examination does not exclude intrathoracic injury. Potentially life-threatening injuries identified on the chest radiograph include pulmonary contusion, rib fractures, hemothorax, tension pneumothorax, thoracic aortic injury, diaphragmatic rupture, esophageal rupture, and tracheobronchial disruption. Many major thoracic injuries are diagnosed by physical examination. Tension pneumothorax must be diagnosed clinically and treated without radiographic confirmation. Massive hemothorax and pneumothorax can be suspected clinically, and if the patient is unstable, tube thoracostomy is performed before chest radiography. Certain other injuries have few if any clinical signs, and chest radiography is essential for their diagnosis. Key examples include traumatic aortic tear and diaphragmatic herniation. CT scanning of the thorax has greater sensitivity for other intrathoracic injuries

such as rib fractures, small pneumothoraces, and small pleural effusions, but these findings rarely change management.[39]

Pulmonary contusion is the most common potentially lethal chest injury seen in blunt thoracic trauma. Typically, the extent of the pulmonary contusion is much larger than shown on initial plain films. It is usually evident on chest films within 6 hours of injury. Management is based on the patient's ventilatory status (Fig. 20-4).

TRAUMATIC AORTIC INJURY. Radiographic evidence of acute traumatic aortic injury (ATAI) is present in over 95% of patients with this condition (Fig. 20-12). There are many plain chest film signs suggestive of aortic injury (Tables 20-5 and 20-6; Fig. 20-6). Clinical suspicion as well as radiographic findings dictate the need for further studies. The key radiographic manifestation of aortic injury is hemorrhage into the mediastinum. Radiographs show widening of the mediastinum, obliteration of normal mediastinal contours, widening of the right paratracheal stripe or left paraspinous line, obliteration of the aorticopulmonary window, or rightward shift of the trachea

TABLE 20-5

Clinical Features Suggestive of Traumatic Aortic Injury

High-speed deceleration injury
Interscapular or retrosternal pain
Interscapular murmur
Hypotension
Diminished or absent pulses
Upper extremity hypertension
Multiple rib fractures or flail chest
Palpable fracture of the thoracic spine
Expanding hematoma at the thoracic outlet
Superior vena cava syndrome
Palpable sternal fracture
Fractures of all three upper ribs
No external signs of thoracic injury (10–25%)

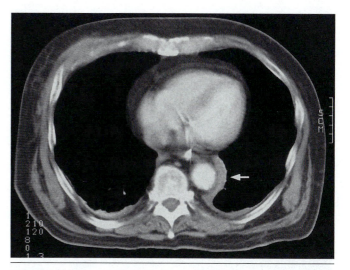

FIGURE 20-13. CT of aortic injury. There is blood adjacent to the descending aorta *(arrow)*. The aorta is opacified by intravenous contrast but a tear of the aortic wall is not seen.

or nasogastric tube. There are various criteria for mediastinal widening, including width greater than 8 cm on a supine film or a ratio of mediastinal to chest width of greater than 25%. The judgment of an experienced radiologist that the mediastinum has an abnormal contour or width correlates best with the presence of hemomediastinum. However, this conclusion is based on work by expert trauma center radiologists when technically suboptimal films were excluded. The difficulty in detecting subtle signs of mediastinal blood is compounded by the suboptimal radiographic technique of the supine portable AP radiographs in the injured patient. In the stable patient, an upright chest radiograph better evaluates the mediastinum. In the patient with stable hemodynamics, no clinical sign of great vessel injury, and a normal chest film, it is prudent to obtain in-

terval chest radiographs at 6 h and again at 24 h, since signs of mediastinal hemorrhage can develop over time.

Neither the clinical presentation nor these numerous chest film signs are diagnostic of aortic injury. Therefore, liberal use of aortography on the basis of an abnormality on the chest film and a history of violent trauma is the wisest approach. Plain-film changes suggesting a mediastinal hematoma are nonspecific for aortic disruption. This is because the source of the mediastinal blood is not the aorta itself but ruptured smaller branch vessels such as the intercostal arteries or veins. A complete through-and-through tear of the aorta is a rapidly fatal injury. Therefore, patients who survive to reach the ED must have an incomplete, nonleaking aortic tear. The presence of mediastinal blood is thus an indirect marker of an aortic injury. In fact, only about one-third of patients with CT-confirmed mediastinal blood have aortic injuries. Because ATAI is an ultimately fatal although treatable injury, aortography is used liberally in suspected cases. Patients undergoing aortography based on clinical suspicion or definite or equivocal radiographic findings have aortic injuries in only 15 to 20% of cases.[40–42]

Chest CT assists in the diagnosis of aortic injury (Fig. 20-13). Unfortunately, the resolution of conventional contrast-enhanced CT is too low to detect intimal irregularities in some cases of aortic injury and therefore is unreliable for excluding aortic injury. Equivocal results occur in up to 25% of studies.[43] In addition, CT can miss injuries to major vessels branching off the aorta. Preliminary results with helical CT, including reconstructed images of "CT angiography," show promise in replacing aortography. CT does provide indirect evidence of aortic injury by demonstrating a mediastinal hematoma. Some centers use mediastinal CT in hemodynamically stable

TABLE 20-6

Chest Radiographic Findings Suggestive of Traumatic Aortic Injury

	SENSITIVITY	SPECIFICITY
Mediastinal widening		
Width >8 cm on spine portable film	82–97%	34–60%
Mediastinum-to-chest ratio >0.25	40–100%	59–75%
Abnormal superior mediastinal contour	53–72%	21–55%
(obliteration of aortic arch or descending aorta)		
Left apical cap	2–62%	75–95%
Obliteration of the aorticopulmonary window	40–100%	56–83%
Left paraspinal stripe widened or extending above aortic	3–83%	89–97%
arch (wide = >5 mm or >2 × distance from the		
spine to the left margin of the descending aorta)		
Widened or obliterated right paratracheal stripe	2–83%	94–99%
Nasogastric tube displacement more than 2 cm to	9–71%	90–96%
the right at T4		
Depression of the left mainstem bronchus		
(shifted >40° below the horizontal)	3–80%	80–99%
Tracheal deviation to the right		
(right of T4 spinous process)	12–100%	80–92%

SOURCE: Mirvis SE, Rodriguez A: Diagnosis in thoracic trauma, in Mirvis SE, Young JWR (eds): *Imaging in Trauma & Critical Care,* Baltimore: Williams & Wilkins, 1992, with permission.

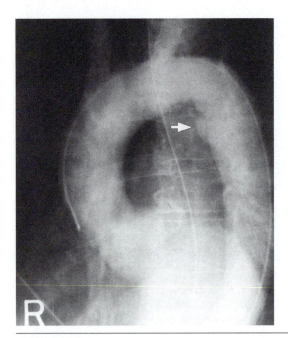

FIGURE 20-14. Aortogram of aortic injury. A small intimal tear and aortic pseudoaneurysm is seen *(arrow).* The angiographic catheter follows the outer contour of the aorta.

patients with a low index of suspicion and an equivocal mediastinum on plain-film chest radiography to screen for mediastinal hematoma. This approach is especially beneficial in the stable patient requiring CT imaging of the abdomen or head. If thoracic CT demonstrates a mediastinal hematoma, thoracic aortography is performed.

Transesophageal echocardiography (TEE) can aid in the diagnosis of ATAI. TEE is rapid (29 min versus 76 min for aortography), and is performed in the trauma suite or operating room. It also evaluates the pericardium, heart valves, and myocardium. Moreover, TEE can identify an intimal flap and false lumen. TEE can also detect hemorrhage surrounding the aorta. Sensitivities for aortic tear vary from 68 to 100% and specificities vary from 88 to 100% for detecting an aortic injury.[44–47] TEE is operator-dependent and requires adequate sedation and airway protection. It is difficult to perform in patients with maxillofacial trauma or significant esophageal disease. The sensitivity and specificity is decreased in patients with extensive aortic atherosclerosis, and TEE provides only limited evaluation

TABLE 20-7

Sensitivity of Various Modalities for Diagnosing Diaphragmatic Rupture

	CXR	DPL	US	CT	UGI
Left-sided	18%	81%	0%	17%	100%
Right-sided	17%	67%	0%	0%	NA
Total	18%	79%	0%	14%	100%

KEY: CXR, chest film; DPL, diagnostic peritoneal lavage; US, ultrasound; CT, computed tomography; UGI, upper gastrointestinal series.
SOURCE: Gelman et al.,[48] with permission.

of the carotid and subclavian vessels. Many centers are unable to perform TEE, and some studies have failed to achieve the requisite high sensitivity of TEE.

Aortography is the procedure of choice for victims of blunt trauma with a high-energy mechanism of injury and an abnormal mediastinum (Fig. 20-14). It can assess other thoracic great vessels (subclavian artery, pulmonary artery, internal mammary artery). Life-threatening intracranial and intraabdominal hemorrhage should be excluded prior to aortography. Shock is a relative contraindication to angiography. MRI and MRA have high sensitivity and specificity for aortic disorders but are impractical in the acute trauma setting.

DIAPHRAGMATIC HERNIATION. Diaphragmatic injuries are uncommon in blunt trauma and can be difficult to diagnose (Table 20-7).[48] Placement of a nasogastric tube and serial AP chest films increases the sensitivity for diaphragmatic herniation. Left-sided diaphragmatic injuries are most common. Both chest radiography and CT scanning can miss this type of injury. Air or fluid containing abdominal viscera or a nasogastric tube tip above the hemidiaphragm are diagnostic (Fig. 20-15). Subtle findings include distortion or elevation of the diaphragm, ipsilateral atelectasis, and contralateral mediastinal displacement. Rupture of the right hemidiaphragm is difficult to identify. Superiomedial displacement of the right hemidiaphragm is a subtle sign.[49] The diagnosis can be made by an oral contrast study, thoracoscopy or laparoscopy, or at laparotomy.

ESOPHAGEAL PERFORATION. Esophageal perforation from blunt neck or chest trauma is uncommon and difficult to diagnose. Virtually all deaths from esophageal injuries result from delayed or missed diagnoses. Esophagography with water-soluble contrast is sensitive for this injury. Low-osmolality contrast materials are used initially, and if negative, are followed by barium. Negative esophagography with barium is followed by endoscopy if a high probability of injury remains.[50]

TRACHEOBRONCHIAL DISRUPTION. Tracheobronchial disruption is a rare injury and is suspected in the patient with extensive mediastinal or subcutaneous emphysema or with a persistent pneumothorax despite a tube thoracostomy. Complete reexpansion of a pneumothorax with tube thoracostomy does not exclude this injury.[51] Disruption usually occurs at the right mainstem bronchus. Up to 10% of patients do not have initial radiographic or physical evidence of the injury. The *fallen lung sign* is diagnostic. The collapsed lung falls away from the hilum laterally and superiorly in the supine patient and inferiorly in the upright position. The position of the lung may change with patient position. An abrupt cutoff of the involved mainstem bronchus may be seen.

BLUNT CARDIAC INJURIES. Cardiac injuries are diagnosed by two-dimensional echocardiography rather than chest radiography. Echocardiographic assessment of pericardial effusion is done rapidly at the bedside with the subxyphoid view. In myocardial contusion, echocardiography shows dyskinesia of the right ventricular free wall. Contused myocardium has increased

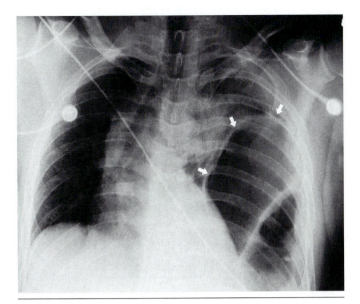

FIGURE 20-15. Diaphragm rupture. The stomach and splenic flexure of the colon have herniated into the thorax *(arrows)*. The heart and trachea are displaced to the right.

echo brightness, increased end-diastolic wall thickness, and impaired regional systolic function.

RIB FRACTURES. The ribs are the most commonly injured component of the adult thoracic cage in blunt trauma. A flail segment occurs if two breaks per rib occur in three or more consecutive ribs or if rib fractures are combined with sternal or costochondral fractures. This is usually palpable and sometimes even visible on examination. Rib fractures are uncommon in the pliable chest of the child (excluding child abuse), but pulmonary contusion is common. Rib films are better able to detect rib fractures but add little to the treatment of thoracic trauma. Rib fractures are clinically significant because they serve as a marker of nearby visceral injuries. Complications like pneumothorax, hemothorax, and pulmonary contusion are more important and are well seen on chest radiography.[52] Contiguous fractures of the first three upper ribs are associated with vascular injury. The association of first- and second-rib fractures and scapular fractures with injury of a major intrathoracic vessel has been questioned.[53] Fractures of the lower three ribs may signify injury to the underlying solid organs like the liver, kidneys, and spleen. The increased use of seat belts with shoulder harnesses has increased the incidence of sternal fractures. The outcome in the patient with a sternal fracture is determined by associated injuries and not by the sternal fracture.[54]

Abdominal Trauma

The primary task in assessing and managing abdominal trauma is not the accurate diagnosis of a specific injury but rather determining that an intraabdominal injury exists that requires emergent operative intervention. Up to 20% of patients with acute hemoperitoneum have a benign physical examination (nontender, nondistended abdomen).[55] Blood is a relatively

weak peritoneal irritant and the abdominal examination is often normal. In addition, abdominal injury can be masked by other painful injuries, central nervous system (CNS) injury, or intoxication. Therefore, a low threshold is maintained for suspecting intraabdominal hemorrhage in a patient with a sufficient mechanism of injury.

In the hemodynamically stable patient with a suspected abdominal injury, abdominopelvic CT is the preferred imaging procedure to evaluate injury to solid organs (Fig. 20-16).[56] CT has a high sensitivity and specificity for intraabdominal injury and allows nonoperative treatment of stable patients with splenic or hepatic injury (Figs. 20-17 and 20-18). It also provides excellent visualization of the kidneys, pelvis, and

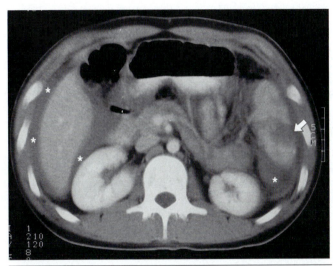

FIGURE 20-16. A splenic laceration and parenchymal hematoma are seen on CT *(arrow)*. There is blood in the splenorenal fossa, surrounding the liver, and in Morison's pouch between the liver and right kidney *(asterisks)*.

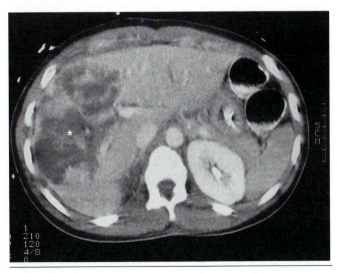

FIGURE 20-17. Extensive liver lacerations and hematoma are seen on CT *(asterisk)*. The intrahepatic hematoma appears darker than the contrast-enhanced liver parenchyma. Without intravenous contrast, the hematoma would have the same radiographic density as the liver parenchyma and would not be visible.

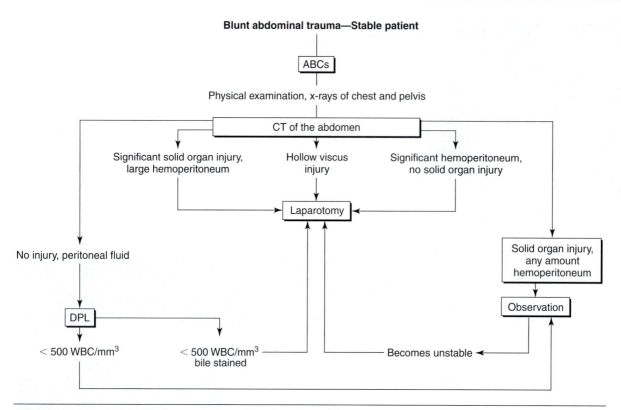

FIGURE 20-18.   Management of blunt abdominal trauma in the stable patient. (From Fabian TC, Croce MA: Abdominal trauma, including indications for celiotomy, in Feliciano DV, Moore EE, Mattox KL (eds): *Trauma,* 3rd ed. Stamford, CT: Appleton and Lange, 1996, with permission.) *ABCs,* airway, breathing and circulation; *DPL,* diagnostic peritoneal lavage.

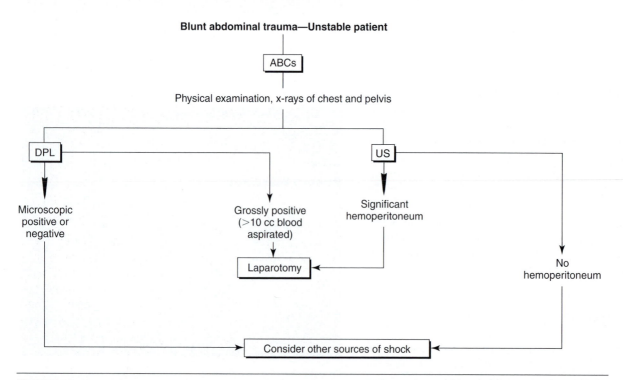

FIGURE 20-19.   Blunt abdominal trauma in the unstable patient. (From Fabian TC, Croce MA: Abdominal trauma, including indications for celiotomy, in Feliciano DV, Moore EE, Mattox KL (eds), *Trauma,* 3rd ed. Stamford, CT: Appleton and Lange, 1996, with permission.) *ABCs,* airway, breathing and circulation; *DPL,* diagnostic peritoneal lavage; *US,* ultrasonography.

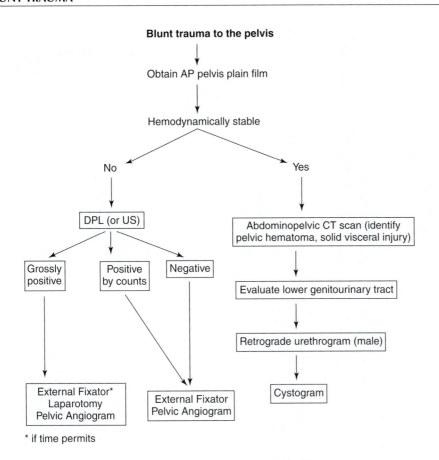

Blunt trauma to the pelvis

↓

Obtain AP pelvis plain film

↓

Hemodynamically stable

No ← → Yes

DPL (or US)

Grossly positive — Positive by counts — Negative

External Fixator* Laparotomy Pelvic Angiogram

External Fixator Pelvic Angiogram

Abdominopelvic CT scan (identify pelvic hematoma, solid visceral injury)

↓

Evaluate lower genitourinary tract

↓

Retrograde urethrogram (male)

↓

Cystogram

* if time permits

FIGURE 20-20. Management of pelvic injury.

retroperitoneum. The abdominopelvic CT is less accurate in detecting hollow viscus and pancreatic injuries. Small bowel perforation is uncommon in blunt trauma, occurring in roughly 3% of patients. Jejunal and duodenal perforations are the most common hollow viscus lesions. CT findings in the small bowel and mesenteric injury in blunt trauma are often subtle and nonspecific.[57] They include free intraperitoneal fluid, mesenteric infiltration, bowel wall thickening, pneumoperitoneum, and extravasated oral contrast. Free fluid in the abdomen in the absence of other identifiable injuries is a sign of injury to the bowel or mesentery.[58] A study without oral contrast is more apt to miss a small bowel mural hematoma or perforation.[59] Ideally, oral contrast (120 mL) is administered 30 to 45 min prior to scanning with an additional 120 to 180 mL given just prior to scanning. This regimen helps to opacify the stomach and small bowel and to distinguish fluid-filled bowel loops from free intraperitoneal fluid. Oral contrast also helps to visualize the borders of the pancreas. If time is crucial, oral contrast can be omitted or scanning can be done sooner after contrast administration. Intravenous contrast enhances solid organs and delineates areas of injury. Early pancreatic injury can be missed on CT because the fracture may not be seen. Subtle findings of increased attenuation of the peripancreatic fat, thickening of the left anterior pararenal fascia, or subtle peripancreatic hemorrhage suggest early injury.[60]

In the unstable patient, immediate DPL or abdominal US is indicated. The treatment delay caused by CT scanning of the abdomen is dangerous in an unstable patient (Fig. 20-19). US

may replace DPL in the emergent evaluation of blunt abdominal trauma. An US examination is rapid, simple, and performed in the resuscitation area. US has a low incidence of indeterminate results, is repeatable, and has a high sensitivity (83 to 99%), specificity (98 to 100%), and accuracy (97%) for detecting hemoperitoneum.[61–64] Patients with a significant amount of intraperitoneal fluid (>2 mm stripe of fluid in Morison's or in the pelvis if the patient is lying supine) usually require laparotomy. Extensive solid organ parenchymal damage is sometimes identified by US.[65] Ultrasound is less sensitive than CT for detecting solid organ injury.[66] Ultrasonography is interpreted cautiously in the pregnant patient because of the distortion of landmarks and the difficulty in differentiating intrauterine and extrauterine fluid. False-positive US results are seen in patients with ascites and on peritoneal dialysis.

Pelvic Trauma

Disruptions of the pelvic ring are potentially lethal because of the associated hemorrhage (Fig. 20-20). Anteroposterior compression, vertical shearing, or combination forces produce the highest rate of bleeding complications. External pelvic fixation can slow or stop bleeding by acting as a splint to tamponade blood loss. This is true even though most fixators do not directly stabilize the posterior pelvis, from which most bleeding emanates. The fixator can be applied in 15 min and is adjusted to allow access for abdominal surgery, CT evaluation, and angiography. The only contraindication is severe fracture with comminution. The fixator is generally placed before pelvic angiography is performed and often controls bleeding (Fig. 20-21). Continued bleeding and hypotension after pelvic fixation prompt angiography.

Angiography with embolization can be lifesaving when there is persistent hypotension despite external fixation and no evidence of major hemorrhage from abdominal or thoracic organs. Smaller arteries are embolized with hemostatic sponges, coils, and other devices. Intravenous pyelography and cystourethrography is avoided prior to pelvic angiography because a bladder filled with contrast or extravasated contrast obscures the pelvic vasculature. A plain abdominal film performed *after* the pelvic angiogram demonstrates the upper urinary tract.

Injury to the urinary tract is seen in up to 20% of patients with significant blunt injury to the anterior pelvis. Displaced fractures of the pubic rami and separation of the symphysis cause injuries to the bladder and urethra. Generally, the likelihood of injury increases with greater displacement and sepa-

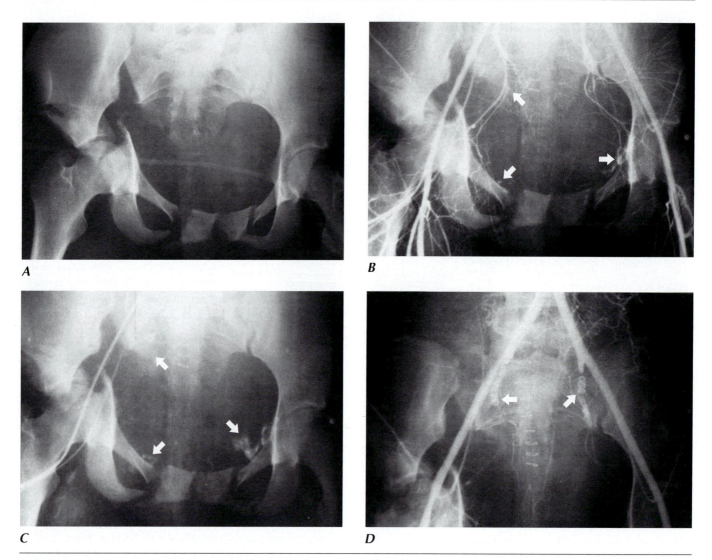

FIGURE 20-21.   Pelvic angiography and embolization. *A.* A complex pelvic fracture is seen in a hypotensive trauma victim. DPL was negative for gross hemorrhage. *B* and *C.* Angiography reveals active extravasation from the left and right internal iliac arteries *(arrows).* *D.* Embolization of both internal iliac arteries with coils *(arrows)* stopped the hemorrhage. (Copyright David T. Schwartz, M.D.)

ration. Nonetheless, significant urinary tract damage can occur with little skeletal disruption.

Urogenital Trauma

Nearly all major urinary tract injuries (renal, bladder, urethral) in adults are associated with gross hematuria. Indications for evaluation of the urinary tract after blunt trauma in adults are gross hematuria or microscopic hematuria in a hypotensive patient, even if the hypotension was transient (Fig. 20-22).[67] Any degree of hematuria in a child is an indication to image the urinary tract. Renal contusions are the most frequent upper urinary tract injuries (70%). Renal lacerations and renal pedicle injuries are infrequent (20 and 10%, respectively). Kidneys with congenital abnormalities are more vulnerable to trauma because of their increased size or abnormal position. Anomalous kidneys are present in 0.1 to 23% of blunt trauma cases.[68]

CT has largely replaced intravenous pyelography (IVP) in the evaluation of renal injury because it provides better imaging of the renal parenchyma and can identify injury to other organs (Fig. 20-23). The order of radiographic studies, CT (or IVP) versus cystography, is based on the degree of suspicion for upper versus lower tract injury. In general, the upper tract is studied first because upper tract injuries may be accompanied by nonurologic organ injuries such as trauma to the liver and spleen. If CT (or IVP) demonstrates a nonfunctioning kidney, a renal arteriogram is indicated in the stable patient. IVP and cystourethrography should not be performed before pelvic angiography. The contrast-filled bladder or extravasated contrast obscures visualization of the pelvic arteries.

Urethral injury in the male is suggested by blood at the urethral meatus, a high-riding or absent prostate, and a perineal or penile hematoma (Fig. 20-24). Posterior urethral injuries are usually associated with pelvic fractures. An anterior urethral injury results from a direct blow. The retrograde urethrogram is performed using a 12- to 16-Fr Foley catheter secured at the meatus with balloon inflation with 3mL sterile water or saline. A supine, preinjection KUB is obtained before urethrography or cystography. Under gentle pressure, 60 mL of undiluted

Urogenital Trauma

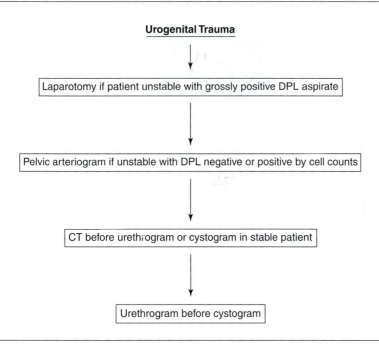

Laparotomy if patient unstable with grossly positive DPL aspirate

Pelvic arteriogram if unstable with DPL negative or positive by cell counts

CT before urethrogram or cystogram in stable patient

Urethrogram before cystogram

FIGURE 20-22. Radiographic priorities for urogenital trauma.

(60%) contrast is instilled over 60 seconds. A frontal film centered on the symphysis pubis is taken during injection. Resistance to contrast flow suggests urethral injury. Although oblique films are helpful in seeing the entire length of the urethra, they require rolling a patient with a pelvic fracture and potentially unstable pelvic hematoma.[69]

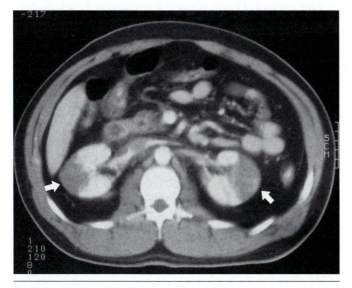

FIGURE 20-23. CT of renal injury. Bilateral wedge-shaped renal injuries are seen.

Gross hematuria, either alone or with a pelvic fracture, suggests a bladder injury. Bladder contusions are the second most common injury to the genitourinary tract, and bladder injury complicates 14% of pelvic fractures. Most pelvic fractures with bladder injury are pelvic ring disruptions. The frequency of extraperitoneal and intraperitoneal rupture is roughly equal (Figs. 20-25 and 20-26). The cystogram requires an indwelling Foley catheter to fill the bladder. On male patients, urethrography is done first. The bladder is filled by instillation of contrast with a bulb or Toomey syringe until bladder contraction is initiated or until 400 mL of contrast is instilled. Then, either a CT or AP and postevacuation plain films are obtained. If bladder injury is strongly suspected (gross hematuria with pelvic ring disruption), an initial AP film after 100 mL is instilled may show rupture, sparing the patient the additional extravasated contrast. Unless the bladder is fully distended, an extraperitoneal rupture may be missed. A CT or IVP cannot be used to exclude bladder injury. If the index of suspicion is high, a delayed KUB can identify intraperitoneal extravasation.

Thoracolumbar Spine Trauma

Injuries of the thoracic and lumbar spine make up a significant proportion of spinal injuries.[70] The greatest number of fractures occur at the T12-L2 junction where the mobile thoracic spine is anchored to the lumbar spine. Most spine injuries affect only a single level, but up to 11% of patients have fractures at multiple levels. Risk factors for thoracolumbar fractures include ejection from a motor vehicle or motorcycle, a vehicular crash at over 40 mph, a fall of at least 10 ft, a GCS score of 8 or less,

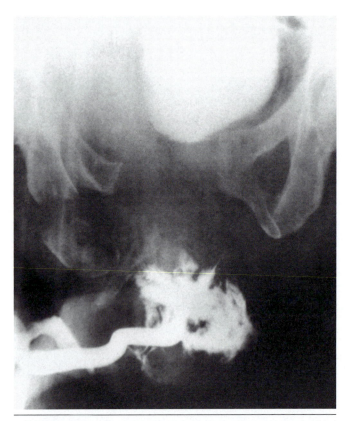

FIGURE 20-24. Retrograde urethrogram showing posterior urethral disruption in a patient with a severe pelvic fracture.

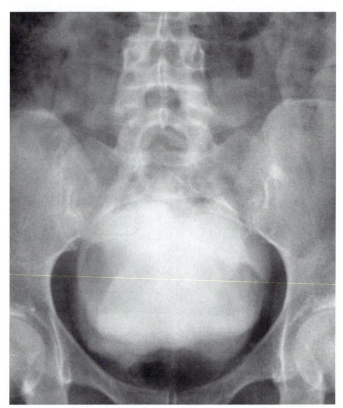

FIGURE 20-25. Cystogram showing intraperitoneal bladder rupture. Extravasated contrast has a smooth contour as it layers in the base of the peritoneal cavity.

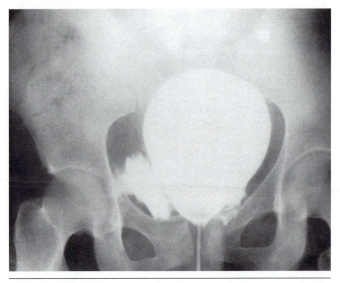

FIGURE 20-26. Cystogram showing extraperitoneal bladder rupture. Characteristic flame-shaped appearance of extravasated contrast adjacent to the bladder.

the presence of concomitant cervical fracture, a neurologic deficit, and back pain or tenderness.[71,72] Significant axial load injuries with fractures of the calcaneus or tibial plateau raise suspicion for thoracolumbar fractures. Evaluation of a thoracolumbar spine injury should follow evaluation and treatment of intracranial, intraabdominal, and intrathoracic injuries. Ini-

tal radiographic studies are AP views of the spine on a chest or abdominal radiograph. A portable cross-table lateral can also be used for imaging thoracolumbar injuries. CT scanning is indicated in burst fractures, suspected posterior element injuries, neurologic defects with no fracture seen on plain film, and equivocal plain films. CT myelography or MRI may be needed if initial studies do not explain a neurologic deficit or if the deficit progresses.

Thoracolumbar spine films are not needed in the awake, non-intoxicated patient with a normal sensorium, no neurologic deficits, no back pain or tenderness, no spine fractures elsewhere, no distracting injuries, and no need of airway support.[73,74] Nonetheless, spine radiographs should be liberally obtained in victims of major blunt trauma who have intraabdominal, intracranial, and intrathoracic injuries.

Extremity Trauma

Radiologic studies of the limbs are the last films undertaken in the course of trauma resuscitation. Signs of peripheral vascular injury include bleeding, expanding hematoma, bruit, absent or abnormal pulses or limb blood pressure, neurologic deficit, impaired distal circulation, decreased sensation, or increasing pain (Table 20-8). The presence of pulses by Doppler examination does not exclude an arterial injury. In patients with obvious and complete arterial occlusion, prompt surgical exploration is considered without waiting for an arteriogram.

Angiography is performed prior to lengthy orthopedic procedures if a patient has a diminished or absent pulse after reduction. High-risk injuries for arterial involvement include fractures and dislocations about the knee and elbow where the popliteal and brachial arteries are injured and fractures of the proximal humerus and lateral scapula with potential trauma to the axillary and brachial arteries (Fig. 20-27).[75] Venography is used selectively in the upper extremity because the sequelae of unrepaired venous thromboses or pseudoaneurysms are rare. Venography is used when injury to the popliteal vein is suspected. Frequent reexamination helps detect the development of a compartment syndrome. Severely traumatized, head-injured, and intoxicated patients are frequently unable to complain of the symptoms of compartment syndrome. Any tense, swollen limb is assessed with compartmental pressures. Significant blood loss (330 to 1300 mL)[76] can occur with a single femoral fracture. Rhabdomyolysis can complicate lower extremity trauma.

Two plain-film views of the limb suspected of fracture or dislocation are obtained in perpendicular planes. The radiographs must include the joint above and below the bone in question. Portable fluoroscopy is attractive because of its speed, but it lacks sufficient sensitivity to exclude simple extremity fractures.[77]

RADIOGRAPHIC EVALUATION OF PENETRATING TRAUMA

Penetrating Torso Trauma

Any stab or gunshot wound (GSW) to the torso has the potential to cause injury to the thorax, abdomen, or retroperitoneum. The diaphragm extends up to the fourth intercostal space in expiration, so that an intraabdominal injury can occur with penetrating chest trauma. With regard to GSWs, the emergency physician should not assume a straight course between entrance and exit wounds because bullets can change direction after striking bone. Stab wounds have a more predictable course, but peritoneal violation may occur several centimeters away from the skin wound.

Penetrating Thoracic Trauma

The portable chest film helps identify a hemothorax, pneumothorax, mediastinal widening, pneumomediastinum, rib fractures, vertebral fractures, and bullet fragments. Whenever possible, an upright chest radiograph better defines intrathoracic pathology following penetrating trauma. On a supine film, a small pneumothorax or hemothorax is often missed, and the mediastinum often appears widened. An expiratory chest radiograph improves the visualization of a small pneumothorax. If the chest radiograph is normal in a patient with a chest stab wound, a repeat radiograph after 4 to 6 hours of observation is obtained prior to discharge (in stable stab-wound patients with initially normal films). The wound tract should not be explored

TABLE 20-8

Signs of Peripheral Arterial Injury

HARD SIGNS	SOFT SIGNS
Pulse absent	History of moderate hemorrhage
Pulsatile bleeding	Stable, non-pulsatile hematoma
Expanding hematoma	Injury in proximity to vessel
Bruit or thrill	Diminished but palpable pulse
Regional ischemia (pale, cool)	Peripheral nerve deficit

to determine penetration of the pleura because this can create a pneumothorax.

The chest radiograph is not useful in the assessment of acute pericardial tamponade because the cardiac silhouette is not expected to be enlarged. The emergency physician must maintain a high index of suspicion for cardiac injury in patients with penetrating injuries in the parasternal region. Unstable patients with penetrating parasternal wounds require an emergent thoracotomy; valuable time must not be spent on an echocardiogram. Emergent pericardiocentesis may be used as a temporary measure. In a stable patient, the echocardiogram is an excellent diagnostic tool to detect pericardial fluid.[78,79] If the US is

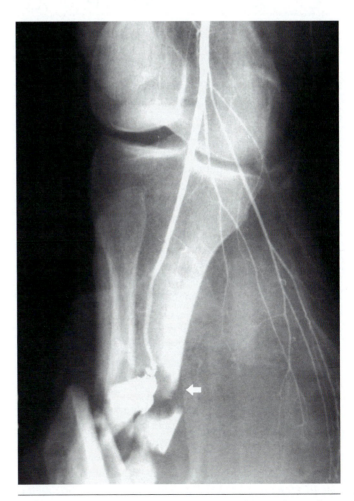

FIGURE 20-27. Arteriogram showing arterial laceration and extravasation complicating fractures of the tibia and fibula (*arrow*).

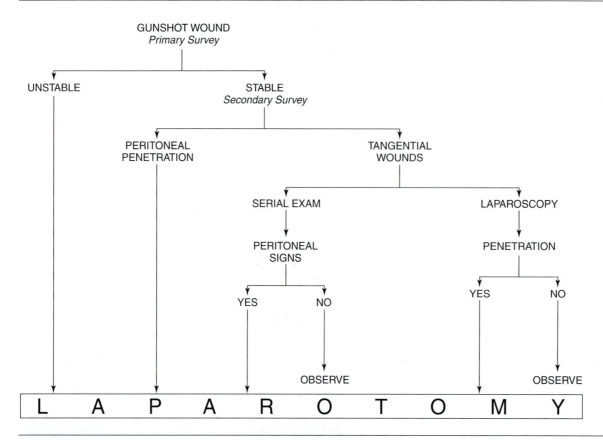

FIGURE 20-28. Evaluation of the patient with an abdominal gunshot wound. (From Cayten CG, Nassoura ZE: Abdomen, in Ivatury RR, Cayten NG (eds): *Textbook of Penetrating Trauma.* Baltimore: Williams & Wilkins, 1996, with permission.)

unavailable or questionable, then a surgical exploration through a subxyphoid window is considered. The diagnosis of hemopericardium must be aggressively pursued because a stable-appearing patient may suddenly suffer cardiovascular collapse.

In addition to cardiac injuries, penetrating trauma to the mediastinum can cause injury to the thoracic great vessels. Unstable patients require immediate operative intervention. If the patient's condition permits, angiography can define the lesion. False-negative arteriograms occur if the injury "seals off" or the radiologic projection fails to demonstrate the false aneurysm. Multiple tangential views are essential if the initial films are negative and the index of suspicion is high.

Penetrating injury to the chest can injure the esophagus, trachea, or diaphragm. Esophagography using water-soluble contrast media is used to diagnose esophageal perforation. If the diagnosis of esophageal injury remains in doubt after a contrast study or if the study cannot be performed, then endoscopy is indicated. Bronchoscopy is the modality of choice in the diagnosis of injury to the trachea or mainstem bronchus.

Penetrating injuries to the diaphragm are difficult to diagnose radiographically. The injury is more often diagnosed on the left side because on the right the liver covers the defect in the diaphragm. The chest radiograph can reveal bowel, stomach, or a nasogastric tube in the thorax. Common radiographic manifestations of diaphragmatic injury include an elevated left hemidiaphragm, a loculated pneumothorax, or a subpulmonic hematoma. Diagnostic modalities to detect diaphragmatic injury include an upper gastrointestinal contrast study or thora-

coscopy. Visceral herniation or strangulation is a delayed complication of a diaphragmatic tear.

Penetrating Abdominal, Flank, and Back Trauma

In patients with a GSW to the abdomen, a chest and abdominal radiograph is used to help locate the bullet, define potential thoracic trauma, and help detect a rare case of bullet embolism in the vasculature. The addition of a one-shot IVP demonstrates the presence of two functioning kidneys. Immediate surgical consultation is essential for GSWs to the anterior abdomen since all such patients require a laparotomy (Fig. 20-28).[80,81] The only possible exception to mandatory exploration is a GSW to the right upper quadrant in the hemodynamically stable patient. Although controversial, it has been suggested that a CT scan of the abdomen and lower chest along with serial physical examinations watching for peritonitis or hemodynamic instability can substitute for operative exploration.[82]

In a patient sustaining a stab wound to the anterior abdomen, the upright chest film is the only radiographic study needed to detect intrathoracic pathology. These patients are best evaluated by serial examinations, local wound exploration, DPL, or laparoscopy.[83] There is little role for a CT scan in these patients. Unstable patients or those with peritonitis require prompt surgery (Fig. 20-29).

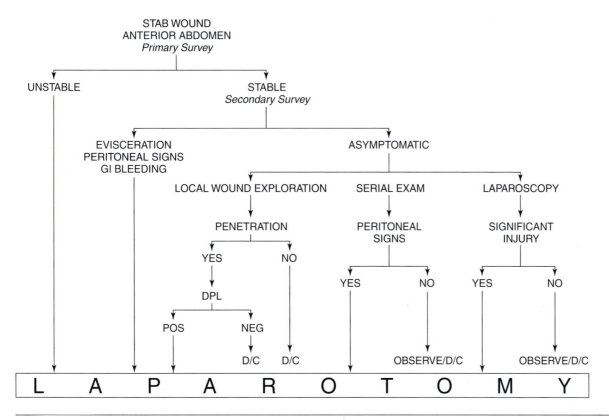

FIGURE 20-29. Evaluation of the patient with a stab wound to the anterior abdomen. (D/C, discharge patients.) (From Cayten CG, Nassoura ZE: Abdomen, in Ivatury RR, Cayten NG (eds): *Textbook of Penetrating Trauma.* Baltimore: Williams & Wilkins, 1996, with permission.)

The anatomic limits of the flank are the anterior and posterior axillary lines, the sixth rib, and the iliac crest. The back is defined as the region between the posterior axillary lines, iliac crest, and the tip of the scapula. Intraabdominal injury occurs in 40% of GSWs to the flank and 25% of stab wounds. GSWs to the back injure abdominal organs 41% of the time, while stab wounds have a 10% rate of abdominal injury. Physical examination is unreliable in wounds to this region, and there can be injuries to the posterior aspect of the colon, kidney, pancreas, spleen, liver, and vascular structures. Patients sustaining penetrating trauma to the back or flank who demonstrate hemodynamic instability, peritonitis, or pneumoperitoneum require emergent laporatomy (Fig. 20-30). A triple-contrast CT scan of the abdomen is indicated for stable patients who do not demonstrate the above findings. In a triple-contrast CT, contrast is administered orally, rectally (to distend the colon), and intravenously.[84–87] If the CT scan is negative, serial examinations are essential, because the patient can still have an injury to a hollow viscus.

Penetrating Neck Trauma

With regard to penetrating injuries, the neck is divided into three zones: Zone I extends from the cricoid cartilage to the clavicle, Zone II is between the cricoid cartilage and the angle of the mandible, and Zone III is above the angle of the mandible to the base of the skull (Fig. 20-31). Clinical findings of vis-

ceral injury in patients with penetrating neck injuries include hemorrhage, hematoma formation, airway compromise, spinal cord or cerebrovascular injury, and difficulty speaking or swallowing. All patients with hypotension, expanding hematomas, uncontrolled bleeding, or airway compromise must be taken directly to the operating room without radiography.

Stable patients with penetrating neck injuries receive cervical radiographs to look for hematomas, tracheal deviation, subcutaneous air, retropharyngeal swelling, or foreign bodies. The use of arteriography in stable patients with clinical evidence of arterial injury is controversial and is done at the discretion of the surgeon. Stable patients without evidence of arterial injury who have a wound in either Zone 1 or 3 are evaluated with an arteriogram (Figs. 20-32 and 20-33). Surgical exploration in these regions is difficult and precise definition of the location and extent of injury is important to the surgeon.[88–91] Laryngoscopy defines injury to the airway and a water-soluble contrast esophagram defines esophageal pathology. Esophagoscopy is indicated if the patient cannot swallow or if the contrast study is nondiagnostic.

Several strategies are proposed for evaluating wounds in Zone 2. Traditionally, all patients required operative exploration if the platysma was penetrated. Many surgeons now use nonoperative evaluation with arteriography, laryngoscopy, and contrast esophagography. Surgery is undertaken selectively if an injury is found on these studies. Another strategy is to follow stable patients clinically with serial physical examinations without using invasive diagnostic studies.[92]

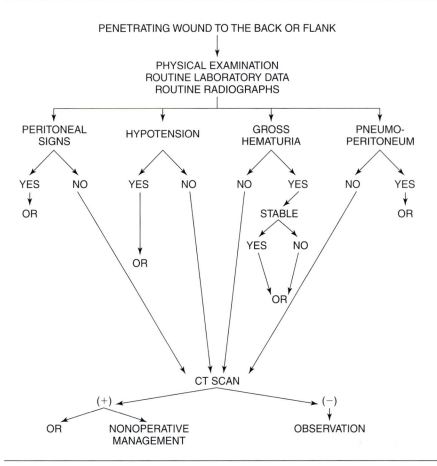

PENETRATING WOUND TO THE BACK OR FLANK

PHYSICAL EXAMINATION
ROUTINE LABORATORY DATA
ROUTINE RADIOGRAPHS

PERITONEAL SIGNS   HYPOTENSION   GROSS HEMATURIA   PNEUMO-PERITONEUM

YES   NO   YES   NO   NO   YES   NO   YES

OR   OR   STABLE   OR

YES   NO

OR

CT SCAN

(+)   (−)

OR   NONOPERATIVE MANAGEMENT   OBSERVATION

FIGURE 20-30.   Evaluation of the patient with penetrating trauma to the flank or back. (Modified from Coppa G: Back and flank, in Ivatury RR, Cayten NG (eds): *Textbook of Penetrating Trauma.* Baltimore: Williams & Wilkins, 1996, with permission.)

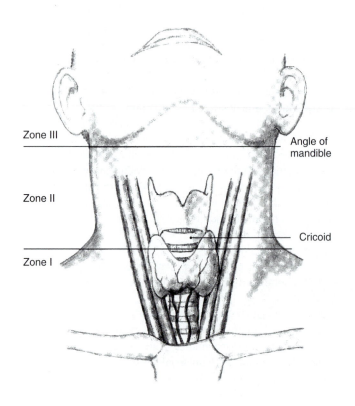

Zone III

Zone II

Zone I

Angle of mandible

Cricoid

Penetrating Peripheral Arterial Trauma

Peripheral vascular injuries occur with both stab wounds and gunshot injuries. The "gold standard" for the evaluation of peripheral arterial injury is the angiogram. The presence of distal pulses does not exclude the diagnosis of proximal arterial pathology, because pulses can be transmitted from collateral flow. Common types of arterial injury include laceration, transection, contusion, segmental spasm, thrombosis, true aneurysm formation, false aneurysm formation, and arteriovenous fistula formation. Physical findings indicating the need for immediate exploration include pulsatile bleeding, an expanding hematoma, a palpable thrill, an audible bruit, or evidence of regional ischemia (e.g., pain, pallor, paralysis, pulselessness, paresthesia) (Table 20-8). With any of these "hard signs," immediate surgical consultation is essential and must not await imaging studies. Arteriography should be considered in patients

FIGURE 20-31.   Zones of the neck. (From Borgstrom D, Weigelt JA: Neck: aerodigestive tract, in Ivatury RR, Cayten NG (eds): *Textbook of Penetrating Trauma.* Baltimore: Williams & Wilkins, 1996, with permission.)

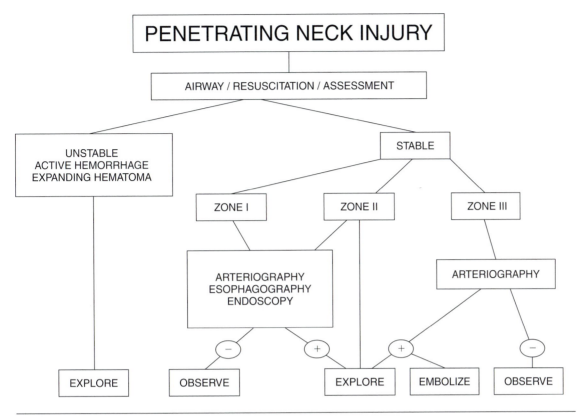

FIGURE 20-32. Evaluation of the patient with penetrating neck trauma. (From Jacobson LE, Gomez GA: Neck, in Ivatury RR, Cayten NG (eds): *Textbook of Penetrating Trauma.* Baltimore: Williams & Wilkins, 1996, with permission.)

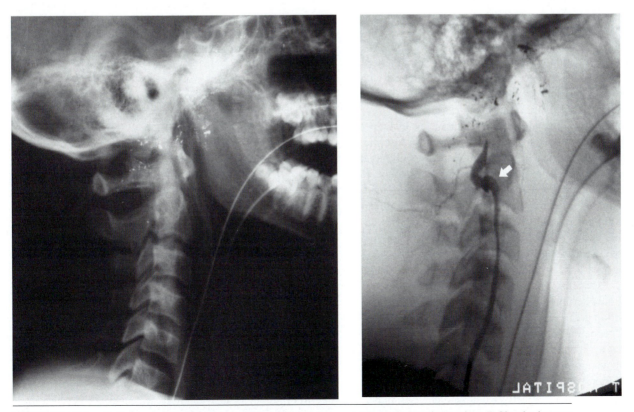

FIGURE 20-33. Bullet wound to the neck. *A.* Bullet fragments are visible at the cervicocranium *B.* Vertebral artery angiogram reveals occlusion of the right vertebral artery and extravasation of contrast *(arrow).*

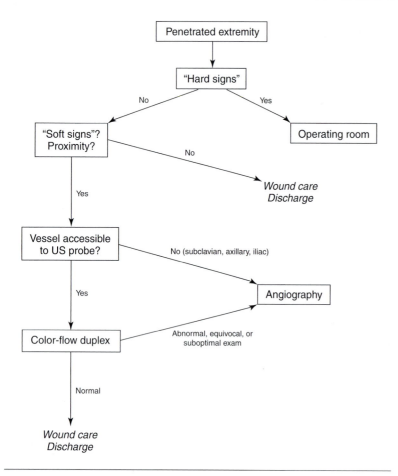

FIGURE 20-34.   Management of penetrating wounds to the extremities.

the next day to avoid late-night studies on low-risk patients. Color-flow duplex US is noninvasive and accurate in determining arterial injury if the vessel is accessible to the probe. This scan combines real-time B-mode US imaging with a Doppler flow detector, allowing vascular imaging and the determination of the velocity spectra of the flowing elements in the vessel. Some vessels are not anatomically suitable for US studies and require angiography (subclavian, axillary, iliac arteries). The largest prospective study comparing color flow duplex ultrasonography with arteriography evaluated 86 penetrating extremity injuries and found that US had a specificity of 99%, sensitivity of 71%, negative predictive value of 98%, and positive predictive value of 83%.[103]

with multiple penetrating wounds in whom the actual site of vascular injury is unknown (shotgun wounds), in patients with a bullet trajectory that spans a long segment of artery, and in those patients with preexisting vascular disease.

"Soft signs" indicating potential vascular injury include a history of moderate hemorrhage, injury in proximity to a major artery, a diminished but palpable pulse, and a peripheral nerve deficit. Controversy exists as to the optimal method to evaluate these patients. Proximity alone is no longer considered an indication for angiography (Fig. 20-34). Some physicians use a Doppler arterial pressure index (API) to help decide on angiography.[93,94] The API is determined by dividing the systolic pressure in the injured limb by the systolic pressure in the normal one. An index of less than 0.9 has a sensitivity of 95%, specificity of 97%, and a negative predictive value of 99% in determining a clinically significant arterial injury. If the API is greater than 0.9 in the presence of soft signs, then patients may either be observed or undergo a duplex scan. If close follow-up is unavailable on an outpatient basis, the patient should have an imaging procedure or be hospitalized for serial examinations.

If the API is less than 0.9 and the patient has "soft signs," then either an arteriogram or a duplex US is performed.[95-102] Many institutions image these patients on a semiurgent basis

REFERENCES

1. U.S. Department of Health and Human Services; Centers for Disease Control and Prevention, National Center for Injury Prevention and Control, *Summary of Injury Mortality Data,* 1986–1992.
2. Rice DP, MacKenzie EJ: *Cost of Injury in the United States: A Report to Congress.* Institute for Health and Aging, University of California, San Francisco and the Injury Prevention Center. Baltimore: Johns Hopkins University, 1989.
3. American College of Surgeons Committee on Trauma: Resource document 2: Prehospital triage criteria, in *Advanced Trauma Life Support Instructor Manual.* Chicago: American College of Surgeons, 1993, p. 328.
4. Feliciano DV: Patterns of injury in trauma, in Feliciano DV, Moore EE, Mattox KL (eds): *Trauma,* 3d ed. Stamford, CT: Appleton & Lange, 1996, pp. 31–40.
5. Hollerman JJ, Fackler ML: Gunshot wounds: Radiology and wound ballistics. *Emerg Radiol* 2:171, 1995.
6. Enderson BL, Reath DB, Meadors J, et al: The tertiary trauma survey: A prospective study of missed injury. *J Trauma* 30:666, 1990.
7. Ben-Menachem Y, Fisher RG: Radiology, in Feliciano DV, Moore EE, Mattox KL (eds.): *Trauma,* 3d ed. Stamford, CT: Appleton & Lange, 1996, pp. 207–236.
8. Hehir MD, Hollands MJ, Deane SA, et al: The accuracy of the first chest x-ray in the trauma patient. *Aust NZ J Surg* 60:529, 1990.
9. MacDonald RL, Schwartz ML, Mirich D, et al: Diagnosis of cervical spine injury in motor vehicle crash victims: How many x-rays are enough? *J Trauma* 30:392, 1990.
10. Woodring JH, Lee C: Limitations of cervical radiography in the evaluation of acute cervical trauma. *J Trauma* 34:32, 1993.
11. Perry NM, Lewars MD: ABC of major trauma. Radiological assessment—I. *BMJ* 301:805, 1990.
12. Holley J, Jorden R: Airway management in patients with unstable cervical spine fractures. *Ann Emerg Med* 18:1237, 1989.
13. Knopp RK: The safety of orotracheal intubation in patients with suspected cervical-spine injury. *Ann Emerg Med* 19:603, 1990.
14. Scannell G, Waxman K, Tominaga G, et al: Orotracheal intuba-

tion in trauma patients with cervical fractures. *Arch Surg* 128:903, 1993.

15. Kreipke KL, Gillespie KR, McCarthy MC, et al: Reliability of indications for cervical spine films in trauma patients. *J Trauma* 29:1438, 1989.

16. Roberge RJ, Wears RC, Kelly M, et al: Selective application of cervical spine radiography in alert victims of blunt trauma: A prospective study. *J Trauma* 28:784, 1988.

17. Hoffman JR, Schriger D, Mower W, et al: Low-risk criteria for cervical spine radiography in blunt trauma: A prospective study. *Ann Emerg Med* 21:1454, 1992.

18. Civil ID, Ross SE, Botehlo G, Schwab CW: Routine pelvic radiography in severe blunt trauma: Is it necessary? *Ann Emerg Med* 17:488, 1988.

19. Cales RH, Trunkey DD: Preventable trauma deaths: A review of trauma care systems development. *JAMA* 254:1059, 1985.

20. Thomason M, Messick J, Rutledge R, et al: Head CT scanning versus urgent exploration in the hypotensive blunt trauma patient. *J Trauma* 34:40, 1993.

21. Wisner DH, Victor NS, Holcroft JW: Priorities in the management of multiple trauma: Intracranial versus intra-abdominal injury. *J Trauma* 35:271, 1993.

22. Beall AC, Crawford HW, DeBakey ME: Considerations in the management of acute traumatic hemothorax. *J Thorac Cardiovasc Surg* 52:351, 1966.

23. Evers BM, Cryer HM, Miller FB: Pelvic fracture hemorrhage: Priorities in management. *Arch Surg* 124:424, 1989.

24. Flint L, Babikian G, Anders M, et al: Definitive control of mortality from severe pelvic fracture. *Ann Surg* 211:703, 1990.

25. Cryer HG, Johnson E: Pelvic fractures, in Feliciano DV, Moore EE, Mattox KL (eds): *Trauma,* 3d ed. Stamford, CT: Appleton & Lange, 1996, pp. 635–660.

26. Seeling JM, Becker DP, Miller JD, et al: Traumatic acute subdural haematoma: Major mortality reduction in comatose patients treated within four hours. *N Engl J Med* 304:1511, 1981.

27. American College of Surgeons Committee on Trauma: Head trauma, in *Advanced Trauma Life Support Instructor Manual.* Chicago: American College of Surgeons, 1993, pp. 159–183.

28. Smirniotopolis JG, Mirvis SE, Wolf A: Imaging of craniocerebral trauma, in Mirvis SE, Young WJR (eds): *Imaging in Trauma and Critical Care.* Baltimore: William & Wilkins, 1992, pp. 23–92.

29. Valadka AB, Narayan RK: *Injury to the Cranium,* in Feliciano DV, Moore EE, Mattox KL (eds): *Trauma,* 3d ed. Stamford, CT: Appleton & Lange, 1996, pp. 267–278.

30. Sweeney TA, Marx JA: Blunt neck injury. *Emerg Med Clin North Am* 11:1, 1993.

31. Davis JW, Phreaner DL, Hoyt DB, Mackersie RC: The etiology of missed cervical spine injuries. *J Trauma* 34:342, 1993.

32. Kirshenbaum KJ, Nadimpalli SR, Fantus R, Cavallino RP: Unsuspected cervical spine fractures associated with significant head trauma: Role of CT. *J Emerg Med* 8:183, 1990.

33. Hills MW, Deane SA: Head Injury and facial injury: Is there an increased risk of cervical spine injury? *J Trauma* 34:549, 1993.

34. Link TM, Schuierer G, Hufendiek A, et al: Substantial head trauma: Value of routine CT examination of the cervicocranium. *Radiology* 196:741, 1995.

35. Freemyer B, Knopp R, Piche J, et al: Comparison of five-view and three-view cervical spine series in the evaluation of patients with cervical trauma. *Ann Emerg Med* 18:818, 1989.

36. Polansky A, Resnick D, Sofferman RA, et al: Hyoid bone elevation: A sign of tracheal transection. *Radiology* 150:117, 1984.

37. Gussack GS, Jurkovich GJ, Luterman A: Laryngotracheal trauma: A protocol approach to a rare injury. *Laryngoscope* 96:660, 1986.

38. Schaider JJ, Dunne P: Head and neck trauma, in Rosen P, Doris PE, Barkin RM, et al (eds): *Diagnostic Radiology in Emergency Medicine.* St. Louis: Mosby, 1992, pp. 25–50.

39. Poole GV, Morgan DB, Cranston PE, et al: Computed tomography in the management of blunt thoracic trauma. *J Trauma* 35:296, 1993.

40. Richardson JD, Wilson ME, Miller FB: The widened mediastinum: Diagnostic and therapeutic priorities. *Ann Surg* 211:731, 1990.

41. Harris JH, Horowitz DR, Zelitt DL: Unenhanced dynamic mediastinal computed tomography in the selection of patients requiring thoracic aortography for the detection of acute traumatic aortic injury. *Emerg Radiol* 2:67, 1995.

42. American College of Surgeons Committee on Trauma: Thoracic trauma, in *Advanced Trauma Life Support Instructor Manual.* Chicago: American College of Surgeons, 1993, pp. 111–127.

43. Fisher RG, Chasen MH, Lamki N: Diagnosis of injuries of the aorta and brachiocephalic arteries caused by blunt chest trauma: CT vs aortography. *AJR* 162:1047, 1994.

44. Buckmaster MJ, Kearney PA, Johnson SB, et al: Further experience with transesophageal echocardiography in the evaluation of thoracic aortic injury. *J Trauma* 37:989, 1994.

45. Kearney PA, Smith DW, Johnson S, et al: Use of transesophageal echocardiography in the evaluation of traumatic aortic injury. *J Trauma* 34:696, 1993.

46. Saletta S, Lederman E, Fein S, et al: Transesophageal echocardiography for the initial evaluation of the widened mediastinum in trauma patients. *J Trauma* 39:137, 1995.

47. Smith MD, Cassidy JM, Souther S, et al: Transesophageal echocardiography in the diagnosis of traumatic rupture of the aorta. *N Engl J Med* 332:356, 1995.

48. Gelman R, Mirvis SE, Gens D: Diaphragmatic rupture due to blunt trauma: Sensitivity of plain chest radiography. *AJR* 156:51, 1990.

49. Baron B, Daffner R. Traumatic rupture of the right hemidiaphragm: Diagnosis by chest radiography. *Emerg Radiol* 1:231, 1994.

50. Beal SL, Pottmeyer EW, Spisso JM: Esophageal perforation following external blunt trauma. *J Trauma* 28:1425, 1988.

51. Burke JF: Early diagnosis of a traumatic rupture of the bronchus. *JAMA* 181:682, 1962.

52. Verma SM, Hawkins H, Coglazier, et al: The clinical utility of rib detail films in the evaluation of trauma. *Emerg Radiol* 2:264, 1995.

53. Stephens NG, Morgan AS, Corvo P, Bernstein BA: Significance of scapular fracture in the blunt-trauma patient. *Ann Emerg Med* 26:439, 1995.

54. Roy-Shapira A, Levi I, Khoda J: Sternal fractures: A red flag or a red herring? *J Trauma* 37:59, 1994.

55. American College of Surgeons Committee on Trauma: Abdominal trauma, in *Advanced Trauma Life Support Instructor Manual.* Chicago: American College of Surgeons, 1993, pp. 141–154.

56. Novelline RA: Abdomen: Traumatic emergencies, in Harris JH Jr, Harris, WH, Novelline RA (eds): *The Radiology of Emergency Medicine*, 3d ed. Baltimore: William & Wilkins, 1993, pp. 640–641.

57. Sherck J, Shatney C, Sensaki K, Selivanov V: The accuracy of computed tomography in the diagnosis of blunt small-bowel per-

foration. *Am J Surg* 168:670, 1994.

58. Rizzo MJ, Federle MP, Griffiths BG: Bowel and mesenteric injury following blunt abdominal trauma: Evaluation with CT. *Radiology* 173:143, 1988.

59. Kinnunen J, Kivioja A, Poussa K, Laasonen EM: Emergency CT in blunt abdominal trauma of multiple injury patients. *Acta Radiol* 35:319, 1994.

60. Fabian TC, Croce MA: Abdominal trauma, including indications for celiotomy, in Feliciano DV, Moore EE, Mattox KL (eds): *Trauma*, 3d ed. Stamford, CT: Appleton & Lange, 1996, p. 456.

61. Hoffmann R, Nerlich M, Muggia-Sullam M, et al: Blunt abdominal trauma in cases of multiple trauma evaluated by ultrasonography: A prospective analysis of 291 patients. *J Trauma* 32:452, 1992.

62. McKenney M, Lentz K, Nunez D, et al: Can ultrasound replace diagnostic peritoneal lavage in the assessment of blunt trauma? *J Trauma* 37:439, 1994.

63. Rothlin MA, Naf R, Amgwerd M, et al: Ultrasound in blunt abdominal and thoracic trauma. *J Trauma* 34:488, 1993.

64. Rozycki GS, Ochsner MG, Jaffin JH, Champion HR: Prospective evaluation of surgeons' use of ultrasound in the evaluation of trauma patients. *J Trauma* 34:516, 1993.

65. Bode PJ, Niezen RA, van Vugt AB, Schipper J: Abdominal ultrasound as a reliable indicator for conclusive laparatomy in blunt abdominal trauma. *J Trauma* 34:27, 1993.

66. Pearl WS, Todd KH: Ultrasonography for the initial evaluation of blunt abdominal trauma: A review of prospective trials. *Ann Emerg Med* 27:353, 1996.

67. Mee SL, McAninch JW, Robinson AL, et al: Radiographic assessment of renal trauma: A 10 year prospective study of patient selection. *J Urol* 141:1095, 1989.

68. Petersson NE: Genitourinary trauma, in Feliciano DV, Moore EE, Mattox KL (eds): *Trauma*, 3d ed. Stamford, CT: Appleton & Lange, 1996, pp. 661–693.

69. Schneider R: Genitourinary trauma. *Emerg Med Clin North Am* 11:137, 1993.

70. Przybylski GJ, Marion DW. Injury to the vertebrae and spinal cord, in Feliciano DV, Moore EE, Mattox KL (eds): *Trauma*, 3d ed. Stamford, CT: Appleton & Lange, 1996, pp. 307–327.

71. Frankel HL, Rozycki GS, Ochsner MG, et al: Indications for obtaining surveillance thoracic and lumbar spine radiographs. *J Trauma* 37:673, 1994.

72. Pal JM, Mulder DS, Brown RA, Fleiszer DM: Assessing multiple trauma: Is the cervical spine enough? *J Trauma* 28:1282, 1988.

73. Samuels LE, Kerstein MD: Routine radiographic evaluation of the thoracolumbar spine in blunt trauma patients. A reappraisal. *J Trauma* 34:85, 1993.

74. Terregino CA, Ross SE, Lipinski MF, et al: Selective indications for thoracic and lumbar radiography in blunt trauma. *Ann Emerg Med* 26:126, 1995.

75. Lee DH, Neviaser RJ: Upper extremity fractures and dislocations, in Feliciano DV, Moore EE, Mattox KL (eds): *Trauma*, 3d ed. Stamford, CT: Appleton & Lange, 1996, 733–790.

76. Lieurance R, Benjamin JB, Rappaport WD: Blood loss and transfusion in patients with isolated femur fractures. *J Orthop Trauma* 6:175, 1992.

77. Jones J, McDonald JH, Smith M, Holt SP: Bedside fluoroscopy to screen for simple extremity trauma in the ED. *J Emerg Med* 13:545, 1995.

78. Aaland MO, Bryan FC III, Sherman R: Two-dimensional echocardiogram in hemodynamically stable victims of penetrating precordial trauma. *Am Surg* 60:412, 1994.

79. Nagy KK, Lohmann C, Kim DO, Barrett J: Role of echocardiography in the diagnosis of occult penetrating cardiac injury. *J Trauma* 38:859, 1995.

80. Feliciano DV, Burch JM, Spjut-Patrinely V, et al: Abdominal gunshot wounds: An urban trauma center's experience with 300 consecutive patients. *Ann Surg* 208:362, 1988.

81. Moore EE, Marx JA: Penetrating abdominal wounds—Rationale for exploratory laparotomy. *JAMA* 253:2705, 1985.

82. Renz BM, Feliciano DV: Gunshot wounds to the right thoraco-abdomen: A prospective study of nonoperative management. *J Trauma* 37:737, 1994.

83. Rosemurgy AS, Albrink MH, Olson SM, et al: Abdominal stab wound protocol: Prospective study documents applicability for widespread use. *Am Surg* 61:112, 1995.

84. McCarthy MC, Lowdermilk GA, Canal DF, Broadie TA: Prediction of injury caused by penetrating wounds to the abdomen, flank, and back. *Arch Surg* 126:962, 1991.

85. Meyer DM, Thal ER, Weigelt JA, Redman HC: The role of abdominal CT in the evaluation of stab wounds to the back. *J Trauma* 29:1226, 1989.

86. Demetriades D, Rabinowitz B, Sofianos C, et al: The management of penetrating injuries of the back. A prospective study of 230 patients. *Ann Surg,* 207:72, 1988.

87. Hauser CJ, Huprich JE, Bosco P, et al: Triple–contrast computed tomography in the evaluation of penetrating posterior abdominal injuries. *Arch Surg* 122:1112, 1987.

88. Asenio JA, Valenziano CP, Falcone RE, Grosh JD: Management of penetrating neck injuries: The controversy surrounding zone II injuries. *Surg Clin North Am* 71:267, 1991.

89. Noyes LD, McSwain NE, Markowitz IP: Panendoscopy with arteriography versus mandatory exploration of penetrating wounds of the neck. *Ann Surg* 204:21, 1986.

90. Miller RH, Duplechain JK: Penetrating wounds of the neck. *Otolaryngol Clin North Am* 24:15, 1991.

91. Fry WR, Dort JA, Smith S, et al: Duplex scanning replaces arteriography and operative exploration in the diagnosis of potential cervical vascular injury. *Am J Surg* 168:693, 1994.

92. Beitsch P, Weigelt JA, Flynn E, Easley S: Physical examination and arteriography in patients with penetrating zone II neck wounds. *Arch Surg,* 129:577, 1994.

93. Lynch K, Johansen K: Can Doppler pressure measurement replace "exclusion" arteriography in the diagnosis of occult extremity arterial trauma? *Ann Surg* 214:737, 1991.

94. Johansen K, Lynch K, Paun M, Copass M: Non-invasive vascular tests reliably exclude occult arterial trauma in injured extremities. *J Trauma* 31:515, 1991.

95. Stain SC, Yellin AE, Weaver FA, Pentecost MJ: Selective management of nonocclusive arterial injuries. *Arch Surg* 124:1136, 1989.

96. Fry WR, Smith RS, Sayers DV, et al: The success of duplex ultrasonographic scanning in diagnosis of extremity vascular proximity trauma. *Arch Surg* 128:1368, 1993.

97. Anderson RJ, Hobson RW II, Lee BC, et al: Reduced dependency on arteriography for penetrating extremity trauma: Influence of wound location and noninvasive vascular studies. *J Trauma* 30:1059, 1990.

98. Dennis JW: New perspective on the management of penetrating trauma in proximity to major limb arteries. *J Vasc Surg* 11:84, 1990.

99. Fry WR, Smith RS, Sayers DV, et al: The success of duplex ultrasonographic scanning in diagnosis of extremity vascular proximity trauma. *Arch Surg* 128:1368, 1993.

100. Bergstein JM, Blair JF, Edwards J, et al: Pitfalls in the use of

color-flow duplex ultrasound for screening of suspected arterial injuries in penetrated extremities. *J Trauma* 33:395, 1992.

101. Panetta TF, Hunt JP, Buechter KJ, et al: Duplex ultrasonography versus arteriography in the diagnosis of arterial injury: An experimental study. *J Trauma* 33:627, 1992.

102. Knudson MM, Lewis FR, Atkinson K, Neuhaus A: The role of duplex ultrasound arterial imaging in patients with penetrating extremity trauma. *Arch Surg* 128:1033, 1993.

103. Edwards JW. Bergstein JM, Karp DL, et al: Penetrating proximity injuries: The role of duplex scanning: A prospective study. *J Vasc Technol* 17:257, 1993.

CHAPTER 21

EMERGENCY DEPARTMENT ULTRASONOGRAPHY

DIETRICH JEHLE / TANVIR DARA / BOBBY ABRAMS

The emergency bedside ultrasound (US) examination differs from the US examination performed in a radiology department owing to a dissimilarity in time constraints, equipment, goals, and operator skill. The emergency department (ED) examination is highly focused and is used in emergency situations to provide quick and accurate yes-or-no answers to a number of specific diagnostic questions. There are six primary conditions for which bedside US is used in the ED: abdominal aortic aneurysms, traumatic hemoperitoneum, ectopic pregnancies, pericardial tamponade, gallstones, and renal colic. The first four are acutely life-threatening emergencies for which any delay in evaluation and treatment must be minimized. US evaluations for acute gallbladder disease and flank pain are both frequent and significant in terms of minimizing patient morbidity and expediting patient management.

Other applications of US can fall into the purview of ED ultrasonography. These include the evaluation of cardiac motion in *pulseless electrical activity* (PEA), assessing fetal viability, and detecting abruptio placentae and placenta previa. In addition, other uses of US are helpful in evaluating the ED patient. These include evaluation of common bile duct obstruction, appendicitis, deep venous thrombosis (DVT), ovarian cysts, ovarian torsion, and aortic dissection.

FUNDAMENTALS OF ULTRASOUND

Diagnostic US equipment uses the *piezoelectric effect* both for generating US waves and receiving the reflected echoes. The piezoelectric effect has two components, both of which are essential to the operation of diagnostic US. First, when a piezoelectric substance is compressed, as by a returning US wave, an electric current is produced. Second, when an alternating electric current is applied to the piezoelectric element, the object vibrates at a stable frequency. That frequency is a characteristic of the material and its thickness. These two properties allow for the transmission and reception of US waves by an US probe or transducer.

Many modifications of the piezoelectric transducer exist. The most frequently used transducer in the ED is the mechanical sector scanner. This uses a single element that oscillates back and forth or rotates within the transducer head. A second type of transducer is the linear array, which comprises a sequential array of piezoelectric elements. Consequently, the transducer head is longer than that of the mechanical sector scanner. The transducer contains numerous crystals that are triggererd electronically in groups to produce an US beam. The electronic sector scanner combines the advantages of the electronic circuitry of the linear-array scanner, but the arrangement of piezoelectric elements allows for a smaller transducer head. The annular (curved) array is another arrangement of transducers, in which the piezoelectric elements are grouped in a curved fashion around a central point. A final type of transducer is the curved linear array, which is capable of providing excellent images, particularly in the near field, because of the convex shape of the head.

The two-dimensional image on an US screen is produced from the electrical information that is generated by the transducer. Usually, the image is displayed so that the area nearest the transducer is at the top of the screen.

Sound waves are transmitted through a medium as a series of compressions and rarefactions. The number of these compressions and rarefactions per second is referred to as *frequency* and is measured in cycles per second, or hertz (Hz). US is defined as any frequency above the range of normal human hearing, generally greater than 20,000 Hz or 0.02 MHz. For most applications of diagnostic US, transducer frequencies range from 3.0 to 7.5 MHz. As a general rule, higher frequencies provide finer resolution in the near field and lower frequencies provide a greater depth of penetration.

Sound waves travel slowly in gases, faster in liquids, and fastest in solids. Structures containing fluid, (e.g., soft tissues) are good transmitters of US waves. Solid structures reflect or absorb most sound waves, while air-filled objects do not transmit the US beam. Therefore, solid and air-filled structures are poorly seen by US.

An object that reflects virtually all the US waves back toward the transducer is "echogenic" and appears white on the US screen. Because this object generates many echoes between itself and the transducer head, it is also referred to as *hyperechoic*. An object that transmits all the US impulses and has no reflected echoes is depicted as black on the screen and is referred to as *anechoic*. Most anechoic structures are cystic. Most structures are neither completely echogenic nor anechoic. Because the majority of bodily organs both transmit and reflect US waves, they are seen as gray on the screen.

Doppler US quantitates flow within blood vessels or the heart. The change in frequency of the reflected US wave is a

TABLE 21-1

Common Ultrasound Artifacts

ARTIFACT	CAUSE	SOLUTION
Pseudosludge (beam-width artifact)	Echoes from adjacent organ (e.g., bowel) projected into nearby organ lumen (e.g., gallbladder) when transducer is placed at center of organ lumen	Variation in patient position
Side lobe artifact	Echoes returning to transducer through side lobes rather than main beam	Alternating angle of transducer head; change type of transducer
Reverberation artifact	Reflection of beam between highly reflective surfaces results in parallel echoes of decreasing intensity	Variation of probe frequency and position
Mirror artifact	Reflection of echoes from liver by diaphragm creates image above diaphragm	Visualization from different position, altering angulation of probe
Gain artifact	Inappropriate gain or time-gain-compensator (TGC) setting	Careful adjustment of gain using region of known echogenicity

function of direction and velocity of flow (see Chap. 19, Fig. 19-53). Color Doppler assigns different colors to different flow velocities, allowing one to visualize flow over an area of the ultrasound image. This powerful but expensive tool is used for vascular, cardiac and aortic scanning. As cost decreases, Doppler and color Doppler may become a routine part of ED ultrasonography.

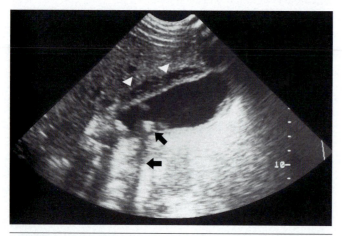

FIGURE 21-1.   Gallbladder with stone. Note the multiple echogenic structures with posterior acoustic shadowing, representing gallstones in a patient with gangrenous cholecystitis *(arrows)*. There are multiple striations and anechoic spaces within the markedly thickened gallbladder wall *(arrowheads)*. (Courtesy of Dietrich Jehle, M.D.)

Many times the US images appear clear and anatomically accurate. At other times, the images are distorted or have potentially misleading findings created by *artifacts* of the US technique. It is important to be familiar with these US artifacts and be able to interpret the images correctly (Table 21-1). In some important instances, US "effects" such as shadowing or posterior enhancement are helpful in interpreting the sonographic images.

ABDOMINAL APPLICATIONS

The Gallbladder and Cholelithiasis

Real-time sonography is the "gold standard" for diagnosing gallstones. The normal gallbladder is a cystic structure whose echogenic walls surround dark, anechoic bile. The normal fasting gallbladder is usually easy to visualize. The US probe is placed under the right costal margin or in an intercostal space. The liver serves as an "acoustic window" over the gallbladder. Patients are usually supine during imaging. Moving the patient into a left posterior oblique and upright positions demonstrates stone mobility. Images are obtained in both longitudinal (long-axis) and transverse (short-axis) planes.

Gallstones are highly echogenic and cast acoustic shadows (Fig. 21-1). Calculi as small as 1 mm can be seen within the gallbladder lumen. Intraluminal stones are easier to see than those lodged in the cystic duct, common bile duct, or the neck of the gallbladder. The acoustic shadow produced by the stone is sometimes easier to see than the stone itself (see Chap. 19, Fig. 19-39).

The mere identification of gallstones, however, does not prove that they are responsible for the patient's symptoms. US signs suggesting acute cholecystitis include the sonographic Murphy sign, gallbladder wall thickening, and pericholecystic fluid. An ultrasonographic Murphy sign is elicited when probe pressure causes tenderness over the gallbladder. The specificity and sensitivity of this sign for acute cholecystitis are about 90%. Pericholecystic fluid or wall thickening greater than 3 mm also suggests acute cholecystitis. Less common biliary tract abnormalities include intraluminal gas (emphysematous cholecystitis) and focal irregularities in the wall of the gallbladder, which may represent microabscess, infarction, hemorrhage, or carcinoma. About 50% of cases of acute cholecystitis have sludge or stasis-related echogenic bile. However, sludge is also seen in bedridden patients with poor oral intake and in individuals after a prolonged fast. Overall, US is approximately 90 to 95% sensitive and 94 to 98% specific in identifying acute cholecystitis.

Despite the fact that US is rapid, accurate, and not limited by critical illness, there can be false-positive and false-negative studies. Common errors include the failure to use the decubitus and erect positions to identify stones or sludge, failure to

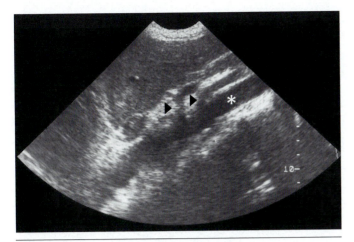

FIGURE 21-2. Normal abdominal aorta—long axis view (*asterisk*). The takeoff of the celiac axis and the superior mesenteric artery are seen in this image (*arrow heads*). (Courtesy of Dietrich Jehle, M.D.)

recognize an impacted stone at the neck of the gallbladder, and the misdiagnosis of a hyperechoic spiral valve in the neck of the gallbladder as an impacted stone. Bowel gas and massive obesity interfere with the sonographic detection of gallstones. Nuclear medicine studies can be helpful in differentiating biliary colic from acute cholecystitis if the clinical presentation and US studies are unable to distinguish between these two entities (see Chap. 19, Fig. 19-40).

US is useful in distinguishing obstructive jaundice from that due to hepatocellular disease. Common bile duct dilation and intrahepatic biliary distention suggest an obstruction due to choledocholithiasis or a tumor at the head of the pancreas. Normally, the common bile duct measures less than 7 mm and the intrahepatic biliary ducts are not prominent.

Abdominal Aorta

Emergency US can diagnose abdominal aortic and iliac artery aneurysms. The clinical presentation of an abdominal aneurysm can range from an incidental discovery in an asymptomatic individual to the hypotensive patient with a pulsatile abdominal mass. In symptomatic patients who are hemodynamically stable, bedside emergency US can provide a rapid diagnosis. Although a second imaging procedure, such as computed tomography (CT) scanning, may be necessary prior to surgery, a rapidly performed bedside US can expedite actions such as notifying the surgeon, arranging for interfacility transportation, or mobilizing the operating room.

CT scanning provides more detailed information regarding the anatomy of the lesion. However, the accuracy of US studies is comparable to that of CT scanning with regard to measuring the diameter of the aneurysm. Therefore, the role of US is to both measure the size of the aneurysm in an asymptomatic patient and to establish the presence of an abdominal aortic aneurysm in a symptomatic patient. US does not directly detect aneurysm leakage. While CT scanning is superior to US in the identification of retroperitoneal leakage, US is faster and

does not require the patient to leave the ED. US is better than the physical examination, which detects as few as 50% of abdominal aortic aneurysms.

The abdominal aorta is visualized by scanning with a standard abdominal transducer from the diaphragm to the iliac bifurcation (Figs. 21-2 and 21-3). The inferior vena cava (IVC) is normally located to the right of the aorta. The distinction between the aorta and IVC is made in several ways. The aorta has thicker walls and a narrower diameter than the IVC. In addition, the aorta is not compressible with probe pressure. Although the aorta is actively pulsatile, transmitted pulsations from both the aorta and the right ventricle create an undulating motion of the IVC, making the differentiation between the two difficult on this basis. The normal aorta is smaller than 3 cm at the level of the diaphragm and gradually tapers to 1.0 to 1.5 cm at the level of the bifurcation. The origins of the celiac axis, the superior mesenteric artery, and the renal arteries are appreciated in both longitudinal and transverse planes. A cross-sectional diameter (measured from the outer walls) larger than 3 cm indicates an abdominal aneurysm. Leakage is unlikely from an aneurysm smaller than 5 cm in diameter unless the aneurysm has "collapsed" following the rupture. The vast majority of abdominal aortic aneurysms are fusiform in shape and are located distal to the renal arteries. Elective operative repair is considered in patients with aortic aneurysm diameters larger than 5 cm.

Kidneys

The US appearance of the kidney is easy to recognize (Fig. 21-4). The echogenic area outlining the kidney represents the Gerota's fascia and perinephric fat. The central collecting tissue is also normally echogenic. In a well-hydrated patient, obstructing calculi result in dilation of the urinary collecting system within this central complex (*hydronephrosis*). The dilation appears as a central echo-free area. Hydronephrosis constitutes

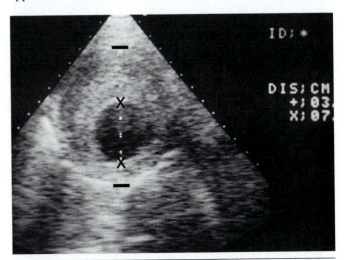

FIGURE 21-3. Abdominal aortic aneurysm—short axis view. There is a 7.8-cm abdominal aortic aneurysm with a large mural thrombus. The internal lumen of the aorta measures only 3.6 cm on this transverse view. (Courtesy of Dietrich Jehle, M.D.)

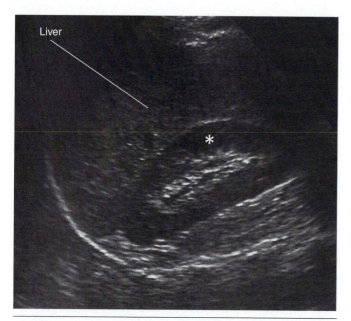

FIGURE 21-4. Normal kidney. The kidney lies below the liver in this image. It is surrounded by a bright echogenic capsule. The renal cortex *(asterisk)* is less echogenic than the liver. The renal cortex surrounds the echogenic central collecting system. (Courtesy of Dietrich Jehle, M.D.)

indirect evidence that a stone is present. Ureteral stones and the normal ureter are difficult to see; however, a dilated ureter, intrarenal calculi, and obstructions of part of the calyceal system by a proximal stone within the pelvis (Fig. 21-5) can be detected.

Generally, the right kidney is more easily imaged than the left because the liver is an acoustic window to the right kidney.

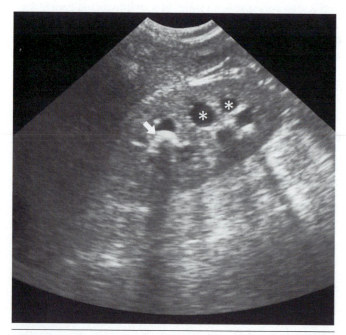

FIGURE 21-5. Intrarenal calculi. There are several centrally located renal stones that are echogenic with posterior acoustic shadowing *(arrow)*. In addition, there is mild hydronephrosis *(asterisks)*. (Courtesy of Dietrich Jehle, M.D.)

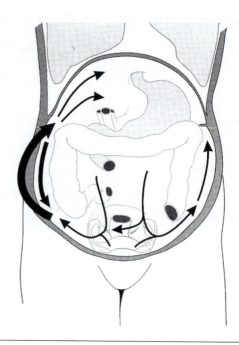

FIGURE 21-6. Abdominal cavity. This illustration demonstrates a pattern of free fluid movement within the abdominal cavity. (From Heller M, Jehle D: *Ultrasound in Emergency Medicine.* Philadelphia: Saunders, 1995. With permission.)

US of the left kidney is more difficult due to interposed air-filled bowel loops and stomach. The spleen is an acoustic window on the left.

Flank pain due to renal colic is the most common manifestation of obstructive uropathy prompting an ED visit. Although this condition is not life-threatening, emergent imaging is useful to confirm the diagnosis. Intravenous pyelography (IVP) and noncontrast CT are the "gold standards" for diagnosing ureteral colic. US is less accurate than IVP or CT in demonstrating obstruction. Nonetheless, US is preferable to IVP or CT in patients who are pregnant. When it is rapidly available in the ED, US provides quick evidence for or against the diagnosis of ureteral colic.

US is useful when the diagnosis of ureteral obstruction is uncertain. The differential diagnosis may include cholecystitis, pyelonephritis, appendicitis, and pelvic inflammatory disease. Since US can be performed within a few minutes at the bedside, the emergency physician can either confirm a diagnosis of obstructive uropathy and treat accordingly or can order an alternative diagnostic study based on the US and clinical information.

Traumatic Hemoperitoneum

The use of US to diagnose hemoperitoneum in the trauma patient is an important application of ED ultrasonography. CT and diagnostic peritoneal lavage (DPL) are the techniques most often used to diagnose traumatic intraabdominal hemorrhage in the United States. The sonographic screening examination is usually performed in less than 1 min. It is noninvasive and rap-

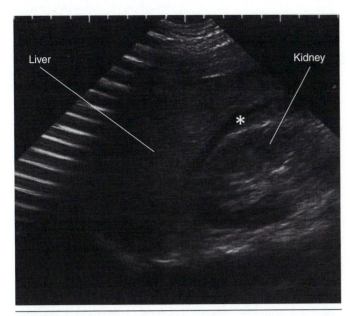

FIGURE 21-7. Hemoperitoneum. There is a large anechoic stripe in Morison's pouch *(asterisk)*. The echogenic areas within the anechoic stripe represent small clots. (Courtesy of Dietrich Jehle, M.D.)

idly detects hemoperitoneum in an unstable patient. Clinical trials in Europe and the United States have demonstrated that US is accurate (86 to 99%) in detecting hemoperitoneum; it may replace DPL in identifying hemoperitoneum in the unstable patient. In addition, US provides a rapid assessment of the thorax and pericardial space.

Free fluid flows to the dependent areas of the abdominal cavity (Fig. 21-6), including Morison's pouch (the potential space between the liver and the right kidney); the left upper quadrant (either in the paracolic gutter surrounding the left kidney or between the spleen and the kidney); and the pelvis in the region of the cul-de-sac. Fresh, unclotted blood appears anechoic. A black "stripe" in these locations is indicative of fluid which, in the trauma patient, is presumed to be blood (Fig. 21-7).

The complete sonographic screening examination in the trauma patient assesses four areas for free fluid (Fig. 21-8). The transducer is placed in the subxyphoid area to look for pericardial blood. The right upper quadrant is then examined for evidence of fluid in the right hemithorax, Morison's pouch, and the right paracolic gutter. The left upper quadrant is examined next for fluid in the left paracolic gutter or between the spleen and the left kidney (Fig. 21-9). Trendelenburg positioning can make the examination of Morison's pouch and the splenorenal space more sensitive. The pelvic cul-de-sac is also assessed for free fluid. Optimal visualization of the pelvis is aided by bladder filling (Fig. 21-10).

The threshold for reliably diagnosing hemoperitoneum is approximately 400 to 500 mL intraabdominally. With large amounts of blood, the fluid is visible from almost anywhere in the abdomen. Although fresh blood initially appears anechoic, fibrin formation during the clotting process results in the creation of variable echoes. Another advantage of US is the ability to perform serial examinations, because the quantity of intraabdominal blood can change rapidly. One limitation of US

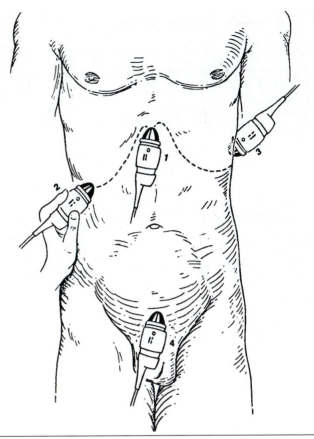

FIGURE 21-8. Four areas for identifying free fluid in the standard trauma examination: (1) subxyphoid areas looking for hemopericardium, (2) right upper quadrant, (3) left upper quadrant, and (4) pelvis. (From Rozycki GS, Ochner MG, Jaffin JH: Prospective evaluation of surgeons' use of ultrasound in the evaluation of trauma patients. *J Trauma* 34:517, 1993. With permission.)

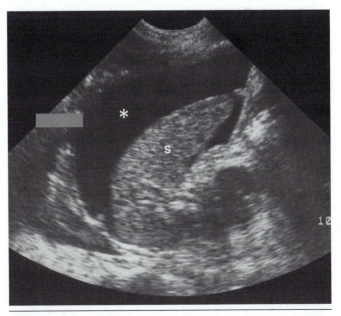

FIGURE 21-9. Perisplenic fluid. There is a large amount of free fluid *(asterisk)* that outlines the border of the spleen *(S)*. (Courtesy of Dietrich Jehle, M.D.)

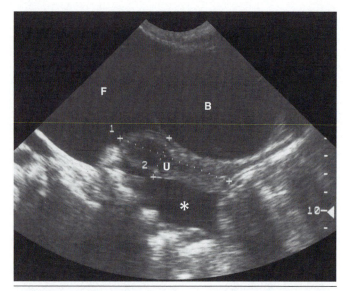

FIGURE 21-10. Cul-de-sac fluid. In this longitudinal view of the pelvis there is a large amount of anechoic fluid below the uterus *(asterisk)*. There is also a large amount of free fluid *(F)* cephalad to the uterus *(U)* and the bladder *(B)*. (Courtesy of Dietrich Jehle, M.D.)

is in diagnosing specific abdominal organ injury, where CT is clearly the preferred study in the stable patient.

Appendicitis

US graded-compression techniques have been used to diagnose appendicitis. Data are encouraging, with sensitivities of approximately 80 to 90% with specificities of 95%. The reliability of US in cases of appendicitis is dependent upon the experience of the operator and the type of equipment used. The US

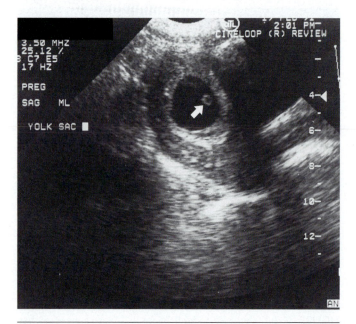

FIGURE 21-11. Yolk sac *(arrow)*. This is the first embryonic structure that is visualized with the chorionic sac. The presence of the yolk sac confirms the diagnosis of an intrauterine pregnancy. (Courtesy of Dietrich Jehle, M.D.)

diagnosis of appendicitis requires special techniques and expertise and falls outside the purview of bedside ED ultrasonography.

When visualized, the diameter of the normal appendix is 6 mm or less. If inflamed, the appendix is increased in diameter and is noncompressible. Appendicoliths, or concretions of fecal matter within the appendix, can also be detected. In fact, many complications of appendicitis—including gangrene, perforation, and phlegmon—have been detected sonographically. In the child with a suspected abdominal emergency, US is useful in differentiating appendicitis from pyloric stenosis or intussusception.

Gynecologic and Obstetric Applications

Pelvic sonography is regularly used to assess pregnant patients with abdominal pain or vaginal bleeding. Both transabdominal and transvaginal sonography are used. Transvaginal sonography uses a higher-frequency transducer (5 to 7.5 MHz), permitting better resolution for identifying small amounts of fluid in the cul-de-sac and an early intrauterine pregnancy. With transabdominal sonography, a 3.5-MHz probe is used, resulting in a better overview of pelvic structures. The transabdominal technique requires bladder filling to serve as an acoustic window. The scan is performed using a series of sagittal, coronal, and oblique images. Transabdominal and transvaginal examinations supplement one another when the initial scanning does not answer the immediate clinical question.

Early Pregnancy

The gestational sac is the earliest sonographic finding of a normal intrauterine pregnancy. It is a small, sonolucent area within the uterine cavity surrounded by a bright echogenic ring. It may contain no identifiable structures when first seen. However, depending on the resolution of the US equipment used, the yolk sac (Fig. 21-11) may be seen by the time the gestational sac reaches 5 to 8 mm in diameter. By the end of the sixth menstrual week, the average diameter of the gestational sac grows by 1 mm each day, the yolk sac is distinct, and cardiac activity may be detectable. The observation of cardiac activity substantiates the presence of a living intrauterine pregnancy. This is usually seen at 5 to 6 weeks using transvaginal equipment and at 7 weeks using a transabdominal technique. The embryo, or fetal pole, is smaller than the yolk sac at this time. During and after the eighth menstrual week, the embryo is much larger and is clearly imaged by both transvaginal and transabdominal scanning.

Ectopic Pregnancy

The emergency physician can generally exclude an ectopic pregnancy by identifying an intrauterine pregnancy. Concomitant intrauterine and extrauterine pregnancy occurs in 1 out of

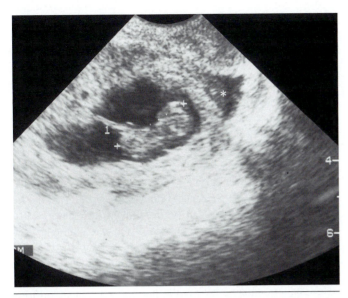

FIGURE 21-12. Ectopic pregnancy. This transvaginal US image demonstrates an ectopic pregnancy. Note the absence of surrounding myometrium and the small amount of anechoic free fluid in the pelvis. *(asterisk).* (Courtesy of Dietrich Jehle, M.D.)

every 30,000 low-risk pregnancies. The incidence of twins or multiple gestations is much higher with the use of assisted reproductive technology.

An ectopic pregnancy is confirmed when the uterus is empty and a living embryo is seen outside the uterus (Fig. 21-12). More commonly, however, an empty uterus (Fig. 21-13) plus clinical findings suggestive of an ectopic pregnancy (positive pregnancy test and lower abdominal pain or vaginal bleeding) make the diagnosis of ectopic pregnancy highly likely. Findings seen with an ectopic pregnancy include an echogenic pelvic mass or free pelvic fluid. An ectopic pregnancy has a complex sonographic appearance containing both echogenic and sonolucent components. Cystic "adnexal rings" can also be encountered with an ectopic pregnancy.

Molar Pregnancy

The sonographic hallmarks of a molar pregnancy (hydatidiform mole) are a "snowstorm" appearance of intrauterine contents with scattered large sonolucent areas in the uterus and associated theca lutein ovarian cysts. Stable patients with this diagnosis do not require any emergency intervention. However, prompt arrangement for follow-up and performance of suction dilation and curettage are mandatory because of the possibility of malignant degeneration into choriocarcinoma.

Ovarian Cysts

Torsion, hemorrhage, and rupture of an ovarian cyst can cause acute pelvic pain. A hemorrhagic ovarian cyst is more echogenic than a simple cyst because of clot formation within the cyst. With ovarian torsion, Doppler studies demonstrate reduced to absent blood flow (see Chap. 19, Fig. 19-53). US di-

agnosis of an ovarian cyst can be difficult and is not usually done in the ED. However, free fluid in the pelvis can be readily identified both by transabdominal and transvaginal US. (Fig. 21-10).

Placenta Previa–Abruptio Placentae

US is the best noninvasive method of establishing a diagnosis of *placenta previa.* The diagnosis is confirmed if the placenta extends into the lower uterine segment when the bladder is empty (Fig. 21-14). Only with an empty bladder can one be sure that the cervix has not been artificially lengthened due to pressure from a distended bladder. The axis of the vagina and cervix may not be longitudinal, and oblique sections may be necessary to show this relationship. If the placenta appears to lie adjacent to the cervix, one should scan transversely at right angles to see whether the placenta is centrally located or lying to one side of the cervix. This relationship is easy to determine if the fetus is breech but more difficult with a cephalic presentation.

In *abruptio placentae,* the primary event is bleeding between the placenta and uterine wall. Blood can also enter the amniotic cavity. Bleeding can be visualized sonographically in both locations. Unfortunately, abruptio may be present without being detectable sonographically. Patients who are more than 24 weeks pregnant (viable fetus) with significant abdominal trauma or painful vaginal bleeding should undergo ultrasound studies in addition to 4 to 6 h of maternofetal monitoring in order to exclude placental abruption.

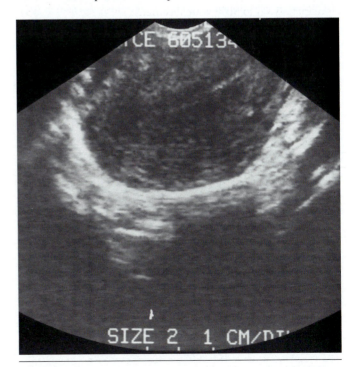

FIGURE 21-13. Empty uterus. The echogenic structure in the center of this transvaginal US image represents endometrium. The thickness and brightness of the endometrial echo varies within the menstrual cycle. There is no evidence of an intrauterine pregnancy. (Courtesy of Dietrich Jehle, M.D.)

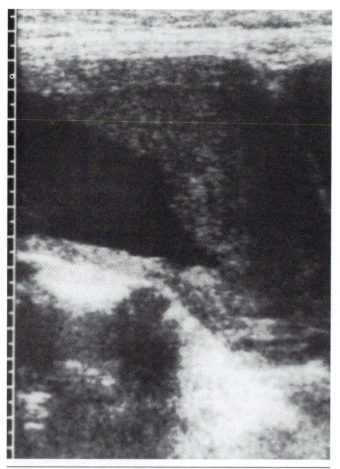

FIGURE 21-14.   Placenta previa. In this third-trimester pregnancy, the placenta covers the entire cervical os. (Courtesy of Dietrich Jehle, M.D.)

CARDIOVASCULAR APPLICATIONS

Cardiac Tamponade

The pericardium is highly echogenic and serves as the sonographic border of the cardiac image. US is highly sensitive for the detection of pericardial fluid, which is easily recognized as an anechoic area between the echogenic pericardium and the heart (Fig. 21-15). Sonography can be used for both traumatic and nontraumatic pericardial effusions.

The simplest view is obtained by placing a 3.5-MHz transducer in the subxyphoid area. Although visualization of the individual heart chambers can be difficult in this view, a pericardial effusion is easily appreciated. Other commonly used views include the left parasternal long- and short-axis views (Fig. 21-16). With the probe just to the left of the sternum in the second through fourth intercostal spaces, the long-axis view is obtained by placing the marker dot in the 4 o'clock position (US machine setup with standard abdominal-pelvic settings). By rotating the probe to the 8 o'clock position, a short-axis view is obtained. These views can detect small pericardial effusions. Clotted blood within the sac is often somewhat echogenic. Anechoic pericardial fat and pleural effusions can occasionally be confused with small pericardial effusions.

Pulseless Electrical Activity (PEA) and Shock

Another use for ED ultrasonography is to determine whether true PEA exists in a patient with apparent cardiac arrest. Although this is usually a straightforward diagnosis, emergency physicians encounter patients who have an electrical cardiac

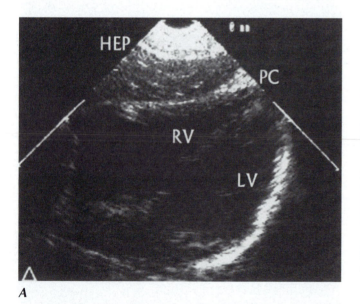

A

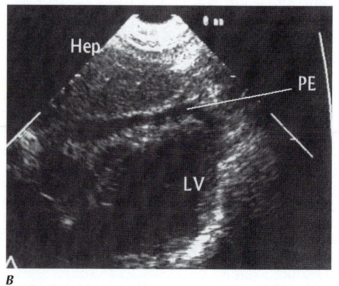

B

FIGURE 21-15.   *A.* Normal heart. Normal subxyphoid view of the heart. HEP, liver; PC, pericardium; RV, right ventricle; LV, left ventricle. (From Heller M, Jehle D: *Ultrasound in Emergency Medicine.* Philadelphia: Saunders, 1995. With permission.) *B.* Heart with pericardial effusion. The anechoic stripe represents fluid in the pericardial space. HEP, liver; PE, pericardial effusion; LV, left ventricle. (From Heller M, Jehle D: *Ultrasound in Emergency Medicine.* Philadelphia: Saunders, 1995. With permission.)

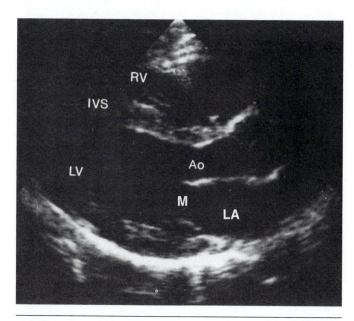

FIGURE 21-16. Long-axis view of the heart. RV, right ventricle; IVS, intraventricular septum; LV, left ventricle; Ao, aortic outflow tract, LA left atrium, M, mitral valve. (From Heller M, Jehle D: *Ultrasound in Emergency Medicine.* Philadelphia: Saunders, 1995. With permission.)

rhythm without a palpable pulse who are simply not generating an adequate perfusion pressure or have severe vascular disease. Such patients can be erroneously presumed to be non-viable. Using the subxyphoid view, a determination of the presence or absence of mechanical cardiac activity and an assessment of overall contractility is made. US provides instantaneous determination as to whether noncardiac causes of PEA are present, including hypovolemia and tamponade. If present, these can be promptly treated.

In a patient in profound shock with a palpable pulse, cardiac US helps distinguish the several possible causes. Global hypokinesis suggests a cardiomyopathy, regional wall motion abnormalities indicate myocardial ischemia or infarction, right ventricular dilation suggests massive pulmonary emboli, large pericardial effusions with end-diastolic chamber collapse imply tamponade, and a hyperkinetic small heart implies hypovolemia.

Doppler US and Duplex Ultrasonography

Acute peripheral vascular obstruction, be it arterial or venous, requires prompt and accurate diagnosis. *Doppler US* is a noninvasive test that is readily available to most EDs. Typically, a transducer frequency between 5 and 10 MHz provides reasonable sensitivity to blood flow while assuring good tissue penetration. It is important to recognize the character of audible signals in differentiating arterial from venous flow and normal from abnormal flow. Normal arterial signals are characterized by brisk, multiphasic sounds that change rapidly in pitch during the cardiac cycle. Normal venous flow signals are low-pitched and more constant in nature. Venous flow varies with

the respiratory cycle. Technique is important to obtain the best possible Doppler flow signals. The best flow signals are obtained if the transducer is aligned along the longitudinal axis of the blood vessel and firmly held at an angle of 45° to the skin surface. There should be minimal direct pressure against the skin.

Duplex ultrasonography combines two-dimensional US images with a Doppler flow probe. It is well suited for screening and follow-up of proximal DVT, with an accuracy equivalent to that of contrast venography. The findings of DVT are an inability to compress the vein with light downward pressure from the probe, echogenic material in the vein lumen, an absence of flow signals from within the lumen of the vein, lack of respiratory variation, and an absence of flow augmentation with calf compression. The results are dependent on the expertise of the sonographer. A portable Doppler examination without the US image has significant limitations and is more strongly examiner-dependent. False-positive duplex examinations can result from such patient-related factors as obesity and muscle guarding. False-negative studies arise from nonocclusive thrombosis and thrombus isolated to the deep veins of the calf. In experienced hands, there is a sensitivity of 96% and a specificity approaching 99% in identifying clot in the femoral and popliteal veins. Serial duplex studies are useful in detecting propagation of calf vein thrombosis to the popliteal and femoral veins.

OTHER APPLICATIONS

Because US is safe, portable, and noninvasive, its uses in the ED are expanding. For example, researchers are currently examining the use of US to aid emergency physicians with certain previously blind procedures. Diagnostic US can be of significant benefit in procedures such as abdominal paracentesis, bladder taps, thoracentesis, guided vascular access, and foreign-body removal. With further technologic advances in US, its common use by emergency physicians in the ED will be realized.

SELECTED READINGS

Branney SW, Wolfe RE, Moore EE, et al: Quantitative sensitivity of ultrasound in detecting free intraperitoneal fluid. *J Trauma* 39:375, 1995.

Chang TS, Lepanto L: Ultrasonography in the emergency setting. *Emerg Med Clin North Am* 10:1, 1992.

Cox GR, Browne BJ: Acute cholecystitis in the emergency department. *J Emerg Med* 7:501, 1989.

Ernst CB: Abdominal aortic aneurysm. *N Engl J Med* 328:1167, 1993.

Grossman SJ, Joyce JM: Hepatobiliary imaging. *Emerg Med Clin North Am* 9:853, 1991.

Heller M, Jehle D: *Ultrasound in Emergency Medicine.* Philadelphia: Saunders, 1995.

Jehle D, Abrams B, Sukumvanich P, et al: Ultrasound for the detection of intraperitoneal fluid: The role of Trendelenburg positioning (abstr). *Acad Emerg Med* 2:407, 1995.

Jehle D, Guarino J, Karamanoukian H: Emergency department ultrasound in the evaluation of blunt abdominal trauma. *Am J Emerg Med* 11:342, 1993.

Johnston DE, Kaplan MM: Pathogenesis and treatment of gallstones. *N Engl J Med* 328:412, 1993.

Lederle FA, Parenti CM, Chute EP: Ruptured abdominal aortic aneurysm: The internist as diagnostician. *Am J Med* 96:163, 1994.

Marston WA, Ahlquist R, Johnston G, Meyer AA: Misdiagnosis of ruptured abdominal aortic aneurysm. *J Vasc Surg* 16:17, 1992.

Rozycki GS, Ochner MG, Jaffin JH: Prospective evaluation of surgeons' use of ultrasound in the evaluation of trauma patients. *J Trauma* 34:517, 1993.

Wellford AL, Snoey ER: Emergency medicine applications of echocardiography. *Emerg Med Clin North Am* 13:831, 1995.

Zeman RK, Garra BS: Gallbladder imaging. *Gastroenterol Clin North Am* 2:127, 1991.

CHAPTER 22

PEDIATRIC CONSIDERATIONS

KEN BUTLER / MARTIN PUSIC

Interpretation of radiographic studies in children differs from that in adults. Because general emergency physicians see fewer pediatric studies than adult studies, it is essential that they understand those radiographic signs in children that indicate conditions associated with substantial morbidity. For example, there are obvious differences between the developing skeleton of the child and the fully mineralized adult skeletal system. Likewise, there are differences in pediatric chest and abdominal radiology. Certain radiographic indicators of disease have different frequencies in adults and children. In acute appendicitis, for example, one is more likely to see an appendicolith in the child than in the adult. Finally, there are certain conditions that occur only in children and have a characteristic radiographic appearance (e.g., the metaphyseal corner fracture as a sign of child abuse).

The emergency physician initially reads most films taken for pediatric emergencies. In one study, subspecialty-trained pediatric emergency physicians were concordant with the radiologists' interpretations in over 90% of cases.[1] Rarely did a misinterpreted radiograph result in an adverse outcome or require a revision of care. In cases when care was amended, half involved a missed fracture. Despite an emergency physician's proficiency in interpreting pediatric radiographs, some patients benefit from routine review by a radiologist. Since physicians in a general emergency department (ED) see fewer children's radiographs, they stand to benefit more from radiologist review.

SKELETAL RADIOLOGY

Skeletal Development

Developing bone differs considerably from adult bone in composition and physical properties. Developing bone is more porous, contains more water, has slightly less mineral, and larger haversian canals. As a result, children's bones are more elastic and stronger.[2] When subjected to traumatic forces, the child's bone tends to bend or buckle rather than fracture completely.

The periosteum is thicker, more elastic, and less firmly bound to the cortex. The periosteum is therefore more likely to remain intact when the bone is fractured. This makes children less likely to have comminuted fractures or fracture nonunion.[2]

Growth of long bones occurs at the epiphyseal growth plate (physis). The cartilagenous growth plates lie between the mineralized metaphysis and the epiphysis. Early in development, the epiphysis is not mineralized and the long bones appear to end at the metaphysis. At this stage, radiographs cannot distinguish the growth plate from the articular cartilage, since both are radiolucent. Later, ossification centers appear in the epiphyses. These mineralized, radiodense ossification centers form between the epiphyseal growth plate and the articular cartilage. They appear in a predictable sequence during a child's growth (Table 22-1).

TABLE 22-1

Approximate Ages of Appearance of Ossification Centers

OSSIFICATION CENTER	BOYS	GIRLS
Hand/foot		
Epiphyses of fingers and toes	1–4 years	9 months–3 years
Sesamoid of first finger	12 years	10 years
Wrist		
Capitate/hamate	3 months	2 months
Triquetrum	29 months	22 months
Lunate	4 years	3 years
Scaphoid	5 years	4 years
Distal epiphysis of radius	12 months	10 months
Distal epiphysis of ulna	7 years	5 years
Elbow		
Capitellum	4 months	3 months
Olecranon	9 years	8 years
Medial epicondyle	6 years	3 years
Lateral epicondyle	11 years	9 years
Shoulder		
Head of humerus	2 weeks	2 weeks
Acromion	13 years	11 years
Greater tubercle of humerus	10 months	6 months
Knee		
Proximal epiphysis of tibia	2 weeks	2 weeks
Tubercle of tibia	12 years	10 years
Patella	4 years	2.5 years
Hip		
Head of femur	4 months	4 months
Greater trochanter	3 years	22 months
Ankle		
Epiphysis of calcaneus	7.5 years	5.5 years

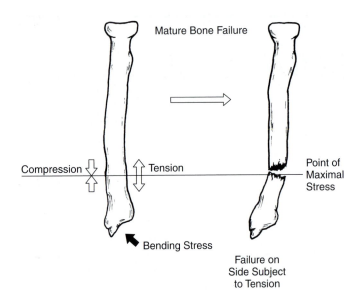

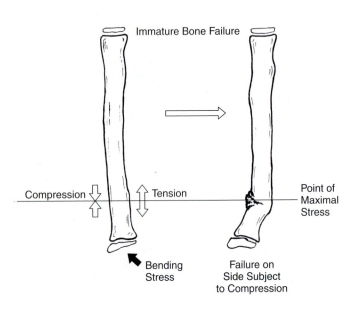

FIGURE 22-1.   Forces that cause bone to fracture—mature and immature bone.

The epiphyseal growth plate is the weakest part of a child's bone and constitutes a "fault line" where a fracture is likely to occur. In children, the joint capsule and ligaments are two to five times as strong as the growth plate.[2] As a result, forces that typically cause a ligamentous injury in an adult are likely to cause a growth plate injury in the child. These fractures are commonly described according to the Salter-Harris classification scheme.[3] The metaphysis is also a zone of weakness of developing bone.

Fracture Types

Factors affecting the response of bone to a mechanical stress include its energy-absorbing capacity, its elasticity, the fatigue strength of the bone, and its density. All of these are greater in children than in adults. Also important is the aforementioned loose attachment of the elastic periosteum to the cortex. The differences in these physical properties lead to different patterns of structural failure when a child's bone is stressed.[4,5]

When a long bone is "bent," typically one side is under tension (stretched) while the other is compressed. These forces deform the bone and determine the fracture pattern. Mature bone is most likely to fail when under tension; developing bone is more likely to fail while under compression (Fig. 22-1). Mature bone breaks first at the surface under tension, then breaks completely, rapidly and cleanly. Immature bone fails first on the surface under compression causing it to buckle. This results in a torus fracture. With greater deformity, the bone breaks incompletely on the opposite side. Greenstick and bowing fractures represent other patterns seen with similar stresses (Fig. 22-2).[5,6]

TORUS FRACTURES.   The torus (buckle) fracture is the most common fracture seen in children. There is abrupt outward bending of the cortical surface. Buckle fractures are most common at the metaphysis (Figs. 22-3 and 22-4). A discrete break in the cortex is usually absent. A torus fracture results when an axial or bending force is applied to a long bone, resulting in compression on one or both sides of the bone. The area of cortex at the transition between metaphysis and diaphysis is the

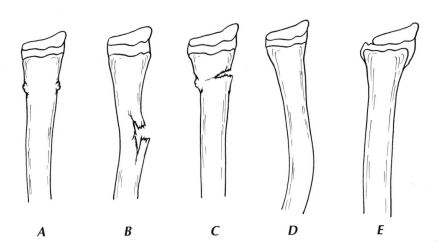

FIGURE 22-2.   Fracture types peculiar to children. *A.* Torus fracture; one or both sides of the cortex are buckled. *B.* Greenstick fracture; an incomplete fracture through only one side of the cortex. *C.* Lead-pipe fracture; an incomplete fracture where the intact side of the cortex is buckled. *D.* Plastic bowing fracture; no discrete fracture line. Innumerable microfractures result in bending of the bone. *E.* Growth-plate fracture; the injury may also involve the adjacent bone. (Rogers LF (ed): *The Radiology of Skeletal Trauma,* 2d ed. New York: Churchill Livingstone, 1992, with permission.)

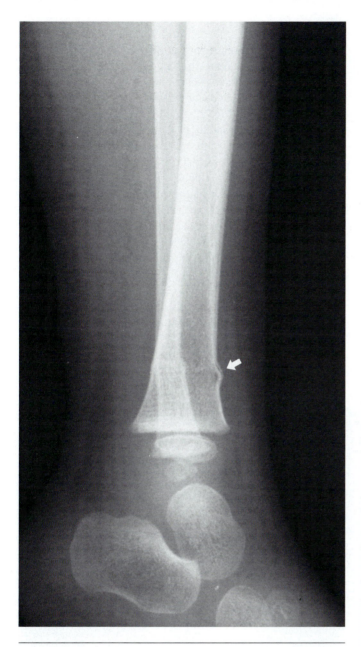

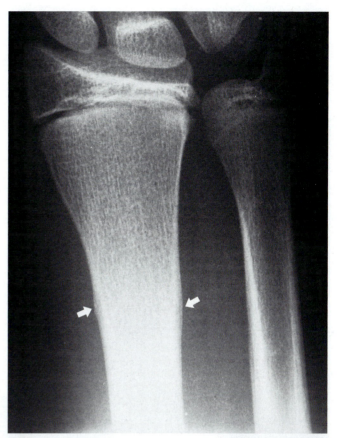

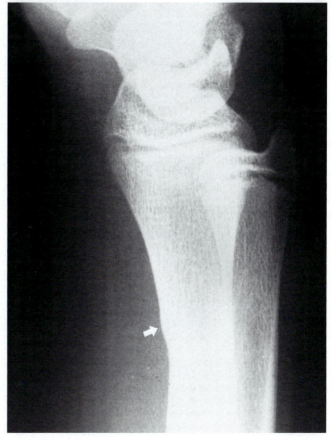

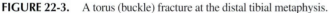

FIGURE 22-3.   A torus (buckle) fracture at the distal tibial metaphysis.

most vulnerable site for a buckle fracture. At the metaphysis, the periosteum is tightly adherent to the cortex and the cortex is thin and relatively weak. At the diaphysis, the periosteum is loosely adherent to the cortex, with dense, strong lamellar bone forming the cortex.

The radiologic appearance of a torus fracture can be subtle. The clinical importance of detecting a subtle torus fracture is uncertain, since displacement or nonunion of minor torus fractures is uncommon.

GREENSTICK FRACTURES.   With a greenstick fracture, only one side of the cortex is fractured. This results from bending forces that cause tension (stretching) on one side of the bone and compression on the other. The structural failure of the immature

FIGURE 22-4.   A subtle torus fracture of the distal radius. Slight buckling of the cortex is seen on the AP and lateral views (*arrows*).

bone occurs on the side of the cortex under tension (Fig. 22-5). Greenstick fractures usually occur in the diaphysis of long bones, where the cortex is relatively thick and strong. A "lead-pipe" fracture combines features of greenstick and torus fractures, in which the buckled cortex fractures (Fig. 22-6).

BOWING FRACTURES. The bowing fracture resembles a greenstick fracture. However, a bowing fracture has no discrete cortical defect. The traumatic stresses are insufficient to cause a complete cortical break. Many microscopic fractures occur along the cortex that is under tension, resulting in diffuse deformity of the bone (Fig. 22-5). Bowing fractures usually occur at the radius, ulna, and fibula. Recognition of a bowing fracture is important because the potential for bone remodeling is poor. Comparison radiographs of the uninjured side are helpful in detecting a bowing fracture. Bowing fractures can cause considerable functional impairment of the forearm, resulting in limited supination-pronation. Timely closed reduction is essential. Often, no periosteal reaction is seen following a bowing fracture. Because of this, follow-up films taken 2 weeks after the injury are not helpful for determining whether or not a bowing fracture has occurred.

AVULSION FRACTURES. In children, ligaments and tendons are stronger than bone. For this reason, avulsion fractures are common. Frequent sites for avulsion fractures include the tibial plateau at the insertion of the posterior cruciate ligament (Fig. 22-7) and the proximal fifth metatarsal. Additional sites of avul-

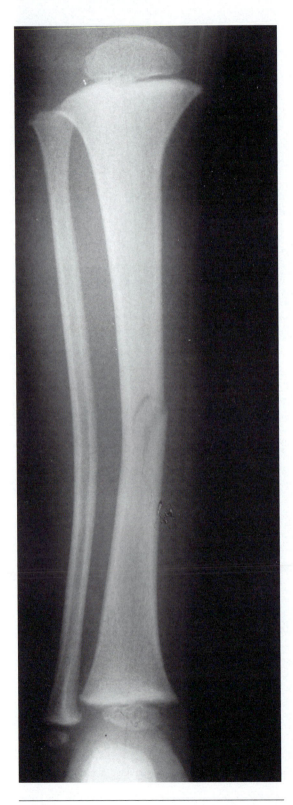

FIGURE 22-5. A greenstick fracture of the midshaft of the tibia. There is a concomitant bowing fracture of the fibula.

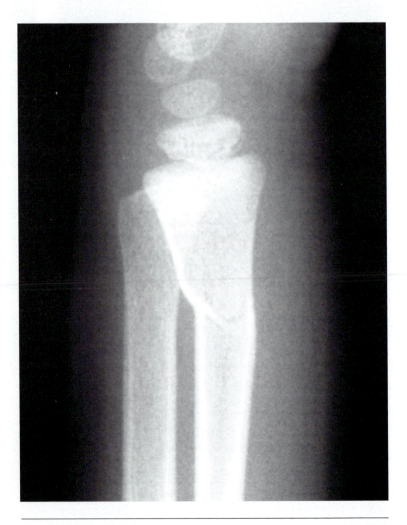

FIGURE 22-6. A "lead-pipe" fracture of the distal radius. There is buckling and an incomplete fracture of one side of the cortex.

sion include the insertion of the sartorius muscle at the anterosuperior iliac spine (Fig. 22-8), the lateral epicondyle of the elbow, and the insertion of the extensor digitorum on the phalanges of the hand.

EPIPHYSEAL GROWTH PLATE FRACTURES.   Injuries to the growth plate can be difficult to detect because the growth plate is radiolucent. An acute fracture involving the physis can occur without any radiographic abnormality. Moreover, mineralized bone fragments are occasionally confused with developing ossification centers. Careful correlation with clinical findings and the selective use of comparison films minimize errors in diagnosis.

The Salter-Harris scheme classifies growth plate fractures (Fig. 22-9). The prognosis is worse with increasing Salter-Harris categories. For example, a Salter-Harris II fracture has a better prognosis than a Salter-Harris V fracture. A Salter-Harris I fracture is most common in the younger child (< 5 years). An acute, nondisplaced Salter-Harris I fracture is difficult to diagnose radiographically. An increased width of the radiolucent growth plate and soft tissue swelling are often the only clues

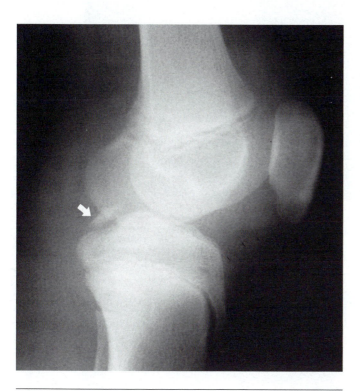

FIGURE 22-7.   An avulsion fracture at the insertion site of the posterior cruciate ligament on the tibial plateau *(arrow).*

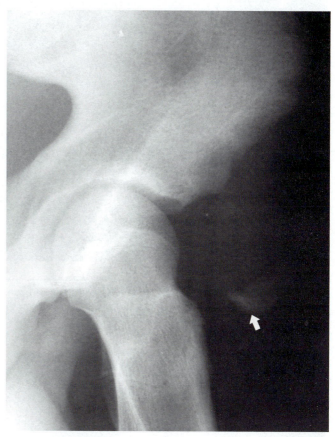

FIGURE 22-8.   An avulsion fracture from the anterior superior iliac spine at the insertion of the sartorius muscle *(arrow).*

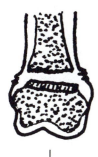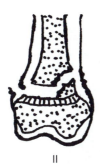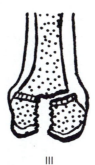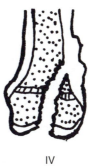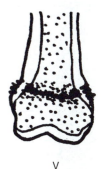

| I | II | III | IV | V |

FIGURE 22-9.   Salter-Harris classification of fractures through the epiphyseal growth plate (physis). In type I, there is a fracture through the growth plate alone. In type II, there is extension of the fracture through the metaphysis. This is a common injury pattern. In type III, the fracture includes the epiphysis. This is an intraarticular fracture.

In type IV, the fracture involves both the epiphysis and metaphysis. In type V, there is a crush injury to the growth plate. In general, the prognosis is poorer for the higher numbers, especially types III through V. Types I through IV may be either displaced or nondisplaced.

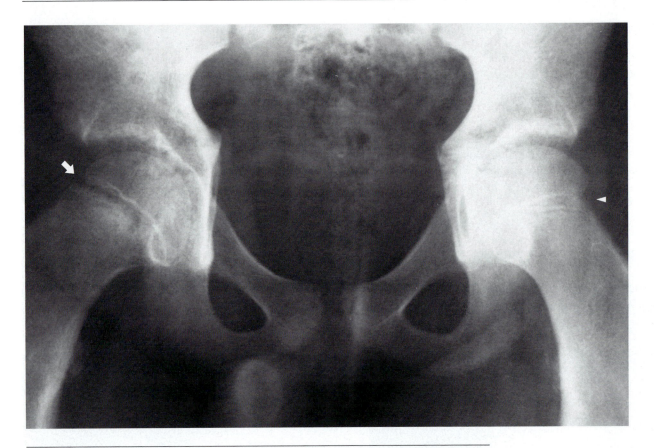

FIGURE 22-10.   A minimally displaced Salter-Harris type I fracture through the growth plate of the femoral head on the right. Widening of the growth plate (*arrow*) is recognized by comparison with the opposite normal side (*arrowhead*). This is known as a slipped capital femoral epiphysis (SCFE).

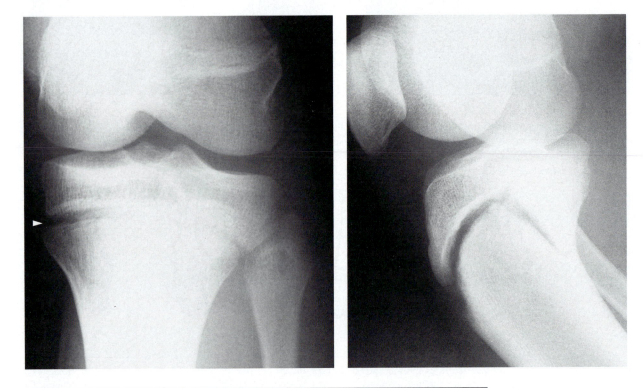

FIGURE 22-11.   A Salter-Harris type II fracture of the proximal tibia. On the AP view, there is slight widening and displacement of the growth plate (*arrowhead*). On the lateral view, extension of the fracture into the metaphysis is seen.

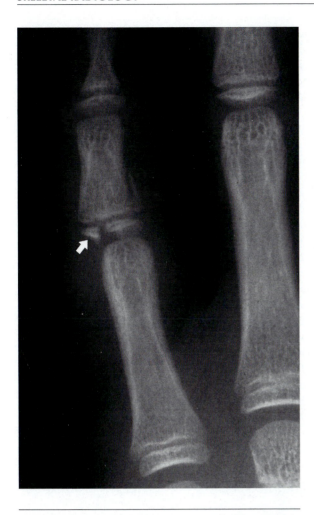

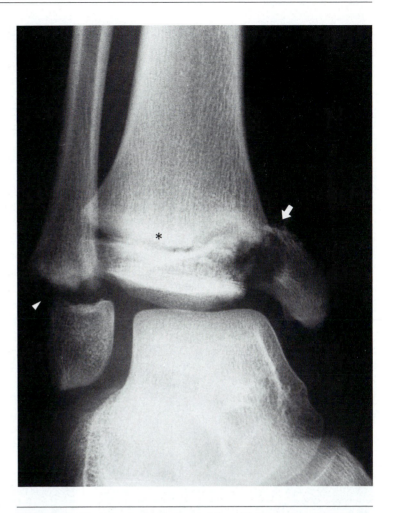

FIGURE 22-12. Salter-Harris type III fracture of the proximal end of the middle phalanx. A thin fracture fragment is also seen on the opposite side involving the metaphysis of the phalanx *(arrow)*.

FIGURE 22-13. A complex fracture of the ankle mortise. A Salter-Harris type III fracture involves the medial malleolus (distal tibial epiphysis)*(arrow)*. There is also a displaced Salter-Harris type I fracture of the distal fibula growth plate (lateral malleolus) *(arrowhead)*. Finally, the central portion of the distal tibia growth plate is crushed (a Salter-Harris type V fracture)*(asterisk)*.

to a Salter-Harris I fracture (Fig. 22-10). Radiographic comparison of the contralateral site and a repeat study in 10 to 14 days can be helpful. In subtle cases, the clinical examination, not the radiographic findings, is the chief factor in making a diagnosis. If there is significant tenderness and swelling over a growth plate suggestive of a Salter-Harris I fracture, the site should be immobilized in a cast and reexamined 1 to 2 weeks later.

Salter-Harris II fractures involving the physis and metaphysis are the most common epiphyseal growth plate injuries (Fig. 22-11).[6] Salter-Harris III and IV fractures are frequently displaced and hence easily detected (Figs. 22-12 and 22-13). Salter-Harris V fractures are crush injuries of the growth plate (Fig. 22-13). Fewer than 0.3% of epiphyseal growth plate fractures are Salter-Harris V fractures.

Comparison Views

There is considerable debate regarding the use of comparison radiographs of the contralateral, unaffected limb to improve di-

agnostic accuracy especially for injuries involving the growth plate or ossification centers. Although ossification centers become calcified at different times in different individuals, there is less variability between the two sides of a given individual. This same principle also applies to the epiphyseal growth plates and the ends of the metaphyses. Comparison views are of most benefit at joints, where anatomic variability is great and where the radiographic appearance of a fracture can be subtle, such as at the elbow.

There is no absolute rule that determines when to obtain contralateral films. Swischuk recommends the liberal use of contralateral films, even for experienced radiologists.[7] Comparison views should not be obtained in all cases, even for the elbow, because the clinical examination coupled with the radiographic findings on the injured side are usually sufficient to guide therapy. Although some investigators have shown that contralateral films do not improve diagnostic accuracy, these reports studied the routine use of contralateral films and not their selective use.[8,9] Comparison films can improve diagnostic accuracy in cases where clinical findings and routine radiographs are inconclusive.

Specific Skeletal Lesions

TODDLER'S FRACTURE.   The child between 1 and 3 years of age who refuses to walk presents a diagnostic challenge. The differential diagnosis includes toxic (transient) synovitis, septic arthritis, osteomyelitis, and fracture. The physical findings are nonspecific, and it is often difficult to localize the exact site of tenderness. In such cases, a toddler's fracture must be considered. A toddler's fracture is an oblique or spiral fracture of the distal tibia (Fig. 22-14). In children older than 3 years, the toddler's fracture can extend proximally. In many cases, the fracture is nondisplaced and not apparent radiographically. A toddler's fracture is usually visible on only one projection. Careful consideration must be given to nonaccidental trauma in

preschool children. A metaphyseal corner fracture is a radiographic sign of abuse.

A bone scan is more sensitive than plain radiography, and can detect increased activity within hours of the injury. Nonetheless, bone scanning is generally unnecessary because the child with a clinically significant injury requires casting irrespective of the radiographic findings.

OSTEOMYELITIS.   The metaphysis of the child is especially prone to osteomyelitis because of its rich capillary network, which favors bacterial growth (see Chap. 2, Fig. 2-11).[10] The bone is seeded by hematogenous spread. In other cases of osteomyelitis, the infection is caused by direct inoculation of the bone (e.g., the calcaneus with a plantar puncture wound) or by spread from an adjoining infected joint. Patients with sickle cell disease are prone to both osteomyelitis and bone infarction.

At the time of initial presentation, plain radiographs are often normal. The earliest radiographic signs of osteomyelitis, seen at 2 weeks, are periosteal elevation and "moth-eaten" radiolucencies involving the metaphysis (Figs. 22-15 and 22-16, and Chap. 2, Fig. 2-13).[11] Bone scanning is more sensitive. However, bone scan is nonspecific in cases where septic arthritis and fracture are also diagnostic considerations.[12] Ultrasound (US) can also be used in the early detection of osteomyelitis. In one small series, the finding of fluid adjacent to bone on US was 100% sensitive for osteomyelitis. However, US could not distinguish septic arthritis from osteomyelitis.[13]

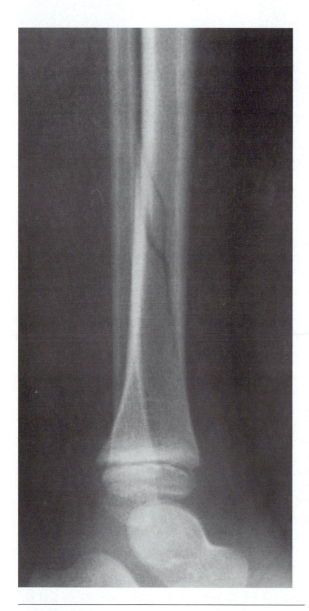

FIGURE 22-14.   A toddler's fracture of the distal tibia.

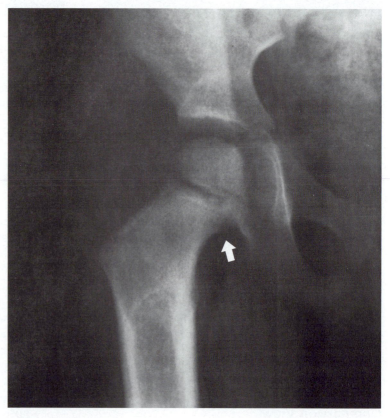

FIGURE 22-15.   Osteomyelitis of the proximal femur. Note the cortical hypodensity involving the medial cortex of the proximal femur (*arrow*). This child has sickle cell disease.

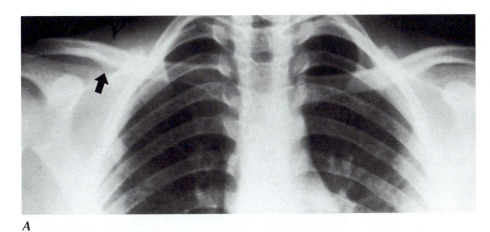

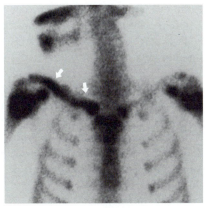

A   *B*

FIGURE 22-16.   Osteomyelitis. *A.* Osteomyelitis of the right clavicle is difficult to see on plain film. There is slight endosteal cortical erosion, pe-riosteal elevation, and new bone formation *(arrow)* in comparison to the left clavicle. *B.* On the bone scan, the osteomyelitis is obvious *(arrows).*

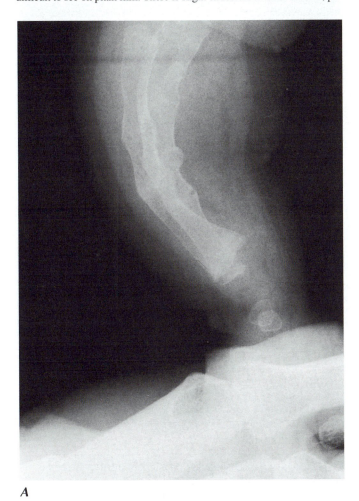

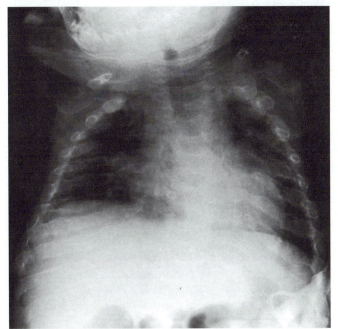

B

FIGURE 22-17.   Osteogenesis imperfecta. Osteogenesis impefecta in a 3-month-old child is demonstrated by the irregular appearance of the bone due to multiple healed fractures and profound osteopenia *(A).* The degree of osteopenia is evident relative to the bone density of the radiology technician's fingers at bottom of figure. The chest film demonstrates multiple healing rib fractures and osteopenia *(B).*

A

Gallium scanning can distinguish soft tissue infection from os-teomyelitis. Computed tomography (CT) and magnetic reso-nance imaging (MRI) are also helpful in difficult cases.[12,14]

OSTEOGENESIS IMPERFECTA.   There are four types of osteogen-esis imperfecta (OI). All are characterized by the failure to form normal collagen and bone fragility. Radiography reveals gen-eralized osteopenia and multiple fractures in different stages of

healing and callus formation (Fig. 22-17). Limb deformities are caused by bowing of the long bones and angulation of old frac-tures. The extent of disease ranges from fatal in childhood to a mild adult-onset form.[15]

Although OI is occasionally confused with child abuse, cer-tain features help to differentiate them. The presence of a clin-ical syndrome (e.g., blue sclera, hearing impairment); the lack of metaphyseal corner fractures; abnormal, osteopenic bone in uninjured areas; and the continued occurrence of fractures in a safe home are most consistent with OI.[16] When these clinical features are taken into account, confusion between OI and abuse should rarely occur.

OSGOOD-SCHLATTER DISEASE. Osgood-Schlatter disease (OS) is painful inflammation at the site of insertion of the patellar tendon. When the tibial tubercle ossifies (at age 10 to 12 years), it is susceptible to repeated microfracture. Radiographically, little is seen other than soft tissue swelling. In advanced cases, irregularity and fragmentation of the tibial tubercle are seen (Fig. 22-18).

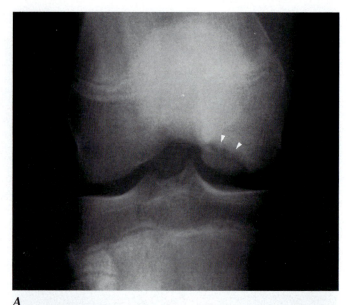

A

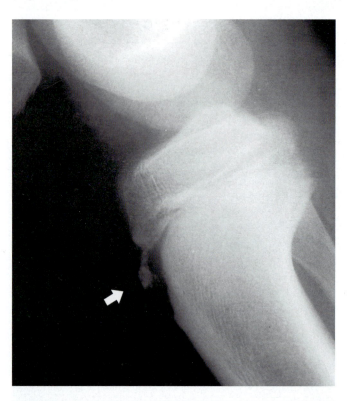

FIGURE 22-18. Osgood-Schlatter disease. There is a fragmented anterior tibial tuberosity.

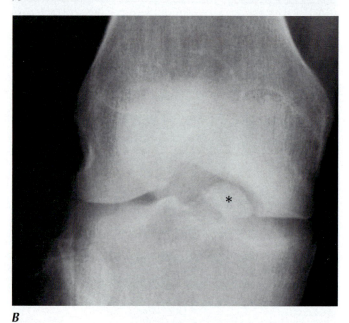

B

FIGURE 22-20. Osteochrondritis dissecans. *A.* Osteochondritis dissecans of the medial femoral condyle is seen a few weeks after the onset of symptoms *(arrowheads). B.* Five years later, the patient has relatively few symptoms despite the well-demarcated fragment involving the distal femur *(asterisk).*

OSTEOCHONDRITIS DISSECANS. Osteochondritis dissecans results from avascular necrosis of a small fragment of bone adjacent to the articular cartilage (Fig. 22-19). The bone fragment occasionally separates from the adjacent cartilage and, rarely, becomes free-floating within the joint. The lateral femoral condyle at the knee is the most common site of osteochondritis dissecans (Fig. 22-20). In its acute stage, the lesion may be undetectable radiographically. Subsequent radiographs reveal a bony defect at the site of avascular necrosis. Later, a free-floating bone-cartilage fragment may be seen within the joint space. Bone scan and MRI can detect the lesion early on but are usually not necessary. The lesion usually heals

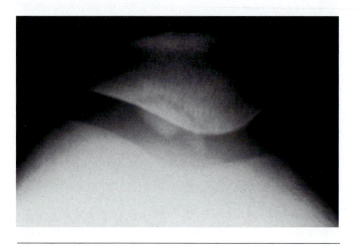

FIGURE 22-19. Osteochondritis dissecans. There are subchondral lesions involving the inferior aspect of the patella.

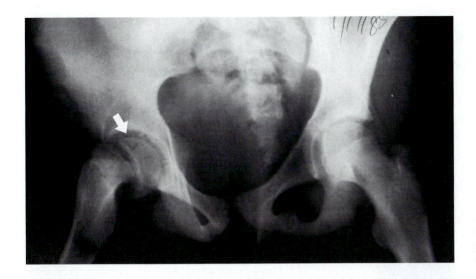

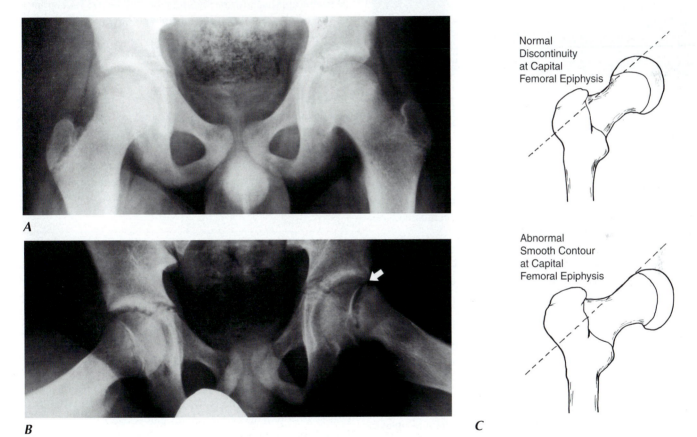

FIGURE 22-21. Slipped capital femoral epiphysis (SCFE). There is moderate displacement on the right.

Normal
Discontinuity
at Capital
Femoral Epiphysis

Abnormal
Smooth Contour
at Capital
Femoral Epiphysis

A

B   *C*

FIGURE 22-22. SCFE can be difficult to detect on the AP view *(A)*. On the frog-leg view, SCFE is often more easily seen *(B)*. A line drawn along the femoral neck should intersect part of the femoral head *(C)*.

spontaneously. If bone fragments enter the joint, surgical removal may be required.[17]

SLIPPED CAPITAL FEMORAL EPIPHYSIS. A separate epiphyseal ossification center called the *capital femoral epiphysis* occurs at the developing head of the femur. Its growth plate is a point of structural weakness. With a *slipped capital femoral epiphysis* (SCFE), the femoral head slips posterolaterally relative to the femoral neck (Fig. 22-21).

SCFE can result in a variable degree of avascular necrosis of the femoral head. It is important to maintain a high index of suspicion for this condition in any adolescent presenting with hip or knee pain. It typically occurs in 10- to 15-year-old obese boys. SCFE often affects the opposite hip within the next 2 years.

Radiographically, the slippage can be subtle. Both hips are compared on both the AP and frog-leg views (Fig. 22-22).

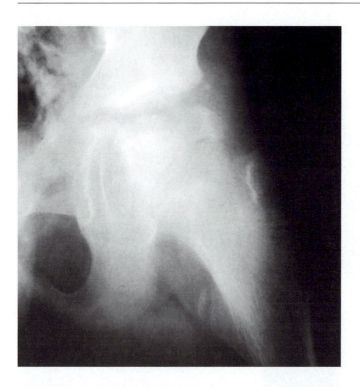

FIGURE 22-23.   Legg-Calvé-Perthes disease. There is marked fragmentation and collapse of the femoral head epiphysis due to avascular necrosis.

Widening of the growth plate on the affected side may be the only radiographic sign. On the AP view, a line drawn along the superior border of the femoral neck normally intersects part of the femoral head. If it does not, especially when compared with the other side, the diagnosis of SCFE is likely.

AVASCULAR NECROSIS.   Avascular necrosis (AVN) is the death of bone tissue due to interruption of its blood supply. Two examples in children are *Legg-Calvé-Perthes disease* (LCP) involving the proximal femur and *Scheuermann disease* involving the vertebral bodies.

LCP is most common among 5- to 9-year-old boys. It causes limping with mild to moderate hip pain. Radiographs taken at the time of onset are often normal. There may be mild joint-space widening. A bone scan is more sensitive, showing a perfusion defect in the ischemic area. Bone scanning is indicated if the diagnosis is in doubt. On the bone scan, increased uptake in an affected hip suggests a septic joint, whereas decreased uptake confirms AVN. Two weeks after the onset of pain, hip radiographs in patients with LCP demonstrate radiolucent (lytic) areas, subchondral lucency (the "crescent sign"), and periosteal reaction (Fig. 22-23). Failure to recognize LCP leads to progressive deformation of the femoral head.[18,19]

CERVICAL SPINE EVALUATION

Clinical Decision Making

The relatively large head and weak cervical muscles make the young child vulnerable to cervicocranial injuries. Jaffe et al. prospectively evaluated all cervical spine radiographs done in

children during a 1-year period. They also retrospectively reviewed all patients with injuries of the cervical spine at their hospital during the previous 10 years.[20] Using these results, they developed clinical criteria indicating the need for cervical spine radiographs. Neck pain, an abnormal neurologic examination, and abnormal mental status were indications for obtaining cervical spine films. Rachesky et al. applied similar criteria retrospectively to 2133 patients and reached similar conclusions.[21] Both authors concluded that completely asymptomatic children do not require radiographic study. On the other hand, up to 20% of children with spinal cord injury will not have a radiographic abnormality.

Radiographic Analysis

A useful approach to the interpretation of lateral radiographs of the cervical spine is the mnemonic ABCD'S: *a*lignment, *b*ones, *c*ount-*c*urvature, *d*ens-*d*isks, and *s*oft tissues (Fig. 22-24). (The reader is referred to Chapter 13 for a complete discussion.)

ADEQUACY.   First, the radiographs must be of adequate technical quality. All seven cervical vertebral bodies must be seen, as well as the superior portion of the T1 vertebral body. A partially rotated film makes assessment of the articular facets difficult. Although some information can be gleaned from suboptimal films, the patient must continue to be managed as though he or she were injured until a full assessment with adequate films is completed.

ALIGNMENT.   Assessment of alignment is useful for detecting subtle fractures. It may be the only means of detecting ligamentous injury. To assess alignment, the anterior and posterior vertebral body lines are carefully examined. Any malalignment prompts a closer inspection for fractures and ligamentous injury.

Children have relatively lax intervertebral ligaments, allowing for some normal variability in the alignment of the cervical spine. Often C2 is displaced anteriorly with respect to C3 (Fig. 22-25). This phenomenon, termed *pseudosubluxation*, can occur to a lesser degree between C3 and C4. Pseudosubluxation is most pronounced in infants and is uncommon after puberty. Pseudosubluxation must be distinguished from true subluxation due to a fracture or ligamentous injury. This is done by drawing a line through the spinolaminar junctions of C1, C2, and C3. These three points should align within 2 mm of a straight line in the presence of pseudosubluxation. If the points do not align and C2 is slipped anteriorly on C3, then the slippage is likely to be a true subluxation. True subluxation is most often due to a fracture at the base of the dens or bilateral fractures through the neural arch of C2 (a hangman's fracture).

BONES.   Each bone of the cervical spine must be carefully inspected. The vertebral bodies are examined first. The vertebral bodies of C3 through C7 should be of a consistent size and shape. In children, the vertebral bodies are rounded or wedge-

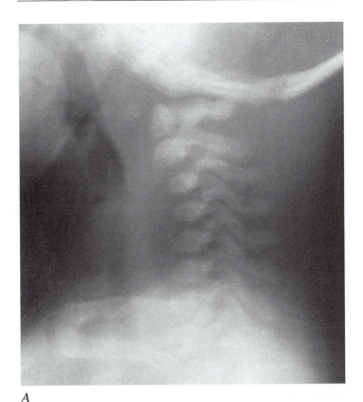
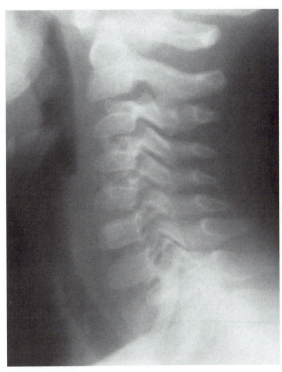

A *B*

FIGURE 22-24. The normal cervical spine of the child. *A.* Eight-week-old child. *B.* Three-year-old child.

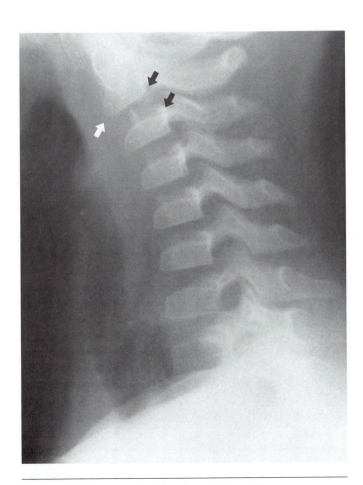

FIGURE 22-25. Pseudosubluxation of C2 on C3.

shaped because the epiphyseal end plates have not yet ossified. An adult appearance is seen by puberty.

The facet joints of a child are shorter and more horizontal than those of an adult. Although it is uncommon for a child to present with dislocated articular facets, each of the facet joints must be examined closely. The laminae and spinous process form the neural arch surrounding the spinal cord.

DENS. The odontoid process is inspected closely. One must distinguish between the normal subdental synchondrosis, which appears as a straight horizontal line at the base of the odontoid, and a fracture through the base of the dens. A normal synchondrosis is perfectly straight, is of uniform width, and does not interrupt the anterior border of C2. In addition, if the subdental lucency is a normal synchondrosis, there is no displacement of the odontoid process relative to the body of C2. The dens synchondrosis is normally open through age 6 years.

The atlantoaxial region is particularly susceptible to injury in children because of the higher fulcrum point and the increased laxity of the transverse and alar ligaments. The distance between the anterior surface of the odontoid process and the anterior portion of C1 (the anterior atlantodental interval or predental space) is an indicator of the integrity of the atlantoaxial joint. In adults, a width of up to 3 mm is normal. However, children have more lax ligaments and can have up to 5 mm between these two surfaces. The open-mouth odontoid view and flexion-extension films can reveal an injury undetected on the lateral view.

SOFT TISSUES. The cervicocranial prevertebral soft tissues normally follow the contour of the vertebral column. In young children, laxity of these tissues allows them to appear abnormally thickened if the child is not properly positioned. If the child's neck is flexed rather than extended or if the child is swallowing or crying at the time of exposure, the prevertebral soft tissues can appear considerably swollen. If clinical suspicion for an injury is low, the radiograph should be repeated with better positioning.

THE PROXIMAL AIRWAY

Adequate radiographic evaluation of the soft tissues of the child's neck usually requires two views—a lateral and an anteroposterior (AP) view. To best demonstrate the soft tissues of the neck, the film is exposed near the end of an inspiration. The neck is fully extended unless a cervical spine injury or epiglottitis is suspected. Neck extension will reduce the thickening of the prevertebral soft tissues in infants and young children, which can simulate a retropharyngeal mass.

Stridor

Stridor is produced by turbulent airflow in the upper airways, usually during inspiration. Stridor is a sign of potentially life-threatening upper airway obstruction. Stridor can occur during inhalation or exhalation. If stridor is heard during inspiration, the lesion is probably in the glottic or paraglottic region. If stri-

dor occurs only during exhalation, the lesion site is below the glottis, usually in the chest. Voice or cry alterations associated with stridor almost always place the obstruction at the glottis. Dysphagia with stridor is associated with lesions in the hypopharynx (e.g., epiglottitis, retropharyngeal abscess, hypopharyngeal tumors). Radiographs for the evaluation of stridor are obtained primarily to detect a retropharyngeal abscess, a pharyngolaryngeal foreign body, subglottic narrowing, and epiglottitis (Table 22-2).

Epiglottitis

Acute epiglottitis is a life-threatening infection of the supraglottic tissues, involving the epiglottis and the aryepiglottic folds. Epiglottitis can occur at any age.[22] Children typically have an acute onset of inspiratory stridor, high fever, dysphagia, and drooling. In contrast to patients with croup, children with epiglottitis rarely cough.[23] The patient suspected of having epiglottitis *should not be sent for radiographic examination unattended* because of the risk of acute airway obstruction.

On the lateral view, epiglottitis is suggested by thickening and edema of the epiglottis and aryepiglottitic folds. In advanced cases, the swollen epiglottis appears as an upward-pointing thumb (the *thumb sign*), and separation of the tracheal and esophageal air columns (Fig. 22-26).

TABLE 22-2

Differential Diagnosis of Stridor in Children

Newborns
    Laryngomalacia
    Subglottic stenosis
    Vocal cord paralysis
    Tracheomalacia
    Vascular anomalies
    Hemangioma
Infants to 1 year
    Congenital anomalies
    Croup
    Retropharyngeal abscess
    Foreign bodies
1 to 2 years
    Croup
    Foreign bodies
    Epiglottitis
3 to 6 years
    Enlarged tonsils and adenoids
    Foreign bodies
All ages
    Angioneurotic edema
    Tumors
    Trauma
    Thermal or chemical inhalation
    Tracheal stenosis

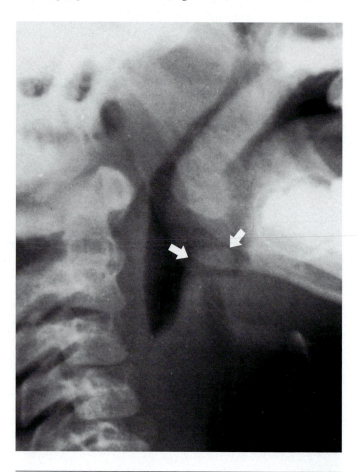

FIGURE 22-26.   Epiglottitis. There is thickening of the epiglottis and ariepiglottic folds *(arrows)*. (Courtesy of Dr. Frank Schneiderman, Sparrow Hospital, Lansing, Michigan.)

Croup

In patients with croup, stridor is heard on inspiration. A barking cough is typical. Croup occurs most commonly in late fall and early winter in children between 6 months and 3 years of age.

Radiographically, there is hypopharyngeal overdistention during inspiration, with a normal epiglottitis and aryepiglottic folds (Fig. 22-27). The vocal cords appear thickened and fuzzy, and the subglottic portion of the trachea is narrowed. On the frontal view, the vocal cords are thickened and funnel-like owing to edema and spasm. Normally, on inspiration, the vocal cords fall away, revealing a wide-open airway. With croup, there is little change in the appearance of the cords between inspiration and expiration; thus, the funnel-shaped or "steeple" configuration is almost always present. Often the steeple sign can be seen on the standard AP chest film, especially if the chin and head are tipped back.

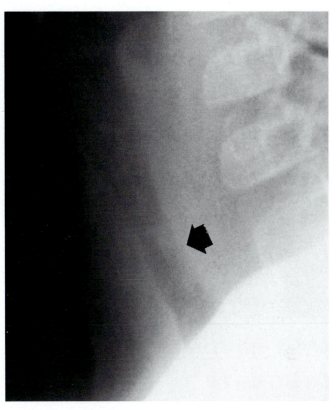

FIGURE 22-28. Bacterial tracheitis. There is a faint cast of mucopurulent material lining the child's airway *(arrow)*. (Courtesy of Dr. A. Oestreich, Children's Hospital Medical Center, Cincinnati, Ohio.)

Bacterial Tracheitis

Bacterial tracheitis ("pseudomembranous croup," "membranous laryngotracheitis") is a bacterial infection of the subglottic airway, causing mucosal swelling at the level of the cricoid cartilage and accompanied by copious thick, purulent sputum.[24] Children with bacterial tracheitis appear toxic, are usually febrile (>38.9° C), have a leukocytosis, and produce purulent airway secretions. Airway obstruction results from subglottic edema and copious mucopurulent secretions. When these secretions become inspissated, they form casts of the bronchopulmonary trunk that can mimic an aspirated foreign body on the lateral radiograph. The epiglottis is normal, there is subglottic narrowing, and the tracheal air column has ragged margins (Fig. 22-28). The chest film may show patchy infiltrates.

Retropharyngeal Abscess

The child below 6 years of age has retropharyngeal lymph nodes that can become infected and form an abscess. A retropharyngeal abscess can also result from perforation of the hypopharynx by a foreign body. On the lateral neck radiograph, a retropharyngeal abscess is suggested by thickening of the

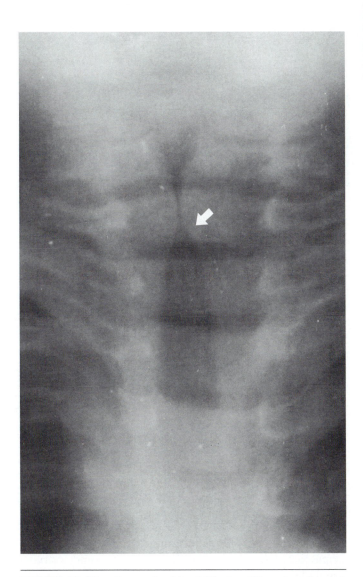

FIGURE 22-27. Croup. In this child, the AP neck radiograph demonstrates smoothly tapered narrowing of the subglottic space, known as the "steeple sign."

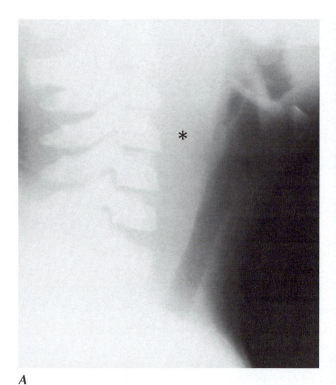

A

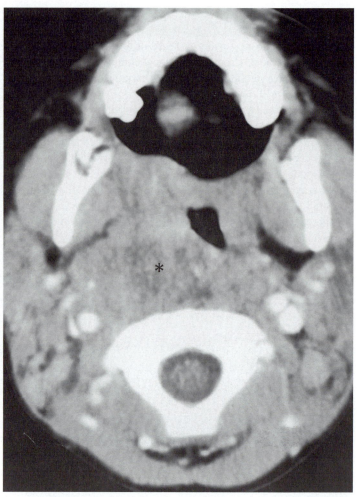

B

FIGURE 22-29. Retropharyngeal abscess. *A.* There is soft tissue swelling anterior to C2 and C3, indicating retropharyngeal abscess *(asterisk)*. *B.* CT confirms the poorly defined abscess *(asterisk)*, which is causing displacement of the airway anteriorly and to the patient's left.

retropharyngeal soft tissues and a forward bulge that encroaches on the airway (Fig. 22-29). There is an increase in the width of the prevertebral soft tissues greater than half the width of the adjacent vertebral body. Streaks of gas may be seen within the retropharyngeal soft tissue mass. Differentiating normal tracheal buckling and prominent lymphoid tissue from true thickening of the retropharyngeal soft tissue can be difficult. With retropharyngeal infection, the normal step-off from the posterior pharyngeal wall to the posterior wall of the trachea is lost.[25] CT and MRI provide additional detail.

Foreign Bodies

Many foreign bodies trapped in the proximal airway are radiopaque and easily seen. Glass, chicken bones, pencils, and polyvinylchloride are radiopaque, whereas some fish bones, wood, and other plant-vegetable foreign bodies are not. Coins most often lodge in the proximal epiglottis. In the AP view, the coin appears *en face*. When in the trachea, the coin appears on edge (AP view). Although the AP view alone is satisfactory in determining coin location (trachea versus esophagus), a lateral view is still obtained to determine the number of foreign bodies (Fig. 22-30). Cervical films are also obtained to demonstrate an-

imal bones. Fish bones are small and may easily be missed on radiographs. Symptomatic fish-bone ingestions often require direct visualization of the oropharynx. On the other hand, poultry bones are of sufficient density to appear on radiographs as a rule. In most patients, the poultry bone is completely swallowed, leaving a residual esophageal abrasion that causes the persistent symptoms.

PEDIATRIC CHEST RADIOGRAPHY

The standard images for evaluating cardiopulmonary conditions in the child are the frontal and lateral radiographs. Because infants and children are often unable to cooperate, an AP frontal view is obtained with the patient in the supine position. The lateral view is a supine cross-table exposure. With the cooperative child, a PA view is taken while the patient is standing. The lateral view is also taken standing. The films are exposed with the breath held at the end of a deep inspiration. Exposure of the film while the child is crying should be avoided, because motion of the chest wall, mediastinum, and diaphragm produces images that are difficult to interpret.

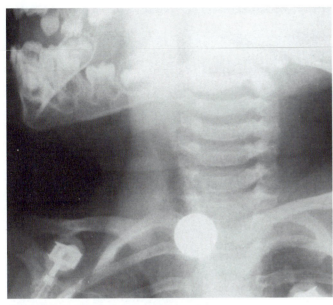

A

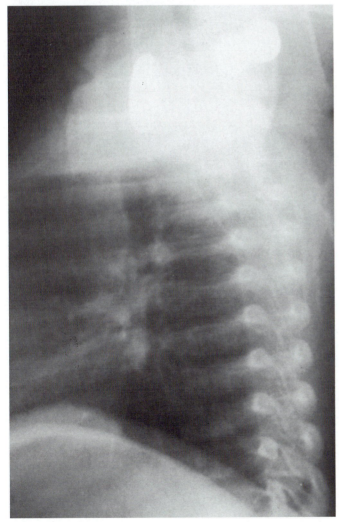

B

FIGURE 22-30. Esophageal foreign body. Esophageal coins are seen *en face* on the AP view *(A)* and on edge on the lateral view *(B)*.

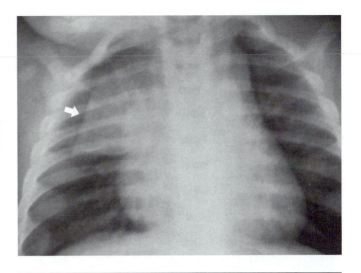

FIGURE 22-31. The thymus. In a young child, the thymic shadow can be mistakenly interpreted as an infiltrate. This is called the "sail sign."

The Thymus. The thymus is a thin, bilobed organ located in the superior mediastinum. The relative size of the thymus increases with expiration and decreases with inspiration. Occasionally, the thymus extends inferiorly to the level of the diaphragm. Because the thymus is a soft organ, overlying ribs can indent it, causing a *wave sign*. The right lobe of the thymus can overlap with the minor fissure, causing a *sail sign* (Fig. 22-31). This is occasionally misinterpreted as a mediastinal mass, pneumonia, or atelectasis. After 3 years of age, the thymus usually involutes, becoming radiographically inapparent.

Viral Pneumonia

Viral lower respiratory tract infections usually affect the tracheobronchial system. This results in bronchitis and peribronchitis rather than an alveolar, consolidative pneumonia. Radiographically, there is parahilar peribronchial infiltration and parahilar prominence or a diffuse reticular pattern. The heart's borders may appear "shaggy" because of the adjacent peribronchial inflammation.

RESPIRATORY SYNCYTIAL VIRUS INFECTION. In young children, after the first few months of life and up to about 5 years of age, most pneumonias are caused by viruses. Respiratory synctial virus (RSV) accounts for most of these infections.[26] RSV has a predictable annual epidemic that lasts from December through early spring. Bronchiolitis, which usually overlaps with RSV pneumonia, is the most common diagnosis in infants hospitalized with RSV infection. Bronchiolitis produces necrosis of the bronchiolar epithelium, submucosal edema, and hypersecretion of mucus. These bronchiolar changes result in mucus plugging, patchy subsegmental atelectasis, and widespread pulmonary hyperinflation. The radiographic findings in RSV bronchiolitis are hyperaeration of the lungs with variable degrees of perihilar interstitial infiltrate or a reticular pattern (Fig. 22-32).

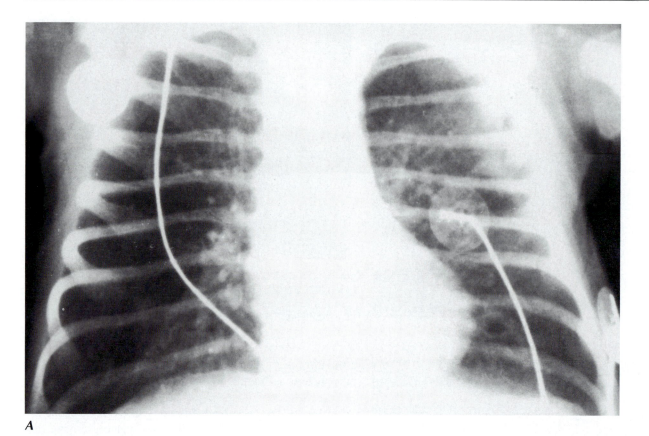

A

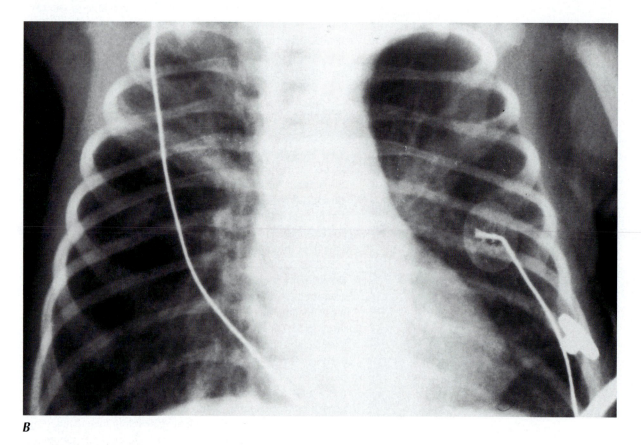

B

FIGURE 22-32. Respiratory syncytial virus pneumonia. *A.* There is an ill-defined reticular pattern in the upper zones of both lungs on the admission chest radiograph. *B.* Two days later, the infiltrates have become more distinct, although the child was improving clinically. (Courtesy of Dr. Ellen Cavanagh, Sparrow Hospital, Lansing, Michigan.)

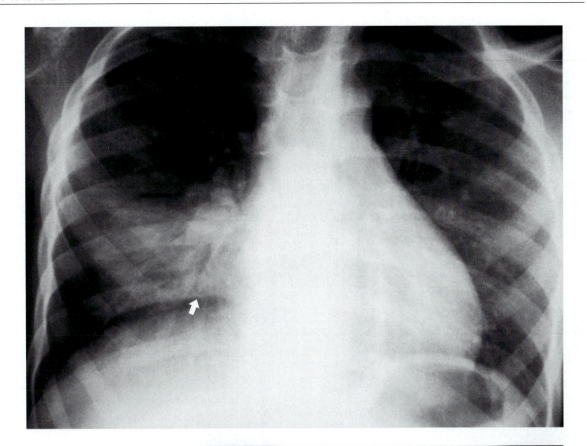

Bacterial Pneumonia

Common causes of acute pneumonia in infants and children are *Streptococcus pneumoniae, Chlamydia trachomatis, Mycoplasma pneumoniae,* and *Haemophilus influenzae.* Pneumococcus causes a "typical" clinical and radiographic pneumonia, whereas *Mycoplasma, Chlamydia,* and viruses are responsible for "atypical" pneumonia. Patients with recurrent or persistent pneumonia should be evaluated for immunologic deficiency, cystic fibrosis, aspirated foreign body, neuromuscular dysfunction, tracheoesophageal fistulas, and central nervous system disorders.

Children with *typical bacterial pneumonia* usually present with an abrupt onset of fever of 39.5 to 40.5° C (103 to 104° F), tachypnea, and cough. Older children may complain of chest or abdominal pain. The radiograph shows a lobar consolidation.

For bacterial pneumonia, auscultatory-roentgenographic correlation is good, unlike that of viral pneumonia. Radiographs usually confirm the location of the clinically suspected pneumonia. Its appearance can range from a small peripheral infiltrate to a completely consolidated lobe, its size being dependent on the duration of the pneumonia (Fig. 22-33).

Pneumonias that are round (similar to a coin lesion) are commonly seen in the pediatric population (Fig. 22-34). These round, spherical, or oval

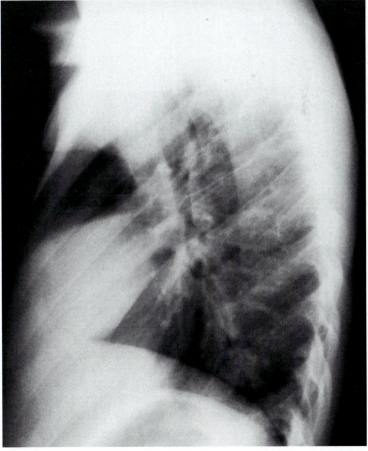

FIGURE 22-33. Lobar pneumonia. This child has a pneumonia involving the right middle lobe. The right heart border is obliterated on the AP radiograph *(arrow).*

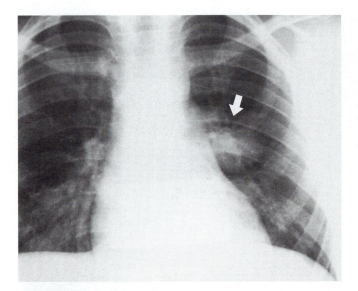

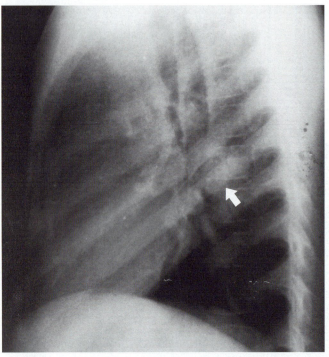

FIGURE 22-34. Round pneumonia. Early in the course of pneumonia, the radiographic infiltrate can appear round, like a coin lesion. This radiographic appearance mimics a tumor. This child has a small pneumonia involving the superior segment of the left lower lobe. (Courtesy of Dr. Ellen Cavanagh, Sparrow Hospital, Lansing, Michigan.)

infiltrates can be misinterpreted as pulmonary or mediastinal masses. In the symptomatic child, round pneumonias usually represent pneumococcal infection in the early consolidative phase. Retrocardiac infiltrates, which can be difficult to see, are most obvious on the lateral radiograph. On the PA or AP view, careful inspection reveals a round radiodensity "behind" the heart.

Atypical pneumonia usually presents with a less abrupt onset and nonrespiratory symptoms including myalgia, coryza,

pharyngitis, and diarrhea. The radiographic picture of mycoplasmal, chlamydial, and viral pneumonia is variable and can appear as a focal consolidation, diffuse or patchy airspace filling, or parahilar peribronchial infiltration.

Foreign-Body Aspiration

When a child has "swallowed" a foreign body followed by immediate coughing and focal wheezing on auscultation, the clinical need for evaluation is obvious. Nonetheless, children can have subtle symptoms long after an unwitnessed aspiration. In fact, the child can present with a history of recurrent pneumonia. The radiographic evaluation of the child with a suspected tracheobronchial foreign body begins with AP (or PA) and lateral chest films. Supplementary views include the forced-expiratory and bilateral decubitus chest views.

Radiographic findings of an aspirated foreign body include an infiltrate or atelectasis involving a distal segment or lobe. Acute infections can present with empyema or ipsilateral hilar lymphadenopathy. Infection is more common with aspirated vegetable matter. Other findings include mediastinal shift due to air trapping.

Expiratory views are used to detect air trapping when the foreign body causes a ball-valve phenomenon. Unfortunately small children (the group at highest risk for aspiration) are unable to cooperate, thus limiting the ability of this technique to detect mediastinal shift. A forced AP expiratory view is accomplished by pressing on the child's abdomen and gently but completely forcing expiration. A lead glove is used to protect the examiner's hand. The inspiratory AP chest is compared with this film to detect air trapping represented by mediastinal shift. This is the preferred plain-film study for foreign-body detection. In the past, bilateral chest decubitus views have been used to detect air trapping, but decubitus studies are not as sensitive as a forced expiratory study. In many cases, fiberoptic bronchoscopy is required to establish the diagnosis.

GASTROINTESTINAL IMAGING

Examination of selected children with acute abdominal pain or bilious vomiting entails supine and upright views of the abdomen and a frontal view of the chest. The principal role of plain abdominal radiography is in the diagnosis of bowel obstruction. Because abdominal pain may be caused by pneumonia in children, many centers do both the AP and lateral chest views. Pneumoperitoneum due to bowel perforation is also detected on chest radiographs, and, if there is a massive amount of free air, a supine abdominal film. If upright views are difficult to obtain because of the patient's condition, a cross-table lateral or lateral decubitus abdominal view is taken.

Appendicitis

After gastroenteritis, appendicitis is the most common acute abdominal inflammatory process in the child. It is frequently undetected until 24 to 48 h after onset and after perforation has occurred.

The history and physical examination usually suggest appendicitis. The role of plain radiographs in appendicitis is threefold. First, radiographs verify the diagnosis when a finding such as an appendicolith is seen. Second, radiographs can detect a nonsurgical condition mimicking appendicitis (e.g., lower lobe pneumonia). Finally, radiologic evaluation excludes other surgical conditions of the abdomen masquerading as or accompanying appendicitis (e.g., perforation, bowel obstruction).

Most children with acute nonperforated appendicitis have diminished air in the gastrointestinal tract. The diminished air pattern is secondary to anorexia, nausea, vomiting, or diarrhea. However, an adynamic ileus causing increased intestinal gas may also be seen. If dilated bowel is present, appendiceal perforation should be considered. Additional signs suggestive of acute appendicitis include lumbar scoliosis with concavity to the right, absence or indistinctness of the right psoas margin, a localized loop of dilated bowel in the right lower quadrant, a calcified fecalith in the proximal appendix, an inflammatory mass or abscess in the right lower quadrant or pelvis, and obliteration of the properitoneal fat line on the right.[27]

Ultrasound (US) is able to provide an imaging diagnosis of appendicitis and to reduce the negative laparotomy rate. In a recent study, the sensitivity and specificity rates of US were higher than 90%. Criteria for a "positive" study include lack of compressibility of the appendix, a cross-sectional diameter that exceeds 6 mm, the presence of a complex mass in the right lower quadrant, and the presence of an appendicolith.[28] CT is also able to accurately make a diagnosis of appendicitis. In some institutions, US is preferred because of its lack of radiation exposure. However, to be successful, US requires a skillful operator and a cooperative child.

Gastrointestinal Obstruction in the Infant

A variety of congenital and developmental conditions cause gastrointestinal obstruction in the newborn and infant. These include duodenal atresia, malrotation with midgut volvulus, pyloric stenosis, and an incarcerated inguinal hernia. Indications for radiographic evaluation include a "surgical" rigid abdomen, bilious vomiting, unremitting emesis, and the absence of a bowel movement. A "double-bubble" sign characterizes duodenal atresia and a duodenal hematoma (Fig. 22-35). There is an air bubble in the stomach as well as in the proximal duodenum. A gastric volvulus appears as a gastric outlet obstruction on plain films. Hirschsprung's disease (aganglionic colon)

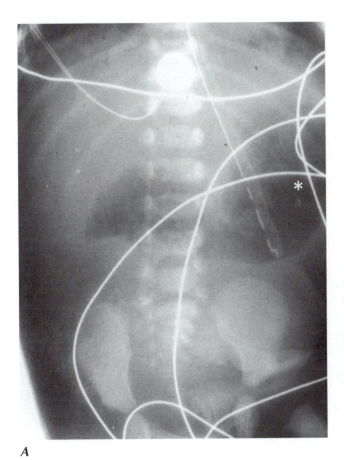

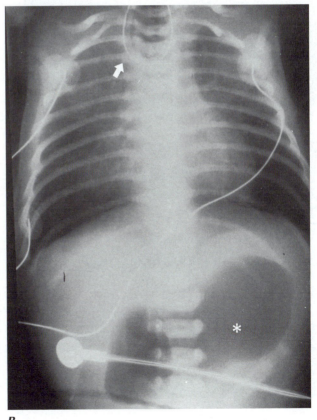

A   *B*

FIGURE 22-35.   Duodenal atresia. *A.* An infant with duodenal atresia. The plain abdominal film shows a massively distended, stomach *(asterisk). B.* Another infant with both duodenal and esophageal atresia. The plain abdominal film shows a massively distended, air-filled stomach *(asterisk).* The nasogastric tube is doubled back and cannot reach the distal esophagus *(arrow).* (Courtesy of Dr. Ellen Cavanagh, Sparrow Hospital, Lansing, Michigan.)

and cystic fibrosis result in constipation. The plain-film findings range from accumulation of stool to a bowel obstruction. In severe cases of Hirschsprung's disease, toxic enterocolitis can occur.

MALROTATION AND MIDGUT VOLVULUS. A midgut volvulus resulting from congenital malrotation of the gut can appear either as a gastric outlet obstruction or a small bowel obstruction with or without an accompanying soft tissue mass. The soft tissue mass is actually a fluid-filled loop of bowel. A contrast upper GI series demonstrates the malrotation (Figs. 22-36 and 22-37).

PYLORIC STENOSIS. Pyloric stenosis is the most common cause of intestinal obstruction in infancy. It results from diffuse hypertrophy and hyperplasia of the smooth muscle of the antrum of the stomach and the circular pyloric muscles. Males are four times more likely to develop pyloric stenosis, the hallmark of which is nonbilious vomiting that commences between the second and sixth weeks of life. The diagnosis is made by palpating an olive-sized mass just to the right of the midline above the umbilicus. Plain films may show a large, gas-filled stomach. In an infant suspected of having pyloric stenosis, US can detect the pyloric smooth muscle mass. If the sonographic findings are diagnostic, no further examination is indicated. On a contrast upper GI study, the most significant radiologic signs are elongation and narrowing of the pyloric channel (Fig. 22-38).

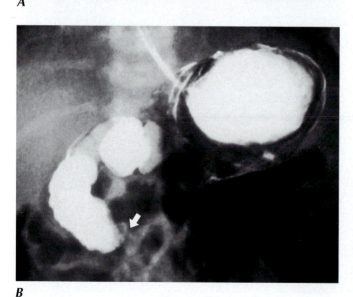

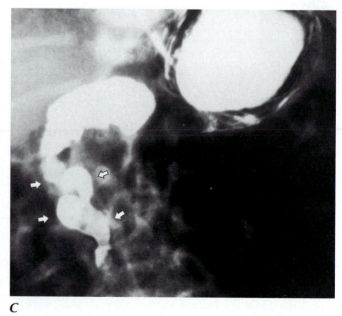

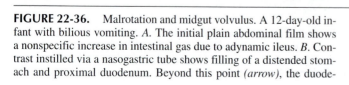

FIGURE 22-36. Malrotation and midgut volvulus. A 12-day-old infant with bilious vomiting. *A.* The initial plain abdominal film shows a nonspecific increase in intestinal gas due to adynamic ileus. *B.* Contrast instilled via a nasogastric tube shows filling of a distended stomach and proximal duodenum. Beyond this point *(arrow)*, the duodenum is compressed by either duodenal bands (Ladd's bands) or the twisted midgut volvulus. *C.* A later film shows contrast entering the distal duodenum and proximal small bowel. There is a pathognomonic spiral pattern due to twisting of the midgut *(arrows)*. (Courtesy of Dr. Ellen Cavanagh, Sparrow Hospital, Lansing, Michigan.)

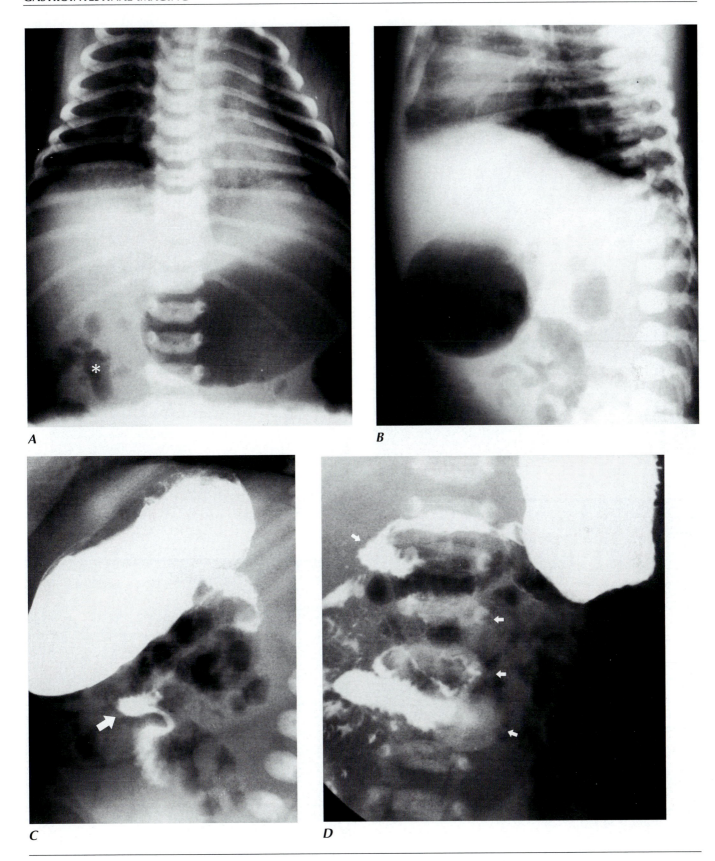

FIGURE 22-37. Malrotation and midgut volvulus. A 6-day-old infant presents with nausea and vomiting. *A.* There is marked distention of the stomach and slight filling of the duodenum and proximal small bowel *(asterisk).* Gastric and duodenal distention is due to extrinsic compression of the third portion of the duodenum either by constricting duodenal bands (Ladd's bands) or by the twisted midgut volvulus itself. *B.* The lateral abdominal film shows an air-filled, distended stomach and air in the proximal duodenum posterior to the stomach. *C* and *D.* Upper GI contrast films show gastric distention. The contrast in the duodenum and proximal small bowel has a spiral appearance where the gut is twisted upon itself *(arrows).* (Courtesy of Dr. Ellen Cavanagh, Sparrow Hospital, Lansing, Michigan.)

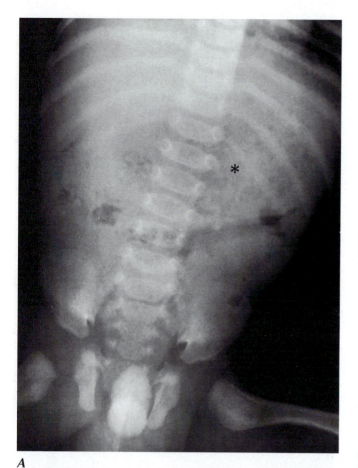

A

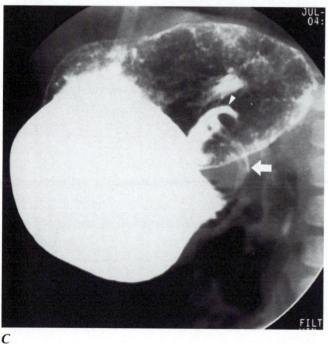

C

INTUSSUSCEPTION.   Intussusception is the most common cause of bowel obstruction in children between the ages of 2 months and 6 years, with a peak incidence between 3 and 36 months. In older children, it may be the presenting feature of cystic fibrosis or lymphoma. The classic triad of symptoms comprises colicky abdominal pain, vomiting, and hematochezia. However, only 10 to 20% of patients with intussusception present with all three symptoms. In some cases, lethargy is the predominant feature.

Plain-film findings of intussusception vary. The radiographic findings depend on the duration of symptoms and the presence

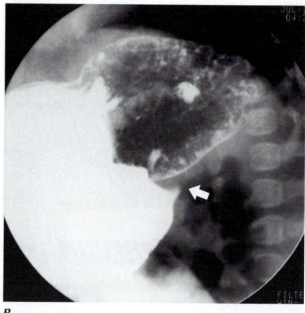

B

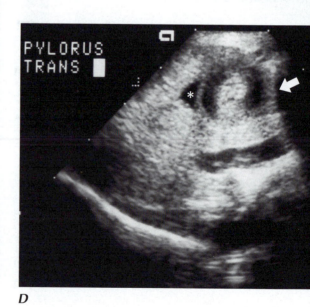

D

FIGURE 22-38.   Pyloric stenosis. *A.* The initial plain abdominal film in an infant with lethargy and poor feeding reveals a stomach massively distended with a mixture of fluid and air *(asterisk).* The transverse colon is displaced inferiorly by the stomach. If the stomach were distended by air, the radiograph would show the "single-bubble" sign. *B.* Contrast upper GI series shows a massively distended stomach that tapers abruptly to a stenotic pylorus. A thin column of contrast is seen passing through the constricted lumen of the pylorus—the "string sign" *(arrow). C.* The string sign is again seen. Contrast has begun to enter the duodenum *(arrowhead). D.* In another patient, abdominal ultrasound reveals a greatly thickened pyloric wall *(arrow).* A small amount of free fluid is seen outside the pylorus *(asterisk).* (Courtesy of Dr. Ellen Cavanagh, Sparrow Hospital, Lansing, Michigan.)

or absence of complications. Immediately after the intussusception occurs, the bowel gas pattern is normal. Eventually, a typical pattern of small bowel obstruction is seen. About half the cases show a soft tissue mass. An upright or lateral decubitus abdominal film may also demonstrate the head (lead point) of the invaginating portion of the intussusception (Fig. 22-39).

Other radiographic findings include lack of definition of the inferior aspect of the liver and the absence of gas in the right

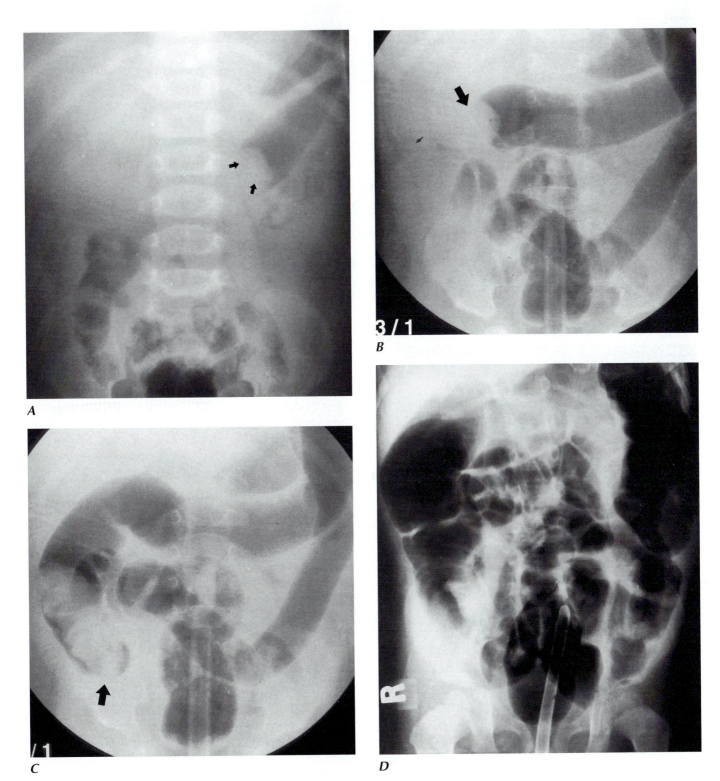

FIGURE 22-39. Intussusception. *A.* Initial plain abdominal film shows an overall paucity of bowel gas. Air in the distal transverse colon abruptly ends at the head of the intussusception, which produces a mass-like filling defect *(arrows)*. *B.* Air enema—initial film. Air is introduced into the sigmoid, descending, and transverse colon until the gas shadow ends at the head of the intussusception *(arrow)*. *C.* As more gas is introduced through the rectal tube, the intussusception is reduced back down the ascending (right) colon. *D.* Reduction of the intussusception is confirmed when air fills the entire colon and small bowel. (Courtesy of Dr. Ellen Cavanagh, Sparrow Hospital, Lansing, Michigan.)

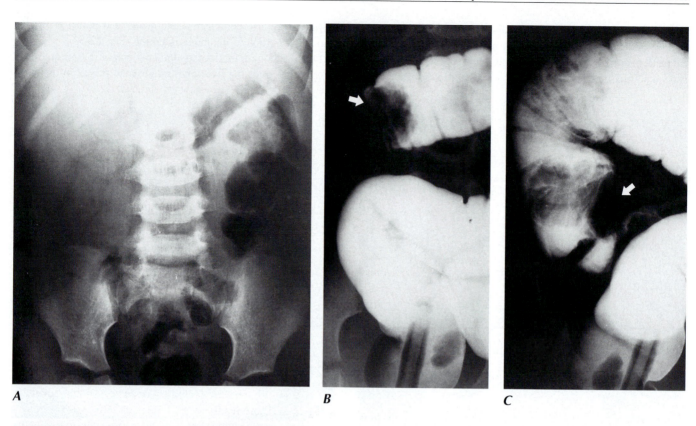

A   *B*   *C*

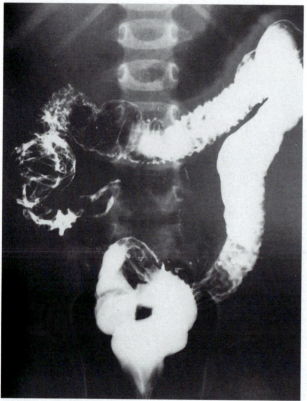

D

FIGURE 22-40.   Intussusception diagnosed and treated by contrast enema. *A.* Initial abdominal film is nonspecific. There is a paucity of gas on the right side of the abdomen. *B.* Contrast enema shows intussusception in the transverse colon. *C.* A later film shows reduction to the ascending colon. *D.* Final film shows filling of entire colon and reflux of contrast into the terminal ileum.

lower quadrant. The liver edge is obscured because, when right-upper-quadrant bowel gas is absent, the normal contrast of the solid liver against adjacent air-filled bowel is lost. Normal plain films do not exclude the diagnosis of an intussusception. If the clinical suspicion is high, additional diagnostic examinations are warranted.

Ultrasound can be used to detect an intussusception. Findings suggestive of intussusception include a layered oval mass on longitudinal views and concentric rings on cross section. A significant amount of free peritoneal fluid raises the suspicion of perforation or bowel necrosis. Color Doppler US can also disclose bowel ischemia, which is susceptible to perforation.

More often, plain-film studies are followed by a contrast enema examination using either barium or air insufflation (Figs. 22-39 and 22-40). Plain abdominal and chest films must be done prior to contrast enema in order to detect intestinal perforation with pneumoperitoneum. Perforation is a contraindication to contrast enema. Before the radiologist attempts reduction with barium enema or air, the surgical service should be notified to be ready to treat perforation or failure of reduction. In the past, reduction of intussusception was accomplished using barium. More recently, air has been used as a reducing agent. A postevacuation film is obtained after reduction is completed as well as a 24-hour follow-up film to determine whether the intussusception has remained, reduced, or recurred. Recurrence rates after nonsurgical reduction range from 4 to 10%. The first recurrence should be treated with repeat contrast enema reduction.

THE RADIOLOGY OF CHILD ABUSE

Tragically, child abuse continues to be a leading cause of death in young children. Radiography plays an important role in case identification, evaluation, and treatment. Imaging studies also serve as legal evidence. Radiographic evidence of child abuse is often the only objective evidence of abuse available to the courts.

Fractures and other injuries that are inconsistent with the alleged mechanism of injury are often the means by which abuse is discovered in the ED. Abuse cases are also identified when fracture patterns pathognomonic of abuse are found on routine radiographs.

The radiographic appearance of fracture healing follows a predictable sequence that allows injuries to be dated. The ability to date fractures allows assessment of the history of injury and often has legal implications. Nonetheless, the ED physician should be wary of attempting to date fractures *precisely*. If there is no evidence of bone healing, the physician can say with certainty only that the injury is less than 2 weeks old.[29] This fact is often useful in determining ED disposition.

The first radiographic evidence of bone healing is the resolution of soft tissue swelling, within 2 to 5 days. After 7 to 10 days, the periosteum becomes radiodense as osteoblasts begin laying down mineralized bone of the callus. In subtle fractures, this may be the only radiographic finding. In the absence of periosteal reaction, a fracture is likely to be less than 2 weeks old.

Callus formation and resorption of the bone along the fracture line is the next radiologic stage of healing, beginning at 10 to 14 days. The callus is visible for up to 3 months. Bone remodeling continues for up to 1 year.[29]

Indications for Imaging

The physically abused child is managed as a victim of major trauma. The investigation of suspected child abuse involves the search for occult injuries undetected during the clinical evaluation. One must ask, "Could the purported mechanism have produced the injury observed?" "Is the extent of injury consistent with the force described?" For example, a twisting mechanism does not explain a transverse fracture. A complete skeletal survey, bone scan, and cranial CT play a role in detecting injuries due to child abuse.

Imaging Modalities

THE SKELETAL SURVEY. Whenever child abuse is suspected in children below 2 years of age, a skeletal survey should be performed.[30] The yield from a skeletal survey drops considerably for children aged 2 to 5 years and is minimal for those older than 5 years.[31] However, the indications for radiography must be individualized. The skeletal survey helps prove child abuse by detecting occult fractures, demonstrating a fracture pattern suggestive of child abuse, and detecting multiple fractures of different ages.

TABLE 22-3

Suggested Films for Skeletal Survey

Lateral view of skull
Lateral of cervical, thoracic, lumbar, and sacral spine
AP of humeri
AP of forearms
PA of hands
AP chest film
Obliques of ribs
AP pelvis
AP femurs
AP tibias
AP feet

The skeletal survey must include an adequate radiograph of every bone of the child's body (Table 22-3). The practice of taking a "babygram," an AP and lateral of the entire child on a large x-ray film, is inadequate. Such radiographs do not provide sufficient detail to detect subtle fractures.

In certain situations, bone scanning may be preferable to the skeletal survey. Generally, a bone scan is a complementary study to the more readily available skeletal survey.[30,32]

Because the skeletal survey can be made up of over twenty radiographs, it is extremely important that the physician resists the tendency to "skim" the films. Each individual film must be evaluated as though that were the only film taken for a complaint originating from the body part studied. In a busy ED, proper evaluation of the skeletal survey may be impossible. Eventually, full evaluation by a radiologist is required.

BONE SCAN. The skeletal survey is not 100% sensitive for detecting fractures. Fractures are most likely to be missed at the ankles and elbows. Furthermore, posterior rib fractures tend to be undetected until callus formation appears at 2 weeks. Salter-Harris type I fractures are also problematic because their radiographic appearance can be normal. All of these fractures are detected on the bone scan. Bone scans remain positive even after "radiographic" healing and can therefore be used to demonstrate fractures older than 2 to 3 months.

While bone scanning is more sensitive than the skeletal survey, it is not as specific.[33] An osseous contusion, infection, or tumor can have the same appearance as a fracture. Normal epiphyseal growth plates appear "hot." Distinction from Salter-Harris type I fractures is made by comparison with the contralateral side. Bone scans are not useful for skull fractures.[34] Metaphyseal fractures can be concealed by uptake in the adjacent epiphyseal growth plate. Given these considerations, bone scanning is best used as an adjunct to the skeletal survey in cases where the skeletal survey is negative but the index of suspicion is high, especially when posterior rib fractures are suspected.[30]

BRAIN IMAGING. Any child suspected of being abused and having altered neurologic status requires brain imaging, since the physical examination is an insensitive indicator of brain injury.[30] In addition, retinal hemorrhages mandate brain imaging even in the absence of an altered neurologic status. Seizures can be the first presentation of head injury due to child abuse.[35] Infants under 1 year of age who have been severely abused may have subtle neurologic findings.[36,37] The indications for brain imaging in asymptomatic children older than 1 year of age are not well established and rely on clinical judgment.

CT of the head without contrast is easily obtained from the ED and detects injuries requiring immediate treatment. However, MRI is more sensitive at detecting brain injury and is useful in cases where the CT is negative but the index of suspicion remains high.[38] CT scanning is better able to detect subarachnoid hemorrhages but is less sensitive than MRI for subdural hematomas, cortical contusion, cerebral edema, white matter injuries, and chronic injuries. MRI is also better able to date injuries. In cases where the initial CT is negative or where not all clinical findings are explained by the CT findings, MRI should be performed.[39]

THORACOABDOMINAL IMAGING.

While thoracoabdominal injuries are relatively uncommon, they are likely to be lethal. The indications for investigation of thoracoabdominal injury in child abuse are similar to those of general trauma.

Injuries Suspicious for Child Abuse

Metaphyseal corner fractures are almost pathognomonic for child abuse. Similarly, rib fractures, especially posterior fractures, mandate a child abuse investigation. Humeral fractures not involving the supracondylar region are strongly associated with child abuse. The vast majority of children's fractures oc-cur in typical locations—torus fractures at the wrist, spiral fractures of the tibia, and clavicular fractures. Children with fractures in unusual locations require close scrutiny (Table 22-4).

If multiple fractures have occurred at different times, the diagnosis of child abuse is strongly suspected. Finally, a discrepancy between the radiographic age of a fracture and the time of injury stated by the caregiver prompts consideration of child abuse.

SHAKEN BABY SYNDROME.

The shaken-baby syndrome (shaken-impact syndrome) results from violent shaking of a small infant.[40] Two types of injury occur during the abusive episode: diffuse injury caused by acceleration-deceleration forces and focal injury caused by direct impact with a hard surface.[40–42] The shaking-impact event results in brain injuries, skull fracture, rib fractures, and retinal hemorrhages (Table 22-5).

METAPHYSEAL CORNER FRACTURES.

Violent shaking, twisting, or pulling across a joint generates shear forces across the epiphyseal growth plate and the spongiosa layer of the metaphysis. These forces result in epiphyseal or, more commonly, metaphyseal fractures. The radiolucent epiphysis and a thin rim of metaphysis is sheared off the remaining metaphysis. Little is seen on the radiograph except a thin "bucket handle" of mineralized metaphysis or, in more subtle cases, small flecks off the corner of the metaphysis (Fig. 22-41). Metaphyseal corner fractures are typically seen at the knees, ankles, elbows, or wrists. Once bone healing has begun, periosteal reaction and callus formation make the injury more apparent. The thick periosteum in children's long bones can deposit a thick layer of new bone, resulting in a "railroad track" radiographic appearance.[43]

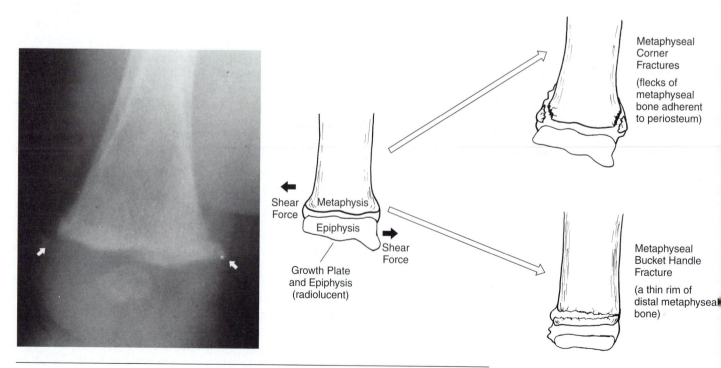

FIGURE 22-41. Metaphyseal corner fracture. Metaphyseal corner fractures are seen at the distal femur in this 5-month-old girl *(arrows)*. A metaphyseal corner fracture is indicative of child abuse. It is caused by violent shaking, which shears off a small fragment of bone from the distal metaphysis.

TABLE 22-4

Fracture Locations Suggestive of Child Abuse

Femoral fractures in nonambulatory children
Humeral fractures away from the supracondylar region
Sternum, sternoclavicular joint
Scapular fractures
Hand and foot fractures in non-weight-bearing children
Spines of vertebrae
Ribs

LONG BONE FRACTURES. The body mass of a child younger than 12 months of age does not generate sufficient force to fracture a normal long bone in a fall from a bed, crib or couch.[44,45] In infants, humeral fractures are strongly associated with abuse.[46,47] In toddlers, nonsupracondylar humeral fractures are associated with abuse, whereas supracondylar fractures are seen in both accidental and abusive injuries. Abuse is highly likely in cases of femoral fracture in nonambulatory children (Fig. 22-42).[48] Spiral fractures of the tibia, especially the distal tibia, tend to be accidental ("toddler's fracture").[49]

RIB FRACTURES. The ribs of a child are extremely pliable, and it takes considerable force to break them. If a fracture does oc-

cur, it does so at one of three sites along the rib. Posteriorly, ribs are likely to fracture at the costovertebral junction. The rib is bent over the transverse process of the vertebra during violent shaking and compression of the chest.[50] Fractures at this site are usually not seen on plain films at the time of injury unless special coned down views are obtained. Posterior rib fractures are detected more easily after callus formation has begun. The second site of rib fracture is at the most lateral point of the thorax. Severe squeezing results in bowing of the rib and a fracture when its elastic capacity is exceeded. The third weak point in the rib is the costochondral junction. Here, the costal cartilage is prone to separation from the rib. Because the cartilage

TABLE 22-5

Possible Brain Injuries in Shaken-Infant Syndrome

Retinal hemorrhage
Acute and/or chronic subdural hemorrhage
Subarachnoid hemorrhage
Brain contusions
Interhemispheric blood
Spinal cord injuries of the cervicomedullary junction
Spinal cord hematomas or contusions
May have neurologic abnormalities without abnormality on brain
    imaging

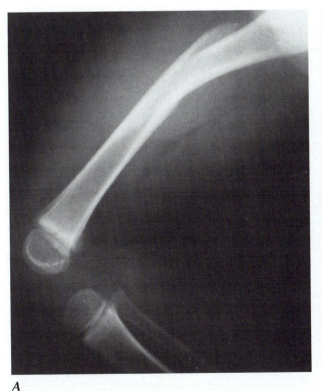

A

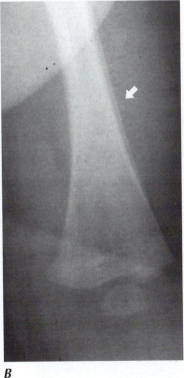

B

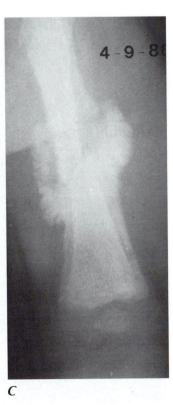

C

FIGURE 22-42. Fractures suggestive of child abuse. Fractures of the femoral shaft are highly unusual in nonambulatory children and suggest nonaccidental trauma. *A.* A relatively recent fracture is seen here. *B.* The layer of periosteal new bone formation along the femoral shaft is characteristic of trauma in a young child. The pe-riosteum is less adherent to the adjacent cortical bone in children and so readily becomes separated during trauma. *C.* Exuberant callous formation is seen in this healing femoral fracture. (*B* and *C* are courtesy of Dr. Ellen Cavanagh, Sparrow Hospital, Lansing, Michigan.)

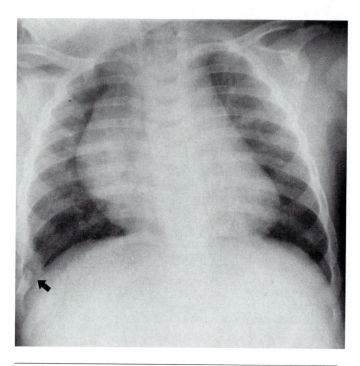

FIGURE 22-43. Rib fracture suggestive of child abuse. Fracture of the lateral right ninth rib in a 4-month-old child *(arrow)*. There is no callous formation in this acute fracture.

is radiolucent, these fractures are not seen at the time of injury but are detected after the callus forms.

The AP chest film is carefully inspected for rib fractures. Posterior rib fractures, seen just lateral to the transverse processes, are pathognomonic for child abuse. It is uncommon to detect these fractures in the acute phase; more commonly, they are seen when callus formation is advanced. They appear as a ballooning of the end of the rib (Fig. 22-43). Lateral rib fractures are detected by assessing the alignment of the lateral border of the rib cage. Fractures make the affected rib protrude with respect to the other ribs. Finally, anterior rib fractures are seen at the costochondral junction.

Chest compression performed during resuscitative efforts are extremely unlikely to cause rib fractures.[51] If any rib fractures are seen, a child abuse investigation should be carried out.

HEAD INJURIES.   Head injuries in children younger than 1 year of age are associated with child abuse.[36] Features of a skull fracture suspicious for child abuse include complex configuration, involvement of more than one bone, nonparietal fracture, and associated intracranial injury (Fig. 22-44).[52]

ABDOMINAL INJURIES.   Hollow viscus injuries (e.g., stomach perforation) and traumatic pancreatic injuries in young children may be due to child abuse.[53,54]

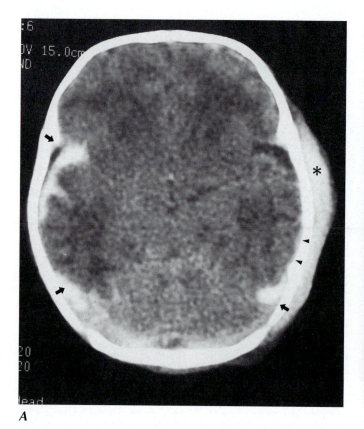

A

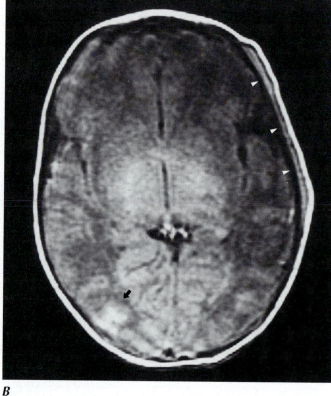

B

FIGURE 22-44. Head injury in a 7-week-old child due to violent shaking. *A.* CT reveals scalp swelling on the left *(asterisk)* and multiple areas of traumatic subarachnoid hemorrhage *(arrows)*. A small subdural hematoma is barely visible in the left parietal region *(arrowheads)*. *B.* MRI better demonstrates the subdural hemorrhage *(arrowheads)*. An intraparenchymal cerebral contusion is seen in the right occipital region *(arrow)*.

REFERENCES

1. Simon HD, Khan NS, Nordenberg DF, Wright JA: Pediatric emergency physician interpretation of plain radiographs: Is routine review by a radiologist necessary and cost-effective? *Ann Emerg Med* 27:295, 1996.

2. Rogers LF: Special considerations in children, in Rogers LF (ed): *The Radiology of Skeletal Trauma,* 2d ed. New York: Churchill Livingstone, 1992:109–148.

3. Salter RB, Harris WR: Injuries involving the epiphyseal growth plate. *J Bone Joint Surg* 45:587, 1963.

4. Wilkins KE: Changing patterns in the management of fractures in children. *Clin Orthop* 254:136, 1991.

5. Light TR, Ogden DA, Ogden JA: The anatomy of metaphyseal torus fractures. *Clin Orthop* 188:103, 1984.

6. Mizuta T, Benson WM, Foster BK, et al: Statistical analysis of the incidence of physeal injuries. *J Pediatr Orthop* 7:518, 1987.

7. Swischuk LE: Extremities, in Swischuk LE (ed): *Emergency Radiology of the Acutely Ill or Injured Child,* 2d ed. Baltimore: Williams & Wilkins, 1986:310–490.

8. Kissoon N, Galpin R, Gayle M, et al: Evaluation of the role of comparison radiographs in the diagnosis of traumatic elbow injuries. *J Pediatr Orthop* 15:449, 1995.

9. Chacon D, Kissoon N, Brown T, Galpin R: Use of comparison radiographs in the diagnosis of traumatic injuries of the elbow. *Ann Emerg Med* 21:895, 1992.

10. Sherk H, Black J: Orthopedic emergencies, in Fleisher GR, Ludwig S (eds): *Textbook of Pediatric Emergency Medicine,* 3d ed. Baltimore: Williams & Wilkins, 1993:1396–1402.

11. Silverman FN: Infections in bone, in Silverman FN, Kliegman RM (eds): *Caffey's Pediatric X-Ray Diagnosis,* 9th ed. St. Louis: Mosby, 1993:1844–1845.

12. Narasimhan N, Marks M: Osteomyelitis and septic arthritis, in Nelson WE, Behrman RE, Kliegman RM, Arvin AM (eds): *Nelson's Textbook of Pediatrics,* 15th ed. Philadelphia: Saunders, 1996:724–727.

13. Nath AK, Sethu AU: Use of ultrasound in osteomyelitis. *Br J Radiol* 65:649, 1992.

14. Azouz EM, Greenspan A, Marton D: CT Evaluation of primary epiphyseal bone abscesses. *Skel Radiol* 22:17, 1993.

15. Hall BD: Inherited osteoporoses, in Nelson WE, Behrman RE, Kliegman RM, et al (eds): *Nelson's Textbook of Pediatrics.* 15th ed. Philadelphia: Saunders, 1996:1978–1980.

16. Silverman FN: Skeletal dysplasias, in Silverman FN, Kuhn JF (eds): *Caffey's Pediatric X-ray Diagnosis,* 9th ed. St. Louis: Mosby, 1993:1676–1681.

17. Thompson GH, Scales PV: The knee, in Nelson WE, Behrman RE, Kliegman RM, et al (eds): *Nelson's Textbook of Pediatrics,* 15th ed. Philadelphia: Saunders, 1996:1936.

18. Thompson GH, Scales PV: The hip, in Nelson WE, Behrman RE, Kliegman RM, Arvin AM (eds): *Nelson's Textbook of Pediatrics,* 15th ed. Philadelphia: Saunders, 1996:1941–1942.

19. Mazur PM, Kornberg AE: Limp, in Fleisher GR, Ludwig S (eds): *Textbook of Pediatric Emergency Medicine,* 3d ed. Baltimore: Williams & Wilkins, 1996:304–309.

20. Jaffe DM, Binns H, Radkowski MA, et al: Developing a clinical algorithm for early management of cervical spine injury in child trauma victims. *Ann Emerg Med* 16:270, 1987.

21. Rachesky I, Boyce WT, Duncan B, et al: Clinical prediction of cervical spine injuries in children: Radiographic abnormalities. *Am J Dis Child* 141:199, 1987.

22. Brilli RJ, Benzing G, Cotcamp DH: Epiglottitis in infants less than two years of age. *Pediatr Emerg Care* 5:16, 1989.

23. Baldwin GA (ed): Acute upper airway obstruction, in *Handbook of Pediatric Emergencies.* Boston: Little, Brown, 1989:59–67.

24. Henry RL, Mellis CM, Benjamin B: Pseudomembranous croup. *Arch Dis Child* 58:180, 1983.

25. Swischuk LE (ed): Upper airway, nasal passages, sinuses, and mastoids, in *Emergency Imaging of the Acutely Ill or Injured Child,* 3d ed. Baltimore: Williams & Wilkins, 1994:171–174.

26. Carlsen KH, Larsen S, Bjerre O, Legaard J: Acute bronchiolitis: Predisposing factors and characterization of infants at risk. *Pediatr Pulmonol* 3:153, 1987.

27. Swischuk LE, Hayden CK Jr: Appendicitis with perforation: The dilated transverse colon sign. *AJR* 135:687, 1980.

28. Ramachandran P, Sivit C, Newman KD, Schwartz MZ: Ultrasonography as an adjunct in the diagnosis of acute appendicitis: A 4-year experience. *J Pediatr Surg* 31:164, 1996.

29. O'Connor JF, Cohen J: Dating fractures, in Kleinman PK (ed): *Diagnostic Imaging in Child Abuse.* Baltimore: Williams & Wilkins, 1987:103–114.

30. American Academy of Pediatrics: Diagnostic imaging of child abuse. *Pediatrics* 87:262, 1991.

31. Merton DF, Radkowski MA, Leonidas JC: The abused child: A radiographical reappraisal. *Radiology* 146:377, 1983.

32. Kleinman PK: Skeletal trauma: General considerations, in Kleinman PK (ed): *Diagnostic Imaging of Child Abuse.* Baltimore: Williams & Wilkins, 1987:5–28.

33. Leonidas JC: Skeletal trauma in the child abuse syndrome. *Pediatr Ann* 12:875, 1983.

34. Kleinhans E, Kentrup H, Alzen G, et al: A false negative bone scintigram in biparietal skull fracture in a case of a battered child syndrome. *Nuklearmedizin* 32:206, 1993.

35. Duhaime AC, Alario AJ, Lewander WJ, et al: Head injury in very young children: Mechanisms, injury types, and ophthalmologic findings in 100 hospitalized patients younger than 2 years. *Pediatrics* 90:179, 1992.

36. Billmire ME, Meyers PA: Serious head injury in infants: Accidents or abuse? *Pediatrics* 75:340, 1985.

37. Mertin DF, Osborne DP: Craniocerebral trauma in the child abuse syndrome. *Pediatr Ann* 12:882, 1983.

38. Sato Y, Yuh WTC, Smith WL, et al: Head injury in child abuse: Evaluation with MR imaging. *Pediatr Radiol* 173:653, 1989.

39. Giangiacomo J, Khan JA, Levine C, Thompson VM: Sequential cranial computed tomography in infants with retinal hemorrhages. *Ophthalmology* 95:295, 1988.

40. Bruce D, Zimmerman R: Shaken impact syndrome. *Pediatr Ann* 18:482, 1989.

41. Hadley MN, Sonntag VK, Rekate HL, Murphy A: The infant whiplash-shake injury syndrome: A clinical and pathological study. *Neurosurgery* 24:536, 1989.

42. Duhaime AC, Gennarelli TA, Thibault LE, et al: The shaken baby syndrome: A clinical, pathological, and biomechanical study. *J Neurosurg* 66:409, 1987.

43. Kleinman PK, Marks SC, Blackbourne B: The metaphyseal lesion in abused infants: a radiologic-histopathologic study. *AJR* 146:895, 1986.

44. Chadwick DL, Chin S, Salerno C, et al: Deaths from falls in children: How far is fatal? *J Trauma* 31:1353, 1991.

45. Helfer RE, Slovic TL, Black M: Injuries resulting when small children fall out of bed. *Pediatrics* 60:533, 1977.

46. Leventhal J, Thomas S, Rosenfield N, Markowitz RI: Fractures in young children: Distinguishing child abuse from unintentional injuries. *Am J Dis Child* 147:87, 1993.

47. Thomas SA, Rosenfield NS, Leventhal JM, Markowitz RI: Long-bone fractures in young children: Distinguishing accidental from child abuse. *Pediatrics* 88:471, 1991.

48. Dalton JH, Slovic T, Helfer RE, Comstock J, et al: Undiagnosed abuse in children younger than 3 years of age with femoral fracture. *Am J Dis Child* 144:875, 1990.

49. Mellick LB, Reesor K: Spiral tibial fractures of children: A commonly accidental spiral long bone fracture. *Am J Emerg Med* 8:234, 1990.

50. Klein PK: Bony thoracic trauma, in Kleiman PK (ed): *Diagnostic Imaging of Child Abuse.* Baltimore: Williams & Wilkins, 1987:67–89.

51. Feldman KW, Brewer DK: Child abuse, cardiopulmonary resuscitation, and rib fractures. *Arch Dis Child* 65:423, 1990.

52. Hobbs CJ: Skull fracture and the diagnosis of abuse. *Arch Dis Child* 59:246, 1984.

53. Kleinman PK, Brill PW, Winchester P: Resolving duodenal-jejunal hematoma in abused children. *Radiology* 160:747, 1986.

54. Orel SG, Nussbaum AR, Sheth S, et al: Duodenal hematoma in child abuse sonographic detection. *Am J Radiol* 151:147, 1988.

SELECTED READINGS—PEDIATRICS

Swischuk LE: *Emergency Radiology of the Acutely Ill or Injured Child,* 3rd ed. Baltimore: Williams and Wilkins, 1992

Silverman FN, Kliegman RM: *Caffey's Pediatric X-Ray Diagnosis,* 9th ed. St. Louis: Mosby, 1993.

Kleinman PK: *Diagnostic Imaging of Child Abuse,* 2nd ed. Baltimore: Williams & Wilkins, 1998.

Rogers LF: Special considerations in children, in Rogers LF (ed): *The Radiology of Skeletal Trauma,* 2nd ed. New York: Churchill Livingstone, 1992:109–148.

CHAPTER 23

TOXICOLOGIC EMERGENCIES

DAVID T. SCHWARTZ

Overdoses, poisonings, and toxin exposures are common problems in emergency medicine. Although diagnostic imaging is not usually considered an important aspect of clinical toxicology, in certain instances radiographic studies make a significant contribution to patient care. Imaging can establish the diagnosis of a specific toxin, assist in patient management, detect complications of the toxin exposure, and exclude alternative diagnoses. In some cases, radiographs detect the toxin itself, whereas in other cases the effects of the toxin on the body are revealed. Occasionally, an imaging study will suggest a toxicologic etiology when one was not initially suspected. Nevertheless, imaging studies are always supplementary to a complete history and physical examination.

The following six cases illustrate the role of radiographic imaging in toxicologic emergencies. The answers for each case are given at the end of each section of the chapter.

CASE 1. A 46-year-old man presents with abdominal pain. He has a depressed level of consciousness and a strong odor of alcohol on his breath. He has mild, diffuse abdominal tenderness. Plain films of the chest and abdomen are negative. Because of his blunted mentation and abdominal pain, a computed tomography (CT) scan of the abdomen is obtained, which reveals multiple tablet-shaped densities within the stomach (Fig. 23-1). What ingested substances can be detected radiographically?

CASE 2. A 2-year-old boy is rushed into the emergency department (ED) by his mother because of vomiting. His emesis contains blood. He is hemodynamically stable and has minimal abdominal tenderness. Although abdominal radiographs are generally not indicated in the diagnosis of gastrointestinal (GI) bleeding, could they be useful in this patient?

CASE 3. A 26-year-old woman complains of progressive pain and numbness of her hands and lower legs that began the day before she came to the ED. She also complains of pleuritic chest pain and abdominal cramping. Her examination is normal except for hypesthesia of the extremities. There is no motor weakness. Laboratory values are normal except for mild proteinuria. She is admitted to the hospital for evaluation and pain management. The next day, two of her friends develop similar but milder symptoms. Six days later, the patient's hair begins to fall out. Can a radiographic study assist in establishing the diagnosis in these patients?

CASE 4. A 3-year-old boy is brought to the ED because he has been irritable and eating poorly for 2 weeks. He was seen 1 week earlier with similar symptoms and was diagnosed as having a viral syndrome. He has had no fever. The child lives with his teenage mother and grandmother in an old building in a low-income section of the city. Laboratory values are remarkable for a mild normocytic anemia (hemoglobin 10.1 g/dL; hematocrit 33%). What radiographic studies can provide clues to the diagnosis in this child?

CASE 5. A 71-year-old man presents with dyspnea and confusion. He has been ill since he was diagnosed with prostate cancer 6 months earlier. He has no history of cardiac or pulmonary disease. On examination, he is frail and in mild respiratory distress. Vital signs are heart rate 100 beats per minute, blood pressure 120/70 mmHg, respiration 24 breaths per minute, and rectal temperature 101.7 °F (38.7 °C). He is alert

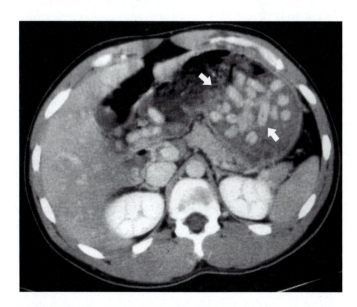

FIGURE 23-1. Case 1. [From Schwartz DT: Toxicologic imaging, in Goldfrank LR, Flomenbaum NE, Lewin NA, et al (eds): *Goldfrank's Toxicologic Emergencies,* 6th ed. Stamford, CT: Appleton & Lange, 1998. With permission.]

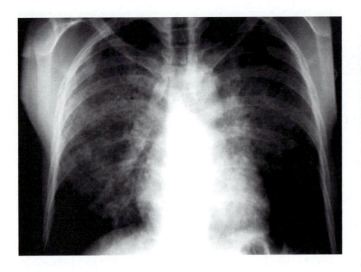

FIGURE 23-2. Case 5.

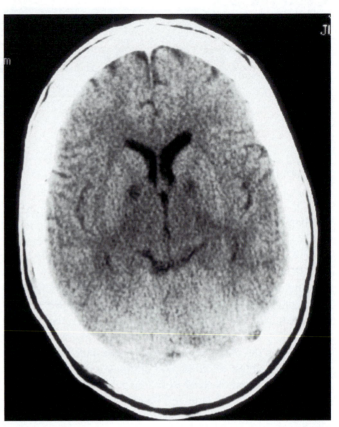

FIGURE 23-3. Case 6. [Courtesy of Paul Blackburn, D.O., Maricopa Medical Center, Phoenix, AZ. From Schwartz DT: Toxicologic imaging, in Goldfrank LR (ed): *Goldfrank's Toxicologic Emergencies,* 6th ed. Stamford, CT: Appleton & Lange, 1998. With permission.]

but mildly confused. The lung exam reveals scattered ronchi. The heartbeat is regular and abdomen nontender. The chest film shows bilateral infiltrates (Fig. 23-2). The arterial blood gas on room air reveals pH 7.38, P_{CO_2} 24, and P_{O_2} 64. Blood cultures are obtained, intravenous antibiotics are given, and he is admitted to the hospital. Are there any problems with this management?

CASE 6. A 65-year-old man is found in his home by his neighbor, not having been seen for several days. He has a history of alcoholism and lives in a small apartment above a busy midtown coffee shop. He is confused and somnolent. There is no evidence of trauma and no focal neurologic deficits are present. An emergency head CT is obtained to determine whether there is a subdural hematoma (Fig. 23-3). What is the cause of his altered mental status as suggested by this study?

INGESTION OF AN UNKNOWN SUBSTANCE

Although plain radiography could theoretically help in the management of a patient who has ingested medications that are radiopaque, the benefit of imaging in this setting is very limited.[1] Several in vitro studies have looked at the radiopacity of various medications in an attempt to determine which might be detected on an abdominal radiograph. Using an experimental water-bath model, a limited number of medications were radiopaque.[2–5] Handy studied 211 medications, of which 15% (32) were moderately radiopaque and 5% (11) were densely radiopaque.[2] The most densely radiopaque were iron preparations, chloral hydrate, and trifluoperazine (Stelazine). O'Brien studied 459 medications and found that 30% (136) were moderately radiopaque and 6% (29) were densely radiopaque (iron preparations, enteric-coated potassium chloride, chloral hydrate, trifluoperazine).[3] Savett studied 312 medications and found that 10% (31) were moderately radiopaque and 1% (4) were densely radiopaque (iron preparations, multivitamins with iron, potassium chloride, calcium carbonate).[4] A simple mnemonic device for recalling radiopaque toxins is: CHIPS [*c*hloral hydrate, *h*eavy metals, *i*ron and *i*odine, *p*sychotropics and *s*ustained-release (enteric-coated) preparations].

Unfortunately, most medications that are radiopaque in vitro are not readily identified within the complex shadows of an abdominal radiograph. In addition, many medications rapidly dissolve in the stomach and become invisible (e.g., chloral hydrate, trifluoperazine). Conversely, when a radiopaque substance is seen on an abdominal radiograph, its appearance is not sufficiently distinctive to determine its identity (Fig. 23-4). Only when the tablets are densely radiopaque and slow to dissolve in the gastrointestinal tract (e.g., iron) is radio-graphic detection clinically useful. Therefore, the use of plain-film radiography in the diagnostic evaluation of a patient with an unknown ingestion is of limited use.

CASE 1. Based on the abdominal CT findings; gastric lavage was planned. Before it could be performed the patient vomited a large amount of whole undigested fava beans. CT is able to detect small, nearly isodense structures such as these, which are undetectable with conventional radiography (Fig. 23-1). However, the radiographic detection of an ingested substance does not permit its toxicologic identification.

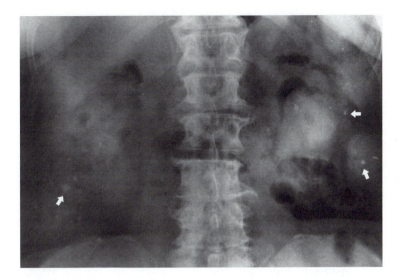

FIGURE 23-4. A 60-year-old woman presents to the ED with abdominal pain and dark stools. Radiopaque fragments are seen scattered throughout the abdomen *(arrows)*. Ingested radiopaque substances that can cause abdominal pain include ferrous sulfate and lead (i.e., paint chips). In this case, the patient had a peptic ulcer associated with *Helicobacter pylori* and was taking bismuth subsalicylate (Pepto-Bismol). Bismuth is radiopaque because of its high atomic number, 83. The radiographic appearance does not enable the clinician to distinguish between these various radiopaque substances.

IRON OVERDOSE

The best use of plain radiography in the detection of an ingested medication is an overdose of iron tablets (ferrous sulfate). Identification of iron tablets helps confirm the diagnosis, estimate the number of tablets ingested, and assess GI decontamination. The ability of radiography to exclude an iron ingestion is limited because some iron preparations do not have consistent radiopacity. Iron formulations that are most difficult to detect are liquid preparations and multivitamin preparations containing iron, especially if they are chewable or in beads ("spansules"). These iron preparations tend to fragment rapidly and disperse after ingestion. Staple and McAlister studied 15 different iron preparations in vitro and in live dogs.[6] Although all were visible initially, after 3 h the tablets were visible in only 6 of the 13 dogs and after 6 h in only 2. Everson et al. studied 54 children who had ingested iron tablets.[7] Thirty (55%) of the children had ingested chewable multivitamins with iron, and in only one of these patients were the tablets visible on an abdominal radiograph.

When iron tablets are identified radiographically, serial abdominal films can be used to follow GI decontamination and detect remaining tablets (Fig. 23-5).[8] In some instances, the

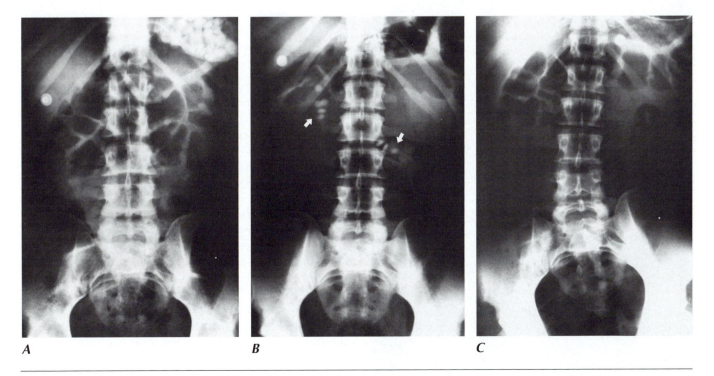

A   *B*   *C*

FIGURE 23-5. *A.* The identification of the large amount of radiopaque tablets confirms the diagnosis in a patient with a suspected iron overdose and permits rough estimation of the amount ingested. *B.* Following whole-bowel irrigation, a second radiograph revealed some remaining tablets and indicated the need for further intestinal decontamination. *C.* A third radiograph after additional bowel irrigation demonstrates clearing of the intestinal tract. (Courtesy David C. Lee, M.D., Division of Toxicology, Medical College of Pennsylvania, Philadelphia.)

iron tablets form a concretion or are adherent to the stomach lining. The persistence of iron tablets in the stomach despite lavage and bowel irrigation mandates surgical or endoscopic removal of the tablets.[9]

CASE 2. This 2-year-old child who presented to the ED with hematemesis had ingested his parents' iron pills. This is common because the pills often look like candy and the parents do not appreciate the toxicity of 2 or 3 iron pills in a young child. In addition, the child often does not tell the parents about the ingestion. This is one situation in which abdominal radiography can be helpful in identifying the cause of gastrointestinal hemorrhage (Fig. 23-6).

HEAVY METALS

Although "heavy metal" is not a proper chemical term, it is used in medical toxicology to refer to metals of high atomic number that cause biological toxicity. Heavy metals include

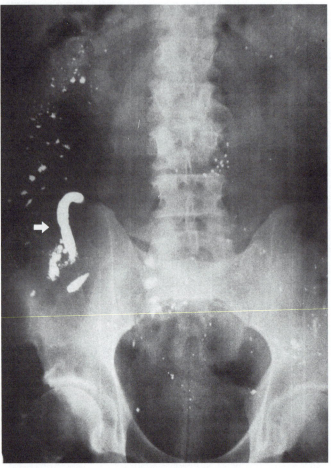

FIGURE 23-7. Mercury introduced into the intestinal tract when the mercury-weighted balloon at the end of a long intestinal tube ruptured. Liquid mercury fills the appendix (arrow).

lead, mercury, arsenic, thallium, cadmium, and chromium. When present in a large enough quantity, a heavy metal can be detected by conventional radiography.[10,11] Radiography is used to detect heavy metals located in the abdomen, imbedded in soft tissues, or outside of the body. The potential for systemic absorption depends on the specific heavy metal involved and the site of contact. Some heavy metals are toxic when ingested, whereas others pass unabsorbed through the GI tract. Mercury is liquid at room temperature and is present in such medical devices as thermometers and long intestinal tubes (Fig. 23-7). When ingested, liquid mercury passes unabsorbed through the GI tract as long as the mucosa is intact. If the mucosa is not intact, such as when glass from a broken thermometer lacerates the intestinal wall, systemic absorption can occur. When liquid mercury is injected, it either remains in soft tissues or disperses intravascularly (Fig. 23-8).[12–14] Subcutaneous deposits must be surgically debrided, and postoperative radiography is used to confirm complete removal.

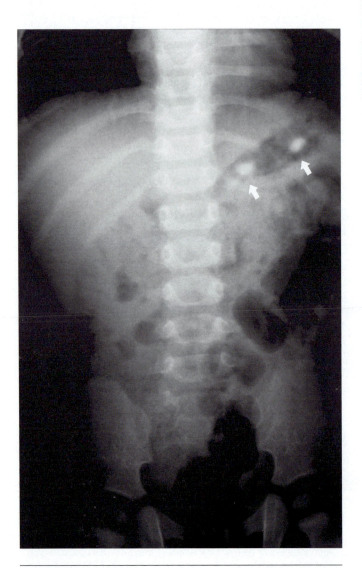

FIGURE 23-6. Case 2.

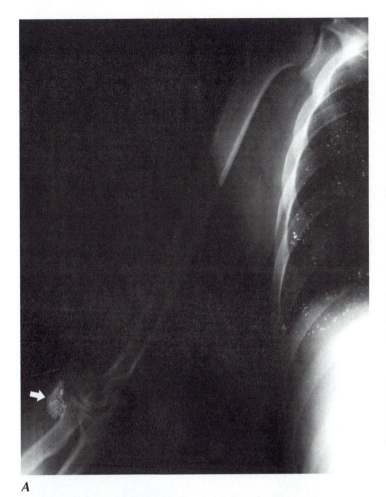

A

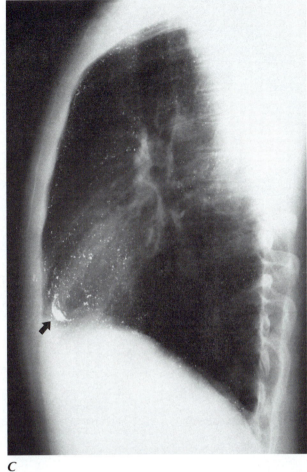

C

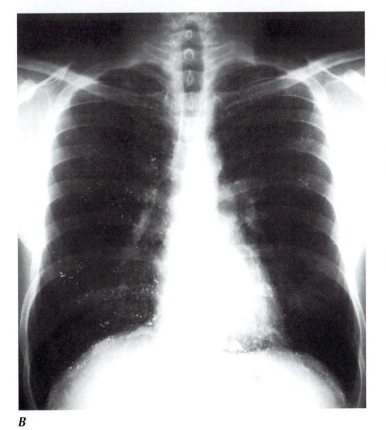

B

FIGURE 23-8. This patient received an intravenous injection of liquid elemental mercury. *A.* Extravasated subcutaneous mercury is seen in the right antecubital fossa *(arrow). B.* Intravascular injection resulted in mercury pulmonary emboli. *C.* Pooling of mercury in the right ventricle is seen *(arrow).* (Courtesy Janet Eng, D.O., Ingham Regional Medical Center, Lansing, MI.)

CASE 3. This patient had an isolated, painful sensory neuropathy for which there is a broad differential diagnosis. The rapidity of onset and clustering of cases suggest a common source for the illness. Potential toxins include solvents, organophosphates, heavy metals, isoniazid, mitotic inhibitors such as colchicine, and chemotheraputic agents such as vincristine. The pronounced painful neuropathy and multisystem involvement (thoracic, abdominal, and renal) suggest heavy metal poisoning. The degree of pain and the alopecia are suggestive of thallium intoxication.

This patient had recently received a box of marzipan candies sent anonymously from Europe. Radiographs of the remaining candies demonstrated their heavy metal content (Fig. 23-9). The patient's urinary thallium levels were markedly elevated. She developed transient total alopecia and had a mild residual peripheral neuropathy. Her friends, the other patients, recovered completely.[15]

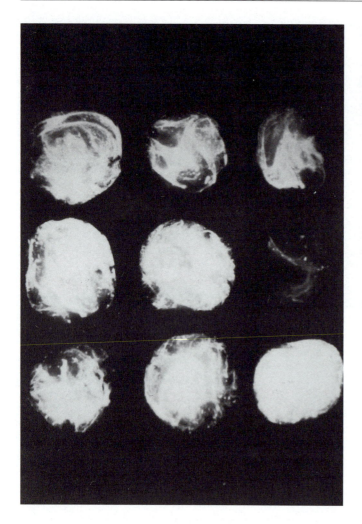

FIGURE 23-9. Case 3. [Courtesy Toxicology Fellowship of the New York City Poison Center. From *Goldfrank's Toxicologic Emergencies,* 6th ed. Appleton & Lange, 1998. With permission.]

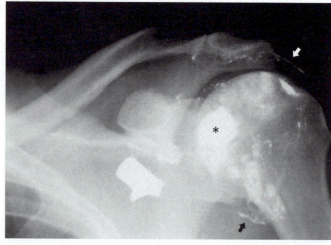

A

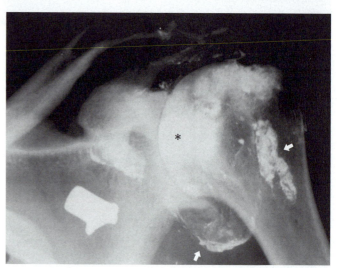

B

FIGURE 23-10. Lead intoxication and a "lead arthrogram" that developed years after a bullet wound to the shoulder (*A* and *B*). The bullet was imbedded in the articular surface of the humeral head. At the time of the initial injury, the portion of the bullet that protruded into the joint space was surgically removed, leaving a portion of the bullet adjacent to the synovial space *(asterisk)*. A second bullet is seen overlying the scapula. Eight years after the injury, the patient presented with shoulder pain, weakness, and anemia. Shoulder radiographs revealed extensive lead deposition throughout the synovium *(arrows)*. The serum lead level was 91 μg/dL. The patient was treated with dimercaptosuccinic acid chelation and surgical debridement of the synovium. [From *Goldfrank's Toxicologic Emergencies,* 6th ed. Appleton & Lange, 1998. With permission.]

Lead Poisoning

Despite considerable efforts to eliminate lead from the environment in gasoline, batteries, and household paint, it remains ubiquitous. When present in large quantities, lead can be detected radiographically. Lead bullets are generally left in place when they are imbedded in soft tissues. However, when the bullet is in contact with synovial fluid in a joint space, chemical and mechanical actions over the course of several years gradually cause fragmentation and systemic absorption of lead. It is therefore generally recommended to remove bullets that are in contact with joint spaces (Fig. 23-10).[16–18]

Lead poisoning in children is usually due to the ingestion of leaded paint chips. An abdominal radiograph may demonstrate radiopaque material.[19,20] In young children, lead poisoning causes dense transverse bands in the metaphyses of rapidly growing bones.[21–24] Radiographic detection of these bands provides provisional evidence of lead poisoning. Metaphyseal bands are due not to the deposition of lead but to "metabolic poisoning" that inhibits resorption of the zone of provisional calcification adjacent to the growth plate. Such metaphyseal bands are also caused by toxic exposure to bismuth (no longer used for medicinal purposes) and yellow phosphorus (formerly in cod liver oil). These bands must be distinguished from the common "stress lines" caused by an intercurrent illness during childhood that temporarily arrests bone growth (Fig. 23-11).

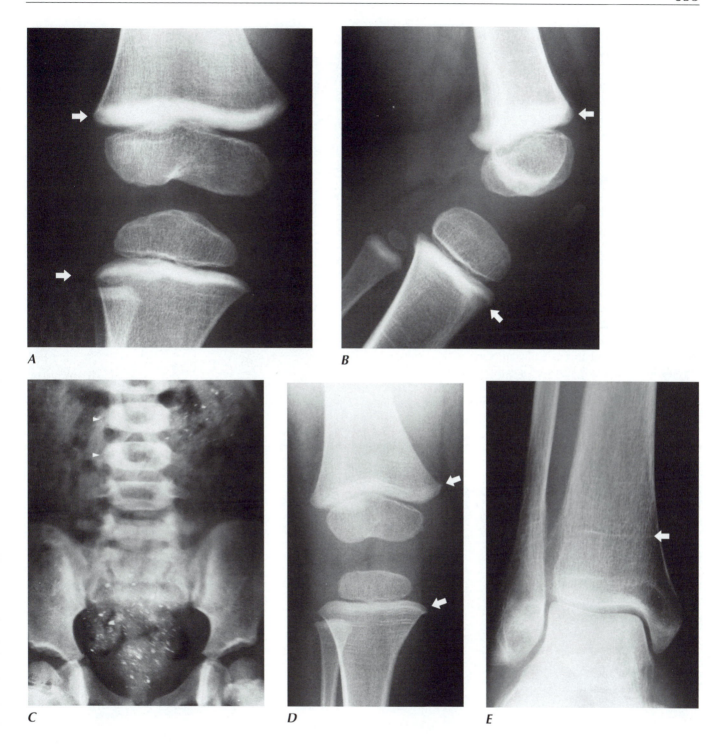

FIGURE 23-11. *A* and *B*. Metaphyseal bands due to lead poisoning. *C*. An abdominal film of another child shows leaded paint chips throughout the abdomen. Note the increased cortical bone density of the vertebral bodies, indicative of lead toxicity *(arrowheads)*. [Courtesy of Nancy Geneiser, M.D., Professor of Radiology, New York University. From *Goldfrank's Toxicologic Emergencies*, 6th ed. Appleton & Lange, 1998. With permission.] *D*. Normal metaphyseal bands can sometimes appear prominent. These should not be mistaken for pathologic lead lines. *E*. "Growth arrest" or "stress" lines. These fine lines represent brief periods of slow bone growth in childhood due to an intercurrent illness, or minor trauma. The lines can persist into adulthood and are of no pathologic significance.

CASE 4. In this child, radiographs of the lower extremities revealed dense transverse metaphyseal bands indicative of lead poisoning (Fig. 23-11*A* and *B*.). A plain film of the abdomen showed no radiodense lead particles. The child's serum lead level was toxic (60 μg/dL), and he was treated with chelation therapy. An investigation of his home environment found significant amounts of old, peeling paint on the walls, which the child had ingested.

RADIOGRAPHIC MANIFESTATIONS OF ILLICIT DRUG USE

Many complications of illicit drug use have radiographic manifestations. The complications depend on the particular drug involved, and the route of administration (ingestion, injection, or inhalation).

Intravenous Drug Use

Complications of intravenous drug use are predominantly infectious and are due to the injection of bacteria or viruses (such as HIV). Injected bacteria cause infective endocarditis and septic emboli. Septic embolization is often amenable to radiographic detection. Embolization from right-sided endocarditis results in septic pulmonary emboli.[25] These appear as multiple ill-defined opacities that often undergo cavitation (Fig. 23-12). Attempted injection into the internal jugular veins of the neck is a common cause of pneumothorax in urban populations.[26] Injection of particulate contaminants such as talc causes a chronic interstitial lung disease known as as *talcosis*.[27]

Osteomyelitis affecting the axial skeleton is typical of injection drug use. Back pain in such patients must be thoroughly investigated for vertebral body osteomyelitis. An epidural abscess can also occur without any plain radiographic abnormality. In

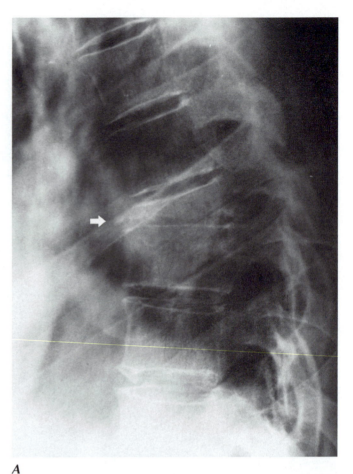

A

FIGURE 23-13. Skeletal complications of intravenous drug use. *A.* Vertebral body osteomyelitis in a patient presenting with back pain and lower extremity weakness. *S. aureus* grew in a specimen obtained

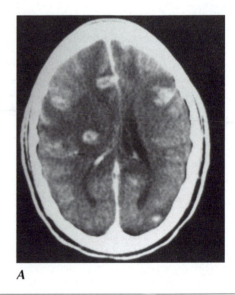

A

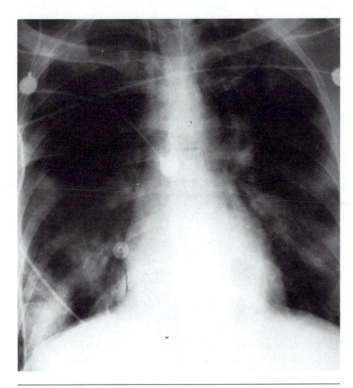

FIGURE 23-12. The chest radiograph of an intravenous drug user who presented with high fever but did not have pulmonary symptoms. There are multiple ill-defined pulmonary opacities throughout both lungs, characteristic of septic pulmonary emboli. His blood cultures grew *Staphylococcus aureus*. (From *Goldfrank's Toxicologic Emergencies*, 6th ed. Appleton & Lange, 1998. With permission.)

FIGURE 23-14. Three patients with ring-enhancing lesions as a complication of intravenous drug use. *A.* Multiple lesions of toxoplasmosis in a patient with AIDS. There is mass effect and midline shift due to a right-sided lesion. *B.* The patient improved rapidly with corticosteroids and antitoxoplasmosis antibiotics. *C.* This AIDS pa-the presence of spinal cord signs or symptoms, magnetic resonance imaging (MRI) or CT should be performed (see Chap. 14, Fig. 14-14). Sternoclavicular and sternomanubrial osteomyelitis and septic arthritis also occurs in these patients (Fig. 23-13).

Septic embolization to the brain is a catastrophic complica-

tion of injection drug use. On CT, emboli appear as ring-enhancing lesions indistinguishable from those of central nervous system (CNS) toxoplasmosis and primary CNS lymphoma, which are complications of AIDS (Fig. 23-14).

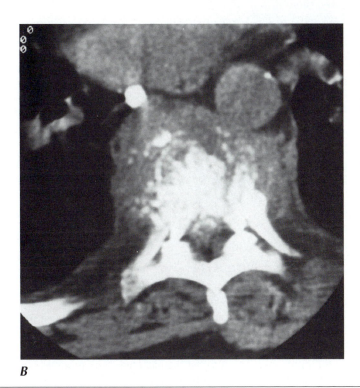

B

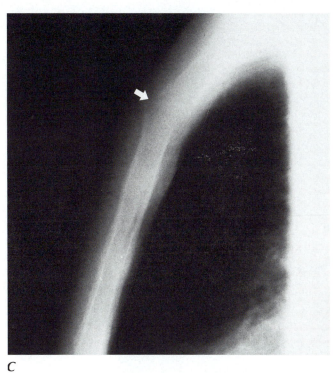

C

during surgical decompression. *B*. CT scan in this patient showing vertebral body destruction. *C*. Osteomyelitis at the manubrial sternal junction, a common site of infection in parenteral drug users. (*C*. from

Goldfrank's Toxicologic Emergencies, 6th ed. Appleton & Lange, 1998. With permission.)

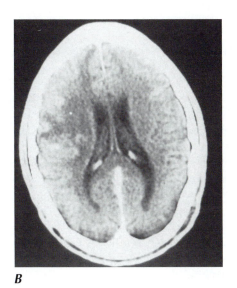

B

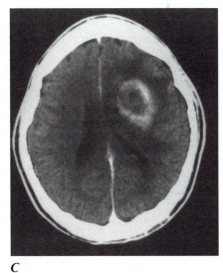

C

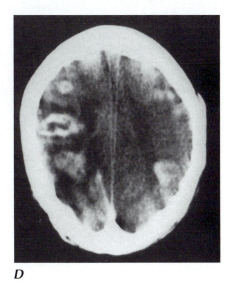

D

tient presented with headache and a ring-enhancing lesion on CT. He failed to respond to antitoxoplasmosis therapy and developed a right hemiparesis. After empiric radiation therapy for primary central nervous system lymphoma, the lesion partially regressed and the

patient improved. *D*. This injection drug user presented with high fever and stupor. The ring-enhancing lesions represent septic emboli secondary to *S. aureus* endocarditis. (From *Goldfrank's Toxicologic Emergencies,* 6th ed. Appleton & Lange, 1998. With permission.)

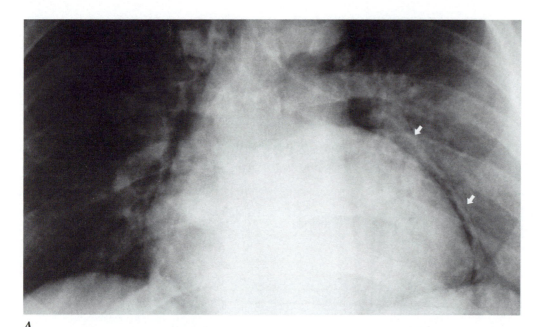

A

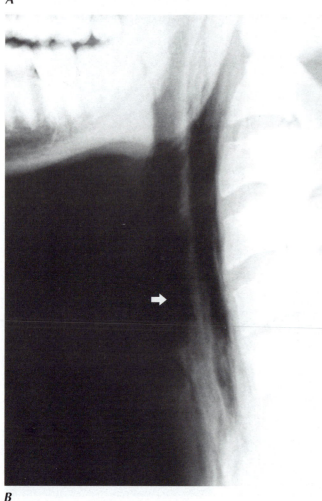

B

FIGURE 23-15. Pneumomediastinum in a patient who presented with chest pain after smoking crack cocaine. *A.* The chest film showed the fine white line of the parietal pleura lifted off of the heart, aorta, and other mediastinal structures by free air in the mediastinum. *B.* Air can be seen extending superiorly from the mediastinum into the pre-vertebral soft tissues.

Inhalational Drug Use

Forceful inhalation while smoking such drugs as crack cocaine and marijuana causes barotrauma resulting in pneumomediastinum (Fig. 23-15). Alveolar air ruptures into the peribronchovascular tissues and leaks along the lung interstitium to the hilum and then into the mediastinum. The prognosis of this form of pneumomediastinum is good.[28–30] Pneumomediastinum is one cause of cocaine-related chest pain that is amenable to radiographic diagnosis.

Abuse of volatile substances (e.g., glue sniffing) can cause noncardiogenic pulmonary edema. Chronic solvent abuse causes a dilated cardiomyopathy.

Illicit Drug Ingestion

Although ingestion is not the usual route of cocaine or opiate use, ingestion of sufficient quantities of the drug can result in serious toxicity. Two settings in which illicit drug ingestion is encountered are the *body stuffer* and the *body packer.* A body stuffer is a person who has hurriedly ingested contraband in an attempt to hide it from law enforcement officials.[31] A body packer is a professional drug smuggler who has swallowed a large quantity of securely sealed containers.[32] Although the body stuffer has generally ingested a smaller quantity of the drug, fatalities have occurred when such substances leak from the poorly sealed containers, typically soft plastic bags. In both instances, it is usually the container rather than the drug itself that is detected radiographically.

When brought to the ED in police custody, the body stuffer usually denies having ingested any drug. In the large majority of patients, the drug is not detected by plain radiography.[33,34] In a few cases, the cocaine "rock" has impurities that are radiodense.[35] Occasionally, the container is detected when it is a hard plastic or glass crack vial (Fig. 23-16).[36] The absence of

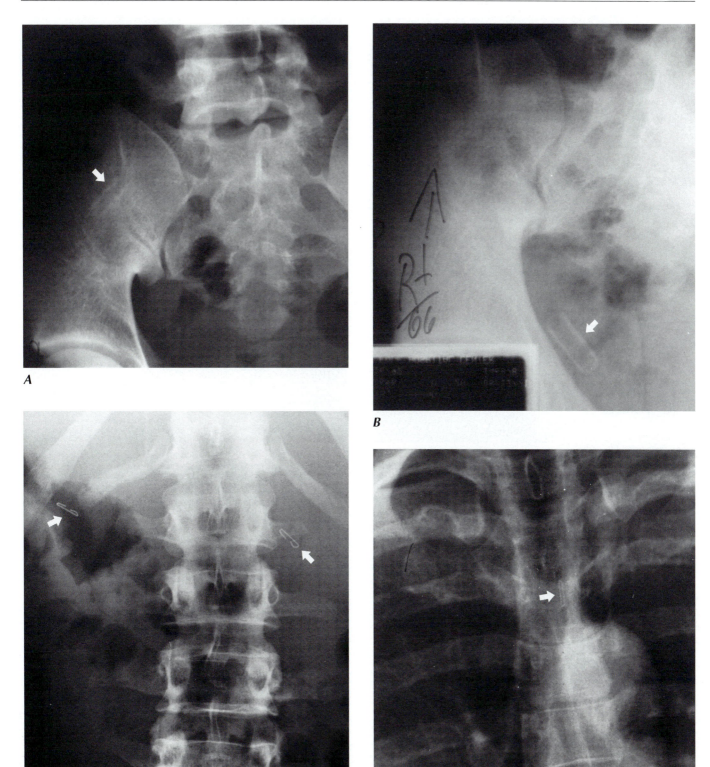

FIGURE 23-16. Two cocaine "body stuffers." Radiography helps with this diagnosis only rarely. *A.* An ingested glass crack vial is faintly seen overlying the right sacral wing on the upright abdominal film. *B.* On the upright film, the crack vial is more easily seen on the right side of the pelvis. Only the tubular container and not the drug is visible. *C.* Another patient in police custody was brought to the ED for allegedly ingesting his drugs. The radiographs revealed "nonsurgical" staples in his abdomen. *D.* His chest radiograph revealed a bag stuck in his esophagus. A second film, taken a short while later, showed that the bag had passed into the abdomen. The patient was treated with whole bowel irrigation. (*B* and *C* from *Goldfrank's Toxicologic Emergencies,* 6th ed. Appleton & Lange, 1998. With permission.)

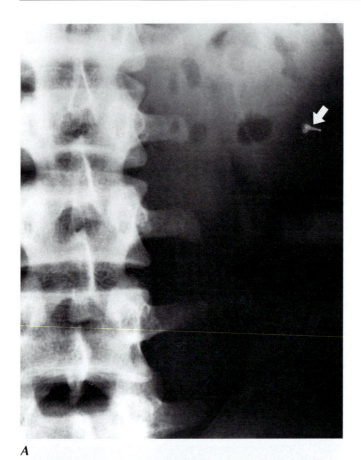

A

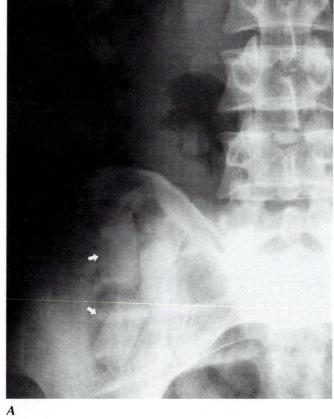

A

FIGURE 23-18. The radiographic appearances of packets ingested by two "body packers." *A.* Multiple solid, oblong packages are seen within the bowel. *B* and *C.* The packets are visible in this patient be-

B

FIGURE 23-17. A contrast CT scan reveals a plastic bag that was ingested in an attempt to conceal illicit drugs. *A.* The initial abdominal radiograph detected a "rock" of crack cocaine that contained radiopaque impurities. A second radiograph failed to disclose the cocaine and a CT scan was performed in an attempt to locate the drug. *B.* On the CT scan, the bag can be seen floating on the layer of contrast material in the stomach. The bag was removed by endoscopy but was empty. (Courtesy Dr. Fred Hachelroad, Pittsburg Poison Center, Pittsburgh, PA.)

such containers on the radiographs does not exclude an ingestion. Abdominal CT has also been used to detect the plastic bags (Fig. 23-17). However, whether the bags still contain any drug is not disclosed by the radiograph.[37,38]

With a body packer, the presence of numerous uniform, well-sealed containers in the GI tract is nearly always detected radiographically.[39–41] Although the drugs themselves are not radiopaque, the oblong packets are seen because they are surrounded by bowel gas or because there is a thin layer of gas or metallic foil in the container wall (Fig. 23-18). Since each packet contains a potentially fatal quantity of drug, it is crucial to remove all of the packets. This is generally accomplished by whole bowel irrigation. The patient usually knows the exact number of packets that have been ingested, and this number is compared with the number of packets recovered. One or two remaining packets are difficult to detect by plain radiography, and enteric contrast can be used to disclose the presence and location of these packets (Fig. 23-19).[42]

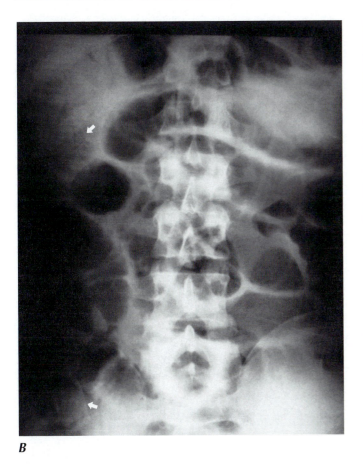

B

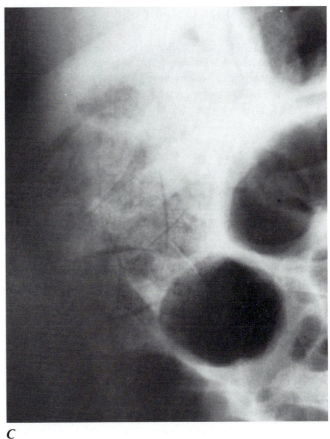

C

cause they are surrounded by a thin layer of air within the walls of the packets. There is diffuse dilation of the bowel. This is probably due to coingestion of antiperistaltic agents that allow the gut to retain

the large number of packets. However, the bowel dilation also raises the possibility of a mechanical obstruction caused by the packets. This patient was successfully treated with whole-bowel irrigation.

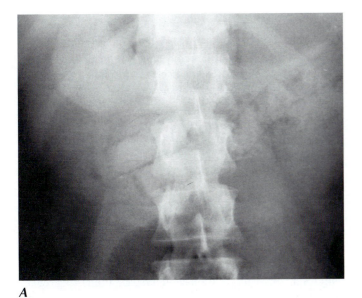

A

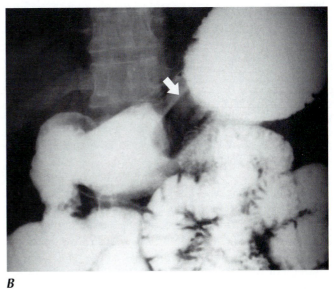

B

FIGURE 23-19. A cocaine body packer was intercepted and arrested at the airport. *A*. The initial film showed numerous packets outlined by air. Whole-bowel irrigation eliminated a large number of packets. Repeat abdominal films were negative. *B*. An upper GI and small bowel contrast study revealed one remaining packet in the stomach.

The packet was removed using flexible endoscopy. (Courtesy of the New York City Poison Control Center, Fellowship Training Program in Toxicology. From *Goldfrank's Toxicologic Emergencies,* 6th ed. Appleton & Lange, 1998. With permission).

Heroin and Other Opioids

Noncardiogenic pulmonary edema can occur following a massive heroin overdose. The onset of pulmonary edema and the attendant radiographic manifestations can be delayed for several hours. Therefore, the patient should be closely monitored to detect delayed-onset pulmonary edema. The mechanism of pulmonary toxicity is unknown.[43]

Cocaine

Chest pain or dyspnea following cocaine use often represents myocardial ischemia. In some cases, the chest radiograph reveals an alternative explanation for the symptoms, such as a pneumothorax or pneumomediastinum.[28] Noncardiogenic pulmonary edema and diffuse pulmonary hemorrhage can also occur with cocaine use.[44,45] Finally, cocaine use can cause acute aortic dissection or rupture of an aortic aneurysm because of its extreme hypertensive effects.[46,47] In such patients, a chest radiograph often shows an enlarged aortic knob, although a contrast CT or transesophageal echocardiography is needed to confirm the diagnosis.

CNS manifestations of cocaine toxicity include both nonhemorrhagic and hemorrhagic strokes. A headache or seizure following cocaine use may be due to subarachnoid or intraparenchymal hemorrhage from rupture of a preexisting aneurysm or vascular malformation (Fig. 23-20).[48,49]

Abdominal pain following cocaine use can be due to peptic ulcer perforation or mesenteric ischemia.[50,51] Bowel ischemia is primarily a clinical diagnosis, although a plain abdominal film may demonstrate an ileus or, rarely, intramural gas. Abdominal CT can detect intramural edema, hemorrhage, or gas.

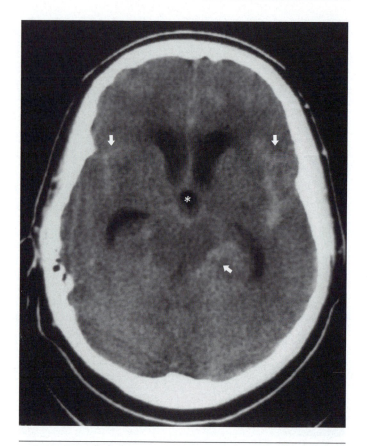

FIGURE 23-20.   Subarachnoid hemorrhage in a patient who smoked "crack" cocaine and developed a severe headache. Hemorrhage can be seen surrounding the brainstem and in the sylvian fissures *(arrows)*. These is communicating hydrocephalus with dilation of the lateral ventricles (frontal and temporal horns) and the third ventricle *(asterisk)*. Cerebral angiography revealed an aneurysm of the anterior communicating artery.

TOXIN AND DRUG-MEDIATED PULMONARY DISEASE

The lung is especially vulnerable to toxin exposure.[52,53] Lung tissue is directly exposed to toxic substances by inhalation or aspiration. Alternatively, toxins can have systemic effects on the lung as the result of direct toxicity on lung tissue or immunologically mediated injury (Table 23-1). Additional factors such as hypoxia, hypotension, respiratory depression, and aspiration of gastric contents due to CNS depression can also cause pulmonary injury.

Many pulmonary pathologic processes are readily detected by conventional radiography because they result in fluid accumulation within the normally air-filled lung. Most toxins are widely distributed throughout the lungs and therefore produce a diffuse or multifocal radiographic abnormality rather than a localized infiltrate. The radiographic appearance is usually not sufficiently distinctive to identify the particular toxin; the clinical circumstances provide the correct diagnosis (e.g., occupational exposure to a toxin). The radiographic findings serve to confirm an exposure, gauge its severity, and estimate prognosis. When a history of exposure is not obtained, the patient may

be misdiagnosed. Pneumonia is a frequent misdiagnosis because infection is considerably more common than toxin-mediated lung damage. In all patients, the physician should consider the possibility of a toxin exposure in the workplace or at home.

There is usually a delay between the time of toxin exposure, the onset of symptoms, and the point where sufficient fluid has accumulated in the lungs to become visible on a radiograph. Therefore, the initial radiograph may not reflect the extent of injury. Furthermore, if the pathologic insult does not cause fluid accumulation, radiographic changes do not develop. The chest radiograph is negative when the toxin exposure causes reactive airways disease or emphysematous parenchymal destruction.

CASE 5.   This elderly patient with prostate cancer presented with fever, confusion, and bilateral airspace filling (Fig. 23-2). His arterial blood gas revealed hypoxia and a mixed metabolic acidosis and respiratory alkalosis. He was admitted to the hospital with a presumptive diagnosis of pneumonia and sepsis. Several hours after admission, he had a generalized seizure. An emergency head CT scan was negative. While in the CT scanner, he began seizing continuously. He was intubated and an

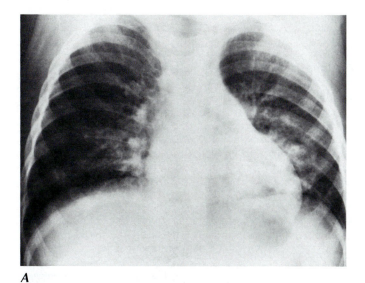

A

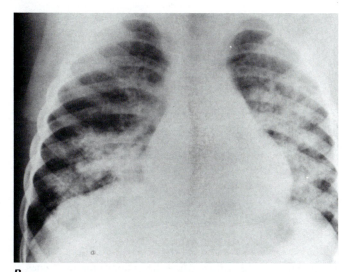

B

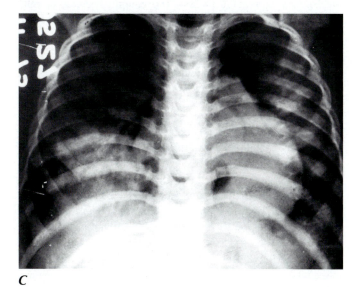

C

TABLE 23-1

Mechanisms of Toxin-Mediated Pulmonary Injury

MECHANISM OF INJURY	EXAMPLES
Inhalation	Irritant gases (low water solubility): silo filler's disease (nitrogen dioxide), allergens (extrinsic allergic alveolitis): farmer's lung (moldy hay), inorganic particulates (pneumoconioses): asbestosis, silicosis
Aspiration	Hydrocarbons (low viscosity, low surface tension): gasoline, kerosene, gastric aspiration (central nervous system depression, seizure)
Systemic toxicity	Medications: chemotheraputic agents (bleomycin), salicylates, illicit drugs: heroin
Immune-mediated	Hypersensitivity pneumonitis Inhaled allergens (extrinsic allergic alveolitis) Medications: nitrofurantoin
Embolization	Particulate injection: talcosis Septic emboli: injection drug use

infusion of phenobarbital was initiated. Soon thereafter he developed ventricular fibrillation and died. A perimortem salicylate level was toxic (74.5 mg/dL). One week earlier he was prescribed salicyl-salicylate, which he had been taking four times daily rather than twice daily as directed. He mistakenly thought it was like aspirin.

The clinical presentation in this patient—pulmonary infiltrates, fever, confusion and a mixed metabolic acidosis–respiratory alkalosis—suggests salicylate intoxication. Not all patients with fever and pulmonary infiltrates have pneumonia.

Inhaled Toxic Gases

Inhaled toxic gases exert their effect by asphyxiation (blocking oxygen delivery to the tissues), by airway irritation and bronchospasm, and by direct cellular injury (Table 23-2). Radiographic abnormalities are seen with low-water-soluble irritant gases such as nitrogen dioxide (silo-filler's disease) and phosgene ($COCl_2$). Low-solubility gases are initially nonirritating, so the victim is unaware of the gas and it is inhaled deeply into

FIGURE 23-21. A young child with severe hydrocarbon aspiration. *A.* The initial film showed patchy densities in the bases of both lungs. *B.* The next day, there were extensive, diffuse alveolar infiltrates. *C.* On day 6, there was dense consolidation of the right lower lobe. (Courtesy of Nancy Geneiser, M.D., Professor of Radiology, New York University. From *Goldfrank's Toxicologic Emergencies,* 6th ed. Appleton & Lange, 1998. With permission.)

TABLE 23-2

Toxic Gases and Fumes

TYPE	EXAMPLES	MECHANISM	RADIOGRAPHIC SIGNS
Simple asphyxiants	Carbon dioxide (CO_2), methane, nitrous oxide (NO), nitrogen, helium	Displace oxygen from inspired air	Normal chest film
Chemical asphyxiants	Carbon monoxide (CO), cyanide (CN), hydrogen sulfide (H_2S), arsine	Prevent oxygen delivery to the cell or use of oxygen by the cell	Normal chest film
Irritant gases (water-soluble)	Ammonia, sulfur dioxide (SO_2), chlorine (intermediate solubility)	Upper airway mucosal irritation	Normal chest film
Irritant gases (water-insoluble)	Nitrogen dioxide (NO_2), phosgene ($COCl_2$)	Pulmonary parenchymal injury	Diffuse airspace filling
Metal fumes	Cadmium, etc.	Fever	Normal chest film Cadmium—delayed pulmonary edema, hemorrhage
CLINICAL SETTINGS			
Farmer	Silo filler (NO_2), farmer's lung (moldy hay—hypersensitivity pneumonitis), H_2S (manure-tank asphyxiation—"dung lung")		
Welder	NO_2, CO_2, CO, O_3 (ozone), phosgene, metal fumes.		
Dwelling fires	CO, CN, SO_2, NO_2, phosgene. Thermal upper airway injury.		

the lung. Within the alveoli, the gas combines with water, producing an acid that causes alveolar damage. Clinical and radiographic findings can be delayed for 4 to 24 h. Noncardiogenic pulmonary edema follows an initial phase of bronchospasm or asphyxiation. If the patient survives, radiographic abnormalities resolve. In some patients, a chronic obstructive airways syndrome *(bronchiolitis obliterans)* develops 3 to 5 weeks after the exposure. With bronchiolitis obliterans, there is plugging of small airways by fibrinous exudate and subsequent organization and fibrosis. The chest radiograph is usually normal but can show a fine nodular interstitial pattern.

Highly water-soluble irritant gases, such as ammonia and sulfur dioxide, cause immediate upper airway irritation that alerts victims to their presence. Pulmonary injury (and radiographic abnormalities) are usually absent unless the exposure is massive or the victim cannot escape, in which case the pulmonary damage is considerable.

Aspiration

The aspiration of liquids causes alveolar damage and intrapulmonary fluid accumulation. Low-viscosity hydrocarbons—which include gasoline, kerosene, turpentine, furniture polish, and pine oil—are often inadvertently aspirated when they are swallowed. The low surface-tension promotes spread along the airways and into the alveoli. The alveolar capillary membrane is damaged and edema fills the airspaces. The infiltrates are lo-

calized to the dependent portions of the lung, usually the lower lobes. If the patient is recumbent at the time of aspiration, the posterior or lateral portions of the lungs are involved. The infiltrates can take several hours to develop; therefore the initial chest film may be normal when the patient initially comes to the ED. Asymptomatic patients (no cough, dyspnea, or rales and negative chest films) should be observed for 6 h. Radiographic resolution of an infiltrate tends to lag behind clinical improvement (Fig. 23-21).[54]

Drugs Causing Pulmonary Disease

A number of medications and illicit drugs cause alveolar and pulmonary endothelial damage (Table 23-3). The radiographic abnormality can be interstitial (reticular or nodular), airspace-filling, or mixed. Mechanisms of injury include direct cellular toxicity, damage due to inflammatory mediators, and hypersensitivity. Various chemotherapeutic agents have direct pulmonary toxicity (busulfan, bleomycin, cyclophosphamide, methotrexate). The onset is insidious and the disease progresses gradually. Symptoms begin several weeks after the start of therapy and are related to the total cumulative dose. Patients develop dyspnea, fever, and pulmonary infiltrates. In addition to drug toxicity, other diagnoses to consider in these patients include opportunistic infection, carcinomatosis, and intrapulmonary hemorrhage. If a medication is suspected of causing pulmonary disease, it is crucial to discontinue the offending medication (Fig. 23-22).

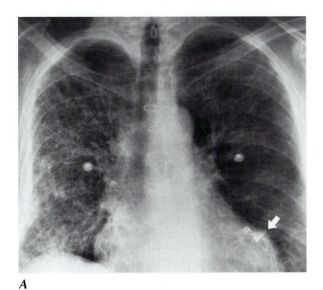
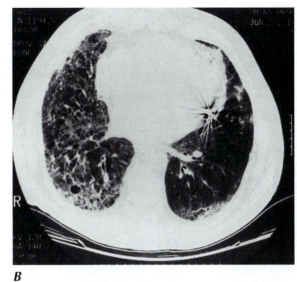

A   *B*

FIGURE 23-22. A patient with a history of malignant ventricular arrhythmias developed shortness of breath. He was being treated with amiodarone and had an implanted automatic defibrillator *(arrow)*. His chest radiograph revealed a reticular interstitial pattern that was initially interpreted as interstitial pulmonary edema *(A)*. The patient's dyspnea did not improve with diuretic medications. A high-resolution CT scan revealed a reticular pattern consistent with amiodarone toxicity *(B)*. His symptoms improved after the medication was stopped. (Courtesy of Georgeann McGuinness, M.D., Department of Radiology, New York University. From *Goldfrank's Toxicologic Emergencies,* 6th ed. Appleton & Lange, 1998. With permission.)

TABLE 23-3

Medications and Drugs Causing Pulmonary Toxicity

DRUG	TOXIC EFFECT	RADIOGRAPHIC FINDINGS
Chemotheraputic agents: bleomycin, busulfan, mitomycin, cyclophosphamide, methotrexate, azanthioprine	Direct cellular toxicity Progressive onset, weeks into the course of therapy Less often, acute or subacute reaction	Interstitial and variable acinar filling infiltrate, fibrosis Distinguish from opportunistic infection in the cancer patient
Nitrofurantoin Less often: sulfonamides, penicillins	Hypersensitivity pneumonitis Occurs within hours in previously sensitized individuals	Diffuse reticular pattern
Amiodarone	Phospholipidosis: accumulation of phospholipids within intracellular organelles	Diffuse reticular and patchy airspace filling Distinguish from congestive heart failure in the cardiac patient
Procainamide, isoniazid, hydralazine, phenytoin	Systemic lupus reaction	Pleural and pericardial effusion
Phenytoin	Pseudolymphoma (hypersensitivity)	Hilar and mediastinal adenopathy
Salicylates (aspirin)	Increased capillary permeability (in overdose) Bronchospasm in sensitive individuals	Noncardiogenic pulmonary edema Normal chest film
Opioids (heroin, etc.)	Increased permeability	Noncardiogenic pulmonary edema
Crack cocaine	Uncertain	Diffuse intrapulmonary hemorrhage or edema

Immunologically Mediated Disorders— Hypersensitivity Pneumonitis

Pulmonary toxicity can be mediated by immediate or delayed immunologic mechanisms. If an inhaled allergen produces immediate hypersensitivity, there is bronchospasm without radiographic abnormalities.

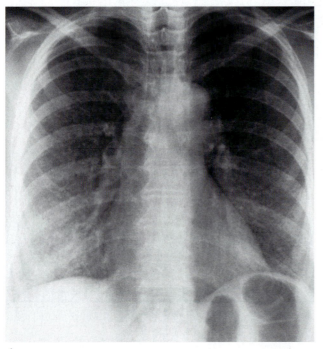

A

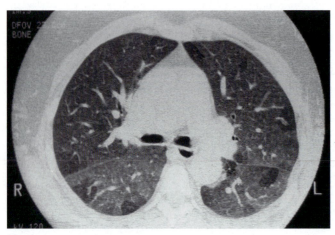

B

FIGURE 23-23. Hypersensitivity pneumonitis—pigeon breeder's lung. This 26-year-old woman presented with a low-grade fever and shortness of breath. Chest auscultation revealed scattered wheezes. *A.* Her chest film showed diffuse fine opacification of both lungs. When questioned, she stated that her brother kept pet pigeons in their backyard. *B.* High-resolution chest CT showed faint "ground-glass" opacification of the airspaces. This is indicative of mild alveolar filling. Air trapping in some peripheral lobules causes less opacification in these regions. Precipitins for avian proteins were markedly elevated. The birds were removed from her home and the patient's symptoms and radiographic findings resolved over several weeks. (Courtesy of Doreen Adrizzo-Harris, M.D., New York University, NY.)

Delayed hypersensitivity to an inhaled toxin, a systemic toxin, or a medication causes *hypersensitivity pneumonitis.* When the allergen is inhaled, hypersensitivity pneumonitis is also known as *extrinsic allergic alveolitis.* Hypersensitivity pneumonitis is caused by sensitization to various organic allergens, e.g., farmer's lung (moldy hay), pigeon breeder's and mushroom handler's disease, and diseases caused by contaminated air filtration systems (Fig. 23-23). Nitrofuration is the medication most often responsible for hypersensitivity pneumonitis.

There are two clinical syndromes of hypersensitivity pneumonitis: an acute recurrent illness and a chronic progressive form. The acute form presents with fever and dyspnea mimicking pneumonia or asthma. The chest radiograph is usually normal although it may show an interstitial pattern or alveolar infiltrate. The diagnosis depends on the history of exposure to an allergen. Typically, symptoms abate when the patient is away from the workplace, and symptoms return with reexposure. With the chronic form of hypersensitivity pneumonitis, the patient has persistent dyspnea, and there is an interstitial pattern on the chest film.

Pneumoconiosis

Inhalation of inorganic particulate matter, usually in an occupational setting, causes chronic interstitial lung disease known as *pneumoconiosis.* The most common offending agents are asbestos, silica, and coal dust. The radiographic abnormality is a linear, nodular, or mixed interstitial pattern. The nodular pattern is the most common.

Pleural disease, particularly calcified pleural plaques, is also associated with asbestos exposure. It develops over many years and can occur even when the exposure was in the distant past. Asbestos-related pleural plaques are generally benign and have only a minor association with malignancy and interstitial lung disease. The pleural plaques should not be called *asbestosis* because that term refers specifically to the interstitial lung disease (Fig. 23-24).

NEUROIMAGING OF THE POISONED PATIENT

The most common neurologic disturbance in the poisoned patient is an alteration in consciousness, causing a depressed level of consciousness, delirium, or confusion. Other neurologic manifestations include seizures, headache, and focal neurologic deficits. In most toxicologic emergencies, there is no radiographically detectable abnormality and an emergency head CT is not indicated. The time and effort involved in obtaining a CT diverts the caregiver from providing therapeutic interventions (see Case 5—salicylate overdose causing seizure). However, in certain toxicologic cases, an emergency head CT is important.[55]

The presence of a focal neurologic deficit is the strongest indication for obtaining a CT scan. The cranial lesion may be a hemorrhage, infarct, tumor, or abscess. However, a focal neurologic deficit can also occur in certain metabolic disturbances, most importantly hypoglycemia. Therefore, a low blood sugar must be excluded in all patients presenting with an apparent "stroke."

Even in the absence of a focal neurologic deficit, a cerebral mass lesion may be present. Mass lesions that do not cause focal neurologic deficits include extraaxial lesions (subdural hematoma, subarachnoid hemorrhage), mass lesions in "silent" areas of the brain, and mass lesions in the frontal lobes that cause

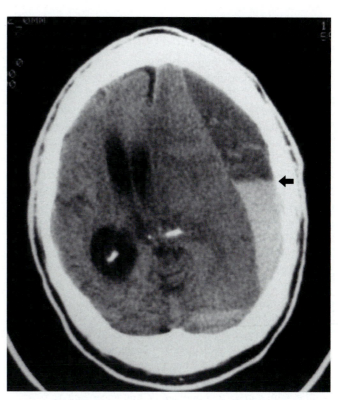

FIGURE 23-25. A subacute subdural hematoma in an alcoholic patient following an alcohol binge. The patient's mental status did not improve during several hours of observation. There were no external signs of head trauma and no focal neurological deficits. A crescent-shaped blood collection is seen between the right cerebral convexity and the inner table of the skull causing compression of the right lateral ventricle. There is a layering "hematocrit" effect in which the more radiopaque heme elements have settled to the inferior level of the hematoma. Alternatively, this finding may represent an acute hemorrhage within a chronic subdural hematoma.

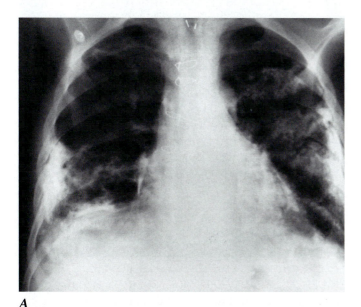

A

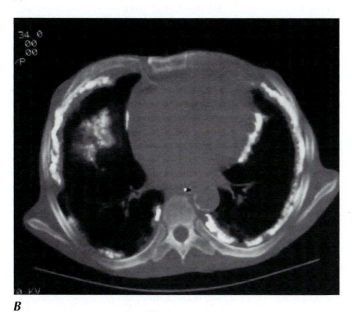

B

FIGURE 23-24. *A.* Calcified pleural plaques typical of asbestos exposure are seen surrounding the lung and on the surface of the diaphragm and heart. The patient was asymptomatic; this was an incidental radiographic finding. *B.* A lower thoracic CT image shows calcified pleural plaques (the diaphragmatic plaque is seen on the right) as well as the absence of any pleural-based tumor or interstitial lung disease ("asbestosis"). (From Schwartz DT: Toxicologic imaging, in Goldfrank LR (ed): *Goldfrank's Toxicologic Emergencies,* 6th ed. Norwalk, CT: Appleton & Lange, 1998. With permission.)

behavioral changes without focality. Therefore, a head CT should be obtained in a patient with altered mental status who does not have a focal neurologic deficit if (1) the cause of the altered consciousness is unexplained by a metabolic toxicologic or disturbance, (2) if there is failure to improve after a period of observation, or (3) if the patient is at high risk for an intracranial mass lesion. Patients at increased risk for mass lesions include the elderly, alcoholics, users of illicit drugs, and patients with AIDS.

Alcoholics are at increased risk for subdural hematoma, as are the elderly and patients on anticoagulants. All of these patients can bleed after minimal trauma (Fig. 23-25). Factors contributing to this risk are a high frequency of falls, cerebral atrophy (stretching the bridging dural veins), coagulopathy, and thrombocytopenia.

Cocaine users are at risk for subarachnoid hemorrhage, intracerebral bleeding, and cerebral infarction. The patient presents with a headache, seizure, or altered mentation (Fig. 23-20). Patients who inject drugs intravenously are also at high risk for intracerebral lesions. These include septic emboli and, if the patient is HIV-infected, AIDS-related toxoplasmosis and CNS lymphoma. These lesions are best demonstrated with a contrast CT. All show a ring pattern of enhancement (Fig. 23-14).

Toxin-Mediated Brain Damage

Ethanol is the most frequently encountered neurotoxin, and chronic ethanol consumption is associated with generalized loss of brain tissue.[56–58] However, the extent of cerebral atrophy seen on CT does not correlate closely with the patient's clinical status (dementia or cerebellar dysfunction). Similar CT findings of cerebral atrophy occur with chronic inhalant abuse (e.g., toluene).[59–61]

Some toxins cause acute brain damage and produce characteristic lesions detectable on CT and MRI. An important example is *carbon monoxide* poisoning. CT scans in patients with neurologic dysfunction following carbon monoxide exposure show symmetrical lucencies in the basal ganglia, particularly the globus pallidus.[62–64] This region is especially sensitive to hypoxic-ischemic damage because of its poorly anastomotic blood supply and its high metabolic requirements. Brain injury following carbon monoxide poisoning is caused by the direct toxic effect of carbon monoxide binding to neuronal cytochrome oxidase, as well as by hypoxia, hypoperfusion, and acidosis. Although basal ganglion lucencies are characteristic of carbon monoxide poisoning, they also occur with poisoning by cyanide, methanol, hydrogen sulfide, and barbiturates as well as with anoxia, hypoglycemia, and encephalitis.[59,65]

Despite initial reports, bilateral lucent lesions of the globus pallidus have only limited correlation to the patient's clinical prognosis.[66–68] Better prognostic correlation has been noted with lesions of the subcortical and periventricular white matter. These regions are also susceptible to injury from hypoxia and hypoperfusion. Patients with neurologic manifestations of carbon monoxide poisoning and normal CT scans have a better prognosis that those with CT abnormalities.

MRI is more sensitive than CT at detecting lesions due to carbon monoxide poisoning.[69,70] The white matter lesions detected on MRI correlate with poor long-term outcome. However, in some patients, white matter lesions improve with time, and this correlates with their clinical improvement. Reversible white matter lesions represent demyelinization with axon preservation rather than irreversible necrosis.

Neuroimaging (CT and MRI) has been used in other causes of toxin-mediated neurologic degeneration. These include methanol, ethanol, ethylene glycol, cyanide, hydrogen sulfide, inorganic and organic mercury, and solvents such as toluene (occupational and illicit use).[65,71–74]

CASE 6.   The CT scan in this obtunded, alcoholic patient was obtained because a subdural hematoma was suspected. Instead, the scan revealed bilateral lucencies in the basal ganglia (Fig. 23-26). Because of the CT findings, a carboxyhemoglobin level was ordered, which was 34%. Further investigation showed that the ventilation in the restaurant below the patient's apartment was faulty, causing carbon monoxide to accumulate in the patient's apartment. Interestingly, a restaurant worker had been hospitalized the day before for syncope. Carbon monoxide poisoning had also caused this second patient's illness.

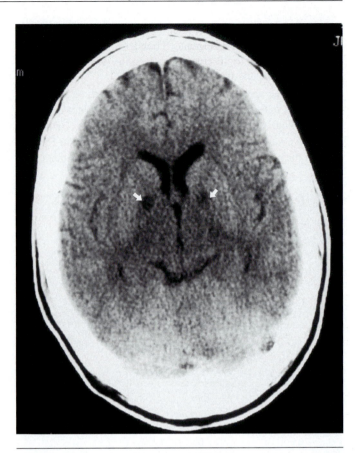

FIGURE 23-26.   Case 6. Bilateral lucencies in the basal ganglia *(arrows).*

ACKNOWLEDGMENTS

Thanks to Dr. Lewis R. Goldfrank for his many helpful suggestions, to the New York City Poison Control Center, Fellowship Training Program in Toxicology, and to Dr. Goldfrank and Appleton & Lange publishers for permission to use material from *Goldfrank's Toxicologic Emergencies.*

REFERENCES

1. American College of Emergency Physicians: Clinical policy for the initial approach to patients presenting with acute toxic ingestion or dermal or inhalation exposure. *Ann Emerg Med* 25:570, 1995.
2. Handy CA: Radiopacity of oral nonliquid medications. *Radiology* 98:525, 1971.
3. Savitt DL, Hawkins HH, Roberts JR: The radiopacity of ingested medications. *Ann Emerg Med* 16:331, 1987.
4. O'Brien RP, McGeehan PA, Helmeczi AW, Dula DJ: Detectability of drug tablets and capsules by plain radiography. *Am J Emerg Med* 4:302, 1986.
5. Tillman DJ, Ruggles DL, Leiken JB: Radiopacity study of extended-release formulations using digitized radiography. *Am J Emerg Med* 12:310, 1994.
6. Staple TW, McAlister WH: Roentgenographic visualization of iron preparations in the gastrointestinal tract. *Radiology* 83:1051, 1964.

7. Everson GW, Oudjhane K, Young LW, Krenzelok EP: Effectiveness of abdominal radiographs in visualizing chewable iron supplements following overdose. *Am J Emerg Med* 7:459, 1989.

8. Everson GW. Bertaccini EJ, O'Leary J: Use of whole bowel irrigation in an infant following iron overdose. *Am J Emerg Med* 9:366, 1991.

9. Foxford R, Goldfrank L: Gastrotomy—A surgical approach to iron overdose. *Ann Emerg Med* 14:1223, 1985.

10. Lee DC, Roberts JR, Kelly JJ, Fishman SM: Whole-bowel irrigation as an adjunct in the treatment of radiopaque arsenic (letter). *Am J Emerg Med* 13:244, 1995.

11. Roberge RJ, Martin TG: Whole bowel irrigation in an acute oral lead intoxication. *Am J Emerg Med* 10:577, 1992.

12. Celli B, Khan MA: Mercury embolism of the lung. *N Engl J Med* 295:883, 1976.

13. Chitkara R, Seriff NS, Kinas HY: Intravenous self-administration of metallic mercury in attempted suicide: Report of a case with serial roentgenographic and physiologic studies over an 18-month period. *Chest* 73:234, 1978.

14. Hohage H, Otte B, Westermann G, et al: Elemental mercurial poisoning. *South Med J* 90:1033, 1997.

15. Meggs WJ, Hoffman RS, Shih RD, et al: Thallium poisoning from maliciously contaminated food. *J Toxicol Clin Toxicol* 32:723, 1994.

16. Switz DM, Elmorshidy ME, Deyerle WM: Bullets, joints and lead intoxication. A remarkable and instructive case. *Arch Intern Med* 136:939, 1976.

17. Dillman RO, Crumb CK, Lidsky MJ: Lead poisoning from a gunshot wound. *Am J Med* 66:509, 1979.

18. Farber JM, Rafii M, Schwartz D: Lead arthropathy and elevated serum lead levels after a gunshot wound of the shoulder. *AJR* 162:385, 1994.

19. McElvaine MD, DeUngria EG, Mattte TD, et al: Prevalence of radiographic evidence of paint chip ingestion among children with moderate to severe lead poisoning, St. Louis, Missouri, 1989 through 1990. *Pediatrics* 89:740, 1992.

20. Kulshrestha MK: Lead poisoning diagnosed by abdominal x-rays. *J Toxicol Clin Toxicol* 34:107, 1996.

21. Blickman JG, Wilkinson RG. Graef JW: The radiologic "lead band" revisited. *AJR* 146:245, 1986.

22. Woolf DA, Riach CF, Derweesh A, Vyas H: Lead lines in young infants with acute lead encephalopathy: A reliable diagnostic test. *J Trop Pediatr* 36:90, 1990.

23. Resnick D: Heavy metal poisoning, in Resnick D, Niwayama G (eds): *Diagnosis of Bone and Joint Disorders,* 2d ed. Philadelphia: Saunders, 1988:3102–3114.

24. Edeiken J, Dalinka M. Karasick D (eds): Osseous manifestations of metal poisoning, in *Edeiken's Roentgen Diagnosis of Diseases of Bone,* 4th ed. Baltimore: Williams & Wilkins, 1990:1401–1406.

25. Heffner JE, Harley RA, Schabel SI: Pulmonary reactions from illicit substance abuse. *Clin Chest Med* 11:151, 1990.

26. Douglass RE, Levison MA: Pneumothorax in drug abusers: An urban epidemic? *Am Surg* 52:377, 1986.

27. Feigen DS: Talc: Understanding its manifestations in the chest. *AJR* 146:295–201, 1986.

28. Eurman DW, Potash HI, Eyler WR, et al: Chest pain and dyspnea related to "crack" cocaine smoking: Value of chest radiography. *Radiology* 172:459, 1989.

29. Panache EA, Singer AJ, et al: Spontaneous pneumomediastinum: Clinical and natural history. *Ann Emerg Med* 21:1222, 1992.

30. Smith BA, Ferguson DB: Disposition of spontaneous pneumomediastinum. *Am J Emerg Med* 9:256, 1991.

31. Roberts JR, Price D, Goldfrank L, Hartnett L: The bodystuffer syndrome: A clandestine form of drug overdose. *Am J Emerg Med* 4:24, 1986.

32. McCarron MM, Wood JD: The cocaine "body packer" syndrome. *JAMA* 250:1417, 1983.

33. Sporer KA, Firestone J: Clinical course of crack cocaine body stuffers. *Ann Emerg Med* 29:596, 1997.

34. Keys N, Wahl M, Aks S, et al: Cocaine body stuffers: A case series (abstr). *J Toxicol Clin Toxicol* 33:517, 1995.

35. Harchelroad F: Identification of orally ingested cocaine by CT scan. *Vet Hum Toxicol* 34:350, 1992.

36. Hoffman RS, Chiang WK, Weisman RS, Goldfrank LR: Prospective evaluation of "crack-vial" ingestion. *Vet Hum Toxicol* 32:164, 1990.

37. Pollack CV, Biggers DW, Carlton FB, et al: Two crack cocaine body stuffers. *Ann Emerg Med* 21:1370, 1992.

38. Cranston PE, Pollack CV, Harrison RB: CT of crack cocaine ingestion. *J Comput Assist Tomogr* 16:560, 1992.

39. Horrocks AW: Abdominal radiography in suspected "body packers." *Clin Radiol* 45:322, 1992. (Comment, 47:219, 1993.)

40. Beerman R, Nunez D, Wetli C: Radiographic evaluation of the cocaine smuggler. *Gastrointest Radiol* 11:351, 1986.

41. Balthazar EJ, Lefleur R: Abdominal complications of drug addiction: Radiologic features. *Semin Roentgenol* 18:213, 1983.

42. Hoffman RS, Smilkstein MJ, Goldfrank LR: Whole bowel irrigation and the cocaine body-packer. *Am J Emerg Med* 8:523, 1990.

43. Smith DA, Leake L, Loflin JR, Yealy DM: Is admission after intravenous heroin overdose necessary? *Ann Emerg Med* 21:1326, 1992.

44. Forrester JM, Steele AW, Waldron JA, Parsens PE: Crack lung: An acute pulmonary syndrome with a spectrum of clinical and histopathological findings. *Am Rev Respir Dis* 142:462, 1990.

45. Hoffman CK, Goodman PC: Pulmonary edema in cocaine smokers. *Radiology* 172:463, 1989.

46. Gadaleta D, Hall MH, Nelson RL: Cocaine–induced acute aortic dissection. *Chest* 96:1203, 1989.

47. Rashid J, Eisenberg MJ, Topol EJ: Cocaine-induced aortic dissection. *Am Heart J* 132:1301, 1996.

48. Levine SR, Brust JCM, Futrell N, et al: Cerebrovascular complications of the use of the "crack" form of alkaloidal cocaine. *N Engl J Med* 323:699, 1990.

49. Landi JL, Spickler EM: Imaging of intracranial hemorrhage associated with drug abuse. *Neuroimag Clin North Am* 2:187, 1992.

50. Cheng CL, Svesko V: Acute pyloric perforation after prolonged crack smoking. *Ann Emerg Med* 23:126, 1994.

51. Kram HB, Hardin E, Clark SR, Shoemaker WC: Perforated ulcers related to smoking "crack" cocaine. *Am Surg* 58:293, 1992.

52. Aronchick JM, Gefter WB: Drug-induced pulmonary disorders. *Semin Roentgenol* 30:18, 1995.

53. Miller WT: Pleural and mediastinal disorders related to drug use. *Semin Roentgenol* 30:35, 1995.

54. Anas N, Namasonthi V, Ginsberg CM: Criteria for hospitalizing children who have ingested products containing hydrocarbons. *JAMA* 246:840, 1981.

55. Lexa FJ: Drug-induced disorders of the central nervous system. *Semin Roentgenol* 30:7, 1995.

56. Hillbom M, Muuronen A, Holm L, Hindmarsh T: The clinical versus radiological diagnosis of alcoholic cerebellar degeneration. *J Neurol Sci* 73:45, 1986.

57. Gilman S, Adams K, Koeppe RA, et al: Cerebellar and frontal hypometabolism in alcoholic cerebellar degeneration studied with positron emission tomography. *Ann Neurol* 28:775, 1990.

58. Wang GJ, Volkow ND, Roque CT, et al: Functional importance of ventricular enlargement and cortical atrophy in healthy subjects and alcoholics as assessed with PET, MR imaging, and neuropsychologic testing. *Radiology* 186:59, 1993.

59. Nelson DL, Batnitzky S, McMillan JH, et al: The CT and MRI features of acute toxic encephalopathies. *AJNR* 8:951, 1987.

60. Hormes JT, Filley CM, Rosenberg NL: Neurologic sequelae of chronic solvent vapor abuse. *Neurology* 36:698, 1986.

61. Rosenberg NL, Kleinschmidt-DeMasters BK, Davis KA, et al: Toluene abuse causes diffuse central nervous system white matter changes. *Ann Neurol* 23:611, 1988.

62. Jones JS, Lagasse J, Zimmerman G: Computed tomographic findings after acute carbon monoxide poisoning. *Am J Emerg Med* 12:448, 1994.

63. Piatt JP, Kaplan AM, Bond RO, Berg RA: Occult carbon monoxide poisoning in an infant. *Pediatr Emerg Care* 6:21, 1990.

64. Pracyk JB, Stolp BW, Fife CE, et al: Brain computerized tomography after hyperbaric oxygen therapy for carbon monoxide poisoning. *Undersea Hyperb Med* 22:1, 1995.

65. Ho VB, Fitz CR, Chuang SH, Geyer CA: Bilateral basal ganglia lesions: Pediatric differential considerations. *Radiographics* 13:269, 1993.

66. Sawada Y, Takahashi M, Ohashi N, et al: Computerized tomography as an indication of long-term outcome after acute carbon monoxide poisoning. *Lancet* 1(8172):783, 1980.

67. Miura T, Mitomo M, Kawi R, Harada K: CT of the brain in acute carbon monoxide intoxication: Characteristic features and prognosis. *AJNR* 6:739, 1985.

68. Vieregge P, Klostermann W, Blumm RG. Borgis KJ: Carbon monoxide poisoning: Clinical, neurophysiological, and brain imaging observations in acute disease and follow-up. *J Neurol* 236:478, 1989.

69. Chang KH, Han MH, Kim HS, et al: Delayed encephalopathy after acute carbon monoxide intoxication: MR imaging features and distribution of cerebral white matter lesions. *Radiology* 184:117, 1992.

70. Horowitz AL, Kaplan R, Sarpel O: Carbon monoxide toxicity: MR imaging in the brain. *Radiology* 162:787, 1987.

71. Finelli PF: Changes in the basal ganglia following cyanide poisoning. *J Comput Assist Tomogr* 5:755, 1981.

72. Aquilonius SM. Bergstrom K, Enoksson P, et al: Cerebral computed tomography in methanol intoxication. *J Comput Assist Tomogr* 4:425, 1980.

73. Hantson P, Duprez T, Mahieu P: Neurotoxicity to the basal ganglia shown by magnetic resonance imaging (MRI) following poisoning by methanol and other substances. *J Toxicol Clin Toxicol* 35:151, 1997.

74. Tumeh SS, Nagel JS, English RJ, et al: Cerebral abnormalities in cocaine abusers: Demonstration by SPECT perfusion brain scintigraphy. *Radiology* 176:821, 1990.

SUGGESTED READINGS

Ansell G: *Radiology of Adverse Reactions to Drugs and Toxic Hazards.* Rockville, MD: Aspen Publishers, 1985.

Dee P: Drug and radiation induced lung disease, in Armstrong P, Wilson AG, Dee P, Hansell DM (eds): *Imaging of Diseases of the Chest,* 2d ed. St. Louis: Mosby–Year Book, 1995:461–483.

Fulkerson WJ, Gockerman JP: Pulmonary disease induced by drugs, in Fishman AP (ed): *Pulmonary Diseases and Disorders,* 2d ed. New York: McGraw-Hill, 1988:793–811.

Goldfrank LR, Flomenbaum NE, Lewin NA, Weisman RS, Howland MA, Hoffman RS (eds): *Goldfrank's Toxicologic Emergencies,* 6th ed. Stamford, CT: Appleton & Lange, 1998. (Schwartz DT: Toxicologic imaging, pp. 77–103)

Warach SJ, Charness ME: Imaging the brain lesions of alcoholics, in Greenberg JO (ed): *Neuroimaging: A Companion to Adams and Victor's Principles of Neurology.* New York: McGraw-Hill, 1995:503–515.

CHAPTER 24

QUALITY IMPROVEMENT IN EMERGENCY RADIOLOGY

CORINNA REPETTO / DAVID T. OVERTON

Techniques for studying health care quality were first developed by manufacturing industries in order to improve productivity and product quality.[1,2] Given the increasing regulatory oversight of health care, the need to contain costs, and the need to maintain and improve quality, the health care industry has adopted similar methodologies.[3]

Neither payers nor society continue to base their decisions solely on the individual practitioner-patient relationship. When dealing with the quality and the cost of health care delivery, physicians are accountable to society as a whole, not just to individual patients.[2] Consequently, physician cost trending and cost profiling[4,5] derived from quality-based research[6] are having a growing impact on medical practice.

Unfortunately, perfection is an elusive and ultimately unattainable goal. Quality can be improved upon but never absolutely guaranteed,[7] which is a difficult concept for a society that has minimal tolerance for errors in health care.

Various medical practice quality techniques, such as quality assurance (QA) and continuous quality improvement (CQI), differ in philosophy and approach. QA methodology traditionally emphasized problem identification and has been viewed by some as a negatively enforced system.[7,8] Under QA, performance standards are established and compliance of individuals with these standards is evaluated.[9] In contrast, CQI attempts to study and improve underlying system processes, deemphasizing individual error.[8] Therefore, when human error does occur, the process rather than the individual is evaluated.[6,7] The focus of CQI is to improve *all* care, not just bad care. In theory, CQI leads to a continuous improvement in patient care.

In the field of emergency radiology, most of the quality literature is discussed in terms of QA rather than CQI. While acknowledging the important underlying differences, in this chapter all such quality management programs will be referred to as *quality improvement* or *QI*.

The radiology services provided in the emergency department (ED) are subject to the same quality scrutiny as any other ED service. In fact, the quality of emergency radiology services has probably received more attention in the medical literature than most other aspects of emergency medicine QI.

QI in emergency radiology is multifaceted. It is necessary to consider the following: (1) the appropriateness of radiograph ordering[10]; (2) the accuracy of radiograph interpretation; (3) the appropriateness and timeliness of follow-up; and (4) patient outcome and satisfaction. In addition, questions about reimbursement may influence these quality considerations.

APPROPRIATENESS OF RADIOGRAPH ORDERING

Utilization Review

Both health insurance and consumer groups have become more selective in the allocation of health care dollars. Increasingly, physicians must prove that they are delivering quality care in a cost-effective manner.[11] In an attempt to contain radiology costs, the emphasis is often on minimizing such expensive procedures as computed tomography (CT) and magnetic resonance imaging (MRI).

However, less expensive, higher-volume services may actually contribute more to the cost of medical care.[12] For instance, almost half of all emergency patients have at least one radiologic study per visit.[13,14] It is estimated that over $1 billion is spent annually on knee radiographs in the United States and Canada.[15] Using guidelines for knee radiographs with a sensitivity of 100% and a specificity of 54% could reduce radiograph use by 28%.[16] This would save $280 million yearly. Thus, the more efficient use of seemingly mundane, low-cost studies can yield tremendous savings, in patient changes as well as in staff and patient time.

Reasons for Overuse

There are a number of reasons why emergency radiology services are overused. One is clinician ignorance of the limitations of a given radiologic study to detect a certain pathologic condition. This is not surprising, as utilization issues have rarely been emphasized in medical education. To the contrary, teaching settings have traditionally rewarded clinicians who performed the most "careful" (meaning exhaustive) patient evaluations.

Another commonly cited reason is defensive medicine, where clinicians may overorder tests to make sure that even a profoundly unlikely disease will be either detected or ruled out. Clinicians may also rationalize that when a battery of tests is performed, patient care will be more legally defensible in the event of an untoward outcome.

Finally, patients commonly present for medical care with the expectation that radiographs will be performed. These expectations are compounded by the patient's perception that he or she is not financially responsible for a particular test, leading to little sympathy for cost-containment practices. Customer dissatisfaction can be defined as "unmet expectations,"[16] perhaps heightened by a lack of trust in the single ED encounter setting. Particularly adroit interpersonal skills are required to maintain patient satisfaction while avoiding unnecessary radiographic testing in this setting.

Clinical Guidelines

Clinical guidelines attempt to unify physicians' approaches to clinical problem solving. Although clinical guidelines can aid in cost containment, some fear that they undermine physicians' clinical judgment, leading to "cookbook medicine"[17,18] and loss of physician autonomy.[18,19] Ideally, guidelines should assist physicians in clinical decision-making.[18] Indeed, physicians constantly formulate their own internal, informal clinical guidelines, based on anecdotal experience, and apply them to clinical decision making. The development of formal, properly researched guidelines could substantially improve upon this process.

The ideal guideline is both easy to use and highly sensitive (sensitivity close to 1.0), leading to an outcome comparable to or higher than that of common clinical practice without the guideline.[16]

Examples of Improved Utilization

Among the examples of clinical guidelines are the Ottawa rules for ankle radiograph selection, which have a reported sensitivity of 1.0 for the detection of malleolar and midfoot fractures.[20–23,23a] Implementation of these rules did not change patient satisfaction with the ED care, yet it decreased patient visit times and reduced total medical costs.[22]

More recent studies have looked at the clinical criteria for knee radiographs.[24] Stiell et al. identified five parameters in the setting of acute knee injury that reached a sensitivity of 100% and a specificity of 54%. Implementation of these guidelines would have reduced radiograph use by 28%.[16]

The utility of several other emergency radiologic studies has been scrutinized and their use in certain circumstances has been questioned. These studies include skull radiographs and head CTs[25–31] as well as radiographs of the abdomen[32–37] ribs,[38,39] nasal bones,[40–42] lumbar spine,[43–45] cervical spine,[46–52] and knee.[16,24,53–56] For instance, abdominal radiographs show a low overall diagnostic yield, yet they may be useful in evaluating bowel obstruction[34] and in the localization of foreign bodies. Nasal and rib films may reveal fractures but generally do not alter treatment.

Although cervical fractures can be excluded in patients without altered level of consciousness, intoxication, neck tenderness, or distracting painful injuries elsewhere,[47] emergency physicians take a liberal approach when ordering such radiographs. Because of the high morbidity and litigation rates associated with the misdiagnosis of cervical fractures, the development of guidelines has been hindered and they have been less readily accepted by the medical community.

ACCURACY OF RADIOGRAPH INTERPRETATION

Emergency Overread Systems

Appropriate procedures must be established and followed to ensure that the most accurate interpretation of radiographic studies guides patient care. In most hospitals, radiologists are the physicians credentialed to render final interpretations of radiographs. A variety of different procedural systems ensure that the radiologist's interpretation guides care.

One common procedure is as follows. A radiographic study is ordered by the emergency physician, who records the clinical indication on a film requisition. Upon completion of the study, the films are returned to the emergency physician, who renders an immediate, preliminary interpretation. This interpretation is recorded on a form that goes into the film jacket with the films. The emergency physician then treats the patient based on this interpretation. The films, together with the requisition and the emergency physician's preliminary interpretation are reviewed ("overread") by a radiologist some time later (hours to days). The radiologist renders a "final" interpretation, and notes any discrepancy between this and the emergency physician's interpretation. If a discrepancy exists, the ED is notified. ED personnel assess the significance of the discrepancy and take any action necessary, such as calling the patient back to the ED or notifying the patient's personal physician. A permanent record of the discrepancy and the action taken is kept.

Many variations on this process may exist. The individual variations are not as important as the fact that a reliable procedure is established and is consistently followed. For instance, many EDs have standing orders by which nonphysician personnel such as nurses, physician assistants, or nurse practitioners may order certain radiographs. Sometimes, emergency and the physicians and other busy clinicians neglect to record the clinical history and the indications for the study. However, diagnostic accuracy improves when a clinical history is provided.[57–60] Ideally, the emergency physician should document these indications rather than defer this task to others.

In some institutions, ED studies are immediately interpreted, either some or all of the time, by radiologists or radiology residents. In academic centers, 66% of EDs have a radiology resident in house overnight, and 8% of all films are read immediately by radiologists.[61] In such circumstances, a written report rather than the actual films may be all that is routinely returned to the ED and available to the emergency physician. If this immediate radiologist interpretation is also the final one, no reconciliation is necessary. However, if the preliminary interpretation is by a radiology resident, an overread by the attending radiologist is still needed and a reconciliation mechanism must be in place.

In many settings, studies such as CT scans and ultrasounds are immediately interpreted by a radiologist, regardless of the time of day. Even in this setting, however, films may still be subject to overreading. For example, an on-call radiologist may render a "preliminary" interpretation, perhaps via teleradiology, that is later overread by another radiologist. In this circumstance, a reconciliation mechanism between the preliminary and final interpretations must be in place.

In addition, many ED physicians have the option, either part or all of the time, to request an immediate radiologist interpretation of a questionable film, even if such films are routinely preliminarily interpreted by the ED physician. A recent study reported an 11% rate of request for radiologist consultation by ED physicians.[62]

In some EDs, the emergency physician's interpretation is not recorded (or is recorded inconsistently), so that all final radiographic interpretations are returned to the ED. In this situation, ED staff must review all interpretations and charts to detect any discrepancies. This process can even be applied when an attending radiologist reviews the interpretations of a radiology resident.

The manner in which the ED is notified of potential discrepancies may also vary. Some hospitals use the same form on which the emergency physicians record their interpretation to note the discrepancy, a copy of which is returned to the ED. This same form may also be used to indicate the action taken to remedy the discrepancy and then placed in the patient's permanent medical record. An exception may occur for a potentially dangerous discrepancy, in which case the radiologist will notify the ED by phone immediately and then follow up in writing. In other hospitals, the radiologists verbally notify the ED by phone of *any* discrepancy. Despite these wide variations in practice, the individual variations are not as important as the fact that a reliable procedure is established and consistently followed.

Emergency Physician Interpretation Variability

A number of studies have examined discrepancy rates between emergency physicians and radiologists in interpreting emergency radiographs. However, these studies use a variety of different methods and definitions that make direct comparison difficult.

In order to determine if a reported discrepancy leads to inappropriate treatment, one must find out whether the discrepancy is clinically significant. "Clinical significance" is inconsistently defined and may vary from the simple need to advise the patient of the findings[63] to the existence of an actual adverse outcome resulting directly from the misinterpretation. One way to define clinical significance is to include all discrepancies that lead to a change in either immediate patient management or prescribed follow-up.[64] For example, although the discovery of an incidental coin lesion on a chest film might not alter acute treatment in the ED, it may change the follow-up and long-term care. Thus it would be considered clinically significant.

One study noted an overall discrepancy rate of 6.4% between emergency physicians and radiologists.[65] Similar rates were reported by Seltzer et al. (6.3%).[66] Most (4.6%) of these errors were underreads (false negatives).[65] In a rural setting where all initial films were read by family practitioners and physician assistants, McLain and Kirkwood[67] reported that interpretative disagreement occurred 9.2% of the time. However, case management and disposition was inappropriate in less than 1%.

When comparing interpretations between radiologists and radiology residents, Rhea et al. reported a discrepancy of 6.2%.[68] In comparing interpretations by house officers who were not radiologists, studies by Gratton et al. and Mayhue et al. found no difference in misinterpretation between resident levels.[63,69]

Overall, reported clinically significant misinterpretation rates for emergency physicians are quite low, ranging from 0.06 to 3.1%.[63,64,67,70–72] In view of such low numbers, radiology interpretation discrepancy rates may be a poor measure of quality in emergency radiology. Misinterpretations might be more important in determining trends and designing educational programs.[63,73]

Radiologist Interpretation Variability

Reported discrepancy rates between different radiologists tend to be higher than those between emergency physicians and radiologists. For instance, 30 to 41% of chest radiograph interpretations are reported to contain significant or potentially significant errors.[74–76] The figure for discordant interpretations between different radiologists was 27% for pediatric ED films.[77] Radiologists agree completely in only 50% of mammogram interpretations, leading to a 65 to 91% variability in recommendation for breast biopsy.[78]

Similarly, MRI (brain, spine, lower extremity) discordance among radiologists is reported to have affected treatment in 22% of cases.[79] Most discrepancies were noted in MRIs of the lower extremity. However, brain MRIs showed a clinically significant misinterpretation rate of 4%. An additional 20% of studies were noted to have inappropriate reports that did not affect patient treatment.[79]

Many discrepancies cited when comparing radiologists involve fine points of limited clinical importance, like "borderline cardiomegaly" or "questionable osteopenia." In contrast, most studies involving emergency physicians report discrepancies related to clinical care or diagnosis. For instance, if an elderly patient has fallen and sustained a hip fracture, an emergency physician might report "fractured right hip" and not comment upon osteopenia and phleboliths. Few radiologists would go to the trouble of sending an overread back to the ED for such findings. However, a radiologist overreading such an interpretation by a fellow radiologist might feel that the osteopenia and phleboliths should have been noted.

Thus, discrepancy rates are difficult to compare between different groups and different studies. Although it is necessary to have systems in place ensuring that the best possible radiograph interpretation is used to guide patient care, raw discrepancy rates are difficult to interpret.

Commonly Misread Films

Surprisingly, there is little consistency in the literature concerning which emergency studies have the highest misinterpretation rates. One study of orthopedic injuries found that the most commonly missed fractures included those of the carpals (scaphoid), elbow, and foot (calcaneus).[73] Among all emergency radiographs, chest films show the highest discordance rates between radiologists and ED physicians.[62,80] In one study, abdominal radiographs showed a clinically significant discrepancy rate in 4.1% of cases.[81] In trauma films, Chan and Ainscow found that fractures of the ankle, knee, and hip were the most commonly missed.[82]

In pediatric extremity radiographs, fractures of the hand, foot (especially phalanges), and elbow, were the most commonly missed.[73,83,84] ED pediatricians most often failed to identify subtle fractures such as epiphyseal, buckle, or avulsion fractures. These pediatricians also frequently overlooked findings such as lead lines in traumatized extremities, opacified sinuses, or prematurely closed skull sutures.[85] Walsh-Kelly et al., in a study of pediatric chest radiographs, reported a misinterpretation rate of 16%, although only 0.8% were regarded as clinically significant.[77]

High-Risk Misread Films

Certain kinds of radiographs, such as those of the cervical spine, are particularly dangerous if misinterpreted. Of cervical spine fractures, 3.9 to 6.7% are missed on initial ED interpretation.[49,63]

Similarly, many institutions rely on emergency physicians for the initial interpretation of head CTs. There is a 38.7% discrepancy rate between emergency physicians and radiologists in interpreting head CTs, with 11.4% potentially clinically significant errors of omission by ED physicians.[72] The most commonly missed diagnosis was cerebral infarction, followed by intracranial mass. However, only 0.6% were mismanaged, largely due to the clinical assessment of the ED physicians. No adverse outcomes were reported. Gratton et al. found only a 3.2% discrepancy rate between emergency physicians and radiologists for head CTs. This most likely reflects their interpretation of "clinically significant."[63]

Although radiograph misinterpretation has the potential for considerable morbidity, the low incidence of actual mismanagement suggests that emergency physicians' assessments are largely based on clinical evaluation, and radiologic studies are often used to confirm rather than refute clinical impressions.

Teleradiology

Teleradiologic technology[86] has provided radiology services in various settings, such as remote or underserved areas, or in circumstances in which a radiologist covers more than one site simultaneously. This technology has also been used in the ED setting. Ultimately, teleradiology has the potential to provide real-time, on-line interpretation anywhere in the world 24 h a day.[86] Concerns regarding image quality continue to be raised. Initial trials of radiograph transmission with closed-circuit television equipment provided a satisfactory image quality in only 80 to 93% of cases.[87,88] The advent of digital equipment greatly improved image and interpretation quality, particularly with CT, MRI, and nuclear scans, all of which are obtained in a digital format.[89] Conventional radiographs, on the other hand, must be digitized before transmission. Digital conversion decreases image quality, and its suitability for adequate interpretation is still debated.[90-93]

For instance, when transmitted and conventional radiographs were interpreted by both radiologists and emergency physicians, accuracy was significantly better with the use of conventional films. A 2.0 to 2.6% discrepancy rate existed between original and digitized formats,[91,94-97] yet differentiation between observer performance and fidelity of the digital display was difficult. Thus, caution should be exercised in adopting teleradiology in the ED.[92] As this technology continues to improve,[89] however, it may change emergency practice and improve care.

APPROPRIATENESS AND TIMELINESS OF FOLLOW-UP

Emergency Radiology Follow-up Systems

It is important to establish reliable systems to ensure emergency radiograph interpretation. It is equally important to make certain that all discrepancies identified are appropriately followed up. Again, different EDs may successfully use different systems, but any system requires the cooperation of both the radiology and emergency departments. Procedures should be written and contained in applicable policy and procedure manuals.

It is important for the radiology department to return copies of the final report to the patient's private physician as well as to the ED. Multiple reporting channels provide a better fail safe system ensuring that abnormal findings will be followed up.

The ED should be notified of any identified discrepancies in writing. Certain discrepancies should also be communicated by phone to the physician. This may be done by the interpreting radiologist at the time the discrepancy is identified, although alternative methods may be used. An identified contact person such as the charge nurse, clerk, or emergency physician in the ED should be consistently used. Clerical or nursing personnel should pull the ED chart, most often from the previous day, and the physician or nursing staff should review the chart and the reported discrepancy to assess its clinical significance and determine any action is needed. In some settings, specific nursing staff may perform the initial screening, with emergency physician consultation only in selected cases. This may be necessary if the radiologist has a low threshold for calling discrepancies, resulting in many reports of limited clinical importance. Actions to be taken may include acknowledging the discrepancy without need for action; notifying the patient to follow up with his or her own doctor or a consultant; contacting the patient in order to prescribe a medication, such as an antibiotic; asking the patient to return to the ED for further evaluation; or notifying the patient's physician of the finding. If the patient cannot be reached, alternative sources (old medical records, phone books, directory assistance) should be pursued and documented. If these efforts fail, a letter is sent to the patient.

Regardless, the reported discrepancy and all actions taken should be permanently documented. This documentation may be kept in the radiograph file jacket or a separate ED log, but is best placed into the patient's actual medical record. Some EDs use a specific form for radiograph rereads, while others have a generic form for all types of follow-ups, including laboratory results. In EDs with dictation systems, physicians may dictate a short addendum to the record.

PATIENT SATISFACTION AND RISK MANAGEMENT

Satisfaction

Quality assurance, risk management, and patient satisfaction are interrelated. Dissatisfaction may be defined as "unmet expectations." Patients often present with preconceived expectations. Occasionally, patients request radiographic studies that may be unwarranted. In an era of cost containment, this is a conundrum for the emergency physician—one that requires as much art as science. In this situation, one might first attempt to preempt the issue by bringing up the subject of radiographs before the patient does. Common clinical settings include mild pediatric head injuries or nasal injuries. One should discuss the lack of usefulness of the radiograph and advise against it, often citing a desire to decrease radiation exposure. The vast majority of times, patients will concur.

If the patient or family brings up the subject first, one should pursue the above discussion in a polite, noncondescending, and nonjudgmental manner. If the patient or family still requests the study, the authors usually gracefully concede. Arguing or refusing is usually a lose-lose situation, since the clinician spends more time arguing than simply obtaining the test. Arguments about cost savings are usually not convincing, either. Such patients may seek care elsewhere until they get the desired test, ultimately spending more money. The clinician also acquires a significant adversary, which is undesirable.

Another problematic situation occurs when the patient has already been advised by another health care professional or individual (private physician, bystander, friend, triage nurse in the ED) that a radiograph is necessary. Regardless of who is right, disagreement pits the opinions against each other. In the patient's mind, this means that someone is wrong. In such cases, it is usually advisable to simply obtain the films, without debate or discussion. One may wish to follow up with the referring individual, clarifying the reasons why radiographs might not be indicated.

However, exceptions to these seemingly lenient policies do exist. Well-meaning attempts to maximize patient satisfaction do not require needlessly exposing patients to substantial risk, regardless of patient desire.

Risk Management

The range of clinically significant discrepancies between radiologists and emergency physicians is between 0.06 and 3.1%. Missed fractures account for many lawsuits against emergency physicians.[88] In a Massachusetts study, missed fractures accounted for the second largest number of closed malpractice claims.[99]

Medicolegally, the responsibility of radiograph interpretation and patient outcome is shared between emergency physicians and radiologists.[100] Emergency physicians are responsible for ordering appropriate films and rendering treatment based on their interpretation. If possible, emergency physicians who doubt their interpretation should consider obtaining a consultation with a radiologist prior to patient disposition.[101] Radiologists are responsible for conveying their reports back to the ED[98] and the patients' attending physicians. Ongoing interdepartmental cooperation and communication are important to assure that a reliable review system is in place.[102] Equally important is documentation of all actions taken and attempts to contact the patient, which can be critical in the event of a legal dispute.

REIMBURSEMENT ISSUES AFFECTING QUALITY

A final issue that may significantly affect these quality control systems involves changes in third-party reimbursement patterns. Rulings by the Health Care Financing Administration (HCFA) now give emergency physicians the latitude to separately report and bill for their radiograph interpretations. According to these HCFA regulations, reimbursement may be based on the "interpretation that contributes to the diagnosis of the patient in the emergency room."[104] Reimbursement is provided for only one radiograph interpretation. A billing emergency physician is required to provide a full written report of the interpretation instead of just a mere notation of normal or abnormal. These less extensive reviews are already included in the "payment for the evaluation and management services rendered" in the ED.

These regulations allow emergency physicians to bill for radiograph interpretations as long as a distinct reading is provided. On the other hand, emergency physicians who do not feel comfortable with this practice should continue to defer the final interpretation to the radiologist, who ultimately will bill for the study. In this case, the emergency physician should not bill for the initial interpretation. The HCFA ruling does not dictate which physician is allowed to bill for the interpretation but does state that only one interpretation will be reimbursed. An exception is that, if an emergency physician furnishes an interpretation necessary for the immediate management of the patient and subsequently a radiologist provides a further unrelated diagnosis, both are entitled to bill for the services.[104]

The HCFA ruling may potentially lead emergency physicians to perform the sole interpretation on some or all films without a radiology overread. As reimbursement moves from fee for service to capitation, such a change might be viewed as a cost saving, although the cost of ED rereads by radiologists is unknown. However, the HCFA ruling deals only with reimbursement and does not address the question of quality.

One possibility for maintaining quality might be for emergency physicians to refer only questionable studies for overreading. This assumes that when physicians have a high level of confidence in their interpretation, clinically significant misinterpretations are unlikely. Although increased interpretative confidence decreases misinterpretation rates, it does not eliminate them.[69]

It seems intuitive that the more times a radiograph is reviewed, the fewer findings will be overlooked. Rhea found that a second reading of the same image uncovered about one-third of the initial errors.[68] It is unknown whether this would be true if emergency physicians rather than radiologists overread each other's radiographs. It seems logical that maximum accuracy occurs when interpretations are performed by both an emergency physician knowing the clinical picture and a radiologist armed with additional training and expertise in interpreting images.

SUMMARY

Radiology services are a key feature of ED operations. The application of quality management techniques has the potential to simultaneously improve quality, decrease costs, and lower legal risk for both the radiology and emergency departments. However, successful emergency radiology QI systems require interdepartmental cooperation. Further research in emergency radiograph interpretation, quality monitoring, and interdisciplinary collaboration is needed.

REFERENCES

 1. Sato N: Quality assurance and risk management in Japan. *Med Biol Eng Comput* 32:411, 1994.
 2. Olsen ED, Ellek DM: Parameters of quality assurance: An evolving science. *Int Dental J* 45:49, 1995.
 3. Levy R, Goldstein B, Trott A: Approach to quality assurance in an emergency department: A one-year review. *Ann Emerg Med* 13:166, 1984.
 4. Sinert R, Ackerman M, Fishkin E: A continuous quality improvement approach applied to emergency department care of asthma patients (abstr). *Ann Emerg Med* 22:231, 1993.
 5. Donabedian A: The quality of care: How can it be assessed? *JAMA* 260:1743, 1988.
 6. Overton DT: Quality-related programs. *Acad Emerg Med* 1:192, 1994.
 7. O'Leary DS: CQI-A step beyond QA. *JCAHO* 2–3:1, 1990.
 8. Berwick DM: Continuous improvement as an ideal in health care. *New Engl J Med* 320:53, 1989.
 9. Wascom KR, Keiser MF: Quality assessment of emergency department activities. *Emerg Med Serv* Jan/Feb:21, 1981.
10. Platin E, Ludlow JB: Knowledge and adoption of radiographic quality assurance guidelines by general dentists in North Carolina. *Oral Surg Oral Med Oral Pathol Oral Radiol Endod* 79(1):122, 1995.
11. Jewell MA: Quantitative methods for quality improvement. *Pharmacotherapy* 15(1 pt 2):27S, 1995.
12. Moloney TW, Rogers DE: Medical technology—A different view of the contentious debate over cost. *New Engl J Med* 301:1413, 1979.
13. O'Leary MR, Smith M, Olmsted WW, et al: Physician assessments of practice patterns in emergency department radiograph interpretation. *Ann Emerg Med* 17:1019, 1988.
14. de Lacey: Letter. *Br J Radiol* 52:332, 1979.
15. *The Ontario Statistical Reporting System, 1991–92.* Toronto, Ontario, Canada: Ontario Ministry of Health, 1992.
16. Stiell IG, Greenberg GH, Wells GA, et al: Derivation of a decision rule for the use of radiography in acute knee injuries. *Ann Emerg Med* 26:405, 1995.
17. Schwartz LR, Overton DT: The management of patient complaints and dissatisfaction. *Emerg Med Clin North Am* 10:557, 1992.
18. Leape L: Are practice guidelines cookbook medicine? *J Arkansas Med Soc* 86(2):73, 1989.
19. Davidson SJ: Practice, malpractice and practice guidelines (editorial). *Ann Emerg Med* 19:943, 1990.
20. Stiell IG, Greenberg GH, et al: A study to develop clinical decision rules for the use of radiography in acute ankle injury. *Ann Emerg Med* 21:384, 1992.
21. Stiell IG, Greenberg GH, et al: Decision rules for the use of radiography in acute ankle injuries: Refinement and prospective validation. *JAMA* 1127, 1993.
22. Stiell IG, McKnight, et al: Implementation of the Ottawa ankle rules. *JAMA* 271:827, 1994.
23. McDonald CJ: Guidelines you can follow and trust: An ideal and an example. *JAMA* 271:872, 1994.
23a. Stiell I, Wells G, Laupacis A, et al. Multicentre trial to introduce the Ottawa ankle rules for use of radiography in acute ankle injuries. Multicentre Ankle Rule Study Group. *BMJ* 311:594, 1995.
24. Weber JE, Jackson RE, Peacock WF, et al: Clinical decision rules discriminate between fractures and non-fractures in acute isolated knee trauma. *Ann Emerg Med* 26:429, 1995.
25. De Lacey GJ, Wignall BK, Bradbrooke S, et al: Rationalizing abdominal radiography in the accident and emergency department. *Clin Radiol* 31:453, 1980.
26. Jennett B: Skull X-rays after recent head injury. *Clin Radiol* 31:463, 1980.
27. Briggs M, Clarke P, Crockard A, et al: Guidelines for initial managment of head injury in adults. Suggestions from a group of neurosurgeons. *Br Med J* 288:983, 1984.
28. Gorman DF: The utility of post traumatic skull x-rays. *Arch Emerg Med* 4:141, 1987.
29. Mikhail MG, et al: Intracranial injury following minor head trauma. *Am J Emerg Med* 10(1):24, 1992.
30. Pasman P, Twijnstra A, Wilmink J, et al: The value of head radiography in patients with head trauma. *JBR-BTR* 78:169, 1995.
31. Lloyd KR, English K, et al: A prospective evaluation of radiologic criteria for head injury patients in a community emergency department. *Am J Emerg Med* 11:327, 1993.
32. Hackney DB: Skull radiography in the evaluation of acute head trauma: A survey of current practice. *Radiology* 181:711, 1991.
33. Campbell JPM, Gunn AA: Plain abdominal radiographs and acute abdominal pain. *Br J Surg* 75:554, 1988.
34. Eisenberg RL, et al: Evaluation of plain abdominal radiographs in the diagnosis of abdominal pain. *Ann Surg* 197:464, 1983.
35. McCook TA, et al: Abdominal radiography in the emergency department: A prospective analysis. *Ann Emerg Med* 11:7, 1982.

36. Rothrock SG, Green SM, Hummel CB: Plain abdominal radiography in the detection of major disease in children: A prospective analysis. *Ann Emerg Med* 21:1423, 1992.

37. Rothrock SG, Green SM, et al: Plain abdominal radiography in the detection of acute medical and surgical disease in children: A retrospective analysis. *Pediatr Emerg Care* 7:281, 1991.

38. Danher J, Eyes BE, Kumar K: Oblique rib views after blunt chest trauma: An unnecessary routine? *B M J* 289:1271, 1984.

39. Cantrill S, Karas S (eds): *Cost-Effectitve Diagnostic Testing in Emergency Medicine: Guidelines for Appropriate Utilization of Clinical Laboratory and Radiology Studies.* Dallas: American College of Emergency Physicians, 1994.

40. Nigam A, Goni A, et al: The value of radiographs in the management of the fractured nose. *Arch Emerg Med* 10:293, 1993.

41. Logan M, et al: The utility of nasal bone radiographs in nasal trauma. *Clin Radiol* 49(3):192, 1994.

42. de Lacey GJ, Chir B, et al: The radiology of nasal injury: Problems of interpretation and clinical relevance. *Br J Radiol* 50:412, 1977.

43. Baker SR, Rabin A, et al: The effect of restricting the indications for lumbosacral spine radiography in patients with acute low back symptoms. *AJR* 149:535, 1987.

44. Gehweiler JA, Daffner RH: Low back pain: The controversy of radiologic evaluation. *AJR* 140:109, 1983.

45. Kelen GD, Noji EK, et al: Guidelines for use of lumbar spine radiography. *Ann Emerg Med* 15:245, 1986.

46. Haines JD: Occult cervical spine fractures. *Postgrad Med* 80:73, 1986.

47. Hoffman JR, Schriger DL, Mower W, et al: Low-risk criteria for cervical-spine radiography in blunt trauma: A prospective study. *Ann Emerg Med* 21:1454, 1992.

48. Cadoux CG, White JD, Hedberg MC: High-yield roentgenographic criteria for cervical spine injuries. *Ann Emerg Med* 16:738, 1987.

49. Ringenberg BJ, Fisher AK, et al: Rational ordering of cervical spine radiographs following trauma. *Ann Emerg Med* 17:792, 1988.

50. Jacobs LM, et al: Prospective analysis of cervical spine injury: A methodology to predict injury. *Ann Emerg Med* 15:85, 1986.

51. Fischer RP: Cervical radiographic evaluation of alert patients following blunt trauma. *Ann Emerg Med* 13:905, 1984.

52. Walter J, Doris PE, Shaffer MA: Clinical presentation of patients with acute cervical spine injury. *Ann Emerg Med* 13:512, 1984.

53. Stiell IG, Greenburg GH, Wells GA, et al: Prospective validation of a decision rule for the use of radiography in acute knee injures. *JAMA* 275:611, 1996.

54. Stiell IG, Wells GA, McDowell I, et al: Use of radiography in acute knee injuries: Need for clinical decision rules. *Acad Emerg Med* 2:966, 1995.

55. Bauer SJ, Hollander JE, Fuchs SH, Thade JC Jr: A clinical decision rule in the evaluation of acute knee injuries. *J Emerg Med* 13:611, 1995.

56. Seaberg DC, Jackson R: Clinical decision rule for knee radiographs. *Am J Emerg Med* 12:541, 1994.

57. Rickett AB, Finlay DBL, Jagger C: The importance of clinical details when reporting accident and emergency radiographs. *Injury* 23:458, 1992.

58. Berbaum KS, El-Khoury GY, Franken EA Jr, et al: Impact of clinical history on fracture detection with radiography. *Radiology* 168:507, 1988.

59. Berbaum KS, Franken EA, El-Khoury GY: Impact of clinical history on radiographic detection of fractures: A comparison of radiologists and orthopedists. *AJR* 153:1221, 1989.

60. Kramer MS, Roberts-Brauer R, Williams RL: Bias and "overcall" in interpreting chest radiographs in young febrile children. *Pediatrics* 90:11, 1992.

62. Walters RS; Radiology practices in emergency departments associated with pediatric residency programs. *Pediatr Emerg Care* 11(2):78, 1995.

63. Gratton MC, Salomone JA, Watson WA: Clinically significant radiograph misinterpretations at an emergency medicine residency program. *Ann Emerg Med* 19:497, 1990.

64. Simon HK, Khan NS, et al. Pediatric emergency physician interpretation of plain radiographs: Is routine review by a radiologist necessary and cost-effective? *Ann Emerg Med* 27:295, 1996.

65. Barber F, Marx JA: Accuracy of emergency radiograph interpretation by emergency physicians. *J Emerg Med* 1:483, 1984.

66. Seltzer SE, Hessel SJ, Herman PG, et al: Resident film interpretations and staff review. *AJR* 137:129, 1981.

67. McLain PL, Kirkwood CR: The quality of emergency room radiograph interpretations. *J Fam Pract* 20:443, 1985.

68. Rhea JT, Potsaid MS, DeLuca SA. Errors of interpretation as elicited by a quality audit of an emergency radiology facility. *Radiology* 132:277, 1979.

69. Mayhue FE, Rust DD, Aldag JC, et al: Accuracy of interpretations of emergency department radiographs: Effect of confidence levels. *Ann Emerg Med* 18:826, 1989.

70. Nitowski LA, O'Connor RE, Reese CL: The rate of clinically significant plain radiograph misinterpretation by faculty in emergency medicine residency program. *Acad Emerg Med* 3:782, 1996.

71. Overton DT: A quality assurance assessment of radiograph reading accuracy by emergency medicine faculty (abstr). *Ann Emerg Med* 16:503, 1987.

72. Alfaro D, Levitt MA, et al: Accuracy of interpretation of cranial computed tomography scans in an emergency medicine residency program. *Ann Emerg Med* 25:169, 1995.

73. Freed HA, Shields NN: Most frequently overlooked radiographically apparent fractures in a teaching hospital emergency department. *Ann Emerg Med* 13:900, 1984.

74. Garland LH: Studies on the accuracy of diagnostic procedures. *Am J Roentgenol* 82:25, 1959.

75. Stevenson CA: Accuracy of the x-ray report. *JAMA* 207:1140, 1969.

76. Herman PG, Gerson DE, Hessel SJ, et al: Disagreements in chest roentgen interpretation. *Chest* 68:278, 1975.

77. Walsh-Kelly CM, Melzer-Lange MD, Hennes HM, et al: Clinical impact of radiograph misinterpretation in a pediatric ED and the effect of physician training level. *Am J Emerg Med* 13:262, 1995.

78. Elmore JG, Wells CK, Lee CH, et al: Radiologists differed in their interpretations of mammograms. *New Engl J Med* 331:1493, 1994.

79. Friedman DP, Rosetti GF, et al: MR imaging: Quality assessment method and ratings at 33 centers. *Radiology* 196:219, 1995.

80. Quick G, Podgorny G: An emergency department radiology audit procedure. *J Am Coll Emerg Phys* 6:247, 1977.

81. Suh RS, Maglinte DD, Lavonas EJ, et al: Emergency abdominal radiography: Discrepancies of preliminary and final interpretation and management relevance. *Emerg Radiol* 2:315, 1995.

82. Chan RNW, Ainscow D: Diagnostic failure in the multiple injured. *J Trauma* 20:684, 1980.

83. Minnes BG, Sutcliffe T, Klassen TP: Agreement in the interpretation of extremity radiographs of injured children and adolescents. *Acad Emerg Med* 2:826, 1995.

84. Chacon D, Kissoon N, et al: Use of comparison radiographs in the diagnosis of traumatic injuries of the elbow. *Ann Emerg Med* 21:895, 1992.

85. Fleisher G, Ludwig S, McSorley M: Interpretation of pediatric x-ray films by emergency department pediatricians. *Ann Emerg Med* 12:153, 1983.

86. Wright R, Loughrey C: Teleradiology. *BMJ* 310:1392, 1995.

87. Jelasco DV, Southworth G, Purcell LH: Telephone transmission of radiographic images. *Radiology* 127:145, 1978.

88. Page G, Gregoire A, Garland C, et al: Teleradiology in northern Quebec. *Radiology* 140:361, 1981.

89. Mun SK, Elsayed AM, Tohme WG, et al: Teleradiology/telepathology requirements and implementation. *J Med Syst* 19:153, 1995.

90. Cox GG, Cook LT, McMillan JH, et al: Chest radiography: Comparison of high resolution digital displays with conventional and digital films. *Radiology* 176:771, 1990.

91. Goldberg MA, Rosenthal DI, Chew FS, et al: New high-resolution teleradiology system: Prospective study of diagnostic accuracy in 685 transmitted clinical cases. *Radiology* 186:429, 1993.

92. Scott WW , Bluemke DA, et al: Interpretation of emergency department radiographs by radiologists and emergency medicine physicians: Teleradiology workstation versus radiograph readings. *Radiology* 195:223, 1995.

93. Slasky BS, Gur D, Good WF, et al: Receiver operating characteristic analysis of chest image interpretation with conventional, laser-printed, and high resolution workstation images. *Radiology* 174:775, 1990.

94. Carey LS, O'Connor BD, Bach DB, et al: Digital teleradiology: Seaforth-London network. *J Can Assoc Radiol* 40:71, 1989.

95. DeCorato DR, Kagetsu NJ, Ablow RC, et al: Off-hour interpretation of radiologic images of patients admitted to the emergency department: Efficacy of teleradiology. *AJR* 165:1293, 1995.

96. Slovis TL, Guzzardo-Dobson PR, et al: The clinical usefullness of teleradiology of neonates: Expanded services without expanded staff. *Pediatr Radiol* 21:333, 1991.

97. Reponem J, Lahde S, Tervonen O, et al: Low cost digital teleradiology. *Eur J Radiol* 19:226, 1995.

98. Goldman B, George JE, Fish RM: Curbing the threat of litigation in the emergency department: A risk management approach. *Emerg Med Rep* 11(2):11, 1990.

99. Karcz A, Holbrook J, Auerbach BS, et al: Preventability of malpractice claims in emergency medicine: A closed claims study. *Ann Emerg Med* 19:865, 1990.

100. Berlin L: Does the "missed" radiographic diagnosis constitute malpractice? *Radiology* 123:523, 1977.

101. Dobbs D: Emergency physician responsibility for the interpretation of x-rays. *Pediatr Emerg Care* 2:197, 1986.

102. Bauman TW, Bauman DH: Quality assurance for the radiology-emergency interface. *Emerg Med Clin North Am* 9:881, 1991.

103. Trautlein JJ, Lambert RL, Miller J: Malpractice in the emergency department—Review of 200 cases. *Ann Emerg Med* 13(pt 1):709, 1984.

104. *Fed Reg* 60(236):63130, 19.

INDEX

Page numbers followed by *f* indicate figures; page numbers followed by *t* indicate tables.

ISBN 0-07-050827-5

90000

9 780070 508279

SCHWARTZ/EMER. RAD.

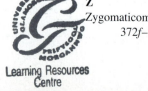

Learning Resources
Centre